S0-BPR-468

THE SPINE

Volume I

THE SPINE

Third Edition

Founding Editors:

Richard H. Rothman, M.D., Ph.D.
James Edwards Professor and Chairman,
Department of Orthopaedic Surgery,
Thomas Jefferson University;
Chairman, The Rothman Institute,
Pennsylvania Hospital, Philadelphia

and

Frederick A. Simeone, M.D.
Professor of Neurosurgery,
The University of Pennsylvania School of Medicine;
Chief of Neurosurgery,
Pennsylvania Hospital;
Director of Neurosurgery,
Elliott Neurological Center of Pennsylvania Hospital, Philadelphia

W. B. SAUNDERS COMPANY
Harcourt Brace Jovanovich, Inc.
Philadelphia London Toronto Montreal Sydney Tokyo

W. B. SAUNDERS COMPANY
Harcourt Brace Jovanovich, Inc.

The Curtis Center
Independence Square West
Philadelphia, PA 19106

Library of Congress Cataloging-in-Publication Data

The Spine / [edited by] Richard H. Rothman,
Frederick A. Simeone.—3rd ed.

p. cm.

1. Spine—Surgery. 2. Spine—Diseases.
3. Spine—Wounds and injuries. 4. Spine—
Abnormalities. I. Rothman, Richard H.
II. Simeone, Frederick A.

[DNLM: 1. Spinal Diseases. WE 725 S759]

RD533.S68 1992 617.5′6—dc20

DNLM/DLC 91–18294

ISBN 0–7216–3203–3 (2 volume set)
ISBN 0–7216–4036–2 (vol. 1)
ISBN 0–7216–4037–0 (vol. 2)

Listed here are the latest translated editions of this book together with the language of the translation and the publisher.

Italian *(1st Edition)*—Aulo Gaggi Editore, Bologna, Italy
Spanish *(2nd Edition)*—Editorial Medica Panamericana, Buenos Aires, Argentina

Editor: W. B. Saunders Staff
Developmental Editor: Hazel N. Hacker
Designer: Maureen Sweeney
Production Manager: Ken Neimeister
Manuscript Editor: W. B. Saunders Staff
Illustration Coordinator: Walt Verbitski
Indexer: Susan Thomas
Cover Designer: Michelle Maloney

The Spine, 3rd edition ISBN 0–7216–3203–3

Printed in the United States of America

Last digit is the print number: 9 8 7 6 5 4 3 2 1

The decision to go forth with this edition of The Spine, *originally conceived and edited by Rothman and Simeone, was initiated three years ago. It was based on our dedication to, respect for, and friendship with Dick Rothman and Fred Simeone and our desire to continue the project they started and knowledge they imparted to us years ago. Since that time many hours have gone into organization, manuscript preparation, editorial responsibility, and periodic crisis resolution. To finally see the culmination of the hours result in the completion of this textbook represents a dream come true and a tribute to Dick and Fred, two important mentors and persons in our lives. It would, however, be a serious omission not to acknowledge those special individuals whose support, understanding, and encouragement provided the boost to keep the fire going.*

HARRY N. HERKOWITZ, M.D.

To my wife Jan and my children Seth Adam and Rachael Helene, whose love and boundless energy have given me the happiest moments of my life.

To Richard H. Rothman, my mentor, my friend, whose presence encourages me to continue to strive for excellence.

To L. Carl Samberg for introducing me to the world of spine surgery.

STEVEN R. GARFIN, M.D.

To my wife Susan, whose love, patience, and loyalty I cherish, and to my children Jessica and Cory, whose achievements provide unlimited joy and inspiration. The successes have been shared by all, while the long hours and occasional disappointments have been endured by strong hearts.

RICHARD A. BALDERSTON, M.D.

To my wife Claudia for her constant love and support and my children Philip and Jessica, who make it all worthwhile.

FRANK J. EISMONT, M.D.

To my wife Emily and my children Andrew, Allison, and April.

To Dr. Charles Herndon for teaching how medicine should be practiced.

GORDON R. BELL, M.D.

To my teachers and professors, particularly Richard H. Rothman, Frederick A. Simeone, Marc Colonnier, and John Pegington. To my wife Kathy for helping to make efforts such as this worthwhile.

SAM W. WIESEL, M.D.

To the chief, Richard H. Rothman—an outstanding professor, true colleague, and good friend.

Contributors

Todd J. Albert, M.D.
Orthopaedic Resident, Thomas Jefferson University Medical School, Philadelphia, Pennsylvania
Spinal Instrumentation

Jean-Jacques Abitbol, M.D.
Assistant Professor, Department of Orthopaedics, University of California, San Diego; Spine Surgeon, UCSD Medical Center, San Diego, California
Complications of Spinal Surgery: Complications Associated with Posterior Instrumentation of the Spine

Marshall B. Allen, M.D.
Chief, Section of Neurosurgery, Medical College of Georgia; Attending Neurosurgeon, Medical College of Georgia Hospital and Clinics and Veterans Administration Hospital, Augusta, Georgia
Intraspinal Infections

Michael J. Aminoff, M.D., F.R.C.P.
Professor of Neurology, School of Medicine, University of California, San Francisco; Attending Physician, University of California Medical Center, San Francisco, California
Electrodiagnosis: Somatosensory and Motor Evoked Potentials

Glenn Amundson, M.D.
Assistant Professor, Uniformed Services University of the Health Sciences, Bethesda, Maryland; Chief, Spine Service, Department of Orthopaedics, Naval Hospital, Portsmouth, Virginia
Spondylolisthesis

Howard S. An, M.D.
Assistant Professor and Director of Reconstructive Spine Surgery, Department of Orthopaedics, Milwaukee Regional Medical Center, The Medical College of Wisconsin; Attending Physician, Milwaukee County Medical Complex, Children's Hospital of Wisconsin, and Froedert Lutheran Memorial Hospital, Milwaukee, Wisconsin
Juvenile Kyphosis

David F. Apple, Jr., M.D.
Associate Clinical Professor of Orthopaedic Surgery, and Clinical Assistant Professor in Rehabilitation Medicine, Emory University School of Medicine; Clinical Professor of Orthopedics, Georgia State University; Medical Director, Shepherd Spinal Center, Atlanta, Georgia
Spinal Cord Injury Rehabilitation

J. Hampton Atkinson, M.D.
Associate Adjunct Professor, Department of Psychiatry, UCSD School of Medicine, La Jolla; Attending Physician, UCSD Medical Center and San Diego Veterans Affairs Medical Center, San Diego, California
Chronic Pain Management: Behavioral Medicine Approaches to Chronic Back Pain

Richard A. Balderston, M.D.
Clinical Professor, Orthopaedic Surgery, and Director, Spine Fellowship Program, Jefferson Medical College; Chief, Scoliosis Services, Thomas Jefferson University Hospital and Pennsylvania Hospital, Philadelphia, Pennsylvania
Juvenile Kyphosis; Spinal Instrumentation

Gordon R. Bell, M.D.
Staff Surgeon, Department of Orthopedics; Surgical Consultant, Center for the Spine; Director, Spinal Fellowship Program, Cleveland Clinic Foundation, Cleveland, Ohio
Differential Diagnosis of Sciatica; Radiology of the Lumbar Spine

Joseph R. Berger, M.D.
Professor of Neurology and Internal Medicine, University of Miami School of Medicine, Miami, Florida
Medical Myelopathies

Mark Bernhardt, M.D.
Clinical Assistant Professor, Department of Orthopaedic Surgery, University of Missouri–Kansas City School of Medicine; Associate in Orthopaedic Surgery, Dickson-Diveley Orthopaedic Clinic; Attending Physician, St. Luke's Hospital, Children's Mercy Hospital, and Truman Medical Center, Kansas City, Missouri
Biomechanical Considerations of Spinal Stability

Joseph Bernstein, M.D.
Orthopaedic Resident, University of Pennsylvania School of Medicine, Philadelphia, Pennsylvania
Metabolic Bone Disorders of the Spine

Kalman D. Blumberg, M.D.
Orthopaedic Surgeon, Ft. Lauderdale, Florida
Surgical Management of Cervical Disc Disease: Indications for Surgery in Cervical Myelopathy: Anterior Versus Posterior Approach

Scott D. Boden, M.D.
Assistant in Orthopaedics, Department of Orthopaedic Surgery, George Washington University School of Medicine and Health Care Sciences, Washington, D.C.
Cervical Disc Disease: Conservative Treatment; The Multiply Operated Low Back Patient; Workers' Compensation as It Affects the Spine: Compensation Low Back and Neck Pain

Henry H. Bohlman, M.D.
Professor, Department of Orthopedic Surgery, Case Western Reserve University School of Medicine; Chief, Reconstructive and Traumatic Spine Surgery Center, University Hospital; Chief, Acute Spinal Cord Injury Service, Veterans Administration Medical Center, Cleveland, Ohio
Spine Trauma in Adults: Spine and Spinal Cord Injuries

Robert E. Booth, Jr., M.D.
Clinical Professor and Vice-Chairman, Orthopaedic Surgery, Thomas Jefferson University; Director, The Rothman Orthopaedic Institute; Co-Chief, Section on Orthopaedic Surgery; Chief, Section on Physical Medicine and Rehabilitation, Pennsylvania Hospital, Philadelphia, Pennsylvania
Arthritis of the Spine; Spinal Stenosis: Nonoperative and Operative Treatment

Michael J. Botte, M.D.
Assistant Professor, Department of Orthopaedics, University of California, San Diego; Chief, Hand and Foot Surgery, UCSD Medical Center; Chief, Department of Rehabilitation Medicine, Veterans Administration Medical Center, La Jolla; Consultant, Muscle Disease Clinic, Children's Hospital and Medical Center, San Diego, California
Spinal Orthoses for Traumatic and Degenerative Disease

Brian C. Bowen, M.D., Ph.D.
Assistant Professor, Division of Neuroradiology, Department of Radiology, University of Miami School of Medicine; Attending Radiologist, Jackson Memorial Medical Center and University of Miami Hospitals and Clinics, Miami, Florida
Syringomyelia

Richard P. Bunge, M.D.
Professor of Neurological Surgery and Cell Biology and Anatomy, University of Miami School of Medicine, Miami, Florida
Experimental Spinal Cord Injury: Pathophysiology and Treatment

J. C. Butler, M.D.
Associate Professor of Orthopaedic Surgery, Tulane University School of Medicine; Staff, Tulane Medical Center Hospital and Clinic,

Charity Hospital–New Orleans, Veterans Administration Hospital–New Orleans, United Medical Center, Pendleton Memorial Methodist Hospital, and Slidell Memorial Hospital, New Orleans, Louisiana
Complications of Spinal Therapy: Postlaminectomy Kyphosis of the Cervical Spine

Jonathan F. Camp, M.D.
Department of Orthopedics, Children's Hospital, Humana Hospital Sunrise, Las Vegas, Nevada
Neuromuscular Scoliosis

Charles R. Clark, M.D.
Professor of Orthopaedic Surgery and Director of Spine Fellowship, University of Iowa, College of Medicine; Attending Physician, University of Iowa Hospitals and Clinics, Iowa City, Iowa
Rheumatoid Arthritis: Surgical Considerations

Mark S. Cohen, M.D.
Clinical Spine Fellow, Department of Orthopaedics, University of California, San Diego, San Diego, California
Anatomy of the Spinal Nerve Roots in the Lumbar and Lower Thoracic Spine

Bradford L. Currier, M.D.
Instructor in Orthopedics, Mayo Medical School; Senior Associate Consultant, Departments of Orthopedics and of Neurologic Surgery, Mayo Clinic and Mayo Foundation, Rochester, Minnesota
Thoracic Disc Disease; Infections of the Spine

William H. Dillin, M.D.
Spinal Surgery Consultant, Kerlan-Jobe Orthopaedic Clinic, Inglewood, California
Back Pain in Children and Adolescents; Cervical Disc Disease: Clinical Syndromes in Cervical Myelopathy; Surgical Management of Cervical Disc Disease: Surgical Management of Cervical Myelopathy: Laminectomy

Dudley S. Dinner, M.D.
Staff, Section of Epilepsy and Sleep Disorders, Department of Neurology, Cleveland Clinic, Cleveland, Ohio
Intraoperative Spinal Cord Monitoring

Thomas B. Ducker, M.D.
Former Professor and Head of Neurosurgery, University of Maryland; Clinical Professor of Neurosurgery, University of Maryland; Associate Professor of Neurosurgery, Johns Hopkins University, Baltimore, Maryland
Spine Trauma in Adults: Spine and Spinal Cord Injuries

Charles C. Edwards, M.D.
Professor of Orthopaedic Surgery, University of Maryland; Director of Spine Section, University of Maryland Hospital, Baltimore, Maryland
Spondylolisthesis

Frank J. Eismont, M.D.
Professor, Department of Orthopedics, and Clinical Professor of Neurologic Surgery, University of Miami School of Medicine; Co-Director of Spinal Cord Injury Service, Jackson Memorial Hospital, Miami, Florida
Thoracic Disc Disease; Infections of the Spine

Hani El-Kommos, M.D.
Fellow, Spine Surgery, Department of Orthopaedic Surgery, William Beaumont Hospital, Royal Oak, Michigan
Spinal Stenosis: Clinical Evaluation and Differential Diagnosis

Ronney L. Ferguson, M.D.
Director of Clinical Research, Shriners Hospitals–Greenville Unit; Associate Clinical Professor, Medical University of South Carolina; Attending Physician, Shriners Hospitals for Crippled Children–Greenville Unit, Charleston, South Carolina
Thoracic and Lumbar Spinal Trauma of the Immature Spine

Ann Marie Flannery, M.D.
Assistant Professor, Department of Surgery, Section of Neurosurgery (Pediatrics), Medical College of Georgia; Attending Neurosurgeon (Pediatrics), Medical College of Georgia Hospital and Clinics and Veterans Administration Hospital–Augusta, Augusta, Georgia
Intraspinal Infections

Steven R. Garfin, M.D.
Professor, Department of Orthopaedics, University of California, San Diego; Chief, Section of Spine Surgery, UCSD Medical Center, San Diego, California
Anatomy of the Spinal Nerve Roots in the Lumbar and Lower Thoracic Spine; Lumbar Disc Disease; Spinal Stenosis: Pathophysiology and *Nonoperative and Operative Treatment; Spondylolisthesis; Complications of Spinal Surgery: Complications Associated with Posterior Instrumentation of the Spine*

Barth A. Green, M.D.
Professor of Neurological Surgery and Clinical Professor of Orthopedics, University of Miami School of Medicine; Director of Spinal Cord Injury Service, Jackson Memorial Medical Center; Attending Neurosurgeon, Veterans Administration Medical Center, Miami, Florida
Thoracic Disc Disease; Experimental Spinal Cord Injury: Pathophysiology and Treatment; Syringomyelia

Edward N. Hanley, Jr., M.D.
Chairman, Department of Orthopaedic Surgery, Carolinas Medical Center, Charlotte, North Carolina
Spinal Fusion: Allograft

James C. Harvell, Jr., M.D.
Clinical Instructor, Department of Surgery, Division of Orthopaedic Surgery, East Carolina University School of Medicine; Active Medical Staff, Pitt County Memorial Hospital, Greenville, North Carolina
Spinal Fusion: Allograft

John G. Heller, M.D.
Assistant Professor of Orthopaedic Surgery, Emory University School of Medicine; Attending Physician, Emory University Hospital, Grady Memorial Hospital, Henrietta Eggleston Children's Hospital, and Atlanta Veterans Administration Hospital, Atlanta, Georgia
Complications of Spinal Surgery: Postoperative Infections of the Spine

Robert N. Hensinger, M.D.
Professor, Section of Orthopaedic Surgery, Department of Surgery, University of Michigan; Chief, Pediatric Orthopaedic Surgery, Mott Children's Hospital, University of Michigan, Ann Arbor, Michigan
Congenital Anomalies of the Cervical Spine

Harry N. Herkowitz, M.D.
Chairman, Department of Orthopaedic Surgery, William Beaumont Hospital; Director, Section of Spine Surgery, Department of Orthopaedic Surgery, William Beaumont Hospital, Royal Oak, Michigan
Surgical Management of Cervical Disc Disease: Surgical Management of Cervical Radiculopathy: Anterior Fusion and *Cervical Laminaplasty; Spinal Stenosis: Clinical Evaluation and Differential Diagnosis, Radiologic and Electrodiagnostic Evaluation,* and *Nonoperative and Operative Treatment; Spinal Fusion: Techniques and Complications*

Kiyoshi Hirabayashi, M.D.
Professor, Department of Orthopaedic Surgery, School of Medicine, Keio University; Chief of Spine Group, Orthopaedic Surgery, Keio Gijuku University Hospital, Tokyo, Japan
Ossification of the Posterior Longitudinal Ligament

Sten Holm, Ph.D.
Associate Professor of Orthopaedic Surgery, University of Gothenburg; Associate Professor, Department of Orthopaedics, Sahlgren Hospital, Gothenburg, Sweden
Pathophysiology of the Intervertebral Disc and Adjacent Neural Structures

Rollin M. Johnson, M.D.
Associate Clinical Professor of Orthopaedics and Rehabilitation, Yale School of Medicine, New Haven, Connecticut; Attending Surgeon, Cooley Dickinson Hospital, Northampton, Massachusetts
Surgical Approaches to the Spine

Alexander M. Jones, M.D.
Staff, Department of Orthopaedic Surgery, and Director, Spine Service, Naval Hospital–Oakland, Oakland, California
Spinal Instrumentation

Neil Kahanovitz, M.D.
Executive Director, National Spine Center at the Anderson Clinic, Arlington, Virginia; Clinical Associate Professor, Orthopedic Surgery, Georgetown Medical Center, Washington, D.C.
Spinal Fusion: Electricity

John P. Kostuik, M.D., F.R.C.S.(C.)
Professor of Orthopedic Surgery, University of Toronto; Director, Dewar Spinal Unit, and Director, Biomechanics Laboratory, Toronto Hospital, Toronto, Ontario, Canada
Adult Scoliosis

Lawrence T. Kurz, M.D.
Attending Orthopaedic Surgeon, Section of Spine Surgery, Department of Orthopaedic Surgery, William Beaumont Hospital, Royal Oak, Michigan
Cervical Disc Disease: The Differential Diagnosis of Cervical Radiculopathy; Spinal Fusion: Techniques and Complications

Joseph M. Lane, M.D.
Professor of Orthopaedic Surgery, Cornell University Medical College; Director, Research Operations, Chief, Metabolic Bone Disease Service, and Orthopaedic Attending, Hospital For Special Surgery; Orthopaedic Attending, Memorial Sloan-Kettering Cancer Center, New York, New York
Metabolic Bone Disorders of the Spine; Spinal Fusion: Principles of Bone Fusion

S. Henry LaRocca, M.D.
Clinical Professor, Orthopaedic Surgery, Tulane University Medical School, New Orleans, Louisiana
Chronic Pain Management: Surgical Procedures for the Control of Chronic Pain

Carlos J. Lavernia, M.D.
Clinical Instructor of Surgery, Department of Orthopedics, UCSD Medical Center, San Diego, California
Spinal Orthoses for Traumatic and Degenerative Disease

Alan M. Levine, M.D.
Professor of Orthopedic Surgery and Oncology, University of Maryland; Associate Chief of Orthopedic Surgery, University of Maryland; Consultant—Spinal Trauma, Maryland Institute for Emergency Medical Services; Chief of Scoliosis Service, Kernan Hospital, Baltimore, Maryland
Spine Trauma in Adults: Surgical Techniques for Thoracic and Lumbar Trauma

Robert M. Levy, M.D., Ph.D.
Associate Professor of Neurosurgery and Physiology, Northwestern University School of Medicine, Chicago, Illinois
Medical Myelopathies

Stephen J. Lipson, M.D.
Associate Clinical Professor of Orthopaedic Surgery, Harvard Medical School; Orthopaedic Surgeon, Brigham and Women's Hospital, Boston, Massachusetts
Spinal Stenosis: Pathophysiology

John E. Lonstein, M.D.
Clinical Associate Professor, Orthopaedic Surgery, University of Minnesota; Staff Surgeon, Minnesota Spine Center, Minneapolis and St. Paul; Staff Surgeon, Spine Service, Gillette Children's Hospital, St. Paul, Minnesota
Juvenile and Adolescent Scoliosis

Hans Lüders, M.D., Ph.D.
Chairman, Department of Neurology, Cleveland Clinic Foundation, Cleveland, Ohio
Intraoperative Spinal Cord Monitoring

Parley W. Madsen, III, M.D., Ph.D.
Assistant Professor, Department of Neurological Surgery, University of Miami School of Medicine; Attending Neurosurgeon, Jackson Memorial Medical Center; Consultant, Neurosurgery, Veterans Administration Medical Center, Miami, Florida
Syringomyelia

Joseph C. Maroon, M.D.
Professor of Neurosurgery, The Medical College of Pennsylvania, Philadelphia; Chairman, Department of Neurosurgery, Allegheny General Hospital, Pittsburgh, Pennsylvania
Alternative Forms of Disc Excision: Percutaneous Automated Discectomy

Lawrence F. Marshall, M.D.
Professor of Surgery, University of California, San Diego; Chief, Neurosurgery, UCSD Medical Center, San Diego, California
Complications of Spinal Surgery: Cerebrospinal Fluid Leaks: Etiology and Repair

Alberto Martinez-Arizala, M.D.
Assistant Professor, The Miami Project, Department of Neurology and Department of Orthopaedics and Rehabilitation, University of Miami School of Medicine; Attending Physician, Jackson Memorial Hospital, Miami, Florida
Experimental Spinal Cord Injury: Pathophysiology and Treatment

Tom G. Mayer, M.D.
Clincal Professor, Department of Orthopedic Surgery, University of Texas Southwestern Medical School; Medical Director, Productive Rehabilitation Institution of Dallas for Ergonomics (PRIDE), Dallas, Texas
Lumbar Musculature: Anatomy and Function; Spine Functional Restoration

Paul C. McAfee, M.D.
Associate Professor of Orthopedic Surgery, Johns Hopkins Hospital; Spinal Reconstructive Surgery, Scoliosis Surgery, and Orthopaedic Surgery with Orthopaedic Associates, P.A., Baltimore, Maryland
Spine Trauma in Adults: Spinal Instrumentation for Thoracolumbar Fractures

John A. McCulloch, M.D., F.R.C.S.(C.)
Professor of Orthopaedics, Northwestern Ohio Universities College of Medicine, Rootstown; Attending Orthopaedic Surgeon, Akron City Hospital, Akron General Medical Center, and St. Thomas Medical Center, Akron, Ohio
Alternative Forms of Disc Excision: Chemonucleolysis and *Microdiscectomy*

Dennis P. McGowan, M.D. M.Sc.
Clinical Fellow in Orthopaedic Surgery, Harvard Medical School; Associate in Orthopaedic Surgery, Daniel E. Hogan Spine Research Fellow, Beth Israel Hospital, Boston, Massachusetts
Biomechanical Considerations of Spinal Stability

R. F. McLain, M.D.
Fellow, Department of Orthopaedics, University of California, Davis, Sacramento, California
Tumors of the Spine

Luis A. Mignucci, M.D.
Clinical Assistant Professor of Neurosurgery, The University of Texas—Southwestern Medical Center at Dallas; Attending Physician, Zale-Lipshy University Hospital, Parkland Hospital, HCA Medical Center of Plano, RHD Memorial Medical Center—Dallas, Richardson Medical Center, Dallas, Texas
Differential Diagnosis of Sciatica

Srdjan Mirkovic, M.D.
Assistant Professor, Department of Orthopaedic Surgery, Northwestern University Medical School; Staff Orthopaedic Surgeon, Northwestern University Medical School Hospital, Chicago, Illinois
Spinal Stenosis: Nonoperative and Operative Treatment

Michael T. Modic, M.D.
Chairman, Division of Radiology, Cleveland Clinic Foundation, Cleveland, Ohio
Radiology of the Lumbar Spine

Scott Mubarak, M.D.
Associate Clinical Professor, Department of Orthopedics, University of California, San Diego; Director, Orthopedic Institute, Children's Hospital, San Diego, California
Neuromuscular Scoliosis

Michael J. Murphy, M.D.
Assistant Clinical Professor, Department of Orthopaedics and Rehabilitation, Yale University School of Medicine; Attending Surgeon, Yale–New Haven Hospital, New Haven, Connecticut
Surgical Approaches to the Spine

George F. Muschler, M.D.
Attending Surgeon, Department of Orthopaedic Surgery, The Cleveland Clinic Foundation, Cleveland, Ohio
Spinal Fusion: Principles of Bone Fusion

Kjell Olmarker, M.D., Ph.D.
Assistant Research Professor, Department of Anatomy, University of Gothenburg; Assistant Research Professor, Department of Orthopaedics, Sahlgren Hospital, Gothenburg, Sweden
Anatomy of the Spinal Nerve Roots in the Lumbar and Lower Thoracic Spine

Gary Onik, M.D.
Associate Professor of Radiology and Neurosurgery, University of Pittsburgh; Staff Physician, Allegheny General Hospital, Pittsburgh, Pennsylvania
Alternative Forms of Disc Excision: Percutaneous Automated Discectomy

Manohar M. Panjabi, Ph.D., D.Tech.
Professor of Biomechanics in Surgery and Director of Bioengineering Research, Department of Orthopaedics and Rehabilitation, Yale University School of Medicine, New Haven, Connecticut
Biomechanical Considerations of Spinal Stability

Wesley W. Parke, Ph.D.
Professor and Chairman, Department of Anatomy, University of South Dakota School of Medicine, Vermillion, South Dakota
Development of the Spine; Applied Anatomy of the Spine

Eric Phillips, M.D.
Active Medical Staff, Lee's Summit Hospital, Lee's Summit, Missouri
Spinal Fusion: Allograft

Richard H. Rothman, M.D., Ph.D.
James Edwards Professor and Chairman, Department of Orthopaedic Surgery, Thomas Jefferson University; Chairman, The Rothman Institute, Pennsylvania Hospital, Philadelphia, Pennsylvania
Lumbar Disc Disease

Björn L. Rydevik, M.D., Ph.D.
Associate Professor, Department of Orthopaedics, University of Gothenburg and Sahlgren Hospital, Gothenburg, Sweden
Anatomy of the Spinal Nerve Roots in the Lumbar and Lower Thoracic Spine; Pathophysiology of the Intervertebral Disc and Adjacent Neural Structures; Spinal Stenosis: Pathophysiology

Eugene L. Saenger, M.D.
Professor Emeritus of Radiology, University of Cincinnati College of Medicine, Cincinnati, Ohio
Discitis

L. Carl Samberg, M.D.
Co-Director, Section of Spine Surgery, Department of Orthopaedic Surgery, William Beaumont Hospital, Royal Oak, Michigan
Spinal Fusion: Techniques and Complications

Kazuhiko Satomi, M.D.
Assistant Professor, Department of Orthopaedics, School of Medicine, Keio University; Co-Chief of Spine Group, Orthopaedic Surgery, Keio Gijuku University Hospital, Tokyo, Japan
Ossification of the Posterior Longitudinal Ligament

Robert W. Shields, Jr., M.D.
Staff Neurologist, EMG Laboratory—Neuromuscular Program, Cleveland Clinic Foundation, Cleveland, Ohio
Intraoperative Spinal Cord Monitoring

Frederick A. Simeone, M.D.
Professor of Neurosurgery, University of Pennsylvania School of Medicine; Chief of Neurosurgery, Pennsylvania Hospital; Director of Neurosurgery, Elliott Neurological Center of Pennsylvania Hospital, Philadelphia, Pennsylvania
Cervical Disc Disease: Cervical Disc Disease with Radiculopathy; Surgical Management of Cervical Disc Disease: Surgical Management of Cervical Radiculopathy: Posterior Approach, Indications for Surgery in Cervical Myelopathy: Anterior Versus Posterior Approach and *Surgical Management of Cervical Myelopathy: Laminectomy; Intradural Tumors; Complications of Spinal Surgery: Vascular Complications in Spine Surgery* and *Neurogenic Complications in Spine Surgery*

Edward H. Simmons, M.D., F.R.C.S.(C.), M.S.(Tor.), F.A.C.S.
Professor, Orthopaedic Surgery, State University of New York at Buffalo; Head, Department of Orthopaedic Surgery, Buffalo General Hospital, Buffalo, New York
Ankylosing Spondylitis: Surgical Considerations

J. Michael Simpson, M.D.
Spine Fellow, The Rothman Orthopaedic Institute, Thomas Jefferson University Medical College; Attending Staff, Pennsylvania Hospital and Thomas Jefferson University Hospital, Philadelphia, Pennsylvania
Arthritis of the Spine

Mark A. Slater, Ph.D.
Assistant Professor, Department of Psychiatry, University of California, San Diego, La Jolla; Director, Pain Management and Behavioral Medicine Program, Veterans Administration Medical Center, San Diego, California
Chronic Pain Management: Behavioral Medicine Approaches to Chronic Back Pain

Susan Snodgrass, M.D.
Assistant Professor of Neurology, University of Miami School of Medicine, Miami, Florida
Medical Myelopathies

Robert A. Solomon, M.D.
Associate Professor of Clinical Neurological Surgery, Columbia University College of Physicians and Surgeons; Associate Attending, Presbyterian Hospital in the City of New York, New York, New York
Arteriovenous Malformations of the Spinal Cord

Wayne O. Southwick, M.D.
Professor, Department of Orthopaedics and Rehabilitation, Yale University School of Medicine; Attending Surgeon, Yale–New Haven Hospital, New Haven, Connecticut
Surgical Approaches to the Spine

Dan M. Spengler, M.D.
Professor and Chairman, Department of Orthopaedics and Rehabilitation, Vanderbilt University Medical Center, Nashville, Tennessee
Workers' Compensation as It Affects the Spine: Newer Assessment Approaches for the Patient with Low Back Pain

Jeffery L. Stambough, M.D.
Associate Professor of Orthopaedic Surgery; Assistant Professor of Neurosurgery; Director, Giannestras Spine Service, University of Cincinnati College of Medicine, Cincinnati, Ohio
Discitis; Complications of Spinal Surgery: Vascular Complications in Spine Surgery and *Neurogenic Complications in Spine Surgery*

Bennett M. Stein, M.D.
Byron Stookey Professor and Chairman, Department of Neurosurgery, Columbia University College of Physicians and Surgeons; Director of Service, Neurosurgery, Presbyterian Hospital in the City of New York, New York, New York
Arteriovenous Malformations of the Spinal Cord

Joanna G. B. Sullivan, M.D.
Assistant Professor of Clinical Anesthesia, University of California, San Francisco
Chronic Pain Management: The Anesthesiologist's Approach to Back Pain

Leslie Sutton, M.D.
Associate Professor of Neurosurgery, University of Pennsylvania School of Medicine; Attending Physician, Children's Hospital of Philadelphia, Philadelphia, Pennsylvania
Congenital Anomalies of the Spinal Cord

Vernon Tolo, M.D.
Professor of Orthopaedics, University of Southern California School of Medicine, Los Angeles, California
Spinal Disorders Associated with Skeletal Dysplasias and Metabolic Diseases

Eric J. Wall, M.D.
Research Spine Fellow, Department of Orthopaedics, University of California, San Diego, California
Anatomy of the Spinal Nerve Roots in the Lumbar and Lower Thoracic Spine

Ay-Ming Wang, M.D.
Clinical Associate Professor of Radiology, University of Missouri–Kansas City; Kansas City, Missouri; Co-Chief, Neuroradiology Division, Department of Diagnostic Radiology, William Beaumont Hospital, Royal Oak, Michigan
Cervical Disc Disease: Radiologic Evaluation

Robert G. Watkins, M.D.
Associate Clinical Professor, University of Southern California Medical School, Los Angeles; Spinal Surgery Consultant, Kerlan-Jobe Orthopaedic Clinic, Inglewood, California
Back Pain in Children and Adolescents; Cervical Disc Disease: Clinical Syndromes in Cervical Myelopathy

J. N. Weinstein, D.O.
Associate Professor, Department of Orthopaedic Surgery, University of Iowa; Director, Spine Diagnostic and Treatment Center, University of Iowa Hospitals and Clinics, Iowa City, Iowa
Tumors of the Spine

Dennis Wenger, M.D.
Associate Clinical Professor, and Chief, Section of Pediatric Orthopaedics, Department of Orthopaedics, University of California, San Diego; Director of Orthopedics, Children's Hospital, San Diego, California
Neuromuscular Scoliosis

David P. Wesolowski, M.D.
Co-Chief, Division of Neuroradiology, Department of Diagnostic Radiology, William Beaumont Hospital, Royal Oak, Michigan
Cervical Disc Disease: Radiologic Evaluation

F. Todd Wetzel, M.D.
Assistant Professor, Division of Orthopaedic Surgery, Milton S. Hershey Medical Center, Pennsylvania State University College of Medicine; Chief, Section of Adult Spinal Surgery, University Hospital, Milton S. Hershey Medical Center, Hershey, Pennsylvania
Chronic Pain Management: Surgical Procedures for the Control of Chronic Pain

Augustus A. White III, M.D., D.Med. Sci.
Professor of Orthopaedic Surgery, Harvard Medical School; Orthopaedic Surgeon-in-Chief, Beth Israel Hospital, Boston, Massachusetts
Biomechanical Considerations of Spinal Stability

T. S. Whitecloud III, M.D.
Professor and Chairman, Department of Orthopaedics, Tulane University School of Medicine; Staff Surgeon, Tulane Medical Center Hospital and Clinic, Charity Hospital–New Orleans, and Veterans Administration Hospital–New Orleans, New Orleans, Louisiana
Complications of Spinal Surgery: Postlaminectomy Kyphosis of the Cervical Spine

Sam W. Wiesel, M.D.
Professor and Chairman, Department of Orthopaedic Surgery, Georgetown University School of Medicine and Medical Center, Washington, D.C.
Cervical Disc Disease: Conservative Treatment; The Multiply Operated Low Back Patient; Workers' Compensation as it Affects the Spine: Compensation Low Back and Neck Pain

Asa J. Wilbourn, M.D.
Associate Clinical Professor (Neurology), Case Western Reserve University School of Medicine; Director, EMG Laboratory, Department of Neurology, Cleveland Clinic, Cleveland, Ohio
Electrodiagnosis: The Electromyographic Examination

Harold A. Wilkinson, M.D., Ph.D
Professor and Chairman, Division of Neurosurgery; Professor of Anatomy/Cell Biology, University of Massachusetts Medical School; Chief, Neurosurgical Service, University of Massachusetts Hospital; Neurosurgical Staff, St. Vincent Hospital and Medical Center of Central Massachusetts, Worcester, Massachusetts
Complications of Spinal Surgery: Adhesive Arachnoiditis

Robert B. Winter, M.D.
Clinical Professor, Orthopaedic Surgery, University of Minnesota; Staff Surgeon, Minnesota Spine Center, Minneapolis and St. Paul; Chief of Spine Service, Gillette Children's Hospital, St. Paul, Minnesota
Juvenile and Adolescent Scoliosis

Ronald J. Wisneski, M.D.
Assistant Professor, Department of Orthopaedic Surgery, Hospital of the University of Pennsylvania; Chief of the Spinal Disorders Service, Hospital of the University of Pennsylvania; Chief, Section of Orthopaedic Surgery, Presbyterian Medical Center of Philadelphia, Philadelphia, Pennsylvania
Lumbar Disc Disease

FOREWORD

Monumental texts on spinal disorders have been rare in the past, with the classic Rothman and Simeone two-volume book as one outstanding exception. Even though today there is a plethora of new books on back problems, few encompass the broad, multidisciplinary approach like this new addition of the old classic. The Rothman and Simeone texts have always been well balanced, and the editorial board of this third edition has again succeeded in giving this fascinating topic a mixture of authors from many different specialties, which is a definite necessity when dealing with diseases of the spine. They have also been able to assemble many of the most prominent researchers in the world on some of the various vertebral topics, augmenting the high standards and excellent reputation of the previous editions. For up-to-date, mature, well-balanced descriptions of the multiplicity of spinal disorders, this third expanded edition of an already classic book will have no comparison and I am certain it will be the standard reference text for the nineties.

ALF L. NACHEMSON, M.D., PH.D.
HON FRCS (ENG), AAOS, SRS, ESDS
Professor and Chairman
Department of Orthopaedics
University of Gothenburg,
Gothenburg, Sweden

SECTION 1

BASIC SCIENCE AND DIAGNOSIS

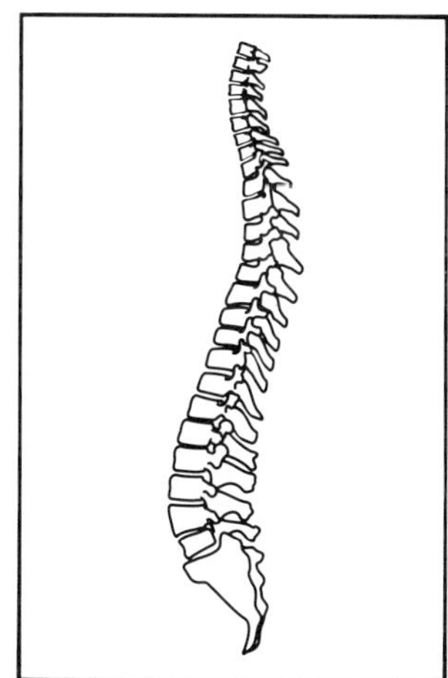

CHAPTER

1

DEVELOPMENT OF THE SPINE

Wesley W. Parke, Ph.D.

The role of metamerism in the evolution of vertebrate morphology is remarkably illustrated in the development of the spine. This biologic principle, whereby the organism is formed by the linear repetition of many anatomically similar segments (metameres), evolved in the higher invertebrates. However, it is only in the chordates that the segments are formed from a series of mesenchymal condensations flanking a longitudinal notochord and dorsal neural tube (Fig. 1–1). The resultant body sections, including their neural and notochordal regions, form the somites.

Primitively, all somites have the same developmental potential, and in the lower aquatic vertebrates they formed a definitive spine that showed minimal regional differentiation. With the evolution of limbs the variety of postures and modes of locomotion required more specific regional differences, and another biologic principle, Stromer's law,[52] was superimposed on the original segmentation. As applied to metamerism, this "law" is actually an observed adaptive trend in which the many similar segments (isomerism) of the primitive animal decrease in number through deletion or fusion, while the remaining segments increase their diverse functional and anatomic specialization (anisomerism).

Despite the evolutionary overlay, the higher vertebrate spine still shows a monotonous similarity of the somites in its early stages of development, and by following the embryologic acquisition of the regional peculiarities, the common homologies of the various components of the different adult vertebrae are revealed. Therefore, the first part of this discussion is devoted to the development of a typical vertebral element, and the regional specialization is discussed subsequently.

Early Development of Somites

The development of the human spine starts with the onset of the triploblastic stage of the embryo and ends in the third decade of life. On the 17th day of human gestation, cells at the center of the dorsal layer of the bilaminar embryonic disc invaginate to form the primitive pit. The cells around this opening form the primitive knot and further proliferate cranially between the ectoderm and endoderm as the tubular notochordal process. The cells underlying the hollow axis of this process and their contiguous layer of endoderm both degenerate, so that the upper half of the notochordal process comes to lie directly in contact with the contents of the yolk sac and forms the flat notochordal plate. Starting cranially, the lateral edges of this plate then curl under

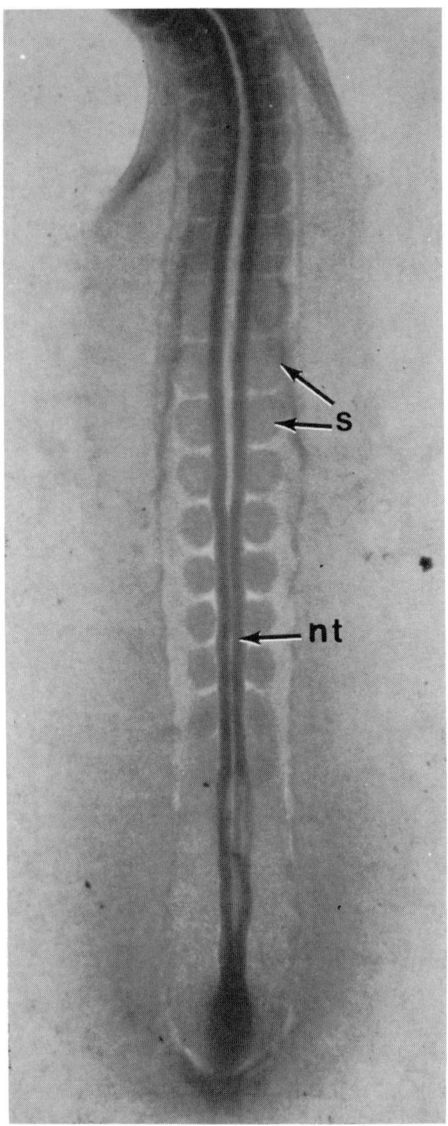

Figure 1–1. Chick embryo at the 20 somite stage. The formation of the cuboidal somites (s) lateral to the neural tube (nt) is apparent. Each somite is separated by the intermyotomic septum.

until they meet. This reunites the endoderm and produces the true notochord. The presence of the notochordal cells induces a thickening in the overlying ectoderm (neurectoderm), which forms the neural plate. On the 18th day the edges of this plate curl upward, and their union creates the dorsal neural tube.

In the higher vertebrates the notochord is primarily a developmental structure that determines the longitudinal axis of the early embryo and induces ectodermal and mesodermal differentiation, but in prevertebrate chordates and the cyclostomes it persists throughout life as a firm, flexible rod that is the essential part of the axial skeleton.

With the elaboration of the notochord and neural tube, the intraembryonic mesoderm lateral to these structures thickens to form two longitudinal columns, the paraxial mesoderm. Further lateral proliferation of this cell mass results in two additional areas, so that by the 19th day three distinct areas of the mesoderm are evident. These consist of the medial paraxial columns, a bilateral pair of intermediate mesodermal columns, and the most lateral mesodermal plates. The lateral mesoderm forms the layers that encase the coelomic cavities, while the intermediate columns give rise to urogenital structures.

The somites arise from the paraxial mesoderm. On approximately the 20th day the cells in the anterior parts of these columns condense into pairs of blocklike segments. The first pair appears just caudal to the rostral end of the notochord, and an additional 38 pairs of somites continue to form in a craniocaudal sequence throughout the next ten days, which is called the somite period. Eventually 42 to 44 somites appear. Externally, they are evident as a series of elevated beads (Fig. 1–5) along the dorsolateral surface of the embryo and, in section, are wedge-shaped with an ephemeral cavity, the myocoele.

During the somite stage the more cranial, older somites show internal specializations. The cells dorsolateral to the myocoele become the dermomyotome. The lateral group of these cells, the cutis plate, will give rise to the integument, and the more medial group, the muscle plate, establishes the dorsal musculature. The ventromedial cell mass, the sclerotome, exhibits cell migration in three directions in anticipation of forming skeletal structures (Figs. 1–2 to 1–6).

The development and migration of these sclerotome cells indicates the formation of the first of three successive vertebral columns. In the precartilaginous stage the sclerogenous mesenchyme that aligns itself along the notochord and neural tube forms the membranous vertebral column (Fig. 1–6). Chondrification results in the cartilaginous column, and endochondral ossification eventually produces the definitive skeleton columns (Figs. 1–6*B*, 1–7).

At this point of the chapter in previous editions of this book, the author began to describe the differentiation of the sclerotome into the various prechondrous cell masses that were destined to become the neurocostal and axial components of the definitive vertebra. This narration included the concept of "resegmentation" wherein the caudal half of one sclerotome was believed to fuse with the cranial half of the subadjacent sclerotome to form a truly intersegmental vertebral body. First postulated by Remak[41] in 1855, this idea was amplified by von Ebner[59] who, in 1889, coined the term "Neugliederung" (resegmentation) and claimed that the process was necessary to account for the alternating arrangement of the definitive muscular and skeletal elements of the spine. Given this initial view, subsequent investigators published various elaborations of the theory until the authority of its antiquity and unquestioned repetition made it a paradigm of the evolution of a scientific dogma. As nearly all extant texts (and the previous versions of this chapter) found that a simplified schema of the resegmentation theory so facilely explained the "problems" of spine devel-

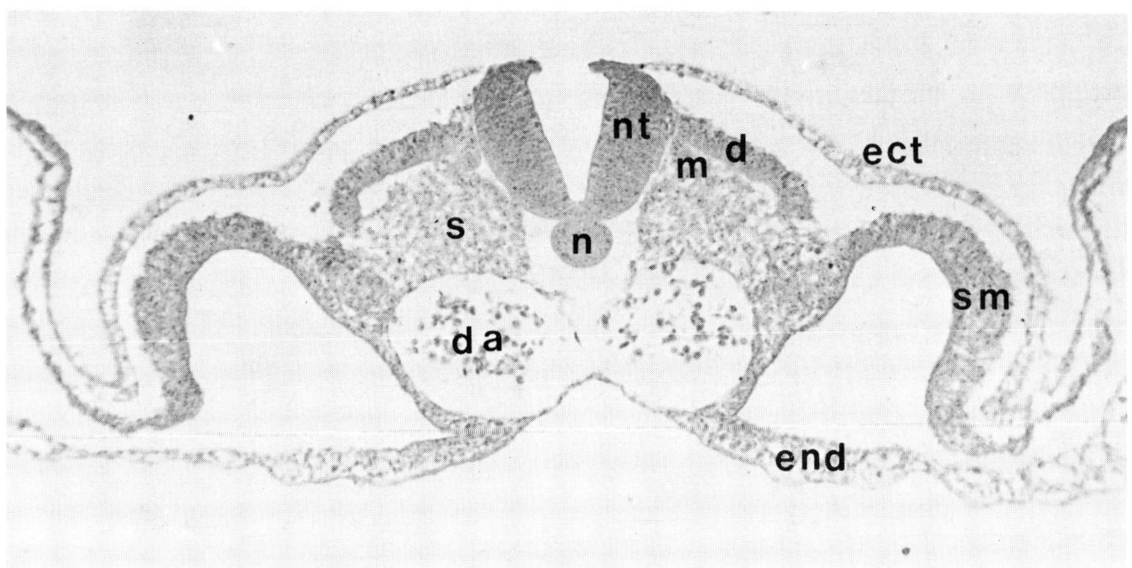

Figure 1–2. Cross section of a thoracic somite in a chick embryo of the 20 somite stage. Notochord (n) underlies neural tube (nt). The somite is divided into dermatome (d), myotome (m), and sclerotome (s). Lateral to this the somatic mesoderm (sm), endoderm (end), and ectoderm (ect) are displayed. Ventral to the sclerotomes lie the paired dorsal aortae (da). Transient myocele is apparent on the right side between the dermatome and myotome.

AM
N
LM
IV
DM
A

CR
CA
CE
DP
ISP
LP
SN
M
N
B

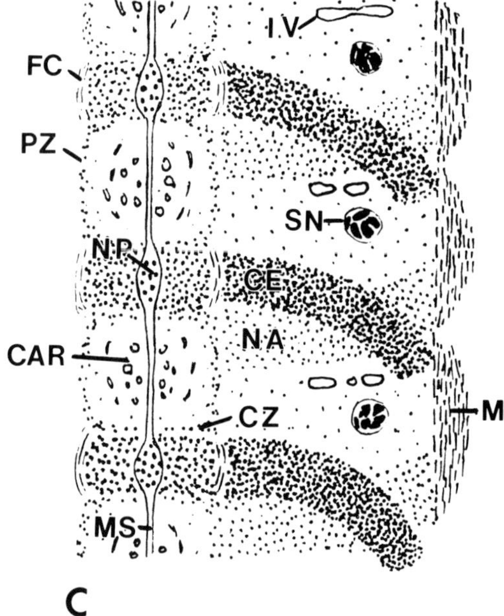

Figure 1–3 *See legend on opposite page*

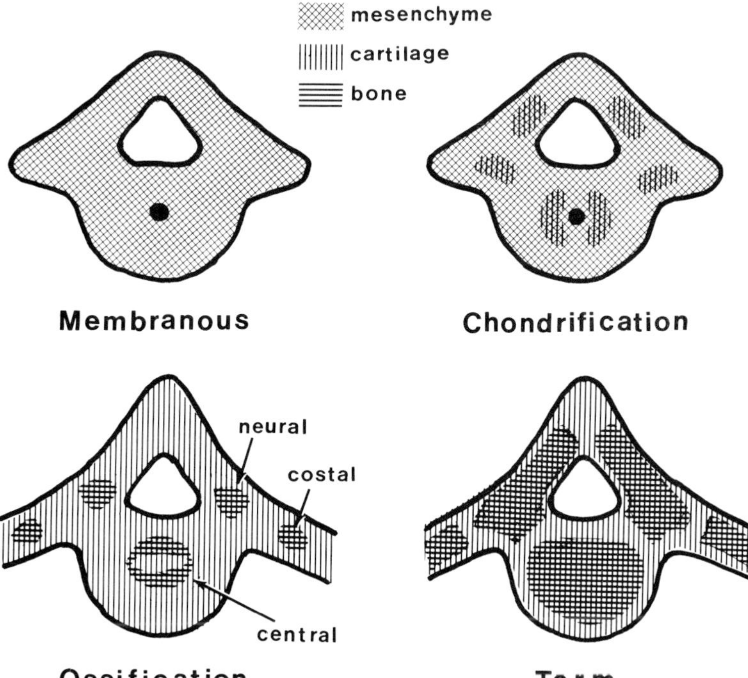

Figure 1–4. Schematic illustration of the sequential development of the typical vertebral element.

opment, it was fortunate that some investigators took the effort to re-examine the data.

Although the resegmentation concept was not accepted without question initially,[16] it was not until 1969 that Baur[4] published an extensive critique that presented considerable contrary evidence. Within the next two decades, Verbout[56] and his associates[11, 58] published a series of observations that left little doubt of the invalidity of the resegmentation theory. This work culminated in 1985 with Verbout's[57] meticulous monograph on the development of the vertebral column using three directional views of sheep embryos in virtually every gradation of early spine development. Verbout's findings received additional support from the independent observations of Dalgleish,[12] who, also in 1985, published his account of spine development in the mouse using autoradiography to identify certain sites of cell proliferation more accurately.

All the above-cited critics claimed that the

Figure 1–3. Schematic representation of the early development of the mammalian vertebrae derived from information provided by Verbout[57] and Dalgleish.[12] *A,* Early organization of mesenchymal columns. Notochord (N) is of uniform diameter and surrounded by loose unsegmented axial mesenchyme (AM) from which vertebral centra and discs will be derived. Lateral sclerotomic mesenchyme (LM) also shows little evidence of segmentation at first. The dermamyotome (DM) retains the original somitic segmentation, and the intersegmental vessels (IV) mark intersclerotomic boundaries. *B,* Axial mesenchyme shows differentiation into dense perichordal disc (DP) and loose perichordal disc (LP). These will become the intervertebral disc and centrum, respectively. The lateral mesenchyme separates into a loose tissue of its cranial sclerotomic region (CR), which accommodates the intervertebral vessels (IV) and the developing spinal nerves (SN), and a dense caudal sclerotomic region (CA) that is precursor to the neural arches. A costal element (CE) organizes lateral to the incipient disc. The intrasclerotomic plane (ISP) is the abrupt demarcation of cell differentiation that may produce spurious "intrasegmental clefts" in histologic preparation. *C,* Here the notochord shows the differentiation into the mucoid streak (MS) and the cell concentration that will contribute to the nucleus pulposus (NP). The disc now shows the development of fibrocartilage (FC), and additional growth is now provided by the perichondral and chondrogenous zones (PZ, CZ). The "crossing" of the membranous precursors of the costal element (CE) and the neural arch element (NA) is a graphic attempt to indicate that the costal elements grow ventrolaterally while the neural arch grows dorsolaterally that was borrowed from Dalgleish. The staggered positions of the myotomes (M) relative to the neural arch elements indicate why "resegmentation" is not required to explain the definitive muscle-bone overlapping.

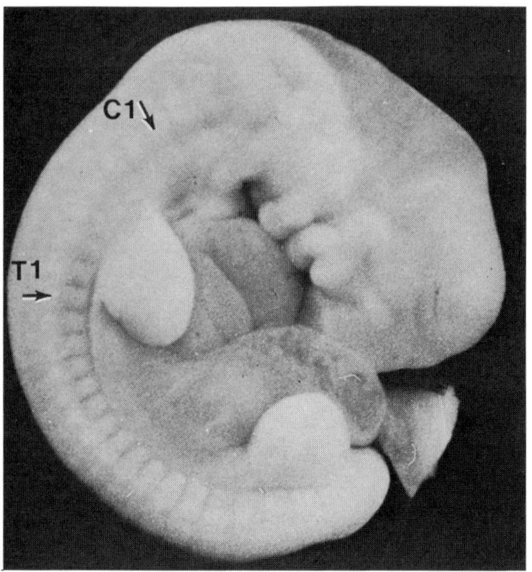

Figure 1–5. Human embryo of 5.5-mm crown-rump length. Note that the somites are externally represented as a series of dorsolateral swellings, and that at least two somites may be discerned rostral to the atlantal (C1) segment.

two major premises of the resegmentation theory (first, the necessity of explaining the alternation of muscle and skeletal components and second, the existence of the intrasclerotomic fissure that indicated the splitting of the original sclerotome) failed to be substantiated in their studies. In fact, von Ebner admitted that the fissures were difficult to demonstrate, and Baur stated that they are simply interfaces between two tissue densities where histologic processing may readily produce a tear.

These same critics were equally concerted in their belief that, in the transformation from the membranous to the cartilaginous stages of development, the diverse histories of the lateral and axial mesenchymal regions must be recognized. The following account is essentially an abstract of their collective investigations.

In the early membranous stages of vertebral column development, the somitic mesenchyme proliferates to first fill the triangular area lateral to the neural tube with bilateral columnar masses of fairly dense mesenchymal cells. By further ventromedial proliferation, another mass of more loosely arranged cells surrounds the notochord and separates it from the ventral aspect of the neural tube and the dorsal aspect of the aorta, to thus form a median column of axial mesenchyme. The columns of lateral mesenchyme are the membranous precursors to the cartilaginous stages of the neurocostal components of the developing vertebrae, while the axial mesenchyme predetermines the intervertebral disc and the cartilaginous vertebral body. At this stage the cell masses of the lateral and axial mesenchyme are continuous with each other ventromedially, and uniform in composition longitudinally, so that they now show no evidence of the initial somitic segmentation. Since the formation of the vertebrae results from the diverse events in the differentiation of these two regions of the primitive mesenchyme, the fate of the axial cell mass will be discussed first.

EARLY MORPHOGENESIS OF VERTEBRAL BODY AND INTERVERTEBRAL DISC

The loose unsegmented tissue originally designated axial mesenchyme first shows an intrinsic proliferation that establishes a more defined cylindric column called the perichordal tube. Dalgleish[12] autoradiographically demonstrated that this proliferation is initially moderate and uniformly distributed within the tube, but subsequently there is evidence of more rapid cell propagation at equidistant intervals. This establishes longitudinal alternations of dense and loose cell aggregates. The dense cell propagation, which first appears ventral to the notochord, rapidly surrounds it and extends laterally. The encircling cells then form the dense perichordal discs that alternate with intervening loose perichordal discs (Fig. 1–3*B*). A thin condensation of cells forms a boundary between these two regions that has been called the intradiscal membrane[2] or the perichondrial zone blastema.[12] Chondrogenesis begins in the center of the loose perichordal disc and constricts the notochordal tissue passing through this area, so that notochordal cells eventually are evident only in the center of the dense perichordal disc.

From the foregoing it is obvious that most of the axial structures of the vertebral column are derived from an unsegmented perichordal mesenchyme. The loose perichordal discs that are proliferated within this mesenchyme give rise to the original cartilaginous centra, while

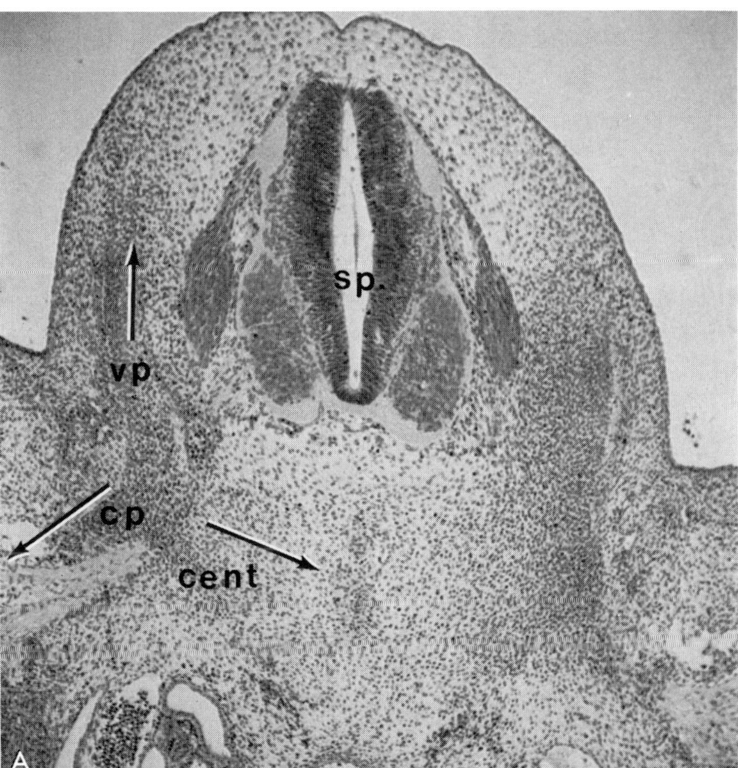

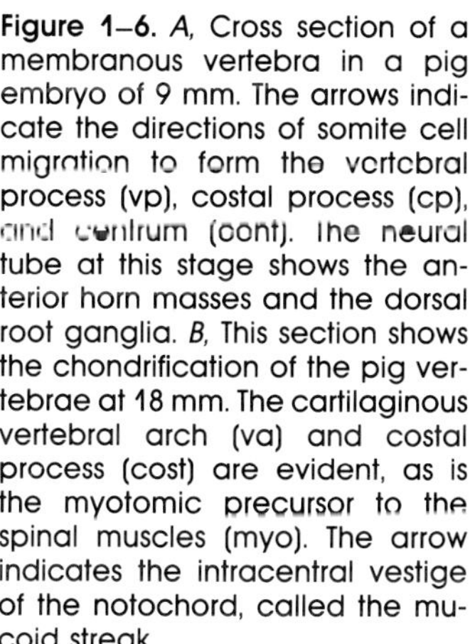

Figure 1–6. *A,* Cross section of a membranous vertebra in a pig embryo of 9 mm. The arrows indicate the directions of somite cell migration to form the vertebral process (vp), costal process (cp), and centrum (cent). The neural tube at this stage shows the anterior horn masses and the dorsal root ganglia. *B,* This section shows the chondrification of the pig vertebrae at 18 mm. The cartilaginous vertebral arch (va) and costal process (cost) are evident, as is the myotomic precursor to the spinal muscles (myo). The arrow indicates the intracentral vestige of the notochord, called the mucoid streak.

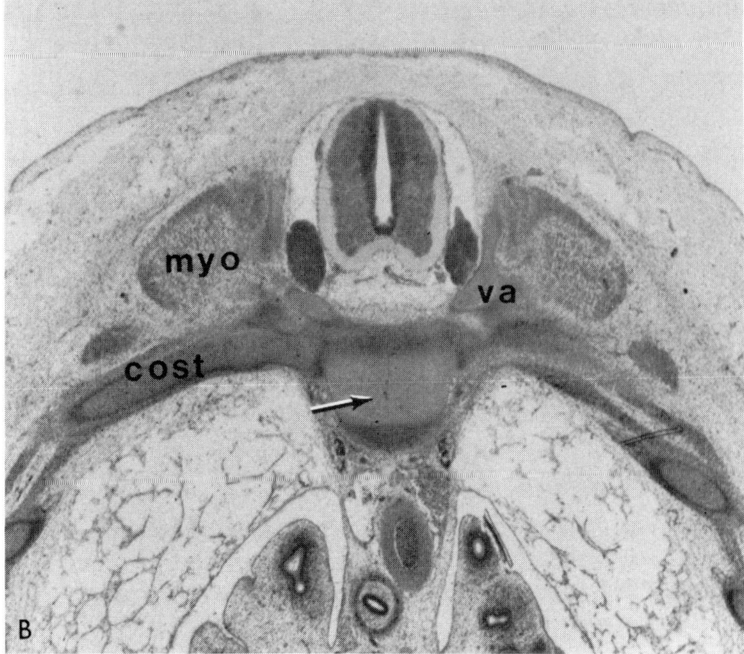

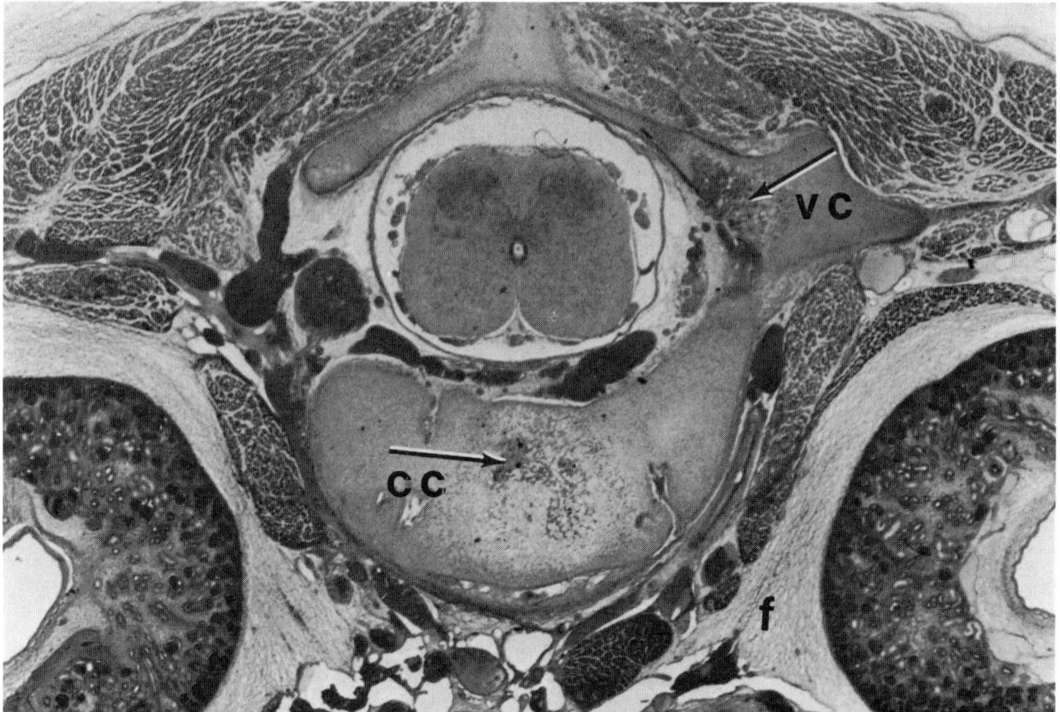

Figure 1–7. A vertebra of a human fetus at 38-mm crown-rump length showing centers of ossification. The section is slightly oblique so that only the right center for the vertebral arch (vc) and the center for the centrum are obvious. Level of section is approximately at T2.

the denser discs form the intervertebral discs. Autoradiographic studies have indicated that when chondrification of the loose perichordal disc is complete, its internal cell proliferation ceases and further growth is then provided by the chondroblasts in the perichondrial zone layers that have come to completely surround the loose disc area (Fig. 1–3*C*).

Early Morphogenesis of Neurocostal Elements

Although the earliest sclerotomic mesenchyme was segmentally arranged along with its respective myotomic elements of the somite and is originally separated from its adjacent counterparts by an intersclerotomic cleft, the ventromedial cell proliferation that forms the axial mesenchyme is also accompanied by a caudal and cranial extension of cells within the lateral mesenchyme. This produces a fusion between the adjacent masses of somitic mesenchyme that obliterates the intersclerotomic cleft, and the originally segmented mesenchyme becomes the continuous lateral column from which the neurocostal contributions to the vertebrae will be derived. However, the intersegmental junctions of the myotomic arcs and the intersegmental vessels continue to mark the relative position of the now vanished intersclerotomic cleft. This lateral column, like the contemporary axial column, initially displays a longitudinally uniform cell density (Fig. 1–3*A*), but the cells lying medial to the cranial half of the myotome soon show a marked diminution in number, either by migration or cell death, and produce a much lighter appearance in this half of the histologically sectioned sclerotome. The intersegmental vessels remain at the superior boundary of this light region, while the associated intersegmental nerve courses within the loose cell mass. Simultaneous with the events described above, the caudal half of the sclerotome exhibits an increased cell density. In the rostromedial part of this caudal hemisclerotome, just lateral to the dense perichordal disc of the axial mesenchyme, a rapid increase in cell concentration signals the formation of the rib primordium.

Caudal to this, the cells of the remaining part of the hemisclerotome proliferate to lie down the membranous precursor of the neural arch (Fig. 1–3*B*). The medial limits of these cell masses at first appear to commingle with the more external cells of the perichordal tube without the intervention of the perichondrial zone layer. However, as chondrification proceeds, the neurocentral synchondrosis eventually develops as a demarcation between these two regions. At this point, it should be emphasized that while the loose-celled axial mesenchyme forms the central component of the vertebral body, the neural arch primordium always contributes substantially to the formation of the definitive body, the greatest contribution (approximately one half the body mass) occurring in the cervical region (Figs. 1–8 to 1–19).

Analysis of the foregoing information will show that the eventual segmentation of the axial mesenchyme and its equivalent lateral sclerotomic cell mass eventually develops a staggered relationship in their longitudinal arrangement. Thus the formation of the intervertebral disc occurs opposite the junction between the loose and dense sclerotomic halves. As this is the reputed location of the elusive intrasclerotomic cleft, one may readily comprehend how this interface could account for an artifactual separation during histologic processing. As the medial part of this junction is also the site of rib blastema formation, especially in the developing thoracic region,

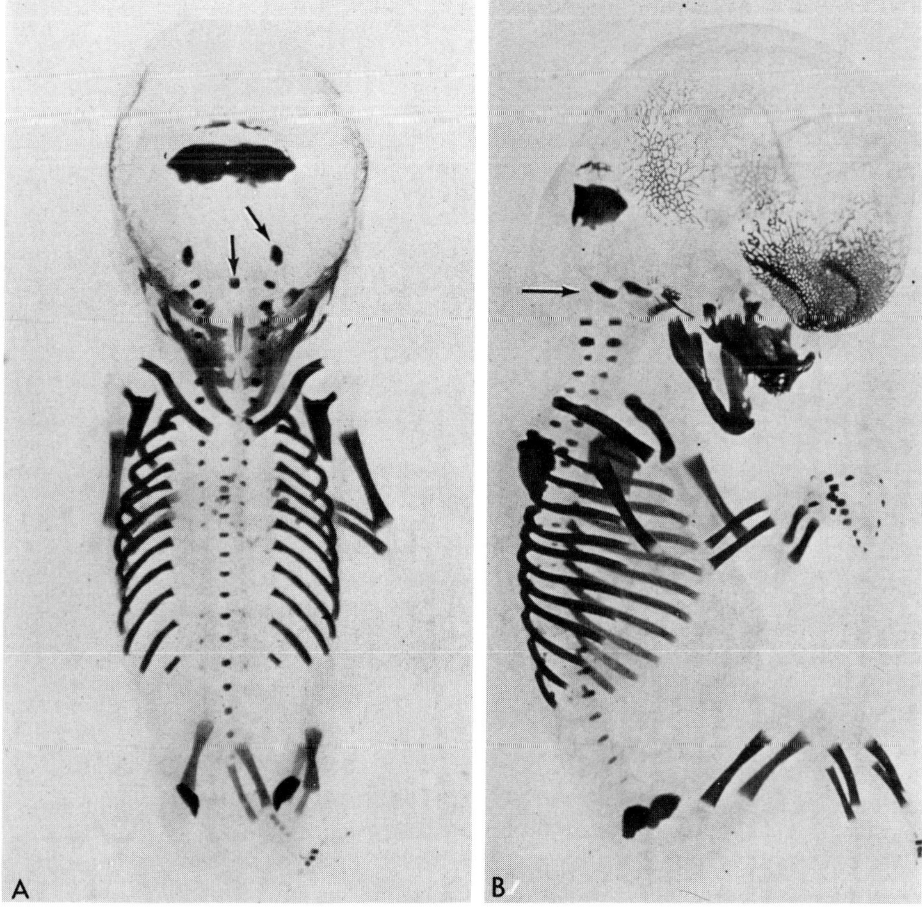

Figure 1–8. *A*, Posterior view of a cleared fetus of 54-mm crown-rump length. Specimen has been stained with alizarin to show areas of ossification. The differential appearance of the central ossification in the lower thoracocolumbar region and the vertebral arch centers in the cervical region are well illustrated. *B*, Lateral view of the same specimen. Arrows in *A* and *B* indicate the ossification of an occipital somite.

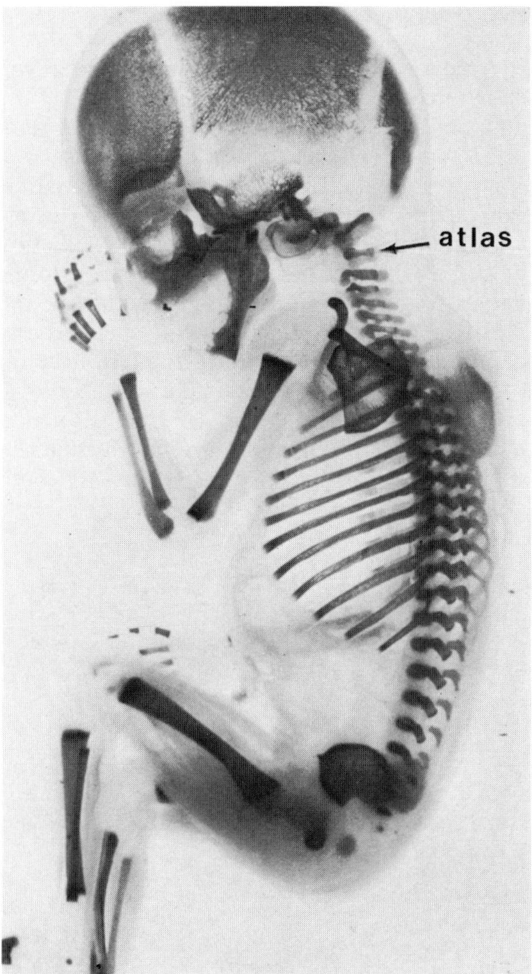

Figure 1–9. An oblique lateral view of a fetus of 125-mm crown-rump length. The separate neural arch and central ossifications are still obvious. Again, note the similarity of occipital and vertebral ossification.

the definitive relationship of the typical rib to a disc and the two adjacent vertebrae becomes obvious. However, the essential concept here is indicated by the fact that the neural arch anlagen forms in the caudal part of the caudal hemisclerotome. During the complex regional differentiations of the axial and sclerotomic mesenchyme, the myotome has maintained its simple arcuate apposition to the entire somite, and the prechondrous components of the neural arch acquire an off-set relationship to the developing myotome. Thus, each myotome comes to extend from a caudal attachment to the caudal edge of its segmentally equivalent neural arch, to the caudal edge of the neural arch of the preceding somite in a shingle-like fashion (Fig. 1–3*C*). This arrangement then obviates the supposed requirement of "Neugliederung" to account for the functional overlapping of the dorsal spinal muscles relative to the vertebrae.

Although recent research has provided a more substantiated concept of vertebral column morphogenesis, there has been little attempt to relate this information to one of the more obscure but very interesting aspects of the phylogeny and ontogeny of the vertebrae:

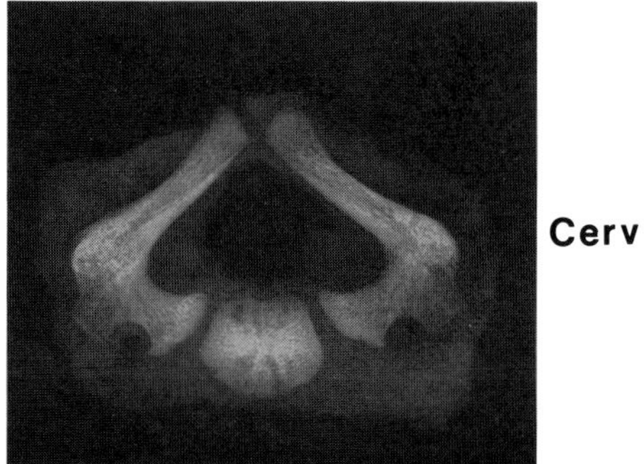

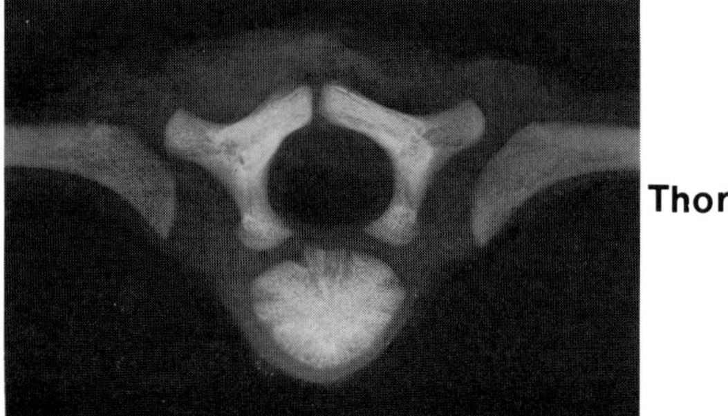

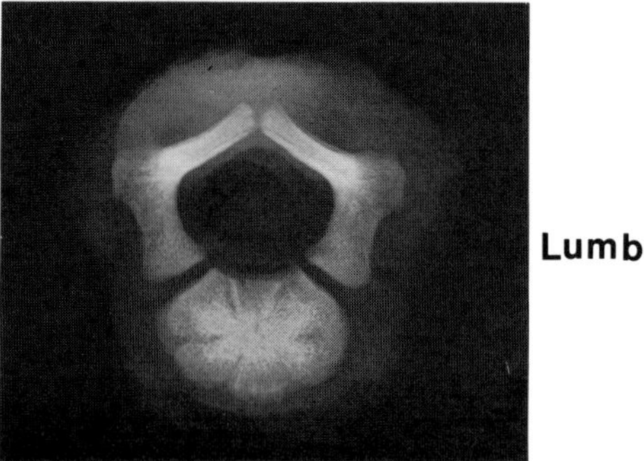

Figure 1–10. Vertical radiograms of individual vertebrae of a 34-week fetus. The contributions of the vertebral arches to the dorsolateral parts of the bodies are apparent. The cartilaginous line between the central ossification and the arches marks the neurocentral synchondroses. The union between the thoracic rib and the vertebral components shows the costovertebral arthroses.

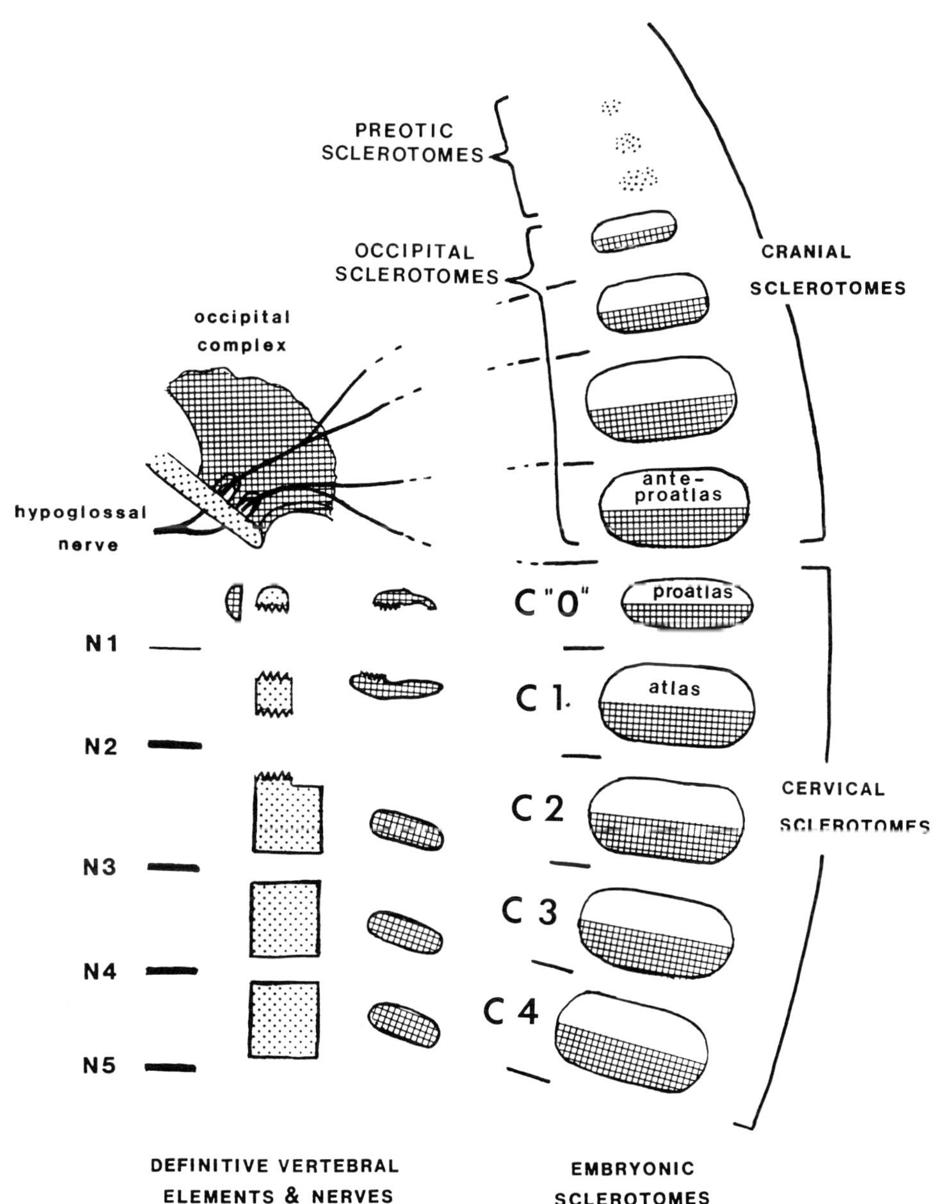

Figure 1–11. Schematic representation of the craniocervical sclerotomes and their segmentally related definitive cranial and vertebral elements and nerves. Note that the cranial and cervical sclerotomes originally formed a continuum. Note also that the axis incorporates three sclerotomic elements, and the atlas ring includes neural arch components of both atlas and proatlas in addition to the hypochordal derivative of the proatlas. The caudal four cranial sclerotomes contribute to the occiput, and their nerves coalesce to form the hypoglossal nerve. This schema shows a double hypoglossal canal in which the membranous strut between the original openings became ossified. This strut is usually a transient contribution from a sclerotome cranial to the ante-proatlas. A developmental basis for the variety of craniocervical anomalies may be readily understood from this schema.

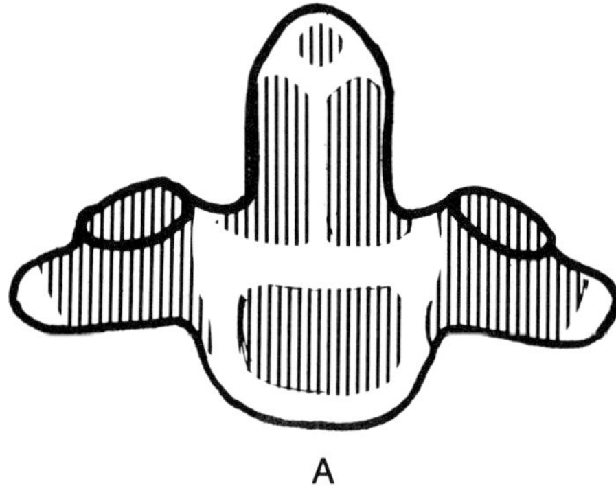

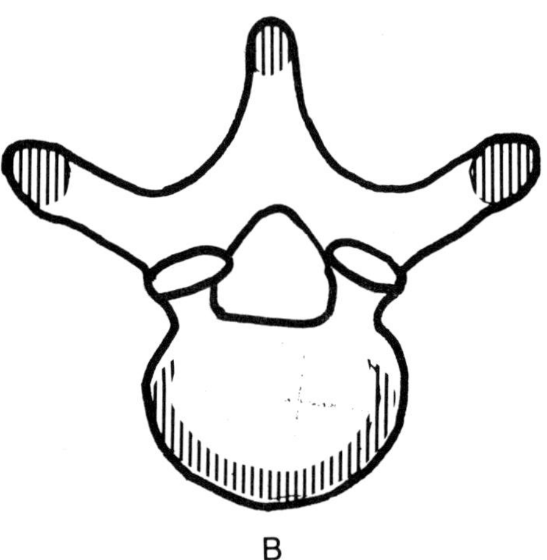

Figure 1–12. *A,* The centers of ossification of the axis. The lateral and central centers for the body of C2 are like those of subsequent vertebrae, but the odontoid shows two bilateral primary centers and a single secondary apical center. *B,* The secondary centers of ossification of a thoracic vertebra. The centers at the tips of the processes appear at 16 years and fuse at approximately 25 years. The ring apophysis at the edge of the centrum ossifies at approximately 14 years and fuses at 25 years.

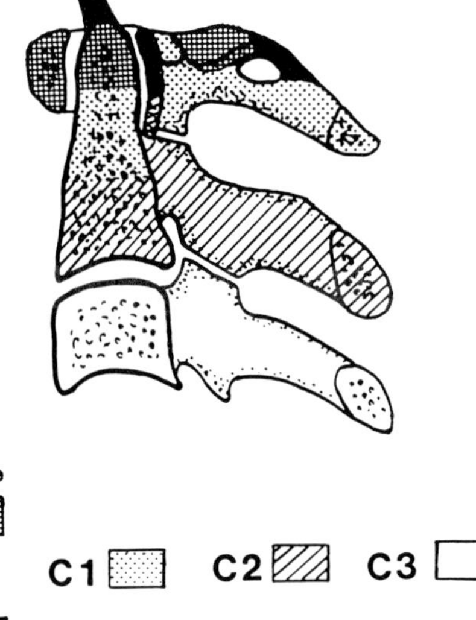

Figure 1–13. This schema shows the definitive contributions from the first three sclerotome segments to the atlantoaxial complex and its syndesmotic relations. The proatlas (C"0") provides the tip of the odontoid process, the hypochordal anterior arch, and the dorsal part of the superior atlas facet as well as the upper half of the transverse ligament and the apical odontoid and retroarticular ligaments, which are indicated in black. The atlas (C1) sclerotome then contributes the remainder of the posterior arch and the inferior major part of the odontoid process.

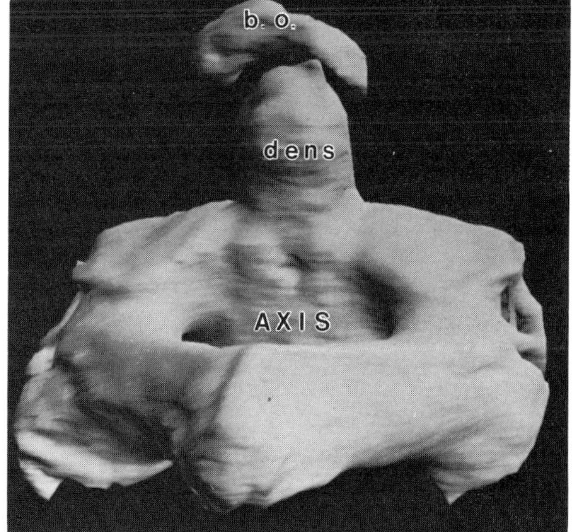

Figure 1–14. A three-dimensional CT reconstruction illustrating a free density assumed to be a Bergmann's ossicle (b.o.) within the dento-occipital joint and superior to an odontoid process of normal configuration.[15] (Photograph courtesy of Dr. H. N Schnitzlein.)

the development of the so-called hypochordal elements. The only constant obvious expression of this embryologic potential in humans is the anterior arch of the atlas, but hypochordal elements are a more common feature in the spinal columns of many lower vertebrates, where they generally constitute the hemal arches. In the tails of some caudate mammals the "chevron bones," like typical hemal arches, developed as ventral counterparts of the neural arches and presumably provide an analogous protection for the contained major vessels (Fig. 1–23). However, anomalous spine conditions suggest that hypochordal elements are an inherent potential of every somitic level, and some alteration in the regionally normal sequences of development in any given vertebral segment may allow their atypical expression. This may be exemplified in cases of the caudal regression syndrome, a condition in which the range of repressed vertebral formation may extend from just a partial sacral agenesis to a complete failure of vertebral development caudal to the thoracic region. This syndrome, although more common in, but not restricted to, the offspring of diabetic mothers, may show at the lower end of its series of normally developed vertebrae a few "transitional" levels of incomplete vertebral components. It appears that when the derivatives of the axial mesenchyme are in default or poorly formed, some lateral column elements, particularly the costal components, may still be partially expressed. In a case known to the author, a pair of costal elements (transverse processes) were radiographically noted caudal to the last fully formed upper lumbar vertebra, and these were *ventrally connected by an osseous bar*. In a personal conversation with Dr. Verbout, he postulated that hypochordal elements are ventral derivatives of the lateral column mesenchyme. It thus appears that an inductive-repressive interplay between the developing elements of any given vertebral level is normally genetically controlled, and the full elaboration of the perichordal tube derivatives may repress further ventral extension of lateral column mesenchyme when these have not acquired or retained genetic "approval." However, if the axial components fail in their normal expression, the inherent hypochordal potential may be variably and atypically manifest. Additional support for this concept may be derived from the occasional occurrence of suspected hypochordal anomalies in the atlanto-occipital region. These are discussed in the section on the treatment of the morphogenesis of this specific area.

Fate of the Notochord

The transition of the notochord from the primary inductive structure of vertebrate axial orientation to its eventual contribution to the formation of the nucleus pulposus has long been generally recognized, but the details of its later fate have been a source of controversy. The very early notochord is closely applied to the neural tube, ovoid in section, and its cells

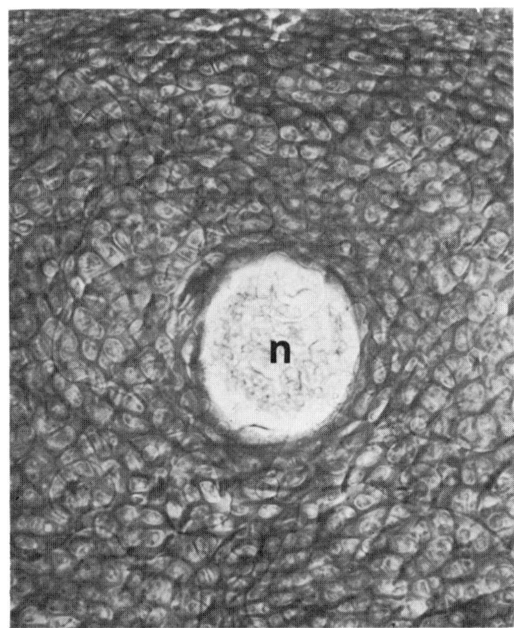

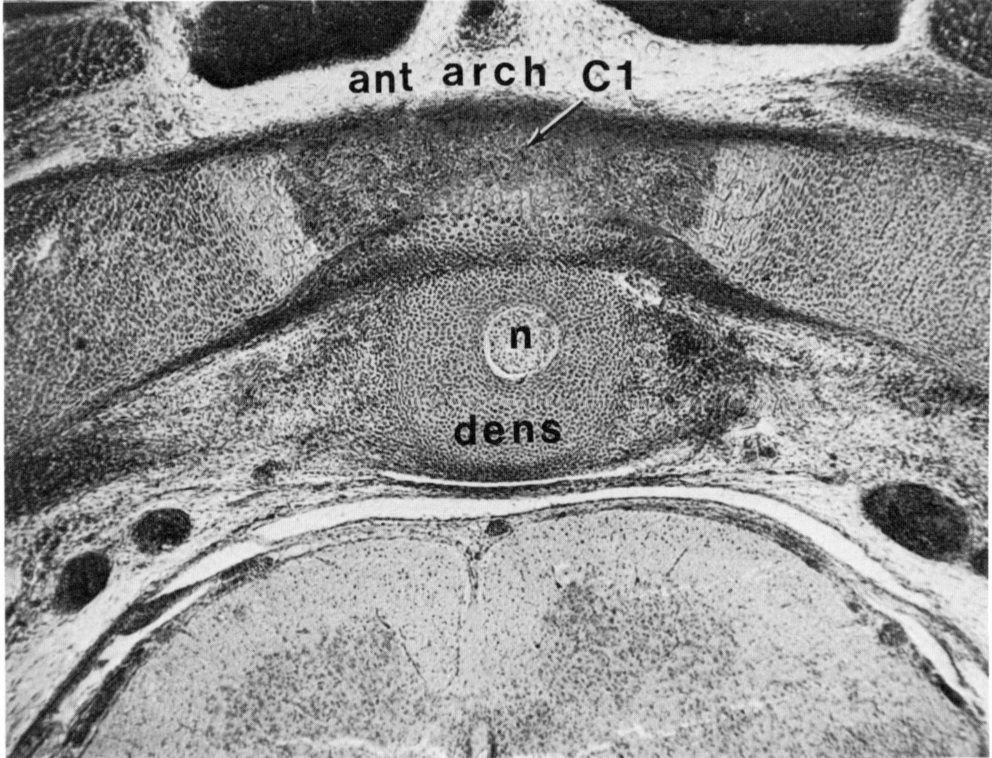

Figure 1–15. Section through the developing odontoid process of the neonatal rat shows the chondrous apex of the process and the ossification of the anterior arch of the atlas. The persistence of the notochord in the odontoid affirms its origin in the homologue of the centrum of C1. The upper illustration shows chondrous cells surrounding loose cellular remnants of notochord.

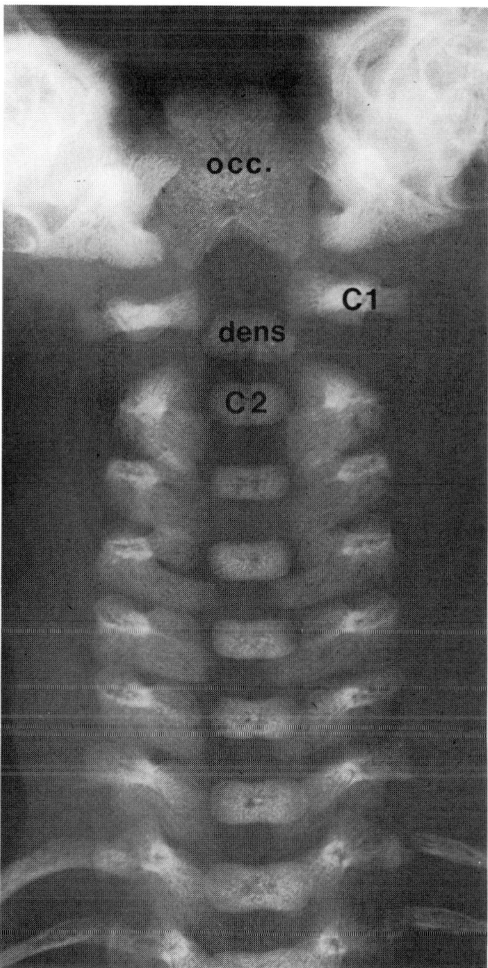

Figure 1–16. Anteroposterior radiogram of the cervical spine of a 30-week fetus. The bilobed ossification of the dens and its separation from the body of C2 are apparent. Fusion of these two elements occurs in the second decade and completes ossification of the axis.

present an epithelial appearance. After it becomes ensheathed by perichordal mesenchyme, the first indication of a segmental influence on the now cylindric chord is the appearance of a series of undulations corresponding to the alternate relations of the dense and light perichordal discs. The cause of these "chordaflexures" is uncertain but apparently related to differential transverse growth rates between the two perichordal disc areas. The change from a fairly uniform rod to an intrinsically segmented structure is evident in the thoracic and lumbar regions of the 20-mm embryo. Here, fusiform enlargements appear in the parts encircled by the dense perichordal disc. At the 30-mm stage this initial indication of segmentation is apparent, to some degree, throughout the entire developing vertebral column, but it is least obvious in the cervical region. The frothy areolar constitution of typical notochordal tissue is now also manifest. With subsequent chondrification and growth of the early vertebral bodies, the expanded notochordal segments within the developing intervertebral discs are drawn farther apart, so that the chord tissue between them is stretched into a "mucoid streak" (Fig. 1–3*C*) that eventually disappears before the formation of the definitive vertebral body.

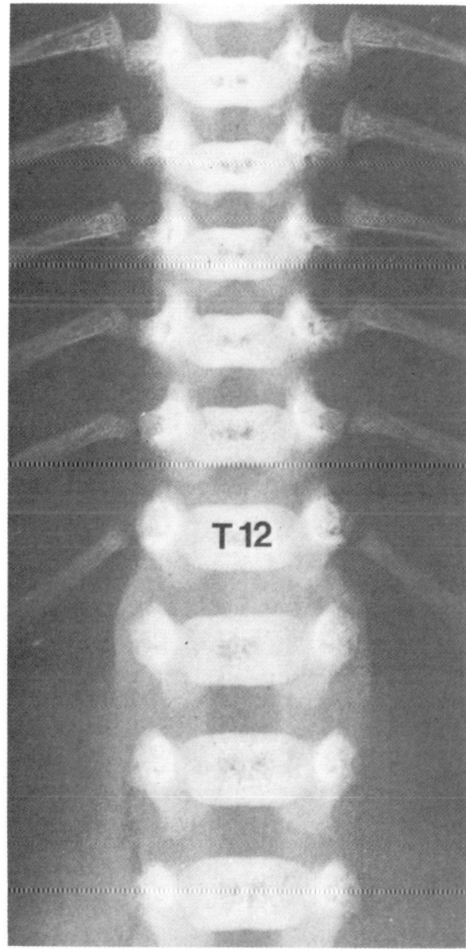

Figure 1–17. Anteroposterior radiogram of the midthoracolumbar region of a 30-week fetus. The oblate spheroid of the central ossification is particularly well illustrated. The costovertebral articulation is shown to form in relation to adjacent vertebrae and their intervening discs. In the region of the fibrocartilaginous anulus, the central radiolucent area indicates the formation of the nucleus pulposus from the notochord.

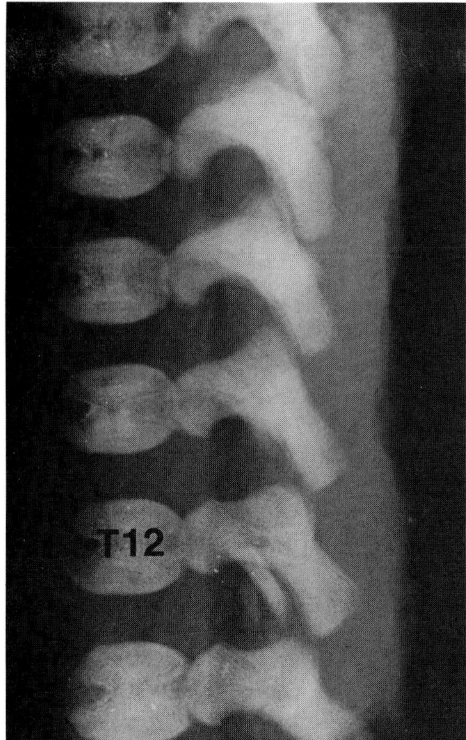

Figure 1–18. Lateral radiogram of a sagittal section of a 34-week spine. The pulley-sheave appearance of the central ossification is due to the ventral and dorsal vascular lakes that almost bisect each centrum. The radiolucent line where the spinal cord was removed marks the position of the spinal canal in relation to the neural arches. Note that the bases of the arches extend ventral to the canal and so contribute to the formation of the vertebral body.

The contribution of the intradiscal expansion of the notochord to the formation of the nucleus pulposus was initially detailed by Luschka.[31] Subsequent authors[26, 61] minimized the role of the notochord in nucleus pulposus development and relegated its significance to only the earliest stages. However, later investigations[53, 65] reconfirmed that the notochord is a major source of the nucleus pulposus, and it has been shown, both histochemically and autoradiographically,[32] that notochordal cells proliferate and remain vital several years after birth. Although it appears that notochordal cells generally are not demonstrable in the human nucleus pulposus of individuals older than 5 years of age, Schwabe[46] reported their survival in the incarcerated discs of the sacrum in a series of specimens ranging from 22 to 45 years in age. The occurrence of chordomas in the adult spine certainly indicates that viable "nests" of notochordal rest cells can persist well into middle age in some individuals. These neoplasms may develop at any point along the original notochordal track, but are usually noted in the more rostral and caudal ends. Slow-growing and locally invasive, chordomas produce prolonged and disastrous neurologic consequences when they occur in their favored locations in the basisphenoid or basiocciput.

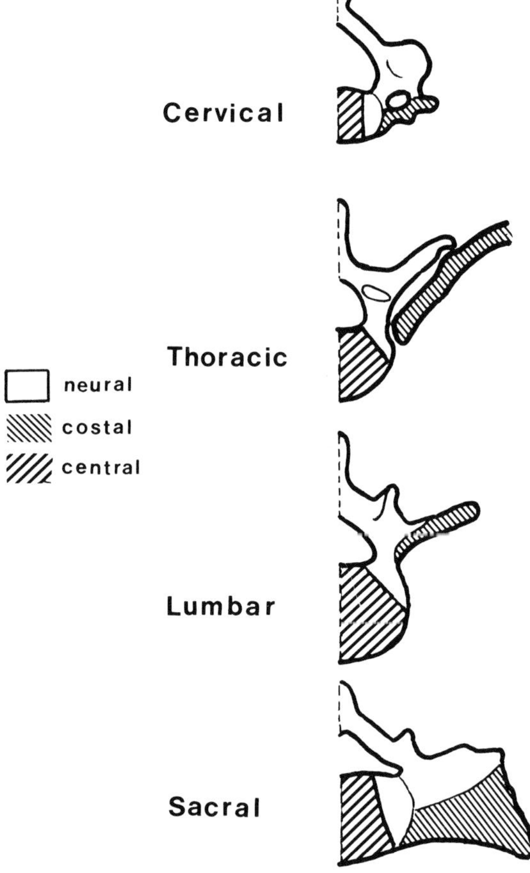

Figure 1–19. Schematic representation of the relative contributions of the ossific centers to the different regional vertebrae. This emphasizes the ever-present rib-bearing potential of all vertebrae. Note that the neurocentral synchondroses lie well within the vertebral body in all cases, but are most medial in the cervical and sacral regions. Normally the costovertebral synchondroses develop a true diarthrosis only in the thoracic region.

Differentiation of the Intervertebral Disc

In the early membranous (blastemal) stage of vertebral column development, the cells of the perichordal disc regions show a greater numerical density in the external circumferential zones, a decrease in cell numbers being evident in the area adjacent to the notochord. Aside from this radial gradient in concentration, the cells otherwise appear to be homogeneous in their initial distribution. As the human embryo exceeds a crown-rump (CR) length of 10 mm, elongating cells of the peripheral zone assume an orientation that suggests an externally curved lamellar arrangement. With the extracellular synthesis of collagen fibers becoming evident between the 20- and 40-mm stages, the characteristic structure of the annulus fibrosus is now anticipated. During later fetal life, there is a marked increase in the fibrous matrix of the future annulus and a simultaneous decrease in the relative cell population of this outer zone. Once the lamellar pattern is established, further growth appears to involve a greater thickening of the individual lamella rather than an increase in the number of layers.[22] The individual lamella is not likely to be continuous around the entire circumference of the disc, but forms part of an interdigitating pattern of incomplete rings that, in their entirety, form the annulus. At the end of the embryonic period (two months), the developing disc shows three regions: an external fibrous zone, an internal hyaline zone around the notochord, and an interposed fibrocartilaginous zone. As the innermost zone does not show any laminar organization, it was labeled a specialized embryonic cartilage by Peacock.[38] Additional growth of the annulus is claimed to be both interstitial and appositional.[7] The former term refers to growth in the transitional zone where the annulus is closely related to the cartilage plates, whereas the latter applies to where the annulus is in close apposition to the developing longitudinal connective tissues of the vertebral column. It has also been observed that a lamellar pattern of fibers extends from the attachments of the inner rings of the developing annulus into the parts of the cartilaginous plates adjacent to the nucleus pulposus. Here, they run parallel to the plates, so that with their attached rings of the annulus they completely encase the early nucleus in a multilayered fibrous container. The attachments of the more peripheral layers of the annulus show a deep embedding into the outer rim of the cartilaginous plate, while those of the most external few lamellae exhibit fiber attachments to the long ligaments and approximate external surfaces of the developing vertebral bodies. In the latter years of the first postnatal decade, the circumferential zone of the cartilaginous plate becomes ossified to form the ring apophysis, and the embedding fibers of the outer annular lamellae become deeply incorporated into this structure. Before this traction apophysis fuses to the vertebral body around the end of the second decade, the cartilaginous interval between the ring and the rim of the vertebral body still provides an entrance for the vessels supplying nutrition to the plate, and, by diffusion, to the inner tissue of the intervertebral disc.

Some classic descriptions include the cartilaginous plates and, hence, the fetal chondroepiphyses as part of the intervertebral disc,[7, 45] whereas other writers and most contemporary texts consider them to be part of the vertebral body. This contention may be a partial source of the controversy over the vascularization of the fetal disc. Undoubtedly, both the fetal and adult disc annulus receives diffusional nutrition from the plexus of vessels within the connective tissues that surround the circumference of both the fetal and adult annulus, but Taylor and Twomney[53] claimed that this plexus sends vessels deep into the fetal annulus, and showed a convincing histologic section to that effect. In contrast, Whalen and colleagues,[63] by the injection and clearing of an extensive series of rabbit and human fetal spines, were able to visualize these vessels only in the outermost lamellae. In the same specimens, however, excellent demonstrations of the cartilage canals of the chondroepiphyses were obtained. It was noted in this work that the so-called cartilage canals (actually, uniquely structured vascular glomeruli) were arranged with a radially geometric precision as they entered the chondroepiphysis from its periphery and angled toward the interface between the cartilage and the developing disc proper (Fig. 1–20). This rather precise spacing supported the suspicions that these vascular organs had specifically defined diffusional territories. A particularly interesting observation showed that these structures never entered the disc proper but would stop

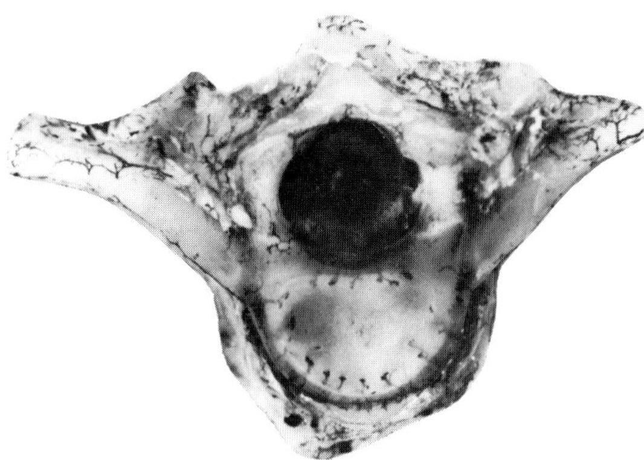

Figure 1–20. Section through the cartilaginous end of the vertebra of 30 weeks. This specimen had been injected to show the coronal vascular pattern in the cartilage. Each tuft consists of a central artery entwined by recurrent veins. It ends in a chondrous lacuna as a terminal arteriovenous anastomotic glomus, from which nutrients diffuse into the surrounding tissue. These vessels do not enter the presumptive disc.

at the interface and spread out along the true disc surface. It is known from studies in other bodily locations that cartilage resists the penetration of a conventional capillary bed by containing an antiangiogenic factor. The glomerular vascular complex of the cartilage canal is evidently capable of penetrating hyaline cartilage by possessing a "drill bit" of chondroclastic cells around its apex. The glomerular tufts never form capillaries of the conventional type, but it appears that their sinusoidal arrangement is uniquely suited to their role as a diffusional organ for a specific topographic region. It may here be stated with reasonable certainty that the deeper parts of the disc proper are never vascularized and depend on diffusional systems in all stages of morphogenesis to provide their metabolic requirements.

Ossification of a Typical Vertebra

As with other bones of the skeleton, ossification of the vertebrae involves both primary and secondary centers. Each vertebra is derived from three primary centers, one for the centrum and two for the vertebral arch. Around the ninth week the preparation for ossification is heralded by anterior and posterior excavations of the chondrous centrum produced by the invasion of pericostal vessels. These vessels produce ventral and dorsal vascular lacunae, which support the initial ossification (Fig. 1–18). What is regarded as a single ossification center for the centrum shows, for a short time, a dorsal and a ventral component briefly separated by an ephemeral plate of cartilage. By the 16th week ossification is well under way, but the centers do not appear simultaneously or follow a craniocaudal sequence as one might expect. The centers for the centra usually appear first in the lower thoracic and upper lumbar regions and develop more rapidly toward the caudal rather than the cranial vertebrae. This is exemplified by the fact that the two vertebral arch centers show well-advanced ossification in the cervical vertebrae much sooner than any detectable ossification in the centra (Fig. 1–8).

Ossification becomes evident in the vertebral arches around the eighth week. Two centers, each forming half of the arch, appear first in the cervical region before the centers for the bodies. However, the laminae of the arches first unite in the lumbar region, and the subsequent unions progress cranially. During the 15th or 16th year secondary centers of ossification appear at the tips of the transverse processes and the spinous processes. These eventually fuse in the middle of the third decade (Fig. 1–12).[36]

The transverse processes of the lower cervical vertebrae, particularly the seventh, may show an additional costal center of ossification that produces the troublesome cervical rib; this reinforces the concept that all vertebrae primitively had the potential of forming ribs.

The upper lumbar vertebrae also exhibit a tendency to extra costal centers, but much less frequently than do the cervical.[34] Lack of fusion of these centers then produces a truly articulated lumbar rib, which may confuse the radiologist in the accurate identification of the vertebral levels. In addition, the lumbar vertebrae show accessory centers for the mamillary processes that surmount the articular projections.

Throughout the vertebrae the eventual fusion of the vertebral arches and the centra occurs well anterior to the pedicles at the site of the neurocentral synchondroses. The definitive vertebral body then includes more than just the bone derived from the ossific center of the centrum, so that the terms "body" and "centrum" are not accurately interchangeable as some writings would indicate (Figs. 1–10, 1–19).

DEVELOPMENT OF SPECIALIZED VERTEBRAL REGIONS

Occipital Complex

It has long been known that the craniocervical region of the mammalian vertebral column has an elaborate evolutionary history that is reflected in the often obscure intricacies of its development. Although the atlantoaxial complex usually receives special treatment in most discussions of spine embryology, the morphogenesis of the neurocranial part of the skull is seldom included. However, it is known that the occipital region and most likely the preotic parts of the skull base are of somitic origin. Thus, some of the anomalies associated with the craniocervical articulations may be better understood if some of the current knowledge of the differentiation of most of the segments involved in the craniocervical complex is included here.

Although there is a contention regarding the sequence of their appearance, four occipital myotomes can be readily identified in the human embryo of 4-mm crown-rump length (CRL).[48] The first is small, the second is of intermediate size, and the third and fourth are equivalent to the succeeding cervical segments. The first cervical nerve and the hypoglossal artery clearly delimit the most caudal occipital segment. Eight rootlets of the hypoglossal nerve can be discerned rostral to the hypoglossal artery, and these usually unite into four, but no less than three, main roots, which confirms the involvement of at least three precervical segments in the formation of the occiput. DeBeer[13] claimed that a total of nine segments might be involved in skull formation. The first four appear very primitive but contribute to the preotic cranium, while the fifth is still very rudimentary and without a myotome. The last four, however, are definite precursors of the occipital complex.

The definitive hypoglossal nerve shows some retention of its multisegmental origins. Its rootlets usually coalesce into two distinct fascicles that exit through separate openings in the dura, and occasionally these do not unite until they have left the skull. The formation of the hypoglossal canal may also indicate a multisegmental relationship. The usual single aperture has been regarded in some texts as homologous to the intervertebral foramen between the neural arch equivalents of two occipital somites, but during chondrification a membranous strut that separates the two main fascicles of the nerve may be discerned. By further chondrification and ossification, a double hypoglossal canal accommodating both strands of the nerve may result. Most likely, this mesenchymal strut is a representative of the membranous neural arch process of an intervening segment, and is a good indicator that at least three somitic levels were involved in forming the part of the occipital bone surrounding the hypoglossal canal.

As a matter of comparative interest, the muscular tongue of amniote vertebrates evolved pari passu with the cranialization of the occipital sclerotomes. Blastemal cells from the four occipital myotomes migrated, taking their segmental innervation with them, into the hypobranchial region to form the musculature of the amniote tongue. The preamniotes (fish and amphibians) do not have a homologous muscular tongue, and their cranial nerve sequence stops with the vagus nerve, since their equivalent somites are still confined to the upper cervical region. For this reason, comparative anatomists refer to the somites associated with the amniote tongue and occipital complex as occipitospinal somites.[23]

Atlantoaxial Complex

Most contemporary texts acknowledge a multisegmental origin for the mammalian axis, but unfortunately most of these describe only a bisegmental history. This is surprising because, for many decades, comparative embryologists in their studies of several mammalian groups have reported the existence of an obscure craniocervical segment, and its contributions to the upper cervical vertebrae have been well documented.

In 1937 Sensenig[49] detailed the previously noted existence of a third centrum in the axis-odontoid complex, and more recently O'Rahilly and Meyer[37] reaffirmed his findings. These latter authors designated the various axis centra as X, Y, and Z in descending order. The apical X component at first projects into the early foramen magnum and forms an occipitoaxial joint, which it retains as a syndesmosis by formation of the alar ligaments. The Y and Z components become the lower part of the odontoid process and the centrum of the axis. Each is related, respectively, to the first three cervical nerves, which explains the redundancy of cervical nerves in relation to the conventional numbering of the cervical vertebrae. Thus, the suboccipital (first cervical) nerve is the segmental nerve of the generally unrecognized sclerotomal precursor to the apical segment of the odontoid process.

Additional (noncentral) derivatives of this cryptic sclerotome may explain other peculiarities in the metameric development of the craniocervical region. Comparative evidence suggests that the mammalian apical odontoid element (the X component of O'Rahilly and Meyer) is the phylogenetic equivalent of the proatlas of reptiles. In most members of this vertebrate class this proatlas fuses to the occiput of the skull, whereas in mammals it becomes fused to the atlantal contribution to the odontoid. In the sphenodon, the only surviving member of a group of primitive reptiles, the proatlas exists as an independent vertebral element with its own neural arch. The confusion of this segment with the true atlantal derivatives in sphenodon has fostered doubts concerning the multisegmental origin of the axis. As a proponent of the now discarded resegmentation theory, Sensenig[49] reconciled this small and exclusively axial contribution as the derivative of only a "sclerotome half," and the resegmentation fissure most probably had relegated the other half of this sclerotome to be the arch component contributions to the occipital condyles.

However, according to Cave[9] and Presley and Hallam,[39] the arch components of the proatlantal sclerotome are retained in the atlantal arch of placental mammals (Fig. 1–13). In humans, these components are expressed as the dorsal part of the superior atlantal articular facet and the contiguous retroarticular ligament, which often ossifies to form a foramen for the vertebral artery. The anterior arch of the atlas is generally regarded as a retained hypochordal bow of an upper cervical vertebra. There is reason to believe that this arch, along with the superior part of the transverse ligament, is also a derivative of the cryptic sclerotome (Fig. 1–11).

The existence of this sclerotome and its contributions to the cranial part of the odontoid also explain the segmental relationship of the "os odontoideum." The fact that this anomaly is manifested as a spherule of bone suspended between the two alar ligaments was difficult to reconcile with a single-centrum origin of the odontoid process, because this would most likely require the separation to occur caudal to the atlantal centrum rather than above it.

Considering the segmental complexities involved in the phyletic and developmental establishment of the normal human craniocervical articulations, the occasional occurrence of anomalous separations, fusions, and intercalated ossicles should not be surprising.

The most frequent manifestation of variant segmentation is the third condyle (basilar tubercle). This structure occurs as a projection on the basion (anterior central point) of the foramen magnum. Some incidences are expressed as a simple rounded tubercle, but in the better developed cases there is actually an articular facet that receives the tip of the odontoid process forming a true diarthrosis. Occasionally, accessory facets lateral to the central projection are in evidence. In a series of 600 skulls, some suggestion of a third condyle was present in 14 per cent.[28]

Toro and Szepe[54] observed that the third condyle often occurs with occipitalization of the atlas. They also believed that it may be the expression of the hypochordal arch of the "ante-proatlas." As they used this term, it appears to designate the most caudal occipital somite (Fig. 1–11). A more complete separation of this ante-proatlas may form a true occipital vertebra. First described by Meckle in 1815, this malformation forms a more or less complete ring inferior to the foramen magnum, and its anterior arch is often fused to the skull, bearing a third condyle. This condition is distinguished from occipitalization of the atlas by the radiologic identification of the true atlas beneath it. Transverse processes of variable relative size may be present in occipital vertebrae, but these do not show a transverse foramen.[20] As bony eminences, bilateral to the third condyle, are common to these structures, they may encroach on the foramen magnum, and neurologic symptomatology may become a complicating factor.

Occipitalization of the atlas occurs in 0.1 to 0.8 per cent of the population according to the series of skulls examined. If the occipitalization is complete, there is no movable atlanto-occipital articulation, and the atlas ring is more constricted. Also, the level of the odontoid tip shows a higher relative position, and the fusion is often asymmetric. Inglemark's[24] series of skulls showed that in 78 per cent of the true congenital cases, the posterior arch was fused to the posterior rim of the foramen magnum, the anterior arch being fused in 54 per cent and lateral fusions showing in 23 per cent.

Toro and Szepe[54] suggested that the variable expressions of fragments of the proatlas arch, which normally form parts of the atlas, may enhance the predilection of this segment to fuse to the skull.

Nonfused "floating" ossicles may occur within the craniocervical syndesmoses. A variably shaped, usually pea-sized, ossification that occurs between the basion and the tip of the odontoid (in the presence of a complete odontoid process) has been labeled Bergmann's ossicle (Fig. 1–14),[6] and is most likely a variant derivative of the ante-proatlas mesenchyme. Putz[40] also recorded the incidence of a small ossicle between the anterior lip of the foramen magnum and the anterior arch of the atlas, and within the anterior atlanto-occipital membrane. He was convinced that this was a manifestation of the hypochordal potential of the last occipital (ante-proatlas) somite.

The Sacrum

Ossification of the bodies of the sacral vertebrae is unique in that, in addition to the single central ossific zone, two true epiphyseal plates later provide accessory ossification to the superior and inferior surfaces of each segment. The central centers for the superior three sacral vertebrae are evident at week nine, whereas these centers for the fourth and fifth segments do not appear until after week 24. Each vertebral arch of the sacrum shows the conventional bilateral centers, but in addition six centers produce the sacral alae. Between weeks 24 and 32 these centers appear anterolateral to the anterior sacral foramina of the upper three sacral vertebrae. They are expressions of the ever-present potential of the vertebral anlagen to produce costal equivalents (Fig. 1–21).

In the early part of the postnatal year the sacral vertebrae are still separated by intervertebral discs, and the lower two are the first to fuse in late adolescence. Before this the ossific centers for the superior and inferior epiphyseal plates of the bodies appear, and between the 18th and 20th years lateral epiphyseal plates form on the auricular surfaces of the sacral alae. By the middle of the third decade the entire sacrum should be fused, although internal remnants of the intervertebral plates remain throughout life. These may be visualized in a sagittal section or in radiograms taken at the appropriate anteroposterior angle.

The coccygeal segments lack neural arch equivalents and form a single ossific center for their bodies. The first usually appears before the fifth year of life, and the succeeding three

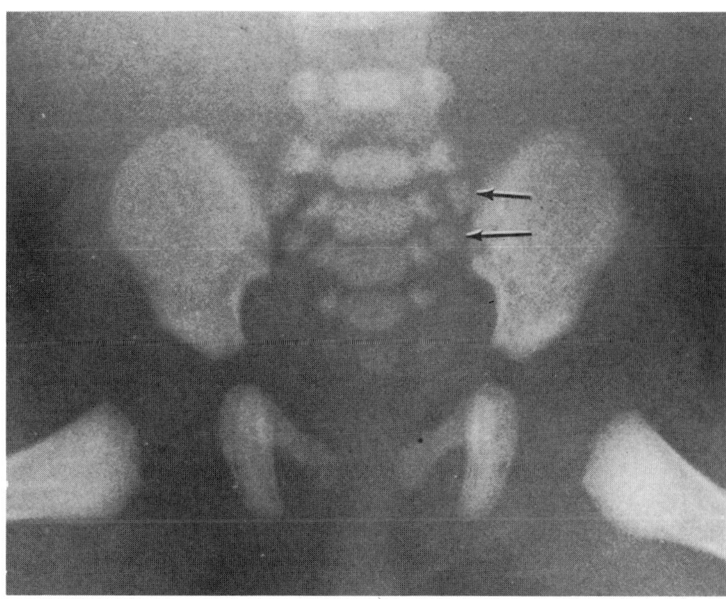

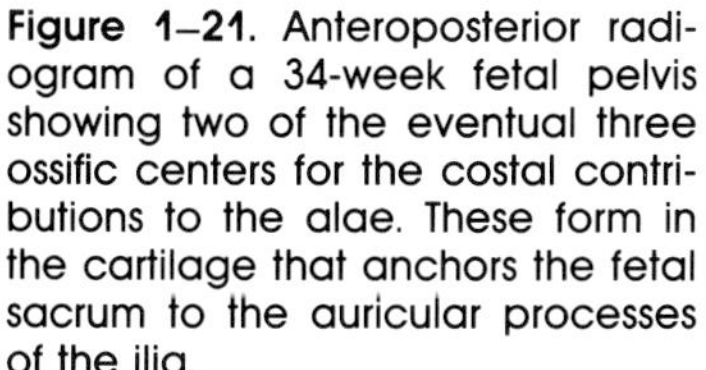

Figure 1–21. Anteroposterior radiogram of a 34-week fetal pelvis showing two of the eventual three ossific centers for the costal contributions to the alae. These form in the cartilage that anchors the fetal sacrum to the auricular processes of the ilia.

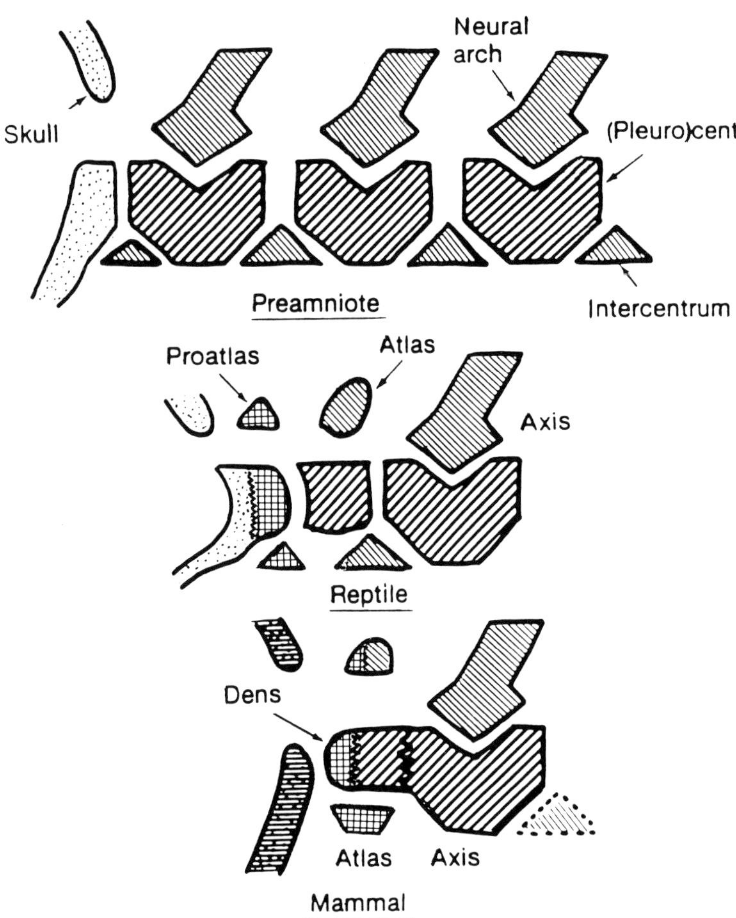

Figure 1–22. Highly schematic depiction of the evolution of the craniocervical articulations. The fact that the primitive cervical segments were incorporated in the formation of the occipital skull has been indicated by the progressive reduction in the number of vertebral elements illustrated. The evolutionary relationship between the intercentrum and hypochordal elements is uncertain. The neural arch of the proatlas and atlas are both depicted in the reptile, as the state of fusion of these varies throughout the class.

then ossify during consecutive five-year intervals.

COMPARATIVE COMMENTS

The earliest evidence of vertebral element formation was found in Agnatha. In the extant members of this group, the cyclostomes, small cartilaginous neural arches surmount the notochord in hagfish, and superior and inferior sheets of cartilage reinforce the caudal notochord of lampreys. Aside from the interposition of accessory arches in the shark, in which they form an uninterrupted conduit over the spinal cord, the neural arch has remained functionally and morphologically constant throughout the vertebrate lineage. A second series of elements, the hemal arches, appear on the ventral aspect of the caudal notochord to provide protection for the dorsal aorta and concurrent vein.

In contradistinction to the straightforward evolution of the arches, the phyletic history of the centrum is a mess, being replete with variations and odd complexities in the preamniotes. It starts out simply enough with four ossicles forming bases for the attachment of the neural and hemal arches to the sides of the notochord. Thus, two *dorsal arch bases* lie superolateral to the notochord, and two *ventral arch bases* lie ventrolateral, as exhibited in the bowfin, *Amia.* These arch bases can be demonstrated developmentally in most forms of fish, in which the definitive spool-shaped centrum results from additional ossification around and between the bases.

In earlier texts the evolution of the centrum from the fish to the amniote involved the postulation of an original four pairs of "arcualia," or primitive ossicles, that through a complex system of rearrangements could account for all the varieties of centrum types encountered. Unfortunately, this concept was more convenient than accurate.

An iteration of the number of types of centra

that have occurred, particularly in the adaptive radiation of the amphibians, is not germane here, but at the risk of oversimplification, a general theme may be traced from the fish to the amniote. Two pairs of ossicles are found lateral to the notochord of the crossopterygian. The ones on each side just below the neural arch are regarded as the equivalent of the *pleurocentrum* of the early amphibian and homologous to the original dorsal arch bases. Inferior to these on the ventral aspect of the notochord, a prism-shaped ossicle represents the *intercentrum* and the derivative of the ventral arch bases. The pleurocentra, through comparative evidence, are assumed to be the antecedents of the true amniote centrum. There is considerable uncertainty about the relationship between the hypochordal elements and the intercentra, for the intercentrum predominates as the major vertebral component in most reptiles and bears the hemal arches. Thus, we arrive at the amniote condition with single centra derived from the pleurocentra and hypochordal elements that may or may not be derived from the intercentra.

Without regard to the development or phyletic composition of the vertebrae, a convenient system of descriptive classification is based on the shapes of the articulating surfaces of the centra. For example, the bodies of the human vertebrae generally articulate through mutually flat surfaces and are therefore called *acelous,* meaning "no cavity" at either end of the centrum. In forms in which much of the notochordal material is still present in spindle-shaped masses between the vertebrae, the centra are biconcave and are designated as *amphicelous*. In many amniotes either the rostral or the caudal end of the body is concave and articulates with a reciprocal convexity of the next element. These are referred to as *procelous* and *opisthocelous* vertebrae, respectively. Most unique are the biaxial articulations seen in the saddle-shaped cervical intervertebral joints of birds, which give these vertebrae the term *heterocelous*.

REGIONAL COMPARATIVE ANATOMY

Atlantoaxial Complex

It has been previously stated that the human embryo exhibits a total of 42 to 44 somites, yet only 33 or 34 segments can be accounted for in the adult spine. Deletion of caudal elements explains the loss of most of these, but the incorporation of rostral somites into the formation of the skull and the evolution of the craniocervical articulations are good examples of Stromer's law.

In the generalized fish, the head and trunk move in unison, and the first vertebra simply articulates with a projection on the skull that resembles the posterior aspect of another centrum. Thus, the range of craniocervical movement is approximately equal to that allowed between the individual vertebrae. With the advent of terrestrial life in the Amphibia, all but the more primitive forms show a splitting of this single projection into two lateral occipital condyles. The resulting articulation provides a hingelike flexion-extension that may have facilitated the raising and lowering of the head to give greater range to jaw movement, but still restricted lateral mobility.

Most reptiles and birds display a single, rounded occipital condyle, but the cranial two vertebrae have been modified into an atlas and axis. The former is a ringlike structure that formed from the union of the neural arch and ventral element of the proatlas sclerotome. The true centrum of C1 tends to remain dissociated from the ring but still does not fuse with C2. Often the proatlas is intercalated between the skull and the atlas. This articulation gives considerable universal motion, but differs from the equivalent joint in mammals in that both the flexion-extension and rotatory actions are achieved between the single condyle and the concave apex of the C1 centrum. The atlantal ring apparently lends stability to the joint by supporting the craniocervical syndesmoses.

In the mammalian atlantoaxial structure, the atlas also represents the neural arch-hypochordal complex. However, the lateral masses of the atlantal ring articulate directly with the bilateral occipital condyles so that most craniocervical flexion-extension is confined to these atlanto-occipital articulations. The homologue of the centrum of the atlas provides the major component of odontoid process. It is capped by a proatlas contribution and becomes fused to the body of C2 to provide the rotatory pivot, but its apex remains free of any axial thrust.

One must not assume that the evolution of the atlantoaxial complex resulted from progressive changes in vertebrae of equivalent segmental levels, for a simultaneous incorporation of rostral somites into the base of the skull accompanied its phyletic development. The fact that the human embryo usually shows four well-defined somites rostral to the definitive level of the craniocervical articulation offers ample evidence of this phenomenon (Figs. 1–5, 1–11). In the cleared specimen of 14 weeks' gestation (Fig. 1–8), illustrating alizarin-stained areas of ossification, what appear to be the ossific centers of the most cranial cervical vertebrae are actually those of the occipital region of the skull.

It is noteworthy that throughout all species of mammals the cervical region always shows seven vertebrae: a remarkable consistency, considering the numerical variations that may be encountered in other regions. This situation is most emphasized in whales and porpoises (Cetacea), in which the return to the aquatic environment reselected the vertebral adaptations of the fish. This does not imply a reverse evolution but rather an adaptive superimposition on the characteristics of higher vertebrates of those that morphologically and functionally meet the requirements of the marine environment. Thus, when the head and trunk again move as a single unit, the cervical vertebrae develop as a stack of seven wafer-thin plates that have the overall dimensions and mobility of a single vertebral element.

Comparative Sacralization

In the evolution of the tetrapod limbs the pectoral girdle of the forelimbs achieves only remote connections with the spine, but the pelvic girdle, from early amphibians on, has established various degrees of direct articulation with vertebrae. The modification of the vertebrae to accommodate this articulation produces the sacrum. In its simplest form, as in the amphibians, only a single vertebral segment became involved, and this usually entailed the modification of a single costal equivalent to form a lateral projection for articulation with the ilium.

In the generalized reptile and all extant legged members of this class, two vertebrae became involved in the spinopelvic articulation. Among the dinosaurs, however, particularly in the ornithischian group, greater numbers of the vertebrae became incorporated. The minimal number of vertebral elements forming the mammalian sacrum is three, additional members being added as adaptive requirements dictated. The Cetacea, in whom the sacrum has been secondarily lost, are an obvious exception.

The results of sacralization reach their epitome in the class Aves (birds), in which not only do those elements regionally associated with the pelvis become fused but also the entire thoracocolumbar spine is rendered rigid by interlocking syndesmoses (although the vertebrae are not fused) to unite with the pelvis as the inflexible *synsacrum*.[44] It is apparent that this rigid fuselage has considerable significance in the dynamics of flight, yet no similar tendency is observed in mammalian bats.

GENETIC CONTROL OF SPINE DEVELOPMENT

Before this decade it was possible to conclude a discussion on the development of the spine without mentioning genetics. Since the late 19th century it was assumed that the informed reader knew that all organs and organisms were the product of an inherited "blueprint" that lay within the chromatin strands mitotically meted to the nucleus of each cell. However, owing to the lack of sufficient detail on the step-by-step processes by which the egg becomes the organism, reference to the genetic control of development was prudently omitted.

The discovery of the chemical basis for the encoding and transfer of genetic information has been the most profound achievement of 20th century biologic research, and any discourse on spine development is now incomplete without a presentation of the recent concepts that the new molecular biology has provided concerning the morphogenesis of segmental body structures.

This chemical basis is a double-stranded molecule of deoxyribonucleic acid (DNA) consisting of two linear phosphate-sugar polymers that allow a sequential bonding of only four different nucleotide bases. These consist of two purines (adenine and guanine) and two pyrimidines (cytosine and thymine). The free end of each of these nucleotides then specifically binds only with one of the other three bases and, in ladder-rung fashion, these base pairs connect the two phosphate-sugar polymers to form an entwined double helix. Under the influence of the appropriate enzymes, these mutual nucleotide bonds may become "unzippered" to expose their binding sites to ambient nucleotides so that the separated complementary half of the linear nucleotide sequence may be resynthesized. Thus, the varieties of nucleotide arrangements may be replicated repeatedly and transferred from cell to cell and generation to generation.

This brief account may indicate how spatially encoded information is transmitted from nucleus to nucleus, but since the DNA molecules are confined within the nuclear envelope, the transfer of the encoded information to the cell plasma and to the extracellular matrices, and how it may influence embryologic elaboration from the single-cell state to the organ system complexes, requires further explanation.

The genetic instructions contained within the DNA molecule govern the synthesis of proteins. Many molecules of DNA, each containing different sets of instructions, reside in each cell nucleus. It is the linear arrangement of the nucleotides that encodes the information, and a specific sequence of nucleotides that establishes the amino acid sequence of a single polypeptide chain is regarded as "the" gene. As there are many genes within a molecule of DNA, a human cell nucleus may contain 60,000 to 100,000 such units of reproducible and transferable information.

Although the information required to synthesize proteins lies within the DNA, this molecule itself is not engaged directly in the construction of the polypeptides. Aside from a small complement of DNA that resides within the mitochondria, almost all these molecules are confined within the nuclear envelope. However, most of the protein synthesis occurs within the cytoplasm. The transfer of the DNA information to the cytoplasmic sites of protein synthesis (the ribosomes) is effected by molecules of ribonucleic acid (RNA). These resemble small sections of one half of the DNA molecule except that the sugar in their phosphate-sugar backbone is ribose rather than deoxyribose, and uracil is substituted for thymine in their nucleotide sequencing. A gene sequence encoded in the nuclear DNA is transcribed to a sequence of RNA nucleotides, and the smaller RNA molecule, now called messenger RNA (mRNA), can leave the nuclear envelope through a nucleopore. It then translates the mRNA information into a specifically arranged polypeptide chain within the cytoplasm. This DNA-to-RNA-to-protein transfer of genetic information has come to be known as the "central dogma" of molecular biology. However, it must be stated at this point that small amounts of proteins are synthesized within the nuclear envelope for the specific purpose of providing a "feedback" modification of the actions of other genes.

It is then apparent that each cell of the developing embryo receives an identical complement of DNA peculiar to its hereditary derivation, yet differing cell lineages rapidly show marked diversification in position and differentiation and eventually assume highly specific functions. It therefore appears obvious that as differentiation proceeds, a feedback influences and selects those parts of the total DNA complement that will be used for a given cellular differentiation, and progressively, more of the total potential sites of DNA protein synthesis become deactivated.

In addition to providing the explanation for the mechanisms of information preservation and transfer, the DNA-to-RNA-to-protein specificity has furnished the molecular biologist with a remarkable probe or tool that reveals the relative time and location of various gene activities during embryogenesis. By the enzymatic removal of segments of nucleotide sequences from a subject species and recombining them into the DNA strands in the plasmids of prokaryotes or in the chromosomes of cultured eukaryotic cells (recombinant DNA), relatively large quantities of a specific monoclonal gene protein product may be recovered. This enables the generation of labeled antibodies that will have binding-sites specific for a given gene product. These then effectively label the embryonic cells in which that particular gene is actively influencing development.

To bring the foregoing information into relevance concerning spine development, another commonality of diverse life forms must be explored. In the introductory paragraphs of this chapter, there was allusion to the fact that many of the ultimate complexities of the human body form had been phyletically derived through the regional modification of a sequential series of original similar somites, and the manifestations of this principle are best exhibited in the developmental and mature morphology of the spine. This concept of segmentation, wherein the definitive body is fabricated by the modulation of a fundamental pattern of repeating units, has been evolved, or independently "reinvented," through many diverse branches of animal phyla. Fortunately, the new techniques developed through molecular biology have revealed how some of the interactions of various genetic principles guide such segmentation and its modulations through a timetable of sequential events, and the gene codes involved show a remarkable similarity throughout the segmented life forms.

The new insights into the control of body segmentation owe much of their origins to an old genetic subject, the fruitfly, *Drosophila.* This animal, like all arthropods, has an exoskeleton and so presents a body plan in which most of the aspects of segmentation are externally visible. Also, unlike higher vertebrates in which evidence of early lethal malformations may be totally lost, the segmented larval stages of *Drosophila* manifest the grosser errors in body organization that allow only the most initial stages of embryogenesis.

The application of classic and molecular genetic techniques to the analysis of *Drosophila* segmental development has been given an excellent review by Akam.[1] The details are too extensive to recount here, but the generalities appear relevant to the embryogenesis of all segmental forms. The most essential concept provided by these studies is the fact that the individual aspects of the advanced stages of development are the result of a sequential action of numerous genes, and the mutation of single-effect genes, whose phenotypic expressions have provided the classic mendelian patterns of heredity, usually show errors in only a single step in this concatenation of events.

Drosophila development shows that a set of *maternal effect* genes (so labeled because they are exclusively derived from the maternal genome) initially establishes the axial symmetry of the body within the ovum. A group of approximately 20 *segmentation* genes then guides cellular construction of the defined segments. Mutations of these genes are manifest as deletions affecting the normal segment number. Most mutations of the segmentation genes are lethal and knowledge of them has been obtained from the doomed larval forms, but as they are commonly recessive, the mutant strain can be propagated for continuous study. Clearly, the equivalent genetic effects would not be so readily observable in vertebrates, but comparative evidence strongly indicates that very similar genetic mechanisms are operable in this group of animals.

Only after the segmental boundaries have been established can the structures regionally characteristic of each segment be determined. These designations are effected by the *homeotic selector genes.* The term "homeotic" (from the Latin *homoeos,* similar) was originally used by Bateson[3] to label the mutant substitution of segment appendages, because he surmised that they indicated a similarity (genetic homology) in their underlying developmental mechanisms. Unlike the segmentation genes whose mutations affect the whole segment, mutations of the homeotic genes are expressed as homologous structures (such as legs and wings) grotesquely appearing on inappropriate segments. It is now known that these homeotic genes are closely grouped in two locations on the third chromosome of *Drosophila's* four chromosomes.

Lewis[29] and Wakimoto and colleagues[60] found that two homeotic gene groups, the *bithorax complex* and the *antennapedia complex,* controlled the appendage specifications for all the *Drosophila* segments. Lewis[30] postulated the existence of a "ground state" or basic plan inherently predetermined in each segment. This was exemplified by the second thoracic segment, which exhibited in basic form the total range of possible appendages. Thus, when modifier transcription units of the normal gene complex were lost by mutation, the moribund embryos of these mutant strains would show a monotonous repetition of the ground state segment in which all the abdominal segments, which normally lack appendages, expressed them.

Another significant outcome of this *Drosophila* genetic research has been the identification of a sequence of nucleotide base pairs that is common to the homeotic selector genes. These were discovered as an area of cross homology between genes of the antennapedia and bithorax complexes.[18] Intergenetic cross homologies of certain gene regions is not unusual, but the relatively small sequence common to these homeotic genes contained only a 180 base-pair unit that could easily be used as a probe to identify the locations of its homologues. This compact genetic fragment was called the *homeobox* by McGinnis and associates[33] in 1984, and the protein it encodes is known as the *homeodomain.* By 1986, more than 29 homeoboxes had been identified, 10

within the homeotic genes in *Drosophila* and 19 within the gene of other species, including amphibian vertebrates, mice, and man.[18]

That the homeobox sequence is a gene-regulatory unit is strongly supported by the fact that the homeodomain proteins for which it is encoded remain within the nuclear envelope and presumably act as enhancers or repressors for other gene units. Because the chance of independent evolution of the same sequence of DNA bases in so many diverse genomes is almost nil, the supposition of Lewis that they are phyletically derived from a primal genome, and have remained highly conserved because of their common functional importance, appears to have considerable validity.

Vertebrate Segmentation

Evolution has appeared to recognize a fundamental advantage in deriving a body plan from the regional diversification of a series of basically similar modules, since virtually all higher organisms develop from some type of segmental organization.

Although vertebrate segmentation is not externally obvious in the postembryonic stages, the sclerotomic contributions to the axial skeleton retain the original metameric organization, and the common neurologic examination based on a knowledge of the myotomic and dermatomic distribution of the cranial and spinal nerves pays perpetual homage to the truth that man and the other vertebrates are, in fact segmentally constructed animals.

As would be expected, the homeobox-containing genes discovered in man[8] and other mammals[17, 21] do not act in exactly the same manner as they do in *Drosophila,* because the types of segmental organization are quite different. Nevertheless, the nucleotide sequence cognates of the *Drosophila* homeobox genes found in mammals appear to have considerable influence in the early establishment of brain stem and spinal cord formation. However, the indication that the segmental pattern formation in both types of organisms is dependent on an analogous hierarchy of sequential gene interactions is obviously inferred. As in the more primitive forms, malfunctions of the genes controlling the more fundamental aspects of segmentation most likely produce early lethal mutations. Since higher vertebrates do not have an autonomous larval stage, the occurrence of such mutations would be lost to general observation. Nevertheless, some gross errors of segmentation that may reach parturition do demonstrate genetic implication. Keynes and Stern[27] listed a number of "segmentation class" gene mutations in mice that are remarkably limited to malformations of the axial skeleton that display a variety of fusions, deletions, and dysplasias.

In humans, congenital vertebral fusions, most commonly manifest in the various "types" of the Klippel-Feil syndrome, serve as a prime example. Many instances of this syndrome appear to result from spontaneous mutations or individual teratogenic accidents in the early developmental sequences, as most reports present single case histories without examination of the extended family and the family's pedigree. Gunderson and colleagues,[19] however, provided substantial evidence that many cases of the Klippel-Feil syndrome would prove to be probands of a familial history of the condition if the examiner were to make the effort to expand the investigation. These authors provided the pedigrees of 11 probands, and of particular interest is their Type II of the syndrome that exhibits fusions limited to the cervical regions at C2–C3 and C5–C6. They concluded that this disorder, which produced segmentation errors at consistent spine levels through several successive generations, strongly indicated a dominant mutant defect of a gene that controls these specific levels of segmentation.

Another class of segmental spinal malformations with indicated genetic import is grouped under the generic term of caudal dysplasias.[62] This covers a spectrum of segmental deficiencies in caudal spinal development (lumbosacral agenesis, caudal regression syndrome, and sacral agenesis.[35, 42, 50, 55]) As examples of this malformation complex have proved to be heritable and have also shown a marked association with maternal diabetes, certain insights into genetic mechanisms of mammalian spinal development may be derived. That some degree of caudal segment regression is a natural phenomenon is shown by the reduction of the original postsacral somites from eight (± 2) to four (± 1) in normal human development, but in the more severe forms of lumbosacral agenesis all vertebral elements as far cephalad as the upper lumbar region may fail to develop. The association with maternal diabetes has been attributed to a teratogenic effect of hyperglycemia, as experimental elevations of blood sugar have produced varying degrees of caudal deficiencies in animals,[35] but similar effects have been induced by a variety of toxic insults during embryogenesis of the spine. Because caudal agenesis is not a consistent occurrence in the offspring of diabetic mothers, a more complex genetic association has been suspected, particularly since both diabetes mellitus and spine defects have been associated with HLA-type histocompatibility genes.[62] This inference has been supported by studies of the T-locus genes in the mouse. This locus appears to be a segment of the mouse chromosomes with a collection of genes that have a profound effect on spine development and other aspects of embryogenesis.[5] The various T alleles fall into two groups (T or t), each showing well-defined dominance or recessiveness. The dominant mutations result in short-tailed heterozygotes (T/+) and lethal homozygotes (T/T), whereas the recessive mutations produce normal-tailed heterozygotes (T/+) or tailless phenotypes (T = tailless) when combined with a dominant mutant allele (T/t). What is most interesting about the genes of the T locus is that their effects are mediated by alterations in the histocompatibility of the various cell lineages in the early embryo. This histocompatibility is of the HLA type that is involved with cell surface antigens that enable differentiating cells to recognize their appropriate groups and lineages and form defined adhesive aggregates at specified locations during development.

There is now evidence that a gene complex, functionally similar to the mouse T locus, may be operable in humans, because an association between histocompatibility antigens of the HLA type and the inheritance of human spinal bifida has been reported.[10] The human HLA antigens are controlled by a cluster of contiguous genes located on the human chromosome 6. As in the mouse T locus, each gene in this group has several alleles, and thus a number of serologically discrete forms of cell surface antigens may be coded by the gene complex. The total ensemble of the HLA antigens produced within an individual determine its HLA "personality." Interestingly, among the Tuaregs, a group of East North African Berbers who are inbred by reason of a tribally required system of first-cousin marriages, the inheritance of the HLA types does not follow the statistically predicted ratios. This indicates that a mutant homozygosity, peculiar to this group, may be lethal.[10] The comparative evidence then suggests that the human HLA complex, because of its defined chromosomal localization, its coding for the HLA antigen complex, and its effect on spine development, is a reasonable candidate for the human analogue of the mouse T locus.

It thus appears that in vertebrates, as in other forms of segmented animals, a definite sequence of genetically controlled events establishes the basic aspects of segment formation. Once this has been accomplished, some analogue of the homeotic system of genes most likely determines the regional specializations of the individual segments. Whatever this system is, it provides an early determination within the vertebrate sclerotome, since these embryonic cell masses exhibit a marked "position effect" before any regional differentiation of the somite is visibly evident. This has been demonstrated in the chick embryo in which the transplantation of an early thoracic sclerotome into the cervical region results in a rib-bearing thoracic vertebra whose specific character development was not modified by its heterotopic location.[27] This early position identity may be due to the fact that vertebrate embryonic patterns are mostly established through early cell-to-cell interactions subsequent to cell cleavages, and these involve the antigen-mediated cell surface recognitions and adhesions as demonstrated by the HLA antigens. Nevertheless, some analogues of the homeotic mechanisms in *Drosophila,* although differing in their modes of expression, must determine whether a given vertebra will exhibit cervical, thoracic, or sacral characteristics.

It is here proposed that the vertebrate somite, like the arthropod segment, most likely possesses a generalized basic plan from which all the regional vertebral variations are genetically determined. This would be analogous to Lewis's "ground-state" arthropod metamere, for like the second thoracic segment of *Drosophila,* the sclerotomic cell mass of each somite should have the inherent potential of elaborating the total range of individual vertebral components exhibited throughout the entire spine and occiput. A schema of this "generic" vertebra is provided in Figure 1–23*A*. Without some analogue of the homeotic types of regional specifications that would repress the various vertebral elements, some basic form of all these potentials would then be expressed.

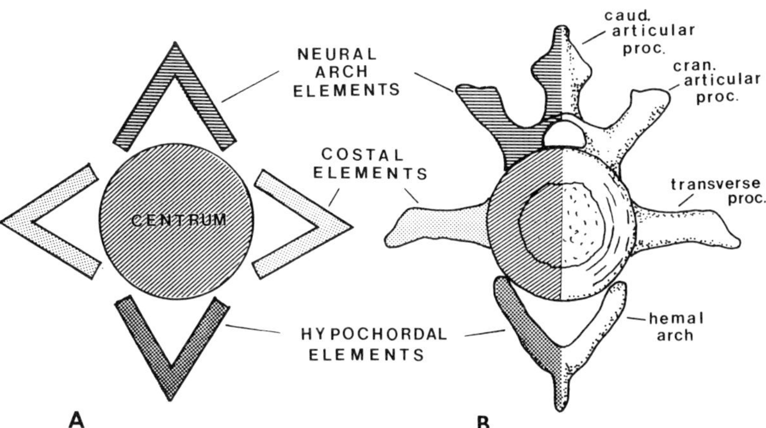

Figure 1–23. *A,* The presumed "ground state" or total potential inherent in the early membranous mammalian sclerotome. In the absence of regional "represser" genetic determinants, any or all of these elements may be expressed. *B,* Sketch of the fourth caudal vertebra of a dog (beagle), showing some form of expression of all the elements inherent in the hypothetical "generic" sclerotome of the mammal.

Unfortunately, the human spine does not present an obvious example of this universal vertebra, but the definitive form of the C1 sclerotome does manifest derivatives of all the basic components. The best mammalian example may be provided by a proximal caudal vertebra. Figure 1–23*B* shows the fourth caudal vertebra of a dog with all the major contributions of the generalized sclerotomic potential indicated.

The range of anomalies observed in the human spine well supports the concept that regional vertebral specification may be the result of a homeotic type of selective repression. In addition to the obvious articulated ribs of the thoracic region, each human vertebral level shows some expression of the costal element potential, but it is usually incorporated as an immovable projection. However, anomalous free or articulated rib components have been observed at virtually every vertebral level including the sacrum and coccyx.[25] However, it is the hypochordal potential that may best indicate the existence of early segmental totipotency in the vertebrates. This component is normally expressed at only the C1 level (and cryptically in the occiput[14, 24, 54]) in man and in the caudal region in other mammals. Should there appear to be some interference in the normal control mechanisms, however, it may also arise at other levels, as hypochordal elements have been observed to occur just below the last normal vertebra in some cases of lumbosacral agenesis.

Unfortunately, much of our knowledge of the genetic control of human spinal development must currently remain in the areas of inference and speculation, but if the recent rate of expansion of our comprehension of molecular biology and its relation to the genetic mechanisms may be extrapolated, a more positive understanding of the normal and abnormal development of the human spine may not be too far in the future.

References

1. Akam, M. E.: The molecular basis for metameric pattern in the *Drosophila* embryo. Development *101*:1–22, 1987.
2. Bardeen, C. R.: Early development of cervical vertebrae and the base of the occipital bone in man. Am. J. Anat. *8*:181–186, 1908.
3. Bateson, W.: Materials for the Study of Variation Treated with the Especial Regards to Discontinuity in the Origin of Species. London, Macmillan, 1894.
4. Baur, R.: Zum Problem der Neugliederung der Wirbelsaule. Acta Anat. *72*:321–356, 1969.
5. Bennett, D.: The T-locus of the mouse. Cell *6*:441–454, 1975.
6. Bergmann, E. von: Die Lehre von den Kopfverletzungen. (Cited by Lang, J.) Stuttgart, Enke, 1880.
7. Bohmig, R.: Die Blutgefassversorg ung der Wirbelbandscheiben das Verhalten des intervertebralen Chordasegments. Arch. Klin. Chir. *158*:374–382, 1930.
8. Cannizzaro, L. A., Croce, C. M., Griffin, C. A., et al.: Human homeobox containing genes located at chromosome regions 2q31–2q37 and 12q12–12q13. Am. J. Hum. Genet. *41*:1–15, 1987.
9. Cave, A. J. E.: The morphological constitution of the odontoid process. J. Anat. *72*:621, 1938.
10. Check, W.: First data for human developmental genes. JAMA *238*:2253–2254, 1977.
11. Christ, B., Verbout, J. A., and Jacob, H. J.: Zur Entwicklung der definitive Korperwandmetamerie: Untersuchungen an Vogel- und Schafsembryonen. Verh. Anat. Ges. *76*:213–214, 1982.
12. Dalgleish, A. E.: A study of the development of the thoracic vertebrae in the mouse assisted by autoradiography. Acta Anat. *122*:91–98, 1985.

13. DeBeer, G. R.: The Development of the Vertebrate Skull. Oxford, 1937, pp. 1–552.
14. Dwight, T.: Concomitant assimilation of the atlas and occiput with the manifestation of an occipital vertebra: II. Notes on a hypochordal brace. Anat. Rec. *3*:321–333, 1909.
15. Engelman, E. D., Schnitzlein, H. N., Hilbelink, D. R., et al.: Imaging anatomy of the cranio-vertebral junction (occipito-atlanto-axial joint). Clin. Anat. *2*:241–252, 1989.
16. Froriep, A.: Zur Entwicklungsgeschichte der Wirbelsaule insbesondere des Atlas und Epistropheus und der Occipitalregion. II. Beobacten an Saugetierembryonen. Arch. Anat. Physiol. Anat. Abt. 69–150, 1886.
17. Gaunt, S. J., Miller, J. R., Powell, D. J., and Duboule, D.: Homeobox gene expression in mouse embryos varies with position by the primitive streak stage. Nature *324*:662–668, 1986.
18. Gehring, W. J., and Hiromi, Y.: Homeotic genes and the homeobox. Ann. Rev. Genet. *20*:147–173, 1986.
19. Gunderson, C. H., Greenspan, R. H., Glasner, G. H., and Lubs, H. A.: The Klippel-Feil syndrome: genetic and clinical reevaluation of cervical fusion. Medicine *46*:491–511, 1967.
20. Hadley, L. A.: Atlanto-occipital fusion, ossiculum terminale and occipital vertebra as related to basilar impression with neurological symptoms. Am. J. Radiol. *59*:511–524, 1948.
21. Holland, P. W. H., and Hogan, B. L. M.: Expression of homeo box genes during mouse development: a review. Genes Dev. *2*:773–782, 1988.
22. Horton, W. G.: Further observations on the elastic mechanism of the intervertebral disc. J. Bone Joint Surg. *40B*:552–561, 1958.
23. Hyman, L. H.: Comparative Vertebrate Anatomy. 2nd ed. Chicago, University of Chicago Press, 1949.
24. Inglemark, B. E.: Über das Craniovertebrale Grenzgebiet beim Menschen. Acta Anat. (Suppl. VI):1–116, 1947.
25. Kaushal, S. P.: Sacral ribs. Int. Surg. *62*:37–38, 1977.
26. Keyes, D. C., and Compere, E. L.: The normal and pathological physiology of the nucleus pulposus of the intervertebral disc. J. Bone Joint Surg. *14A*:897–905, 1932.
27. Keynes, R. J., and Stern, C. D.: Mechanisms of vertebrate segmentation. Development *103*:413–429, 1988.
28. Lang, J.: Clinical Anatomy of the Head (translated by Wilson, R. R. and Winstanley, D. P.). Berlin, Springer-Verlag, 1983.
29. Lewis, E. B.: A gene complex controlling segmentation in *Drosophila.* Nature *276*:565–570, 1978.
30. Lewis, E. B.: Regulation of the genes of the bithorax complex in *Drosophila.* Cold Spring Harbor Symp. Quant. Biol. *50*:155–164, 1985.
31. Luschka, H. von: Die Halbgelenke des Menschlichen Korpers. Berlin, Reimer, 1858.
32. Malinski, J.: Histochemical demonstration of carbohydrates in human intervertebral discs during postnatal development. Acta Histochem. *5*:120–126, 1958.
33. McGinnis, W., Garber, R. L., Wirz, J., et al.: A homologous protein-coding sequence in *Drosophila* homeotic genes and its conservation in other metazoans. Cell *37*:403–408, 1984.
34. Meyer, D. B.: The appearance of cervical ribs during early human fetal development. Anat. Rec. *190*:481, 1978.
35. Miller, P., Herndon, W. A., and Yngve, D. A.: Lumbosacral agenesis. Orthopedics *8*:1297–1298, 1985.
36. Noback, C. R., and Robertson, G. C.: Sequence of appearance of ossification centers in the human skeleton during first five prenatal months. Am. J. Anat. *89*:1–28, 1951.
37. O'Rahilly, R., and Meyer, D. B.: The timing and sequence of events in the development of the vertebral column during the embryonic period proper. Anat. Embryol. *157*:167–176, 1979.
38. Peacock, A.: Observations on the prenatal development of the intervertebral disc in man. J. Anat. *85*:260–275, 1951.
39. Presley, R., and Hallam, L. A.: A pro-atlas arch in mammals. J. Anat. *131*:209–210, 1980.
40. Putz, V. R.: Zur Manifestation der hypochordalen Spangen im cranio-vertebralen Grenzgebiet beim Menschen. Anat. Anz. *137*:65–74, 1975.
41. Remak, R.: Untersuchungen über die Entwicklung der Wirbeltiere. Berlin, Reimer, 1855.
42. Renshaw, T. S.: Sacral agenesis. J. Bone Joint Surg. *60A*:373–383, 1978.
43. Romer, A. S.: The Osteology of Reptiles. Chicago, Chicago University Press, 1956.
44. Schufeldt, R. W.: Osteology of birds. Bull. N.Y. State Mus. *130*:5–81, 1909.
45. Schmorl, G., and Junghanns, H.: The Human Spine in Health and Disease. 2nd ed. New York, Grune & Stratton, 1971.
46. Schwabe, R.: Untersuchungen über die Ruckbildung der Bandscheiben im Menschlichen Kreuzbein. Virchows Arch. *287*:651–665, 1933.
47. Sensenig, E. C.: The early development of the human vertebral column. Contr. Embryol. Carneg. Inst. *33*:21–51, 1949.
48. Sensenig, E. C.: The development of the occiput and cervical segments and their associated structures in human embryos. Contr. Embryol. Carneg. Inst. *36*:143–151, 1957.
49. Sensenig, E. C.: The origin of the vertebral column in the deer-mouse, *Peromyscus maniculatus rufinus.* Anat. Rec. *86*:123–141, 1943.
50. Stanley, J. K., Owen, R., and Koff, S.: Congenital sacral anomalies. J. Bone Joint Surg. *61B*:401–409, 1979.
51. Strasmann, T.: Axiale Mesenchymstrukturen in der Anlage der Halswirbelsaule des Menschen. Acta Anat. *130*:197–212, 1987.
52. Stromer, E.: Gesicherte Ergebnisse der Palaozoologie. Abh. Bayer. Akad. Wissensch. *54*:1–144, 1944.
53. Taylor, J. R., and Twomney, L. T.: The development of the human intervertebral disc. *In* Ghosh, P. (ed.): The Biology of the Intervertebral Disc. Vol. I. Boca Raton, FL, CRC Press, 1988.
54. Toro, I., and Szepe, L.: Untersuchungen über die Frage der Assimilation und Manifestation des Atlas. Z. Anat. Entwickl. *111*:186–200, 1942.
55. Treble, N. J., Owen, R., and Rickwood, A. M. K.: Classification of congenital abnormalities of the sacrum. Acta Orthop. Scand. *59*:412–416, 1988.
56. Verbout, A. J.: A critical review of the "Neugliederung" concept in relation to the development of the vertebral column. Acta Biotheoret. *25*:219–258, 1976.
57. Verbout, A. J.: The development of the vertebral

column. Adv. Anat. Embryol. Cell Biol. *90*:1–122, 1985.

58. Verbout, A. J., and Huson, A.: The resegmentation of the embryonic vertebral column. Proc. 3rd Europ. Anat. Congress, Manchester, England, 1973, pp. 215–217.
59. von Ebner, V.: Urwirbel und Neugliederung der Wirbelsaule. Sitzungber. Akad. Wiss. Wein *III/101*:235–260, 1889.
60. Wakimoto, B. T., Turner, F. R., and Kaufman, T. C.: Defects in embryogenesis in mutants associated with the antennapedia gene complex of *Drosophila melanogaster*. Dev. Biol. *102*:147–172, 1984.
61. Wamsley, R.: The development and growth of the intervertebral disc. Edin. Med. J. *60*:341–364, 1953.
62. Welch, J. P., and Alterman, K.: The syndrome of caudal dysplasia. Pediatr. Pathol. *2*:313–327, 1984.
63. Whalen, J. L., Parke, W. W., Mazur, J. M., and Stauffer, E. S.: The intrinsic vasculature of developing vertebral end plates and its nutritive significance to the intervertebral disc. J. Pediatr. Orthop. *5*:403–410, 1985.
64. Williams, E. E.: Gadow's arcualia and the development of tetrapod vertebrae. Qt. Rev. Biol. *34*:1–32, 1959.
65. Wolfe, H. J., Putschar, W. G., and Vickery, A. L.: Role of the notochord in human intervertebral discs. I. Fetus and infant. Clin. Orthop. *39*:205–215, 1965.

CHAPTER

2

APPLIED ANATOMY OF THE SPINE

Wesley W. Parke, Ph.D.

The spine is the segmental column of vertebrae that constitutes the major subcranial part of the axial skeleton. Its individual elements are united by a series of intervertebral articulations to form a firm but flexible shaft that supports the trunk and its appendages while providing a protective covering for the spinal cord. The entire column typically consists of 33 vertebrae. Seven cervical, 12 thoracic, and five lumbar vertebrae compose the movable presacral section of the spine; five fused elements form the inflexible sacrum that articulates with the pelvic girdle. Caudal to the sacrum, four or five irregular ossicles make up the coccyx.

THE VERTEBRAE

Since 97 diarthroses and an even greater number of amphiarthroses are involved in the movements of the spine, the individual vertebra must bear multiple processes and surface markings that indicate the attachments of the numerous ligamentous and tendinous structures. Yet, despite the fact that these characteristics may vary considerably from one region to the next, the homologous segmental origin of the vertebrae provides that a single generalized description can be applied to the basic morphology of all but the most superior and inferior elements.

The typical vertebra consists of two major components: a roughly cylindric ventral mass of cancellous bone, the body, and the dorsal vertebral arch. The vertebral bodies vary considerably in size and sectional contour, but exhibit no salient processes or unique external features other than the facets for rib articulation in the thoracic region. Contrarily, the vertebral arch has a more complex structure. It is attached to the dorsolateral aspects of the body by two stout pillars, the pedicles. These are united dorsally by a pair of arched flat laminae that are surmounted in the midline by a dorsal projection, the spinous process. The pedicles, laminae, and dorsum of the body thus form the vertebral foramen, a complete osseous ring that encloses the spinal cord.

Near the junction of the pedicles and the laminae are found the lateral transverse processes and the superior and inferior articular processes. The transverse processes extend from the sides of the vertebral arches, and as all vertebrae are phyletically and ontogenetically associated with some form of costal element, they either articulate with or incorporate a rib component.

The articular processes (zygapophyses) form

The vascular studies presented here were supported by N.I.H. research grant HL-14035.

the paired diarthrodial articulations between the vertebral arches. The superior processes (prezygapophyses) always bear an articulating facet whose surface is directed dorsally to some degree, and complementarily the inferior articulating processes (postzygapophyses) direct their articulating surfaces ventrally. Variously shaped bony prominences (mamillary processes or parapophyses) may be found lateral to the articular processes and serve in the multiple origins and insertions of the spinal muscles.

The superoinferior dimensions of the pedicles are roughly half that of their corresponding body, so that in their lateral aspect the pedicles and their articulating processes form the superior and inferior vertebral notches. As the base of the pedicle arises somewhat superiorly from the dorsum of the body, the inferior vertebral notch appears more deeply incised. In the articulated spine, the opposing superior and inferior notches form the intervertebral foramina that pass the neural and vascular structures between the corresponding levels of the spinal cord and their developmentally related body segments.

Regional Characteristics

Although the 24 vertebrae of the presacral spine are divided into three distinct groups, in which the individual members may be recognized by one or two uniquely regional features, there is also a gradual craniocaudal change, so that in a number of ways the vertebrae found above and below the point of regional demarcation will be transitional and bear some of the characteristics of both areas.

Cervical Vertebrae

Of the seven cervical vertebrae, the first two and the last require special notation, but the third to the sixth are fairly uniform and can be covered by a common description.

As the cervical vertebrae bear the least weight, their bodies are relatively small and thin with respect to the size of the vertebral arch and vertebral foramen. In addition, their diameter is greater transversely than in the anteroposterior direction. The lateral edges of the superior surface of each body are sharply turned upward to form the uncinate processes that are characteristic of the cervical region. However, the most obvious diagnostic feature of the cervical vertebrae is the transverse foramina that perforate the transverse processes

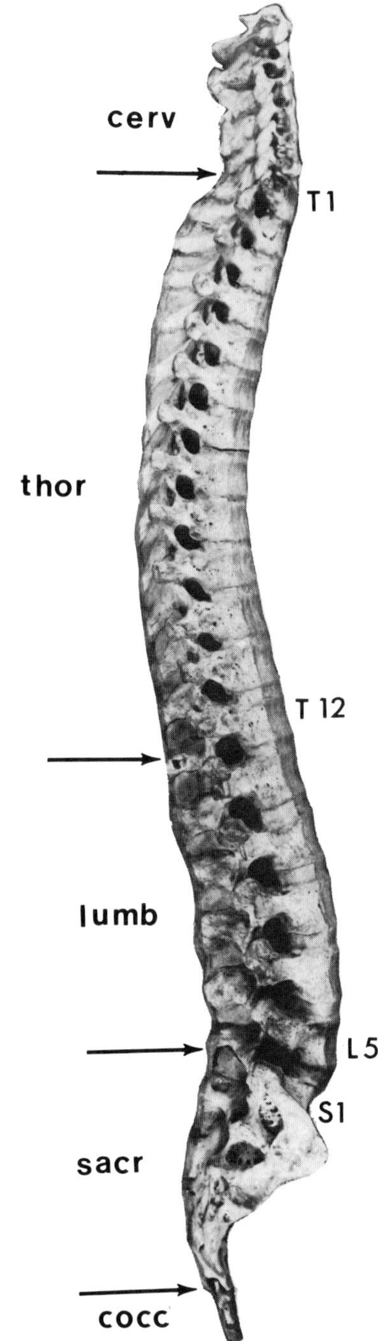

Figure 2–1. Lateral view of dried preparation of the spine with anterior longitudinal and supraspinous ligaments intact.

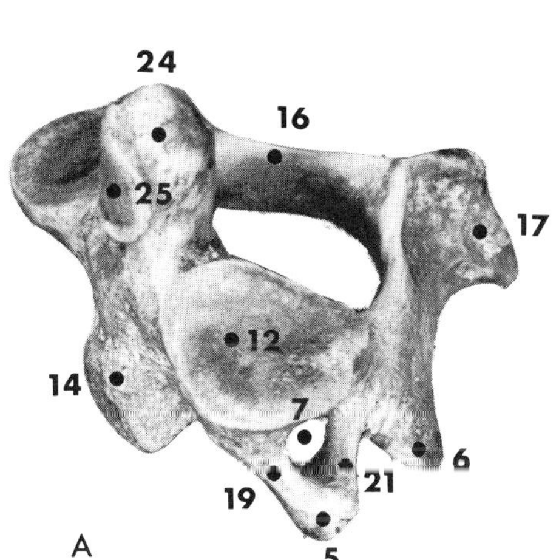

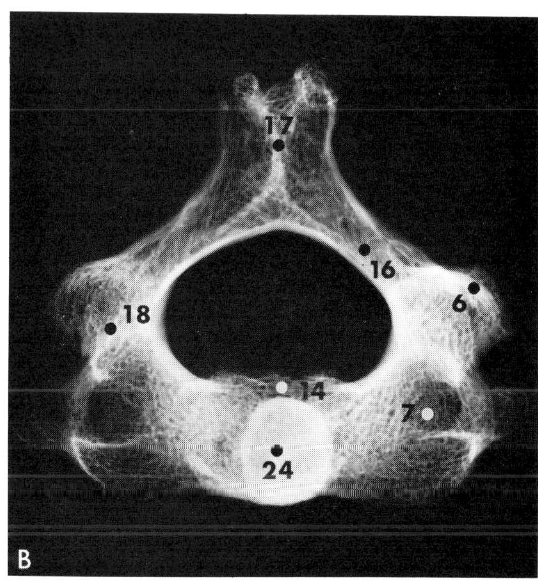

Figure 2–2. The atlas, the axis, and a typical vertebra of each region are illustrated photographically and radiographically. The following numerical key is applicable to all subdivisions of this figure. *A,* Oblique view of atlas. *B,* Ventral radiographic view of atlas.

1. lateral mass of atlas
2. superior articulating process
3. posterior arch
4. anterior arch
5. transverse process
6. inferior articulating process
7. transverse foramen
8. alar tubercle
9. groove for vertebral artery
10. neural arch element of transverse process
11. costal element of transverse process
12. superior articulating process
13. pedicle
14. body
15. uncinate process
16. lamina
17. spinous process
18. articular pillar
19. anterior tubercle of transverse process
20. neural sulcus
21. posterior tubercle of transverse process
22. superior demifacet for head of rib
23. inferior demifacet for head of rib
24. odontoid process
25. articular facet for anterior arch of atlas

Illustration continued on following page

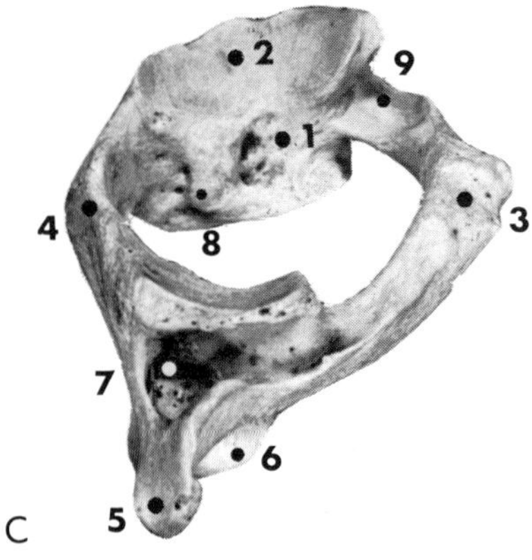

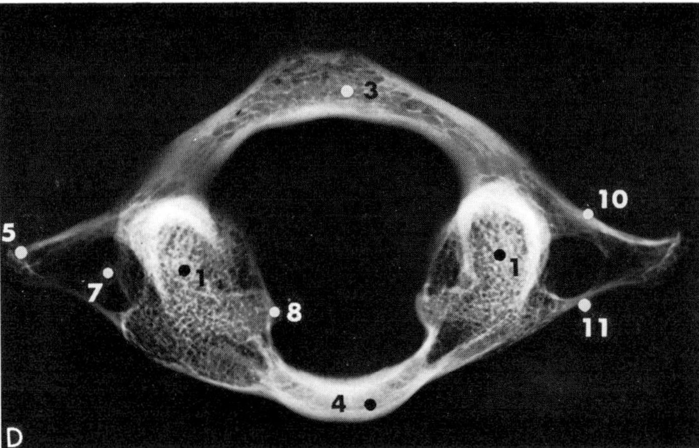

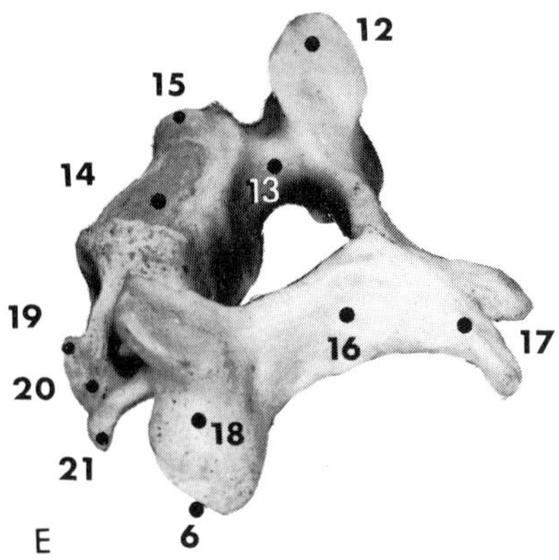

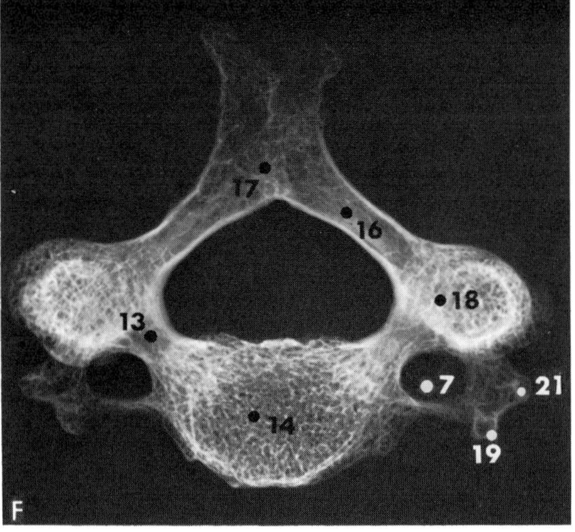

Figure 2–2 *Continued C*, Oblique view of axis. *D*, Vertical radiographic view of axis. *E*, Oblique view of typical (fourth) cervical vertebra. *F*, Vertical radiographic view of typical cervical vertebrae.

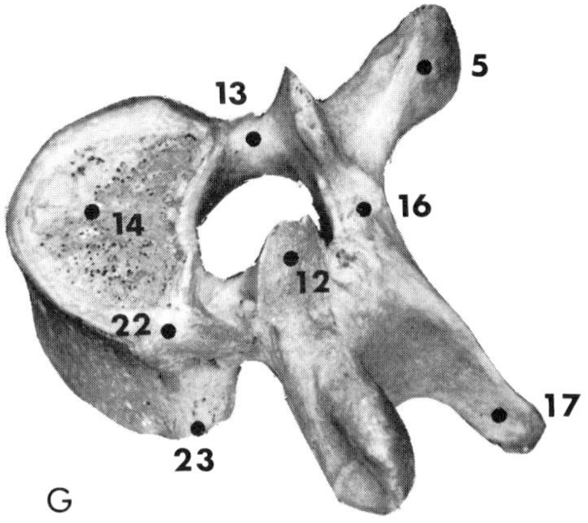

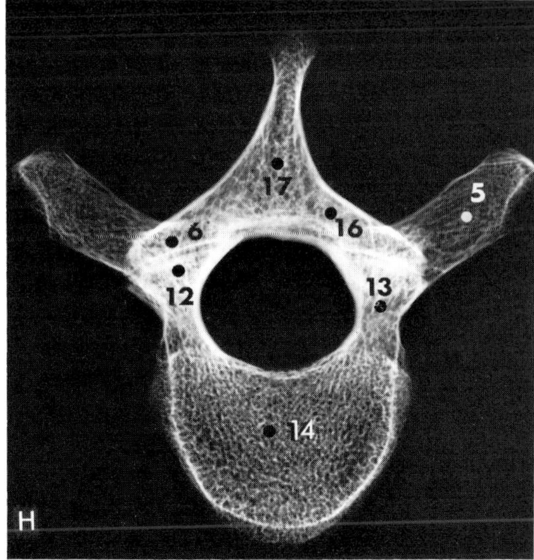

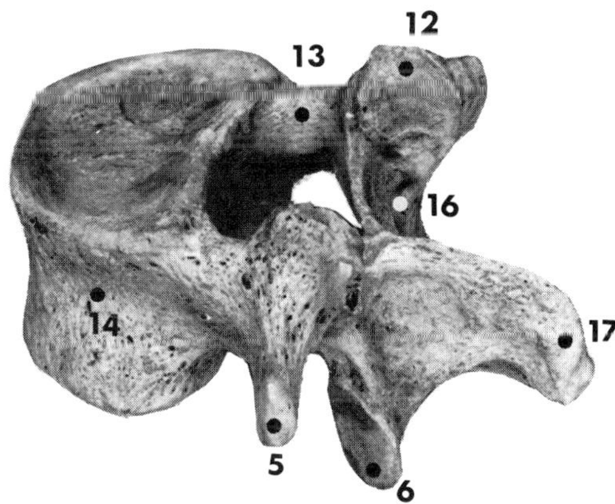

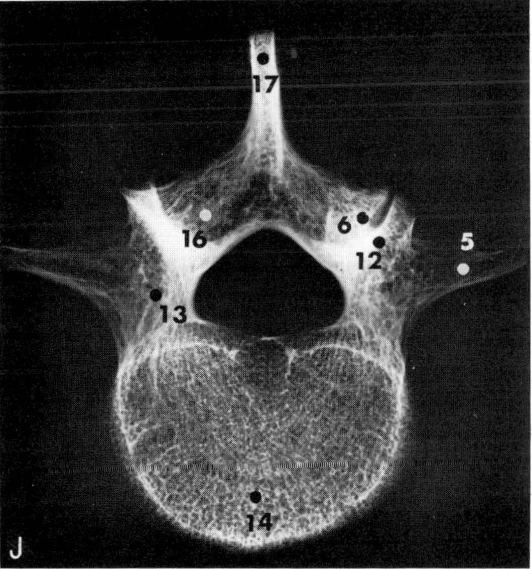

Figure 2–2 *Continued G,* Oblique view of typical (fifth) thoracic vertebra. *H,* Vertical radiographic view of thoracic vertebra. Note that the plane of the articular facets would readily permit rotation. *I,* Oblique view of typical (third) lumbar vertebra. *J,* Vertical radiographic view of lumbar vertebra. Note that the plane of the articular facets is situated to lock the lumbar vertebrae against rotation.

and transmit the cervical arteries. The anterior part of the transverse processes represents fused costal elements that arise from the sides of the body. The lateral extremities of the transverse processes bear two projections, the anterior and posterior tubercles. The former serve as origins of anterior cervical muscles; the latter provide both origins and insertions for posterior cervical muscles. A deep groove between the upper aspects of the tubercles transmits the cervical spinal nerves.

Both the superior and inferior articular processes appear as obliquely sectioned surfaces of short cylinders of bone that, when united with the adjacent vertebrae, form two osseous shafts posterolateral to that of the stacked vertebral bodies. Thus, the cervical vertebrae present a tripod of flexible columns for the support of the head.

The laminae are narrow and have a thinner superior edge, and at their middorsal junction they bear a bifid spinous process that receives the insertions of the semispinalis cervicis muscles.

Atlantoaxial Complex

The first two cervical vertebrae are structurally and developmentally peculiar. Together they form a complex articular system that permits both the nutational and rotational movements of the head. The first cervical vertebra, or atlas, is a bony ring consisting of an anterior and a posterior arch, which are connected by the two lateral masses. Close inspection, however, reveals that it has all the homologous features of a typical vertebra with the exception of the body. The lateral masses correspond to the combined pedicles and articular pillars of the lower cervical vertebrae, but both the superior and inferior articular facets are concave. The superior articular surfaces face upward and internally to receive the occipital condyles of the skull, whereas the inferior articulating surfaces face downward and internally to rotate on the sloped "shoulders" of the axis.

The posterior arch consists of modified laminae that are more round than flat in their sectional aspect, and a posterior tubercle that represents an attenuated spinous process and gives origin to suboccipital muscles. Immediately behind the lateral masses on the superior surface of the posterior arch, two smooth grooves serve to pass the vertebral arteries as they penetrate the posterior atlanto-occipital membrane. These arteries take a tortuous course from the transverse processes of the atlas. The anterior arch, which is of uncertain homology, forms a short bridge between the

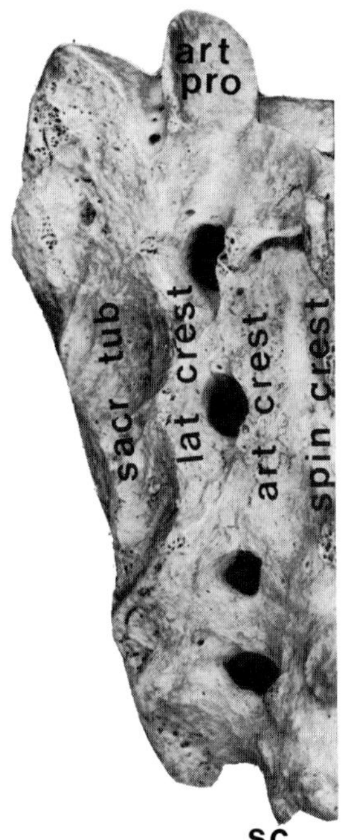

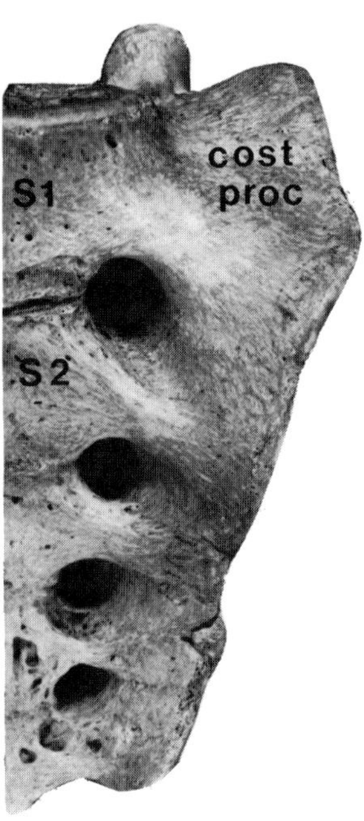

Figure 2–3. Composite anteroposterior view of the sacrum. The roughened crests on the dorsum (*left side of illustration*) indicate longitudinal fusions of vertebral arch structures. Note that the articular process is directed backward to buttress the vertebral arch of the fifth lumbar vertebra.

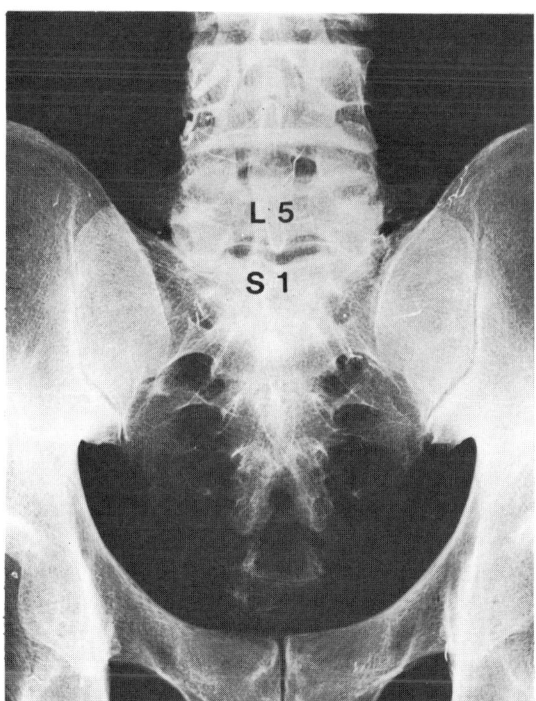

Figure 2–4. Anterior radiographic view of the lumbosacral and sacroiliac articulations. The load transfer from the lumbar spine to the iliac bones via the costal processes of the first and second sacral segments is obvious.

anterior aspects of the lateral masses and bears an anterior tubercle that is the site of insertion of the longus colli muscle. On the posterior surface of the anterior arch, a semicircular depression marks the synovial articulation of the odontoid process, and internal tubercles on the adjacent lateral masses show the attachments of the transverse atlantal ligaments that hold the odontoid against this articular area.

The second cervical vertebra, or axis, provides a bearing surface on which the atlas may rotate, but its most distinctive characteristic is the vertically projecting odontoid process that serves as a pivotal restraint against horizontal displacements of the atlas. This bony prominence represents the phyletically purloined centrum of the first cervical vertebra. It exhibits a slight constriction at its neck and an anterior facet for its articulation with the anterior arch of the atlas. Posteriorly, a groove in the neck of the odontoid marks the position of the strong transverse atlantal ligament.

The apex of the odontoid process is slightly pointed and is the attachment of the apical ligament. Posterior to the apex, two lateral roughened prominences indicate the attachments of the alar ligaments. These structures and the apical ligament connect the odontoid process to the base of the skull. The superior articulating surfaces of the axis are convex and are directed laterally to receive the direct thrust of the lateral masses of the atlas. The inferior articulating surfaces, however, are typical of those of the cervical vertebrae and serve as the commencement of the articular columns. The lateral processes of the axis are directed downward, and their posterior or noncostal elements are often quite thin. Anteriorly, the inferior aspect of the body of the axis forms a liplike process that descends over the first intervertebral disc and the body of the third cervical vertebra.

The seventh cervical vertebra is transitional, and the inferior surface of its body is propor-

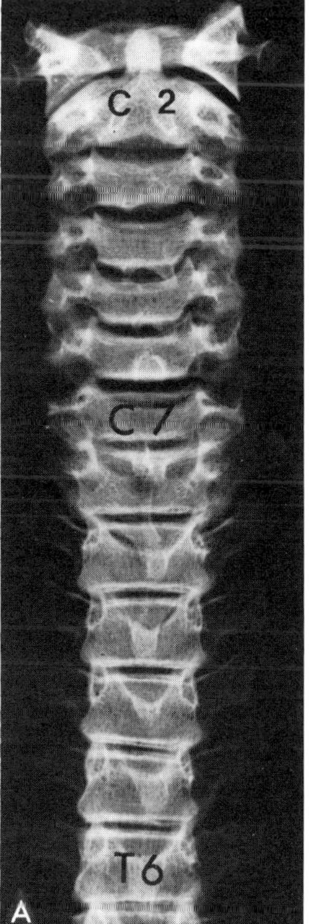

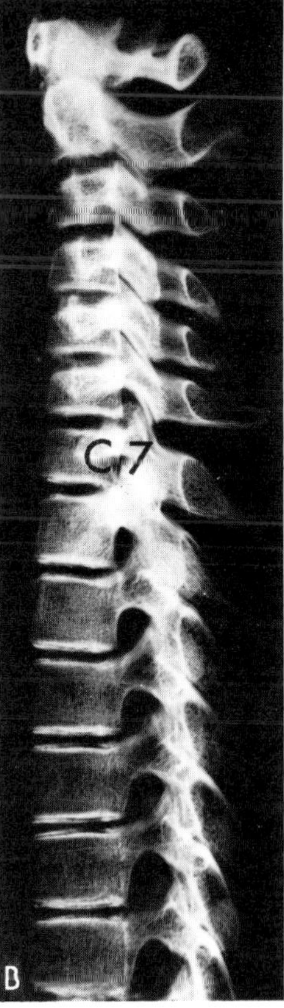

Figure 2–5. Anteroposterior radiograph of dried preparation of cervical and upper thoracic spine. Note the greater relative thickness of the cervical discs and the more lateral disposition of the cervical articular pillars. *B*, Lateral view of preceding specimen. Unfortunately, the normal curvatures did not survive the preparation, but the gradual increase in size of both the bodies and the intervertebral foramina is well illustrated.

tionately larger than the superior surface. It bears a long, distinct spinous process that is easily palpable in the living body. The superior and inferior articulating facets are more steeply inclined and presage the form of these structures in the thoracic region. Blunt transverse processes show heavy posterior roots and much lighter anterior roots that surround transverse foramina that are often bilaterally unequal and seldom pass the vertebral arteries. Not infrequently, one or both of the anterior roots realize their true potential as a costal element and develop into the often troublesome cervical rib.

Thoracic Vertebrae

All 12 thoracic vertebrae support ribs and thus show facets for the diarthrodial articulations of these structures. The first and last four have specific peculiarities in the manner of costal articulations, but the second to the eighth may be covered by a common description.

The body of a midthoracic vertebra is heart shaped, and its length and width are roughly halfway between that of the cervical and lumbar centra. Often a flattening of the left side of the body indicates its contact with the descending aorta. In the midthorax the heads of the ribs form a joint that spans the intervertebral disc, so that the inferior lip of the body of one vertebra and the corresponding site of the superior lip of the next inferior element share in the formation of a single articular facet for the costal capitulum. Thus, the typical thoracic vertebra bears two demifacets on each side of its body.

The thoracic vertebral arch encloses a small, round vertebral foramen that will not admit the first joint of the index finger, even when the specimen is derived from a large adult. Because the pedicles arise more superiorly on the dorsum of the body than they do in the cervical region, the inferior vertebral notch

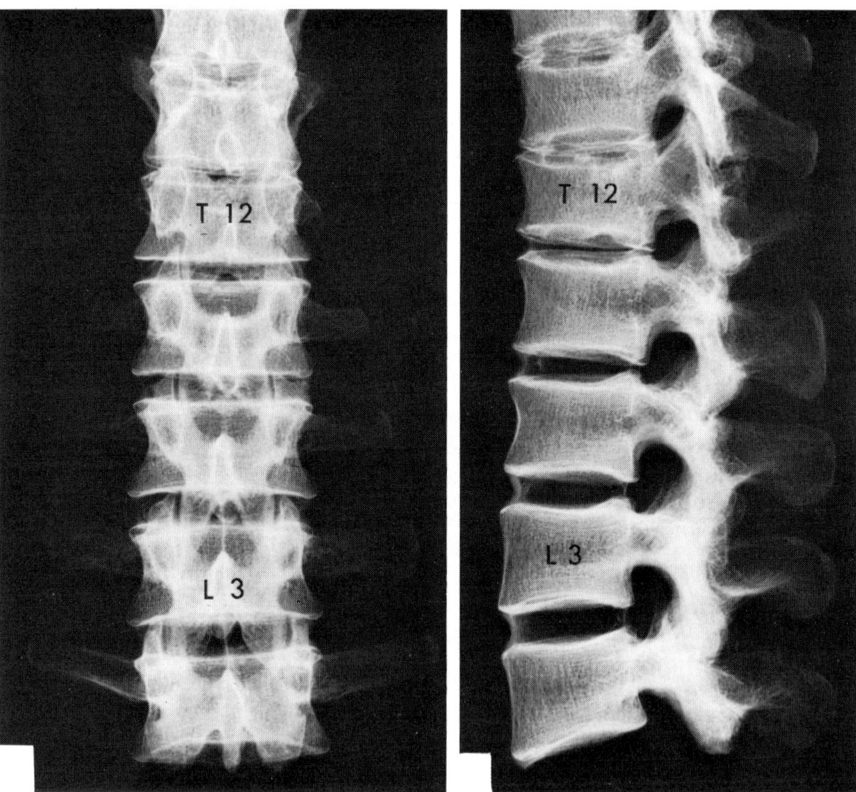

Figure 2–6. Anteroposterior and lateral radiographs of lower thoracic–upper lumbar region of articulated dried preparation.

forms an even greater contribution to the intervertebral foramen. The superior articular facets form a stout shelflike projection from the junction of the laminae and the pedicles. Their ovoid surfaces are slightly convex and almost vertical in their plane of articulation. They face dorsally and slightly superolaterally, and in bilateral combination present the segment of an arc whose center of radius lies at the anterior edge of the vertebral body. They thus permit a slight rotation around the axis of this radius. The inferior articular facets are borne by the inferior edges of the laminae, and the geometry of their articular surfaces is complementary to that of the superior processes.

On the ventral side of the tip of the strong transverse processes, another concave facet receives the tuberculum of the rib whose capitulum articulates with the superior demifacet of the same vertebra. The spinous processes of the thoracic vertebrae are long and triangular in section. Those of the upper four are more bladelike and are directed backward at an angle of about 40 degrees from the horizontal. The middle four thoracic spines are longer but directed downward at an angle of 60 degrees, so that their spines completely overlap the next lower segment. The four most inferior spines resemble the first four in direction and shape.

The first thoracic vertebra exhibits a complete facet on the side of its body for the capitulum of the first rib and an inferior demifacet for the capitulum of the second rib. The costal articulations of the ninth to 12th thoracic vertebrae again tend to confine themselves to the sides of the bodies of their respective segments. On the last two thoracic vertebrae, transitional characteristics are evident in the diminution of the transverse processes and their failure to buttress the last two ribs.

Lumbar Vertebrae

The lumbar vertebrae are the lowest five of the presacral column. All their features are expressed in more massive proportions, but their essential diagnostic characteristics are negative; that is, they may be easily distinguished from other regional elements by their lack of a transverse foramen or costal articular facets. The body is large, having a width greater than its anteroposterior diameter, and is slightly thicker in front than behind. All structures associated with the vertebral arch are blunt and stout. The thick pedicles are widely placed on the dorsolateral aspects of the centrum, and with their laminae they enclose a triangular vertebral foramen. Although the inferior vertebral notch is deeper than the superior, both make substantial contributions to the intervertebral foramen. The transverse processes are flat and winglike in the upper four lumbar segments, but in the fifth they are presented as thick, rounded stumps. Aside from their relative size, the lumbar vertebrae may always be recognized by their articular processes. The superior pair arise in the usual manner from the junction of the pedicles and laminae, but their articular facets are concave and directed dorsomedially, so that they almost face each other. The inferior processes are extensions of the laminae that direct the articulating surfaces ventrolaterally and thus lock themselves between the superior facets of the next inferior vertebra in an almost mortise-and-tenon fashion. This arrangement obviously restricts both rotation and flexion in the lumbar region. The lumbar segments also have the most pronounced mamillary processes for the origins and insertions of the thick lower divisions of the epaxial muscles.

Sacral Vertebrae

The sacrum consists of five fused vertebrae that form a single triangular complex of bone that supports the spine and forms the posterior part of the pelvis. It is markedly curved and tilted backward, so that its first element articulates with the fifth lumbar vertebra at a pronounced angle (the sacrovertebral angle).

Close inspection of both the flat, concave ventral surface and the rough, ridged convex dorsal surface reveals that, despite their fusion, all the homologous elements of typical vertebrae are still evident in the sacrum. The heavy, laterally projecting alae that bear the articular surfaces for articulation with the pelvis are fused anterior costal and posterior transverse processes of the first three sacral vertebrae. These lateral fusions require that separate dorsal and ventral foramina provide egress for the anterior and posterior divisions of the sacral nerves. The ventral four pairs of sacral foramina are larger than their dorsal counterparts as they must pass the thick sacral contributions to the sciatic nerve. Although the ventral surface of the sacrum is relatively smooth, since it must accommodate the birth canal and pelvic viscera, it still displays four transverse ridges that mark the fusions of the vertebral bodies and enclose cryptic remnants of the intervertebral discs. Lateral to the bodies of the second, third, and fourth elements, the ridges of bone that separate the anterior sacral foramina are quite prominent and give origin to the piriformis muscle.

The dorsal aspect of the sacrum is convex, rough, and conspicuously marked by five longitudinal ridges. The central one, the middle sacral crest, is formed by the fusion of the spinous processes of the sacral vertebrae. On either side, a sacral groove separates it from the medial sacral articular crest that represents the fused articular process. The superior ends of these crests, however, form the functional superior articular processes of the first sacral vertebra, which articulate with the inferior processes of the fifth lumbar vertebra. They are very strong, and their facets are directed dorsally to resist the tendency of the fifth lumbar vertebra to be displaced forward at the sacrovertebral angle. Inferiorly, the articular crests terminate as the sacral cornua, two rounded projections that bracket the inferior hiatus where it gives access to the sacral vertebral canal. More laterally, the lateral crests and sacral tuberosities form uneven elevations for the attachments of the dorsal sacroiliac ligaments.

The sacrum and its posterior ligaments lie ventral to the posterior iliac spines and form a deep depression that accommodates and gives origin to the inferior parts of the epaxial muscles that extend the spine. The grooves between the central spinous crest and the articular crests are occupied by the origins of the multifidus muscles, while dorsal and lateral to these are attached the origins of the iliocostal and iliolumbar muscles.

Coccyx

The coccyx is usually composed of four vertebral rudiments, but one fewer or one greater than this number is not uncommon. It is the vestigial representation of the tail or caudal vertebrae of the human.

The first coccygeal segment is larger than the succeeding members and resembles to some extent the inferior sacral element. It has an obvious body that articulates with the homologous component of the inferior sacrum, and it bears two cornua, which may be regarded as vestiges of superior articulating processes. The three inferior coccygeal members are most frequently fused and present a curved profile continuous with that of the sacrum. They incorporate the rudiments of a body and transverse processes but possess no components of the vertebral arch.

The coccyx contributes no supportive function to the spine but serves as an origin for the gluteus maximus posteriorly and the muscles of the pelvic diaphragm anteriorly.

ARTHROLOGY OF THE SPINE

The articulations of the spine include the three major types of joints: synarthroses, diarthroses, and amphiarthroses. The synarthroses are found during development and the first decade of life. They are best represented by the neurocentral synchondrosis, a type of nearly immovable joint in which a thin plate of cartilage joins two bones. The neurocentral joints are the two unions between the centers of ossification for the two halves of the vertebral arch and that of the centrum. They are usually obliterated during the second decade. The early unions between the articular processes of the sacral vertebrae also form ephemeral synchondroses.

The diarthroses are the true synovial joints, formed mostly by the articular processes and costovertebral joints, but also include the atlantoaxial and sacroiliac articulations. All the spinal diarthroses are of the arthrodial or gliding type, with the exception of the trochoid or pivot joint found in the median atlantoaxial articulation.

The nonsynovial, slightly movable connective tissue joints are of two types: the symphysis, as exemplified by the fibrocartilage of the intervertebral disc, and the syndesmosis, as represented by all the ligamentous connections between both the adjacent bodies and the adjacent arches.

Articulations of the Vertebral Arches

The joints formed by the articular processes of the vertebral arches possess a true joint capsule and are capable of a limited gliding articulation. The capsules are therefore thin and lax and are attached to the bases of the engaging superior and inferior articulating processes of opposing vertebrae. Since it is mostly the plane of articulation of these joints that determines the types of motion characteristic of the various regions of the spine, it would be expected that the fibers of the articular capsules would be longest and most loose in the cervical region and become increasingly taut in an inferior progression.

The syndesmoses between the vertebral arches are formed by the paired sets of the ligamenta flava, the intertransverse ligaments, the interspinous ligaments, and the unpaired supraspinous ligament.

The ligamenta flava bridge the spaces between the laminae of adjacent vertebrae from the second cervical to the lumbosacral interval. The lateral extent of each half of a paired set commences around the bases of the articulating processes and can be traced medially where they nearly join at the roots of the spines. This central deficiency serves to transmit small vessels and facilitates the passage of a needle during lumbar punctures. The fibers of the ligamenta flava are almost vertical in their disposition but are attached to the ventral surface of the upper lamina and to the superior lip of the next lower one. This shingle-like arrangement conceals the true length of the ligaments because of the overlapping of the superior lamina. Therefore, their morphology is best appreciated from the ventral aspect as in Figure 2–7*B*. The yellow elastic fibers that give the ligamenta flava their name maintain their elasticity even in embalmed specimens, in which, if a series of three or four laminae and their intervening ligaments are removed intact, they will still stretch and retract to a surprising degree. It has been stated in some texts that the elasticity of the ligamenta flava serves to assist in the maintenance of the erect posture. However, a more probable reason for this property is simply to keep the ligament taut during extension, where any laxity would permit redundancy and infolding toward the ventrally related nervous structures.

The intertransverse ligaments are fibrous connections between the transverse processes. They are difficult to distinguish from extensions of the tendinous insertions of the segmental muscles, and in reality may be just that in some regions. Between the cervical transverse processes they appear as a few tough, thin fibers, and in the thoracic area they blend with the intercostal ligaments. Being most distinct between the lumbar transverse processes, they may be isolated here as membranous bands.

The interspinal ligaments (Fig. 2–7*A*) are membranous sets of fibers that connect adjoin-

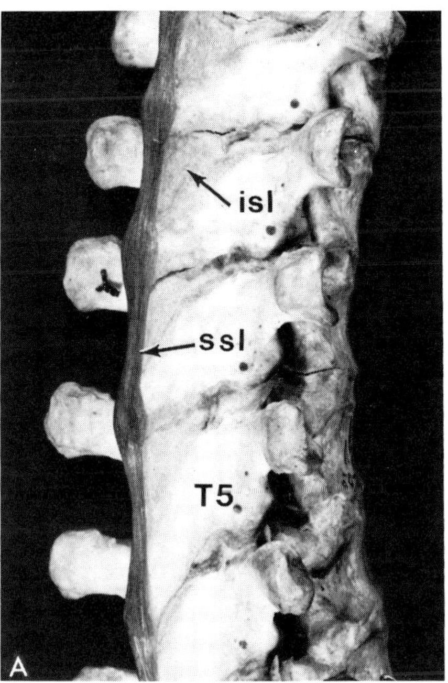

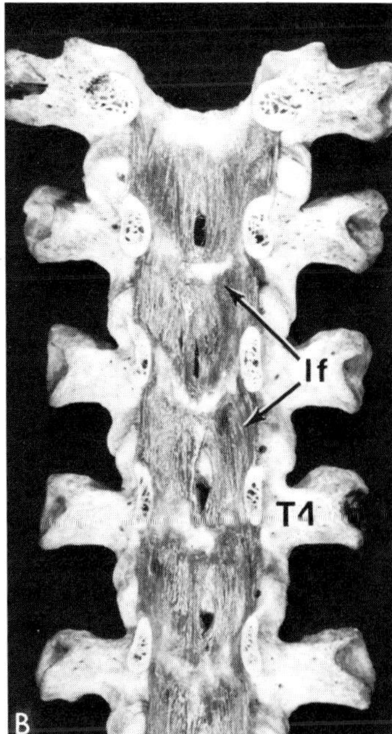

Figure 2–7. *A*, Dried preparation of the thoracic vertebrae showing the supraspinous ligament (ssl) and interspinous ligaments (isl). *B*, Anterior view of the upper thoracic vertebral arches showing the disposition of the ligamenta flava (lf).

ing spinous processes. They are situated medial to the thin pairs of interspinal muscles that bridge the apices of the spine. The fibers of the ligaments, however, are arranged obliquely so that they connect the base of the superior spine with the superior ridge and apex of the next most inferior spinous process. When we realize that virtually all somatic segmented structures are bilateral in origin, it is less surprising that these midline ligaments are found in pairs with a distinct dissectible cleft between them.

The supraspinal ligament (Fig. 2–7*A*) is a continuous fibrous cord that runs along the apices of the spinous processes from the seventh cervical to the end of the sacral spinous crest. Like the longitudinal ligaments of the vertebra, the more superficial fibers of the ligament extend over several spinal segments, while the deeper, shorter fibers bridge only two or three spines. In the cervical region the supraspinal ligament assumes a distinctive character and a specific name, the ligamentum nuchae. This structure is bowstrung across the cervical lordosis from the external occipital protuberance to the spine of the seventh cervical vertebra. Its anterior border forms a sagittal fibrous sheet that divides the posterior nuchal muscles and attaches to the spinous processes of all cervical vertebrae. The ligamentum nuchae contains an abundance of elastic fibers, and in quadripeds it forms a strong truss that supports the cantilevered position of the head.

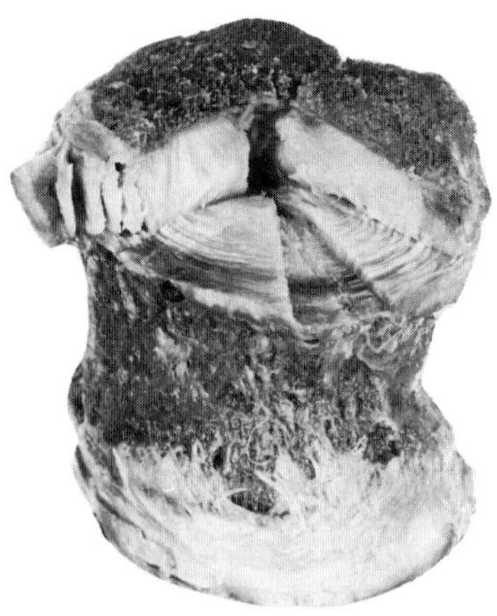

Figure 2–8. Photograph of a dissected third lumbar disc. Note that lamellar bands are still visible when the section is cut deep into bony apophyseal ring. A layer of spongiosa was left attached to the superior surface of the disc to show that only a thin chondral plate intervenes between the vascular trabeculae and the disc. The inward buckling of the lamellae near the cavity of the extirpated nuclear material is well shown (male specimen, 52 years old).

Special Articulations

The atlanto-occipital articulation consists of the diarthrosis between the lateral masses of the atlas and the occipital condyles of the skull, and the syndesmoses formed by the atlanto-occipital membranes. The articular capsules around the condyles are thin and loose and permit a gliding motion between the condylar convexity and the concavity of the lateral masses. The capsules blend laterally with ligaments that connect the transverse processes of the atlas with the jugular processes of the skull. Although the lateral ligaments and the capsules are sufficiently lax to permit nodding, they require that the atlas and skull must rotate as a unit.

The anterior atlanto-occipital membrane is a structural extension of the anterior longitudinal ligament that connects the forward rim of the foramen magnum to the anterior arch of the atlas and blends with the joint capsules laterally. It is dense, tough, and virtually cordlike in its central portion.

The posterior atlanto-occipital membrane is homologous to the ligamenta flava and unites the posterior arch of the atlas. It is deficient laterally where it arches over the groove on the superior surface of the arch. Through this aperture the vertebral artery enters the neural canal to penetrate the dura. Occasionally the free edge of this membrane is ossified to form a true bony foramen around the artery.

The median atlantoaxial articulation is a pivot (trochoid) joint with an intriguing developmental and evolutionary history (Figs. 2–9, 2–10). The essential features of the articulation are the odontoid process (dens) of the axis and the internal surface of the anterior arch of the atlas. The opposition of the two bones is maintained by the thick, straplike transverse atlantal ligament. Both the ligament and the arch of the atlas have true synovial cavities intervening between them and the odontoid process. Alar expansions of the transverse ligament attach to tubercles on the lateral rims of the foramen magnum, and a single, unpaired cord, the apical odontoid ligament, attaches the apex of the process to the anterior rim of the foramen. The entire joint is covered

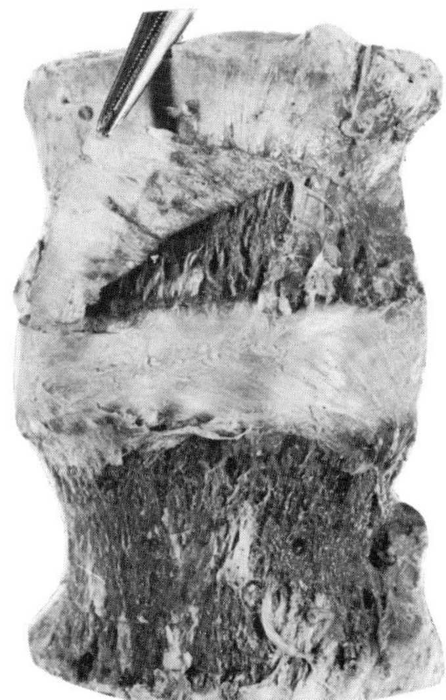

Figure 2–9. Bodies of the third and fourth lumbar vertebrae from a 58-year-old male. The spiral course of fibers of the outer lamellae is evident. The periosteal attachment of the reflected anterior longitudinal ligament is well shown, in addition to the delineation of the loosely attached area raised from the surface of the disc.

posteriorly by a cranial extension of the posterior longitudinal ligament that takes the name membrana tectoria in this region. Since the atlas freely glides over the superior articulating facets of C2, the atlantoaxial pivot is essential for preventing horizontal displacements between C1 and C2. Thus, fracture of the odontoid or, less likely, rupture of the transverse ligament produces a very unstable craniospinal articulation.

Articulations of the Vertebral Bodies

The vertebral bodies are connected by the two forms of amphiarthroses. Symphyses are represented by the intervertebral discs, and syndesmoses are formed by the anterior and posterior longitudinal ligaments.

Intervertebral Disc

The intervertebral disc is the fibrocartilaginous complex that forms the articulation between the bodies of the vertebrae. Although it provides a very strong union, ensuring the degree of intervertebral fixation that is necessary for effective action and the protective alignment of the neural canal, the summation of the limited movements allowed by each disc imparts to the spinal column as a whole its characteristic universal motion. The discs of the various spinal regions may differ considerably in size and in some detail, but they are basically identical in their structural organization. Each consists of two components: the internal semifluid mass, the nucleus pulposus, and its laminar fibrous container, the annulus fibrosus.

Nucleus Pulposus. Typically, the nucleus pulposus occupies an eccentric position within the confines of the annulus, usually being closer to the posterior margin of the disc. Its most essential character becomes obvious in either transverse or sagittal preparations of the disc where, as evidence of internal pressure, it bulges beyond the plane of section. Palpation of a dissected nucleus of a young adult shows that it responds as a viscid fluid under applied pressure, but it also exhibits considerable elastic rebound and assumes its original physical

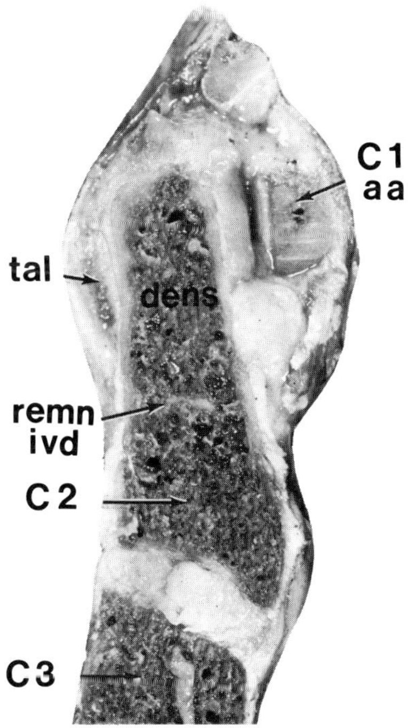

Figure 2–10. Sagittal section through adult odontoid process showing articular relationships with the anterior arch of the atlas (aa) and transverse atlantal ligament (tal). Despite the fact this patient was over 50 years old, a cartilaginous remnant of the homologue of an intervertebral disc may be discerned. Radiologically this might be confused with fracture or a nonunion status.

state upon release. It is somewhat surprising to find that these properties may still be demonstrated in the spine of a cadaver that has been embalmed for many months.

Histologic analysis provides a partial explanation for the characteristics of the nucleus. As the definitive remnant of the embryonic notochordal tissue, it is similarly composed of loose, delicate fibrous strands embedded in a gelatinous matrix. In the center of the mass these fibers show no geometric preference in their arrangement but form a felted mesh of undulating bundles. Only those fibers that are in approximation to the vertebral chondral plates display a definite orientation. These approach the cartilage at an angle, and become embedded in its substance to afford an attachment for the nucleus. A considerable number of cells are suspended in the fibrous network. Many of these are fusiform and resemble typical reticulocytes, but vacuolar and darkly nucleated chondrocytes are also interspersed in matrix. Even in the absence of vascular elements, the profusion of cells should accentuate the fact that the nucleus pulposus is composed of vital tissue.

There is no definite structural interface between the nucleus and the annulus. Rather, the composition of the two tissues blends imperceptibly, a fact that frustrates any attempt to cleanly extirpate the entire nucleus in a fresh dissection.

Annulus Fibrosus. The annulus is a concentric series of fibrous lamellae that encase the nucleus and strongly unite the vertebral bodies. Whereas the essential function of the nucleus is to resist and redistribute compressive forces within the spine, one of the major functions of the annulus is to withstand tension, whether the tensile forces be from the horizontal extensions of the compressed nucleus, from the torsional stress of the column, or from the separation of the vertebral bodies on the convex side of a spinal flexure. Without optical aid, simple dissection and discernment will reveal how well the annulus is constructed for the performance of this service. On horizontal section it is noted that an individual lamella encircling the disc is composed of glistening fibers that run an oblique or spiral course in relation to the axis of the vertebral column. Since the disc presents a kidney- or heart-shaped horizontal section, and the nucleus is displaced posteriorly, these lamellae are thinner and more closely packed between the nucleus and the dorsal aspect of the disc. The bands are stoutest and individually more distinct in the anterior third of the disc, and here when transected they may give the impression that they are of varying composition, because every other ring presents a difference in color and elevation with reference to the plane of section. However, teasing and inspection at an oblique angle will show in the freed lamellae that this difference is due to an abrupt change in the direction of the fibers of adjacent rings. Previous descriptions of the annulus have claimed that the alternating appearance of the banding is the result of the interposition of a chondrous layer between each fibrous ring.[4] Contrarily, our personal observations have shown that the alternations of glistening white lamellae with translucent rings result from differences in the incidence of light with regard to the direction of the fiber bundles. This repeated reversal of fiber arrangement within the annulus has obvious implications in the biomechanics of the disc that will be discussed later.

The disposition of the lamellae on sagittal section is not consistently vertical. In the regions of the annulus approximating the nucleus pulposus, the first distinct bands curve inward, with their convexity facing the nuclear substance. As one follows the successive layers outward, a true vertical profile is assumed, but as the external laminae of the disc are approached, they may again become bowed, with their convexity facing the periphery of the disc.

The attachment of the annulus to its respective vertebral bodies deserves particular mention. This is best understood when a dried preparation of a thoracic or lumbar vertebra is examined first. In the adult the articular surface of the body presents two aspects: a concave central depression that is quite porous and an elevated ring of compact bone that appears to be rolled over the edge of the vertebral body. Often a demarcating fissure falsely suggests that the ring is a true epiphysis of the body, but postnatal studies of ossification have indicated that it is a traction apophysis for the attachment of the annulus and associated longitudinal ligaments.[5]

In life the depth of the central concavity is filled to the level of the marginal ring by the presence of a cribriform cartilaginous plate. Unlike other articular surfaces, there is no closing plate of compact osseous material intervening between this cartilage and the can-

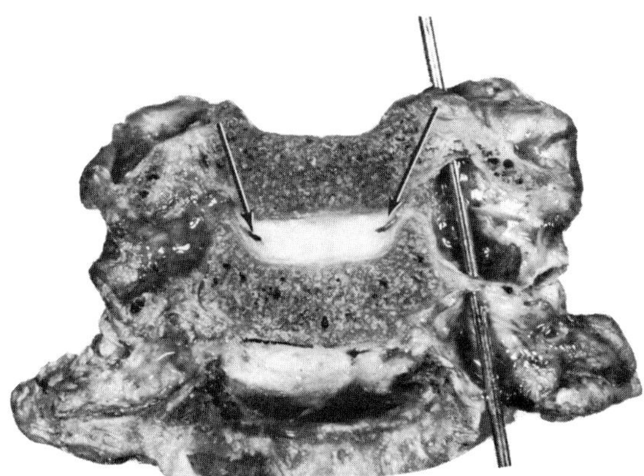

Figure 2–11. Frontal section through the fourth to fifth cervical vertebrae showing a typical cervical disc and its joints of Luschka (*arrows*). A probe has been passed through the vertebral arterial canal to show its relations to the uncovertebral joints.

cellous medullary part of the bone, but the trabeculations of the spongiosa blend into the internal face of the chondrous plate, while fibers from the nucleus and inner lamellae of the annulus penetrate its outer surface. As intimate as this union between the central disc and vertebra may appear, it is the outer bony ring that affords the disc its firmest attachment, for the stoutest external lamellar bands of fibers actually penetrate the ring as Sharpey's fibers, and scraping the disc right down to the bone will show the concentric arrangements reflecting the different angles at which the fibers insert (Fig. 2–12). The fibers of the outermost ring of the annulus have the most extensive range of attachment, for they extend beyond the confines of the disc and blend with the vertebral periosteum and the longitudinal ligaments.

Regional Variations of the Disc. The discs in aggregate make up approximately one fourth of the length of the spinal column exclusive of the sacrum and coccyx, but their degree of contribution is not uniform in the various regions. According to Aeby,[2] the discs provide more than one fifth of the length of the cervical spine, approximately one fifth of the length of the thoracic column, and approximately one third of the length of the lumbar region.

The discs are smallest in the cervical spine, and their lateral extent is less than that of the corresponding vertebral body because of the uncinate processes. Here, as in the lumbar region, they are wedge shaped, the greatest width being anterior. The thoracic discs are somewhat heart shaped on section, the nucleus pulposus being more centrally located than in the lumbar region. Both the thickness and the horizontal dimensions of the thoracic disc increase caudally with the corresponding increase in size of the vertebral bodies. The normal thoracic kyphosis results from a disparity between the anterior and posterior heights of the vertebral bodies as the discs are of uniform thickness. The lumbar discs are reniform and are both relatively and absolutely the thickest in the spine. The progressive caudal increase in the degree of lumbar lordosis is due to the equivalent increase in a differential between the anterior and posterior thickness of the disc, a situation that makes the disc of the lumbosacral union the most wedge shaped.

Anterior Longitudinal Ligament

The anterior longitudinal ligament is a strong band of fibers that extends along the ventral surface of the spine from the skull to

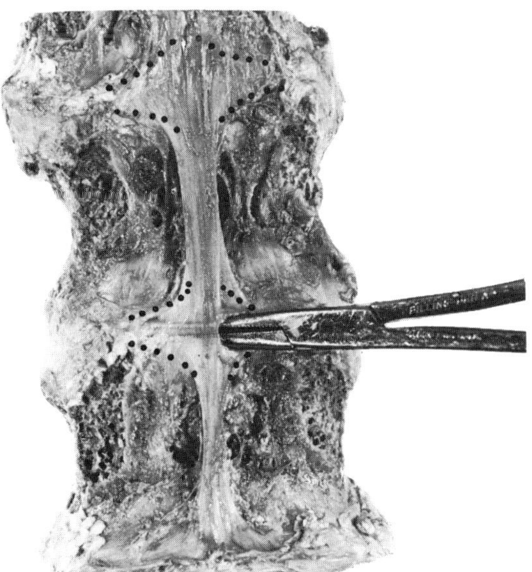

Figure 2–12. Photographic illustration of the posterior longitudinal ligament traversing the bodies of the third and fourth lumbar vertebrae. The central strap of long fibers can be seen passing over the hemostat. The lines of strong attachment of the fibers of the lateral expansions are indicated by the black dots as they outline the rhomboid area, where the fibers are readily dissected from the dorsal surface of the disc. In this case the instrument was inserted into an actual fascial cleft, and the points show the weakest area of the lateral expansion.

the sacrum. It is narrowest and cordlike in the upper cervical region, where it is attached to the atlas and axis and their intervening capsular membranes, but it expands in width as it descends the column to the extent, in the lower lumbar region, of covering most of the anterolateral surfaces of the vertebral bodies and discs before it blends into the presacral fibers. The anterior longitudinal ligament is not uniform in its composition or manner of attachment. Its deepest fibers, which span only one intervertebral articulation, are covered by an intermediate layer that unites two or three vertebrae and a superficial stratum that may connect four or five articular units. Where the ligament is adherent to the anterior surface of the vertebra, it also forms its periosteum, but it is most firmly attached to the articular lip at the end of each body. It is most readily elevated at the point of its passage over the midsection of the discs, where it is loosely attached to the connective tissue band that encircles the annulus (Fig. 2–8).

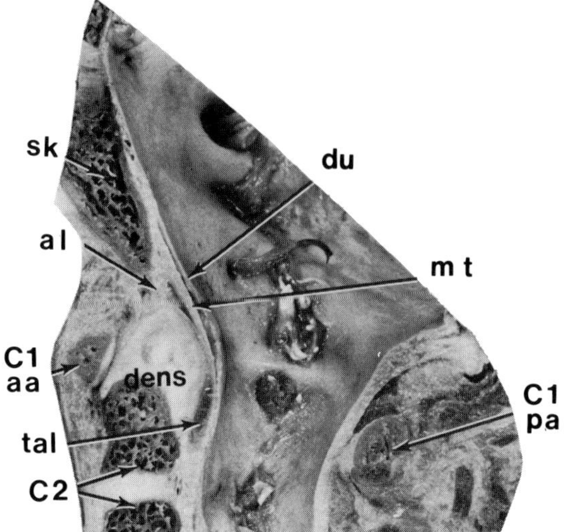

Figure 2–13. Sagittal section through the atlantoaxial articulation of a 4-year-old. Note that the major ossific centers of the odontoid process are still separated from the body of C2 by a well-differentiated disc. The cartilaginous apex of the process shows a condensation marking the apical ossific center. C1aa and C1pa mark the anterior and posterior atlantal arches. The dura (du) overlies the membrana tectoria (mt), a superior extension of the posterior longitudinal ligament. The transverse atlantal ligament (tal) and apical ligament (al) are also indicated.

Posterior Longitudinal Ligament

The posterior longitudinal ligament differs considerably from its anterior counterpart with respect to the clinical significance of its relations to the intervertebral disc. Like the anterior ligament, it extends from the skull to the sacrum, but being within the vertebral canal its central fiber bundles must diminish in breadth as the size of the spinal column increases. The segmental denticulate configuration of the posterior longitudinal ligament is one of its most characteristic features. Between the pedicles, particularly in the lower thoracic and lumbar regions, it forms a thick band of connective tissue that is not adherent to the posterior surface of the vertebral body. Instead, it is bowstrung across the concavity of the dorsum of the body and permits the large vascular elements to enter and leave the medullary sinus located beneath its fibers.

In approximating the dorsum of the disc, the posterior longitudinal ligament displays two strata of fibers. The superficial, longer strands form a distinct strong strap whose filaments bridge several vertebral elements. A second, deeper stratum spans but two vertebral articulations and forms lateral curving extensions of fibers that pass along the dorsum of the disc and out through the intervertebral foramen. It is these deeper intervertebral expansions of the ligament that have the most significant relationship with the disc.

We have found that these fibers are most firmly fixed at the margins of their lateral expansions. This produces a central rhomboidal area of loose attachment or in some cases an actual fascial cleft of equivalent dimensions on the dorsum of the disc. At dissection this characteristic may be readily demonstrated by inserting a blunt probe beneath the intervertebral part of the longitudinal ligament and exploring the area to define the margins of the space where the fibers are strongly inserted (Fig. 2–12). This situation is particularly pertinent to problems involving dorsal or dorsolateral prolapse of the nucleus pulposus. With a dorsocentral protrusion of a semifluid mass, the strong midline strap of posterior longitudinal fibers tends to restrain the herniation. However, if an easily dissectible cleft offers a space for lateral expansion, the mass then extends to either side, dissecting the loose attachment with interruption of numerous nerve fibers. The thinnest part of the lateral expansion of the posterior longitudinal ligament occurs at the convergence of its lines of attachment, and here it is most likely to permit a more dorsal protrusion from internal pressures.

Trabeculations of connective tissue bind the dura to the dorsal surface of the posterior longitudinal ligament, this attachment being the firmest along the lateral edges of the long superficial strap of fibers. Numerous venous cross connections of the epidural sinuses pass between the dura and the ligament, accounting for the fact that venous elements are the most ubiquitous structures among the components related to the vertebral articulations.

Relations of the Roots of the Spinal Nerves

The dorsal and ventral nerve roots pass through the subarachnoid space and converge to form the spinal nerve at approximately the level of its respective intervertebral foramen. Owing to the ascensus spinalis—the apparent developmental rise of the spinal cord resulting from the delayed caudal differential growth of the lower parts of the vertebral column—the course of the nerve roots becomes longer and more obliquely directed as one approaches the lower segments. Therefore, in the cervical region the nerve root and the spinal nerve are both posteriorly related to the same corresponding intervertebral disc, but because of the peculiarity of cervical nerve nomenclature, the nerve designation is one number greater than that of the disc. In the lumbar region, however, a different situation prevails. The nerve roots contributing to the cauda equina travel an almost vertical course over the dorsum of one intervertebral disc to exit with the spinal nerve of the foramen one segment lower. Thus, in both the cervical and lumbar regions, dorsal protrusions of disc material affect the nerve root that is designated one number greater than that of the offending disc, but not for a consistent anatomic reason.

Once the meningeal coverings blend with the epineurium, the nerve components become extrathecal. The actual point of this transition is variable but usually occurs in relation to the distal aspect of the dorsal root ganglion.

Anatomic Relations Peculiar to the Lower Lumbar Spinal Canal

A constrictive alteration in the dimensions of the spinal canal has been termed "spinal stenosis" (Greek *stenos,* narrow) by Verbiest. Its clinical severity is predicated on the original regional tolerances provided between the neural contents and the walls of the canal and the degree of encroachment caused by pathologic processes. Certain spinal regions, such as the lower cervical[66] and the lower lumbar, are dimensionally predisposed to stenotic syndromes whose variant symptomatology reflects the functions of the neural structures compressed.

Since the spinal canal below the second lumbar vertebra contains only the roots of the lumbosacral nerves, subjective evidence of a lower lumbar stenosis usually presents as some form of radiculopathy. In cross section the cavity of the lower lumbar canal usually appears as a triangle with a ventral base. The ventrolateral angles of this configuration form the lateral recesses, which longitudinally accommodate the lumbosacral nerve roots in an already restricted space bounded by the subarticular part of the ligamentum flavum dorsally and the dorsolateral aspects of the disc ventrally. Unfortunately, the points of most frequent failure of the annulus in the degenerating lumbar disc are at the positions ventral to the lateral recesses on either side of the central strap of the posterior longitudinal ligament. At these points, if the external rings of the failing annulus are just pushed dorsally by the herniating nucleus pulposus (bulging disc) or actually rupture to allow nucleus material to press against the dura (protruded nucleus), the end result is a lateral stenosis that may produce varying degrees of radiculopathy. Since the disc lies ventral only to the inferior half of the foramen, the common type of dorsal encroachment usually misses its segmentally equivalent nerve but compromises the next most lateral nerve elements, which at this point are roots of the immediately inferior segmental nerve.

Of particular interest is the distribution of fat around and within the intervertebral foramen. Seldom mentioned in detailed anatomic descriptions, this fat mass is often regarded as an adventitial filler of epidural and intervertebral spaces. However, a study of the various sections of these regions shows that this fat has a rather firm character and forms a mechanically supportive "bushing" for structures entering and leaving the spinal canal. A prominent extension of this fat body also follows the inferior and ventral surfaces of each lumbar nerve, and is thus interposed between this

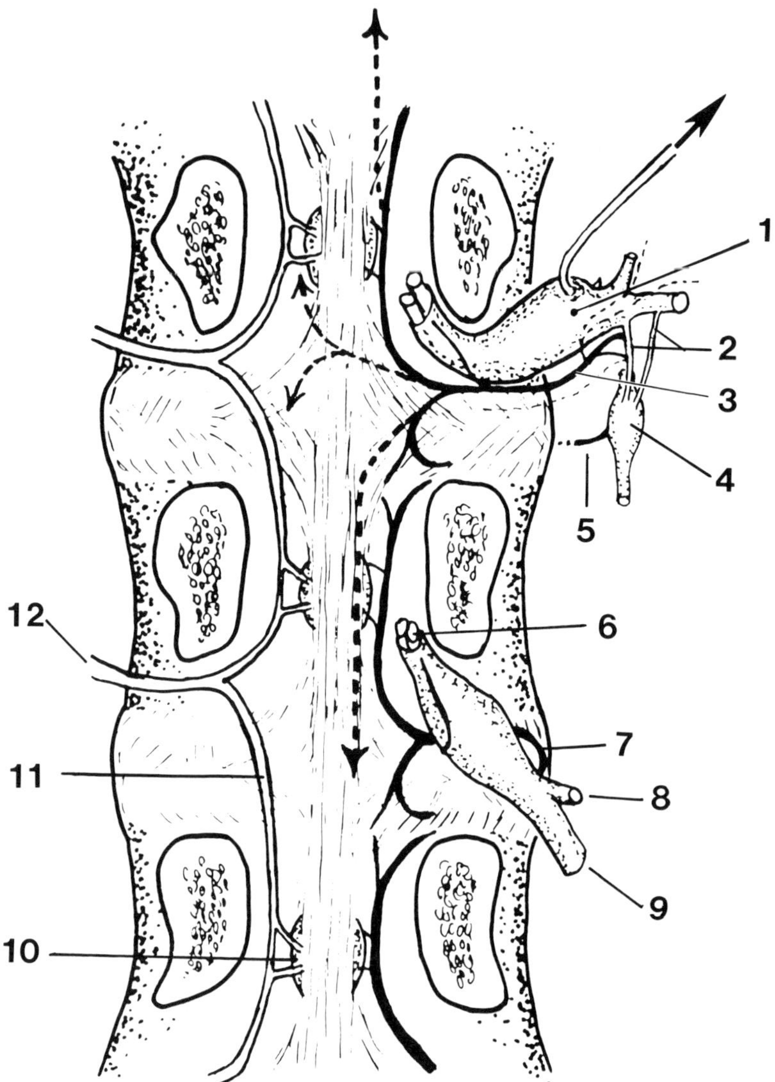

Figure 2–14. Schema of major intraspinal distribution of the dorsal central branches of the segmental vertebromedullary arteries and the distribution and source of the sinuvertebral nerves. The pattern of the nerve shown entering the superior foramen is derived from the data provided by Groen and colleagues. The dotted lines show a composite of the variant ranges (arrows indicate two or more segments) and ramifications tabulated by these authors. The nerve entering the inferior foramen shows the extent and distribution described in previous reports.

1. dorsal root ganglion
2. rami communicantes
3. sinuvertebral nerve and its origin according to Groen and colleagues
4. autonomic ganglion
5. nerve to anterior longitudinal ligament
6. spinal nerve roots
7. sinuvertebral nerve arising from distal pole of ganglion (thought to be its most common source before report of Groen and colleagues)
8. dorsal primary ramus of spinal nerve
9. ventral primary ramus of spinal nerve
10. arteries entering basivertebral sinus to supply cancellous bone
11. descending dorsal central branch of vertebromedullary (spinal) artery
12. ventral branch of vertebromedullary artery

structure and the external surfaces of the pedicle and vertebral body that define the inferior part of the intervertebral foramen. Its amelioration of the downward and ventral distraction of the nerve that accompanies the spine and lower limb motions is obvious. The consistency and uniformity of this intervertebral fat mass indicate that it is not just another deposition of metabolic reserve tissue but is a definite anatomic structure with a biomechanical purpose.

Intervertebral Foramen

The intervertebral foramen is the aperture that gives exit to the segmental spinal nerves and entrance to the vessels and nerve branches that supply the bone and soft tissues of the vertebral canal. It is superiorly and inferiorly bounded by the respective pedicles of the adjacent vertebrae, but its ventral and dorsal relations involve the two major intervertebral articulations. The dorsum of the intervertebral disc, covered by the lateral expansion of the posterior longitudinal ligament, provides a large part of its ventral boundary, while the joint capsule of the articular facets and the ligamentum flavum contribute the major parts of its dorsal limitation. For obvious reasons the caliber of the foraminal opening is larger than the collective size of the structures that pass through it. The remaining space is then obturated by loose areolar tissue and fat to accommodate the slight relative motions of these components (Fig. 2–15).

However ample the overall dimensions of the intervertebral foramen may be, it is its elliptic nature that is responsible for many of its relational problems. In the lumbar region the vertical diameter of the foramen varies from 12 to 19 mm. This undoubtedly accounts for the fact that a complete collapse of the disc may produce little or no evidence of nerve compression. However, the transverse diameter, from the ligamentum flavum to the vertebral body and disc, may be as little as 7 mm. Since the diameter of the fourth lumbar nerve can be just slightly less than 7 mm, the tolerance for pathologic alteration of the bony or connective tissue relations is very restricted.[44]

The existence of any additional ligamentous elements in relation to the intervertebral foramen could be critical. Unfortunately, such structures, known as the transforaminal ligaments, are frequently found in the lumbar region.[24] The transforaminal ligaments are strong, unyielding cords of collagenous tissue that pass anteriorly from various parts of the neural arch to the body of the same or the adjacent vertebra, and may be as much as 5 mm wide.

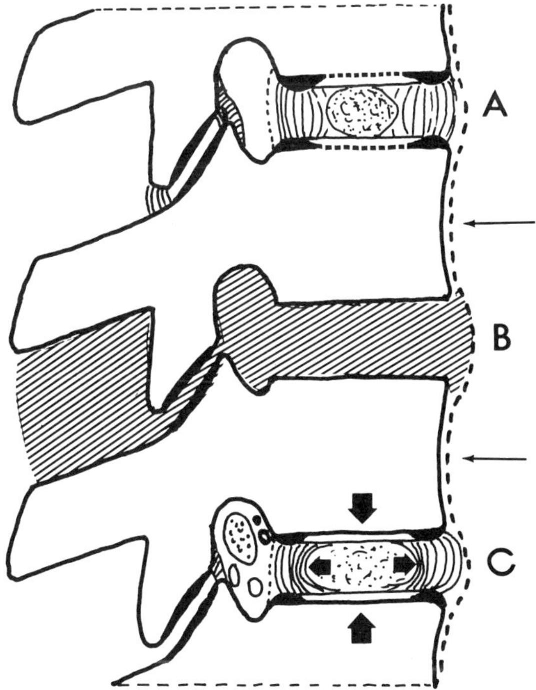

Figure 2–15. Schematic representation showing three aspects of the relational anatomy of the disc. *A* shows the topographic arrangement of the normal disc with the apophyseal ring and perforated chondral plate in relation to the nucleus pulposus and the annulus. *B* indicates, in the cross-hatched area, the inclusions of the motor segment as originally described by Junghanns. The arrows define the limits of the motor segment proposed here. *C* indicates the dissipation by the lateral thrust in a compressed disc. The related anatomy of the intervertebral foramen is also indicated. The two structures passing ventral to the spinal nerve are the sinuvertebral nerve and the artery. The other vessels are veins.

Lumbosacral Nerve Root Variations

In most instances of disc herniation, lumbosacral radicular symptoms provide a fairly reliable indication of the vertebral level involved. However, a sufficient number of cases occur in which the neurologic findings are ambiguous or frankly misleading, and additional diagnostic procedures should always be used to confirm the segmental level(s) of the lesioned disc(s).

A number of anatomic variations in the relations of the lumbosacral roots may be responsible for inconclusive neurologic indications. The most common would involve atypical origins or foraminal exits of individual lumbosacral roots. Although myelographic studies have indicated only a 4 per cent incidence of such lumbosacral root anomalies, an anatomic study by Kadish and Simmons[38] raised this figure to 14 per cent, the L5–S1 level being most commonly involved. These authors' observations provided four types of variations: (1) intradural interconnections between roots at different levels, (2) anomalous levels of origin of nerve roots, (3) extradural connections between roots, and (4) extradural division of nerve roots.

An interesting source of confusing neurologic findings may relate to the variant anatomy of the *furcal nerve.* This name has been applied to the fourth lumbar nerve because it exhibits a prominent bifurcation to contribute to both the lumbar plexus (femoral and obturator nerves) and sacral plexus (lumbosacral trunk). However, Kikuchi and Hasue[41] found that it is often indefinite in its intradural affinities, frequently exhibiting two dorsal root ganglia that have distinct root sources at the conus medullaris. They proposed that when symptoms indicate the involvement of two levels, suspicion should be directed toward four possible causes: (1) two roots compressed by a single lesion, (2) the presence of two lesions, (3) anomalous emergence of two roots through the same foramen, or (4) the existence of the peculiarly doubled components of the furcal nerve.

Infrequently, variant "fixation" alters the expected sequences of nerve root exit. In a *prefixed* lumbosacral plexus, the furcal nerve (the division between the lumbar and sacral plexuses) exits through the third lumbar foramen, and the preceding and subsequent nerves exit one vertebral level higher than in the conventional distribution. Conversely, in the *postfixed* plexus, the furcal nerve exits the L5–S1 foramen, and the lumbosacral nerve sequence is then all one level lower than usually described.[74]

Although Kadish and Simmons[38] noted that the existence of anomalous interconnections between nerve root levels dispels any notion of "absolute innervation," a more recent discovery has shown that there is a consistent system of intersegmental connections between the roots of the lumbosacral nerves. Parke and Watanabe[68] described an epispinal system of motor axons that courses among the meningeal fibers of the conus medullaris and virtually ensheaths its ventral and lateral funiculi between the L2 and S2 levels. These nerve fibers apparently arise from motor neuron cells of the ventral horn gray matter and join spinal nerve roots caudal to their level of origin. In all the spinal cords studied, many of these axons comingled at the cord surface to form an irregular group of ectopic rootlets that could be visually traced to join conventional spinal nerve roots at one to several segments inferior to their original segmental level (Figs. 2–17, 2–18). On occasion, these ventral ectopic rootlets course dorsocaudally to join a dorsal (sensory) nerve root. Although the function and clinical significance of this epispinal system of axons have yet to be explained, it definitely demonstrates that a given segmental level of motor nerve cells may contribute fibers not only to an adjacent segment, but to nerve roots of multiple inferior levels.

An additional variant aspect of the lumbosacral nerve roots concerns the relative location of their dorsal root ganglia. Almost all anatomic illustrations depict the lumbosacral dorsal root ganglia in an intraforaminal position, the central part of the ganglion lying between the adjacent pedicles. However, Hasue and colleagues,[28] by a method of nerve root infiltration,[42] demonstrated that the lumbosacral dorsal root ganglia may also be positioned internal or external to their foramina. They designated the internal positions as *subarticular* or *sublaminar,* depending on their relation to these structures roofing the spinal canal, and found that approximately one third of the L4 and L5 ganglia are in the subarticular position. It is obvious that if the ganglion is subarticular, it is in the lateral recess and subject to the direct consequences of a discogenic lateral spinal stenosis. When the ganglion is thus spatially compromised, there is no mystery about the source of the radicular pain, for it has been established that the ganglion is very mechanosensitive and initiates nerve discharges under even slight external pressures.

INNERVATION OF THE SPINE

The distribution of the medial branches of the dorsal ramus of the spinal nerve to the external periosteum, facet joints, and ligamentous connections of the neural arches, and the general ramification of the "recurrent" sinuvertebral nerve (nerve of Luschka) (*ramus meningeus*) to structures related to the spinal canal, have been known for over a century. However, the recognition that degenerative disease of the intervertebral disc and its consequences are a major cause of low back pain has recently stimulated more serious inquiries. Over the past five decades, a number of investigations have attempted to delineate the origins, terminal ramifications, and nerve ending types of the sinuvertebral nerve, often with contradictory results. The more comprehensive works[7, 8, 30, 34, 53, 61, 76, 91] have agreed on the general source and composition of this nerve and have described it as variously branching from the distal pole of the dorsal root ganglion, the initial part of the spinal nerve, or the dorsal sections of the rami communicantes. It was recognized that a multiple origin is common, especially in the lumbar region, and small autonomic branches often pursue a separate course to enter the intervertebral foramen independently. However, the extent and complexity of the relations of the sinuvertebral nerve within the spinal canal has engendered much argument, particularly concerning the segmental range of the individual nerve ramifications. The source of this diversity of opinion rests in the fragmentary nature of the information provided by various methods of investigation. In illustrations based on dissections, Bogduk and associates[7] and Parke[61] agreed that each nerve supplies two intervertebral discs by means of superiorly and inferiorly directed branches, the inferiorly directed branch ramifying over the dorsum of the disc at the level of entry, and the longer superiorly directed branch coursing along the edge of the posterior longitudinal ligament to reach the disc of the next superior level (Fig. 2–14). However, it is obvious that dissection would favor mainly the larger ramifications, and conventional methods of staining using silver or lipotrophic stains, because of a lack of specificity, have also given controversial results.

Recently, Groen and colleagues,[26] using a highly specific acetylcholinesterase (AChE) staining method on large cleared sections of fetal human spines, have resolved many conflicts concerning the ramifications of the nerves supplying spinal structures. They found that, in contrast to most previous reports, the human sinuvertebral nerves were almost exclusively derivatives of the rami communicantes close to their connections with the spinal nerves. These origins were fairly consistent throughout the length of the thoracolumbar sympathetic trunk, but in the cervical region they were also derived from the perivascular plexus of the vertebral artery.

As many as five sinuvertebral nerves had been observed passing into one intervertebral foramen, but, typically, the group consisted of one thick nerve (the one seen in conventional dissections?) and several fine fibers. However, it was noted that the thick or predominant sinuvertebral nerve is often absent in the upper cervical and sacral regions. The major sinuvertebral element enters the foramen ventral to the spinal ganglion and gives off some fine branches at this point. As the nerve enters the spinal canal, the major branch usually divides into rami that course in approximation of the distribution of the posterior central branches of the segmental artery, thus showing a long ascending element and a shorter descending one. From these branches, one to three coiled rami were shown to supply the ventral dura.

The AChE technique used by Groen and associates[26] made it possible to delineate the plexus of the posterior longitudinal ligament to reveal detail never achieved by other methods. The work of these authors supports the idea that the posterior longitudinal ligament is highly innervated by an irregular plexiform distribution of fibers that show a greater density in the ligament expansions dorsal to the discs. Since this method permitted accurate tracing of the nerve fibers, these authors were able to note the primary direction, length, and "termination area" of the branches of a single segmental sinuvertebral nerve, and classified the variations of individual nerves as follows: (1) ascending one segment, (2) descending one segment, (3) dichotomizing toward one segment caudal and one segment cranial or horizontal, (4) ascending *two or more* segments, and (5) descending *two or more* segments (Fig. 2–14). The existence of these latter two categories, although they are not as common as the others, effectively lays to rest the claim that the sinuvertebral nerve supplies no more than two adjacent segmental levels. Thus, a basis for the poor pain localization of an offending disc may be related to the rather generous distribution possible in the individual sinuvertebral nerve. The large totomounts treated with AChE also showed that the patterns of sinuvertebral nerve distribution to the posterior longitudinal ligament did not display significant regional variations apart from an expected pronounced diminution in the plexus density in the immovable lower sacral region.

The posterior longitudinal ligament is highly innervated with complex encapsulated nerve endings and numerous low-myelinated free nerve endings (Fig. 2–16), but few investigators have emphasized the fact that the lateral expansion of the posterior longitudinal ligament extends laterally through the intervertebral foramen covering all the dorsal and most of the dorsolateral aspects of the disc. Undoubtedly, the elevation of this thin, highly innervated strap of connective tissue may provide a significant component of the pain manifest in acute disc protrusions.

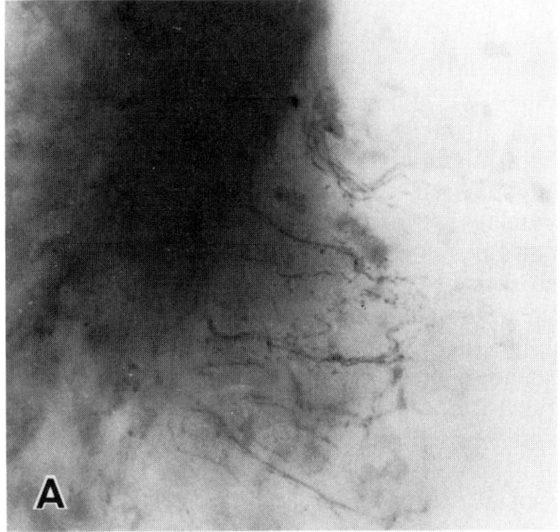

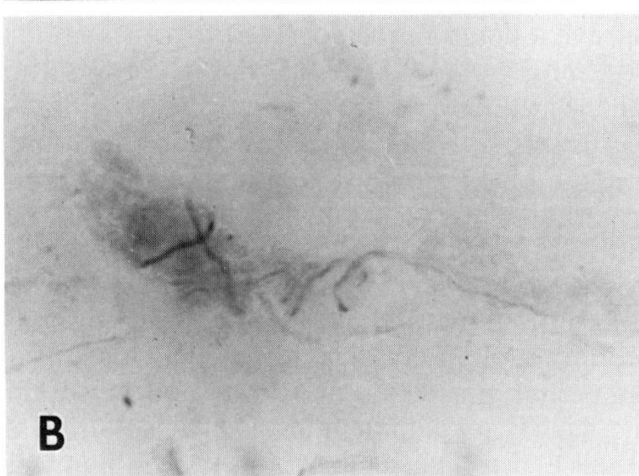

Figure 2–16. Photomicrographs of nerve endings in the posterior longitudinal ligament of a dog. (Methylene blue vital tissue stain.) *A*, Section of the ligament dorsal to a lumbar intervertebral disc. The dark area is the central strap of the ligament and the light area the thin lateral expansion over the dorsum of the disc. These fine nerve endings are characteristic of those in known nociceptors. (×300.) *B*, Complex nerve ending from the posterior longitudinal ligament. This type of ending is believed to be a transducer of mechanical deformation for postural senses. (×500.)

The probable range of diverse functions of the sinuvertebral nerve may be indicated by the analysis of its cross-sectional composition. Stained preparations taken from a section near the nerve origin showed many small myelinated fibers, but some myelin sheaths were in excess of 10 μm in diameter.[72] There is little doubt that many of the smaller fibers are postganglionic efferents from the thoracolumbar autonomic ganglia that mediate the smooth muscle control of the various vascular elements within the spinal canal, and a number of the larger fibers are involved in proprioceptive functions. Concerning the latter, Hirsch and associates[30, 31] and Parke[65] (Fig. 2–16*B*) found numerous complex encapsulated nerve endings in the posterior longitudinal ligament; it is assumed that these may be associated with the larger myelinated fibers whose postganglionic axons enter the cord to mediate postural reflexes, since similar fibers in the cervical region of cats have been shown to be important in tonic neck reflexes.[57]

It appears, however, that the smaller fibers making up the bulk of the sinuvertebral nerve are afferents associated with simple, nonencapsulated, or "free" nerve endings that are generally regarded as nociceptive (Fig. 2–16*A*).

The fact that the sinuvertebral nerve carries pain fibers has been amply demonstrated by both clinical and laboratory experimentation. Direct stimulation of tissues known to be served by the nerve has been shown to elicit back pain in humans. Pedersen and colleagues[72] showed that stimulation of these tissues in decerebrate cats resulted in blood pressure and respiratory changes similar to those elicited by noxious stimuli to known pain receptors in other areas of the body. The essential question remaining, then, is in which components of the spinal motion segment are the nociceptors responsible for so-called discogenic pain?

There existed a major disagreement over whether the annulus itself was innervated, and if so, how extensively. The classic work of Hirsch and associates[31] claimed that nerve endings may be demonstrated only in the dorsal aspect of the most superficial layer of the annulus, and these were presumably from branches of the same nerve fibers that innervated the overlying expansions of the posterior longitudinal ligament.

Pedersen and associates,[72] Stilwell,[81] and Parke[65] had also failed to demonstrate nerve endings in the annulus, and since the connective tissue structures intimately related to the disc show a profusion of nerve endings, Parke assumed that their disruption alone could account for discogenic pain. It now appears that inappropriate methodology may account for the failure to demonstrate intradiscal nerves, because Malinsky,[53] Bogduk and colleagues,[7, 8] and Yoshizawa and colleagues[94] published accounts demonstrating nerve fibers in the outer lamina of the annulus. This has now been supported by the highly specific AChE method of Groen and associates.[26]

Most descriptions of the sinuvertebral nerve indicate that the major meningeal fibers to the spinal dura are distributed to its ventral surface. The median dorsal dural surface has been regarded as virtually free of nerve fibers, a convenience that permits its painless penetration during needle puncture. Although Cyriax[14] claimed that irritation of the ventral dura during protrusion of the nucleus may contribute to discogenic pain, a sufficient distortion of the nerve fibers on the movable or unattached dura does not appear likely. In fact, the coiled configuration of these dural contributions of the sinuvertebral nerve noted by Groen and associates[25] may indicate a compensation to permit a degree of dural movement without placing traction on these nerves. However, Parke and Watanabe[70] observed that the ventral lower lumbar dura is often fixed to the ventral canal surface by numerous connective tissue fibers, and most firmly fixed at the margins of the lower lumbar discs. These apparently acquired adhesions are not to be confused with the ligaments of Hofmann, which are normal straps of tissue connecting the dura to the ventral canal surface that have been obliquely positioned by the developmental craniad traction of the dura and its contents. The above observation has been supported by a series of dissections by Blikra,[6] who was seeking a rationale for lower lumbar intradural disc protrusions. His analysis showed that the dura in some cases may be sufficiently fixed to the ventral surface of the canal, particularly at the L4–L5 levels, for protruding nucleus material to actually rupture the ventral dura. Parke and Watanabe,[70] by microscopic analysis of sections of the dura that had been forcibly freed from these adhesions overlying the fourth or fifth lumbar disc, showed disruption of the nerve fibers bound in the adhesion. Thus, in the high number of cases in which such adhesions are present, the forceful elevation of the dura by a disc protrusion may provide an adjunctive source of the discogenic pain.

SPINAL MOTION SEGMENT

With respect to a single vertebral level, the inclusion of all articular tissue, the overlying spinal muscles, and the segmental contents of the vertebral canal and intervertebral foramen into a single functional and anatomic unit was first suggested by Junghanns.[37, 79] Originally called the "motor" segment, this unit represents a useful concept that stresses the developmental and topographic interdependence between the fibrous structures that surround the intervertebral foramen and the functioning of the structures that pass through it. Although the 23 or 24 individual motion segments must be considered in relation to the spinal column as a whole, no congenital or acquired disorder of a single major component of a unit can exist without affecting first the functions of the other components of the same unit and then the functions of other levels of the spine.

Although Junghanns defined the unit primarily in terms of the movable structures making up the intervertebral articulations, a logical, if not necessary, extension of the motion segment concept should include some aspect of the vertebral elements. DePalma and Rothman[15] included both adjacent vertebrae in their illustration of the unit, but we believe that the unit concept would be improved by incorporating only the opposing superior and inferior halves of each vertebra, thus eliminating redundancy (Fig. 2 15).

In visualizing the motion segment unit as a musculoskeletal complex surrounding a corresponding level of nervous structures, it must be realized that the intervertebral disc is but one form of the articulations involved. The articular facets form the diarthrodial joints of the arthrodial or gliding type. All other intervertebral articulations are generically amphiarthroses. The interosseous fibrous connections that include the interspinous, intertransverse, costovertebral, and longitudinal ligaments as well as the ligamentum flavum are varieties of syndesmoses. In view of the semiliquid nature of the nucleus pulposus and the vacuities that may be demonstrated in the nucleus of aging specimens, von Luschka[50] attempted to classify the intervertebral disc as a diarthrosis in which the vertebral chondral plates were the articular cartilages, the annulus provided the articular capsule, and the fluid and ephemeral spaces within the nucleus corresponded to the synovia and the joint cavity. Although the intervertebral disc forms a joint that should be classified in its own exclusive category because its development, structure, and function are generally different from those of any other joint, it most closely conforms to an amphiarthrosis of the symphysis type.

The cervical intervertebral discs have also been a source of controversy because of the so-called joints of Luschka or uncovertebral joints. These articular modifications are found on both sides of the cervical discs as oblique, cleftlike cavities between the superior surfaces of the uncinate processes and the corresponding lateral lips of the interior articular surface of the next superior vertebra. Since they initially appear in the latter part of the first decade and are not universally demonstrable in all cervical spines, or even in all subaxial discs of the same cervical spine, it is preferable to call them "accommodative joints" that have developed in response to the shearing stresses of the torsions of cervical mobility (Fig. 2–11).

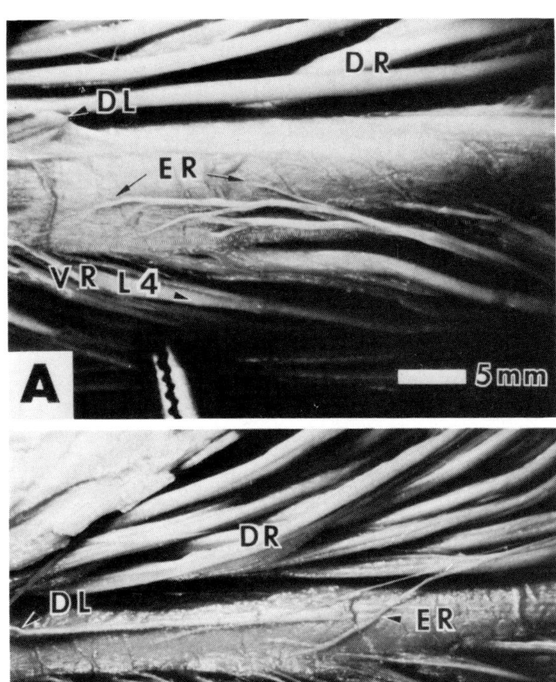

Figure 2–17. *A*, Lateral surface of a human conus medullaris showing the ectopic rootlets (ER) that receive axons from cells in the ventral horn nuclei. Note the origin of some fibers at the level of L4 motor nuclei that extend caudally to join the S1 root. *B*, Photomicrograph showing ectopic nerve rootlets (ER) passing dorsally to join a dorsal (sensory) nerve root (DR). DL indicates the last denticulum of the denticulate ligament.

Nutrition of the Intervertebral Disc

Most descriptive accounts of the intervertebral disc dismiss the subject of its vascular nutrition with a brief mention of the general agreement that the normal adult disc is avascular. Unfortunately, the demonstrable truth of this statement may give the impression that the substance of the disc is rather inert biologically. In fact, experimental evidence has indicated that the normal disc tissue is quite vital and has a demonstrable rate of metabolic turnover.[11, 56] Unlike the nonvascular cartilage in the diarthroses, the cellular elements of the disc cannot receive the blood-borne nutrients through the mediation of the synovial fluid, but must rely on a diffusional system with the vessels that lie adjacent to the disc.

During the past two decades, knowledge of the qualitative and quantitative aspects of the diffusional nutrition of the disc has been considerably advanced, mainly by a series of publications variously coauthored by Maroudas, Urban, Nachemson, Holm, and their associates.[32, 33, 55, 56] A brief review of their findings, primarily based on in vivo studies in the dog, follows.

The peripheral vascular plexus of the annulus and the vessels adjacent to the hyaline cartilage of the bone-disc interface provide the two sources for the diffusion of metabolites into the disc. Although the interface shows an average permeability of 40 per cent, there is a decreasing centrifugal gradient that starts with

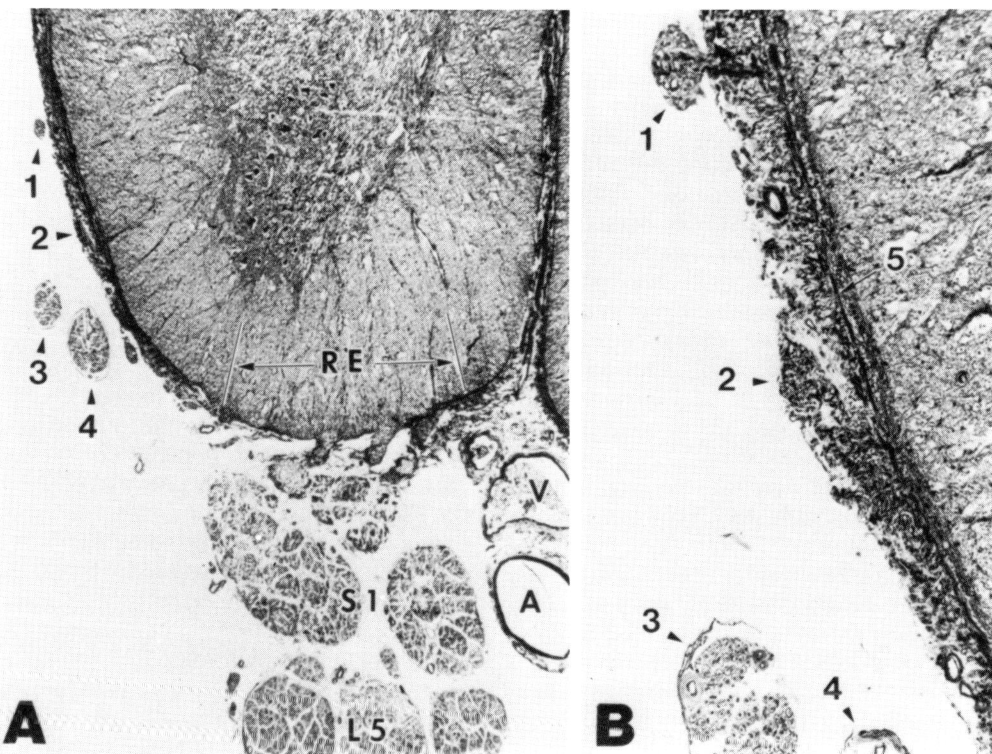

Figure 2–18. Photomicrographs of a 5-μ cross section from the conus medullaris at the S1 level showing ectopic rootlets in various stages characteristic of their emergence from the ventrolateral surface of the cord. From Parke and Watanabe[26]. *A,* Rootlets just appearing on the pial surface (1,2) will eventually join free rootlets (3,4) that have originated from higher levels. The conventional roots of L5 and S1 nerves have emerged from the typical zone of rootlet emergence (RE). A and V, Anterior spinal artery and vein. (×33.) *B,* Higher-power photomicrograph of the preceding section showing greater detail of rootlet emergence. Note that the entire ventrolateral pia is intertwined with epispinal axons, of which only a few form ectopic rootlets. A dense circular band of pial straps (5) is characteristic of the region of the epispinal fibers. (×133.)

an 80 per cent permeability at the center. Because diffusion is the major mechanism that carries small solutes through the disc matrix, the two main parameters affecting this flow are the *partition coefficient* that defines the equilibrium between the solutes within the plasma and those within the disc, and the *diffusion coefficient* that characterizes the solute mobility. The partition coefficient varies with the size and charge of the solute particle. Thus, small uncharged solutes show a near-equilibrium between their plasma and intradiscal concentrations, but since the disc matrix has a predominantly negative charge, anionic solutes show a lower intradiscal concentration in relation to the plasma, whereas the reverse is true for positively charged solutes whose intradiscal concentration is greater than that of the plasma. As the range of these effects depends on the concentration of the fixed, negatively charged, larger molecular aggregates (proteoglycans), the partition coefficient is regionally variable within the disc matrix and especially pronounced in the inner annular lamellae and nucleus where the concentration of proteoglycans is the highest.

Solute mobility (the diffusion coefficient) within the disc is slower than in the plasma because the presence of solids in the form of collagen and proteoglycans impedes diffusional progress. Without regard to charge, the diffusion coefficient within the disc is 40 to 60 per cent of free diffusion within water, and mobility is greatest in the inner annulus and nucleus where the water concentrations are the highest.

Owing to the regional differentials in the densities of the fixed charges within the disc, the two vascular sources for disc nutrition vary in their significance in the supply of certain solutes. With respect to the small uncharged particles, there is little difference in the transport potential of either the peripheral or end plate vascular routes, but because of the greater collective negative charge within the central substances of the disc, the interface vasculature is a greater source of cationic solutes, whereas the anions would gain easier access through the peripheral vessels.

The effect of fluid "pumping" under changes in the load applied to the disc is minimal with respect to the transport of small solutes, since the matrix has a low hydraulic permeability relative to their higher rates of diffusion. With regard to the larger solutes, however, the pumping may have some effect.

Metabolic turnover, as indicated by proteoglycan synthesis in dog discs, is age variable and within the range of two to three years. It is thus roughly equivalent to that of articular cartilage. The central disc tissues show a low oxygen tension and a very high concentration of lactic acid, indicating that the inner disc cell respiration is primarily anaerobic. Since this type of respiration is heavily dependent on glycolytic energy requirements, the interface vasculature must deliver the needed glucose to maintain the central disc cell viability.

Because this interface exchange is precariously dependent on the integrity of the fine vasculature subjacent to the cartilaginous end plate, any change from the optimal state occasioned by age-dependent vagaries in the intrinsic vertebral vasculature may partly explain the marked predisposition to degenerative changes characteristic of the aging disc.

BLOOD SUPPLY OF THE VERTEBRAL COLUMN

The descriptions and terminology of the nutritional vessels of the vertebrae vary considerably in the current anatomy texts. Generally, like the reports they are based on, the texts illustrate and discuss the vascularity of a typical thoracic or lumbar vertebra and show a lack of agreement on such basic issues as whether the vertebral body does (Ferguson[19]) or does not (Willis[92]) receive an anterior supply. In addition, discussions of the vascularization of the atypical (craniocervical, cervical, and sacral) vertebral regions are either superficial or entirely lacking. Therefore, much of the information presented here is the result of a de novo investigation by the author and associates, and the terminology ascribed to the vessels is derived from a selection of what appear to be the most descriptive names previously used in other reports and our own contributions. It is hoped that the resulting system of terminology is both comprehensible and comprehensive.

Shortly after the publication of the first edition of this chapter, Crock and Yoshizawa[13] released a photographically illustrated volume showing many injection preparations of the vertebral column and spinal cord. Owing to the similarity of methods used, the high degree of agreement in their depiction of the vascular patterns should not be unexpected, although the independence of the two investigations understandably produced some disparity in the terminology. A major value of this type of work lies in the fact that the reader may visualize the actual specimens rather than interpretive schematizations.

Despite the fact that regional variations may at first appear to thwart the perception of a common pattern of vertebral vascularization, the homologous origin of all vertebral elements nevertheless provides a certain constancy that may be expressed as follows.

From a segmental artery or its regional equivalent, each vertebra receives several sets of nutritional vessels, which consist of anterior central, posterior central, prelaminar, and postlaminar branches. The first and last of these are derived from vessels external to the vertebral column, whereas the posterior central and prelaminar branches are derived from spinal branches that enter the intervertebral foramina and supply the neural, meningeal, and epidural tissues as well. In the midspinal region the internal arteries (i.e., the posterior central and prelaminar branches) provide the greater part of the blood supply to the body and vertebral arch, but reciprocal arrangements may occur, particularly in the cervical region.

This general pattern of the vasculature is best demonstrated in the area between the second thoracic and fifth lumbar vertebrae, where the segments are associated with paired arteries that arise directly from the aorta (Fig. 2–19). Typically, each segmental artery leaves the posterior surface of the aorta and follows a dorsolateral course around the middle of the vertebral body. Near the transverse processes

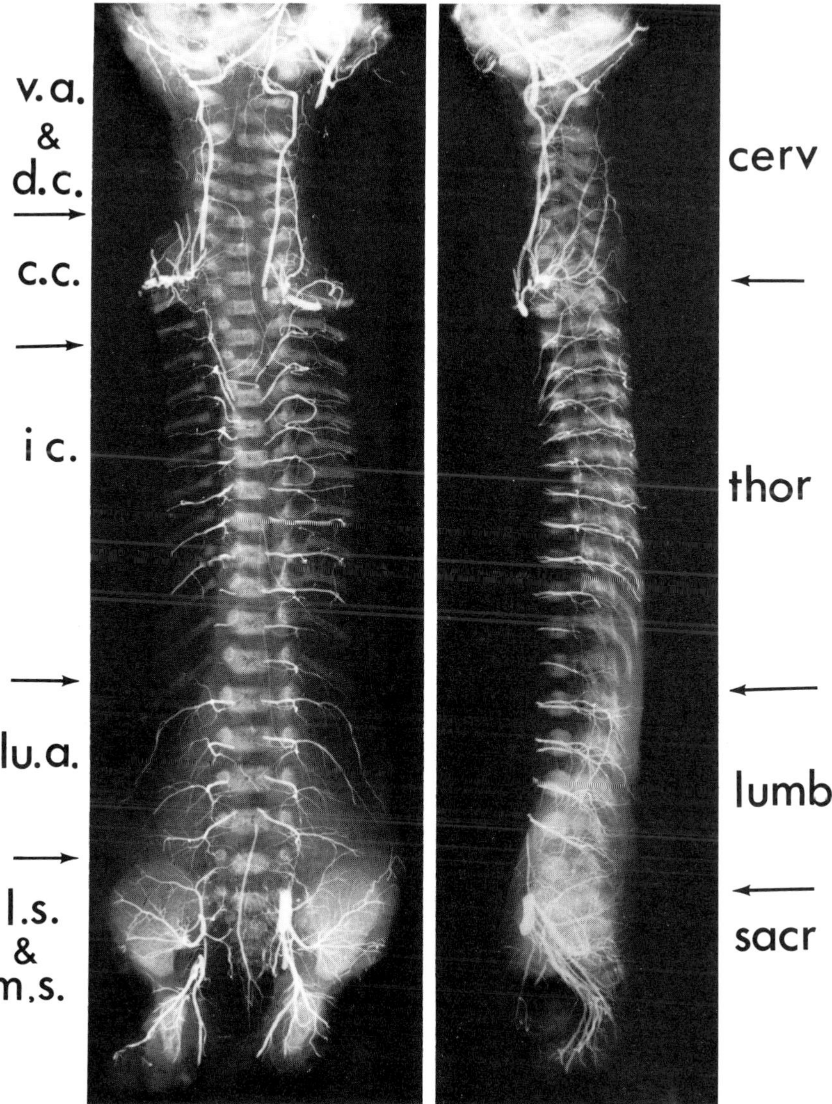

Figure 2–19. Anteroposterior and lateral radiography of spine of 8-month fetus injected with finely divided barium sulfate. The traditional regional subdivisions of the spine are indicated on the left, and the regional arteries that provide the segmental branches to the individual vertebrae on the right. The upper cervical region is supplied by vertebral and deep cervical arteries (v.a. & d.c.). The lower cervical and upper two thoracic segments are supplied by the costocervical trunk (c.c.), while the remaining thoracic vertebrae receive intercostal vessels (i.c.). The lumbar arteries (lu.a.) supply their regional vertebrae, and the sacral segments are provided with branches from lateral sacral (l.s.) and middle sacral (m.s.) arteries.

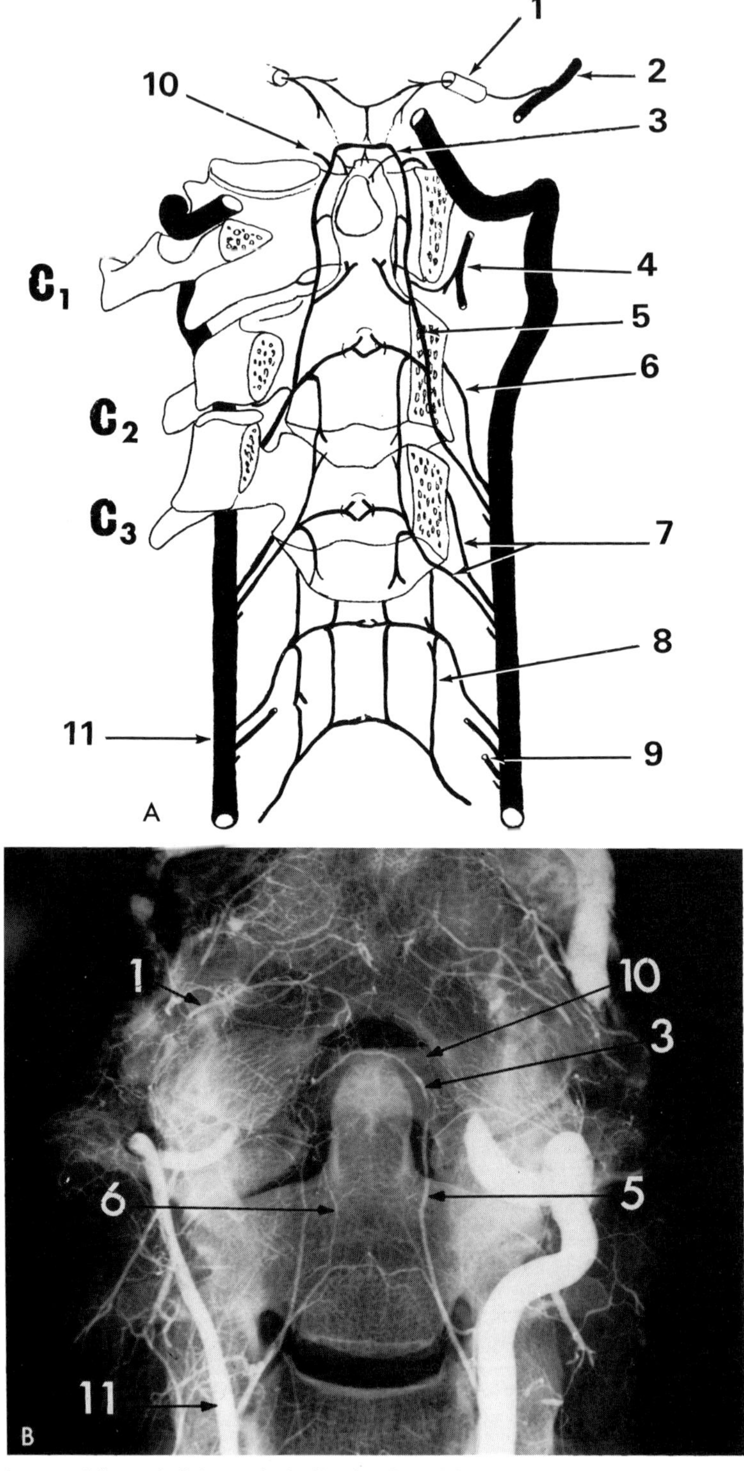

Figure 2–20. *A,* Schema of the arterial supply to the bodies of the upper cervical vertebrae and the odontoid process. Numerical designations apply to the same structures in *B.* 1, Hypoglossal canal passing meningeal artery. 2, Occipital artery. 3, Apical arcade of odontoid process. 4, Ascending pharyngeal artery giving collateral branch beneath anterior arch of atlas. 5, Posterior ascending artery. 6, Anterior ascending artery. 7, Precentral and postcentral arteries to typical cervical vertebral body. 8, Anterior spinal plexus. 9, Medullary branch of vertebral artery. Radicular, prelaminar, and meningeal branches are also found at each level. 10, Collateral to ascending pharyngeal artery passing rostral to anterior arch of atlas. 11, Left vertebral artery.

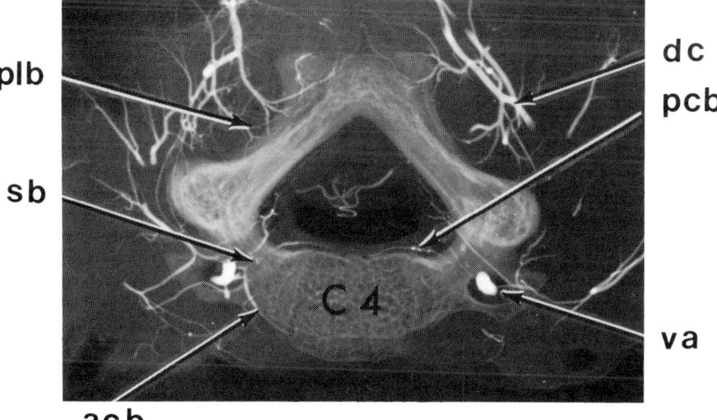

Figure 2–21. Vertical radiograph of section through fourth cervical vertebra of a 6-year-old, showing vascularity. The deep cervical artery (dc) provides the posterior laminar branches (plb). The vertebrals show numerous anastomoses with other cervical arteries, and send spinal branches (sb) that form posterior central branches (pcb) of the body and anterior lamina branches of the arch. The anterior central branches (acb) may arise independently from the vertebral arteries (va).

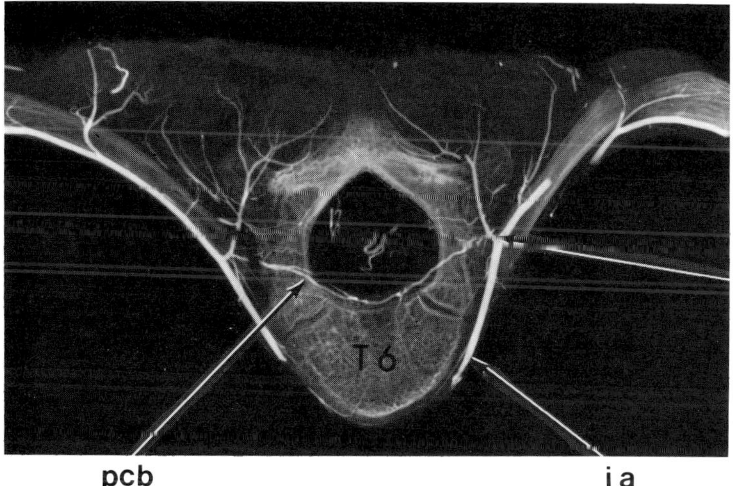

Figure 2–22. Ventral radiograph of a section through T6 of a specimen from a 6-year-old injected with barium sulfate. The intercostal arteries (ia) give rise to dorsal branches (db) that provide spinal branches to the vertebral canal and posterior branches to the arch and dorsal musculature. The posterior central branches (pcb) are well shown as they send vessels into the vertebral body. Fine anterior central and anterior laminar and posterior laminar vessels can be seen. Note the neurocentral synchondrosis.

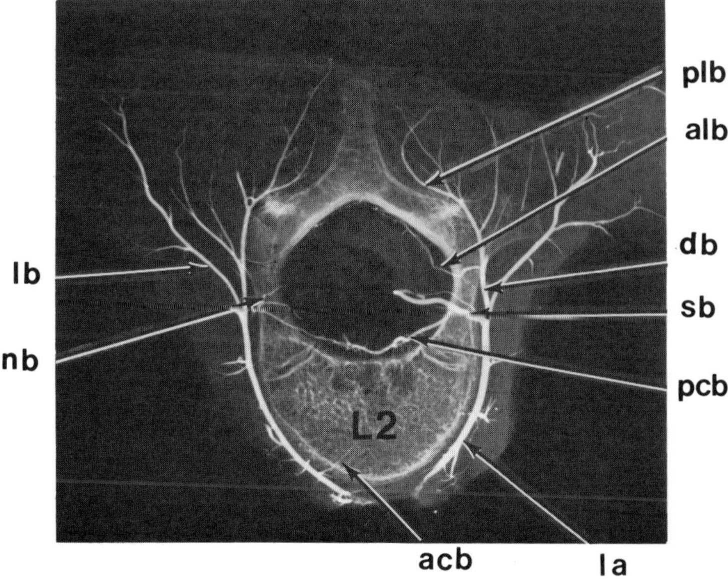

Figure 2–23. Vertical radiograph of a section through the lumbar vertebra of a 6-year-old. The vascularity of the lumbar vertebra may be regarded as the archetypal pattern from which other regions evolved variations. The segmental lumbar artery (la) gives rise to a number of anterior central branches that penetrate the cortical bone of the body. The spinal branch (sb) sends prominent posterior central branches to the dorsum of the body, while the dorsal branch (db) supplies both the anterior (alb) and posterior (plb) laminar branches. Neural branches (nb) follow the nerve roots to the cord. In this section the arteria radicularis magna is seen as a neural branch on the right side. lb, Lumbar branches.

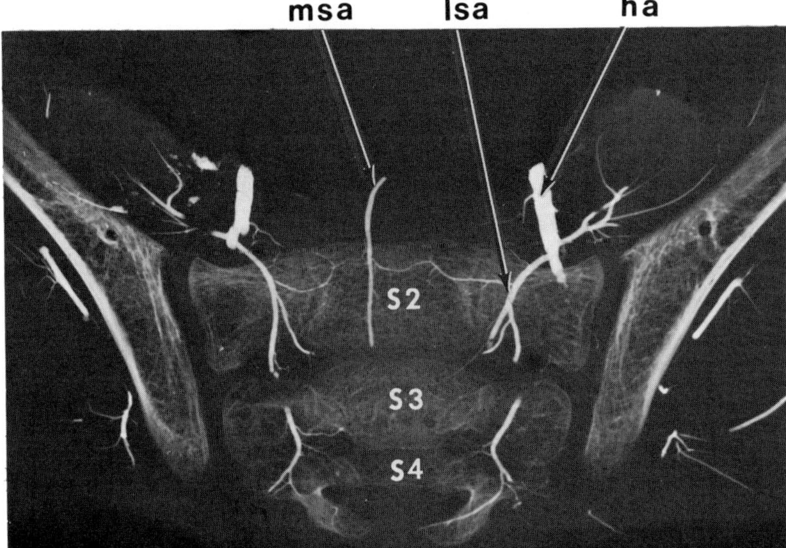

Figure 2–24. Radiograph of a horizontal section through the sacroiliac joint. The natural curvature of the sacrum provided oblique sections through segments 2, 3, and 4. The hypogastric artery (ha) gives off the lateral sacral artery (lsa) that sends anastomotic branches to join the middle sacral artery (msa); from these the sacral segments receive the penetrating anterior central branches. The dorsal branches pass into the anterior sacral foramina to provide posterior, central, neural, and prelaminar branches. The dorsal branches then leave through the posterior sacral foramina to supply the muscles and posterior laminar branches.

it divides into a lateral (intercostal or lumbar) and a dorsal branch. The dorsal branch runs lateral to the intervertebral foramen and the articular processes as it continues backward between the transverse processes to eventually reach the spinal muscles. Since the segmental artery is closely applied to the anterolateral surface of the body, its first spinal derivatives are two or more anterior central branches that directly penetrate the cortical bone of the body and that may be traced radiologically into the spongiosa (Figs. 2–22, 2–23). The same region of the segmental artery also supplies longitudinal arteries to the anterior longitudinal ligament (Fig. 2–27).

After the segmental artery divides into its

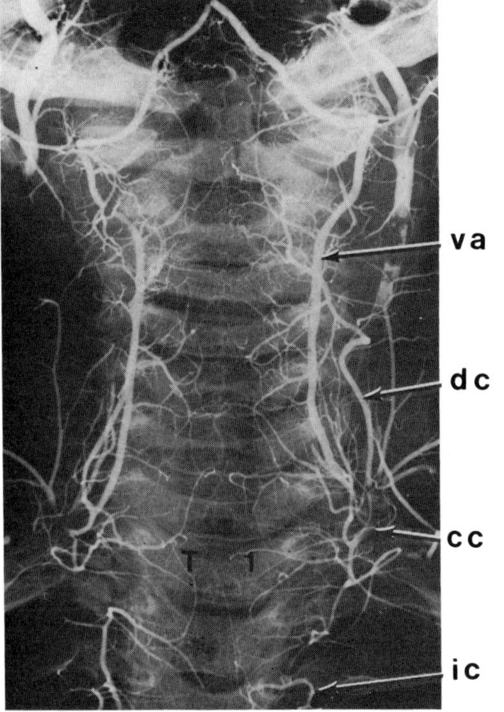

Figure 2–25. Arteriogram of the cervical and upper thoracic regions of the 6-year-old spine seen in Figures 2–21 to 2–23. Note that both the vertebral artery (va) and the deep cervical branch (dc) of the costocervical trunk (cc) supply segmental branches to each vertebra. The costocervical artery also typically supplies T1 and T2, but in this case T2 receives a high intercostal (ic) branch on the left side.

dorsal and lateral branches, the dorsal component passes lateral to the intervertebral foramen, where it gives off the spinal branch that provides the major vascularity to the bone and contents of the vertebral canal. This branch may enter the foramen as a single vessel, or it may arise from the dorsal segmental branch as a number of independent rami. In either case, it ultimately divides into a triad of posterior central, prelaminar, and intermediate neural branches. The posterior central branch passes over the dorsolateral surface of the intervertebral disc and divides into a caudal and a cranial branch, which supply the two adjacent vertebral bodies. Coursing in the same plane as the posterior longitudinal ligament, these branches vascularize the ligament and the related dura before entering the large concavity in the central dorsal surface of the vertebral body. It is apparent, then, that the dorsum of each vertebral body is supplied by four arteries derived from two intervertebral levels. As these vessels tend to converge toward the dorsal central concavity, where they are cross-connected with their bilateral counterparts, their connections with other vertebral levels give the appearance of a series of rhomboid anastomotic loops (Fig. 2–26) that illustrate the extent of collateral supply to a single vertebra.

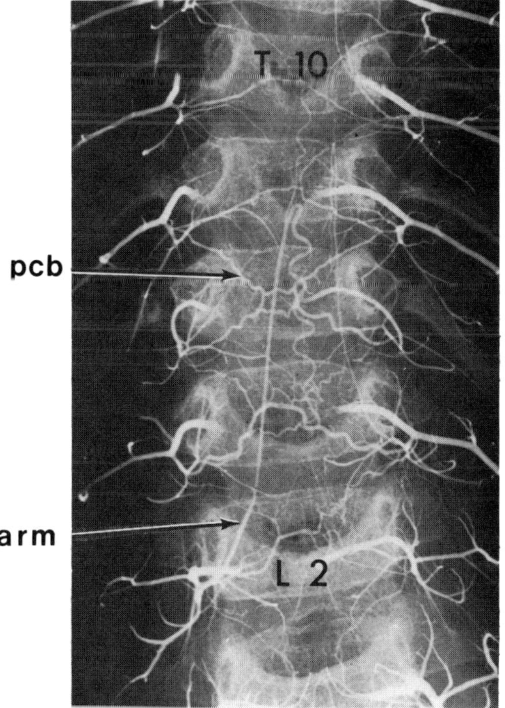

Figure 2–26. Anteroposterior arteriogram of the lower thoracic and upper lumbar vertebrae in a 6-year-old. The interlocking anastomotic pattern formed by the posterior central branches (pcb), and the manner in which four branches converge over the center of the dorsum of the body of each vertebra, are well shown. The arteria radicularis magna, which forms a major contribution to the anterior spinal artery of the cord, can be seen arising at L2.

The prelaminar branch of the spinal artery follows the inner surface of the vertebral arch, giving fine penetrating nutrient branches to the laminae and ligamenta flava while also supplying the regional epidural and dorsal tissue.

The neural branches that enter the intervertebral foramen with the above-described vessels supply the pia-arachnoid complex and the spinal cord itself. In the fetus and the adult the neural or radicular branches are not segmentally uniform in their size or occurrence. Although all spinal nerves receive fine twigs to their ganglia and roots, the major contributions to the cord are found at irregular intervals. Several larger radicular arteries may be discerned in the cervical and upper thoracic regions, but the largest, the arteria radicularis magna, is an asymmetric contribution from one of the upper lumbar segmental arteries. It travels obliquely upward with a ventral spinal root to join the anterior spinal artery in the region of the conus medullaris. Radicular contributions to the dorsal spinal plexus may usually be distinguished by their more tortuous course. Unusual illustrations of the segmental vascularity to the lower spinal cord may be seen in Figures 2–26 and 2–27.

After the dorsal branch of the segmental artery has provided the vessels to the intervertebral foramen, it passes between the transverse processes, where it gives off a fine spray of articular branches to the joint capsule of the articular processes. Immediately distal to this point, it divides into dorsal and medial branches; the larger, dorsal branch ramifies in the greater muscle mass of the erector spinae, while the medial branch follows the external contours of the lamina and the spinous process. This postlaminar artery supplies the musculature immediately overlying the lamina and also sends fine nutrient branches into the bone. The largest of these branches penetrates the lamina through a nutrient foramen located just dorsomedial to the articular capsule.

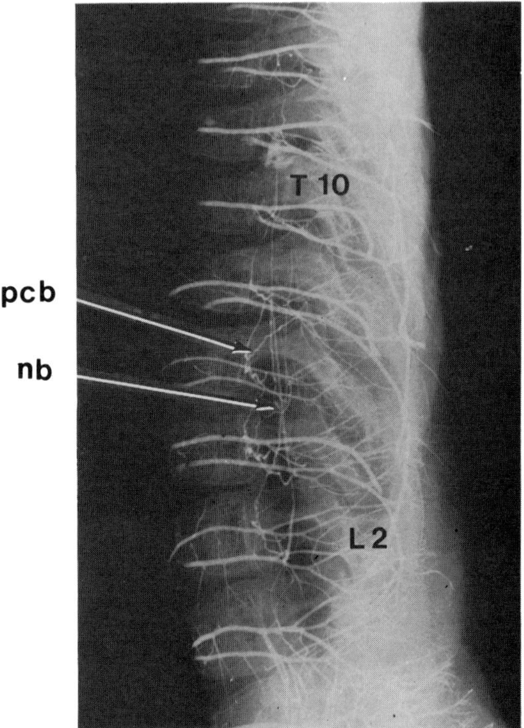

Figure 2–27. Lateral view of the preceding illustration. The longitudinal anastomoses of the posterior central branches (pcb) can be appreciated, and the disposition of neural branches (nb) is clarified. The lumbar arteries also supply small longitudinal branches to the anterior longitudinal ligament.

Regional Variations in Spinal Vasculature

In an overview of the vascular sources to the spine, it becomes apparent that only those vertebrae that are related to the aorta have access to direct segmental branches. Thus, the cervical, upper thoracic, and sacral regions have different patterns in their segmental supply that affect to various extents the arrangements of the finer vessels. In the arteriogram of the entire fetal spine (Fig. 2–19), it can be seen that the greater part of the cervical region is supplied by the vertebral arteries and the deep cervical arteries. An intermediate area that usually includes the lower two cervical and upper two thoracic vertebrae is supplied by costocervical branches of the subclavian that are of variable pattern and often bilaterally dissimilar. From T2 to L5 the typical segmental arrangement prevails, but in the sacral area lateral sacral branches of the hypogastric artery and branches of the middle sacral assume the function of supporting the nutritional vasculature to the vertebral elements.

Cervical Region

The general pattern of the arterial supply with respect to the typical cervical vertebrae is schematically represented in Figure 2–20*A*.[62] Here it can be noted that the vertebral arteries represent a lateral longitudinal fusion of the original segmental vessels, and provide a ventrally coursing anterior central artery and a medially directed posterior central artery to each subaxial vertebral element. The anterior spinal plexus is most greatly developed in the cervical region, where it exhibits a rectangular mesh of vessels in which the transverse members (anterior central arteries) run along the upper ventral edges of their respective intervertebral discs. The conspicuousness of this plexus reflects the fact that it also serves the cervical prevertebral musculature. The thyrocervical and costocervical trunks assist in the lower cervical region, and the upper cervical part of the plexus receives contributions from the ascending pharyngeal arteries.

Atlantoaxial Complex

With their complex phyletic and developmental history, the components of the atlantoaxial articulation display the most atypical vascular pattern of all the vertebrae. Although the odontoid process represents the definitive centrum of the first cervical vertebra, it develops and remains as a projecting process of the axis that is almost completely isolated from the rest of the atlas by synovial joint cavities. Its fixed position relative to the rotation of the atlas and the adjacent sections of the vertebral arteries prevents formation of a major vascularization by direct branches at its corresponding segmental level. One might assume that the nutrition of its tissues would easily be accomplished by interosseous vessels derived from the spongiosa within the supporting body of the axis. It is axiomatic, however, that the vascular patterns of bones were developmentally established to supply the original ossification centers within the nonvascular cartilage matrices, and despite the eventual obliteration of the separating cartilage, the original patterns of vascularity generally prevail throughout life. The transient cartilaginous plate, which represents an incipient intervertebral disc between the atlas and axis, does not calcify until the latter half of the first decade and effectively prevents the development of any significant vascular communication between the axis centrum and the odontoid process. Occasionally, noncalcified remnants of this plate may persist in the adult, and although there may be a stable union between the two elements, a radiolucent area may suggest a fracture nonunion or a "false" os odontoideum.

In light of the foregoing facts, it was not unexpected that the investigations of Schiff and Parke[27, 78] should reveal that the odontoid process was supplied primarily by pairs of anterior and posterior central branches that coursed upward from the surfaces of the body of the axis and were derived from the vertebral arteries at the level of the foramen of the third cervical nerve. The posterior ascending arteries are the larger members of these two sets of vessels and usually arise independently from the posteromedial sides of their respective vertebral arteries. The individual artery enters the vertebral canal through the foramen between the second and third vertebrae, and trifurcates on the dorsum of the axis body. The typical posterior central perforators are sent medially to pass deep to the posterior longitudinal ligament (called the tectorial membrane in the craniocervical region) to penetrate deep into the spongiosa of the axis, and a small descending branch is sent downward to anastomose with vessels of the next lower segment. The major part of the posterior ascending artery crosses the dorsal surface of the transverse ligament of the atlas about 1.5 mm lateral to the neck of the odontoid process (Fig. 2–20). Continuing dorsal to the alar ligament, it sends an anterior anastomotic branch over the cranial edge of this ligament to form collateral connections with the anterior ascending artery. The posterior ascending artery then continues on a medial course to meet its opposite counterpart and thus to form the apical arcade that arches over the apex of the odontoid process.

The smaller anterior ascending arteries arise from the anteromedial aspect of the vertebral arteries and pass to the ventral surface of the axis body. Fine medial branches send perforators into the substance of the vertebral body and then meet in a median anastomosis typical of the anterior central branches of the lower cervical region. The rostral continuance of the anterior ascending arteries brings them dorsal to the anterior arch of the atlas. Here each artery sends a number of fine perforators into the anterolateral surfaces of the neck of the odontoid process and terminates in a spray of vessels that supply the synovial capsule of the median atlantoaxial joint.

Fine branches from the anterior and posterior ascending arteries also assist in the nutrition of the syndesmotic relations of the atlantoaxial and craniovertebral articulations, but the main blood supply to the atlanto-occipital joint is provided by a complex of vessels derived from the vertebral and occipital arteries.

In the original observations of Schiff and Parke,[78] it was noted that collateral vessels passed both over and under the anterior arch of the atlas to anastomose with the apical arcade and ascending arteries, respectively. It was correctly assumed that these were derived from some component of the external carotid system, but since the studies were done with trimmed specimens of the upper cervical spine, they were cautiously referred to as "cleft perforators," implying that they originated anterior to the retropharyngeal cleft. In later observations on injected specimens of the entire neck region of fetuses near term, it was seen that these vessels were actually branches of the ascending pharyngeal artery and that they did not perforate the cleft. Instead, the ascending pharyngeal artery, which has a nearly ubiquitous distribution in the upper pharyngeal region, sends a branch along the inner aspect of the carotid sheath that, on reaching the base of the skull, becomes recurrent and descends deep to the prevertebral fascia to supply the upper prevertebral cervical muscles and anastomose with the anterior spinal plexus. These observations also showed that the numerous small-bore vessels that descend from the rim of the foramen magnum to anastomose with the apical arcade are not also cleft perforators as originally labeled but derivatives of a meningeal branch of the occipital artery that enters the skull through the hypoglossal canal (Fig. 2–20). Its descending branches supply not only the periforaminal dura but also the tectorial membrane and alar and apical ligaments and the fine anastomoses to the arcade.

Sacroiliolumbar Arterial System

From the second thoracic to the fourth lumbar vertebra, the spine and its regionally related structures are supplied by pairs of segmental arteries that are direct branches of the aorta. However, since the aorta terminates in a bifurcation ventral to the fourth lumbar vertebral body, the vertebrae and the associated tissues caudal to this point must rely on an arterial complex derived mostly from the internal iliac (hypogastric) arteries. Although this "sacroiliolumbar system," consisting of contributions from the fourth lumbar artery, the iliolumbar artery, and the middle and lateral sacral arteries, is of considerable functional significance, it has received only cursory mention in most anatomic texts and is almost never exposed in the routine dissections of medical anatomy classes.

With the increasing use of percutaneous approaches to the lower lumbar discs, however, this infra-aortic system of vessels has assumed a greater surgical significance, particularly because, unlike the conventional segmental supply to the more superior vertebrae, its major components are longitudinally related to the dorsolateral surfaces of the discs most frequently involved in these procedures. Therefore, the conscientious operator should be aware of their presence, positions, and variability.

Fourth Lumbar Arteries

The peculiarities of the sacroiliolumbar system of arteries may best be understood if compared with the pattern of distribution of the typical aortic segmental branches. The ramifications of the fourth lumbar arteries were selected for this purpose as they not only exemplify the conventional segmental distribution, but often are involved in the nutrition of the next lower segments by variable contributions to the iliolumbar vessels.

Although extant texts fail to acknowledge some of the unusual features of the fourth lumbar arteries, the observations conducted for this chapter have shown that these vessels often may be twice the caliber of their more cephalad homologues because of a greater muscular and intersegmental distribution.

As depicted in Figures 2–29 and 2–34, the distribution of the major ramifications is very similar to that of the thoracic segmental vessels with the exception of the additional branches that supply the psoas and quadratus lumborum muscles. Unfortunately, the drawing in Figure 2–29 separates the main segmental branch from the surface of the vertebral body for graphic clarity, but it must be realized that all the segmentals are immediately adherent to the surface of the anterior longitudinal ligament and the vertebral periosteum until they reach the region lateral to the intervertebral foramen. The lateral muscular branch (equivalent of the thoracic intercostals) may be quite large at the fourth lumbar level where, in contrast to the other lumbar laterals, it passes anterior rather than posterior to the quadratus lumborum. It then continues to supply the lower posterolateral abdominal wall as it courses superior to the crest of the ilium. As can be seen in Figures 2–28 and 2–29, it may be equivalent in size to the iliac branch of the iliolumbar artery, and its position superior to the crest indicates that it is more liable to be encountered by percutaneous instrumentation than is the latter vessel.

The dorsal musculocutaneous branch of the fourth lumbar artery is equivalent in distribution to that of other thoracolumbar segmentals, as it usually displays a medial branch that supplies the external aspects of the facet joints

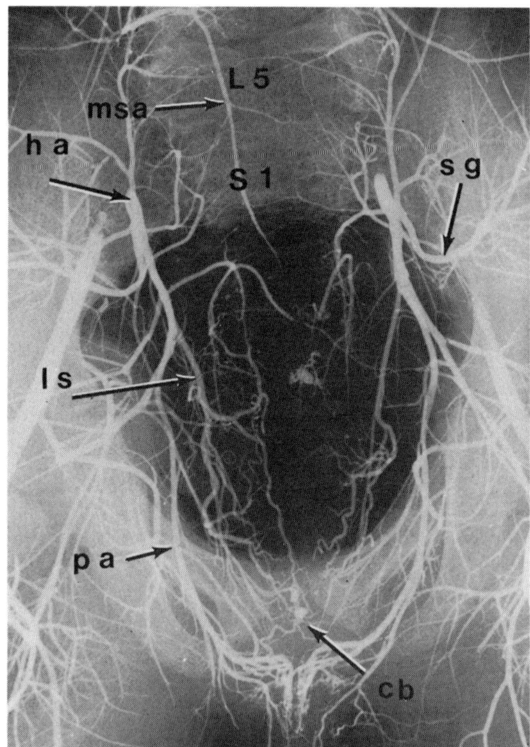

Figure 2–28. Anteroposterior arteriogram of the sacral region in a 7-year-old. The lateral sacral arteries (ls) can be seen coming from the hypogastric vessels (ha). The middle sacral artery (msa) is atypical in this specimen because it stops at S1. Just anterior to the coccyx the coccygeal bodies (cb) are indicated as small knots of arteriovenous anastomoses. Pudendal arteries (pa) are well injected.

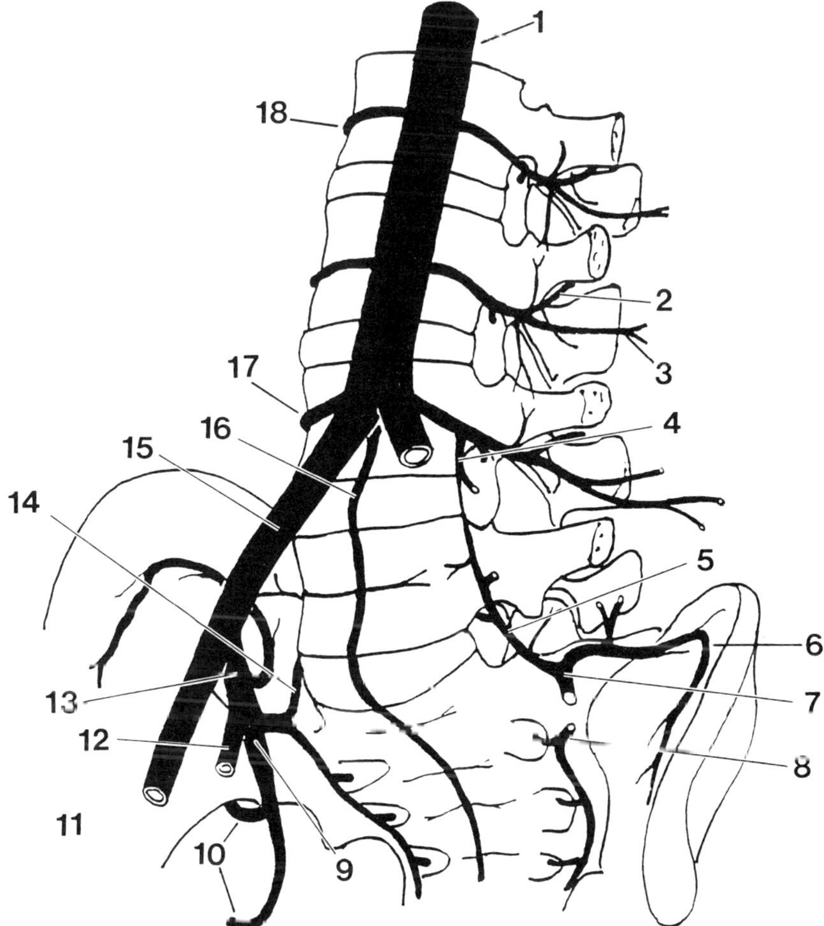

Figure 2–29. Graphic rendering of the distribution and major variations of the sacroiliolumbar system of arteries that supply the vertebrae and their associated structures inferior to the fourth lumbar vertebra. These patterns of the vessels were derived from radiographs of perinatal specimens and dissections of adults, and then drawn against a tracing of the lumbosacral region taken from a left anterior oblique radiograph of an adult male. Note that the aorta lies to the left of center as it approaches the bifurcation ventral to the fourth lumbar vertebra. This schema shows the more frequent arrangement of the sacroiliolumbar system on the right side of the illustration where the iliolumbar vessel (7) has a single origin from the dorsum of the posterior division of the (removed) internal iliac artery. The left side shows the common variation where the iliac artery and the lumbar artery (14) are derived separately. The middle sacral artery (16) is in its typical position, and the anastomotic contribution from the fourth lumbar artery (4) shows its most frequent form.

1. aorta
2. musculocutaneous branch of third lumbar artery
3. muscular branch to posterior abdominal wall
4. anastomotic contribution of fourth lumbar artery to sacroiliolumbar system
5. lumbar branch of iliolumbar artery
6. iliac branch of iliolumbar artery
7. iliolumbar artery
8. left lateral sacral artery
9. posterior division of internal iliac artery
10. superior and inferior gluteal arteries
11. external iliac artery
12. anterior (visceral) division of internal iliac artery
13. internal iliac artery
14. variant origin of lumbar branch of iliolumbar artery from lateral sacral artery
15. common iliac artery
16. middle sacral artery
17. left fourth lumbar segmental artery
18. left second lumbar segmental artery

and neural arch components and the transversospinal group of muscles, and a lateral branch to the transversocostal group of the erector spinae. The vertebromedullary (spinal) branches of the fourth lumbar artery are also similar to those of other segmentals. As can be seen in the radiograph of barium-injected vessels of a perinatal fourth lumbar vertebra (Fig. 2–34), they are a group of vessels of variable caliber that may generally be sorted into three divisions: (1) the ventral periosteal and osseous branches that supply the posterior longitudinal ligament, the periosteum, and the cancellous bone of the vertebral body; (2) the radiculomedullary division that provides the irregularly located medullary arteries of the cord and the constant distal radicular arteries to all the roots; and (3) the dorsal division that supplies fine articular branches to the deep aspects of the facet joints and the periosteum of the deep surfaces of the laminae and their associated ligaments. The first two divisions usually originate from a common branch of the segmental artery and enter the intervertebral foramen just rostral to their respective vertebral pedicle and ventral to the dorsal root ganglion, whereas the dorsal division arises from the musculocutaneous branch of the segmental artery and enters the foramen dorsal to the nerve components. All the vertebromedullary branches may provide fine branches to the spinal dura.

The aortic segmental arteries course around their respective vertebral body at its narrowest circumference and thus come to be positioned almost equidistant between the adjacent discs. Hence, these parts of the arterial distribution are relatively safe from instrumentation properly positioned to enter the discs.

A major peculiarity of the fourth lumbar artery is its proclivity toward providing a relatively large, caudally directed intersegmental branch that arises near the level of the intervertebral foramen and becomes reciprocally involved with the lumbar branch of the iliolumbar artery. Thus, when this latter vessel is small or absent, the descending branch of the fourth lumbar artery may be sufficiently large to provide the predominant nutritional system to as many as two vertebral segments caudal to its origin (Fig. 2–34).

Iliolumbar Artery

As opposed to the mostly visceral distribution of the anterior division of the internal iliac (hypogastric) artery, the posterior division is essentially a somatic artery giving rise to gluteal, iliolumbar, and lateral sacral branches. The iliolumbar artery most frequently is the first branch of this dorsal division and is directed dorsosuperiorly to pass close to the ventrolateral surface of the first sacral vertebral segment. It then passes superiorly dorsal to the obturator nerve and ventral to the lumbosacral trunk. Lateral to the inferior margin of the disc, the iliolumbar artery usually divides into a laterally directed iliac artery and an ascending lumbar artery. The first of these crosses the sacroiliac joint to reach the iliac fossa of the pelvis, where it courses inferior to the iliac crest and usually deep to the muscle to provide muscular branches to the iliac muscle and articular twigs to the acetabulum, and eventually anastomoses with the deep circumflex branch of the femoral artery. The lumbar artery ascends posterolateral to the L5–S1 disc, still between the obturator nerve and the lumbosacral trunk, to provide the vertebromedullary vessels to the L5–S1 intervertebral foramen (Figs. 2–29, 2–34). In most cases a branch of this vessel continues rostrally to anastomose with the descending branch of the fourth lumbar artery. The lumbar branch of the iliolumbar artery provides regional branches to the psoas and quadratus lumborum muscles, but is reciprocal in this function to the relative size of the contributions of the descending fourth lumbar branch and/or the first lateral branches of the middle sacral artery.

Sacral Arteries

Lateral Sacral Arteries. These vessels usually form the second branch of the dorsal division of the internal iliac arteries, and course down the pars lateralis on each side of the sacrum. Opposite the sacral foramina they give off medial branches that dorsally enter the foramina, and after providing the typical vertebromedullary derivatives, their dorsal muscular branches exit through the dorsal sacral foramina to supply the sacral origins of the erector spinae muscles.

Middle Sacral Artery. This median unpaired vessel is the last branch of the aorta, usually derived from its dorsal median surface just above the carina of the bifurcation. It descends down the ventral surface of the anterior longitudinal ligament over the fourth and fifth lumbar bodies and down the ventral sacrum to terminate at the sacrococcygeal junction in a vascular glomus (sacrococcygeal body) in tailless mammals, or continues ventral to the coccygeal (caudal) vertebrae in the tailed mammals as the caudal artery. In humans this is a variable vessel, being totally absent in some cases or replaced by a branch of one of the lateral sacrals. Where it is a significant component of the sacroiliolumbar system, its first lateral branches on the ventral surface of the fifth lumbar body may entirely replace this segment's contributions from the iliolumbar or fourth lumbar vessels and provide its osseous, muscular, and vertebromedullary requirements.

Where it is conspicuously present in the sacral region, it may also contribute a vertebromedullary branch to each anterior sacral foramen; when it is totally absent, these ventral sacral territories are provided with segmental medial branches from the lateral sacral arteries.

Functional Significance

The sacroiliolumbar system, despite its complexity and seemingly endless combinations of reciprocal substitutions, supplies the lower lumbosacral elements of the spine and the inferior half of the lumbosacral spinal nerve roots (cauda equina) as well as the back musculature inferior to the L4 level. It is also a major contributor to the vasa nervorum of the lumbosacral plexus. As demonstrated in the radiograph in Figure 2–34, the distal radicular arteries define the positions of the lumbosacral roots by their injected contrast medium. Although significant medullary branches to the spinal cord are seldom found below L4, they do occur, and from the preceding descriptions it is obvious why the ligation of both internal iliac arteries during radical cystoprostatectomy has resulted in spinal cord ischemia.[40]

Venous System of the Vertebral Column

Both an external and an internal plexus of veins are associated with the vertebral column, and the distribution of the two systems roughly coincides with the areas served by the external and internal arterial supplies. Thus, the external venous plexus also consists of an anterior and a posterior set of veins. The small anterior external plexus is coextensive with the anterior central arteries and receives tributaries that perforate the anterior and lateral sides of the vertebral body, while the more extensive posterior external veins drain the regions supplied by posterior (muscular and postlaminar) branches of the segmental artery. The posterior external veins form what is essentially a paired system, which lies in the two vertebrocostal grooves but has cross anastomoses between the spinous processes. It is a valveless venous complex that receives the draining segmental tributaries of the internal veins through the intervertebral foramina, and communicates ultimately with the lumbar and intercostal tributaries of the caval and azygos system. The posterior external plexus becomes most extensive in the posterior nuchal region, where it receives the intraspinous tributaries via the vertebral veins, and drains into the deep cervical and jugular veins.

The internal venous plexus is of more functional and anatomic interest. This plexus is essentially a series of irregular, valveless epidural sinuses that extends from the coccyx to the foramen magnum. Its channels are embedded in the epidural fat and are supported by a network of collagenous fibers, but their walls are so thin that their extent or configuration cannot be discerned by gross dissection. This latter property may account for the fact that the epidural venous sinuses have been periodically "rediscovered," and it is relatively recently that their functional aspects have been generally appreciated. Although the epidural vertebral veins were known to Vesalius and his contemporaries and were described and beautifully illustrated in the first part of the 19th century by Breschet,[10] it has been only within the past several decades that Batson,[3] Clemens,[12] and others have made the functional and pathologic significance of these vessels apparent (Fig. 2–30).

The plexus does not entwine the dura in a completely haphazard fashion but is arranged in a series of cross-connected expansions that produce anterior and posterior ladder-like configurations up the vertebral canal. The main anterior components of the epidural plexus consist of two continuous channels that course along the posterior surface of the vertebral bodies just medial to the pedicles. These channels expand medially to cross-anastomose over the central dorsal area of each vertebral body

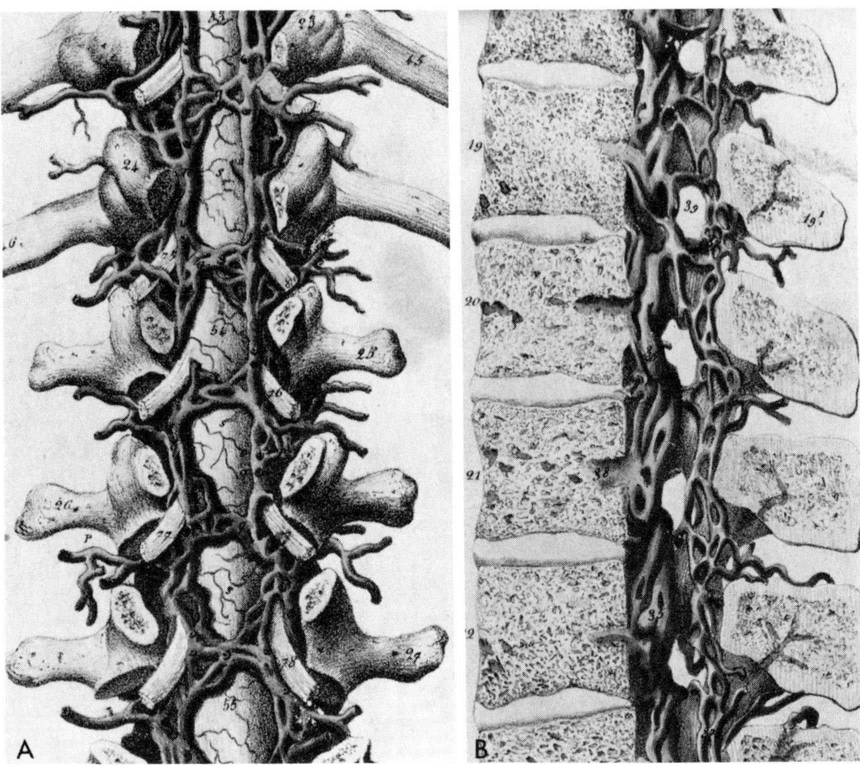

Figure 2–30. *A, B,* Posterior and lateral illustrations of the spinal epidural venous plexus taken from hand-colored copies of Breschet's original work. (ca. 1835, Courtesy of Scott Memorial Library, Jefferson Medical College.)

and are thinnest where they overlie the intervertebral discs. Thus, when injected with a contrast medium, the main channels may appear as a segmental chain of rhomboid beads. Where the main anterior sinuses cross-connect they receive the large unpaired basivertebral sinus that arises within the dorsal central concavity of the spongiosa, and drains the intraosseous labyrinth of sinusoids. Regional visualization of the epidural plexus can be accomplished by introducing a radiopaque medium directly into the spongiosa or the cancellous bone of the spinous process (intraosseous venography). Many drawn cross-sectional illustrations of the vertebral body and its veins show large venous channels passing directly through the spongiosa to connect the basivertebral sinus with veins of the anterior external plexus.

The major external connections of the epidural plexus consist of the veins that pass through the intervertebral foramen and eventually empty into the segmentally available intercostal or lumbar veins. However, since these sinuses are valveless, one cannot refer accurately to directions of drainage and flow, because the greatest functional significance of these vessels lies in their ability to pass blood in any direction according to the constantly shifting intra-abdominal and intrathoracic pressures. Breschet[10] surmised that the epidural plexus served as a collateral route for the valveless caval and azygos systems, and this ability has been amply demonstrated by the experimental ligation of either the superior or inferior venae cavae. In addition, the Queckenstedt maneuver, which tests the patency of the spinal subarachnoid space by compressing the jugulars or intra-abdominal veins, causes an increase in cerebrospinal fluid pressure through dural compression from the expansion of the collaterally loaded epidural plexus. The plexus is evidently capable of passing large quantities of blood without developing varices. Clemens claimed that this feature was due to the intricate network of collagenous fibers that supports the thin walls of the sinuses. Also, passive congestion of the spinal cord is prevented by minute valves in the radicular branches draining the spinal cord.[12] This latter fact is anatomically unique, since valves exist nowhere else in the venous channels associated with the central nervous system.

An ancillary function of the epidural plexus may be to act in a mechanical capacity as a hydraulic shock-absorbing sheath that helps buffer the spinal cord during movements of the vertebral column.

The vertebral sinuses are largest in the suboccipital and upper cervical region. Here they also receive numerous nerve endings from the sinuvertebral nerves and are associated with glomerular arteriovenous anastomoses, which suggests a possible baroceptive function.[71] The patency of these anastomoses is most easily demonstrated in the fetus, in which arterial injections of a contrast medium may also fill the upper cervical epidural sinuses. Similarly, the coccygeal bodies of the same specimen pass the arterial injection directly into the epidural veins of the lower sacral region.

The detrimental aspects of the vertebral epidural veins have been well stated by Batson.[3] Retrograde flow from venous connections to the lower pelvic organs provides an obvious route of metastasis for pelvic neoplasms, both to the spine itself and to the regions of the trunk associated with valveless connections to the plexus. Batson claimed that direct metastatic transfer can occur between the pelvic organs and the brain via the vertebral epidural route.

Another extraspinal-intraspinal venous connection implicated in the transfer of pathologic processes involves the pharyngovertebral veins described in 1984.[67] These vessels constitute a system that drains the superior posterolateral regions of the nasopharynx and coalesces into two to several veins that penetrate the anterior atlanto-occipital membrane to discharge into the venous complex surrounding the median and lateral atlantoaxial joints. As posterior pharyngeal infections have been linked with the atlantoaxial rotatory subluxions characteristic of Grisel's syndrome,[89] it is believed that the pharyngovertebral veins are instrumental in transporting infectious processes that may produce a hyperemic relaxation of the atlantoaxial ligaments. The existence of this venous

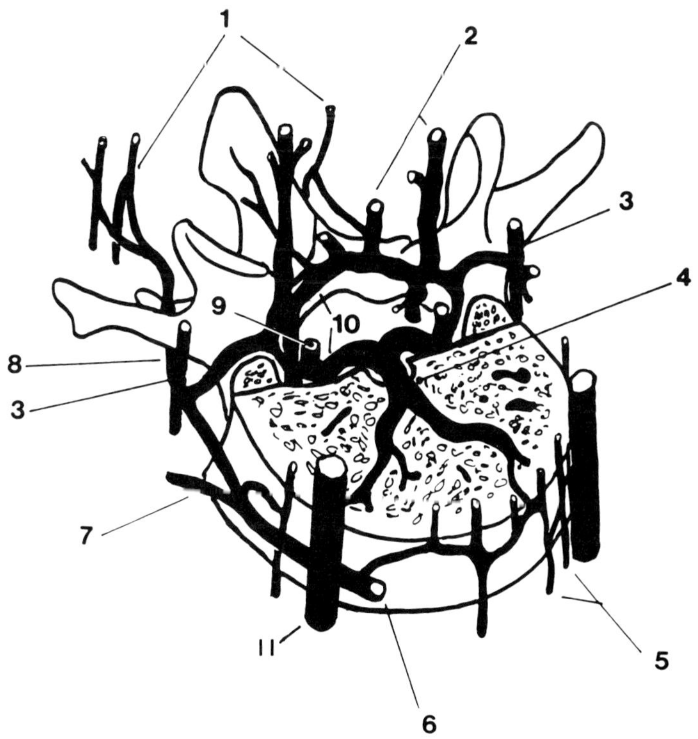

Figure 2–31. Schema showing the venous relations of a lumbar vertebra. Engorgement and a relative venous hypertension in the epidural vessels exacerbate neuroischemic conditions in the lumbosacral roots.

1. dorsal external vertebral plexus
2. dorsal epidural plexus
3. ascending lumbar veins
4. basivertebral vein
5. ventral external vertebral plexus
6. lumbar segmental vein
7. muscular vein from posterior abdominal wall
8. circumferential channels (sinuses) of epidural plexus

system would also explain the ease in transfer of superior pharyngeal metastatic processes to the upper cervical epidural veins.

BLOOD SUPPLY OF THE SPINAL CORD

Throughout the length of the spinal cord a system of three longitudinal vessels receives blood from the irregularly located medullary branches of the segmental spinal arteries and distributes it to the substance of the cord. This system consists of the single median ventral anterior spinal artery (ASA) and two smaller dorsolateral spinal arteries (DSAs) (Fig. 2–32).

The ASA originates from two converging branches of the vertebral arteries just caudal to their formation of the basilar artery, and courses along the ventral median fissure. Although it may be continuous, it is not, functionally, a single artery but consists of a series of anastomotic connections of regional vessels that vary widely in caliber, and within which the direction of the blood flow is dependent on their relationship to their regional medul-

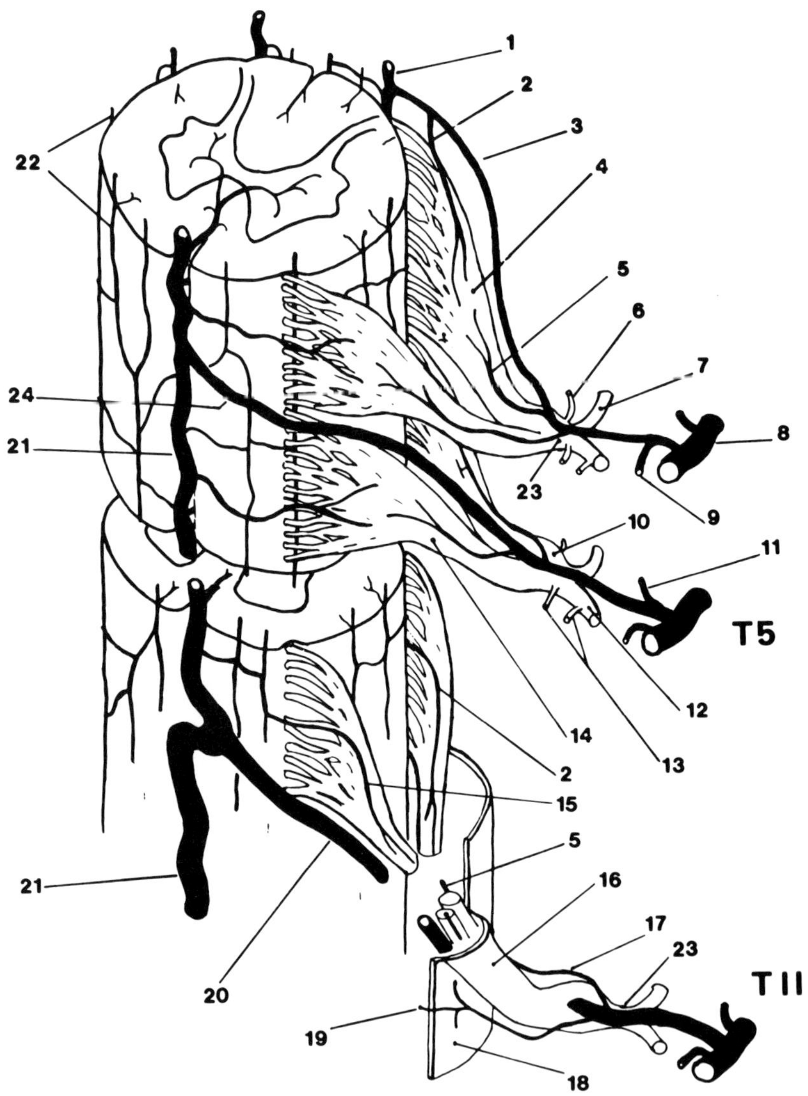

Figure 2–32. *See legend on opposite page*

lary artery. In all regions of the cord, the ASA provides the nutrition to approximately 75 per cent of the cord tissue and all of its gray matter. The ventral position of this vessel and its nutritional importance make it a significant consideration in the consequences of the spinal stenoses. Particularly in the lower cervical region, its compression by dorsal osteophytes and cartilaginous protrusions occasioned by cervical disc degeneration may lead to the neurologically disastrous ASA syndrome.[66] The medullary feeder arteries that supply the ASA may arise from any spinal segmental artery. However, studies by Dommisse[16] showed that there are statistical preferences for certain segmental levels. There are usually three anterior medullary arteries for the cervical region, one or two for the thoracic, and a conspicuous medullary vessel (the arteria radicularis magna of Adamkiewicz) for the lumbosacral cord region. The levels of origin for all these vessels center around certain "average" locations in each region. The ASA is usually of greatest caliber in the lumbosacral part of the cord where it must supply the considerable tissue mass of the proximal cauda equina in addition to the lumbosacral cord intumescence.

The DSAs arise from the posterior inferior cerebellar vessels and are of lesser caliber and nutritional significance. They also are less likely to be longitudinally continuous and often present a more plexiform distribution over the dorsum of the cord. However, they show a greater frequency of smaller medullary sources.

The larger intradural spinal arteries are unusual in that, like the cerebral arteries, they show no significant vasa vasorum. In all other regions of the body, a vessel with an external diameter approaching 1 mm shows a fine vascular plexus (vasa vasorum) on its external surface that nutrifies its outer layers of tissue. Since the cerebral and spinal vessels are bathed in the highly nutrient cerebrospinal fluid, their external layers presumably derive metabolic exchange from this source.

Lateral Spinal Arteries of the Cervical Cord

The highest three to four segments of the cervical spinal cord receive blood from a unique pair of vessels, the lateral spinal arteries. Although, ontogenetically, these appear to be the most rostral expressions of the DSAs, they have a more extensive distribution and are without equivalents in other levels of the cord. They usually arise from the intradural

Figure 2–32. Composite schema of the blood supply to the spinal cord and nerve roots showing two regions of the cord. Note the distinction between medullary arteries and true radicular arteries and that the medullary arteries usually run a course that is independent of the roots.

1. dorsolateral longitudinal artery
2. proximal radicular artery (of dorsal root)
3. dorsal medullary artery
4. dorsal root of thoracic spinal nerve
5. distal radicular artery (of dorsal root)
6. sinuvertebral nerve
7. dorsal ramus of spinal nerve
8. segmental artery
9. dorsal central artery
10. dorsal root ganglion
11. anterior laminar artery
12. ventral ramus of spinal nerve
13. rami communicantes
14. ventral root of spinal nerve
15. proximal radicular artery of ventral root
16. periradicular theca of dura
17. dorsal meningeal branch of vertebromedullary artery
18. dura
19. ventral meningeal plexus
20. great ventral medullary artery (great "radicular" artery of Adamkiewicz)
21. anterior (ventral) spinal artery
22. vasa corona of spinal cord
23. spinal nerve
24. ventral medullary artery of thoracic cord

parts of the vertebral arteries near the origins of the posterior inferior cerebellar arteries (PICAs), or they may arise from the proximal sections of the PICAs themselves. Their typical course carries them anterior to the posterior roots of the cervical spinal nerves C1 to C4, dorsal to the denticulate ligaments, and parallel to the spinal components of the 11th cranial nerve. Their general distribution is to the dorsolateral and ventrolateral cord regions caudal to the olives.

Although these vessels were observed in the later 19th century, they were usually regarded as variants and their functional significance was not appreciated. Lasjaunias and associates[48] compiled an extensive report on the variations and selective angiography of these important vessels.

Intrinsic Vascularity of the Spinal Cord

The tissues of the spinal cord are supplied by two systems of vessels that enter its substance. The first is a centripetal arrangement of arteries that supplies the superficial tracts of the ventral and lateral funiculi, all of the dorsal funiculus, and the extremities of the dorsal horns. They are radially penetrating branches of the vasa corona and the dorsolateral spinal arteries, which serve only a little more than one fourth of the cord. The greater part of the cord and almost all of its gray matter is supplied by a second centrifugal system of vessels derived from the sulcal (or central) arteries. These arteries are a repetitive series of branches derived from the dorsal aspect of the ASA that penetrate the depths of the anterior median fissure. In the midsagittal plane they form a close palisade of vessels that occur with a frequency of three to eight arteries per centimeter in the cervical region and two to six per centimeter in the thoracic cord; they are densest in the lumbar region, where they number five to 12 per centimeter of the ASA. Not surprisingly, the average diameters of the sulcal arteries are greater in the cervical (0.21 mm) and lumbosacral (0.23 mm) regions than in the thoracic cord (0.14 mm).[27] As these vessels approach the anterior commissure, most turn to either the right or left and supply only the corresponding side of the cord. This unilateral proclivity reflects their origins in the early embryonic stages when the ASAs first condensed from a primitive plexus as a symmetric pair of longitudinal vessels, each supplying its respective half of the cord. In subsequent development these two vessels fused in the midline to form the definitive single median ASA, but their sulcal branches retained their original unilateral affinities. However, the earlier reports[22, 29, 39] claiming that all the sulcal arteries are exclusively either right or left in their distribution have been proved incorrect, since 9, 7, and 14 per cent of the cervical, thoracic, and lumbar vessels, respectively, have been shown to have a bilateral distribution.[27, 85]

Although the sulcal arteries may give infrequent branches to the septomarginal white fibers as they extend into the median anterior fissure, their major distribution is derived after they enter the substance of the cord just ventral to the anterior white commissure. Here the individual right and left arteries subdivide into dorsal and ventral branches. A group of ventral branches then supplies the ventral horns and, through more radial extensions, provides vessels to Clarke's column and the deeper fibers of the anterior and lateral funiculi. The smaller, more dorsal group of branches supplies the gray commissure and the ventral one half to two thirds of the dorsal horns. A few second- or third-order branches form anastomotic arcades with their counterparts of adjacent sulcal artery territories. All these vessels then provide the finer arterioles that eventually charge the spinal capillary beds.

The obviously greater metabolic requirements of the spinal gray matter, in contrast to the funicular tissue, are dramatically reflected in their relative capillary densities. Quantification of the microvascularity in the spinal cord has shown that the capillary density of the gray matter is four to five times as great as that of the white.[35] However, the capillary distribution within the gray matter is not homogeneous but varies with the regional concentrations of the nuclei. The nuclei of the dorsal horn are fairly uniformly distributed, but the ventral horn shows segmental nuclear clusters that in turn display distinct nerve cell groups in the cross-sectional aspect. By appropriate techniques of vascular injection and clearing, the locations of these groups may be identified solely by the regional concentrations of their surrounding capillaries.

As noted by Feeney and Watterson,[18] the capillary densities of the white and gray matter of the central nervous system are established at a level that is minimally requisite for the metabolic needs of the given tissue. This is unlike most other body tissues that have a capillary "reserve" and normally function with only part of their capillary channels open. They are thus able to vary their intrinsic vascular resistance by dilation of the accessory channels. Nevertheless, despite the lack of this method of control, the spinal cord exhibits a remarkable range of blood flow autoregulation that has been monitored in a variety of mammals (sheep, dog, monkey) by gas clearance methods and the use of isotope-labeled microspheres.[44, 49, 54] All reports have shown that the intrinsic cord vasculature maintains a constant blood flow throughout a wide range of systemic blood pressure alterations, although each species has a definite upper and lower limit to the systemic blood pressure at which the regulation decompensates. As transection of the upper cervical cord has no effect on this autoregulative capacity, it may be assumed that this reflex is local and independent of autonomic nerve control, but no report has proposed a vascular mechanism or regional localization for this regulation. However, cleared specimens of thick (1 mm or more) parasagittal and cross sections of human lumbosacral cord, vascularly injected with various polymerizing media, revealed that numerous third-order branches of the sulcal arteries communicate directly with veins through convoluted anastomoses. These vascular structures are located primarily in the area that divides the ventral two thirds of the dorsal horn from the dorsal one third and in the more central regions of the ventral horn. They show a paucity of contractile elements and instead exhibit an "epithelioid" type of intima that appears capable of swelling and diminishing its thickness. Since this action could rapidly control the caliber of the anastomotic lumina in immediate response to local metabolic changes, these anastomotic convolutions may be the site of the reflex adjustment in the flow resistance of the spinal cord vasculature.[63]

Perhaps the most essential part of knowledge of the vascular supply of the spinal cord is awareness of the ranges of individual variability. The numerous successful surgical cases in which the arteria medullaris magna has been inadvertently interrupted without producing a disastrous spinal cord ischemia certainly give the impression that an adequate collateral vascularity may protect the cord in most individuals when a single major artery is compromised. However, in procedures involving the interruption of blood flow in numerous consecutive segmental branches of the aorta, such as aortic cross clamping for abdominal vascular surgery, the maintenance of adequate spinal cord blood flow, particularly in the thoracic area, appears to be more dependent on the regional competence of the ASA than on the number of collateral sources to the cord. Spinal cord injury after cross clamping without adjunctive vascular support has been reported to vary between 15 and 25 per cent, depending on the series of cases reviewed.[58, 86] Proximal-to-distal aortic shunting may alleviate both the undesirable hypertension in the aortic distribution proximal to the first clamp, and the hypotension in the segments distal to the second clamp. However, the work of Molina and colleagues[58] on dogs indicated that the shunt capacity should provide more than 60 per cent of the baseline descending aortic flow and have a diameter greater than one half that of the descending aorta to be effective.

Of particular significance was the study by Svensson and associates[82] on the blood flow in the baboon spinal cord and its implications in aortic cross clamping. This animal was chosen because its spinal vascularity was similar to that in humans in that its ASA is a continuous vessel without the occasional interruptions noted in some quadrupeds. Nevertheless, the work of these authors indicated that in the baboon, as in man, the caliber of the ASA is often critically narrowed where the thoracic ASA joins the lumbar segment of this vessel at their common junction with the arteria medullaris magna. The functional implication here is that the shunting of the cross-clamped aorta may help maintain an adequate flow in the lumbosacral sections of the cord, but is of little help to the supply of the lower sections of the thoracic cord owing to the marked discrepancy that usually exists between the ASA diameters above and below the junction of the arteria medullaris magna. In accordance with the hemodynamic principles of Poiseuille's equation, the resistance to blood flow upward from the arteria medullaris magna junction was over 50 times greater than the flow resistance downward into the lumbosacral ASA in the baboon. Since a series of direct measurements showed that this discrepancy in the ASA diameters was even greater in humans, Svensson and associates concluded that even the lowest segments of the thoracic cord were dependent on a blood flow from the superior end of the thoracic ASA in spite of the shunting.

Intrinsic Venous Drainage of the Spinal Cord

Compared with the arterial anatomy, the structural and functional aspects of the venous drainage of the spinal cord have been relatively neglected. Unlike other organ systems in which the equivalent orders of veins and arteries tend to course in a common vascular bundle, the veins of the central nervous system are generally less numerous than the arteries, they are larger than their corresponding efferent vessels, the larger branches may not show a pattern concurrent with the arterial distribution, and they are not accompanied by lymphatics.

The internal substance of the dorsal half of the cord drains by a centrifugal arrangement of intrinsic vessels that are tributaries, by way of a venous vasa corona, to a large median dorsal longitudinal spinal vein; the ventral half sends tributaries to sulcal veins that empty into a large median ventral longitudinal vein that runs parallel to the ASA. Both of these longitudinal vessels are circumferentially connected by a prominent venous vasa corona. This entire system drains into the epidural venous plexus by medullary (previously called radicular) veins that are as infrequent and capricious in their distribution as the medullary arteries.[23] It should be noted that the proximal sections of the spinal nerve roots drain centripetally into the vasa corona and longitudinal veins of the cord, and thence to the epidural system via the medullary veins.

Vascularization of the Spinal Nerve Roots

Although it has been generally recognized that much of the pain consequent to degenerative changes in the spinal motion segment results from compression or tension on the spinal nerve roots, the mechanisms that initiate the actual nerve discharge have remained obscure. As experimental studies on peripheral nerves and observations on numerous cases of neurogenic claudication have suggested that much of the pain may have a neuroischemic basis, a series of investigations were undertaken to determine the nature of the intrinsic vascularity of the spinal nerve root and its response to localized compression or tension. Unfortunately, the nerve roots had long been regarded as part of the peripheral nervous system and were viewed as histologically and vascularly similar to peripheral nerves. Consequently, research on the latter was often uncritically extrapolated to apply to the nerve roots.

The very long roots of the lumbosacral spinal nerves appeared to be particularly vulnerable, because their vascularity was initially believed to be supplied only from their distal ends without the access to the frequent collateral support that is characteristic of peripheral nerves. Since the nerve root fasciculi do not have a strong connective tissue support, it also

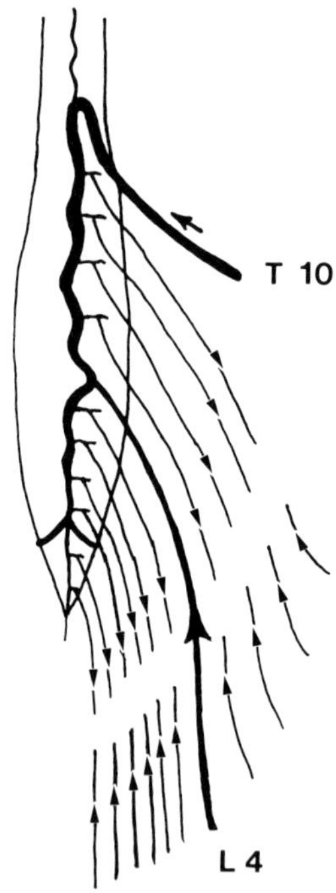

Figure 2–33. Schema indicating the directions of normal blood flow in the cauda equina. Note that the anterior spinal artery of the lumbosacral part of the cord is supplied by medullary arteries, and in turn supplies 75 per cent of the cord substance and the upper parts of the cauda equina via the proximal radicular arteries. This accounts for the enlargement of the anterior spinal artery in the lumbosacral region.

appeared that the fine vascularity they possessed would be at risk from the repeated tension and relaxation resulting from the flexion and extension of the spine. However, Parke and colleagues[64] and Parke and Watanabe[69] showed by vascular injection that the roots receive their arterial supply from both ends (Figs. 2–32, 2–33), a fact physiologically confirmed by Yamamoto.[93] The existence of many redundant coils along the branches of the true radicular arteries ameliorates the stresses that would result from the interfascicular movements that accompany the repeated stretch and relaxation. A most significant finding was of the occurrence of numerous and relatively large arteriovenous anastomoses throughout the length of the root (Figs. 2–35, 2–36). These vascular cross connections apparently allow a blood flow to be maintained in sections of the root both above and below a point of compression. Of particular significance to root nutrition is the work of Rydevik and associates[77] who, using isotopically labeled methylglucose, demonstrated that approximately 50 per cent of the root nutrition is derived from the ambient cerebrospinal fluid; this necessitates a gauzelike architecture of the radicular pia-arachnoid sheath.

A study by Watanabe and Parke[87, 88] of chronically compressed roots indicated that the compressed segment is most likely metabolically deprived, and it has been strongly indicated that the pain is related to radicular ischemia, since the reduction of oxygen intake in patients with neurogenic claudication exacerbates the symptoms.[17] However, the arterial side of the vasa radiculorum appears to be well compensated and maintains a continuity in spite of rather severe chronic compression. Further study has indicated that it is the venous side of the radiculomedullary circulation that is more vulnerable.[88] Since the roots are part of the central nervous system, the relationships of the arteries to the veins more resemble that of the brain than those of peripheral nerves, because the radicular veins do not follow the arterial pattern but are fewer in number and run a separate and usually deeper (more central) course. Being thin walled, they are more liable to the spatial restrictions imposed by degenerative changes in the dimensions of the spinal canal and intervertebral foramina, and show complete interruption in the chronically compressed root. The metabolically deprived or inflamed nerve root becomes hypersensitive

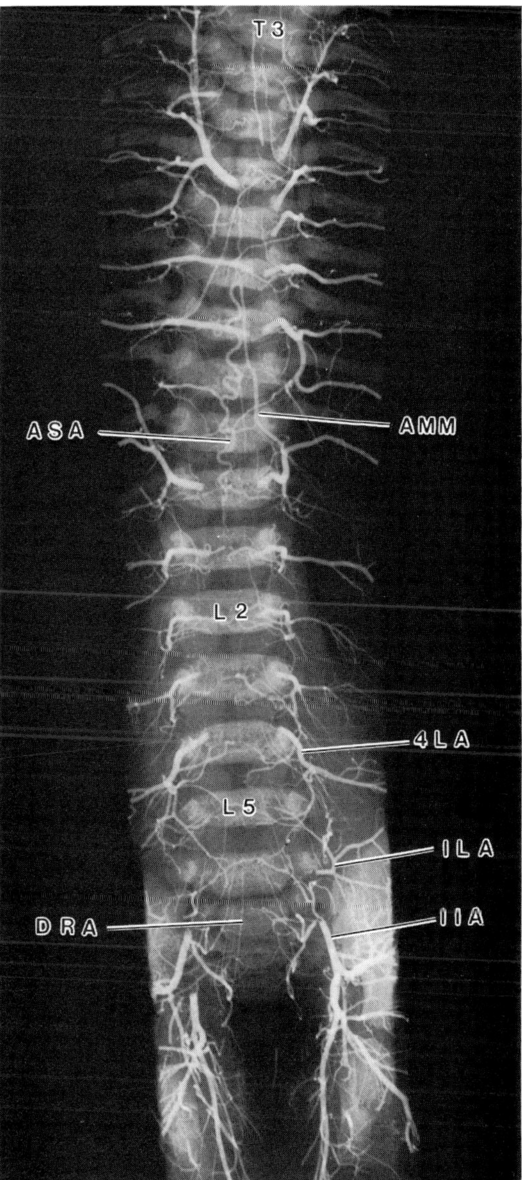

Figure 2–34. Anteroposterior radiograph of a spine from a perinatal cadaver injected with barium sulfate. The aorta and common iliac vessels have been removed before radiography. This specimen was chosen because it showed considerable variation between the two sides of the sacroiliolumbar system. Note that on the right side of the illustration both a small lumbar branch and a descending branch from the fourth lumbar artery (4LA) enter the L5–S1 intervertebral foramen. On the left side, there is no lumbar branch, and a descending branch of the L4 artery supplies all of the vessels to the L5–S1 foramen. Also, the middle sacral artery is absent and other branches of the system supply its domain. The radicular branches of the vertebromedullary vessels supply the distal radicular arteries (DRA) and reveal the positions of the lower ends of the lumbosacral nerve roots.

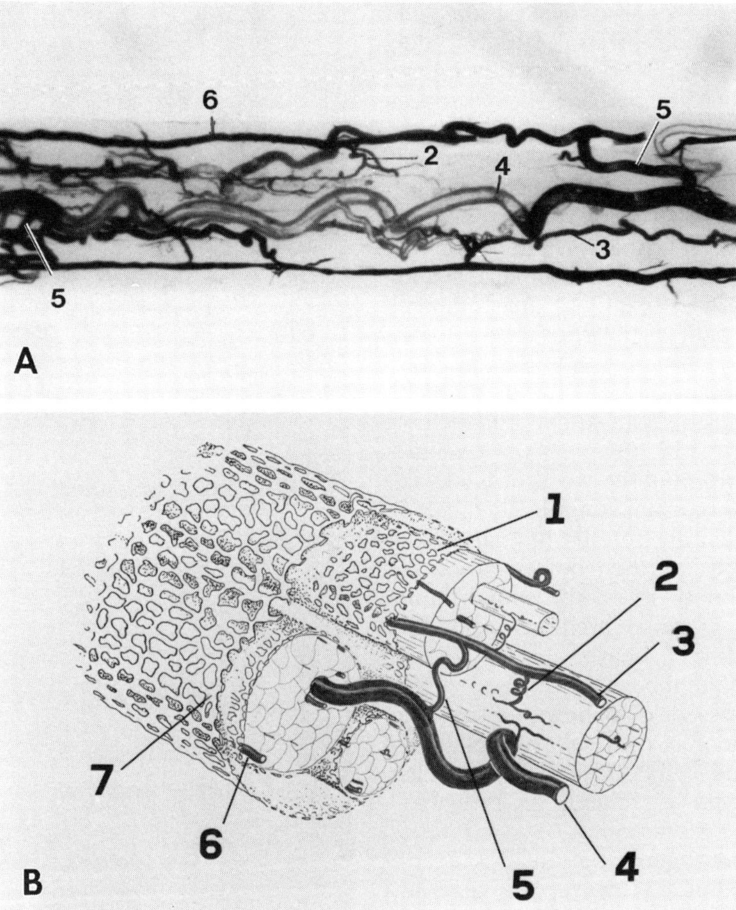

Figure 2–35. *A*, Low-power (×20) transillumination photomicrograph of a midsection from part of an L4 nerve root that had been treated with hydrogen peroxide after vascular injection with latex–India ink, but before clearing in a solution of tributyl-tricresyl phosphates. The peroxidases within the residual blood elements inflated the radicular veins (4) to provide a temporary contrast medium. Note the frequency of the large arteriovenous anastomoses (5) that permitted the latex–India ink to enter the veins. *B*, Graphic compilation showing the structure of a typical lumbosacral nerve root derived from data obtained by injection studies and scanning electron microscopy (see Fig. 2–36). The gauzelike pia-arachnoid membranes permit the cerebrospinal fluid (CSF) to percolate into nerve tissues and assist metabolic support. Numbers in both *A* and *B* are common to equivalent structures.

1. fascicular pia
2. inter- and intrafascicular arteries showing compensating coils to allow interfascicular movement
3. longitudinal radicular artery
4. large radicular vein (does not course with arteries)
5. arteriovenous anastomosis
6. collateral radicular artery
7. gauzelike pia-arachnoid that permits percolation of CSF to assist in metabolic support

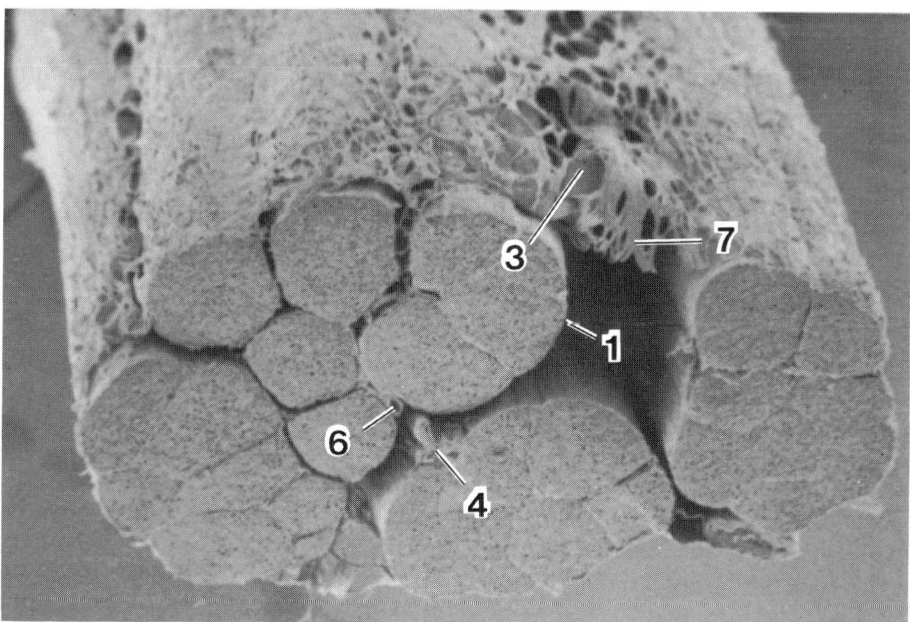

Figure 2–36. Scanning electron photomicrograph of a section of a proximal part of an L5 ventral nerve root. The gauzelike pia-arachnoid sheath is very evident. The numbers correspond to the structures labeled in Figure 2–35. (× 50.)

to any mechanical deformation, and any additional insult to such a nerve may initiate ectopic impulses that produce pain. However, impedance of the radiculomedullary venous return can occur without topographically related venous constriction. The exacerbation of neurogenic pain in cases in which spinal stenosis has been associated with venous hypertension has been recorded by clinical investigators. LaBan[45] and LaBan and Wesolowski[46] noted that patients with diminished right heart compliance and spinal stenosis may eventually show neurogenic pain even in static or recumbent situations. This they attributed to an increased external pressure on the already sensitized roots by the engorgement of the epidural venous sinuses (Fig. 2–31), but the venous hypertension alone may be sufficient to impede the venous return from an already compromized radicular circulation. Madsen and Heros[52] showed that "arterialization" of spinal veins by abnormal arteriovenous shunts in the region of the conus medullaris exacerbates the neurogenic pain in patients with spinal stenosis. Their hypothesis suggested that a variable combination of increased mechanical constriction by dilated epidural veins, and the direct increased resistance to the radicular circulation by the venous hypertension, could contribute to the elicitation of pain. Aboulker and colleagues[1] also concluded that epidural venous hypertension alone may produce radicular and/or cord symptoms without adjunctive stenotic compression.

Thus, it appears that if the intrinsic circulation of the nerve root is impeded in either its arterial input or its venous outflow, the net effect is the same: a neuroischemia of the compressed root segment(s) that may enhance the generation of ectopic nerve impulses.

A phenomenon that could be related to radicular venous stasis is the swelling of the disc-distorted nerve root that Takata and associates[83] well demonstrated in computed tomography (CT) myelograms. This is difficult to explain, since extravasated fluids in the root tissues should have free access to the surrounding cerebrospinal fluid. Nevertheless, the fluid balance of the root tissues appears to be altered, particularly in the segment proximal to the level of the offending disc, but the intricacies of the hemodynamic relationships responsible for this change remain unknown.

The role of the ubiquitous arteriovenous anastomosis in autoregulation of the intrinsic radicular vasculature also offers a fertile field for clinical investigations. Since these vascular shunts are mostly without contractile elements, but appear instead to control their lumina by the thickening response of an epithelioid endothelium, they probably react to chemical changes in the blood within their lumina and therefore offer an immediate local reflex to alterations in the nerve root metabolism.

BIOMECHANICS OF THE SPINE

The biomechanics of the spine constitute a very complex and extensive subject. A comprehensive coverage is not appropriate here, so the reader is directed to the work of White and Panjabi,[90] generally regarded as the major book in this field. However, as an appreciation of the essential functional relationships of the spinal components does enhance an understanding of their anatomy, a brief overview follows.

The spine is capable of ventroflexion, extension, lateral flexion, and rotation. This remarkable universal mobility may seem at odds with the fact that its most essential function is to provide a firm support for the trunk and appendages. The apparent contradiction may be resolved when one realizes that the total ranges of motion are the result of a summation of limited movements permitted between the individual vertebrae and that the total length of the spine changes very little during its movements. The role of the musculature in the performance of the supportive functions cannot be minimized, as the disastrous scolioses that result from their unilateral loss in a few motor segment units may attest.

Obviously, the degree and combination of the individual types of motion described above vary considerably in the different vertebral regions. Although all subaxial-presacral vertebrae are united in a tripod arrangement consisting of the intervertebral disc and the two zygapophyseal articulations, the relative size and shape of the former and the articular planes of the latter determine the range and types of motion that an individual set of intervertebral articulations will contribute to the total mobility of the spine. In general, flexion is the most pronounced movement of the vertebral column as a whole. It requires an anterior compression of the intervertebral disc and a gliding separation of the articular facets, in which the inferior set of an individual vertebra tends to move upward and forward over the opposing superior set of the adjacent inferior vertebra. The movement is checked mainly by the posterior ligaments and epaxial muscles. Extension tends to be a more limited motion, producing posterior compression of the disc, with the inferior articular process gliding posteriorly and downward over the superior set below. It is checked by the anterior longitudinal ligament and all ventral muscles that directly or indirectly flex the spine. Also, the laminae and spinous processes may sharply limit extension. Lateral flexion is accompanied by some degree of rotation. It involves a rocking of the bodies on their discs, with a sliding separation of the diarthroses on the convex side and an overriding of those related to the concavity. The rotational component brings the anterior surface of the bodies toward the convexity of the flexure and the spinous processes toward its concavity. This phenomenon is well illustrated in a dried preparation of a scoliotic spine.

Lateral flexion is checked by the intertransverse ligaments and the extensions of the ribs or their costal homologues.

Pure rotation is directly proportional to the relative thickness of the intervertebral disc and is mainly limited by the geometry of the planes of the diarthrodial surfaces. The architecture of the disc, while permitting limited rotation between the bodies, also serves to check this movement by its resistance to compression. The consecutive layers of the annulus fibrosus have their fibers arranged in an alternating helical fashion, and rotation in either direction can be accompanied only by increasing the angularity of the opposing fibers to the horizontal, which in turn requires compression of the disc.

The entire vertebral column rotates approximately 90 degrees to either side of the sagittal plane, but most of this traversion is accomplished in the cervical and thoracic sections. It flexes nearly the same amount, using primarily the cervical and thoracic regions. Roughly a total of 90 degrees of extension is permitted by the cervical and lumbar regions, while lateral flexion with rotation is allowed to the extent of 60 degrees to both sides, again primarily by the cervical and lumbar areas.

Specific Regional Considerations

The atlanto-occipital joints mostly permit flexion and extension with a limited lateral action, all being checked by the suboccipital musculature and the atlanto-occipital ligaments. The atlantoaxial articulations allow only rotation, the pivoted joint being stabilized and checked by the alar ligaments and the ligaments forming the capsules of the atlantoaxial diarthroses.

One half of the rotational mobility of the entire cervical region takes place between the atlas and the axis, and the remainder is distributed among the joints of the subaxial vertebrae. The atlanto-occipital joint also accounts for approximately half of the cervical flexion. However, the remaining 50 per cent is not evenly distributed among the cervical vertebrae but is greater in the upper section.

The subaxial part of the cervical region shows the freest ranges of motion of all the presacral vertebrae. The discs are quite thick in relation to the heights of the vertebral bodies and contribute about one fourth of the height of this part of the column. In addition, a sagittal section shows the middle part of the cervical disc to be lenticular in shape, so that the anteroinferior lips of the bodies are more capable of sliding slightly forward and overriding one another. The range of spinal flexion is greatest in the cervical region, and although the posterior nuchal ligaments and muscles may tend to resist this motion, it is ultimately checked by the chin coming to rest on the chest.

The cervical spine is normally carried in a moderately extended position and shows a median variation of 91 degrees between extension and flexion. Extension is checked by the anterior longitudinal ligament and the combined resistances of the anterior cervical musculature, fascia, and visceral structures, all three of which may be traumatized in hyperextension injuries.

Cervical lateral flexion is quite limited by the articular pillars and the intertransverse ligaments, and thus most lateral motion involves considerable rotation. The nearly horizontal position of the planes of the cervical articular facets provides good supportive strength to the articular pillars but increases the lateral rigidity, so that hyperextension injuries may be more disastrous if the head is rotated at the time of impact from the rear.

The mobility of the thoracic region is also not uniform throughout its length. Although the upper segments resemble the cervical vertebrae in respect to the size of the bodies and the discs, the ribs attached to the sternum greatly impair the ranges of motion. The circumferential arc of the plane of the articular facets shows that rotation is the movement least restricted by these structures.

Flexion and extension become freer in the lower thoracic region, where the discs and vertebral bodies progressively increase in size, and the more movable become less restrictive. However, the last few thoracic vertebrae are transitional in respect to the surfaces of the articular facets. These begin to turn more toward the sagittal plane and tend to limit rotation and permit greater extension.

The articulations of the lumbar region permit ventroflexion, lateral flexion, and extension, but the facets of the synovial joints lie in a ventromedial to dorsolateral plane that virtually locks them against rotation. This lumbar nonrotatory rigidity is a feature shared with most mammals, and achieves its greatest manifestation in certain quadrupeds in which the inferior articulation fits like a cylindric tenon into the semicircular mortise of the corresponding superior process of the vertebra below. It thus provides a gliding action that only permits the neural arches to separate or approximate each other during extension and flexion. The morphology of the joints can be well appreciated in an appropriate cut of loin chop or T-bone steak.

The synovial articulations at the lumbosacral junctions are unique. Unlike the more superior lumbar joints, the facets of the inferior articulating processes of the fifth lumbar vertebra face forward and slightly downward, to engage the reciprocally corresponding articular processes of the sacrum. Because of the position of these joint surfaces, a certain amount of rotation should be possible between the fifth lumbar segment and the sacrum, but the presence of the strong iliolumbar ligaments quite likely restricts much motion of this type.

The most essential function of the synovial lumbosacral articulations involves their role as buttresses against the forward and downward displacement of the fifth lumbar vertebra in relation to the sacrum. When one considers that each region of the spine has its own characteristic curvature, the tracing of the vertical line indicating the center of gravity shows that it intersects the column through the bodies of the transitional vertebrae. Therefore, the normal cervical lordosis places most of the cervical vertebrae anterior to the center of gravity, and the compensating thoracic kyphosis places the thoracic vertebrae posterior to the center of gravity. Again, the lumbar lordosis brings the middle lumbar vertebrae anterior to the line. Thus, the transitional vertebrae between each region intersect the center of gravity and appear to be the most unstable regions of the spine. This is emphasized by the fact that disc problems and fractures most frequently occur in the transitional vertebrae.

Because the sacrovertebral angle produces the most abrupt change of direction in the column, and the center of gravity, which passes through the fifth lumbar body, falls anterior to the sacrum, there is a marked tendency for the thick, wedge-shaped fifth lumbar disc to give way to the shearing vector that the lumbosacral angularity produces. The resulting condition, spondylolisthesis, most frequently reveals a deficiency in the laminae (spondylolysis) that fails to anchor the fifth vertebral body to the sacrum and allows its forward displacement. There has been considerable discussion as to whether spondylolysis is congenital or acquired, but the spondylolisthesis seldom occurs without the laminar deficiencies as a preceding condition.

Biomechanics of the Intervertebral Disc

It is axiomatic in mechanical engineering that a well-designed machine will automatically reveal its function through the analysis of its structure. There are few instances in biologic circumstances in which this statement is more applicable than in the case of the intervertebral disc. Even when the disc is simply divided with a knife and examined grossly, it is apparent that one is dealing with an organ that is remarkably constructed to simultaneously alleviate shock and yet transmit forces from every conceivable combination of vectors. Moreover, this appreciation of the functional competency of the disc increases as its structure is analyzed at the finer levels of organization.

The internal composition of the disc has evolved to withstand great stresses through the liquid and elastic properties of nucleus and annulus acting in combination. The nucleus is distorted by compression forces, but being liquid in nature it is in itself incompressible. It serves to receive primarily vertical forces from the vertebral bodies and redistribute them radially in a horizontal plane. It is, therefore, the distortion of the annulus by the internal pressure of the nucleus that gives the disc its compressibility, and its resilience makes possible the recovery from pressure.

Were the nucleus pulposus simply a cavity filled with water, it would momentarily act in the same capacity, but the ability to maintain the appropriate quantity of fluid during the continual compression and recovery cycle would be lacking. It is this ability to absorb and retain relatively large amounts of water that is the unique property of the living tissue of the nucleus. It is known that the essential compound involved in this process is a protein-polysaccharide gel, which through a high imbibition pressure will bind nearly nine times its volume of water. It is apparent that the hydrophilia is not a form of biochemical bonding, because a quantity of water can be expressed from the nucleus by prolonged mechanical pressure. This accounts for the diurnal decrease in the total length of the spine and its recovery in the supine position at night.

The annulus must receive the ultimate effects of most forces transmitted from one vertebral body to another. Since the major loading of the intervertebral disc is in the form of vertical compression, it may seem paradoxic that the annulus is best constructed to resist tension, but the nucleus transforms the vertical thrust into a radial pressure that is resisted by the tensile properties of the lamellae. Although the basic plan of alternating bands of fibers is one of the obvious sources of the tensile strength of the annulus, this arrangement is not uniform with respect to the directions of the fibers or the degrees of resistance and resilience encountered throughout the annulus. The fibers generally become longer, and the angle of their spiral course becomes more horizontal near the circumference of the disc, for it is here that the shearing stresses of vertebral torsions would be most effective. Experimental analysis has also shown that various parts of the annulus do not respond equally to the same degree of tension, and the discrepancies were related to the plane of section and the location of the sample.[20] The annulus proved to have the greatest resistance and the greatest recovery in horizontal sections of the peripheral lamellae, whereas both vertical and more medial sections were more distensible.

Because the spine acts as a flexible boom to the guy-wire actions of the erector spinae muscles, it is essentially the fulcrum of a lever system of the first class, in which the loading has a considerable mechanical advantage. Pure vector analysis has indicated that a theoretical pressure of approximately three fourths of a ton could be applied to a disc when 100 lb is lifted by the hands,[9] but this is considerably in excess of the actual pressures achieved. Increased intrathoracic and intra-abdominal pressures alleviate much of the fulcrum compression of the discs by effectively counteracting the load of the anterior lever arm.

The actual pressure variations occurring with postural changes have been recorded by inserting transducers into the third lumbar disc.[56] This procedure indicated that the internal disc pressure increases from approximately 100 kg in a standing position with the spine erect to 150 kg when the trunk is bent forward, and to 220 kg when a 70-kg man lifts a 50-kg weight. It was particularly revealing that the pressure showed a considerable increase when the equivalent maneuvers were repeated in a sitting position, and the weight lifting ultimately created a pressure of 300 kg on the third lumbar disc.

The disc is also "preloaded." The inherent tensions of the intervertebral ligaments and the annulus exert a pressure of about 15 kg, since this weight is required to restore the original thickness of the disc after the ligaments have been divided.[69] From a comparative standpoint this preloading probably offers increased stability to the spine as a functional flexible rod. One is almost induced unconsciously to use teleologic thinking in terms of the vertical thrust resistance when regarding the structure of the disc. In perspective, however, the intervertebral disc shows a rather consistent morphology in all mammals, yet man is the only species that truly stands erect. Although analysis of muscular action would most likely show that all mammalian discs must dissipate and transfer axial thrusts, the preloading would enhance the "beam strength" that is obviously necessary in the vertebral column of quadrupeds.

References

1. Aboulker, J., Bar, D., Marsault, C., et al.: L'hypertension veineuse intra-rachidienne par anomalies multiples du système cave: une cause majeure de souffrance médullaire. Clin. Obstet. Gynoecol. *103*:1003–1015, 1977.
2. Aeby, C.: Die Alterverschiedenheiten der menschlichen Wirbelsaule. Arch. Anat. Physiol. (Anat. Abst.) *10*:77, 1879.
3. Batson, O. V.: The function of the vertebral veins and their role in the spread of metastases. Am. Surg. *112*:138–145, 1940.
4. Beadle, O. A.: The Intervertebral Discs. London, Medical Research Council, Special Report No. 160, 1931, pp. 6–9.
5. Bick, E. M.: The osteohistology of the normal human vertebra. J. Mt. Sinai Hosp. *19*:490–527, 1952.
6. Blikra, G.: Intradural herniated lumbar disc. J. Neurosurg. *31*:676–679, 1969.
7. Bogduk, N., Tynan, W., and Wilson, A. S.: The nerve supply to the human lumbar intervertebral disc. J. Anat. *132*:39–56, 1981.
8. Bogduk, N., Windsor, M., and Inglis, A.: The innervation of the cervical intervertebral discs. Spine *13*:2–8, 1988.
9. Bradford, D. L., and Spurling, R. G.: The Intervertebral Disc. Springfield, IL, Charles C Thomas, 1945.
10. Breschet, G.: Essai sur les Veines der Rachis. Paris, Mequigon-Morvith, 1819.
11. Brown, M. D.: The pathophysiology of the intervertebral disc: anatomical, physiological and biomedical considerations. Doctoral thesis, Jefferson Medical College, Philadelphia, 1969.
12. Clemens, H. J.: Die Venesysteme der menschlichen Wirbelsaule. Berlin, Walter de Gruyter, 1961.
13. Crock, H. V., and Yoshizawa, H.: The Blood Supply of the Vertebral Column and Spinal Cord in Man. New York, Springer-Verlag, 1977.
14. Cyriax, J.: Dural pain. Lancet *1*:919–921, 1978.
15. DePalma, A. F., and Rothman, R. H.: The Intervertebral Disc. Philadelphia, W. B. Saunders Co., 1970.
16. Dommisse, G. F.: The Arteries and Veins of the Human Spinal Cord from Birth. Edinburgh, Churchill-Livingstone, 1975.
17. Evans, J. G.: Neurogenic intermittent claudication. Br. Med. J. *2*:985–987, 1964.
18. Feeney, J. F., and Watterson, R. L.: The development of the vascular pattern within the walls of the central nervous system of the chick embryo. J. Morphol. *78*:231–303, 1946.
19. Ferguson, W. P.: Some observations on the circulation in fetal and infant spines. J. Bone Joint Surg. *32*:640–645, 1950.
20. Galante, J. O.: Tensile properties of the human lumbar annulus fibrosus. Acta Orthop. Scand. (Suppl.) *100*:1–91, 1967.
21. Giles, L. G. F., and Taylor, J. R.: Innervation of lumbar zygapophyseal joint synovial folds. Acta Orthop. Scand. *58*:43–46, 1987.
22. Gillilan, L. A.: The arterial blood supply of the human spinal cord. J. Comp. Neurol. *110*:75–103, 1958.
23. Gillilan, L. A.: Veins of the spinal cord. Neurology *20*:860–868, 1970.
24. Golub, B. S., and Silverman, B.: Transforaminal ligaments of the lumbar spine. J. Bone Joint Surg. *51A*:947–956, 1969.
25. Groen, G. J., Baljet, B., and Drukker, J.: The innervation of the spinal dura mater: anatomy and clinical implications. Acta Neurochir. *92*:39–46, 1988.

26. Groen, G. J., Baljet, B., and Drukker, J.: The nerves and nerve plexuses of the human vertebral column. Am. J. Anat. 1990 (in press).
27. Hassler, O.: Blood supply to human spinal cord. Arch. Neurol. *15*:302–307, 1966.
28. Hasue, M., Kunogi, J., Konno, S., and Kikuchi, S.: Classification by position of dorsal root ganglia in the lumbosacral region. Spine *14*:1261–1264, 1989.
29. Herren, R. Y., and Alexander, L.: Sulcal and intrinsic blood vessels of human spinal cord. Arch. Neurol. Psychiat. (Chic.) *41*:678–683, 1939.
30. Hirsch, C.: Studies on mechanism of low back pain. Acta Orthop. Scand. *22*:184–231, 1953.
31. Hirsch, C., Inglemark, B., and Miller, M.: The anatomical basis for low back pain. Acta Orthop. Scand. *33*:1–17, 1963.
32. Holm, S., Maroudas, A., Urban, J. P. G., and Nachemson, A.: Nutrition of the intervertebral disc: an in vivo study of solute transport. Clin. Orthop. *178*: 1977.
33. Holm, S., Maroudas, A., Urban, J. P. G., et al.: Nutrition of the intervertebral disc: solute transport and metabolism. Connect. Tissue Res. *8*:101–110, 1981.
34. Humzah, M. D., and Soames, R. W.: Human intervertebral disc: structure and function. Anat. Rec. *220*:337–356, 1988.
35. Ireland, W. P., Fletcher, T. F., and Bingham, C.: Quantification of microvasculature in the canine spinal cord. Anat. Rec. *200*:103–113, 1981.
36. Jung, A., and Brunschwig, A.: Recherches histologiques sur l'innervation des articulations et des corps vertebreaux. Presse Med. *40*:316–317, 1932.
37. Junghanns, H.: Der Lumboscralwinkel. Dtsch. Z. Chir. *213*:332, 1929.
38. Kadish, L. J., and Simmons, E. H.: Anomalies of the lumbosacral nerve roots. J. Bone Joint Surg. *66B*:411–416, 1984.
39. Kadyi, H.: Über die Blutgefasse des menschlichen Ruckenmarkes. Nach einer im XV Bande der Denkschriften d. math-naturw. Cl. d. Akad. d. Wissensch. in Krakau erschienen Morphology, aus dem Polnischen Ubersaatz vom Verfasser. Lemberg, Grubrnowicz & Schmidt, 1889.
40. Kaisary, A. V., and Smith, P.: Spinal cord ischemia after ligation of both internal iliac arteries during radical cystoprostectomy. Urology *25*:395–397, 1985.
41. Kikuchi, S., and Hasue, M.: Anatomic features of the furcal nerve and its clinical significance. Spine *11*:1002–1007, 1986.
42. Kikuchi, S., and Hasue, M.: Combined contrast studies in lumbar spine diseases. Spine *13*:1327–1331, 1988.
43. Kimmel, D. L.: Innervation of the spinal dura and the dura of the posterior cranial fossa. Neurology (Minn.) *11*:800–809, 1986.
44. Kobrine, A. I., Doyle, D. F., and Rizzoli, H. V.: Spinal cord blood flow as affected by changes in systemic arterial blood pressure. J. Neurosurg. *44*:12–15, 1976.
45. LaBan, M. M.: "Vesper's curse"—night pain—the bane of Hypnos. Arch. Phys. Med. Rehabil. *65*:501–504, 1984.
46. LaBan, M. M., and Wesolowski, D. P.: Night pain associated with diminished cardiopulmonary compliance. Am. J. Phys. Med. Rehabil. *67*:155–160, 1988.
47. Larmon, A. W.: An anatomic study of the lumbosacral region in relation to low back pain and sciatica. Ann. Surg. *119*:892, 1944.
48. Lasjaunias, P., Vallee, B., Person, H., et al.: The lateral artery of the upper cervical spinal cord. J. Neurosurg. *63*:235–241, 1985.
49. Lobosky, J. M., Hitchon, P. W., Torner, J. C., and Yamada, T.: Spinal cord autoregulation in the sheep. Curr. Surg. *41*:264–267, 1984.
50. von Luschka, H.: Die Halbgelenke des menschlichen Korpers. Berlin, Karpess, 1858.
51. von Luschka, H.: Die Nerven des menschlichen Wirbelkanales. Tubingen, H. Laupp, 1850.
52. Madsen, J. R., and Heros, R. C.: Spinal arteriovenous malformations and neurogenic claudication. J. Neurosurg. *68*:793–797, 1988.
53. Malinsky, J.: The ontogenetic development of nerve terminations in the intervertebral discs of man. Acta Anat. *38*:96–113, 1959.
54. Marcus, M. L., Heistad, D. D., Ehrhardt, J. C., and Abboud, F. M.: Regulation of total and regional spinal cord blood flow. Circ. Res. *41*:128–134, 1977.
55. Maroudas, A., Nachemson, A., Stockwell, R. A., and Urban, J. P. G.: Factors involved in the nutrition of human lumbar intervertebral disc: cellularity and diffusion of glucose in vitro. J. Anat. *120*:113–130, 1975.
56. Maroudas, A.: Nutrition and metabolism of the intervertebral disc. *In* Ghosh, P. (ed.): The Biology of the Intervertebral Disc. Vol. II. Boca Raton, FL, CRC Press, 1988.
57. McCouch, G. P., During, I. D., and Ling, T. H.: Location of receptors for tonic reflexes. J. Neurophysiol. *14*:191–195, 1951.
58. Molina, J. E., Cogordan, J., Einzig, S., et al.: Adequacy of ascending-descending aorta shunt during cross-clamping of the thoracic aorta for prevention of spinal cord injury. J. Thorac. Cardiovasc. Surg. *90*:126–136, 1985.
59. Nachemson, A.: The load on lumbar discs in different positions of the body. Clin. Orthop. *45*:107–122, 1966.
60. Nade, S., Bell, S., and Wyke, B. D.: The innervation of the lumbar spine joints and its significance. J. Bone Joint Surg. *62B*:225–261, 1980.
61. Parke, W. W.: Applied anatomy of the spine. *In* Rothman, R. H., and Simeone, F. A. (eds.): The Spine. 2nd ed. Vol. I. Philadelphia, W. B. Saunders Co., 1982, pp. 18–51.
62. Parke, W. W.: The vascular relations of the upper cervical vertebrae. Orthop. Clin. North Am. *9*:879–889, 1978.
63. Parke, W. W.: Arteriovenous anastomoses in the spinal cord: probable role in blood flow autoregulation. Anat. Rec. *223*:87A, 1989.
64. Parke, W. W., Gammel, K., and Rothman, R. H.: Arterial vascularization of the cauda equina. J. Bone Joint Surg. *63A*:53–62, 1981.
65. Parke, W. W.: Paper delivered at the international symposium on percutaneous lumbar discectomy, Graduate Hospital, Philadelphia, November 1987.
66. Parke, W. W.: Correlative anatomy of cervical spondylotic myelopathy. Spine *13*:831–837, 1988.
67. Parke, W. W., Rothman, R. H., and Brown, M. D.: The pharyngovertebral veins: an anatomic rationale for Grisel's syndrome. J. Bone Joint Surg. *66A*:568–574, 1984.
68. Parke, W. W., and Watanabe, R.: Lumbosacral in-

tersegmental epispinal axons and ectopic ventral nerve rootlets. J. Neurosurg. *67*:269–277, 1987.

69. Parke, W. W., and Watanabe, R.: The intrinsic vasculature of the lumbosacral spinal nerve roots. Spine *10*:508–515, 1985.
70. Parke, W. W., and Watanabe, R.: Adhesions of the ventral lumbar dura: an adjunct source of discogenic pain? Spine 1990 (in press).
71. Parke, W. W., and Valsamis, M. P.: The ampulloglomerular organ: an unusual neurovascular complex in the suboccipital region. Anat. Rec. *159*:193–198, 1967.
72. Pedersen, H. E., Blunck, C. F. J., and Gardner, E.: The anatomy of the lumbosacral posterior rami and meningeal branches of spinal nerves (sinu-vertebral nerves). J. Bone Joint Surg. *38A*:377–391, 1956.
73. Petter, C. K.: Methods of measuring the pressure of intervertebral discs. J. Bone Joint Surg. *15*:365, 1933.
74. Piasecka-Kacperska, A., and Gladykowska-Rzeczycka, J.: The sacral plexus in primates. Folia Morphol. (Warsz.) *31*:21–31, 1972.
75. Puschel, J.: Der Wassergehalt normaler and degenerierter Zwischenwirbelscheiben. Beitr. Path. Anat. *84*:123–130, 1930.
76. Roofe, P. G.: Innervation of anulus fibrosus and posterior longitudinal ligament. Arch Neurol. Psych. *44*:100–103, 1940.
77. Rydevik, B., Holm, S., and Brown, M. D.: Nutrition of spinal nerve roots: the role of diffusion from the cerebrospinal fluid. Transactions of the 30th Annual Meeting of the Orthopaedic Research Society, Atlanta, GA, February 1984.
78. Schiff, D. C. M., and Parke, W. W.: The arterial supply of the odontoid process. Anat. Rec. *172*:399–400, 1972.
79. Schmorl, G., and Junghanns, H.: The Human Spine in Health and Disease. New York, Grune & Stratton, 1959.
80. Siberstein, C. E.: The evolution of degenerative changes in the cervical spine and an investigation into the "joints of Luschka." Clin. Orthop. *40*:184–204, 1965.
81. Stilwell, D. L., Jr.: The nerve supply of the vertebral column and its associated structures in the monkey. Anat. Rec. *125*:139–169, 1956.
82. Svensson, L. G., Rickards, E., Coull, A., et al.: Relationship of spinal cord blood flow to vascular anatomy during thoracic aorta cross-clamping and shunting. J. Thorac. Cardiovasc. Surg. *91*:71–78, 1986.
83. Takata, K., Inoue, S., Takashi, K., and Ohtsuka, Y.: Swelling of the cauda equina in patients who have herniation of a lumbar disc. J. Bone Joint Surg. *70A*:361–368, 1988.
84. Tsukada, K.: Histologische Studien über die Zwischenwirbelscheibe des Mesnschen. Alterveranderungen Akad. Kioto *25*:1–29, 207–909, 1939.
85. Turnbull, I. M., Brieg, A., and Hassler, O.: Blood supply of cervical spinal cord in man. J. Neurosurg. *24*:951–965, 1966.
86. Wadouh, F., Arndt, C-F., Opperman, E., et al.: The mechanism of spinal cord injury after simple and double aortic cross-clamping. J. Thorac. Cardiovasc. Surg. *92*:121–127, 1986.
87. Watanabe, R., and Parke, W. W.: The vascular and neural pathology of lumbosacral spinal stenosis. J. Neurosurg. *65*:64–70, 1986.
88. Watanabe, R., and Parke, W. W.: Structure of lumbosacral spinal nerve roots: anatomy and pathology in spinal stenosis. J. Clin. Orthop. Surg. (Japan) *22*:529–539, 1987.
89. Wetzel, F. T., and LaRocca, H.: Grisel's syndrome. a review. Clin. Orthop. *240*:141–152, 1989.
90. White, A., and Panjabi, M.: Clinical Biomechanics of the Spine. Philadelphia, J. B. Lippincott, 1978.
91. Wiberg, G.: Back pain in relation to nerve supply of intervertebral disc. Acta Orthop. Scand. *19*:211–221, 1949.
92. Willis, T. A.: Nutrient arteries of the vertebral bodies. J. Bone Joint Surg. *31*:538–541, 1949.
93. Yamamoto, H.: Quantitative measurements of blood flow in cauda equina in spinal cords of monkeys by using radioactive microspheres. J. Jap. College Angiol. *22*:35–42, 1982.
94. Yoshizawa, H., O'Brien, J. P., Thomas-Smith, W., and Trumper, M.: The neuropathology of intervertebral discs removed for low back pain. J. Pathol. *132*:95–104, 1980.

CHAPTER

3

LUMBAR MUSCULATURE: ANATOMY AND FUNCTION

Tom G. Mayer, M.D.

Muscles are the dynamic stabilizers of the spine, with functions identical to those performed in other parts of the skeleton. In their ability to control movement and provide stability, the muscles must be seen not as isolated structures, but as part of a system including ligaments, joints and their capsules, in an intricate neurologic feedback mechanism we generally term "coordination." Much of our understanding about the importance of this entire system, and specifically of the muscular component, comes from the extremities, where there are accessible, easily visualized structures and a contralateral side for comparison. Measurement in the spine is considerably more difficult, but new technology involving quantitative assessment, electromyography, and mathematical modeling is rapidly increasing the level of knowledge about the spinal musculoligamentous system.

PHYSIOLOGY

Muscle, the dynamic control mechanism of the skeletal system, consists of long cells specifically adapted for shortening. Voluntary, or skeletal, muscle is by far the muscle type of greatest volume in humans. The musculature involved in spinal movement and control is in turn the largest complex of skeletal muscles in the body. The axial muscle fibers may be only a few millimeters in diameter but may extend 5 cm or more in length. The muscle fiber is surrounded by an external layer known as the *sarcolemma,* which connects one fiber to adjacent fibers or tendons, and is sharply indented by a nerve fibril at the *myoneural junction.* The muscle fiber is filled with many nuclei and smaller myofibrils aligned longitudinally in such a way that alternating light and dark striations are formed ("striated muscle"). The myofibrils are made up of even smaller myofilaments of two varieties: one formed with the protein *myosin,* and the other consisting of *actin.*[18]

Under normal circumstances, contraction of striated muscle does not occur without neural stimulus; this is a necessary condition for skeletal muscle, whereas contraction of cardiac and most smooth muscle fibers can trigger the firing of adjacent fibers without neural stimulation. The cellular mechanics of contractions are relatively simple: actin filaments (light band) slide over the myosin filaments until, with complete contraction, they are completely overlapped and the light bands of the resting muscle are visually eliminated. The biochemical reactions, however, are far more complex. Contraction is initiated by release of acetylcholine at the myoneural junction, probably changing the permeability of the sarcolemma to sodium and potassium ions through depolarization. The contraction that follows is energized by conversion of adenosine triphosphate (ATP) to adenosine diphosphate (ADP), which in turn is powered by the hydrolysis of glucose into water and oxygen. This process requires oxygen. In a situation in which adequate oxygen cannot be supplied (such as vigorous exercise), glucose is converted to lactic acid, producing less energy per unit substrate and an "oxygen debt." The higher the concentration of lactic acid produced, the more time is required for the metabolic breakdown product to be removed, lengthening recovery time.

Over the past 20 years, it has been recognized that distinctly different motor units are present within a muscle. One type has a slow twitch with good fatigue resistance and low tension development. Its muscle fibers have rich capillary beds and high concentrations of mitochondrial enzymes with relatively low concentrations of glycogen and myosin ATPase. They appear ideally suited for aerobic activity with fatigue resistance (Group I). These functions appear in areas with aerobic or endurance demands. A second type (Group II) shows a fast twitch with good strength, but poor endurance. These fibers have contrasting biochemical characteristics and appear organized for high-intensity, short-duration bursts; they are found in muscles used for short-term, high-energy demands requiring a rapid response. Finally, there is also an intermediate variety of fiber, melding the characteristics of both fast- and slow-twitch fibers. Muscles dominated by the capillary-rich, slow-twitch or Group I fibers (as well as the intermediate fibers) tend to be dark in color, whereas the fast twitch–dominated muscles tend to be pale by comparison.

The interrelationship between the biomechanical and histochemical properties of muscle fibers is a fascinating area for study. It is now clear that the use to which a muscle is put can adapt the muscle by selectively stressing one of the types of motor units. However, the concept of actual conversion of one motor unit type to another remains highly controversial. Furthermore, fiber type composition in the spinal musculature is only now beginning to be studied.[6]

In view of the long human gestation period, an infant is probably born with its full complement of muscle fibers. It appears that the growth in muscle size is due to an increase in size of the fibers, rather than an increase in numbers. The strength of contraction, however, appears to be related not only to muscular factors such as muscle size, fiber type, and fiber number, but also (and perhaps to a greater extent) to neural factors. The specific characteristics that affect motor unit firing include the frequency, extent, order, and synchrony of stimulation, which determine fiber recruitment, as well as control of function through the pyramidal tract. Training may affect several of these factors, as does the effect of certain anabolic hormones (both endogenous and exogenous); the characteristic rapid increase in strength and muscle diameter under the hormonal influence of puberty is a specific example. Muscle hypertrophy appears to occur through two processes that may proceed simultaneously: myofibrillar hypertrophy or splitting. The degree and sequence in which these changes occur are under study, but it appears clear that isometric contraction (in which the contracting muscle is not permitted to shorten) is far more effective in increasing muscle bulk than concentric (isotonic or isokinetic) contractions. By contrast, various pathologic factors such as denervation, starvation, or immobilization may produce muscle atrophy. Thus, we may surmise that multiple factors, including a functional nerve supply, good nutrition, and periodic muscle activity, are all necessary to maintain and increase muscle bulk.

ANATOMY

The spine consists of a series of bilaterally symmetric joints phylogenetically adapted for protection of the neural communications network linking brain to periphery.[9] The critical role of the spine musculature in dynamically protecting and vitalizing these articulations with their passive ligamentous supports and accompanying neural transmission lines is currently only partially understood. Our understanding of the evolutionary changes in the role of spine musculature has been greatly enhanced by the work of Gracovetsky and Farfan.[7] Greatly simplified, their theory begins with the concept that the large paravertebral spine muscles were developed to provide lateral flexion for propelling a body through water, best exemplified by the lateral tail motion of the fish. This form of locomotion ultimately evolved to the predominantly flexion-extension mode of propulsion that occurs in the better-adapted four-footed land animals. More recently, the special adaptation of man to a bipedal stance necessitated a lordotic lumbar spine for balance and ambulation. In this regard, Gracovetsky and Farfan proposed a human machine model to describe ambulation.[7] They postulated that, just as laterally bending a segmented curved rod produces torsion at the ends of the rod, so the lateral bend of the lordotic spine powers the progressive advancement of the hips, thus driving the lower extremities during locomotion. In this way, their theory contradicts a more commonly held assumption that the legs drive the trunk.

Another unique factor for humans involves bipedal balance and the need to bend efficiently to allow the hands to touch the ground. A stable "biomechanical chain" is necessary to transfer forces from hands through arms, shoulder girdle, spine, pelvis, legs, and feet to make renewed ground contact (Fig. 3–1).

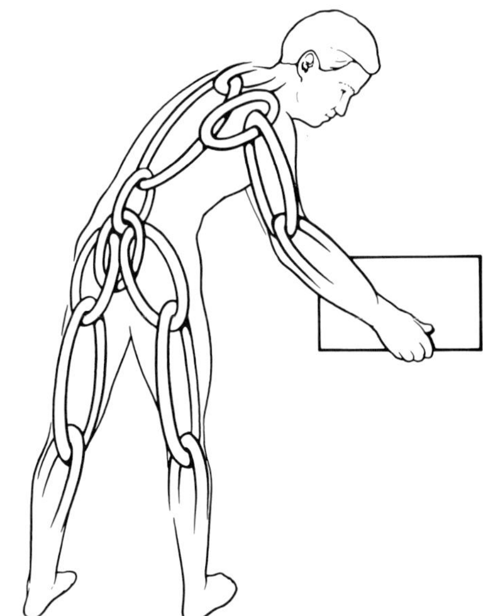

Figure 3–1. The "biomechanical chain" for permitting manual handling of objects while maintaining balance over bipedal base, transmitting forces through the four functional units: (1) upper extremities, (2) shoulder girdle/thoracic spine, (3) lumbar spine/pelvic unit, and (4) lower extremities. (From Mayer, T. G., and Gatchel, R. J.: Functional Restoration for Spinal Disorders: The Sports Medicine Approach. Philadelphia, Lea & Febiger, 1988.)

It is inefficient to control static forward bending with muscles alone, and the space required for the abdominal-thoracic contents imposes size restrictions on spine muscles. The evolutionary solution is twofold: (1) strong, elastic posterior spinal ligaments (midline ligaments, joint capsules, and lumbodorsal fascia) producing passive restraint to spine flexion and allowing static "hanging on the ligaments" subject only to slow "creep," without muscular effort; and (2) an "external power pack" of pelvic motors and stabilizers in extension and abduction. This combination of a posterior ligamentous complex and critical muscles of the buttocks and posterior thigh (along with the psoas muscle controlling the degree of lordosis) permits the spine to function in a way not generally recognized; i.e., as a crane whose boom is the ligament-stabilized flexed spine, whose fulcrum is the hips, and whose engine is the pelvic extensor musculature. This work is discussed in greater detail in the treatise cited earlier.[7] It is supported by work on lumbar spine mobility demonstrating the pattern of spine and hip mobility through a full forward bend, in which the spine flexes first to "hang on its ligaments" with only gradual engagement of the hip flexion mechanism, allowing efficient, limited use of the lumbar paravertebral spine musculature.[17] This underlying mechanism is further confirmed by the appearance of an electromyographically "silent period," when the spine is fully flexed in forward bend, a seeming paradox since the sagittal movement is quite large in this position.

It is beyond the scope of this chapter to discuss these concepts in greater depth, but it is intended to promote an appreciation of the spinal musculature as a component of a "functional unit" encompassing paravertebral, abdominal, buttock, and hamstring muscles critical for bipedal stance, locomotion, and balance. Moreover, this spine-pelvis module is inextricably linked to the cervicothoracic–shoulder girdle–upper extremity modules and to the lower extremity module, providing a complete biomechanical chain that allows manual handling tasks by the upper extremities to be performed while a stable foot-ground contact is maintained.

The small interconnecting vertebrae with their multiplanar motions and "coupling" through the three-joint complex make it difficult to assign specific uniaxial functions to individual groups of muscles. For instance, the erector spinae group of muscles are generally thought of as extensors of the spine. However, functioning unilaterally, they may also be powerful abductors or lateral stabilizers (assisting with locomotion) and have also been shown to function to some extent in spine derotation.[17] Similarly, the lateral abdominal musculature (internal and external oblique and transversus abdominis) may act both as spine flexors and extensors (working through the lumbodorsal fascia).[7] These muscles, forming the anterolateral portion of the soft tissue "barrel-like" lumbar support structures, are powerful spine rotators, and assist in abduction and lateral stabilization.

In describing the gross anatomy of the spinal muscular functional unit, it must be emphasized that long-ignored posterior stabilizers are of extreme importance in spinal functional integrity. The intrinsic lumbar musculature is only a part of the functional unit. The lumbodorsal fascia, interspinous ligaments, and facet joint capsules are important intrinsic stabilizing structures. In fact, the cavalier surgical handling of these collagenous and elastic structures may be as responsible as mishandling of muscles for the high rate of recurrences of lumbar dysfunction in postoperative patients.

Through evolution, the spine musculature has developed certain characteristics. The most superficial layers are truly extensions of the shoulder girdle "functional unit" and include muscles such as the serratus posterior and latissimus dorsi. Their proximal function is confirmed by their innervation from the proximal spinal cord. The true spinal muscles, by contrast, have segmental innervations that arise from the posterior rami of the contiguous spinal nerves (the same nerves that receive sensory input from facet capsules, posterior ligaments, and peripheral annulus). Although the true spinal muscles function together, their most characteristic differentiating factor is length. The deepest muscles, such as the interspinalis, span only a single segment, while the most superficial muscles may traverse a large portion of the entire spinal column. Controlled local action of individual vertebrae is a critically important part of spine function, and loss of appropriate musculoligamentous control may contribute to various pathologic syndromes such as segmental instability and degenerative disc-facet syndromes. However, we are as yet too unsophisticated to detect discrete intersegmental aberrations and must rely on measurements of function in several contiguous segments. On the one hand, this is as crude as measuring the function of a leg, rather than of the hip, knee, or ankle separately; on the other, it is a step forward from having no assessment capability or understanding of functional capacity whatsoever.

MUSCULATURE OF THE SPINAL FUNCTIONAL UNIT

Intrinsic Muscles

Erector Spinae. This large and superficial muscle lies just deep to the lumbodorsal fascia and arises from an aponeurosis on the sacrum, iliac crest, and thoracolumbar spinous processes.[9] The muscle mass is poorly differentiated but divides into three sections in the upper lumbar area: (1) the *iliocostalis,* which is most lateral and inserts into the angles of the rib; (2) the intermediate column, the *longissimus,* which inserts onto the tips of the spinous processes of thoracic and cervical vertebrae; and (3) the *spinalis,* which is most medial and inserts onto the spinous processes of the cervical and thoracic vertebrae (Fig. 3–2).

Multifidi. This series of small muscles, best developed in the lumbar spine, originates on the mamillary processes of the superior facets and runs upward and medially for two to four segments, inserting on the spinous processes (Fig. 3–3). This orientation produces greater capacity for rotation and abduction, in addition to extension.

Quadratus Lumborum. This most lateral of the lumbar musculature (Fig. 3–2) originates on the iliac crest and iliolumbar ligament and runs obliquely to insert into the lowest rib and transverse processes of the upper four lumbar vertebrae.

Deep Muscles. The *interspinalis* are pairs of deep muscles spanning one segment on either side of the strong and elastic interspinous ligaments. The *intertransversarii,* in the lumbar spine, consist of a pair of muscles on each side, spanning the transverse processes of ad-

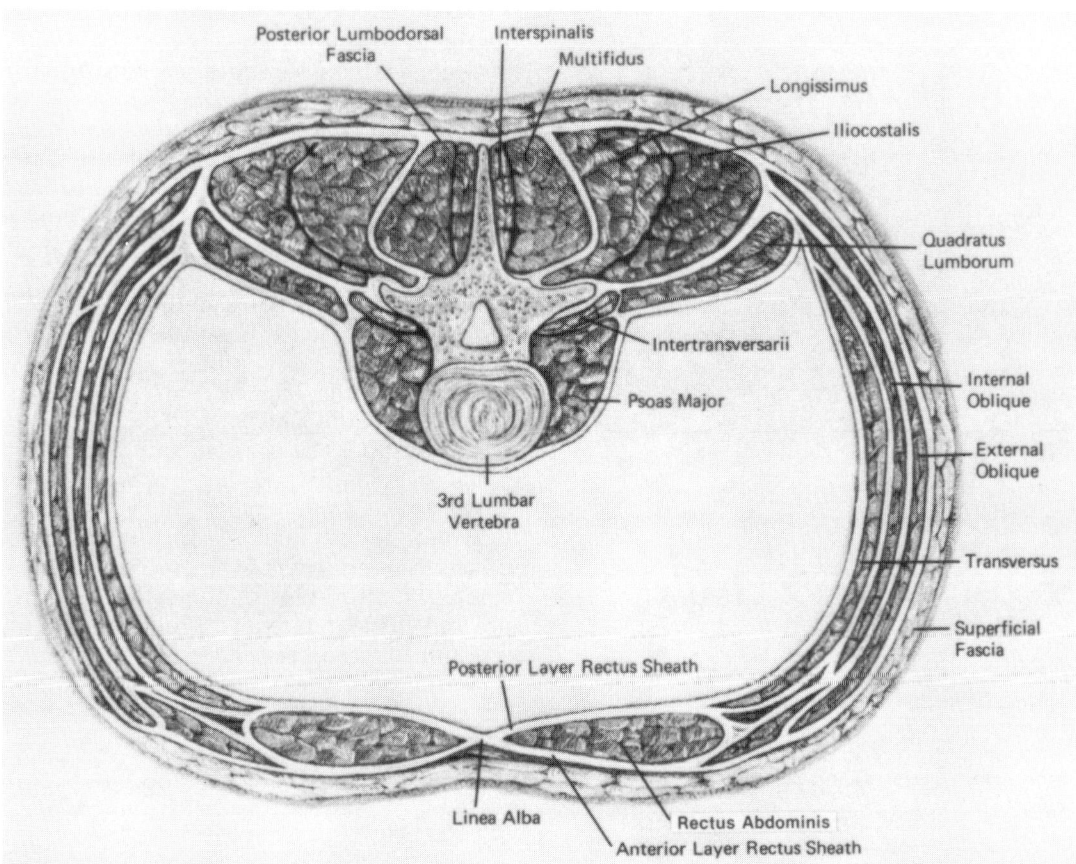

Figure 3–2. Cross section of body musculature and fascia through L3 showing intrinsic spinal musculature. Abdominal muscles also function in containing viscera and respiration. (From Finneson, B. Low Back Pain, 2nd ed. Philadelphia, J. B. Lippincott Co., 1977.)

jacent vertebrae. Each side has dorsal and ventral slips.

Psoas Muscles. The psoas major, although usually thought of primarily as a hip flexor, has a direct section on the vertebral column as it originates bilaterally from the lumbar vertebral bodies and posterior aspects of the transverse processes, thus providing the only muscle acting anterior to the sagittal axis. Paradoxically, however, the psoas is usually an intersegmental extensor in the midlumbar spine, even as it flexes at the lumbosacral junction in the process of increasing lumbar lordosis. It is an important spine stabilizer in sitting and standing.[18] Acting asymmetrically, the psoas may produce ipsilateral abduction concentrically or contralateral abduction resistance eccentrically to maintain coronal balance.

Extrinsic Muscles

Abdominal Musculature. There are four important abdominal muscles in spine function. The *rectus abdominis* is primarily a flexor, spanning the anterior abdomen from its origin on the pubic crest to its insertion on the anterior rib cage between the fifth and seventh ribs. The obliquely oriented abdominal muscles are, from superficial to deep, the *external oblique, internal oblique,* and *transversalis abdominis,* and may all act to produce rotation or abduction, as well as assisting both flexion and extension under different circumstances.[7] The fibers of the external oblique run in an anterointerior direction from attachments on the lower eight ribs to insert along the anterior rectus sheath and anterior wall of the iliac crest (Fig. 3–4). The internal oblique fibers are almost perpendicular in direction to those of the internal oblique fibers. This muscle courses transversely only in its lowermost portion, with most of the muscle running anteriorly and proximally from its origins from the lumbodorsal fascia and anterior two thirds of the iliac crest. It inserts on the lower three ribs and rectus sheath anteriorly. The transversalis

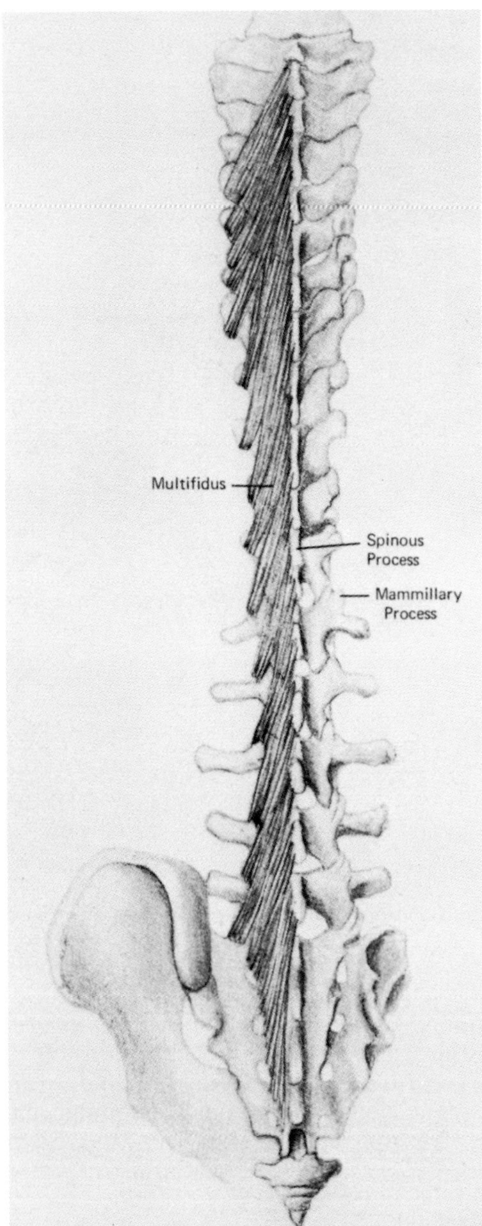

Figure 3–3. The multifidi consist of numerous small muscle slits that arise from small bony prominences on the articular facet. (From Finneson, B. Low Back Pain, 2nd ed. Philadelphia, J. B. Lippincott Co., 1977.)

abdominis, the deepest muscle of the group, runs transversely like a horizontal girdle from the lumbodorsal fascia, anterior iliac crest, and inner surface of the lower six ribs. The main mass of the muscle inserts into the linea alba in the midline. It is probable that in the act of flexion, the abdominal muscles not only act to create a ventral movement, but also stabilize the spine posteriorly through their action on the lumbodorsal fascia.

Gluteal Muscles. The large muscles of the buttocks, chiefly the *gluteus maximus, gluteus medius,* and *gluteus minimus,* act variously as hip extensors and abductors. As such, they act as motor to the spinal "boom" in forward bending and twisting movements. They also provide the "spinal engine" for locomotion (Fig. 3–5).[7, 9]

Posterior Thigh Musculature. Muscles attached to the ischial tuberosity, such as the hamstrings, are also strong pelvic extensors acting about the hip fulcrum. As such, they provide powerful assistance to the musculature of the buttocks in raising and lowering the pelvis. The hamstrings also provide efficient passive restraint on pelvic flexion when the knees are locked in extension. In the absence of active contraction of the posterior thigh and spinal extensor musculature, the hamstrings are the inferior restraint providing the most efficient forward flexion.

ELECTROPHYSIOLOGY

Electromyography (EMG) has been used for some time to analyze normal function and

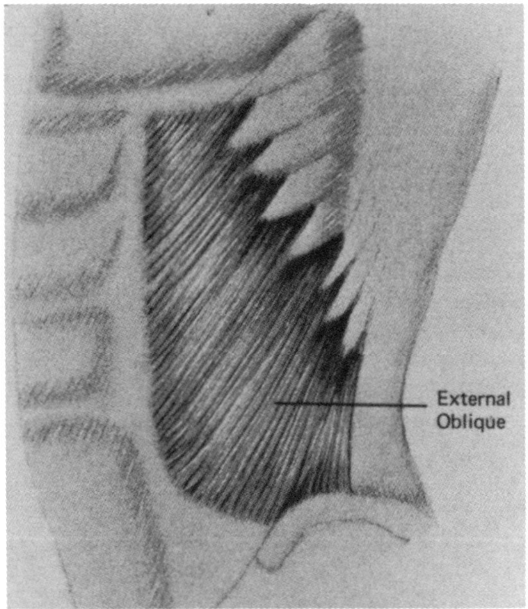

Figure 3–4. External oblique muscle. (From Finneson, B. Low Back Pain, 2nd ed. Philadelphia, J. B. Lippincott Co., 1977.)

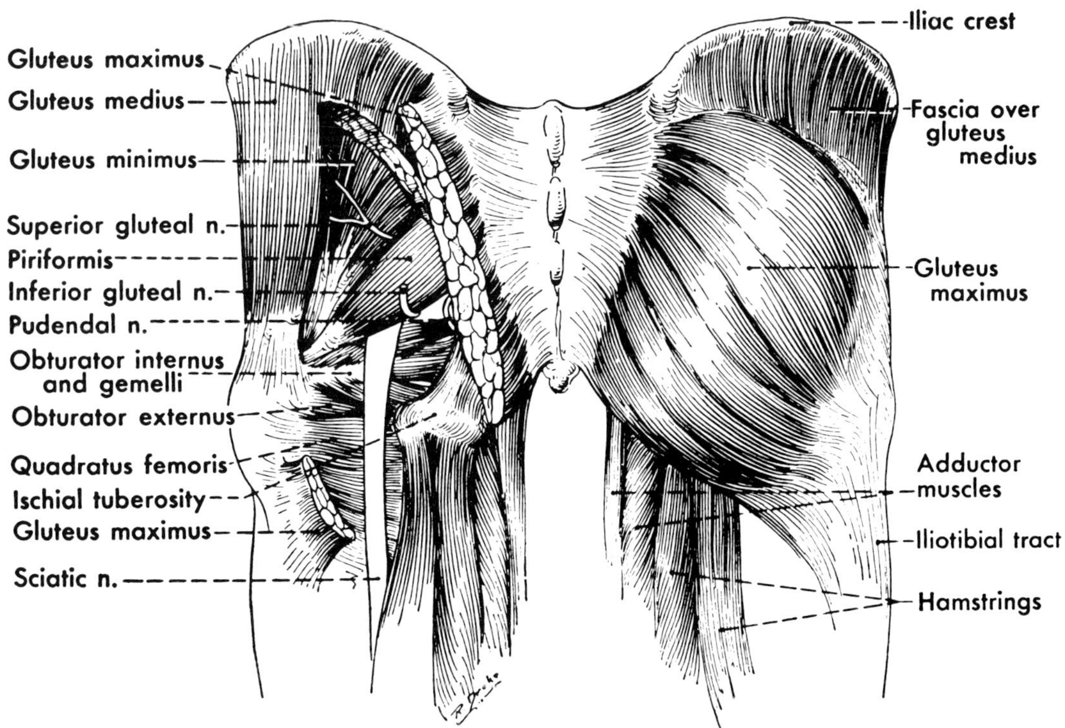

Figure 3–5. Musculature of the buttocks and proximal thigh. (From Hollinshead, W. H. Anatomy for Surgeons, Vol. 3, 3rd ed. Philadelphia, J. B. Lippincott Co., 1982.)

pathologic conditions in the spinal musculature. Trunk stabilization and initiation of motion are two particular patterns of EMG activity that have been clearly identified in trunk movements.[1, 5, 19, 21] Different movements recruit muscles in varying patterns of activity. However, most spinal intrinsic musculature is involved in the initiation of most movements, as well as the maintenance of posture.

The longissimus and other paravertebral muscles are frequently quiet in the "flexion-relaxation" position, in which the flexed spine is "hanging on its posterior ligaments." They are also relatively quiet in gentle extension of the spine, but with full extension, lateral bend, or torsion, the role of the intrinsic musculature as a "balancer" of the spine is demonstrated by its prominent activity.[5] Recently, it has been found that loading of the flexed spine in the posture that normally produces EMG silence leads to an increase in myoelectric activity in the intrinsic spine musculature in proportion to the loads applied. This is similar to the changes seen in loading the spine in the upright position.[21] Presumably, these increasing loads stress and stretch the posterior ligamentous structures sufficiently to require compensatory muscle firing. The multifidus and rotator muscles have similar activity in sagittal plane movements, but they are active in rotation to the contralateral side, in conjunction with bilateral abdominal muscular contraction.[16] These muscles, however, also achieve flexion-relaxation in silence when the spine is in the ligamentous support phase.

It is interesting to note that early investigators[4] discovered that the slouching or full flexion seated posture (often considered "bad posture") is in reality quite comfortable for prolonged periods and that EMG silence is generally maintained in the erector spinae.

Contractions of the abdominal musculature, particularly muscles attaching to the lumbodorsal fascia, are also important in maintaining flexed postures and initiating extension. The lateral pull on the lumbodorsal fascia has two effects: creating a tightening of the cranial-caudal dimension in the lumbar spine and "encapsulating" the intrinsic spine musculature to provide greater efficiency. In so doing, the abdominal mechanism also serves to extend the flexed spine and/or resist flexion loads.[7]

The raw EMG signal has predominated in the literature on spine muscular activity, estimates of loads being made on the basis of integrated EMG (iEMG) or root mean square (RMS) EMG. Recently, observation of the myoelectric spectrum through computerized mean power frequency (MPF) analysis has yielded information about fatigue resistance or endurance of spine musculature, and promises to be a useful tool for future clinical applications and understanding of functional interrelationships.[12]

TRUNK MUSCLE STRENGTH

The obvious relationship between the joints of an extremity and the strength of its contiguous musculature, in both supernormal (athletic) and pathologic (traumatic, arthritic, or immobilized) situations, has stimulated many investigators to study similar relationships in the spine.[4, 11, 17] The early investigators were limited to the use of cable tensiometers, and isometric and isotonic machines. More recent work has been done using individually modified isokinetic dynamometers in various positions.[10, 22, 23] Current technology has provided computerized isokinetic devices for separately measuring isolated lumbar trunk strength in the sagittal and axial planes.[13, 15, 16]

Cady and colleagues[2] demonstrated a relationship between physical fitness and back injury rates, which has been confirmed through isometric lifting testing in several industrial environments. While joint range of motion appears to be an independent variable in trunk function, musculature factors such as trunk strength, endurance, and neuromuscular coordination appear to be critical factors in maintaining the integrity of the lumbar spine.

Tests of isokinetic trunk strength in the sagittal plane have revealed a typical gaussian distribution of strength in the normal population. Normalization of strength by body weight narrows the width of the distribution curve, but use of lean body mass does not appear to offer greater advantages. When genders are compared using body weight as a normalizing factor, males appear to be 10 to 20 per cent stronger than females and to have greater ability to sustain strength at high speeds. Age through the fifth decade does not seem to be a critical variable.

Similar findings are noted when isolated axial strength is measured. Ability to generate torsional torques within the same individual is generally symmetric, although there is a trend toward slightly greater strength rotating to the dominant side in males, which may be due to training in pulling activities. There appears to be a greater tolerance for applying loads at high speeds in the axial plane. This may be due to the greater fast-twitch fiber–type composition of the lateral abdominal musculature, which is primarily responsible for axial plane lumbar spine movements, although work in this area is only in its infancy.

In the pathologic state, significant decrements of muscle strength are frequently noted. Populations with chronic back pain show a selective loss of extensor strength compared with flexors and an inability to maintain strength at high speeds.[15] In rotation, there is also a substantial decrement in strength, but it appears to be relatively symmetric in the chronic state and less subject to high-speed variation.[15] Most work up to this time has been based on peak torque measurements, but advances in computerization make measurements of work performed, power consumed, and curve analysis possible. The latter is important in assessment by allowing variability determination (average points variance). Since only maximal muscular effort is truly reproducible, variability of curve shape and height becomes an excellent measure of effort. In the absence of visual feedback of trunk muscle function to the clinician, these measures become exceedingly important in documenting optimal functional capacity and effort.[8]

By contrast, supernormal individuals who have been studied, such as ballet dancers, appear to exceed mean torque–body weight strengths for the normal population by 15 to 40 per cent. Unlike the pathologic and normal populations, they show almost no "high-speed dropoff," i.e., decreased torque output at high speeds. They also maintain a very stable ratio of extensor-to-flexor strength.

The factors that contribute to decreased strength in the pathologic state are not entirely understood. While muscle atrophy undoubtedly occurs with prolonged disuse and deconditioning, pain may inhibit neuromuscular function through feedback-reflex mechanisms. Similarly, various psychosocially induced phenomena, such as anxiety, fear of reinjury, or depression, may unconsciously attenuate effort, producing submaximal measurements. At this time, it does not appear that techniques are available for assessing subject motivation, although curve variability appears to be a promising tool for identifying attempts to consciously produce submaximal output.[14]

SUMMARY

Trunk musculature is among the most complex in the body. Great strides have been made in the last two decades in analyzing the relationship between the structure and function of spine musculature, but difficulty with visual feedback to the system makes progress slow. New diagnostic and treatment capabilities have been developed that are accelerating our rate of acquisition of knowledge. By inference, many of the treatment protocols used in the extremities can be applied to the low back. Potential implications of trunk muscle strength for surgery, rehabilitation, and the industrial setting must be considered in the light of new information.

References

1. Basmajian, J.: Muscles Alive: Their Functions Revealed by Electromyography. 4th ed. Baltimore, Williams & Wilkins Co., 1978.
2. Cady, L., Bischoff, D., O'Connell, E., et al.: Strength and fitness and subsequent back injuries in firefighters. J. Occup. Med. *21*:269–272, 1979.
3. Finneson, B.: Low Back Pain. 2nd ed. Philadelphia, J. B. Lippincott Co., 1977.
4. Flint, M.: Effect of increasing back and abdominal muscle strength on low back pain. Res. Q. *29*:160–171, 1955.
5. Floyd, W., and Silver, P.: The function of the erector spinae muscles in certain movements and postures in man. J. Physiol. (Lond.) *129*:184–203, 1955.
6. Gonyea, W., Moore-Woodward, C., Moseley, B., et al.: An evaluation of muscle pathology in idiopathic scoliosis. J. Pediatr. Orthop. *5*:323–329, 1985.
7. Gracovetsky, S., and Farfan, H.: The optimum spine. Spine *11*:543–573, 1986.
8. Hazard, R., Reid, S., Fenwick, J., and Reeves, V.: Isokinetic trunk and lifting strength measurements: variability as an indicator of effort. Spine *13*:54–57, 1988.
9. Hollinshead, W.: Anatomy for Surgeons. 3rd ed. Vol. 3. Hagerstown, MD, Harper & Row, 1982, pp. 19–23.
10. Langrana, N., and Lee, C.: Isokinetic evaluation of trunk muscles. Spine *9*:171–175, 1984.
11. Mayer, L., and Greenberg, B.: Measurement of the strength of trunk muscles. J. Bone Joint Surg. *24*:842–856, 1942.
12. Mayer, T., Kondraske, G., Mooney, V., et al.: Lumbar myoelectric spectral analysis for endurance assessment: a comparison of normals with deconditioned patients. Spine *14*:986–991, 1989.
13. Mayer, T., and Gatchel, R.: Functional Restoration for Spinal Disorders: The Sports Medicine Approach. Philadelphia, Lea & Febiger, 1988.
14. Mayer, T., Gatchel, R., Kishino, N., et al.: Objective assessment of spine function following industrial injury: a prospective study with comparison group and one-year follow-up. 1958 Volvo award in clinical sciences. Spine *10*:482–493, 1985.
15. Mayer, T., Smith, S., Keeley, J., and Mooney, V.: Quantification of lumbar function. Part 2: Sagittal plane trunk strength in chronic low back pain patients. Spine *10*:765–772, 1985.
16. Mayer, T., Smith, S., Kondraske, G., et al.: Quantification of lumbar function. Part 3: Preliminary data on isokinetic torso rotation testing with myoelectric spectral analysis in normal and low back pain subjects. Spine *10*:912–920, 1985.
17. Mayer, T., Vanharanta, H., Gatchel, R., et al.: Comparison of CT scan muscle measurements and isokinetic trunk strength in postoperative patients. Spine *14*:33–36, 1989.
18. McComas, A.: Neuromuscular Function and Disorders. 1st ed. Boston, Butterworth, 1977.
19. Morris, J., Benner, G., and Lucas, D.: An electromyographic study of the intrinsic muscles of the back in man. J. Anat. *196*:509–502, 1962.
20. Schultz, A., Haderspeck-Grib, K., Sinkora, G., and Warwick, D.: Quantitative studies of the flexion-relaxation phenomenon in the back muscles. J. Orthop. Res. *3*:189–197, 1985.
21. Nachemson, A.: The possible importance of the psoas muscle for stabilization of the lumbar spine. Acta Orthop. Scand. *39*:47–57, 1968.
22. Smidt, G., Herring, T., Amundsen, L., et al.: Assessment of abdominal and back extensor function: a quantitative approach and results for chronic low-back patients. Spine *8*:211–219, 1983.
23. Suzuki, N., and Endo, S.: A quantitative study of trunk muscle strength and fatigability in the low-back-pain syndrome. Spine *8*:69–74, 1983.

CHAPTER

4

ANATOMY OF THE SPINAL NERVE ROOTS IN THE LUMBAR AND LOWER THORACIC SPINE

Mark S. Cohen, M.D.
Eric J. Wall, M.D.
Kjell Olmarker, M.D., Ph.D.
Björn L. Rydevik, M.D., Ph.D.
Steven R. Garfin, M.D.

The spinal nerve roots are the structural link between the central and peripheral nervous systems. The microanatomy of the spinal nerve roots is closer to the central than to the peripheral nervous system, but in considering their functional properties they are better correlated with the peripheral nervous system. The spinal nerve roots do not have the same organization of protective connective tissue sheath as the peripheral nerves. They are, however, well protected from external trauma by the bony spinal column. Their gross and histologic organization within the dural envelope (intrathecal) and between their exit from the thecal sac and the intervertebral foramen (extrathecal) are described below.

GROSS ANATOMIC CONSIDERATIONS

In the early embryonic stages of development, the spinal cord is the same length as the bony vertebral column. However, the spinal column outgrows the neural elements, and in a fully grown individual the spinal cord ends most frequently at the level of the first and second lumbar intervertebral disc.[16, 19, 22, 23, 30, 32] This termination is referred to as the "conus medullaris." A nerve root that leaves the spinal canal through an intervertebral foramen in the lumbar or sacral spine therefore has to pass from the point where it separates from the spinal cord, which is in the lower thoracic spine, to the point of its exit in the lumbar or sacral spine (Fig. 4–1). Since the spinal cord is not present below approximately the first or second lumbar vertebra, the nervous elements of the spinal canal below this level consist only of the lumbosacral nerve roots. It has been suggested that this "bundle" of nerve roots within the lumbar and sacral part of the spinal canal resembles a horse's tail; it is therefore termed the "cauda equina."

Within the region of the conus medullaris and cauda equina the nerve roots are divided

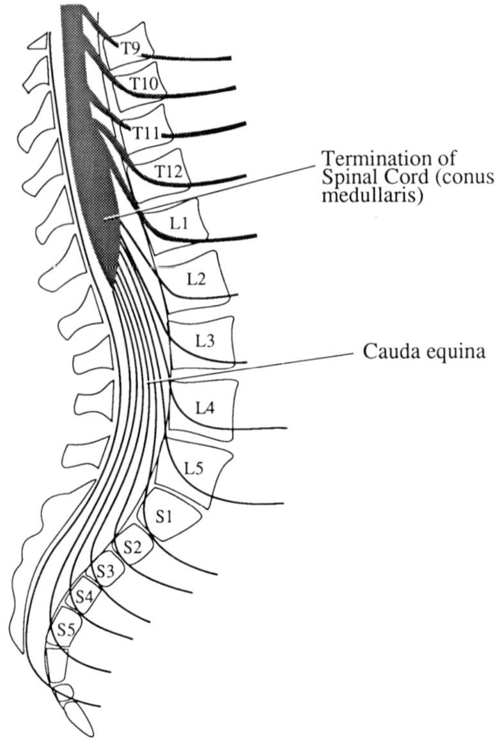

Figure 4–1. Schematic diagram depicting the lower end of the spinal cord, the conus medullaris, and the collection of spinal nerve roots in the lumbar spine referred to as the cauda equina.

into ventral and dorsal components. The ventral roots consist mainly of efferent or motor axons and contain only a small portion of afferent axons.[2, 3] The cell bodies of the motor axons are in the anterior horns of the gray matter of the spinal cord. These roots originate from the ventral aspect of the spinal cord as a collection of tiny rootlets or "fila radicularia." The dorsal roots are composed primarily of afferent or sensory axons and originate on the

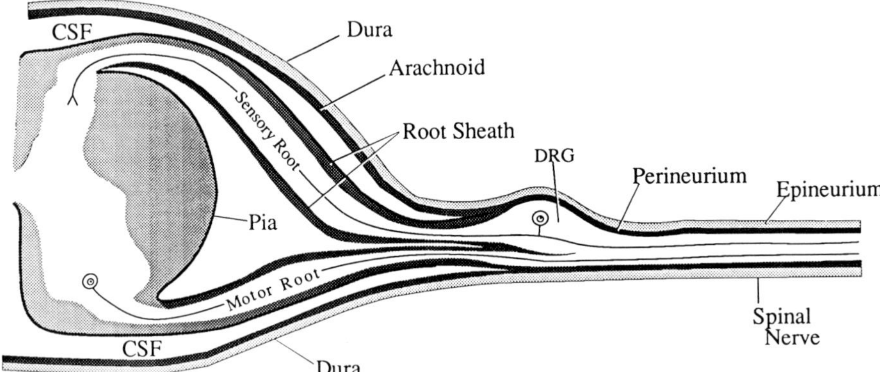

Figure 4–2. Cross section of the spinal cord and a spinal nerve root. The cell bodies of the dorsal (sensory) roots are in the dorsal root ganglion (DRG). The cell bodies of the ventral (motor) roots are in the anterior horn of the gray matter of the spinal cord. The ventral and dorsal roots are bathed in cerebrospinal fluid (CSF). They travel together in the root sleeve and combine distal to the DRG to form the spinal nerve proper. The spinal cord is covered with pia mater. This layer continues out onto the nerve roots as the root sheath. The arachnoid membrane reflects back on the nerve roots to form the outer layer of the root sheath. The inner layer of the root sheath combines with the inner layer of the dura (neurothelium) to form the perineurium of the peripheral nerves. The dura continues as the epineurium of the peripheral nerves.

dorsal aspect of the spinal cord as afferent rootlets. The cell bodies of the sensory axons are in a "dorsal root ganglion," which is a prominence in the region of the intervertebral foramen (see below).

Within the vertebral canal the spinal nerve roots are enclosed by a firm dural cylinder. The nerve roots sequentially exit the thecal sac in separate extensions of spinal dura called root sleeves. In each root sleeve there is a pair of motor and sensory nerve roots from the same spinal cord segment. The root sleeve, between the thecal sac exit and the intervertebral foramen, is often described surgically as the "nerve root" proper. It has also been referred to as the extrathecal nerve root[4, 10, 20, 27] or the nerve root complex.[22, 25] Beyond the dorsal root ganglion, the motor and sensory nerve roots are no longer separate and combine to form the mixed spinal nerve (Fig. 4–2).

MICROSCOPIC ANATOMIC CONSIDERATIONS

The axons of the spinal nerve roots are enclosed in endoneurial tissue, which is very similar to the endoneurium of the peripheral nerves.[6, 17] In addition to axons, there are collagen fibers, fibroblasts, and blood vessels in the endoneurium.[7] The amount of collagen in the nerve roots is one fifth that of the peripheral nerves.[29] It remains unknown whether there are lymphatic vessels in the nerve roots.

Microscopically, there are two very different regions of the nerve roots at their spinal cord origin. Closest to the spinal cord there is a "central glial" segment that contains astrocytes, oligodendrocytes, and microglial cells and thus resembles the organization of the central nervous system (CNS).[31] Several millimeters from the spinal cord this glial segment is replaced by a nonglial segment at a "dome-shaped" junction.[2, 31] Distal to this junction the nerve roots are organized with predominantly Schwann cells (similar to peripheral nerves) with only small islets of glial cells.

Separating the axons within the endoneurium and the cerebrospinal fluid (CSF) is the "root sheath," a thin layer of connective tissue, which is the structural analogue to the pia mater that covers the spinal cord. There are usually three to four cellular layers in the root sheath.[9, 28] The outer layers of the proximal part of the root sheath are composed of cells similar to the pia cells of the spinal cord. More distally, the outer cell layers are more like the arachnoid cells of the spinal meninges.[15] The inner layers of the distal root sheath contain cells similar to the perineurium of the peripheral nerves. These inner layers serve as a diffusion barrier between the endoneurium of the nerve roots and the CSF. This barrier is relatively weak and may serve only to prevent the passage of certain macromolecules.

The spinal dura encloses the nerve roots and CSF. When the two layers of cranial dura enter the spinal canal, the outer layer blends with the periosteum of the cervical laminae within the canal, and the inner layer joins the arachnoid and becomes the spinal dura. Unlike the root sheath, the dura provides a strong diffusion barrier due to the "neurothelium," which is a connective tissue sheath between the dura proper and the arachnoid.[1] Like the inner layer of the root sheath, this neurothelium histologically resembles the perineurium of the peripheral nerves, and these two layers blend to form the perineurium proper in the region of the dorsal root ganglion when the nerve root merges into the peripheral nerve.[1, 15] The dura in turn becomes continuous with the epineurium of the peripheral nerves (Fig. 4–2).[10, 30]

Unlike the nerve roots, the dorsal root ganglia are not completely enclosed by CSF, as the subarachnoid space ends at the proximal ganglia margin, although this is somewhat variable.[10, 30] The covering of the ganglia is composed of a multilayered connective tissue, similar to the perineurium of the peripheral nerves, and the epineurium.[1, 15] With the content of sensory cell bodies and tight enclosure, the dorsal root ganglia have been shown to be mechanosensitive and at risk for intracapsular pressure increases secondary to edema.[8, 12, 25, 26] These ganglia are presently implicated as possible anatomic factors in the pathophysiology of spinal pain syndromes.[11, 13, 14, 33, 36]

INTRATHECAL NERVE ROOT ORGANIZATION

The arrangement of the individual spinal nerve roots around the lower end of the spinal cord (conus medullaris) and in the cauda equina has recently been elucidated.[34, 35] Previously thought to be randomly arranged, the roots have been shown to form an organized overlapping pattern at the level of the conus, separating into reproducible layers in the lower lumbar spine. The roots are not free floating but are held in relation to one another and the dural envelope by an intricate web of arachnoid (Fig. 4–3, see color plate).[10, 18, 21, 34, 35] The patterns shown in the accompanying illustrations represent composite drawings, with the conus ending between the first and second lumbar vertebrae. A low terminating conus would cause slightly more spinal cord to be present in relation to nerve roots at a given level; a high terminating conus would cause the opposite.

T10–T11. At the interspace between the 10th and 11th thoracic vertebrae, the spinal cord is flanked only by the T11 and T12 nerve roots (Fig. 4–4, see color plate). The nerve roots cephalad to T11 have already exited the dural sac, while the lumbar roots originate caudal to this level.

T11–T12. At this disc level the lower spinal cord is surrounded by the 12th thoracic to the third lumbar nerve roots (Fig. 4–5, see color plate). The ventral aspect of the cord is almost completely covered by the ventral roots, while a portion of the dorsal cord remains uncovered (approximately 20 to 25 per cent of the total cord circumference). The nerve roots overlap in a consistent organized fashion around the cord, with the motor and sensory components of the lumbar roots separated at this level.

T12–L1. At the junction between the thoracic and lumbar vertebral bodies the spinal cord begins to taper and is surrounded by the first to the fifth lumbar nerve roots (Fig. 4–6, see color plate). While the entire L1 root is situated laterally, the remaining lumbar ventral and dorsal roots are separated and encircle the lower aspect of the spinal cord in an overlapping fashion. Approximately 10 to 15 per cent of the cord circumference remains uncovered dorsally.

L1–L2. At the interspace between the first and second lumbar vertebrae the spinal cord ends and becomes the filum terminale. This terminal portion of the cord is surrounded by the second lumbar to the fifth sacral nerve roots (Fig. 4–7, see color plate). While the first sacral dorsal and ventral roots remain slightly separated at this level, the L2–L5 motor and sensory roots come together to form organized, nearly vertical layers. The lower sacral roots converge and encircle the terminal cord.

L2–L3. At this interspace the first sacral dorsal root has converged with its ventral counterpart. It now lies adjacent to the third through the fifth lumbar root layers, which all rotate slightly to form oblique layers (Fig. 4–8, see color plate). These layers are observed in the remainder of the cauda equina. Within each root layer the motor bundle sits anterior and medial to its respective sensory bundles. The lower sacral roots (S2–S5) at this level and caudally occupy the dorsal aspect of the cauda equina.

L3–L4. At the third and fourth lumbar vertebral interspace the third lumbar root has exited the thecal sac, and the fourth lumbar to the fifth sacral roots are present (Fig. 4–9, see color plate). The oblique-layered pattern can be appreciated with the single motor bundle consistently anterior and medial to its multifascicular sensory bundle within each layer.

L4–L5. At this interspace the fifth lumbar to the fifth sacral roots are present, with the fifth lumbar root situated anterolaterally before exiting the thecal sac (Fig. 4–10, see color plate). The lower sacral roots remain in the dorsal midline of the cauda equina.

L5–S1. At the transition between the lumbar and sacral vertebrae the first sacral root is positioned anterolaterally (Fig. 4–11, see color plate). The lower sacral roots now spread and form a crescent pattern along the dorsal thecal sac.

The abovementioned nerve root patterns of the cauda equina can be appreciated on current contrast-enhanced computed tomographic (CT) and surface-coil magnetic resonance imaging (MRI) scans (Fig. 4–12).[5] Advances in imaging technology may make these observations of considerable clinical relevance in future studies of lumbosacral disorders (Fig. 4–13, see color plate).

EXTRATHECAL NERVE ROOT ORGANIZATION

The macroscopic organization of the nerve root complex lateral to the thecal sac with regard to the take-off angle of the nerve root sleeve, the relative position of the motor and sensory bundles within the sleeves, and the

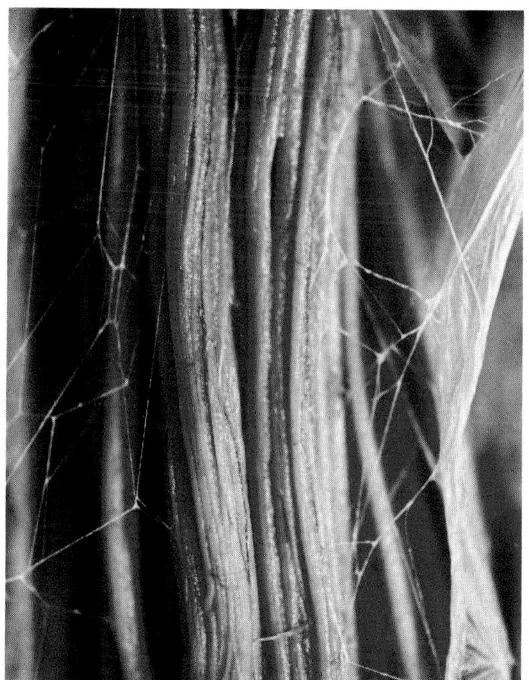

Figure 4–3. Cadaveric specimen showing the arachnoid web connecting individual nerve roots to the surrounding membrane. Arachnoid invaginations and septations help maintain the nerve roots in a fixed relation to one another. (From Wall, E. J., Cohen, M. S., Abitbol, J. J., and Garfin, S. R.: Intrathecal nerve root organization at the level of the conus medullaris. J. Bone Joint Surg. *72A*:1495–1499, 1990.)

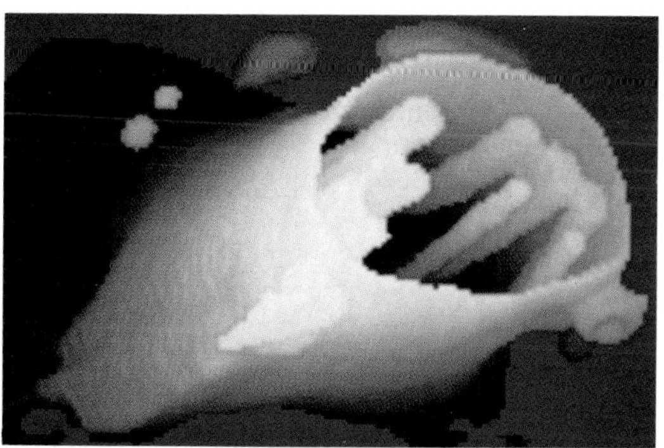

Figure 4–13. Three-dimensional reconstruction from a CT scan of a cadaveric specimen, depicting the intrathecal cauda equina nerve roots at the L3–L4 level. These in vitro reformations allow contiguous tracing of individual nerve roots through the thecal sac. With advances in medical imaging, identification and tracing of individual roots may aid in the understanding and treatment of lumbosacral spine disorders. (From Cohen, M. S., Wall, E. J., Kerber, C. W., et al.: The anatomy of the cauda equina on CT scans and MRI. J. Bone Joint Surg. *73B*:381–384, 1991.)

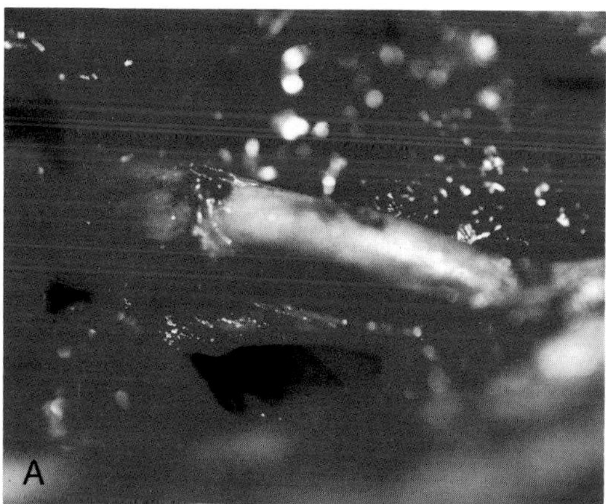

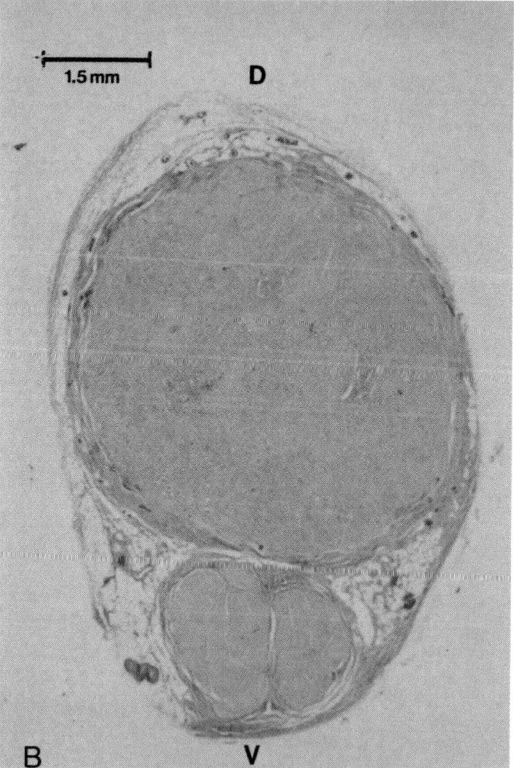

Figure 4–16. *A,* Cadaveric specimen showing the S1 nerve root with the outer sheath removed showing the ventral position of the motor root and the dorsal sensory root and ganglion. *B,* Axial histologic section of the S1 nerve root showing the relationship between the dorsal root ganglion and the smaller ventral motor root. D, dorsal: V, ventral (Masson's trichrome stain.) (From Cohen, M. S., Wall, E. J., Brown, R. A., et al.: Cauda equina anatomy: extrathecal nerve roots and dorsal root ganglia. Spine *15*:1248–1251, 1990.)

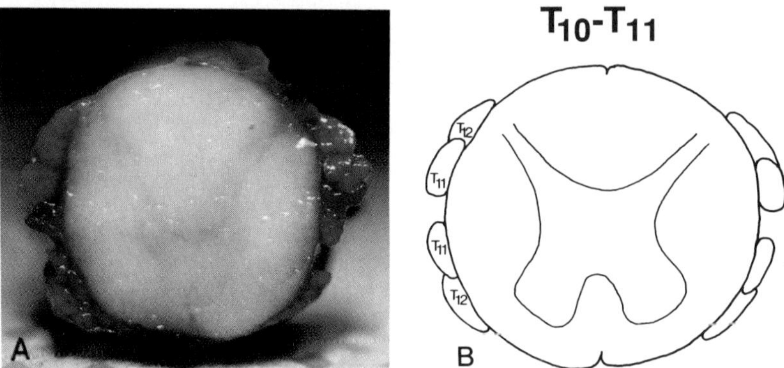

Figure 4–4. *A,* Representative cross-sectional anatomic section of the lower spinal cord at the T10–T11 intervertebral level. The cord is flanked by the T11 and T12 nerve roots (top = dorsal). *B,* Schematic representation of the spinal cord and flanking nerve roots at the T10–T11 disc level. Upper (dorsal) T11 and T12 are sensory roots; lower (ventral) T11 and T12 are motor roots. (From Wall, E. J., Cohen, M. S., Abitbol, J. J., and Garfin, S. R.: Intrathecal nerve root organization at the level of the conus medullaris. J. Bone Joint Surg. *72A*:1495–1499, 1990.)

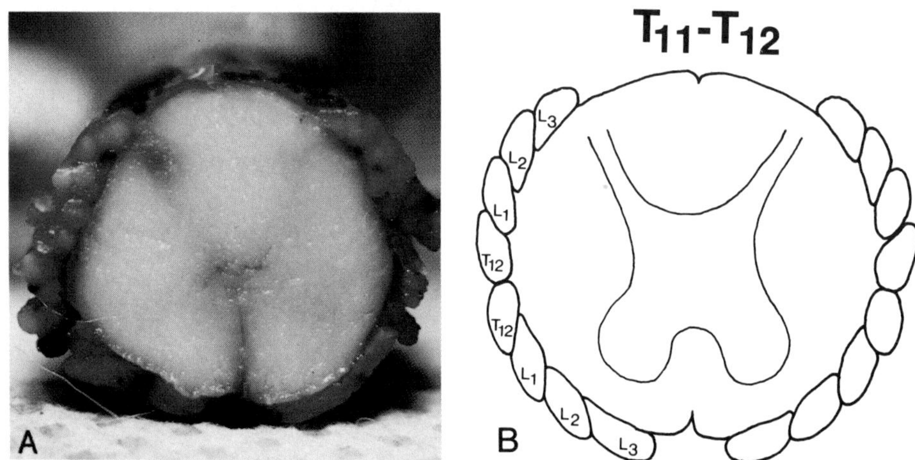

Figure 4–5. *A,* Representative axial section at the T11–T12 intervertebral space. Note that the dorsal aspect of the cord is not covered by nerve roots (top = dorsal). *B,* Schematic representation of the spinal cord, conus, and nerve roots at the T11–T12 interspace. The upper components of the labeled roots are sensory; the lower, or ventral, roots are motor. (From Wall, E. J., Cohen, M. S., Abitbol, J. J., and Garfin, S. R.: Intrathecal nerve root organization at the level of the conus medullaris. J. Bone Joint Surg. *72A*:1495–1499, 1990.)

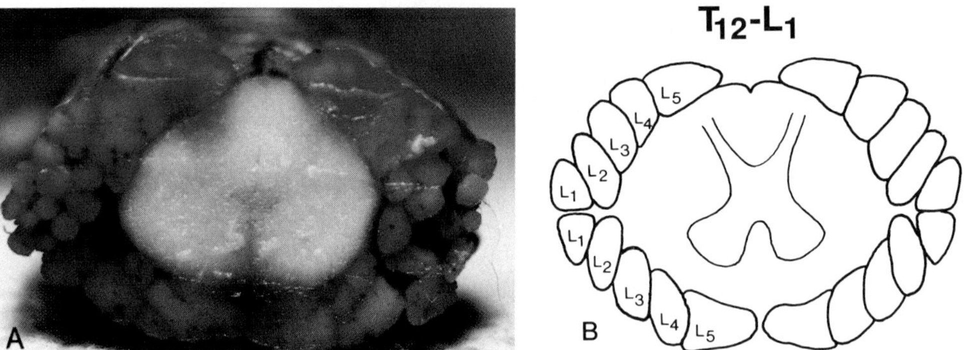

Figure 4–6. *A,* Representative cross-sectional view of the conus medullaris and roots at the T12–L1 disc level (top = dorsal). *B,* Schematic diagram depicting the nerve root pattern surrounding the lower spinal cord at the T12–L1 disc level. The upper root components are sensory; the lower neural elements are motor. (From Wall, E. J., Cohen, M. S., Abitbol, J. J., and Garfin, S. R.: Intrathecal nerve root organization at the level of the conus medullaris. J. Bone Joint Surg. *72A*:1495–1499, 1990.)

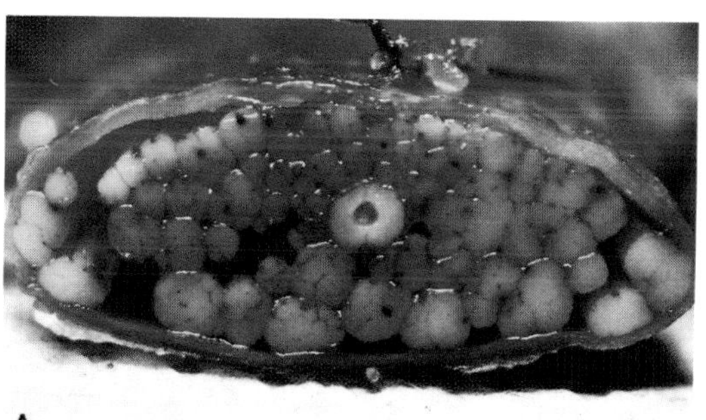

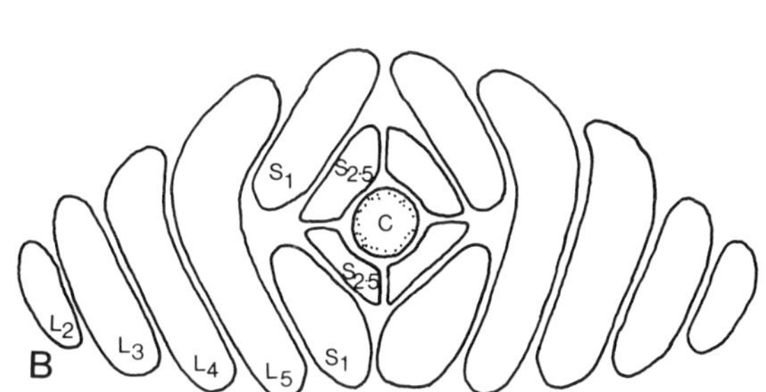

Figure 4–7. *A,* Representative axial anatomic section at the L1–L2 intervertebral level. The terminal spinal cord (central) is surrounded by nerve roots (top = dorsal). *B,* Schematic diagram of the nerve root pattern at the L1–L2 intervertebral level. The L2–L5 roots form nearly vertical layers while the sacral roots encircle the terminal spinal cord. The upper roots are sensory; the lower roots are motor. C, Termination of spinal cord. (From Wall, E. J., Cohen, M. S., Abitbol, J. J., and Garfin, S. R.: Intrathecal nerve root organization at the level of the conus medullaris. J. Bone Joint Surg. *72A*:1495–1499, 1990.)

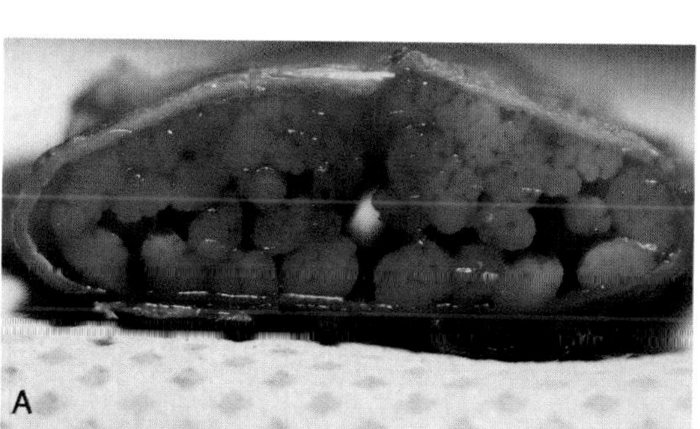

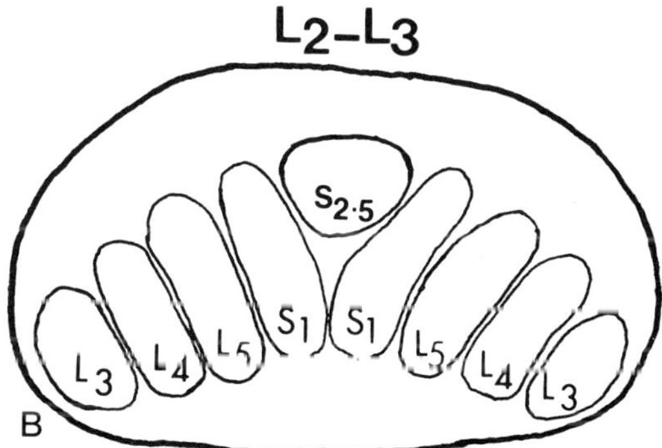

Figure 4–8. *A,* Cross-sectional view through the L2–L3 disc level. The L3–S1 roots form an oblique layered pattern with the lower sacral (S2–S5) roots occupying the dorsal aspect within the thecal sac (top = dorsal). *B,* Schematic depicting the cross-sectional layered pattern of roots at the L2–L3 intervertebral level. (From Wall, E. J., Cohen, M. S., Massie, J. M., et al.: Cauda equina anatomy: intrathecal nerve root organization. Spine *15*:1244–1247, 1990.)

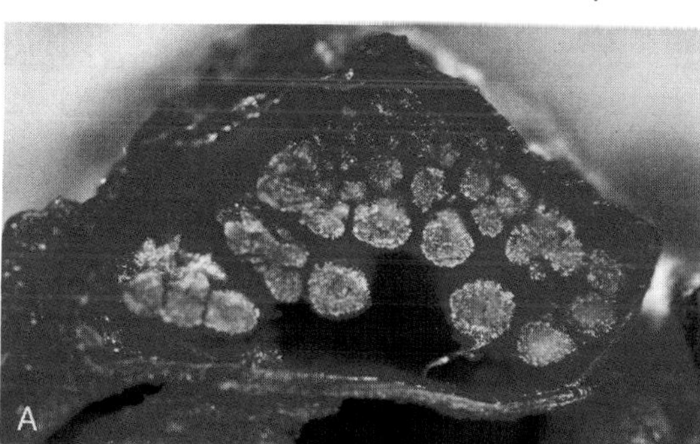

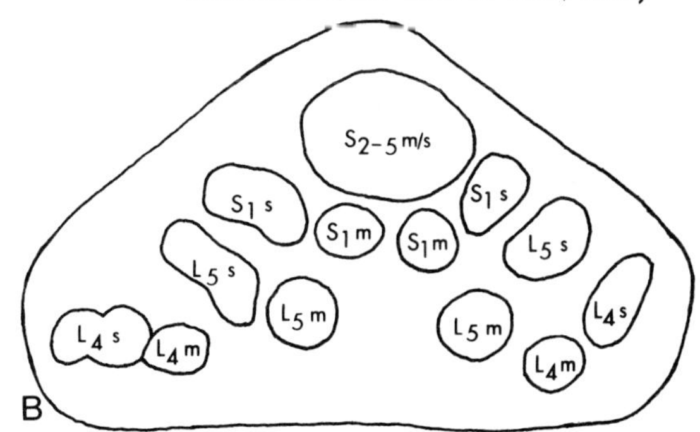

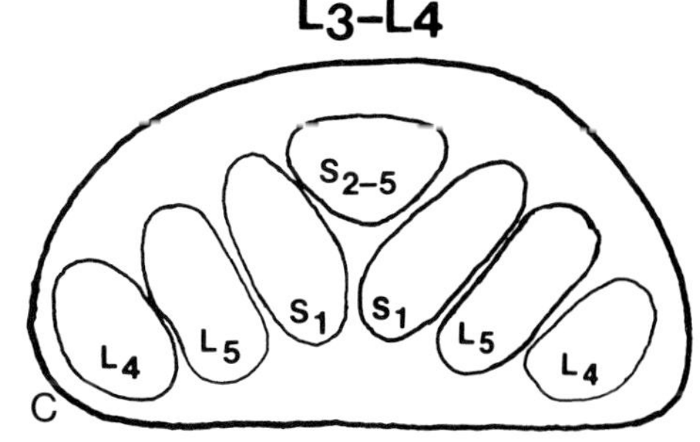

Figure 4–9. *A,* Cross-sectional view through the L3–L4 disc level. An oblique layered configuration of the roots is evident bilaterally. *B,* Schematic diagram depicting single motor bundle (m) medial and ventral to multifascicular sensory bundle (s) within each layer. S2–S5 roots remain dorsal (top = dorsal). *C,* Schematic representation of cross-sectional root organization at the L3-L4 disc level. (From Wall, E. J., Cohen, M. S., Massie, J. M., et al.: Cauda equina anatomy: intrathecal nerve root organization. Spine *15*:1244–1247, 1990.)

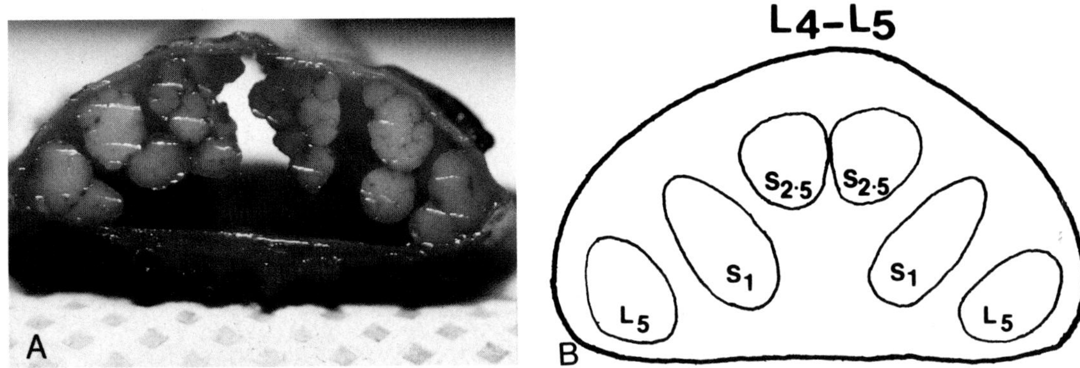

Figure 4–10. *A,* Cross-sectional view at the L4–L5 disc level revealing the L5 root in the anterolateral position. The S1 root is situated medially, forming a diagonal layer. The S2–S5 roots remain in the dorsal midline (top = dorsal). *B,* Schematic representation of the individual roots at the L4–L5 cross-sectional disc level. (From Wall, E. J., Cohen, M. S., Massie, J. M., et al.: Cauda equina anatomy: intrathecal nerve root organization. Spine *15*:1244–1247, 1990.)

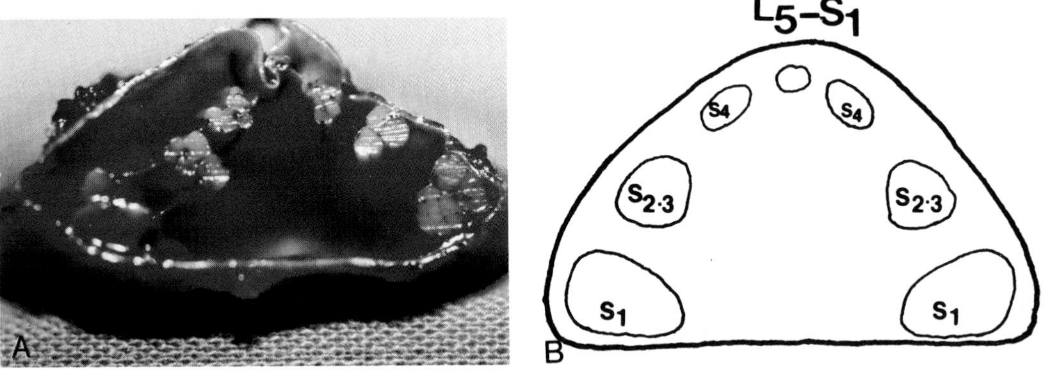

Figure 4–11. *A,* Cross-sectional view through the L5–S1 disc level revealing the S1 root anterolaterally and the crescent-shaped pattern of lower sacral roots (top = dorsal). *B,* Schematic diagram depicting the pattern of sacral root orientation at the L5–S1 intervertebral level. (From Wall, E. J., Cohen, M. S., Massie, J. M., et al.: Cauda equina anatomy: intrathecal nerve root organization. Spine *15*:1244–1247, 1990.)

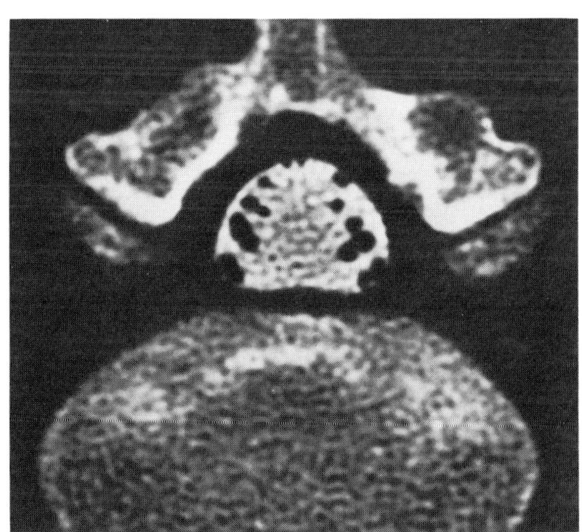

Figure 4–12. Contrast-enhanced CT scan of a live patient at the L4–L5 intervertebral level. Note the anterolateral position of the L5 root. The more dorsal and medial S1 root forms an oblique layer with the motor bundle of S1 anterior and medial to its sensory bundle (see Fig. 4–10). The S2–S5 roots occupy the dorsal midline. (From Cohen, M. S., Wall, E. J., Kerber, C. W., et al.: Computerized tomographic and magnetic resonance imaging of intrathecal cauda equina nerve roots. J. Bone Joint Surg. *73B*:381–384, 1991.)

position and size of the dorsal root ganglia are outlined below (Fig. 4–14).[4]

Nerve Root Sleeve Angulation. The lumbar nerve root sleeves exit the thecal sac at mean angles of approximately 40 degrees (Fig. 4–15). The nerve root take-off angle changes acutely at the first sacral root, which exits at an average angle of 22 degrees. The lower sacral take-off angles progressively decline.

Motor and Sensory Bundle Orientation. In contrast to the abovementioned intrathecal relationship (where the motor bundle of each nerve root is situated anteromedial to its sensory component), within the extrathecal root sleeve the motor bundle lies directly anterior to its sensory counterpart (Fig. 4–16, see color plate). As previously mentioned, distal to the dorsal root ganglion the motor and sensory roots combine to form the mixed spinal nerve.

Dorsal Root Ganglia Size. The size of the dorsal root ganglia varies with vertebral level, increasing from the first lumbar to the first sacral level (which measures a mean of 13 mm in length and 6 mm in width) and decreasing in size thereafter (Fig. 4–17).

Dorsal Root Ganglia Position. The mean length of the spinal nerve root sleeve, as measured from its origin to the proximal margin of the dorsal root ganglion, also varies with vertebral level, from as short as 6 mm at the first lumbar level to 15 mm at the second sacral level (Fig. 4–18). The center of the ganglia lies directly below the vertebral pedicle in 90 per cent of cases, with 8 per cent located inferolateral to the pedicle and 2 per cent medial to the pedicle within the lateral recess. In addition, the center of the lumbar ganglia overlies a lateral portion of the lateral intervertebral

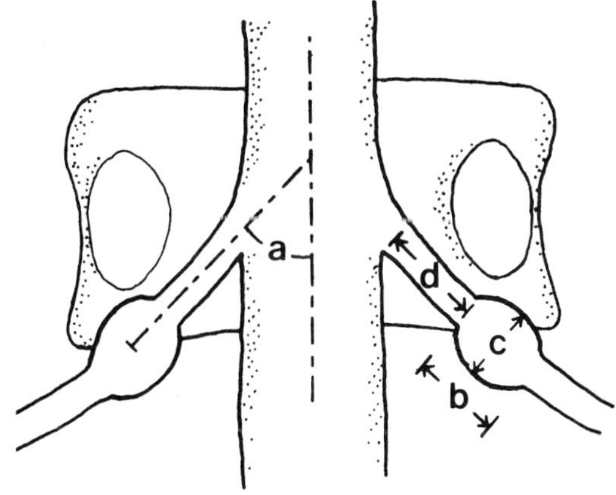

Figure 4–14. Schematic drawing showing measurement of root take-off angle (a); dorsal root ganglia length (b); dorsal root ganglia width (c); and distance of the proximal ganglia border from the nerve root axilla (d). (From Cohen, M. S., Wall, E. J., Brown, R. A., et al.: Cauda equina anatomy: extrathecal nerve roots and dorsal root ganglia. Spine *15*:1248–1251, 1990.)

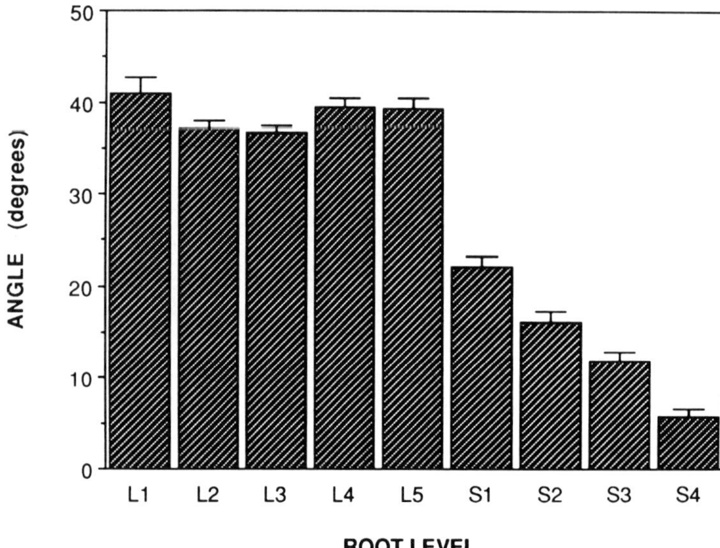

Figure 4–15. Graph showing relationship of root take-off angle in the coronal plane to the vertebral level (mean ± S.E.). The nerve root angles remain approximately 40 degrees from L1 to L5, decreasing acutely to 22 degrees at S1. The lower sacral root angles progressively decrease thereafter. (From Cohen, M. S., Wall, E. J., Brown, R. A., et al.: Cauda equina anatomy: extrathecal nerve roots and dorsal root ganglia. Spine *15:*1248–1251, 1990.)

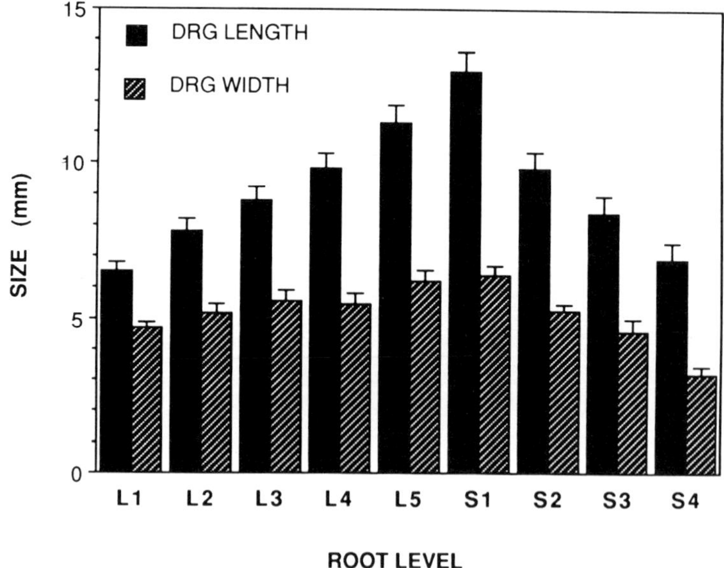

Figure 4–17. Graph showing the relationship between dorsal root ganglia length and width and vertebral level (mean ± S.E.). The length and width of the ganglia progressively increase from the L1 to the S1 level, and then progressively decrease in size at the lower sacral levels. (From Cohen, M. S., Wall, E. J., Brown, R. A., et al.: Cauda equina anatomy: extrathecal nerve roots and dorsal root ganglia. Spine *15:*1248–1251, 1990.)

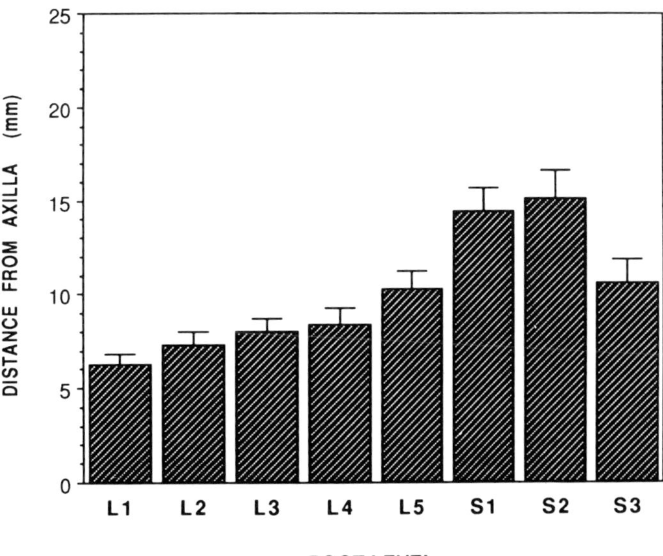

Figure 4–18. Graph of the location of the dorsal root ganglia depicted as the distance from the nerve root axilla to the proximal margin of the ganglia. The proximal ganglia margin is only 6 mm from the nerve root axilla at L1, increasing to 15 mm at the S2 root level. (From Cohen, M. S., Wall, E. J., Brown, R. A., et al.: Cauda equina anatomy: extrathecal nerve roots and dorsal root ganglia. Spine *15*:1248–1251, 1990.)

disc (e.g., the L3 ganglia would overlie a portion of the L3–L4 intervertebral disc) in one third of cases.

This chapter has reviewed the gross and microscopic organization of the thoracic, lumbar, and sacral spinal nerve roots. Knowledge of these recently defined relationships will assist future understanding and treatment of the pathoanatomic processes of the thoracolumbar spine.

References

1. Andres, K. H.: Über die Feinstruktur der Arachnoidea und Dura mater von Mammalia. Z. Zellforsch. *79*:272–295, 1967.
2. Berthold, C. H., Carlstedt, T., and Corneliuson, O.: Anatomy of the nerve root at the central-peripheral transitional region. *In* Dyck, P. J., Thomas, P. K., Lambert, E. H., and Bunge, R. (eds.): Peripheral Neuropathy. Vol. 1. Philadelphia, W. B. Saunders Co., 1984, pp. 156–170.
3. Coggeshall, R. E., Coulter, J. D., and Willis, W. D., Jr.: Unmyelinated axons in the ventral roots of the cat lumbosacral enlargement. J. Comp. Neurol. *153*:39–58, 1974.
4. Cohen, M. S., Wall, E. J., Brown, R. A., et al.: Cauda equina anatomy: extrathecal nerve roots and dorsal root ganglia. Spine *15*:1248–1251, 1990.
5. Cohen, M. S., Wall, E. J., Kerber, C. W., et al.: Computerized tomographic and magnetic resonance imaging of intrathecal cauda equina nerve roots. J. Bone Joint Surg. *73B*:381–384, 1991.
6. Gamble, H. J.: Comparative electron-microscopic observations on the connective tissues of a peripheral nerve and a spinal nerve root. J. Anat. (Lond.) *98*:17–25, 1964.
7. Gamble, H. J., and Eames, R. A.. Electron microscopy of human spinal-nerve roots. Arch. Neurol. *14*:50–53, 1966.
8. Grieve, G. P.: Common Vertebral Joint Problems. Edinburgh, Churchill Livingstone, 1981, pp. 1–157.
9. Haller, F. R., and Low, F. N.: The fine structure of the peripheral nerve root sheath in the subarachnoid space in the rat and other laboratory animals. Am. J. Anat. *131*:1–20, 1971.
10. Hollinghead, W. H.: Anatomy for Surgeons. Vol. 3. The Back and Limbs. 3rd ed. Philadelphia, Harper & Row, 1982, pp. 167–193.
11. Hokfelt, T., Ljungdahl, A., Terenius, L., et al.: Immunohistochemical analysis of peptide pathways possibly related to pain and analgesia: enkephalin and substance P. Proc. Natl. Acad. Sci. *74*:3081–3085, 1977.
12. Howe, J. F., Loeser, J. D., and Calvin, W. H.: Mechanosensitivity of dorsal root ganglia and chronically injured axons: a physiological basis for the radicular pain of nerve root compression. Pain *3*:25–41, 1977.
13. Kerr, F. W. L., and Wilson, P. R.: Pain. Ann. Rev. Neurosci. *1*:83–102, 1978.
14. Marx, J. L.: Brain peptides: is substance P a transmitter of pain signals? J. Sci. *205*:886–889, 1979.
15. McCabe, J. S., and Low, F. N.: The subarachnoid angle: an area of transition in peripheral nerve. Anat. Rec. *164*:15–34, 1969.
16. McCotter, R. E.: Regarding the length and extent of the human medulla spinalis. Anat. Rec. *16*:559–564, 1916.
17. Murphy, R. W.: Nerve roots and spinal nerves in degenerative disk disease. Clin. Orthop. *129*:46–60, 1977.
18. Nauta, H. J. W., Dolan, E., and Yosargil, M. G.: Microsurgical anatomy of the spinal subarachnoid space. Surg. Neurol. *19*:431–437, 1983.
19. Needles, J. H.: The caudal level of termination of the

spinal cord in American whites and American negroes. Anat. Rec. *63:*417–435, 1935.
20. O'Connell, J. E. A.: Sciatica and the mechanism of the production of the clinical syndrome in protrusions of the lumbar intervertebral discs. Br. J. Surg. *30:*315–327, 1943.
21. Parke, W. W., Gammell, K., and Rothman, R. H.: Arterial vascularization of the cauda equina. J. Bone Joint Surg. *63A:*53–62, 1981.
22. Rauschning, W.: Normal and pathologic anatomy of the lumbar root canals. Spine *12:*1008–1019, 1987.
23. Reimann, A. F., and Anson, B. J.: Vertebral level of termination of the spinal cord with report of a case of sacral cord. Anat. Rec. *88:*127–138, 1944.
24. Roth, M.: Caudal end of the spinal cord. Acta Radiol. Diagn. *3:*177–187, 1965.
25. Rydevik, B., Brown, M. D., and Lundborg, G.: Pathoanatomy and pathophysiology of nerve root compression. Spine *9:*7–15, 1984.
26. Rydevik, B., Myers, R. R., and Powell, H. C.: Pressure increase in the dorsal root ganglion following mechanical compression. Closed compartment syndrome in nerve roots. Spine *14:*574, 1989.
27. Spencer, D. L., Irwin, G. S., and Miller, J. A. A.: Anatomy and significance of fixation of the lumbosacral nerve roots in sciatica. Spine *8:*672–679, 1983.
28. Steer, J. M.: Some observations on the fine structure of rat dorsal spinal nerve roots. J. Anat. *109:*467–485, 1971.
29. Stodieck, L. S., Beel, J. A., and Luttges, M. W.: Structural properties of spinal nerve roots: protein composition. Exp. Neurol. *91:*41–51, 1986.
30. Sunderland, S.: Avulsion of nerve roots. *In* Vinken, P. J., and Bruyn, G. W. (eds.): Handbook of Clinical Neurology. Vol. 25. New York, Elsevier, 1975, pp. 393–435.
31. Tarlov, I. M.: Structure of the nerve root. Nature of the junction between the central and the peripheral nervous system. Arch. Neurol. Psychiat. *37:*555–583, 1937.
32. Thompson, A.: Fifth annual report of the Committee of the collective investigating of the Anatomical Society of Great Britain and Ireland for the year 1893–1894. Vol. 29, 1894, pp. 35–61.
33. Vanderlinden, R. G.: Subarticular entrapment of the dorsal root ganglion as a cause of sciatic pain. Spine *9:*19–22, 1984.
34. Wall, E. J., Cohen, M. S., Abitbol, J. J., and Garfin, S. R.: Intrathecal nerve root organization at the level of the conus medullaris. J. Bone Joint Surg. *72A:*1495–1499, 1990.
35. Wall, E. J., Cohen, M. S., Massie, J. M., et al.: Cauda equina anatomy: intrathecal nerve root organization. Spine *15:*1244–1247, 1990.

CHAPTER

5

DIFFERENTIAL DIAGNOSIS OF SCIATICA

Luis A. Mignucci, M.D.
Gordon R. Bell, M.D.

Pain radiating from the back, into the buttock, and into the lower extremity is called *sciatica*.[6, 77] Although disc herniation is one common cause of sciatica, newer radiologic imaging tools and refinements of electrophysiologic studies have identified many other lesions as potential causes.[1, 6, 21, 22, 25, 32, 34, 37, 40, 42, 43, 46, 49, 52–56, 58, 59, 60, 63, 64, 67, 69, 70, 77, 81, 83, 85] Differentiating sciatica due to lumbar disc protrusion from that due to other pathologic conditions, such as tumor or neuropathy, can be a very difficult diagnostic dilemma. Sciatica can originate peripherally or centrally. It can be elicited by any irritative lesion originating anywhere along the course of any nerve of the lower extremity or within the lumbosacral plexus or lumbosacral roots (peripheral).[4, 7, 22, 32, 34, 37, 40–43, 46, 53, 55, 58, 60, 67, 81, 83] It may also be caused by lesions involving the spinothalamic tract of the spinal cord[6, 26, 56] or the thalamus (central).[6] A sciatic type of pain may also be referred from bony lesions of the spine,[19, 35] sacroiliac joint,[36, 77] or hip joint[10, 52] or may be caused by peripheral vascular disease (Fig. 5–1). Finally, a functional etiology must also be considered.[74]

The ensuing discussion of the differential diagnosis of sciatica will follow a distal-to-proximal sequence.

PERIPHERAL NERVE LESIONS

Lower extremity nerves are mixed nerves composed of sensory, motor, and autonomic fibers.[3, 30, 75] Trauma, entrapment, ischemia, infiltration, or compression by tumors, infection, or inflammation may involve any or all components of the nerve and produce pain, paralysis, muscle wasting, reflex changes, or sensory changes. Characteristics of the pain and physical examination findings aid in the diagnosis, which can be corroborated by electrophysiologic[16, 39, 45, 67, 75] or radiologic[12, 60, 62, 63, 84] studies.

Entrapment Neuropathy

Pain or paresthesias due to distal compression anywhere along the course of a peripheral nerve characterize entrapment neuropathies.[11, 24, 28, 54] They may present as a painless, progressive weakness[11] or may masquerade as a

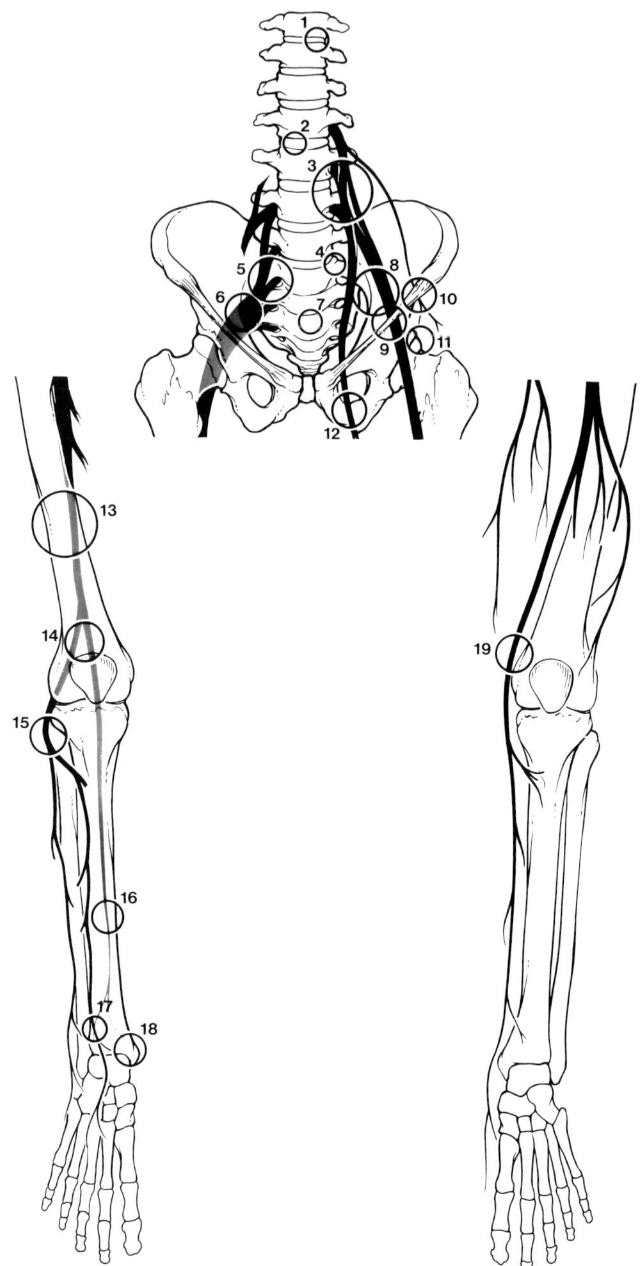

Figure 5–1. Schematic representation of common lesion locations.

1. Central (spinothalamic tract) lesions (thoracic tumor, disc herniation, and arteriovenous malformation)
2. Lumbosacral root lesions (stenosis, arachnoiditis, cyst, tumor)
3. Retroperitoneal lumbar plexus lesions/psoas lesions
4. Sacroiliac joint disease (ankylosing spondylitis, ulcerative colitis)
5. Retroperitoneal/pelvis sacral plexus lesions (tumor, endometriosis)
6. Sciatic nerve entrapment at sciatic notch (piriformis syndrome)
7. Intrasacral lesions (tumor, occult meningocele)
8. Intrapelvic femoral nerve lesions (trauma, tumor infiltration, neuropathy)
9. Femoral nerve entrapment (hernia)
10. Lateral femoral cutaneous nerve entrapment
11. Hip joint disease
12. Obturator nerve entrapment (hernia, trauma)
13. Sciatic nerve lesions (tumor, femur fracture)
14. Common peroneal/tibial nerve lesions at popliteal space (ganglion cyst, hypertrophied gastrocnemius tendon)
15. Peroneal nerve lesions (entrapment, infection)
16. Tibial nerve entrapment
17. Anterior tarsal tunnel syndrome
18. Posterior tarsal tunnel syndrome
19. Saphenous nerve entrapment

painful radiculopathy. Saal and colleagues reported a series of patients with a "pseudoradicular syndrome" in which the sole cause of leg pain was a peripheral entrapment neuropathy diagnosed by electromyography (EMG).[67] The compressive lesions were classified as femoral (proximal to inguinal ligament), saphenous (at the knee), peroneal (at or above the fibular head), or tibial (popliteal space). More than 44 per cent of the patients had positive nerve root tension signs, range of motion abnormalities, or back pain suggesting an intraspinal location of neural compression, as might be seen with a disc herniation. In these cases, the EMG was diagnostic.

Other entrapment neuropathies may also present as radicular pain.[11, 24, 39, 71] These include lesions of the obturator, ilioinguinal, lateral femoral cutaneous, and sciatic nerves. There may be a history of back and leg pain in these patients, which can lead to confusion in diagnosis and management. Saal and colleagues suggested that this "pseudoradicular syndrome" is due to chronic nociceptor stimulation of the dorsal root ganglion leading to an increase in the release of the pain neurotransmitter *substance P* from the dorsal root ganglion to the dorsal root entry zone in the spinal cord, and into the subarachnoid space overlying the superficial dorsal horn of the spinal cord.[67] The release of substance P leads to an increased sensitivity of the dorsal root ganglion and nerve roots to any stimulus, whether noxious or not.

A careful history and physical examination and judicious use of electrophysiologic studies may help distinguish entrapment neuropathy from a typical radiculopathy due to disc herniation. *Obturator nerve* entrapment may be due to a large obturator hernia containing bowel or fat[9] within the obturator canal and may present as medial thigh pain or paresthesia.[11, 24, 39, 77] The pain is characteristically aggravated by activities that increase intra-abdominal pressure and also by thigh extension. It may be bilateral. Weakness is not common but may be present and involve the hip adductor muscles. Brown described a series of such patients operated on via an intraperitoneal abdominal approach in which removal of herniated fat and repair of the obturator canal resulted in relief of symptoms.[9] Obturator nerve lesions are more commonly traumatic in origin. Differential diagnosis includes a high lumbar disc herniation that may also present as weakness of either hip flexion or thigh adduction.

Pain along the medial aspect of the leg and foot, commonly aggravated by walking or climbing stairs and improved by rest, may be seen with entrapment of the *saphenous nerve*.[11, 24, 39] This nerve is a purely sensory nerve that travels in the subsartorial (Hunter's) canal where it can be compressed as it exits through the subsartorial fascia.[41] Digital pressure over the saphenous opening in the subsartorial fascia (5 to 6 cm above the medial femoral condyle) with the knee in extension and the thigh adducted typically increases the pain.[39]

Femoral nerve entrapment beneath the inguinal ligament may mimic the type and distribution of pain seen with saphenous nerve compression.[11, 39] In addition, however, there may be weakness of hip flexors or quadriceps, leading to difficulty in walking and climbing stairs.[24, 25] A positive femoral stretch test is frequently noted, and a positive Tinel sign over the femoral canal may be seen where the nerve enters the thigh beneath the inguinal ligament, lateral to the femoral sheath and vessels.[67] An inguinal hernia may also contribute to femoral nerve entrapment in some instances.

Groin pain that is relieved by hip flexion may be due to *ilioinguinal nerve* entrapment.[11, 24, 39, 75] Although mainly supplying sensation to the root of the penis and scrotum, this nerve does supply a small area of the thigh below the medial end of the inguinal ligament. Nerve compression frequently occurs near the anterior superior iliac spine and has been associated with earlier lower abdominal surgery or previous inguinal hernia repair. This neuropathy can easily be confused with a high lumbar disc herniation causing L1 or L2 root compression.

Paresthesias or pain in an oval area in the anterolateral aspect of the thigh due to the entrapment of the *lateral femoral cutaneous nerve* is called meralgia paresthetica.[11, 39] Symptoms are often produced by walking or standing for long periods and are relieved by sitting.[75] The lateral femoral cutaneous nerve is a purely sensory nerve that supplies sensation to the lateral aspect of the thigh. Paresthesias may occur along the course of the nerve, but the area of sensory loss is usually limited. The hypesthesic area is usually in the anterolateral thigh, similar to the location of a pocket in a pair of pants. Entrapment may occur where the nerve emerges from the pelvis and enters the thigh beneath the lateral end of the inguinal ligament, or it may be compressed where it passes through the fascia lata 10 cm distal to the anterior superior iliac spine. A Tinel sign may be present at the site of entrapment. Edelson and Nathan in cadaveric dissection of 90 adult and 20 fetal lateral femoral cutaneous nerves, found that 51 per cent of adult specimens had a significant enlargement of the nerve (pseudoganglion) in the area where it passed under the inguinal ligament.[18] Microscopic examination revealed connective tissue thickening of the lateral femoral cutaneous nerve. These changes were not found in fetal nerves, suggesting an acquired phenomenon due to chronic compression.

Common predisposing factors in meralgia paresthetica include obesity, chronic cough, and long-time wearing of corsets, tight-fitting pants, and tight belts or binders. The differential diagnosis of meralgia paresthetica includes femoral neuropathy or high lumbar disc herniation. As with other entrapment neuropathies, EMG is useful in differentiating this condition from nerve root lesions or femoral nerve lesions.[11, 24, 67, 75] Conservative management includes weight reduction and avoidance of constricting garments.

Sciatic nerve entrapment at any point along its course may present as a weakness of knee flexion or of calf and foot muscles.[11, 39, 75] The clinical picture is often one of multiple root involvement, making compression by a disc herniation a less likely etiology since the latter usually involves a single root only. Multiple root involvement, however, often affects muscles with differing nerve supply such as the quadriceps (innervated by the femoral nerve) or the paraspinal muscles (innervated by the posterior rami of spinal nerves). Sciatic nerve entrapment has also been described with pentazocine-induced muscle fibrosis, myofascial bands in the distal portion of the thigh between the biceps femoris and adductor magnus, and rheumatoid Baker's (popliteal) cysts.[39] Sciatic nerve entrapment by the piriform muscle (piriformis syndrome) has been the subject of much debate.[6, 39, 71] Pain in this condition is typically in the buttocks with occasional radiation into the thigh, calf, or foot. Kopell and Thompson described entrapment at the sciatic notch secondary to a hip flexion contracture resulting in compensatory hyperlumbar lordosis and neural compression by the hip external rotators.[39] In 6 per cent of postmortem examinations an abnormal relationship between the piriform muscle and sciatic nerve was discovered.[6, 39] This was said to predispose the nerve to compression by rotation of the hip, particularly by internal rotation. Good scientific studies of this condition are lacking, however, so that many clinicians doubt its existence.

Chronic compression of the *peroneal nerve* may present either as pain or paresthesia radiating along the anterolateral aspect of the leg and dorsum of the foot.[11, 39, 75] There may also be weakness of ankle dorsiflexion and foot eversion. The condition may be differentiated from a lumbar radiculopathy by the occasional presence of a positive Tinel sign at the fibular neck or elsewhere along the path of the nerve and by sparing of foot inversion strength.[11, 75] Weakness of foot dorsiflexion from tibialis anterior involvement may be due either to a peroneal nerve lesion or to an isolated L5 radiculopathy. Although the definitive and ultimate diagnosis depends on the EMG, clinical examination is often helpful.[24] The tibialis anterior muscle is innervated by the deep peroneal nerve, which has L4 and L5 root contributions. Therefore, an isolated L4 or L5 root lesion, although producing weakness of foot dorsiflexion, rarely produces a profound footdrop owing to partial sparing of its root innervation. A peroneal neuropathy, on the other hand, usually presents with more profound weakness due to a more complete disruption of the nerve supply to the tibialis anterior. Also, in an isolated L5 root lesion there are other clinical findings such as weakness of hip abduction due to L5 innervation of the gluteus medius.

Tibial nerve entrapment often presents as burning pain in the sole of the foot and in the toes.[11, 39] This pain can also be referred proximally along the course of the sciatic nerve as described by Saal and colleagues.[67] This phenomenon is thought to be due to neural activation of the dorsal root ganglion by chronic nociceptive stimuli. Tibial nerve compression may occur proximally in the popliteal space (for example, by a hypertrophic gastrocnemius tendon, a Baker's cyst, or knee capsule fibrosis) or distally within the tarsal tunnel. A burning quality of the pain, the presence of paresthesias and a positive Tinel sign suggest this diagnosis, which can be confirmed by electrophysiologic studies.

Trauma

Three types of peripheral nerve injury may be associated with trauma: neurapraxia, axonotmesis, and neurotmesis.[30]

Neurapraxia is an incomplete, transient, and reversible loss of function without loss of anatomic integrity.

Axonotmesis is the immediate and complete loss of all motor, sensory, and autonomic function due to complete interruption of the axon and its myelin sheath with preservation of the connective tissue stroma. Potential for recovery depends on the distance between the lesion and the end organ, the degree of recovery being inversely proportional to the length of nerve regeneration required.[30, 75]

Neurotmesis is complete anatomic disruption of neural and connective tissue elements and is incompatible with spontaneous recovery.

Several potential causes of traumatic peripheral nerve injuries have been identified and reported by Gentili and Hudson.[30] These include direct injury by laceration, contusion, traction, compression ischemia (e.g., by tourniquet), heat (e.g., thermal injury from methyl methacrylate during total hip arthroplasty), electricity, or injection. A common example of the last-named is a misdirected intragluteal injection. Direct intrafascicular injection is particularly damaging to the nerve, the extent of damage being related to the nature of the chemical injected.[30, 75] Substances such as benzylpenicillin, diazepam, or chlorpromazine create a severe nerve injury even with extrafascicular injection.

All nerve injuries are followed by an attempt at healing. Regeneration of a sensory or mixed peripheral nerve may be associated with unpleasant dysesthesias. These abnormal sensations may involve ongoing pain and intermittent electric shocks in the distribution of the affected nerve. As regeneration continues, the dysesthesias may subside. Occasionally, however, regeneration can lead to development of a painful neuroma that may occur in continuity with an incomplete nerve injury. The diagnosis of distal peripheral traumatic nerve injuries is usually obvious, but the diagnosis of proximal injuries may be confused with an acute radiculopathy from a disc herniation.

Focal traumatic lesions to mixed peripheral nerves can sometimes be followed by *causalgia,* which is a burning type of pain associated with hyperpathia and an increased threshold to light touch along the distribution of the injured nerve. There seems to be a predilection for the sciatic nerve, perhaps because of its large number of sympathetic fibers. This pain is often exacerbated by emotional stress, which results in increased sympathetic outflow from the affected nerve. Abnormal nonsynaptic lateral contact between nociceptive afferent and sympathetic efferent fibers leading to abnormal nerve conduction (ephaptic cross excitation) has been proposed to explain this phenomenon.[30] When diagnosis is in doubt, relief of symptoms by sympathetic block is diagnostic.

Ischemic Neuropathy

Vascular lesions causing neuropathy may be divided in two groups: (1) large artery disease (acute or chronic) due to embolism, arterial wall trauma, intra-arterial injection of toxic drugs, or atherosclerosis of the aorta or its branches; (2) small artery disease due to diabetes, arteritis, amyloidosis, or blood viscosity disorders.[3, 16]

These conditions may affect the nerve anywhere along its path, including the peripheral nerve, the lumbosacral plexus, and the lumbosacral roots. Vascular pain in the lower limbs is frequently described as "burning" in nature and the neural lesion has been termed "ischemic neuritis."[75] A vascular etiology is suggested by a rapid onset of pain and neurologic deficit, the absence of pulses in the extremity, and temperature and skin changes in the leg and foot. The diagnosis is aided by documentation of impaired blood flow through invasive or noninvasive vascular studies.

Diabetes mellitus and polyarteritis nodosa are common etiologic factors in small vessel ischemic neuritis.[16] Diabetes mellitus may present as either a focal or a multifocal neuropathy.[3] Such neuropathic conditions include cranial mononeuropathies, truncal neuropathies, proximal asymmetric motor neuropathy, or distal symmetric (primary sensory) polyneuropathy. The last-named often presents with hypoesthesia or anesthesia in an irregular stocking distribution. Proximal asymmetric motor neuropathy is also known as "diabetic amyotrophy," a term originally used to describe the prominent muscle weakness and atrophy seen in this condition but which has since been abandoned because of its ambiguity.[25] It can mimic a lumbar radiculopathy, the patient presenting with a mixture of signs and symptoms due to nerve hyperactivity or inactivity. Pain, paresthesias, cramps, fasciculations, and excessive autonomic activity indicate hyperactivity of the affected nerves. Diminished or absent tendon reflexes and an increased threshold for sensation indicate hypoactivity of the nerves.

Pain, which is almost always present in proximal asymmetric motor neuropathy, is usually severe, deep, aching, and constant in nature. It is typically worse at night and may have a burning quality. The pain may start in the lower back or buttocks and may radiate to the thigh or knee on the affected side, and in this respect may mimic a lumbar radiculopathy. The onset of symptoms is usually acute but may be subacute, with pain evolving over several days or weeks. The pain may be so severe that narcotics are required for control. As weakness and wasting of muscles appears, the pain often remits.[3, 16] Muscle wasting is prominent and most frequently involves the quadriceps, iliopsoas, or adductors of the thigh.[25, 75] Other involved muscles include the gluteus, hamstring, and gastrocnemius. The prognosis for recovery within six to 12 months is good.

The underlying pathophysiology of small artery ischemic neuropathy is widespread arteriolar and capillary thickening leading to microinfarctions in the proximal nerve trunk, with consequent axonal loss and varying degrees of demyelination.[3] The lesions are not restricted to the nerve trunk but also affect the more proximal lumbosacral plexus and upper lumbar roots. This entity is more commonly seen in diabetics over the age of 50. The duration and severity of the underlying diabetes is variable, many patients exhibiting other complications of the underlying diabetes. Rarely the neuropathy may occur in individuals with mild or previously undetected diabetes. Involvement of multiple roots suggests a more diffuse process than is seen with lumbar disc herniation.

Ischemic neuropathy can be difficult to differentiate from other lumbosacral lesions such as pelvic tumor, hematoma or lumbar canal stenosis. The sudden onset and progression of symptoms, the presence of other associated entities such as primary sensory distal polyneuropathy or cranial mononeuopathies (e.g., Bell's palsy or third nerve palsy), abnormality of blood glucose, and abnormal electrophysiologic study results help to establish the diagnosis.

Sciatic nerve dysfunction may occur only during exercise, recovering after rest. This is thought to be due to insufficiency of arterial supply to the nerve, which may be correctable by vascular surgery ("claudication of sciatic nerve").[75] This pain has some of the features of a compartment syndrome but its exact cause is unclear.

Infiltration or Compression by Tumors

Peripheral nerve tumors are relatively uncommon lesions. Neoplasms or masses along the course of the sciatic nerve can produce pain or progressive nerve dysfunction resulting in diagnostic confusion.[6, 60, 62, 63, 84] These tumors may be classified as either *extra-* or *intra*neural and may be benign or malignant. The two most common benign extraneural tumors are lipoma and ganglion cyst. The latter has been reported to cause compression of the common peroneal nerve at the knee and the posterior tibial nerve at the ankle.

Intraneural tumors are classified as:

I. Peripheral *nerve sheath* tumors (e.g., schwannoma, neurofibroma, hemangioma, hemangioblastoma, malignant schwannoma).

II. Peripheral *neuron* tumors (e.g., ganglioneuroma).

III. Infiltrative tumors of non-neural origin (e.g., lymphoma, multiple myeloma, or carcinoma).

The spectrum of clinical presentation of peripheral nerve tumors is varied, depending on their location. They may present as sciatica, tarsal tunnel syndrome, progressive leg numbness or leg weakness, footdrop, or a tender mass.[62] Diagnosis depends on maintaining a high index of suspicion and on confirmation by electrophysiologic or radiologic studies such as computed tomography (CT) or magnetic resonance imaging (MRI).[60, 62] Atypical radicular pain with failure to respond to conventional treatment should raise clinical suspicion.

Although normal results from conduction studies on nerve sheath tumors such as sciatic nerve schwannomas have been reported, they are usually abnormal when there are infiltrative lesions.

Other Neuropathies

Axonal or "dying back" neuropathies may be seen with nutritional deficiencies (e.g., beriberi, cachexia), toxins (e.g., lead, alcohol), or metabolic derangements (e.g., hypothyroidism, uremia, hepatic failure).[75] Symptoms may include pain, paresthesias, and distal muscle weakness and may be acute or chronic in duration. Dysesthesias or paresthesias are usually in a stocking distribution. Recovery usually occurs once the precipitating disturbance has been corrected.

The combination of long-standing excessive alcohol consumption and dietary deficiency may lead to a peripheral neuropathy. Patients may present with a dull constant ache in the legs and feet that is occasionally lancinating in character and is of short duration. Muscle weakness may be mild or severe and may even present as a footdrop. Painful paresthesias elicited by light skin contact are commonly seen.

Infectious neuropathy is not as frequent in the United States as in other parts of the world, but must be considered in the differential diagnosis of neuropathic lesions. Leprosy is the most common treatable cause of neuropathy throughout the world.[68] Bacillary invasion of the nerves (usually superficial nerves), skin, upper respiratory tract, eye, and testes has been well described. It frequently involves the peroneal nerve in the leg, enlarging it and causing tenderness to palpation. Typical skin changes and biopsy are diagnostic. Parasitic nerve involvement (e.g., by cysticercus, schistosome) has also been described as a cause of infectious peripheral neuropathy.[75]

One of the initial presenting symptoms in patients with acquired immunodeficiency syndrome (AIDS) is a painful inflammatory neuropathy.[12, 70] These neuropathies usually occur in a clinical subgroup of human immunodeficiency virus (HIV)–infected patients who either are asymptomatic for systemic illness or have only lymphadenopathy. The cause is thought to be a cell-mediated immune response. Patients may present with a burning discomfort in the toes and associated weakness of the extensor hallucis longus or an absent ankle reflex.[70] Plasmapheresis may induce partial clinical remission.[12]

LUMBOSACRAL PLEXUS LESIONS

The lumbosacral plexus is formed by the anterior primary rami of L1–S4.[41] It lies within the posterior wall of the abdominal cavity and pelvis and is retroperitoneally located. The *lumbar plexus* is formed from the anterior primary rami of L1–L4. It is situated anterior to the transverse processes of the lumbar vertebra and is deeply within the psoas major muscle. The *sacral plexus* is formed by the merging of the anterior primary rami of L4 and L5, forming the lumbosacral trunk, with the anterior primary rami of S1–S4. It lies on the piriform muscle. The lumbosacral plexus may be involved by several pathologic processes, and lesions of the plexus may present as pain or impairment of lower extremity function. These processes include compression or infiltration by tumor or aneurysm, postradiation fibrosis, trauma, infection, and ischemia.

Tumors and Aneurysms

The frequency and nature of lumbosacral plexus tumor involvement remains uncertain.[6] Tumors may arise from any adjacent structure including nerve, pelvic viscera, or abdominal viscera. Nerve sheath tumors of the lumbosacral plexus are rare, but giant sacral schwannomas causing low back pain and lower extremity pain have been reported.[1, 22] They may present as an intrapelvic mass and may erode the adjacent anterior aspect of the sacrum. The presence of skin stigmata of neurofibromatosis (café au lait spots) should alert the clinician to the possibility of a nerve sheath tumor in patients presenting with leg pain and weakness.

Visceral tumors such as large uterine fibroids, uterine fibrosarcomas, leiomyomas, malignant tumors of the inferior pole of the kidney, retroperitoneal lymphomas, or pelvic endometriosis have been reported as causes of extrinsic lumbosacral plexus compression.[6, 77, 81] Carcinomas (e.g., prostate, cervical) may involve the plexus by direct extension and invasion of the lymphatic and perineural spaces. Lymphoma and multiple myeloma typically infiltrate the nerves diffusely.[72]

Aneurysms of the abdominal aorta and pelvic arteries (common iliac and hypogastric) can compress the lumbosacral plexus. Rupture of the wall of an aortic aneurysm into the iliopsoas muscle may create a false aneurysm that can compress the lumbar plexus and result in leg pain. Aneurysms of the pelvic arteries can also produce posterior leg pain by the same mechanism or may even cause a sciatic nerve palsy. A pulsatile mass may sometimes be palpated on rectal examination. Abdominal, rectal, and vaginal examination are therefore important tools in the diagnosis of these lesions, which can be confirmed by sonography, angiography, CT, MRI, or EMG.

Radiation

The treatment of abdominopelvic tumors frequently requires radiation therapy, which itself can result in back or leg pain from radiation plexopathy. Distinguishing this from plexus involvement by tumor can be very difficult. Postradiation changes involving the cauda equina and distal spinal cord also present a very confusing clinical picture. Numbness and paresthesias from postradiation fibrosis usually develop within the first year after radiation therapy and slowly progress to weakness and muscle wasting. The presence of myokymia (spontaneous tetanic motor unit contraction) suggests a radiation-induced plexopathy rather than tumor involvement.[72]

Trauma

Trauma to the lumbosacral plexus most often occurs after complex pelvic fractures and is often associated with serious urogenital, vascular, or rectal injuries. Retroperitoneal or psoas hematomas may compress the lumbar or lumbosacral plexus and may present a clinical picture suggesting a plexopathy or radiculopathy. The lumbosacral plexus can also be injured by gunshot and knife wounds. Diagnosis and localization of the lesion is aided by EMG. The prognosis for recovery from direct plexus injury is poor.

Infection

Iliacus and iliopsoas abscess can present as back pain with radiation to the groin or thigh. This condition often results from adjacent vertebral osteomyelitis. A clue to the localization of this condition is a positive femoral nerve stretch test, an elevated sedimentation rate, positive blood cultures, and positive radionuclide studies suggesting infection. MRI is the diagnostic procedure of choice and clearly delineates both the relationship of the abscess to adjacent structures and the presence of neural compression.[51]

Ischemic Plexopathy

Chronic small vessel occlusive disease can lead to vascular insufficiency and nerve dysfunction of the lumbosacral plexus (diabetic polyradiculoplexopathy). The patient may present with a sudden or insidious onset of leg pain and paresthesias, followed by muscle weakness and wasting in the femoral, obturator, or occasionally sciatic nerve distribution.[16, 72] The pain is typically described as "burning" in nature and is usually constant. The absence of a straight leg raising (SLR) sign, lack of a positive femoral nerve stretch test, lack of back pain, and absence of paraspinal muscle denervation on EMG help to differentiate this condition from other intraspinal lesions.

LUMBOSACRAL NERVE ROOT LESIONS

The lumbar and sacral roots are contained within the spinal canal and arise from the distal portion of the spinal cord at the thoracolumbar junction. They travel in the lumbar subarachnoid cistern to pierce the dura and exit via the foramen intertransversalis several centimeters below their site of origin. Injury to the nerve roots may occur at any point along this course.

The dorsal roots carry sensory information to the spinal cord, while the ventral roots transmit primarily motor impulses. Injury to the nerve roots may involve motor, sensory, or mixed (sensorimotor) fibers. Careful clinical examination, although helpful in localizing the site of the lesion, is not always diagnostic. Disc herniation and other extrinsic neural compressive lesions are the most common cause of radiculopathy, but other etiologies must be considered. Such lesions can be classified as either *extra-* or *intra*dural (Fig. 5–2).

Extradural Lesions

Tumors. Metastatic lesions make up the majority of intraspinal extradural tumors, and most metastases involve the vertebral body. It has been estimated that 75 per cent of vertebral metastases originate from the breast, prostate, kidney, or thyroid or from myeloma or lymphoma.[31, 35, 77] Metastatic lesions may be the initial presentation of an unknown malignancy in 10 per cent of cases, with tumor cells reaching the spine and epidural space via hematogenous spread.[5, 8] Tumor pain is typically worse at night and is not relieved by recumbency. Radicular pain and motor or sensory deficit may be present. Tumor therefore must always be considered in the differential diagnosis of radiating or nonradiating low back pain that is worse at night, is not relieved by recumbency, and involves several nerve roots.

Sacral and presacral tumors often present with low back and radiating leg pain.[22] The diffuse nature of the pain and the nonspecific nature of the symptoms may result in a diagnosis of coccydynia. Delay in making the correct diagnosis is common owing to the nonspecific symptoms and the absence of neurologic signs. X-ray findings are often missed because of overlying bowel gas and feces that can obscure the underlying lesion. Delay in diagnosis often leads to tumor progression with resultant sacral neural deficits involving perineal numbness or bowel and bladder dysfunction. Detailed sensory examination of sacral dermatomes and a careful rectal examination may give a clue to the diagnosis of these rare tumors. High-resolution CT is the preferred diagnostic imaging study of choice to define details of bony destruction; MRI is best to delineate neural compression and spread of tumor into the lumbar canal and soft tissues. Angiography is a useful adjunct, particularly when surgery is contemplated.

Spinal Epidural Lipomatosis. Pathologic overgrowth of epidural fat has been described in patients after chronic use of glucocorticoids (e.g., in rheumatoids, in transplant recipients, and in systemic lupus erythematosus patients) and in obese individuals.[23] This condition may present with typical radicular pain or as a myelopathy, depending on the size and location of the lesion. Myelography, postcontrast CT, or MRI usually show the lesion, although MRI shows the size and extent of the lesion most effectively.

Infection. Discitis, osteomyelitis, and epidural abscess usually present with back pain that can radiate down the leg.[38] The back examination reveals percussion tenderness, guarding, loss of lumbar lordosis, and marked limitation of motion.[42] Systemic signs of infection may be present and should be sought. In patients with leg pain, the SLR sign may be positive if there is neural compression from abscess or granulation tissue. An elevated sedimentation rate, a positive bone scan, and characteristic changes on MRI are helpful in establishing the diagnosis.[77]

Lumbar Synovial Cyst. Dorsolateral root compression from an adjacent facet joint synovial cyst may mimic radiculopathy from lumbar disc herniation.[40, 48, 58] There is usually nothing in the history to suggest this etiology for leg pain. Many patients have a history of chronic back pain with recent onset of leg pain. Diagnosis is confirmed by CT or MRI, which shows neural compression by a lesion contiguous with the facet joint.

Lumbar Canal Stenosis. Chronic compression of the cauda equina from gradual spinal canal narrowing may lead to back, buttock, or leg pain provoked by prolonged walking or by standing (neurogenic claudication).[43, 78] This compression may be due to congenital (developmental) or acquired factors and may be focal, segmental, or generalized in scope. The end result of this compression is nerve ischemia induced either by inadequate arterial supply to the nerve or by venous hypertension due to impaired venous drainage.[66, 76] The usual symptom is leg or buttock pain, but motor weakness, numbness, or paresthesias may also be present.

Patients with lumbar canal stenosis are typically over 50 years of age and usually present with a history of chronic back pain and a more recent onset of radiating leg pain. Neurogenic claudication usually starts in the low back area and radiates into buttocks, thighs, or calves. Patients have difficulty with walking or prolonged standing because these positions in-

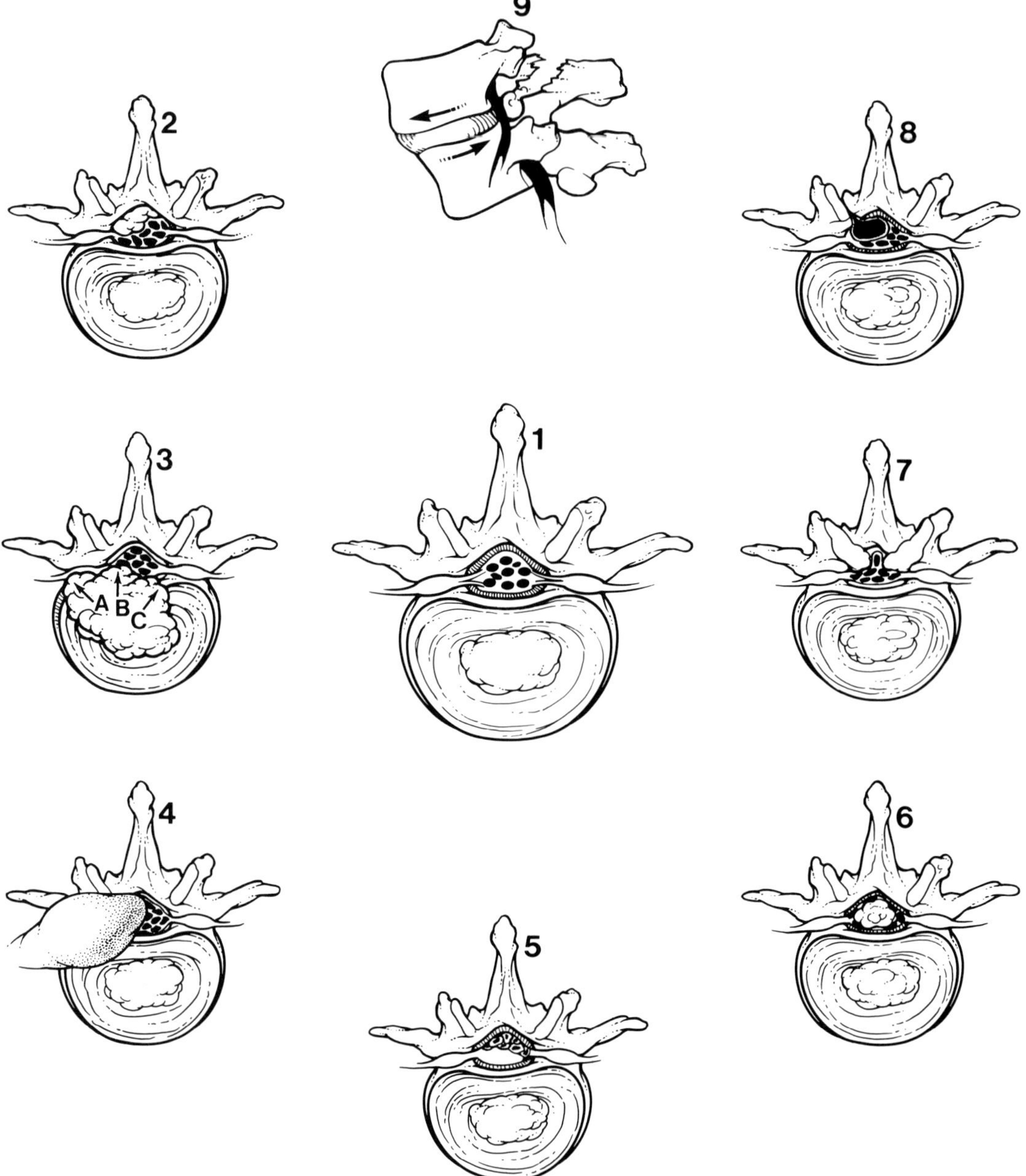

Figure 5–2. Schematic representation of intradural and extradural spinal lesions

1. Normal
2. Epidural tumor/masses
3. Intervertebral disc herniation
   a. extreme lateral
   b. posterolateral
   c. central
4. Spinal nerve tumors
5. Inflammatory/infectious lesions (arachnoiditis)
6. Intradural tumors
7. Lumbar canal stenosis
8. Synovial cyst
9. Spondylolisthesis/spondylolysis

crease lumbar lordosis, which accentuates canal and foraminal narrowing and results in nerve compression. Patients therefore prefer to assume a flexed posture that minimizes lumbar lordosis and decreases canal and foraminal narrowing. A helpful historical feature is the presence of a positive "shopping cart sign": the patient leans over a cart while grocery shopping in order to accentuate foraminal enlargement. There may be complaints of lower extremity weakness, but sensory symptoms usually predominate. The leg pain of neurogenic claudication can be distinguished from that due to vascular claudication by the fact that relief in the latter condition can be obtained merely by cessation of walking, whereas in the former relief is obtained only by a change in position, typically by sitting or by bending forward.[43] Dyck and colleagues described the Van Gelderen bicycle test in which patients with vascular claudication develop leg pain with bicycling, whereas patients with neurogenic claudication do not.[16] The reason for this is that neural compression due to spinal stenosis is relieved by sitting owing to enlargement of the neural foramina.[76]

Resting physical examination of patients with spinal stenosis is usually unremarkable, although there may be loss of lumbar lordosis or restriction of spinal motion. Leg symptoms may, however, be elicited by lumbar extension. Mild leg weakness, patchy areas of hypoesthesia, and diminished or absent deep tendon reflexes may sometimes be elicited after prolonged walking or standing. Weakness of the extensor hallucis longus is the most common motor finding since the condition is most common at the L4–L5 level and therefore affects the L5 root most commonly. The SLR sign is negative, and pulses in the lower extremities are typically present. Discriminating features of the history and physical examination of patients with neurogenic and vascular claudication are listed in Table 5–1.

Spondylolisthesis. Anterior displacement of a vertebral body in relation to its inferior adjacent vertebra can cause root compression with resultant leg pain and weakness. Low back and leg pain is usually mechanical, often aggravated by walking or standing. A pure monoradicular pattern of entrapment may be seen, symptoms frequently being bilateral. With L5–S1 isthmic spondylolisthesis, it is the L5 nerve root that is usually involved by entrapment of the root at the level of the pars defect, although S1 involvement may be seen with high-grade slips. Spondylolisthesis with an intact posterior arch (degenerative spondylolisthesis) can lead to compression of the cauda equina and a clinical picture of intermittent neurogenic claudication. Typically, degenerative spondylolisthesis involves L4–L5 and commonly affects the L5 nerve root.

Intraspinal Extradural Cyst. Intrasacral extradural arachnoid cyst, also called occult intrasacral meningocele, is a rare clinical condition that must be considered in the differential diagnosis of patients with low back and buttock pain.[14, 29] This lesion is not a true meningocele but rather a sac of fibrous tissue resembling dura and lined by arachnoid. It is connected to the caudal aspect of the lumbar cistern by a pedicle that permits flow of cerebrospinal fluid (CSF) by a ball-valve mechanism. The cyst grows gradually, probably by trapping or secreting CSF.[33] This slow enlargement may gradually erode sacral bone and may compress adjacent roots. Pain produced by such cysts is typically aggravated by the Valsalva maneuver, which increases the pressure within the cyst. It may present as a persistent sensation of fullness in the perineum or pelvis. Motor weakness involving S1 may be present as well as perianal or saddle anesthesia. Lateral radio-

Table 5–1. DISCRIMINATING FEATURES OF NEUROGENIC AND VASCULAR CLAUDICATION

	Neurogenic	Vascular
Pulses	Present	Decreased or absent
Palliative factors	Bending over or sitting	Stopping
Provocative factors	Going downhill (increased lumbar lordosis)	Going uphill (increased metabolic demand)
Neurologic evaluation after walking	Diminished reflexes; increased weakness; sensory changes	Unchanged
Van Gelderen bicycle test	No leg pain	Leg pain
"Shopping cart sign"	Present	Absent

graphs of the sacrum may suggest enlargement of its canal. The cyst usually fills during myelography. MRI reveals the cyst as a high-signal-intensity lesion that is isodense with CSF.

Perineural cysts of sacral or coccygeal nerve roots were originally described by Tarlov as arising between the layers of connective tissue covering the nerve roots.[73] A communication between the cyst and the subarachnoid space may be present. The cysts are usually discovered incidentally during myelography and are generally asymptomatic, although several cases associated with radicular pain have been reported. Differential diagnosis of these lesions includes neurofibroma and schwannoma of the sacral region (nerve sheath tumors).

Intradural Lesions

Intradural Tumors. These lesions, uncommon in the lumbosacral area, may arise by direct extension from local structures or may be the result of "dropped metastases" from higher lesions in the central nervous system (CNS).[59] Intradural tumors, insidious in their clinical presentation, elude diagnosis for an average of two years after onset of symptoms. Back pain is the usual initial symptom and is typically worse at night. Nocturnal symptoms are thought to be due to venous pooling and engorgement associated with the supine position during sleep. Neurologic symptoms may involve single or multiple roots and usually present as sensory or motor disturbances with occasional bowel and bladder dysfunction. A history of unremitting, constant back or leg pain, often worse at night, with gradual evolution of neurologic deficit, should suggest to the astute clinician the possibility of neoplasm. MRI, with or without gadolinium, defines the extent and anatomic relationship of the lesion to neural structures and is currently the preferred diagnostic imaging technique, although myelography and CT also show the lesion. Urodynamics and cystometrography may be useful if there is bladder involvement.

Some of the reported intradural tumors include nerve sheath tumors (e.g., schwannomas, neurofibromas), ependymomas (tumors of the conus medullaris and filum terminale) (Fig. 5–3), epidermoid tumors,[44] dermoids, teratomas, lipomas, meningiomas, and "dropped metastases" (e.g., primitive neuroectodermal tumors such as medulloblastomas, high-grade gliomas, germinomas).

Infections and Inflammatory Lesions. Any infectious or inflammatory condition affecting

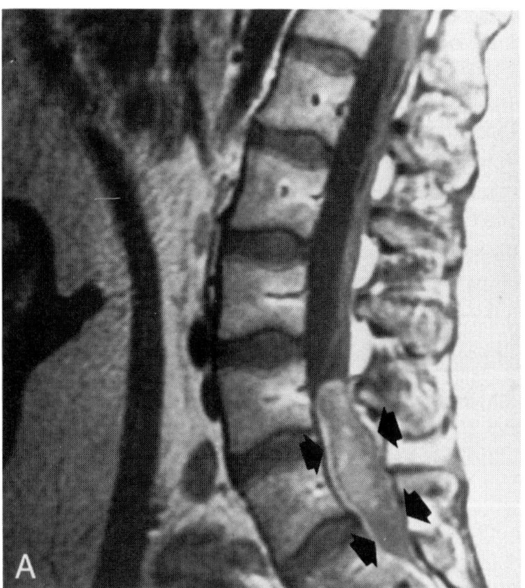

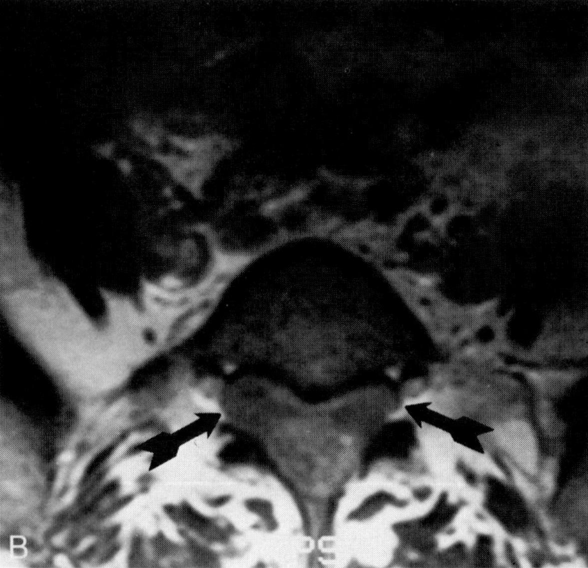

Figure 5–3. Ependymoma. A 41-year-old female with an eight-year history of low back pain, worse over the preceding six months. She presented with numbness in the buttocks and posterior thigh and difficulty with urination. Examination revealed bilateral sacral hypoesthesias, diminished rectal tone, normal strength, and a negative straight leg raising (SLR) sign. Sagittal MRI *(A)* revealed a large intradural lesion *(arrows)* within the enlarged spinal canal. Axial MRI *(B)* revealed complete filling of the canal by the lesion *(arrows)*.

the CSF may also involve the neural elements, which can be damaged by infiltration, compression, or vascular abnormalities. Sensory, motor, or sensorimotor involvement may occur.

Parasitic diseases, very common in underdeveloped countries, must be considered in areas with large immigrant populations. Patients with spinal schistosomiasis, for example, may present with lower extremity pain and weakness as well as bladder or rectal sphincter involvement.[53] Although clinical examination may suggest a disc herniation, CSF analysis typically shows pleocytosis and protein elevation.

Chronic inflammation of nerve roots secondary to long-standing infection may induce secondary inflammation and fibrosis of the adjacent meninges (arachnoiditis) leading to painful and often disabling leg pain.[83] This syndrome may be difficult to distinguish from other sciatic conditions because of a lack of characteristic physical findings. The pain, usually aggravated by activity, is not fully relieved by rest and in this respect is not typical of the mechanical pain usually seen with other sciatic syndromes. Patients often describe a burning sensation or a sensation of small insects crawling over the skin (formication). Myelography and MRI have been useful in the diagnosis of this entity. The axial T1-weighted sequence appears to be the most efficient for imaging arachnoiditis.[65] Infection, subarachnoid hemorrhage, trauma, previous spinal surgery, intradural steroids, or spinal anesthesia have been described as etiologic factors and should be sought in the history. Bilaterality of symptoms, multiplicity of nerve root involvement, and characteristic radiologic findings help to establish the diagnosis.

HIGHER CENTRAL NERVOUS SYSTEM LESIONS (CENTRAL ORIGIN)

Pain information from the lower extremities arises from nociceptors that send electrical impulses to the dorsal horn of the spinal cord. The impulses ascend for a couple of segments ipsilaterally and then cross to the contralateral ventral funiculus to join the spinothalamic tract. Pain and temperature sensation from the lower extremities is carried in the most ventral and lateral portion of the spinal cord, the upper extremities being more medially represented. The relatively superficial location of the spinothalamic tract within the spinal cord makes it prone to injury that can result in ipsilateral motor dysfunction and contralateral sensory disturbances below the level of the lesion. Dysesthesias may occur and are usually diffuse and poorly localized; they are frequently described as "burning" in character. This type of sensation has been termed "tract pain," which usually lacks the sharpness and precision of localization seen with peripherally induced lesions. This phenomenon is thought to represent a disinhibition of normal ascending pain-producing spinal pathways that normally inhibit pain signals, thereby permitting the brain to interpret the lack of normal inhibition as pain.[26] This theory probably explains the radicular type of lower extremity pain seen in patients with spinal cord lesions. Such sciatica-like lower extremity pain has been described with many lesions, including intradural extramedullary tumors, disc herniation, and arteriovenous malformations.[6]

Physical examination usually reveals long tract signs that suggest a lesion at the spinal cord level, but these signs are not always present; the clinical examination may reveal hypoactive reflexes and motor weakness suggesting a lesion within the cauda equina rather than the spinal cord.

An advantage of MRI and myelography over CT in the diagnosis of spinal diseases is their visualization of the thoracolumbar junction and their capability of identifying unsuspected pathology at that level. This is particularly true for MRI, with which the entire spine can be imaged sagittally (Fig. 5–4).

REFERRED PAIN

Referred pain is a dull, aching discomfort commonly felt in the low back, buttocks, or legs. It is due to stimulation of mesodermal structures such as ligaments, periosteum, joint capsule, or annulus fibrosus. The pain is referred along the sclerotome, as opposed to true radicular pain, which has a dermatomal distribution. The dull, deep-boring, poorly localized discomfort of referred pain contrasts with the sharper and better localized pattern of radicular pain.[64] A common example of referred pain in the upper extremity is the

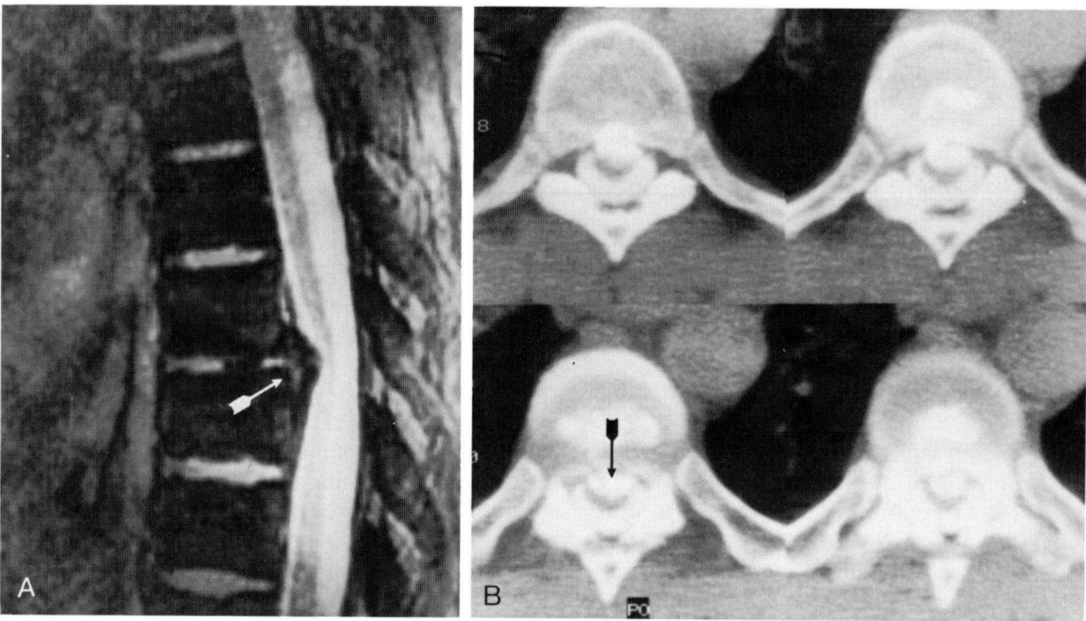

Figure 5–4. Thoracic (T7–T8) disc herniation. A 48-year-old male with back pain and left leg pain who presented with left extensor hallucis longus (EHL) weakness, a negative straight leg raising (SLR) sign, and hypoactive lower extremity weakness. Although initial clinical presentation suggested a lumbar radiculopathy, and myelography suggested a small L5 nerve root filling defect, the major pathology was at T7–T8 where T2-weighted MRI *(A)* revealed a large thoracic disc herniation *(white arrow)*. Metrizamide CT *(B)* revealed a large, central, partially calcified disc herniation at T7–T8 *(black arrow)*. Relief of symptoms followed transthoracic excision of the disc herniation.

shoulder and arm pain seen with angina pectoris. A similar phenomenon in the lower extremity has been demonstrated experimentally by the injection of hypertonic saline into the mesodermal structures of the back, resulting in pain that typically radiates into the low back, buttocks, or legs.

Patients with hip joint disease frequently present with pain that radiates along the anterior aspect of the thigh to the knee, thus mimicking an L4 radiculopathy.[10, 52] This is explained by the fact that the sensory innervation of the hip derives partially from the anterior division of the obturator nerve and partially from the femoral nerve, both of which have a predominant L4 contribution.[41] In some patients with concomitant hip and spine disease, the predominant source of pain can be difficult to determine. Offierski and MacNab[52] described this as the *hip-spine syndrome* and classified it into three categories: (1) *simple hip-spine syndrome* in which the cause of the pain was easily determined by history and physical examination; (2) *complex hip-spine syndrome* in which the symptoms and clinical examination gave a confusing picture, making it difficult to determine the primary source of the disability—these patients often required nerve root infiltration and intra-articular hip joint injections to confirm the diagnosis; and (3) *secondary hip-spine syndrome* in which lumbar radicular symptoms from changes in the lumbar spine were aggravated by pathologic changes in the hip. Such hip pathology included flexion-contracture causing secondary compensatory lumbar hyperlordosis and resultant lumbar nerve root compression and sciatica. Failure to recognize this referred pain pattern in degenerative hip joint disease may lead to misdiagnosis and erroneous treatment.

CONCLUSION

Establishment of the correct diagnosis and proper treatment for a patient with sciatica requires a knowledge of the potential pathologic processes that can affect the nervous structures supplying the lower extremities. The most important information involved in formulating the differential diagnosis comes from an accurate history. A precise physical examination further refines and narrows the diagnostic possibilities. Finally, the judicious use of diagnostic tests builds on information obtained by the history and physical examination and further defines the most likely cause of the condition. A high level of suspicion should arise in patients who present with atypical pain or multiple root involvement, or those who do not respond as expected to the usual treatment.

References

1. Abernathey, C. D., Onofrio, B. M., Scheithauer B., et al.: Surgical management of giant sacral schwannomas. J. Neurosurg. *65:*286–295, 1986.
2. Aoki, S., Barkovich, A. J., Nichimura, K., et al.: Neurofibromatosis types 1 and 2: cranial MR findings. Radiology *172:*527–534, 1989.
3. Asbury, A. K.: Focal and multifocal neuropathies of diabetes. *In* Dyck, P. J., Thomas, P. K., Asbury, A. K., et al. (eds.): Philadelphia, W. B. Saunders Co., 1982, pp. 45–55.
4. Baringer, J. R., and Townsend, J. J.: Herpesvirus infection of the peripheral nervous system. *In* Dyck, P. J., Thomas, P. K., Lambert, E. H., and Bunge, R. (eds.): Peripheral Neuropathy 2nd ed. Vol. II. Philadelphia, W. B. Saunders Co., 1984, pp. 1941–1954.
5. Batson, O. V.: The function of vertebral veins and their role in the spread of metastasis. Ann. Surg. *112:*138, 1940.
6. Bay, J. W.: Other Causes of Low Back Pain and Sciatica: Lumbar Disc Disease. R. W. Hardy Seminars Neurological Surgery. New York, Raven Press, 1932, pp. 203–215.
7. Bilge, T., Kaya, A., Alatle, M., et al.: Hemangioma of the peroneal nerve: case report and review of the literature. Neurosurgery *25:*649–652, 1989.
8. Black, P.: Spinal epidural tumors. *In* Wilkins, R., and Renganchary, S. (eds.): Neurosurgery. New York, McGraw-Hill Book Co., 1989, pp. 1062–1068.
9. Brown, C. W.: Obturator nerve pain. Contributed paper at Annual Meeting of Federation of Spine Associations, New Orleans, LA, February 1986.
10. Callaghan, J. J., Brand, R. A., and Pederson, D. R.: Hip arthrodesis. J. Bone Joint Surg. *67A:*1328–1325, 1985.
11. Dawson, D., Hallet, M., and Millender, L. H.: Entrapment Neuropathies. 1st ed. Boston, Little, Brown & Co., 1983.
12. de la Monte, S. M., Garbuzda, D. H., Ho, D. D., et al.: Peripheral neuropathy in the acquired immunodeficiency syndrome. Ann. Neurol. *23:*485–492, 1988.
13. de Toffol, B., Cotty, P., Gaymord, B., and Velut, S.: Progressive necrosis of the conus medullaris: magnetic resonance imaging and surgical findings. Neurosurgery *26:*147–149, 1990.
14. Doty, J. R., Thompson, J., Simonds, G., et al.: Occult intrasacral meningocele: clinical and radiographic diagnosis. Neurosurgery *24:*616–625, 1989.
15. Dupuis, R. R., Cassidy, J. D., and Kirkaldy-Willis, W. H.: Radiologic diagnosis of degenerative lumbar spinal instability. Spine *10:*262–276, 1985.
16. Dyck, P. J., Katnes, J., and O'Brien, P. C.: Diagnosis, staging and classification of diabetic neuropathy and associations with other complications. *In* Dyck, P. J., Thomas, P. K., Asbury, A. K., et al. (eds.): Diabetic Neuropathy. Philadelphia, W. B. Saunders Co., 1987, pp. 36–45.
17. Eckard, J. J., Kaplan, D. D., Batzdorf, V., and Dawson, E. G.: Extraforaminal disc herniation simulating a retroperitoneal neoplasm. J. Bone Joint Surg. *67A:*1275–1277, 1985.
18. Edelson, J. G., and Nathan, H.: Meralgia paresthetica. An anatomical interpretation. Clin. Orthop. *122:*255–262, 1977.
19. Edgar, M. A., and Ghadially, J. A.: Innervation of the lumbar spine. Clin. Orthop. *115:*35–41, 1976.
20. Epstein, N. E., Epstein, J. A., and Mauri, T.: Treatment of fractures of the vertebral limbus and spinal stenosis in five adolescents and five adults. Neurosurgery *24:*595–604, 1989.
21. Eyster, E. F., and Scott, W. R.: Lumbar synovial cysts: report of eleven cases. Neurosurgery *24:*112–115, 1989.
22. Feldenzer, J. A., McGanley, J. L., and McGillicuddy, J. E.: Sacral and presacral tumors: problems in diagnosis and management. Neurosurgery *25:*884–891, 1989.
23. Fessler, R. G., Johnson, D. L., Brown, F. D., et al.: Epidural lipomatosis in steroid-treated patients. Contributed paper at 6th Annual Meeting of the Joint Section on Disorders of the Spine and Peripheral Nerves AANS/CNS, Captiva Island, FL, February 1990.
24. Fisher, M. A., and Corelick, P. B.: Entrapment neuropathies: differential diagnosis and management. Postgrad. Med. *77:*160–174, 1985.
25. Flatow, E. L., and Michelsen, C. B.: Diabetic amyotrophy. J. Bone Joint Surg. *67A:*1132–1135, 1985.
26. Friedmann, A. H., and Nashold, B.: Spinal injury pain. *In* Long, D. (ed.): Current Therapy in Neurological Surgery. St. Louis, C. V. Mosby Co., 1985, pp. 203–205.
27. Friedmann, A. H., and Nashold, B.: Post-herpetic neuralgia. *In* Wilkins, R., and Renganchary, S. (eds.): Neurosurgery. New York, McGraw-Hill Book Co., 1985, p. 2367.
28. Gateless, D., and Gilroy, J.: Tight-jeans neuralgia: hot or cold? J.A.M.A. *252:*42–43, 1984.
29. Genest, A. S.: Occult intrasacral meningocele. Spine *9:*101–103, 1984.
30. Gentili, F., and Hudson, A.: Peripheral nerve injuries: types, causes, and grading. *In* Wilkins, R., and Renganchary, S. (eds.): Neurosurgery. New York, McGraw-Hill Book Co., 1985, pp. 1802–1811.
31. Gilbert, R. W., Kim, J. H., and Posner, J. B.: Epidural spinal cord compression from metastatic tumor: diagnosis and treatment. Ann. Neurol. *3:*40–51, 1978.
32. Graham, J. J., and Yang, W. C.: Vertebral hemangioma with compression fracture and paraparesis treated with preoperative embolization and vertebral resection. Spine *9:*97–101, 1984.
33. Gwan, K., Houthoff, H. J., Hartsviker, J., et al.: Fluid secretion in arachnoid cyst as a clue to cerebrospinal fluid absorption at the arachnoid granulation. J. Neurosurg. *65:*642–648, 1986.
34. Haddad, S. F., Hitchon, P. W., and Godersky, J. C.: Epidural spinal lipomatosis. Contributed paper at 6th Annual Meeting of Joint Section on Disorders

of the Spine and Peripheral Nerves AANS/CNS, Captiva Island, FL, February, 1990.

35. Harrington, K.: Metastatic disease of the spine. J. Bone Joint Surg. *68A:*1110–1115, 1986.
36. Hodgson, B. F.: Pyogenic sacroiliac joint infection. Clin. Orthop. *246:*146–149, 1989.
37. Isu, T., Iwasaki, Y., Akino, M., et al.: Mobile schwannoma of the cauda equina diagnosed by magnetic resonance imaging. Neurosurgery *25:*968–971, 1989.
38. Kemp, H. B. S., Jackson, J. W., Jeremiah, J. D., et al.: Pyogenic infections occurring primarily in the intervertebral discs. J. Bone Joint Surg. *55B:*698–714, 1973.
39. Kopell, H. P., and Thompson, W. A.: Peripheral entrapment neuropathies. 1st ed. Baltimore, Williams & Wilkins Co., 1963.
40. Kurz, L. T., Garfin, S. R., Unger, A. S., et al.: Intraspinal synovial cyst causing sciatica. J. Bone Joint Surg. *67A:*365–871, 1985.
41. Last, R. J.: Anatomy, Regional and Applied. London, J. A. Churchill, 1970, pp. 213–214.
42. Lonstein, J. E.: Diagnosis and treatment of postoperative spinal infections. Surg. Rounds Orthop. October 1989, pp. 25–32.
43. Lipson, J. J.: Spinal stenosis: definitions. Clinical diagnosis. Semin. Spine Surg. *1:*135–137, 143–144, 1989.
44. Lunardi, P., Missori, P., Gagliardi, F., and Fortuna, A.: Long-term results of the surgical treatment of spinal dermoid and epidermoid tumors. Neurosurgery *25:*860–864, 1989.
45. Lusk, M. D., Kline, D. G., and Garcia, C. A.: Tumors of the brachial plexus. Neurosurgery *21:*439–453, 1987.
46. Madsen, J., and Iveros, R.: Spinal arteriovenous malformations and neurogenic claudication. J. Neurosurg. *68:*793–797, 1988.
47. Malis, L. I.: Spinal arteriovenous malformation. *In* Long, D. (ed.): Current therapy in neurological surgery 1985–1986. St. Louis, C. V. Mosby Co., 1985, pp. 162–164.
48. Maresca, L., Meland, N. B., Maresca, C., and Field, E. M.: Gangion cyst of the spinal canal: case report. J. Neurosurg. *57:*140–142, 1982.
49. Maroon, J. C., Kopitnick, T. A., Schulhof, L. A., et al.: Diagnosis and microsurgical approach to far-lateral disc herniation in the lumbar spine. J. Neurosurg. *72:*378–382, 1990.
50. Medical Research Council Working Party on Tuberculosis of the Spine—Eighth Report. A ten-year assessment of a controlled trial, comparing debridement and anterior spinal fusion in the management of tuberculosis of the spine in patients on standard chemotherapy in Hong Kong. J. Bone Joint Surg. *64B:*393–398, 1982.
51. Modic, M., Feiglin, D. H., Piraino, D. W., et al.: Vertebral osteomyelitis: assessment using MR. Radiology *157:*157–166, 1985.
52. Offierski, C. M., and MacNab, I.: Hip-spine syndrome. Spine *8:*316–321, 1983.
53. Ortiz, H. J.: Parasitic disease of the brain and spinal cord. *In* Long, D. (ed.): Current therapy in neurological surgery. St. Louis, C. V. Mosby Co., 1985, pp. 130–134.
54. Orton, D.: Neuralgia paresthetica from a wallet. J. A. M. A. *252:*3368, 1984.
55. Pagni, C. A., Canaveros, S., and Forni, M.: Report of a cavernoma of the cauda equina and review of the literature. Surg. Neurol. *33:*124–131, 1990.
56. Pappas, C. T. E., Rigamonti, D., Sonntag, V. K., et al.: Herniated thoracic disc. BNI Q. *4:*7–11, 1988.
57. Paris, S. V.: Physical signs of instability. Spine *10:*277–279, 1985.
58. Pendleton, B., Carl, B., and Pollay, M.: Spinal extradural benign synovial or ganglion cyst: case report and review of the literature. Neurosurgery *13:*322–326, 1983.
59. Pezeshkpour, G. H., Henry, J. M., and Armbrustmacher, V. W.: Spinal metastases. A rare mode of presentation of brain tumors. Cancer *54:*353–356, 1984.
60. Pillay, P. K., Hardy, R. W., Wilbourn, A. J., et al.: Solitary primary lymphoma of the sciatic nerve: case report. Neurosurgery *23:*370–371, 1988.
61. Postacchini, F., and Montanaro, A.: Extreme lateral herniations of lumbar disks. Clin. Orthop. *130:*222–227, 1979.
62. Powers, S. K., Norman, D., and Edwards, M. S. B.: Computerized tomography of peripheral nerve lesions. J. Neurosurg. *59:*131–136, 1983.
63. Prusick, V. R., Herkowitz, H. N., Favidson, D. D., et al.: Sciatica from a sciatic neurilemoma. J. Bone Joint Surg. *68A:*1456–1457, 1986.
64. Rabau, M. Y., Werbin, N., and Rabey, J. M.: Sciatic-like referred pain after rubberband haemorrhoidal ligation. Lancet. *1:*924–925, 1987.
65. Ross, J. S., Masaryk, T. J., Modic, M. T., et al.: MR imaging of lumbar arachnoiditis. Am. J. Rheumatol. *149:*1025–1032, 1987.
66. Rydevick, B. L., Hansson, T. H., and Garfin, S.: Pathophysiology of cauda equina compression. Semin. Spine Surg. *1:*139–142, 1989.
67. Saal, J. A., Dillingham, M. F., Gamburd, R. S., and Fanton, G. S.: The pseudoradicular syndrome: lower extremity peripheral nerve entrapment masquerading as lumbar radiculopathy. Spine *13:*926–930, 1988.
68. Sabin, T. D., and Swift, T. R.: Leprosy. *In* Dyck, P. J., Thomas, P. K., Lambert, E. H., and Bunge, R. (eds.): Peripheral neuropathy. 2nd ed. Vol. II. Philadelphia, W. B. Saunders Co., 1984, pp. 1955–1987.
69. Smythe, H.: Referred pain and tender points. Am. J. Med. *81:*90–92, 1986.
70. So, Y. T., Holtzman, D. M., Abrams, D. I., and Olney, R. K.: Peripheral neuropathy associated with acquired immunodeficiency syndrome. Prevalence and clinical features from a population-based survey. Arch. Neurol. *45:*945–948, 1988.
71. Solheim, L. F., Siewers, P., and Paus, B.: The piriformis muscle syndrome. Acta Orthop. Scand. *52:*73–75, 1981.
72. Stevens, J. C.: Lumbosacral plexus lesions. *In* Dyck, P. J., Thomas, P. K., Lambert, E. H., and Bunge, R. (eds.): Peripheral neuropathy. 2nd ed. Vol. II. Philadelphia, W. B. Saunders Co., 1984, pp. 1425–1434.
73. Tarlov, I. M.: Sacral nerve root cysts: another cause of the sciatic or cauda equina syndrome. Springfield, IL, Charles C Thomas, 1953.
74. Waddell, G., McCulloch, J. A., Kunnel, E., and Venner, R. M.: Nonorganic physical signs in low-back pain. Spine *5:*117–125, 1980.

75. Walton, Sir J.: Disorders of peripheral nerves. *In* Brain's Diseases of the Nervous System. 9th ed. Oxford, Oxford University Press, 1985, pp. 492–522.
76. Watanabe, R., and Parke, W.: Vascular and neural pathology of lumbosacral spinal stenosis. J. Neurosurg. *64:*64–70, 1986.
77. Watson, T. C., and Benson, D. R.: Nondiscogenic back and leg pain. *In* Youmans, J. R. (ed.): Neurological Surgery. 3rd ed. Philadelphia, W. B. Saunders Co., 1990, pp. 2629–2963.
78. Watts, C.: Spinal stenosis. *In* Rosenberg, R. N., Grossman, R. G., and Schochet, S. S. (eds.): The Clinical Neurosciences, 1st ed. Vol. II. New York, Churchill Livingstone, 1983, pp. 1459–1467.
79. Wiley, A. M., and Trueta, J.: The vascular anatomy of the spine and its relationship to pyogenic vertebral osteomyelitis. J. Bone Joint Surg. *41B:*796, 1959.
80. Wilke, W. S., and Corbo, D. D.: Fibrositis/fibromyalgia: causes and treatment. Comp. Ther. *13:*47–57, 1989.
81. Wilkes, L. L., Cannon, C. L., and Ham, D. E.: Malignant tumors of the pelvic girdle, mimicking the herniated disc syndrome. Clin. Orthop. *138:*217–221, 1979.
82. Wilkins, R.: Intraspinal cyst. *In* Wilkins, R., and Renganchary, S. (eds.): Neurosurgery. New York, McGraw-Hill Book Co., 1985, pp. 2061–2070.
83. Wilkinson, H. A.: Lumbar adhesive arachnoiditis. *In* Long, D. (ed.): Current therapy in neurological surgery. St. Louis, C. V. Mosby Co., 1985, pp. 198–200.
84. Wolock, B. S., Baugher, W. H., and McCarthy, E. J.: Neurilemoma of the sciatic nerve mimicking tarsal tunnel syndrome. J. Bone Joint Surg. *71A:*932–934, 1989.
85. Zaleske, D. J., Bone, H. H., Benz, R., and Krishnamoorthy, K. S.: Association of sciatica-like pain and Addison's disease. J. Bone Joint Surg. *66:*297–298, 1984.
86. Zuzuki, K., Ishida, Y., Ohmori, K., et al.: Redundant nerve roots of the cauda equina: clinical aspects and consideration of pathogenesis. Neurosurgery *24:*521–528, 1989.

CHAPTER

6

RADIOLOGY OF THE LUMBAR SPINE

Gordon R. Bell, M.D.
Michael T. Modic, M.D.

Intervertebral disc degeneration is a complex and poorly understood process that begins early in life and generally proceeds relentlessly throughout life. The methods used to detect this physiologic process have become more sophisticated as medical technology has become more complex. The fact that radiographic findings of disc degeneration are present in both asymptomatic and symptomatic populations underscores the problem of ascribing a clinical symptom to a radiographic finding.[3, 12, 13, 22–24, 31, 40, 53, 56, 61]

The biochemical events and underlying pathophysiology preceding the observed gross morphologic changes are beyond the scope of this chapter and are discussed elsewhere.[2, 3, 6, 45] The subsequent radiographic findings in the lumbar spine, however, reflect relatively later changes in the three-joint complex. As will be seen later, newer and more sophisticated diagnostic tools such as magnetic resonance imaging (MRI) enable investigators to see these physiologic changes much earlier in the course of the degenerative process.[42] Indeed, the changes seen with MRI give information about the state of hydration of the disc and therefore allow inferences to be drawn regarding proteoglycan content.[42]

The potential causal relationship between an abnormal radiographic finding and a clinical symptom such as low back pain or sciatica is sometimes very difficult to determine but is of paramount importance. From a surgical perspective, accurate diagnosis of lumbar disorders is as important as surgical expertise in determining outcome. Spangfort showed that the degree of disc herniation is the single most important factor in determining the surgical result after discectomy.[52] Specifically, patients found to have a very large herniation causing definite neural compression had a 90.3 per cent chance of complete relief of sciatica after discectomy and a 99.5 per cent chance of at least partial relief, while those in whom the exploration was negative had only a 38.4 per cent chance of obtaining any relief at all. From these data it is clear that a key factor in determining surgical outcome is accurate preoperative prediction of those patients with definite neural compression who will benefit from decompressive surgery.

Although such preoperative determinations are heavily dependent on radiographic diagnostic testing, they are by no means solely dependent on them. Clinical data are equally important in making such determinations. Hakelius reported a 63 per cent correlation between clinical findings and surgically proved pathology.[16] Hirsch and Nachemson reported a 55 per cent correlation between objective neurologic signs and the presence of a disc herniation.[21] When a positive straight leg raising (SLR) sign was combined with objective neurologic findings, diagnostic accuracy increased to 86 per cent. When a positive water-soluble myelogram was correlated with both a positive SLR sign and an objective neurologic deficit, diagnostic accuracy increased to 95 per cent (Fig. 6–1). Overemphasis of one of these parameters at the expense of the other two can result in surgical failure. Under such circumstances the failure is primarily one of diagnosis rather than surgical technique.

It is important always to bear in mind the intimate relationship that must exist between objective clinical findings and positive radiographic findings if one is to ascribe the former to the latter. Without such correlation, it cannot be certain whether radiographic abnormalities are the cause of symptoms. Many studies have attempted to determine the incidence of abnormal radiographic findings in both symptomatic and asymptomatic individuals.[3, 12, 13, 22, 24, 32, 44, 56, 61] An abnormal radiographic finding in the latter has been termed the "false-positive" rate for that test. Such a term is not entirely accurate since a true "false-positive" would imply the complete absence of disease and would of necessity require a negative surgical exploration for confirmation. In the following discussion, various radiographic diagnostic techniques are analyzed with regard to their potential usefulness in the diagnosis of symptomatic lumbar disc disease, and the problem of "false-positive" findings is addressed.

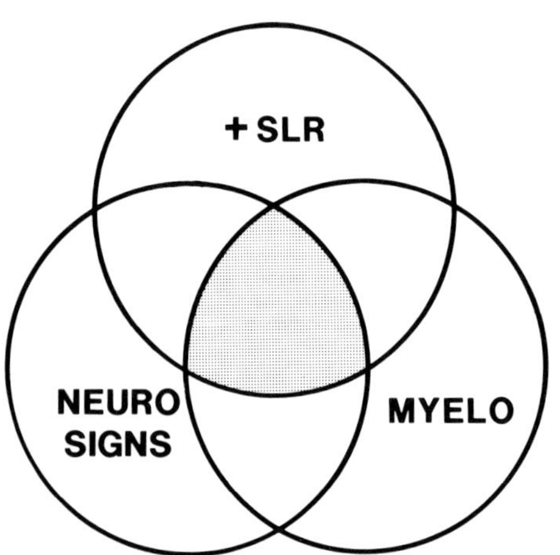

Figure 6–1. Venn diagram illustrating the logic involved in surgical decision making for degenerative lumbar spine surgery. When a patient presenting with predominantly leg pain has a positive straight leg raising (SLR) sign, neurologic findings (neuro signs), and a correlative objective radiologic test (e.g., myelogram), the chance of finding neurologic compression from a disc herniation at surgery is very high and is represented by the shaded area of the diagram.

ROUTINE RADIOGRAPHY

The role of routine x-ray examination of the lumbar spine in the diagnosis of painful low back conditions has been a source of much controversy. O'Connor, for example, reported in 1946 that routine pre-employment lumbar x-rays were helpful in reducing the incidence of low back strains by allowing better job selection.[47] Subsequent investigations cast much doubt on the usefulness of such x-ray findings.[12, 13, 24, 35, 44, 53, 56] Nachemson stated that only one of every 2500 radiographic examinations is useful in providing clinically unsuspected positive findings in patients 20 to 50 years old.[44]

Part of the problem with plain radiography is that radiographic findings of facet joint arthritis and disc degeneration are common, if not ubiquitous, in the general population. Kellgren and Lawrence found radiographic disc degeneration in 83 per cent of males and 72 per cent of females between the ages of 55 and 64 years of age, regardless of symptoms.[31] In the lumbar spine, 66 per cent of males and 45 per cent of females showed radiographic disc degeneration, while 30 per cent of males and 27 per cent of females showed x-ray evidence of facet arthritis. Radiographic disc degeneration and facet arthritis, like facial wrinkles, are age related and are not necessarily indicative of any underlying symptoms.

The disc itself is not directly visible on routine radiography, and inferences about its physiologic state can be made only indirectly by the presence or absence of disc space narrowing and marginal osteophytes. The latter are relatively later changes in disc degeneration, and plain x-ray findings of disc narrowing are therefore rather insensitive indicators of disc degeneration.

The issue of the potential relationship between radiographic disc degeneration or facet arthritis and back pain has been addressed by many investigators.[5, 12, 13, 16, 23, 24, 40, 44, 53, 56, 58] Several studies reported no association between disc space narrowing and low back pain.[23, 24, 40, 53] More recently, the relationship between disc height and pain on discography has been studied.[58] Disc height was found to be an insensitive method of detecting early painful disc degeneration. An association between disc space narrowing and low back pain has been reported by some authors.[12, 56] Torgerson and Dotter compared lumbar x-rays of a consecutive group of symptomatic low back pain patients with supine intravenous pyelography (IVP) films of patients asymptomatic with regard to low back pain.[56] They found lumbar disc space narrowing in 22 per cent of the asymptomatic group versus 56 per cent of the symptomatic back pain group. Although disc space narrowing was clearly an age-related finding, being more common in the seventh decade than in the fifth decade regardless of symptoms, it was more prevalent in symptomatic patients than in asymptomatic individuals. These data indicated that disc degeneration was highly probable if symptoms were present.

Frymoyer and colleagues compared standing lumbar spine radiographs of 292 randomly selected males between the ages of 18 and 55 who were divided into three groups based on the presence or absence of back pain.[12] They found that disc space narrowing only at the L4–L5 level was significantly correlated with low back pain and leg symptoms. Attempts to quantitate such disc narrowing, however, were not fruitful and its diagnosis was based on the radiologist's visual assessment.

Associations between other radiographic findings and back pain have also been studied.[5, 12, 13, 16, 23, 24, 40, 53, 56, 58] Frymoyer and colleagues reported no association between low back pain and transitional vertebrae, Schmorl's nodes, lumbar lordosis, disc vacuum sign, claw spurs, disc space narrowing at levels other than L4–L5, scoliosis, level of pelvic intercristal line, disc space wedging, relative lengths of L3 and L5 transverse processes, or spina bifida occulta.[12] Torgerson and Dotter found no association between back pain and spondylosis (osteophyte formation) or lumbar lordosis.[56] Reported positive associations between low back pain and radiographic findings include the presence of traction spurs at L4–L5[12] and the presence of spondylolysis or spondylolisthesis.[23, 56] Much of this evidence was summarized by Nachemson.[44] From the data relating radiographic findings and low back pain, it appears that plain radiography is of little value in determining the causes of low back pain or in predicting who is at risk in the industrial population group.

WATER-SOLUBLE MYELOGRAPHY

The diagnosis of extradural neural compression by myelography is inferred indirectly by changes in the contour of normal contrast-filled structures and spaces rather than by direct visualization of the compressing agent (Fig. 6–2).[42] The benefit of contrast examination of the spinal canal has been well recognized and was reported as early as 1919 by Dandy, who injected air into the spinal canal to visualize tumors.[6] Since that time, various contrast agents have been used to detect intracanal lesions. Other negative contrast agents such as oxygen have also been used. Positive contrast agents include oil-based agents such as Pantopaque (ethyl iodophenylundecylate) and water-soluble agents. The historical background of negative contrast agents and oil-based positive contrast agents is discussed eloquently elsewhere.[9]

Because of concern regarding the docu-

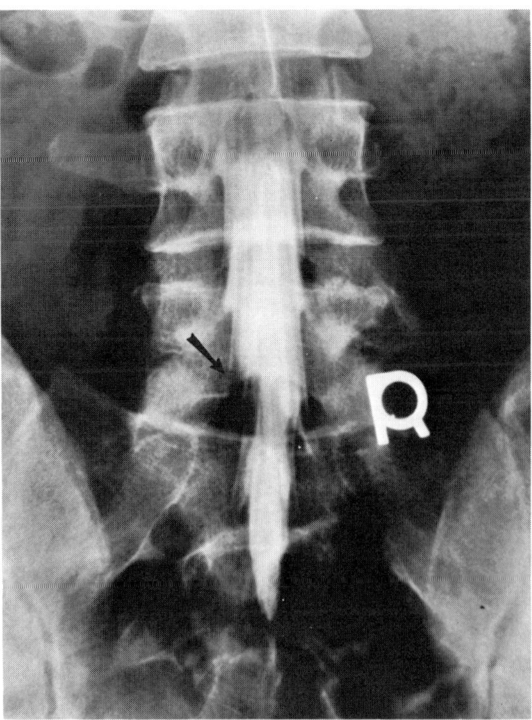

Figure 6–2. Water-soluble myelogram of a patient with a left S1 radiculopathy showing incomplete filling of the left S1 nerve root *(arrow)*. Note in particular the asymmetry between the right and the left S1 nerve roots.

mented relationship between oil-based agents such as Pantopaque and arachnoiditis,[54] attention turned to less toxic water-soluble agents. These include meglumine iothalamate (Conray), meglumime iocarmate (Dimer X), metrizamide (Amipaque), iohexol (Omnipaque), and iopamidol (Isovue). The advantages of such water-soluble agents include higher sensitivity to subtle pathology owing to better definition of nerve root sleeves, less toxicity, and less arachnoiditis. In addition, their absorption through the lumbar theca and parasagittal arachnoid villi makes removal of the agent unnecessary, thereby eliminating the most uncomfortable aspect of oil-based myelography.

The importance of myelography as an adjunct to lumbar disc surgery has been shown by Hirsch and Nachemson, who reported the relationship between neurologic signs and water-soluble contrast myelography in 289 patients operated on for suspected lumbar disc herniation.[21] In this series, 90 per cent of patients in whom the myelogram was positive were found to have a definite disc herniation verified at surgery, thus indicating the high sensitivity of the test. Similar data were reported by Spangfort, who described more than twice as many negative explorations when myelography was not performed preoperatively than when it was.[52]

The importance of not basing surgical decisions exclusively on any imaging test, to the exclusion of clinical findings, was demonstrated by Hitselberger and Witten.[22] Three hundred patients who were asymptomatic with respect to low back pain or leg pain underwent contrast examination of the cervical and lumbar spines while receiving posterior fossa myelography for suspected acoustic neurilemoma. Overall, 37 per cent had myelographic disc abnormalities in the cervical spine, the lumbar spine, or both. In the lumbar spine alone, 24 per cent of patients showed some myelographic abnormality. Clearly, the presence of a myelographic abnormality should not be the sole determinant in surgical decision making.

Although the value of myelography as an aid in patient selection is well accepted, recent controversy has revolved around its risks, limitations, and inaccuracies compared with other studies. Because it is invasive, myelography has potential risks, including headache, nausea, vomiting, urinary problems, seizures, and psychic disturbances.[9, 19] The advent of newer water-soluble agents has diminished such side effects, although their reported incidence, even with agents such as metrizamide, ranges from 23 to 64 per cent.[19]

Interestingly, such side effects have been shown to bear a definite relationship to the presence or absence of objective parameters on which the decision to perform the myelogram is made.[19] Herkowitz and associates reported a twofold increase in headache, nausea, and vomiting in patients in whom the myelogram was normal and who had only subjective complaints, compared with those showing objective clinical findings. This study emphasizes the importance of establishing objective clinical findings before proceeding with myelography.

Myelography has purported disadvantages aside from the issue of toxicity. It has been shown to be less accurate at the L5–S1 level than at higher levels because of the larger anterior epidural space at this level.[9, 52] It is also less accurate for extreme lateral disc herniations than for more central herniations because the lumbar nerve root sheath terminates near the dorsal root ganglion, and myelographic dye therefore cannot penetrate beyond this point to the more distal site of compression.[26, 28, 30, 34] Anatomically the dorsal root ganglion is at a level immediately below the pedicle,[5] so that any herniation lateral to the pedicle escapes myelographic recognition. In spite of these limitations, however, the reported accuracy of water-soluble myelography is 67 to 100 per cent.[1, 19, 26, 27, 43, 49, 51, 55]

COMPUTED TOMOGRAPHY

Computed tomography (CT) is a noninvasive diagnostic imaging tool that allows direct visualization of potential neural compressing structures (Fig. 6–3). In this respect it differs radically from myelography, in which compression is inferred by changes in the contour of contrast-filled neural structures. Purported advantages of CT over myelography include better visualization of lateral pathologic conditions such as foraminal stenosis and lateral disc herniations (Fig. 6–4),[18, 26, 49, 62] less radiation,[55] no known adverse reactions, and the fact that it can be performed on an outpatient basis. In addition, it allows discrimination between neural compression due to soft tissue (e.g., disc) and compression due to bone (e.g.,

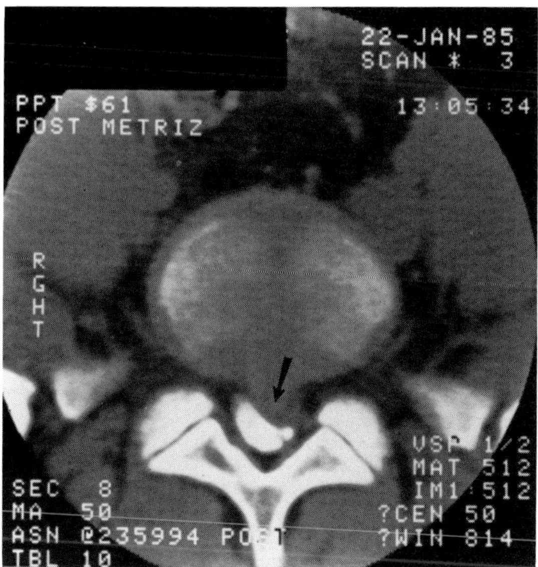

Figure 6–3. Computed tomogram (CT) of the patient shown in Figure 6–2 with a left S1 radiculopathy from a left-sided L5–S1 disc herniation *(arrow)* compressing the contrast-filled thecal sac.

facet joint hypertrophy). In this respect CT is superior to even MRI for its ability to distinguish bone from soft tissue. Unlike myelography, CT can provide two orthogonal views and thus adheres to a basic tenet of radiologic imaging. Additional information can be obtained with multiple parasagittal images and their subsequent reformatting to allow better visualization of the neural foramina. Three-dimensional surface reformation from contiguous axial computed tomograms (3D-CT) permit further imaging of bone architecture (Fig. 6–5). Although more useful in delineating complex pathologic states such as pelvic and acetabular fractures, 3D-CT has been used in the lumbar spine.[25, 48] The data it provides are not new but are presented in a slightly different manner.[48] Typically, 24 images are reconstructed in such a way that the spine can be rotated and bisected in the sagittal plane. Twelve images are rotated around the Y axis in 30-degree increments to visualize a complete revolution of the spine (Fig. 6–5*A*). Each image is then bisected sagittally to visualize the interior of the spinal canal and the neural foramina (Fig. 6–5*B*). Such reformations are useful for visualizing bony architecture and its contribution to neural compression, although, as typically performed, 3D-CT does not actually visualize the neural structures themselves, nor other soft tissue elements such as the intervertebral disc.

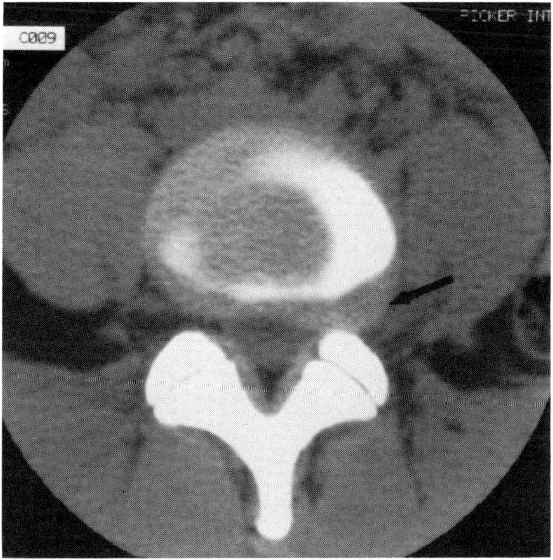

Figure 6–4. CT scan of a patient presenting with a left L4 radiculopathy due to compression of the L4 nerve root by a very lateral herniation of the L4–L5 disc *(arrow)*. Myelography of extreme lateral disc herniations does not reveal the compressive lesion, since the lesion is lateral to the contrast-filled thecal contents.

The history of CT in degenerative spinal conditions has been well documented.[14] The current generation of CT scanners routinely employ contiguous images 4 mm thick, although thinner slices may be obtained. It is important to obtain axial images parallel, rather than oblique, to the plane of the disc and end plates in order to avoid image distortion and thus to minimize false-positive interpretations. To facilitate this, the gantry of the scanner can be tilted up to 20 degrees. In patients with excessive lumbar lordosis, even this maneuver may not permit imaging parallel to the disc, and under such circumstances inaccuracy can occur. Other potential technique-related problems include difficulty in imaging morbidly obese patients owing to size restrictions of the scanner itself, and uncomfortable feelings of claustrophobia experienced by some patients.

An inherent drawback of CT is its routine axial imaging of only the lower three lumbar levels, and the consequent possibility of missing an unsuspected high lumbar lesion or even a thoracolumbar tumor (Figs. 6–6, 6–7). Both myelography and MRI routinely provide sagittal imaging up to and including the thoraco-

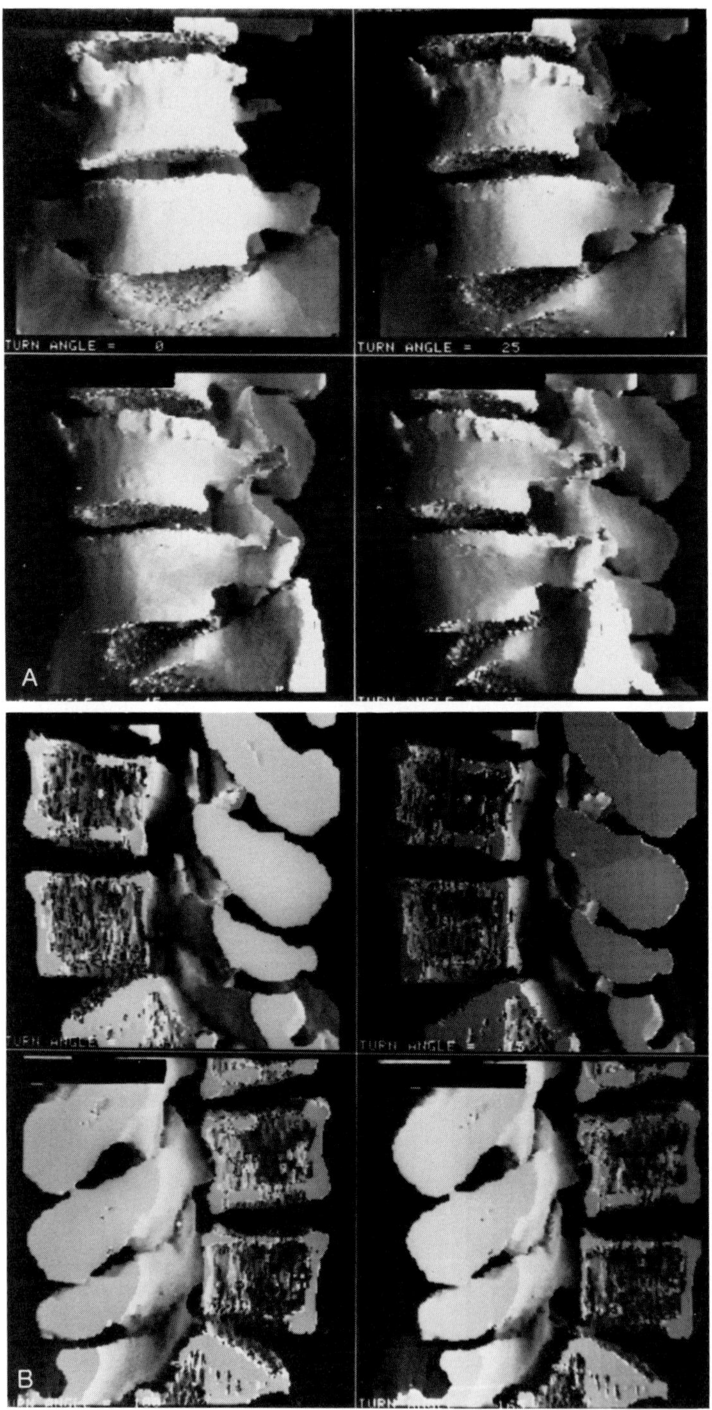

Figure 6–5. Three-dimensional CT scan of the lumbar spine. *A,* Sagittal view at turn angles of 0, 25, 45, and 65 degrees to show the L4 and L5 lumbar vertebrae. By rotating the spine around the Y axis, the entire spine may be visualized, including the neural foramina. *B,* Bisected sagittal view of the lumbar spine at turn angles of 0, 15, 180, and 165 degrees showing the interior of the spinal canal and neural foramina.

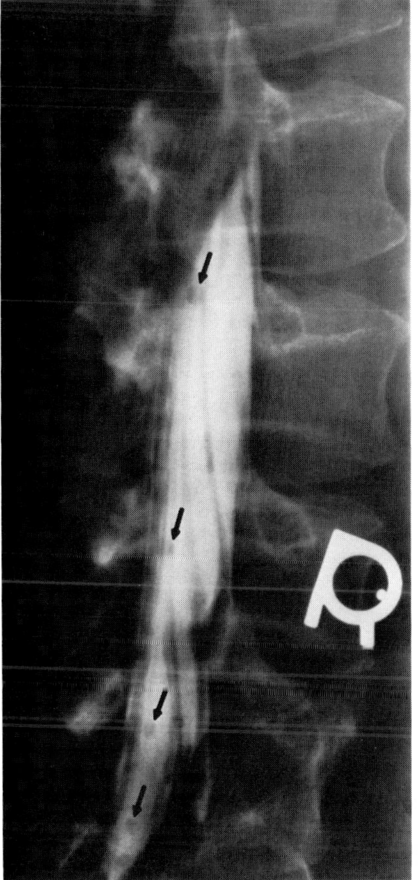

Figure 6–6. Oblique view of water-soluble lumbar myelogram of a patient presenting with left-sided leg pain consistent with a left S1 radiculopathy. The CT scan revealed a typical left-sided L5–S1 disc herniation (not shown). The myelogram, however, revealed multiple filling defects *(arrows)*, which subsequently proved to be intradural metastases from a lung carcinoma. If only the CT scan had been performed, these lesions would not have been recognized.

lumbar junction and therefore minimize the risk of missing a lesion at this location.

Another difficulty with CT is the homogeneity of disc and neural structures as seen on noncontrast CT. When there is canal narrowing at the level of the disc, it can be difficult to distinguish thecal contents from disc material (Fig. 6–8). The use of contrast agents and subsequent postcontrast CT obviates this problem.

The diagnosis of lumbar disc herniation by CT depends on demonstration of an asymmetric ventral density within the spinal canal. When this causes neural compression, it is accompanied by distortion of normal neural anatomy and loss of the epidural fat that normally surrounds the neural structures. In most patients this compression occurs at the level of the disc and is contiguous with the parent disc. In cases of disc sequestration, however, the disc fragment may be at some distance from the intervertebral disc itself and may present a confusing diagnostic picture on the axial images. Under such circumstances, MRI provides valuable information about the presence and location of the sequestered fragment as well as its disc of origin.[41] The MRI characteristics of sequestered disc fragments are discussed later but were delineated by Masaryk and colleagues, who reported MRI to have an 89 per cent sensitivity, an 82 per cent specificity, and an overall accuracy of 85 per cent in the diagnosis of sequestered lumbar disc herniation.[41]

The reported accuracy of CT in the diagnosis of lumbar disc herniation is 48 to 100 per cent.[5, 15, 17, 26, 29, 43, 48, 49, 51, 55, 62] The design flaws in many of these studies have been well documented.[1] More recent studies have addressed these issues, comparing blind CT readings with documented surgical pathology.[26, 27] The importance of blind CT interpretation was emphasized by Eldevik and associates, who showed that a correct diagnosis was more likely

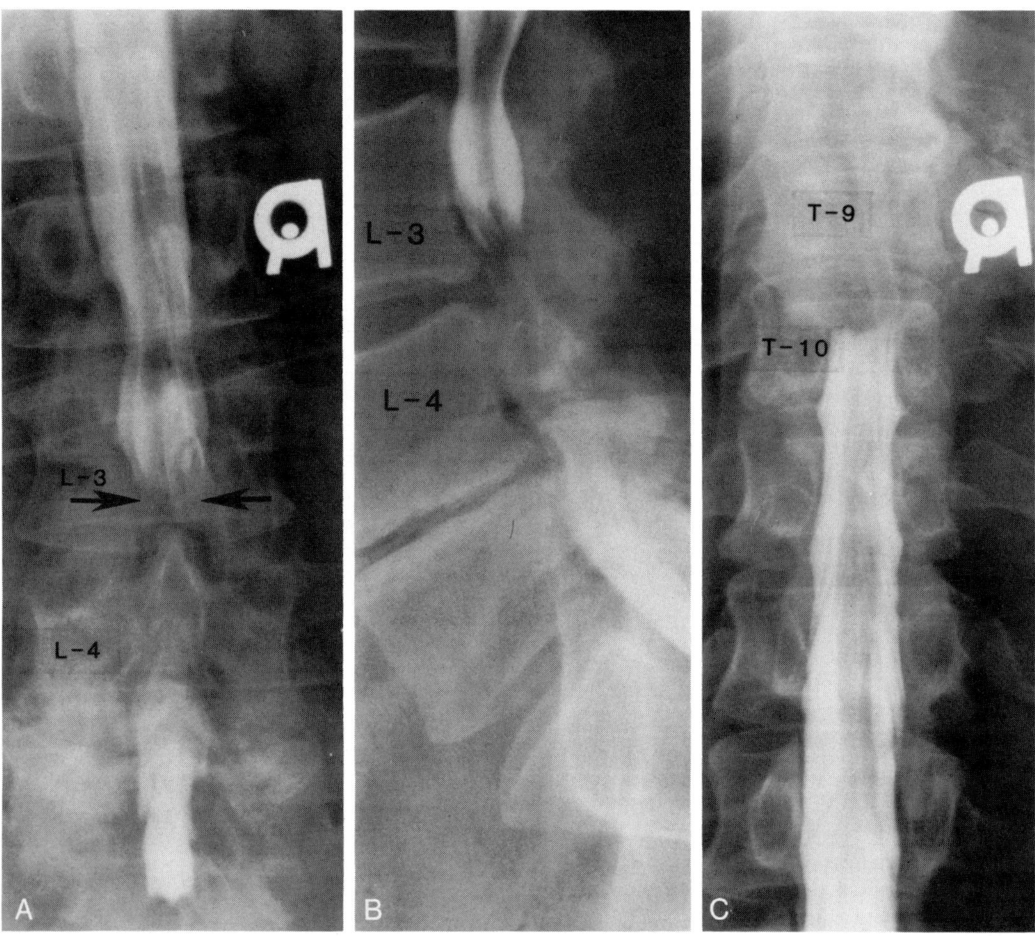

Figure 6–7. *A,* Anteroposterior water-soluble lumbar myelogram of a patient presenting with typical symptoms of spinal stenosis. Note the cut-off of dye at the L3–L4 junction *(arrows). B,* Lateral view showing the block at the L3–L4 level. *C,* It was noted, however, that when the dye was run up to the lower thoracic area, there was a block at the T9–T10 level with an appearance suggesting an intradural lesion on the anteroposterior myelogram.

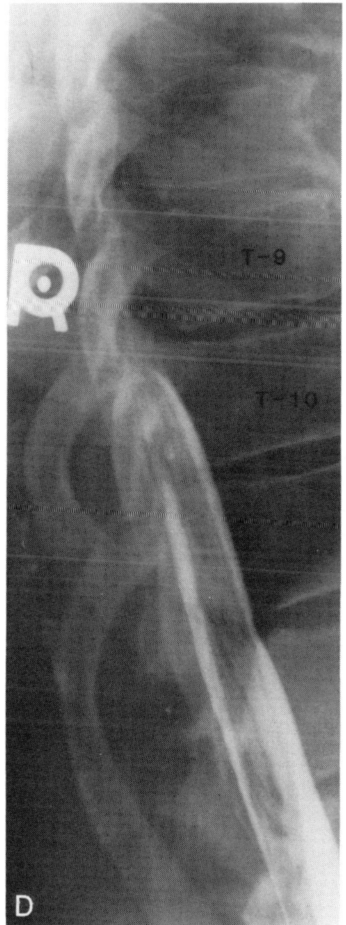

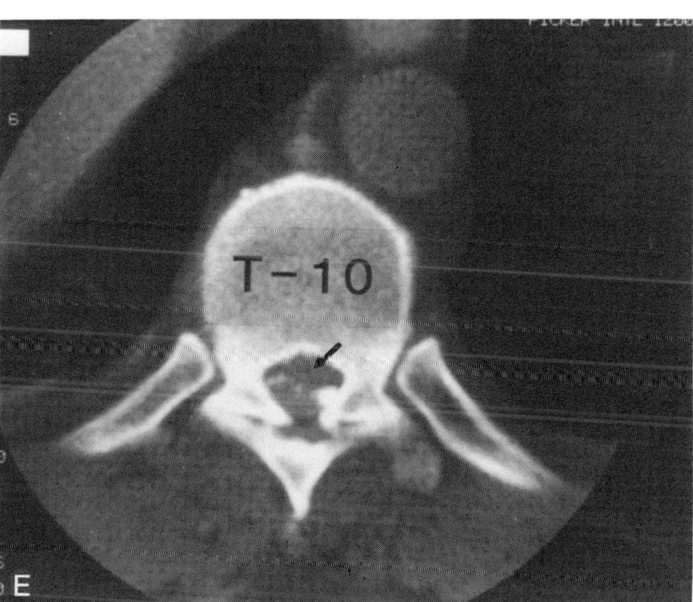

Figure 6–7 *Continued D,* Lateral myelogram showing a complete block to the passage of the dye at T9–T10. *E,* CT scan at the top of T10 showing the contrast-enhanced thecal sac compressed by what appears to be an extradural lesion. At surgery an intradural thoracic disc herniation was found. In this case a routine CT scan of the lower lumbar spine would have detected the compressive lesion at L3–L4 but would have missed the more significant lesion at T9–T10.

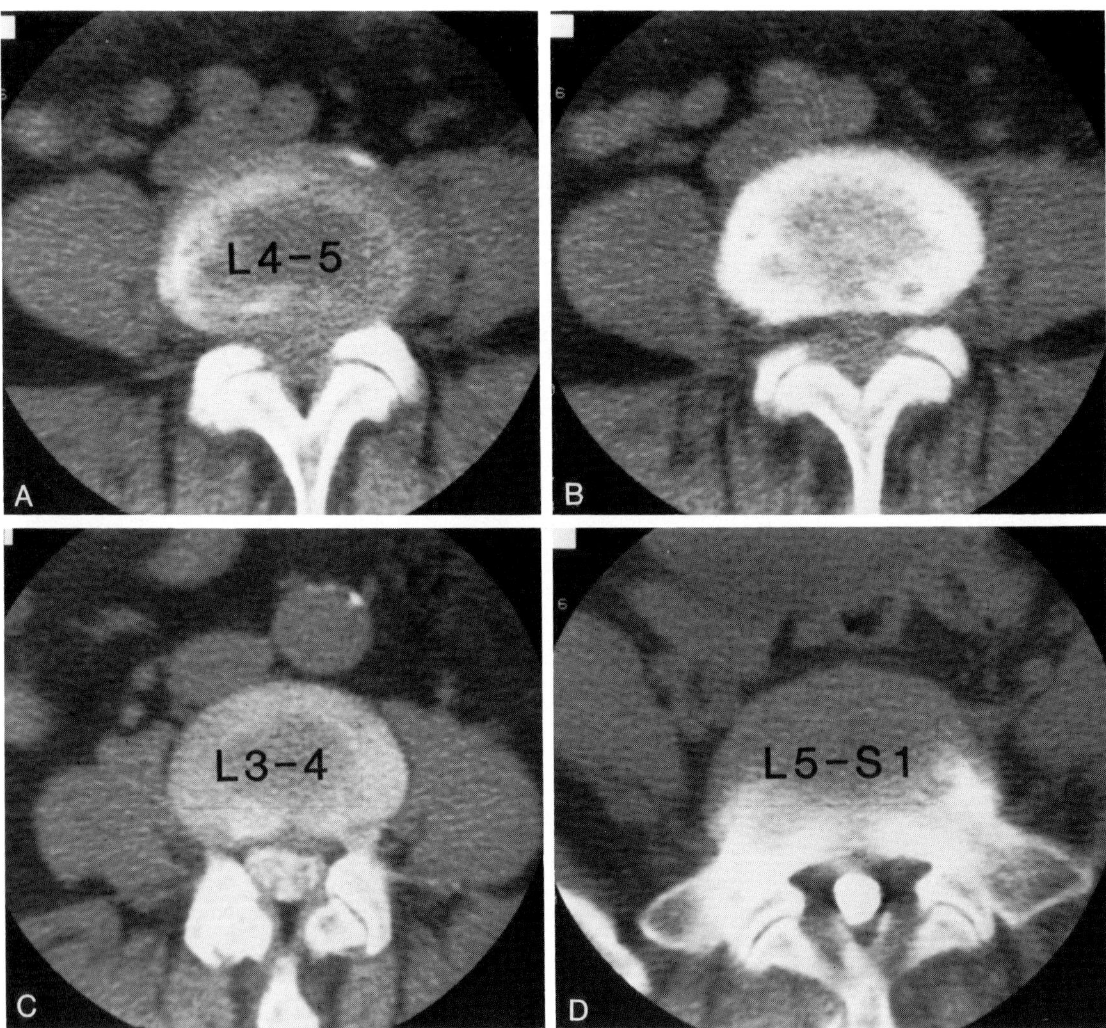

Figure 6–8. *A*, CT scan at L4–L5 showing homogeneity of the L4–L5 disc with the thecal contents. *B*, At the bottom of the L4 vertebral end plate the thecal contents are visualized and appear essentially normal. This is typical of the type of CT scan that is routinely obtained without contrast enhancement. *C*, *D*, In fact, this study was performed after contrast enhancement, as can be seen from the views at the L3–L4 and L5–S1 levels.

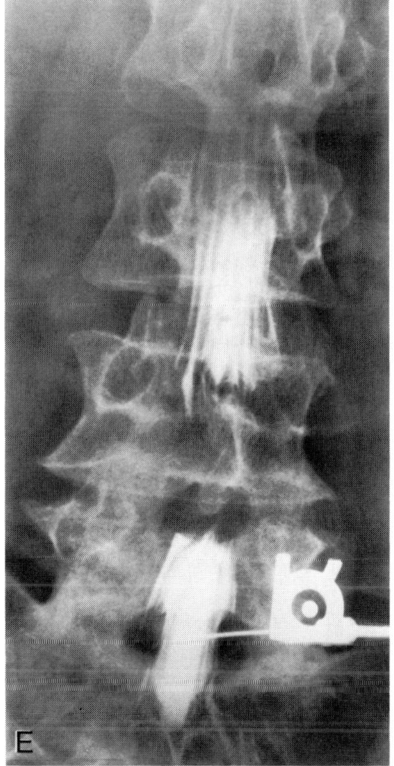

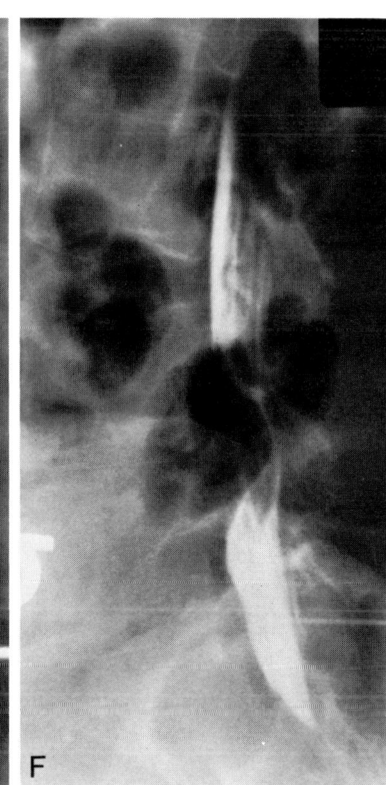

Figure 6–8 *Continued E,* The anteroposterior water-soluble myelogram shows the full extent of the lesion, which was found to be a huge, sequestrated L4–L5 disc fragment. *F,* The lateral view shows a generous amount of dye above and below the lesion, but only a small amount of dye passing at the L4–L5 level.

without clinical information than with it.[8] The addition of clinical information was shown to increase the number of false-positive, and decrease the number of false-negative, interpretations. Using such strict criteria, Jackson and colleagues reported a 74 per cent accuracy of CT in the diagnosis of lumbar disc herniation, with false-positive and false-negative rates of 19 and 29 per cent, respectively.[26] This accuracy was comparable with that of Bell and colleagues, who, using similar stringent diagnostic criteria and blinded CT interpretation, reported 72 per cent accuracy.[1]

CT has been particularly valuable in the diagnosis of extreme lateral or foraminal lumbar disc herniation (Fig. 6–4).[18, 26, 27, 49, 62] Jackson and colleagues reported a 71 per cent accuracy of CT in the diagnosis of foraminal disc herniation compared with only 58 per cent for metrizamide myelography.[26] The anatomy of the lumbar nerve root sheath and its relationship to the dorsal root ganglion, the pedicle and the lateral aspect of the intervertebral disc are well documented.[5, 26, 28, 30, 34] The fact that the nerve root sheath terminates at the dorsal root ganglion proximal to the site of compression from a lateral disc herniation[26, 28, 30, 34] explains the insensitivity of myelography in the diagnosis of lateral disc herniations.

Some authors have suggested that CT may be too sensitive to normal age-related degenerative changes in the lumbar spine.[1, 61] Wiesel and associates,[61] in a CT study similar to the myelography study of Hitselberger and Witten,[22] reported the incidence of positive CT scans in an asymptomatic population. They found an overall 35.4 per cent incidence of abnormal CT scans in their asymptomatic group. Furthermore, such findings were more common in patients over 40 (50 per cent) than in those under 40 (19.5 per cent). Such data underscore the importance of correlating radiographic abnormalities with objective neurologic findings in clinical decision making.

The addition of a water-soluble contrast agent in conjunction with CT imaging increases the accuracy of the study. Jackson and colleagues compared several diagnostic tests with surgical findings in order to determine the sensitivity, specificity, and accuracy of each test.[26, 27] Although not achieving statistical significance, CT myelography was more sensitive than (78 vs. 71 per cent), equally specific to (76 vs. 76 per cent), and slightly more accurate than (77 vs. 74 per cent) CT in the diagnosis of lumbar disc herniation.

Studies have suggested that CT after discography (disco-CT) may be particularly valuable in the diagnosis of lumbar spine disorders.[7, 10, 26–28, 33, 37, 50, 57–59] Plain CT examination depends on the relative densities of the thecal contents, disc material, epidural fat, ligamentum flavum, bone, and scar tissue. Diagnostic inaccuracy can occur when the density of the disc is similar to that of adjacent structures. The injection of contrast agents into the disc allows better distinction between the disc and other structures on subsequent CT examination. Jackson and colleagues reported disco-CT to be more accurate (87 per cent) than either myelography (70 per cent), CT (74 per cent), or myelo-CT (77 per cent) in the diagnosis of lumbar disc herniation. Its usefulness in the diagnosis of foraminal disc herniation and lateral stenosis has been confirmed by several authors.[7, 26–28, 33] Compared with either CT, myelography, or myelo-CT, disco-CT seems to be more accurate in the diagnosis of foraminal disc herniation. Only MRI was shown to be preferable to disco-CT in the diagnosis of lumbar disc herniations.[27]

References

1. Bell, G. R., Rothman, R. H., Booth, R. E., et al.: A study of computer-assisted tomography. Spine *9*:552–556, 1984.
2. Bell, G. R., and Simeone, F. A.: The pathophysiology of disc degeneration. *In* Crockard, A., Hayward, R., and Hoff, J. (eds.): Neurosurgery. The Scientific Basis of Clinical Practice. Boston, Blackwell Scientific Publications, 1985.
3. Boden, S. D., Davis, D. O., Dina, T. S., et al.: Abnormal magnetic-resonance scans of the lumbar spine in asymptomatic subjects. A prospective investigation. J. Bone Joint Surg. *72A*:403–408, 1990.
4. Carrera, G., Williams, A., and Haughton, V.: Computed tomography in sciatica. Radiology *137*:433–437, 1980.
5. Cohen, M. S., Wall, E. J., Brown, R. B., et al.: Cauda equina anatomy: extrathecal nerve roots and dorsal root ganglia. Presented at Fifth Annual Meeting of Federation of Spine Associations (FOSA), New Orleans, LA, February 1990.
6. Dandy, W. E.: Roentgenography of the brain after injection of air into the spinal canal. Ann. Surg. *70*:397, 1919.
7. Edwards, W. C., Orme, T. J., and Orr-Edwards, G.: CT discography: prognostic value in the selection of patients for chemonucleolysis. Spine *12*:792–795, 1987.
8. Eldevik, O. P., Dugstad, G., Orrison, W. W., and Haughton, V. M.: The effect of clinical bias on the interpretation of myelography and spinal computed tomography. Radiology *145*:85–89, 1982.
9. Epstein, B.: The Spine. A Radiological Text and Atlas. Philadelphia, Lea & Febiger, 1976.
10. Forristall, R. M., Marsh, H. O., and Pay, N. T.: Magnetic resonance imaging and contrast CT of the lumbar spine. Spine *13*:1049–1054, 1988.
11. Frey, J., Hendin, B., and Stern, L.: Computed tomography in the diagnosis of lumbosacral disc herniation. Ariz. Med. *38*:839–842, 1981.
12. Frymoyer, J. W., Newberg, A., Pope, M. H., et al.: Spine radiographs in patients with low-back pain. J. Bone Joint Surg. *66A*:1048–1055, 1984.
13. Fullenlove, T. M., and Williams, A. J.: Comparative roentgen findings in symptomatic and asymptomatic backs. Radiology *68*:572–574, 1957.
14. Gargano, F. P.: Axial tomography. *In* Rothman, R. H., and Simeone, F. A.: The Spine. 2nd ed. Philadelphia, W. B. Saunders Co., 1982, p. 464–470.
15. Gulati, A., Weinstein, R., and Studdard, E.: CT scan of the spine for herniated discs. Neuroradiology 22:57–60, 1981.
16. Hakelius, A.: Prognosis in sciatica. Acta Orthop. Scand. (Suppl.) *129*:1–76, 1970.
17. Harley, W., Sava, G., and Fleming, R.: Computerized tomography in the evaluation of lumbar disc herniation. Conn. Med. *45*:349–353, 1981.
18. Haughton, V. M., Eldevik, O. P., Magnaes, B., and Amundsen, P.: A prospective comparison of computed tomography and myelography in the diagnosis of herniated lumbar disks. Radiology *142*:103–110, 1982.
19. Herkowitz, H., Romeyn, R., and Rothman, R.: The indications for metrizamide myelography. Relationship with complications after myelography. J. Bone Joint Surg. *65A*:1144–1149, 1983.
20. Herkowitz, H. N., Wiesel, S. W., Booth, R. E., Jr, and Rothman, R. H.: Metrizamide myelography and epidural venography. Their role in the diagnosis of lumbar disc herniation and spinal stenosis. Spine *7*:55–64, 1982.
21. Hirsch, C., and Nachemson, A.: The reliability of lumbar disk surgery. Clin. Orthop. *29*:189–195, 1963.
22. Hitselberger, W. E., and Witten, R. M.: Abnormal myelograms in asymptomatic patients. J. Neurosurg. *28*:204–206, 1968.
23. Horal, J.: The clinical appearance of low back disorders in the city of Gothenburg, Sweden. Acta Orthop. Scand. (Suppl.) *118*:7–109, 1969.
24. Hult, L.: Cervical dorsal and lumbar spinal syndromes. Acta Orthop. Scand. *24*:174–175, 1954.
25. Hunter, J. C., et al.: Three-dimensional CT imaging of the lumbar spine. *In* Gennant, H. (ed.): Spine Update 1987. Radiology Research and Education Foundation, U.C.S.F. Press, San Francisco, 1987.
26. Jackson, R. P., Cain, J. E., Jacobs, R. R., et al.: The neuroradiographic diagnosis of lumbar herniated nucleus pulposus: I. Spine *14*:1356–1361, 1989.
27. Jackson, R. P., Cain, J. E., Jacobs, R. R., et al.: The neuroradiographic diagnosis of lumbar herniated nucleus pulposus: II. Spine *14*:1362–1367, 1989.
28. Jackson, R. P., and Glah, J. J.: Foraminal and extraforaminal lumbar disc herniation: diagnosis and treatment. Spine *12*:577–585, 1987.
29. Jenkinson, D.: CT beats myelography for lumbar spine diagnoses. J.A.M.A. *246*:2112–2113, 1981.

30. Johansen, J.: Computed tomography in assessment of myelographic nerve root compression in the lateral recess. Spine *11*:492–495, 1986.
31. Kellgren, J. H., and Lawrence, J. S.: Osteo-arthrosis and disk degeneration in an urban population. Ann. Rheum. Dis. *17*:388–397, 1958.
32. Knutsson, F.: The vacuum phenomenon in the intervertebral discs. Acta Radiol. *23*:173–179, 1942.
33. Kornberg, M.: Computed tomography of the lumbar spine following discography. Spine *12*:823–825, 1987.
34. Kornberg, M.: Extreme lateral lumbar disc herniations. Spine *12*:586–589, 1987.
35. La Rocca, M., and Macnab, I.: Value of pre-employment radiographic assessment of the lumbar spine. Can. Med. Assoc. J. *101*:383–388, 1969.
36. Lipson, S., and Muir, H.: Proteoglycans in experimental intervertebral disc degeneration. Spine *6*:194–210, 1984
37. McCutcheon, M. E., and Thompson, W. C.: CT scanning of lumbar discography. Spine *11*:257–259, 1986.
38. Macnab, I.: Backache. Baltimore, Williams & Wilkins Co., 1977.
39. Magnusson, W.: Über die Bedingungen des Hervortretens der Wirklichen Gelenkspalte auf dem Röntgenbilde. Acta Radiol. 18:733–741, 1937.
40. Magora, A., and Schwartz, A.: Relation between the low back pain syndrome and x-ray findings. I. Degenerative osteoarthritis. Scand. J. Rehabil. Med. *8*:115–125, 1976.
41. Masaryk, T. J., Ross, J. S., Modic, M. T., et al.: High-resolution MR imaging of sequestered lumbar intervertebral disks. A.J.N.R. *9*:351–358, 1988.
42. Modic, M. T., Masaryk, T. J., Ross, J. S., and Carter, J. R.: Imaging of degenerative disk disease. Radiology *168*:177–186, 1988.
43. Moufarrij, N., and Hardy, R.: Computed tomographic, myelographic and operative findings in patients with suspected herniated lumbar discs. Neurosurgery *12*:184–188, 1983.
44. Nachemson, A.: Towards a better understanding of low-back pain. A review of the mechanics of the lumbar disc. Rheum. Rehab. *14*:129–143, 1975.
45. Naylor, A.: Intervertebral disc prolapse and degeneration: the biochemical and biophysical approach. Spine *1*:108–114, 1976.
46. Nebel, G., Dihlmann, W., Lingg, G., and Hering, L.: Computed tomography in the diagnosis of prolapsed intervertebral disc. Eur. J. Radiol. *1*:158–162, 1981.
47 O'Connor, R. B.: Physical Capacities Appraisal of Industrial Back. Indust. Med. *15*:639–640, 1946.
48. Pate, D., Resnick, D., Sartorius, D. J., and Andre, M.: 3D CT of the spine: practical applications. Appl. Radiol. *16*:86–94, 1987.
49. Raskin, S., and Keating, J.: Recognition of lumbar disk disease: comparison of myelography and computed tomography. Am. J. Neuroradiol. *3*:215–221, 1982.
50. Sachs, B. L., Vanharanta, H., Spivey, M. A., et al.: Dallas discogram description. A new classification of CT/discography in low-back disorders. Spine *12*:287–294, 1987.
51. Sachsenheimer, W., Hamer, J., and Muller, H.: The value of spinal computed tomography in diagnosis of herniated lumbar discs. Acta Neurchir. *60*:107–114, 1982.
52. Spangfort, E.: The lumbar disc herniation. Acta Orthop. Scand. (Suppl.) *142*:4–95, 1972.
53. Splithoff, C. A.: Lumbosacral junction. Roentgenographic comparison of patients with and without backaches. J.A.M.A. *152*:1610–1613, 1953.
54. Symposium: Lumbar arachnoiditis: nomenclature, etiology and pathology. Spine *3*:21–92, 1978.
55. Tchang, S. P., Howie, J. L., Kirkaldy-Willis, W. H., et al.: Computed tomography versus myelography in diagnosis of lumbar disc herniation. J. Can. Assoc. Radiol. *33*:15–20, 1982.
56. Torgerson, W. R., and Dotter, W. E.: Comparative roentgenographic study of the asymptomatic and symptomatic lumbar spine. J. Bone Joint Surg. *58A*:850–853, 1976.
57. Vanharanta, H., Sachs, B. L., Spivey, M. A., et al.: The relationship of pain provocation to lumbar disc deterioration as seen by CT/discography. Spine *12*:295–298, 1987.
58. Vanharanta, H., Sachs, B. L., Spivey, M. A., et al.: A comparison of CT/discography, pain response and radiographic disc height. Spine *13*:321–324, 1988.
59. Vanharanta, H., Guyer, R. D., Ohnmeiss, D. D., et al.: Disc deterioration in low-back syndromes. Spine *13*:1349–1351, 1988.
60. Weisz, G.: Value of computerized tomography in diagnosing diseases of the lumbar spine. Med. J. Aust. *1*:216–219, 1982.
61. Wiesel, S. W., Tsourmas, N., Fetter, H. L., et al.: A study of computer-assisted tomography. I. The incidence of positive CAT scans in an asymptomatic group of patients. Spine *9*:549–551, 1984.
62. Williams, A., Haughton, V., and Syvertsen, A.: Computed tomography in the diagnosis of herniated nucleus pulposus. Radiology *135*:95–99, 1980.

DISCOGRAPHY

Discography is a reliable means of evaluating the integrity of the intervertebral disc. The normal annulus fibrosus offers fair resistance to distention, and the normal disc accepts only 1 to 1.5 ml of contrast media. The degenerated disc is often injected without difficulty. The easy accommodation of 2 ml or more of contrast medium by a disc is a sign of some degree of degeneration within the annulus fibrosus and nucleus pulposus. Extravasation of contrast medium occurs through fissures and tears of the annulus and may be seen with both degeneration and herniation.[1, 2, 6] Coupled with CT, discography can delineate fissures and defects in the annulus as well as herniation.[1, 2, 6]

Proponents of discography feel strongly that the morphologic assessment of the intervertebral disc can be complemented by the critical physiologic induction of pain that is recognized by the patients as similar or identical to their complaint.[8]

The question that remains is why an abnormal discogram is painful in one patient and not in another. It has been suggested that the concomitant pain sometimes associated with an abnormal discogram image may in part be related to the chemical environment in the intervertebral disc and the sensitized state of its annular nociceptors, a key distinction from the situation in asymptomatic patients with similar morphologic derangement.[11] In addition, the high percentage of false-positive results noted in previous studies has been called into question by a study of ten normal volunteers that suggests that discography had a false-positive rate of 0 and a specificity of 100 per cent.[10]

However, efforts to determine whether a particular disc is symptomatic have never been successful.[7] In fact, a prospective study by Esses and colleagues appeared to indicate that discography has little value in predicting the outcome of spinal surgery such as fusion.[3] Furthermore, as with other tests, it is generally accepted that in many patients a degenerative pattern and pain are commonly seen in asymptomatic discs, which limits the tests' clinical usefulness.[4, 5]

The current role of discography remains controversial because of the inability to prove a cause-and-effect relationship. This leads us back to Holt's original contention: "How do we tell if an internal derangement is sufficiently symptom producing to be of therapeutic objective, especially a surgical one, or whether it represents anything more than an aging process?"[4] The majority opinion is that discography adds little if anything to a diagnostic work-up when CT and MR imaging are available.[9]

References

1. Brodsky, A. E., and Binder, W. F.: Lumbar discography: its value and diagnosis and treatment of lumbar disk lesions. Spine *4*:110–120, 1979.
2. Collis, J. S., and Gardner, W. J.: Lumbar discography: an analysis of 1,000 cases. J. Neurosurg. *19*:452–461, 1962.
3. Esses, S. I., Botsford, D. J., and Kostuik, J. P.: The role of external spine skeletal fixation in the assessment of low-back disorders. Spine *14*:594–601, 1989.
4. Holt, E. P., Jr.: Fallacy of cervical discography: report of 50 cases in normal subjects. J.A.M.A. *188*:799–801, 1964.
5. Holt, E. P., Jr.: The question of lumbar discography. J. Bone Joint Surg. *58*:720–726, 1968.
6. Lindbloom, K.: Backache and its relation to ruptures of the intervertebral discs. Radiology *57*:710–719, 1951.
7. Nachemson, A.: Editorial comment: Lumbar discography—where are we today? Spine *14*:555–557, 1989.
8. Position statement on discography. Executive Committee of the North American Spine Society. Spine *13*:1343, 1988.
9. Shapiro, R.: Current status of lumbar diskography (letter). Radiology *159*:815, 1986.
10. Walsh, T. R., April, C. N., Montgomery, W. J., et al.: Lumbar discography: a controlled prospective study in normal volunteers to determine the false positive rate. Paper 105, American Academy of Orthopaedic Surgeons, February 1989.
11. Weinstein, J., Claverie, W., and Gibson, S.: The pain of discography. Spine *13*:1344–1348, 1988.

RADIONUCLIDE IMAGING (BONE SCANS)

Bone scanning (scintigraphy) uses radiation emitted from radiopharmaceuticals to detect abnormalities in the skeletal system by virtue of its sensitivity to any disturbance in vascularity or osteogenesis. Its primary use is the evaluation of neoplastic, infectious, ischemic, traumatic, and metabolic disorders of the spine; it has a limited role in degenerative disease.

The major limitation of scintigraphy is its lack of specificity, since a number of pathophysiologic disorders have similar appearances. It should always be used in conjunction with pertinent historical information and correlative radiographic data such as conventional radiography, CT, and MRI. The lesion generally must be metabolically active to be detected, although "cold spots" in areas of altered vascularity may be identifiable. It has little if any value in the evaluation of the intervertebral disc or cartilaginous lesions.

Technetium-99m Phosphate

Technetium-99m is the most commonly employed agent in bone scintigraphy.[4, 5] This radiopharmaceutical has a half-life of six hours and emits gamma radiation, but has a low radiation exposure. Any process that disturbs the normal balance of bone production and reabsorption can produce an abnormality on a technetium bone scan. Increased osteoblastic activity is associated with a greater uptake of the radionuclide. An interruption of the blood flow or lack of metabolic activity results in decreased accumulation. Diagnostic imaging can be performed two to four hours after intravenous injection or in a dynamic fashion earlier to determine the rate of uptake.

Increased activity is identified in areas of trauma, degenerative change, infection, and neoplasm. This technique is particularly useful for screening the entire skeleton for abnormal activity, and in circumstances in which radiographic changes may lag behind bone activity, such as in the detection of metastatic disease. Paget's disease, aseptic necrosis, and certain of the hemoglobinopathies also demonstrate abnormal activity.

Gallium

Gallium-67 citrate is most commonly employed as an adjunct to bone scintigraphy in an effort to increase specificity in the detection of inflammatory processes.[1, 2] Gallium has an affinity for the intracellular protein lactoferrin and the lysozomes of neutrophils and thus accumulates in areas of ongoing infection. It is usually the first of all the modalities to revert to normal with successful treatment. An absence of gallium uptake can be detected in this situation, whereas plain films, bone scintigraphy, and MRI studies remain unchanged. Delayed imaging with gallium is the rule and the examination can take anywhere from 24 to 72 hours. The intestinal mucosa becomes the major route of excretion, and in the spine it is best coupled with single-photon emission computed tomography (SPECT) for better spatial localization.

Although more specific than bone scintigraphy, gallium has been reported to accumulate in tumors, most notably hepatomas and lymphomas. There is also some overlap in accumulation relative to areas of new bone formation. Compared with technetium, there is an increased radiation dosage from this radiopharmaceutical because of its long half-life and relatively high energy.

Indium

White blood cells can be labeled with this radiopharmaceutical to provide more specific and earlier localization of inflammatory sites than with gallium or technetium.[3, 6] The major advantage of this agent is that it is selectively accumulated in areas of infection versus areas of new bone formation or reactive change. The sensitivity and specificity for inflammatory processes is higher than with gallium. As would be expected, it is more sensitive to an acute infection than to a chronic one. Another disadvantage is that the study may take 18 to 24 hours. Some accumulation is noted in the spleen and liver, which may make evaluation of the thoracolumbar junction difficult.

References

1. Armas, R. R., and Goldsmith, S. J.: Gallium scintigraphy in bone infarction: correlation with bone imaging. Clin. Nucl. Med. *9*:1–3, 1984.
2. Bruschwein, D. A., Brown, M. L., and McLeod, R. A.: Gallium scintigraphy in the evaluation of disk-space infections: concise communication. J Nucl. Med. *21*:925–927, 1980.
3. Coleman, R. E., and Welch, D.: Possible pitfalls with clinical imaging of indium-111 leukocytes: concise communication. J. Nucl. Med. *21*:122–125, 1980.
4. Lin, D. S., and Alavi, A.: Bone scan evaluation of degenerative joint disease of the spine. Int. J. Nucl. Med. Biol. *9*:63–64, 1982.
5. Muroff, L. R.. Optimizing the performance and interpretation of bone scans. Clin. Nucl. Med. *6*:68–76, 1981.
6. Raptopoulos, V., Doherty, P. W., Goss, T. P., et al.: Acute osteomyelitis: advantage of white cell scans in early detection. AJR *139*:1077–1082, 1982.

MAGNETIC RESONANCE IMAGING

MRI is similar to CT in that it provides cross-sectional images based on a matrix of numbers each assigned a shade of gray and each representing a physical property of the tissue and voxel it represents. In CT the property measured is x-ray attenuation. In MRI the signal represents the intensity of a radiowave signal emanating from the tissue in which hydrogen nuclei have been perturbed by a characteristic radiofrequency (RF) pulse.

The basis of MRI relates to the property of the hydrogen proton in the presence of a superimposed magnetic field and external RF pulse.[6, 27] Nuclei having an odd number of protons or neutrons act as a charge particle and have a net magnetic dipole moment. The hydrogen atoms with their single unpaired proton are the most abundant element in the body and make it ideal for imaging purposes. In the absence of an external magnetic field, the magnetic dipoles of the hydrogen atoms are randomly oriented with a net magnetization of

0. When a strong external magnetic field is superimposed, these magnetic dipoles orient along the direction of the magnetic field or opposite it. Random interaction then takes place between the dipoles and their surrounding environment, which causes them to move back and forth between lower (parallel) and higher (antiparallel) energy states.

Although the net direction of their alignment is parallel or antiparallel to the field, in reality they "precess" in a fashion similar to that of a spinning top. The rate of precession is determined by the strength of the magnetic field and determines the frequency of electromagnetic radiation necessary to excite these nuclei, and the subsequent signal generated by the patient. The relationship between the magnetic field strength and the precessional frequency is called the Larmour frequency.

An externally applied RF pulse at this frequency can tip the magnetization into the plane perpendicular to the static magnetic field called the transverse plane. The 90-degree pulse in the MRI experiment is the precipitating factor that tips the longitudinal magnetization into the transverse plane where it can be measured. Once this pulse is turned off, the net magnetization realigns itself with the external field. The exponential regrowth of this longitudinal magnetization is due to interaction between individual dipoles and nearby molecules and is described as the longitudinal or spin-lattice relaxation time, T1. This is tissue specific, and T1 describes the length of time required for two thirds of the longitudinal magnetization to recover.

After the RF pulse, the transverse magnetization decays rapidly in strength and this is primarily related to a loss of coherence among magnetic dipoles. A small part of the loss is due to reorientation of dipoles along the direction of the static magnetic field. Dipoles precess faster in higher magnetic fields than in weaker fields. This difference in precessional frequency leads to a loss of coherence and is characterized by the relaxation time T2.

T1 may be thought of as a recovery process, while T2 is a decayed process. Thus, a tissue with a short T1 is likely to result in a higher signal intensity than a tissue with a short T2, which has a lower signal intensity.

In imaging, several intrinsic factors affect the signal intensity and/or contrast between tissues in an image. These include the proton density, T1, T2, movement of spins, and contrast media. To manipulate the signal intensity and contrast, a variety of operator-selectable parameters are available in formulating the MR examination. These include the pulse sequence, design (e.g., GE, SE), repetition time (TR), echo time (TE), flip angle, and voxel size. Voxel size influences the signal intensity by altering the volume and therefore the number of hydrogen nuclei in each voxel. Smaller voxels with fewer protons therefore result in a lower signal-to-noise ratio (SNR).

To date, the most commonly used pulse sequence is the spin echo (SE). An initial 90-degree RF pulse tips the tissue magnetization into the transverse plane where it can be measured. The SE experiment requires a rephasing of the magnetization precessing in the transverse plane by applying a 180-degree rephasing pulse after the initial 90-degree pulse. This helps to correct for static magnetic field inhomogeneities. An equal time after the 180-degree pulse, reversible effects are rephased and the signal output or echo is measured. TR represents the interval between the 90-degree pulse, and TE is the time between the middle of the 90-degree pulse and the maximal signal output or echo measured.

Variations in the repetition and echo time allow contrast manipulation. T1 contrast can be magnified by keeping both TR and TE short. These sequences are most useful for anatomic detail. T2-weighted contrast can be obtained by lengthening the echo time and repetition time. While the SNR is usually lower than for a T1-weighted sequence, T2 contrast predominates, which is important in looking for specific tissue pathology. A proton density–weighted sequence employes a short echo time and a long repetition time.

Gradient echo (GE) sequences differ from SE in that a gradient reversal replaces the 180-degree pulse. These can be used in combination with initial RF pulses that flip the longitudinal magnetization less than 90 degrees, leaving an appreciable amount of longitudinal magnetization in the direction of the static magnetic field so that there is no need to wait for T1-induced recovery. Using partial flip angles, pulse sequences may be repeated as soon as the signal measurement is completed. Thus, TR values of tens of milliseconds and total imaging times of seconds are possible. Under these circumstances, signal intensity is related not only to TR and TE but also to the initial flip angle used. The major advantages

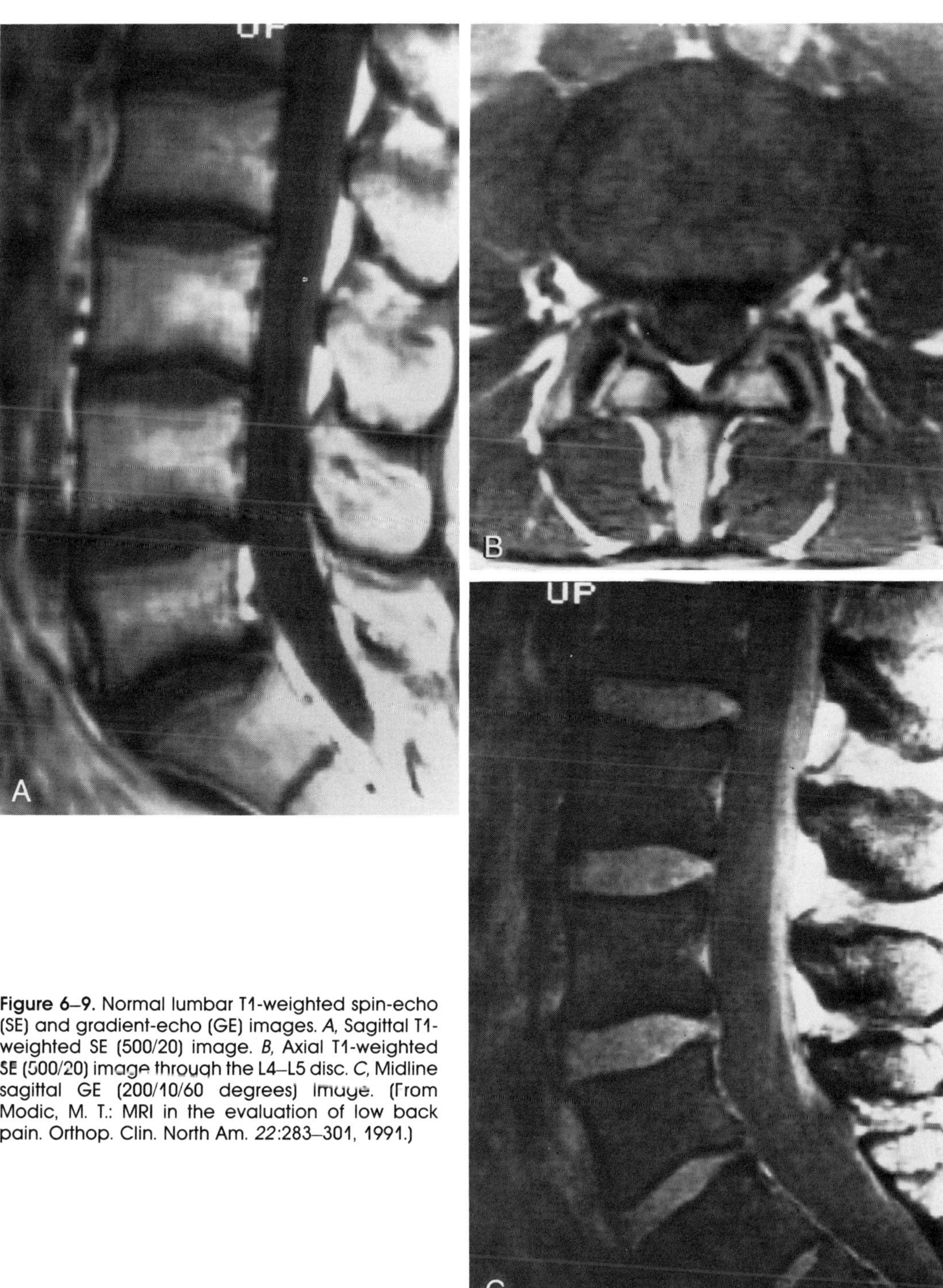

Figure 6–9. Normal lumbar T1-weighted spin-echo (SE) and gradient-echo (GE) images. *A*, Sagittal T1-weighted SE (500/20) image. *B*, Axial T1-weighted SE (500/20) image through the L4–L5 disc. *C*, Midline sagittal GE (200/10/60 degrees) image. (From Modic, M. T.: MRI in the evaluation of low back pain. Orthop. Clin. North Am. *22*:283–301, 1991.)

of these sequences are their rapid acquisition time and their ability to be used in 3D sequences.

In the lumbar spine, most examinations are carried out with a combination of planes and pulse sequences. Orthogonal imaging is the rule with both sagittal and axial images of no more than 4 mm slice thickness. In the main, T1-weighted sequences in the axial and sagittal plane with a GE sequence in the sagittal plane suffice and can be performed in 30 minutes or less (Fig. 6–9). GE 3D sequences with short TRs and short TEs have shown promise in their ability to provide data sets that can be acquired in a short time and can be reconstructive in any plane. T2-weighted sequences are usually reserved for suspected osteomyelitis (Fig. 6–10).[10] Paramagnetic contrast agents are routinely employed in the postoperative spine, but their use in the unoperated spine remains experimental at this time.

Discovertebral Complex

The regions of cortical bone and vertebral end plates have a decreased signal intensity on both T1- and T2-weighted images, reflecting a relatively low mobile proton density. On T1-weighted images the central portion of the disc has a slightly decreased signal intensity compared with the peripheral portion, which blends with an area of even further decreased signal intensity, representing the outer layers of the annulus fibrosus, that is confluent with the longitudinal ligaments (Fig. 6–9*B*). A similar appearance is noted on T2-weighted images, although the signal intensities are reversed (Fig. 6–10*B*). On T2-weighted SE sequences the normal disc has a central portion of high signal intensity and a peripheral portion of decreased signal intensity. The signal intensity differences are related to the difference in hydration as well as the state of water, reflect-

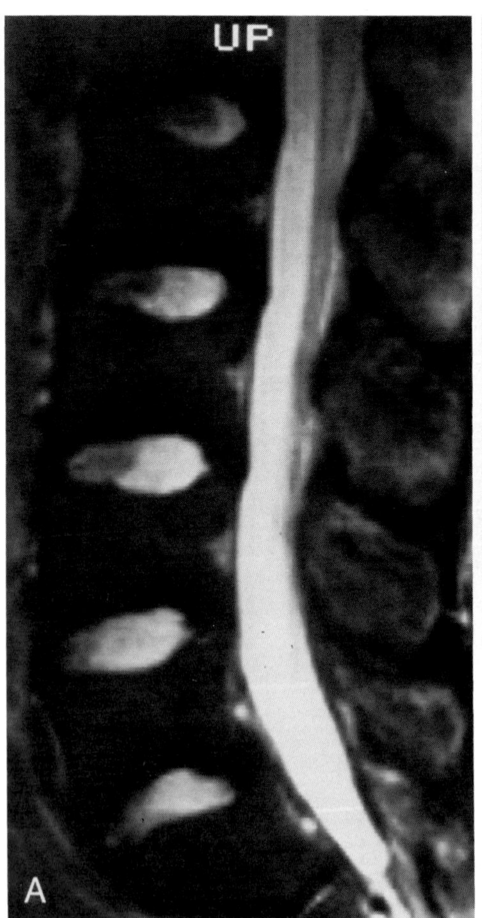

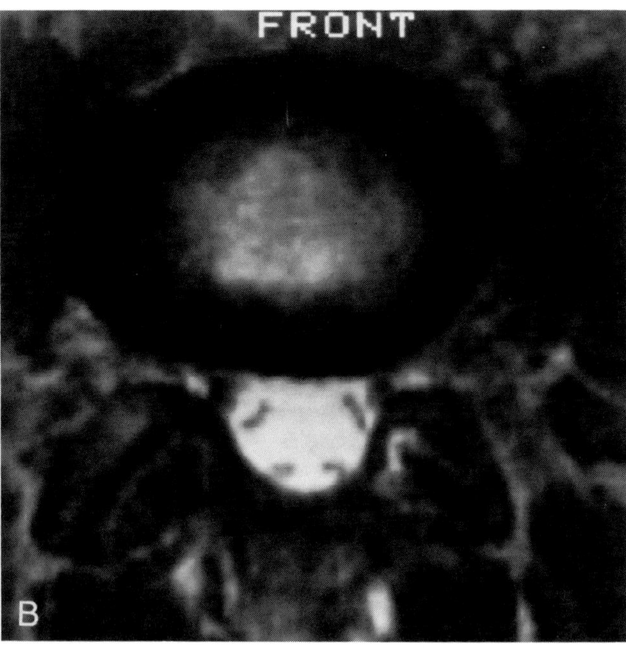

Figure 6–10. Normal T2-weighted SE images of the lumbar spine. *A*, Sagittal midline SE (2000/90) image. *B*, Axial T2-weighted SE (2000/90) image. Note the high signal intensity of the central portion of the disc. Nerve roots are seen as filling defects within the high signal intensity of the CSF. (From Modic, M. T.: MRI in the evaluation of low back pain. Orthop. Clin. North Am. *22*: 283–301, 1991.)

ing a longer T1 and T2 centrally. On images that are more T2 weighted, there is often an area of variable size and decreased signal intensity within the central portion of the disc, creating a notch or biconcave appearance of the disc similar to that seen at discography (Fig. 6–10*A*).[1]

Osseous structures appear as areas of relative signal void, reflecting a paucity of mobile hydrogen protons. Cortical bone, which is dense on CT, is low in intensity on MRI. Cancellous bone, owing to the fat within the marrow with a short T1, is of relatively high signal intensity. In children the signal intensity of the vertebral body and disc may be isointense, while in adults the signal intensity of the vertebral bodies is higher than that of the intervertebral disc on T1-weighted images because of the relative increase in lipid to hematopoietic elements. Pedicles, facet, and lamina appear as structures of high signal intensity. The spinal ligaments are usually intermediate, the longitudinal ligaments appearing decreased in signal intensity and the ligamenta flava of a higher signal intensity (Figs. 6–9, 6–10).

Degeneration

Signal intensity changes in vertebral body marrow adjacent to the end plate of degener-

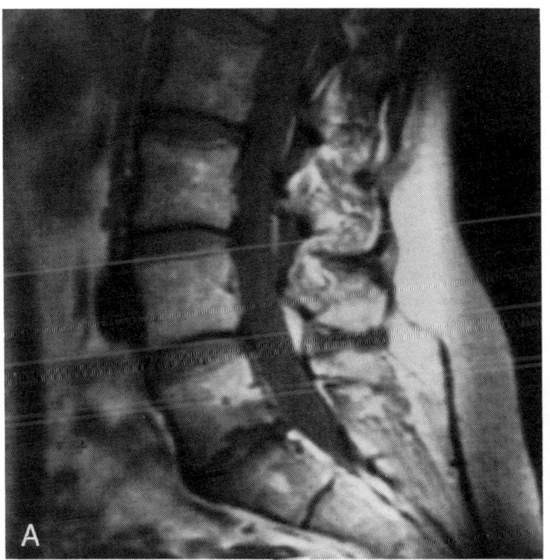

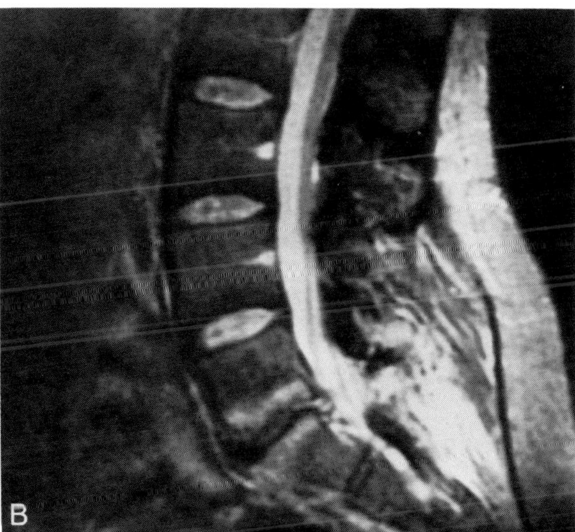

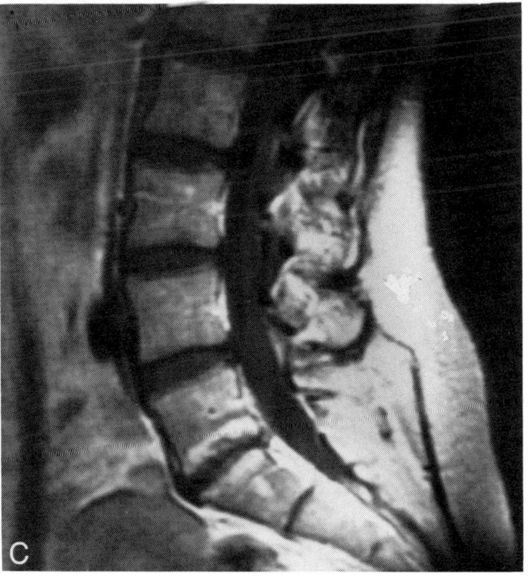

Figure 6–11. Type I vertebral body degenerative changes. *A*, Midline sagittal T1-weighted SE image. Note the decreased signal intensity of the adjacent portions of the L5 and S1 vertebral bodies. There is narrowing of the intervertebral disc space consistent with degenerative disease. *B*, Sagittal T2-weighted SE image. Note the high signal intensity of the adjacent portions of the L5 and S1 vertebral bodies. There is decreased signal intensity of the disc space consistent with degenerative disease. *C*, Sagittal midline T1-weighted SE image after injection of gadolinium-DTPA. Note the enhancement of the adjacent portions of L5 and S1, which were decreased on the unenhanced T1-weighted SE images. (From Modic, M. T.: MRI in the evaluation of low back pain. Orthop. Clin. North Am. *22*:283–301, 1991.)

ative discs are commonly observed on MRI.[2, 5, 8, 11] These take three main forms. The first, Type I, demonstrates a decreased signal intensity on T1-weighted and increased signal intensity on T2-weighted images (Fig. 6–11). There is enhancement of this region with gadolinium-DTPA (Gd-DTPA). Type II changes demonstrate an increased signal intensity on T1-weighted and an iso- or slightly hyperintense signal on T2-weighted images (Fig. 6–12). Histopathologic sections of Type I changes demonstrate disruption and fissuring of the end plate and vascularized fibrous tissue within the adjacent marrow, producing prolongation of T1 and T2. Type II changes are a reflection of yellow marrow replacement in the adjacent vertebral body. Type III changes are represented by decreased signal intensity on both T1- and T2-weighted images, which appear to correlate with extensive bony sclerosis on plain radiographs. The MRI signal intensity is a reflection of the marrow elements, normal hematopoietic tissue, fibrovascular tissue, and lipid (or lack thereof) between trabeculae. The lack of signal in Type III no doubt reflects the relative absence of marrow. All three of these changes are always associated with degenerative disc disease. Type I may reflect a more subacute process; Type II represents a degenerated, albeit more stable, discovertebral complex.

The signal intensity changes of Type I may be similar to those seen in vertebral osteomyelitis, but the distinguishing factor is the involvement of the intervertebral disc, which shows an abnormally high signal intensity and abnormal configuration on T2-weighted images with pyogenic infections. Tuberculosis or brucellosis infections may be confined more to the vertebral body itself and may not involve adjacent disc spaces. Both of these lesions also may skip vertebral bodies and be difficult to distinguish from neoplasm.[21, 22]

Although the annulus fibrosus may play a key role in the pathophysiologic changes of disc degeneration, imaging changes have been poorly characterized. High signal intensity has been noted on T2-weighted images within the annulus fibrosus in the absence of obvious herniation, which appears anatomically to correlate with annular tears (Fig. 6–13).

T2-weighted SE sequences are the most sensitive for characterizing changes within the disc itself that are secondary to degeneration and

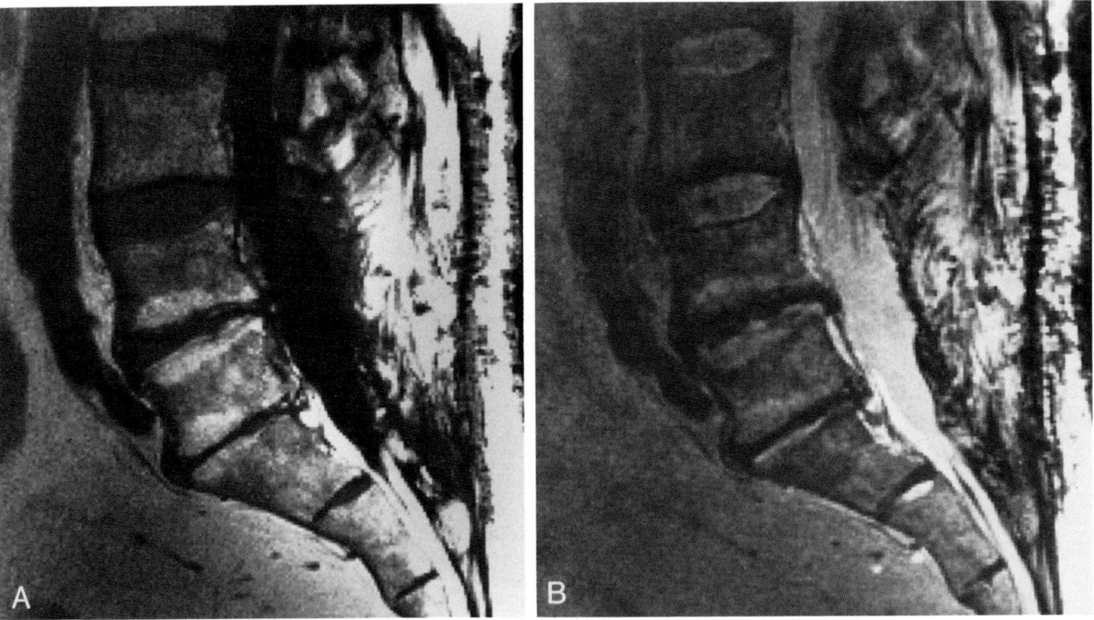

Figure 6–12. Type II vertebral body degenerative changes. *A*, Sagittal midline T1-weighted SE image. Note the high signal intensity of the adjacent portion of the L4 and L5 vertebral bodies and narrowing of the intervertebral disc space. A similar high signal intensity is seen in the adjacent portions of L5 and S1. *B*, Sagittal T2-weighted SE images. There is only a mildly increased signal intensity of the adjacent portions of the L4–L5 and L5–S1 vertebral bodies. There is decreased signal intensity of the L4–L5 and L5–S1 disc consistent with degenerative disease.

6–16) by the presence of continuity with the parent disc (Fig. 6–17). They are often attached by a thin pedicle of tissue. As on CT, lateral disc herniations are well seen (Fig. 6–17).

Related spinal structures, which can be adversely affected by changes within the disc itself, can also be well appreciated on MRI. In particular, changes of lumbar canal stenosis, ligamentous hypertrophy, and facet disease can be evaluated in a fashion analogous to assessment with high-resolution CT (Fig. 6–18). CT probably remains the most accurate means of evaluating bone changes and facet joint disease, but MRI has an advantage in evaluation of the articular cartilage itself because it can be directly assessed, especially on GE images.

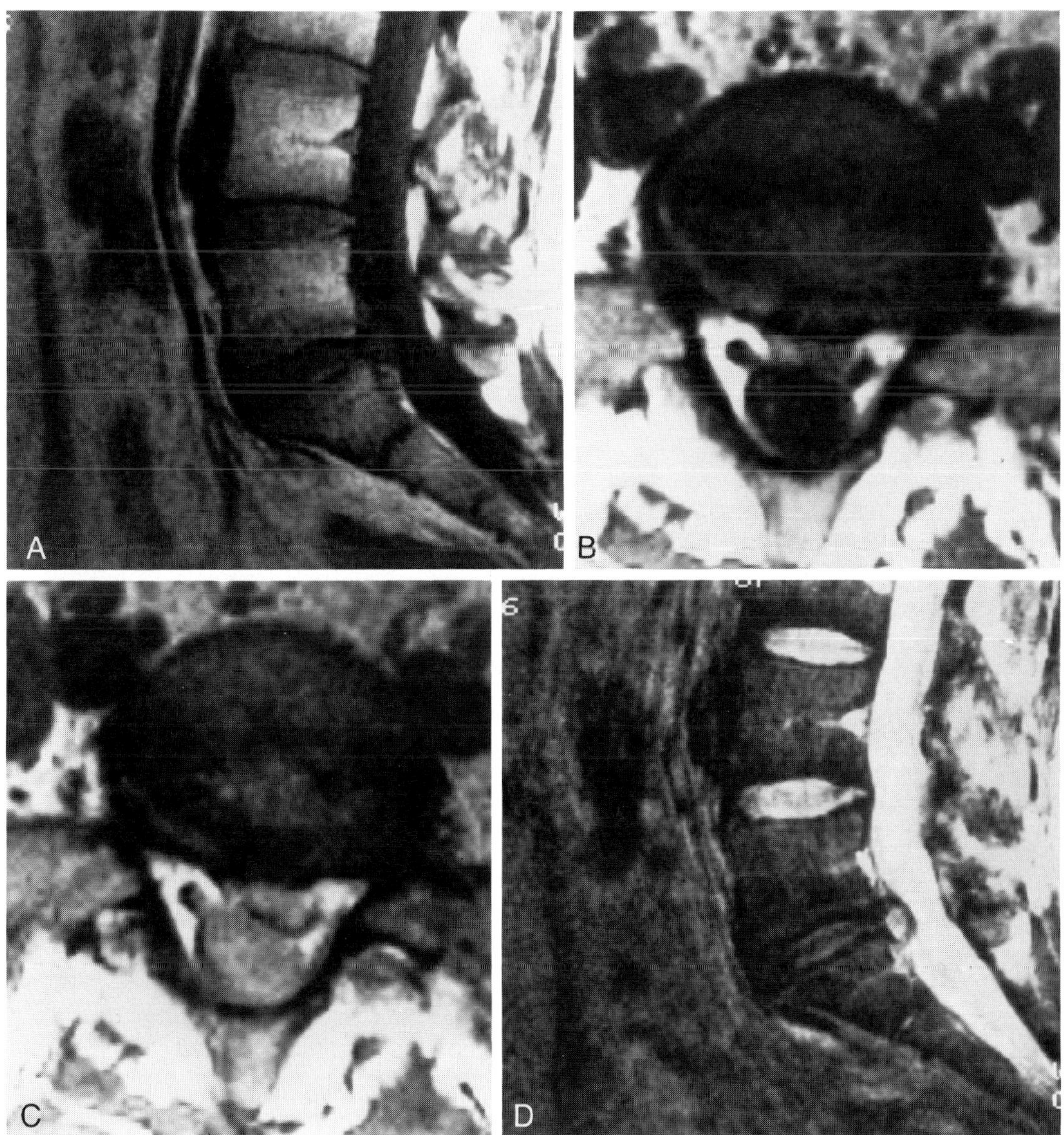

Figure 6–16. Extruded disc. *A,* Sagittal T1-weighted SE image demonstrating a disc extrusion at the L5–S1 level. *B,* Axial T1-weighted SE image through the L5–S1 disc space. The disc herniation is seen central and slightly to the left. *C,* Axial intermediate (2000/20) image through the L5–S1 disc. Note that the herniated disc is partially outlined by an area of decreased signal intensity thought to represent areas of the annulus and longitudinal ligament. *D,* Sagittal T2-weighted SE image. The L5–S1 herniated disc shows a high signal intensity relative to the decreased signal intensity of the parent degenerated disc.

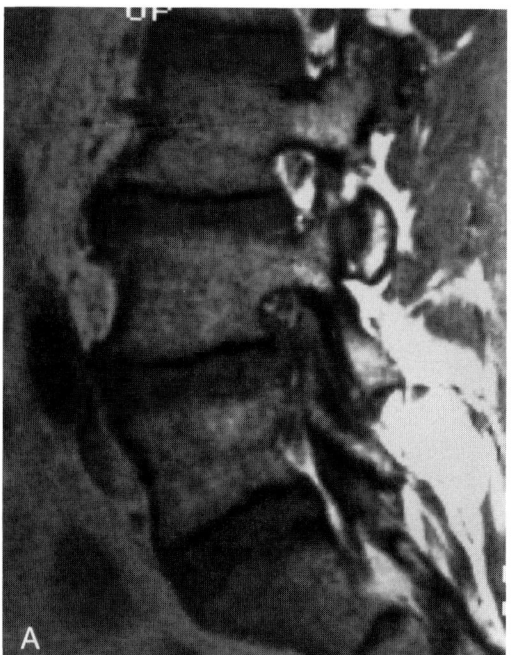

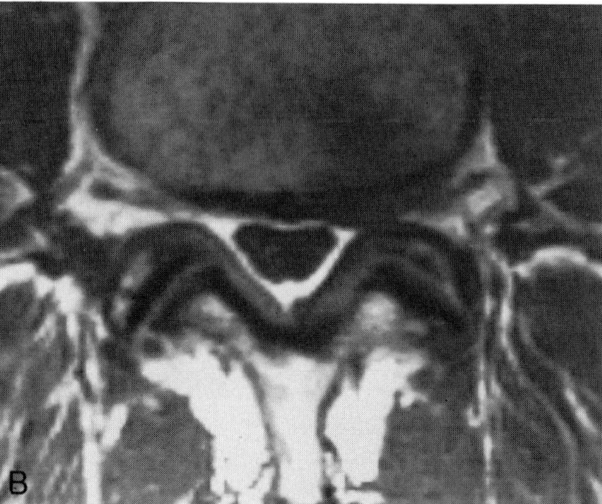

Figure 6–17. Lateral disc herniation. *A*, Parasagittal T1-weighted SE image of the lumbar spine. There is obliteration of the normal epidural fat signal at the L4–L5 level compared with the L5–S1 and L3–L4 levels. *B*, Axial T1-weighted SE image demonstrates left lateral disc herniation with obliteration of the normal epidural fat plane in the neural foramen.

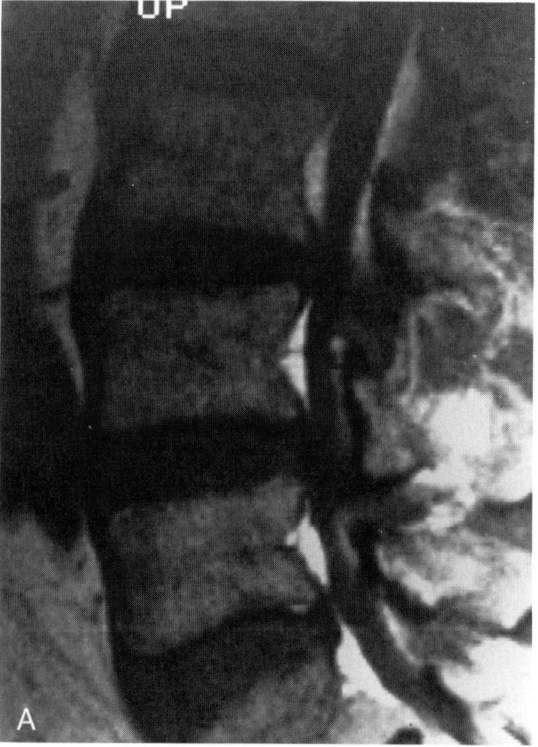

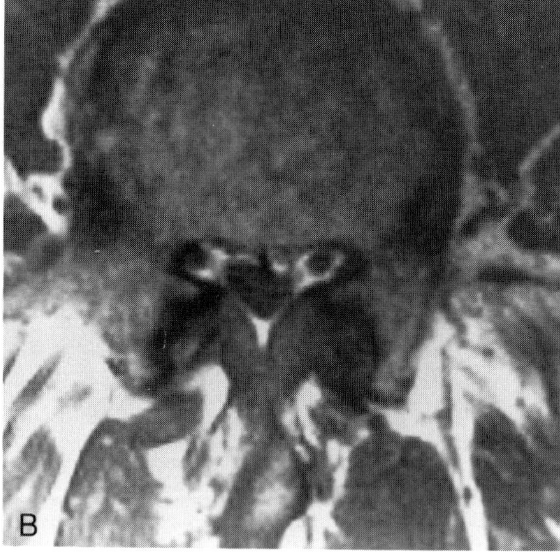

Figure 6–18. Lumbar canal stenosis. *A*, Sagittal T1-weighted SE image showing diffuse central canal stenosis. *B*, Axial T1-weighted SE image through the L5 vertebral body. Note the diffuse central stenosis and thickened posterior ligament.

Paramagnetic Contrast Material Studies

Gadolinium-DTPA is the only currently approved contrast agent for MRI sanctioned for use by the Federal Drug Administration (F.D.A.) for both brain and spine. The current recommended dose is 0.1 mmol. per kg.

Studies of the spine to date have resulted in several well-established applications, which can be conveniently grouped into the conventional categories of exradural, intradural-extramedullary, and intramedullary.

After administration of Gd-DTPA, the epidural venous plexus shows some enhancement, which usually persists for at least 20 to 30 minutes.[16] Variable degrees of enhancement can be noted in the region of the ventral and dorsal nerve root ganglia, especially in the lumbar region. The normal cord, nerve roots, and intervertebral disc do not enhance.

Intramedullary

Assuming good-quality MRI, unenhanced T1- and T2-weighted images are sensitive to intramedullary pathology, identifying changes in cord or nerve root size and signal intensity. Despite the fact that contrast material does not appear to increase the sensitivity of the unenhanced examination, most investigators consider it critical for lesion characterization.[24] This is especially true in cases of neoplasm where contrast improves the localization of tumor nidus and separation from edema (particularly important with hemangioblastomas and metastasis). Furthermore, it aids in differentiating benign or reactive processes from neoplasms.

In addition to neoplasms, enhancement may be seen in other intramedullary disorders when there is disruption of the blood-brain barrier and evidence of an active lesion. Examples include inflammatory disorders such as AIDS myelopathy, sarcoid, and demyelinating disease, in which, as in the brain, not all lesions with a high signal on T2-weighted images enhance.

Intradural-Extramedullary

Although large lesions such as meningiomas, neurofibromas, and schwannomas can usually be identified without difficulty on unenhanced scans, smaller or diffuse lesions may have signal intensity characteristics similar to that of the surrounding CSF and neural structures. This is especially true of lesions spreading via the subarachnoid space or the leptomeninges. Lymphomas, primitive neuroectodermal tumors, ependymomas, glioblastomas, metastases, and inflammatory disease all enhance dramatically, markedly increasing their conspicuity.[3, 25] Occasionally, very mild enhancement is noted of the traversing nerve roots that otherwise appear normal, and in some cases of arachnoiditis. This is rarely a problem of differential diagnosis because of the dramatic enhancement seen with neoplastic or active inflammatory processes.

Extradural

Experience to date has centered primarily on neoplastic and degenerative changes. Unlike the other compartments, routine T2-weighted images are not always obtained and assessment has been primarily morphologic. Gd-DTPA is not routinely used for the evaluation of metastatic disease. Tumor involvement is usually predicted on the basis of marrow or epidural fat infiltration, and studies to date do not indicate that enhanced MRI facilitates the detection of tumors in the extradural compartment (Fig. 6–19). In fact, some lesions become isointense compared with surrounding bone marrow and become difficult to see.[23, 26] An exception may be the patient with a large extradural soft tissue mass and adjacent bony changes in the contours of the lateral recess. Although the situation is uncommon, free disc fragments have been shown to be associated with bony changes, and an enhanced scan should distinguish a tumor that would enhance diffusely from a free fragment with surrounding granulation tissue.[20]

In degenerative disease, Gd-DTPA was first applied to the postoperative spine. Current data suggest that Gd-DTPA has a 96 per cent correlation with surgery in separating epidural fibrosis from disc material and suggest it should be used routinely in the postoperative spine.[7, 17] It seems likely that Gd-DTPA diffuses rapidly into the extravascular space of epidural scar through a "leaky" cellular junction in areas of endothelial discontinuity (Fig. 6–20). Herniated disc, on the other hand, typically does not enhance early, but is often "wrapped in scar" and may enhance on delayed studies

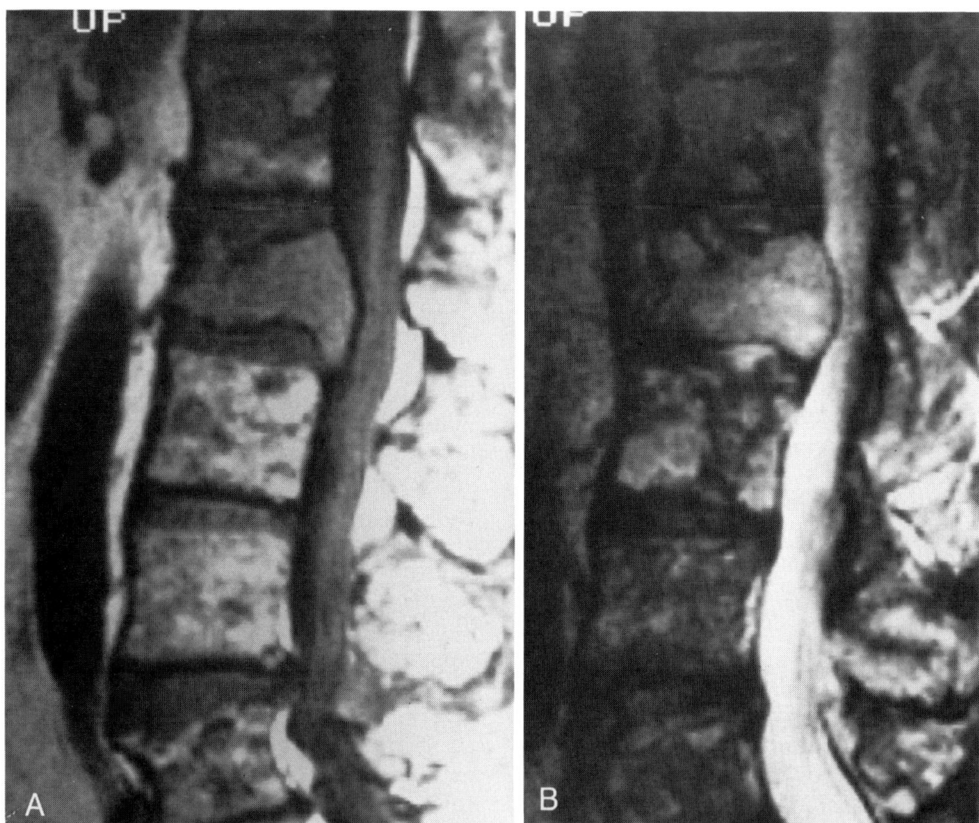

Figure 6–19. Metastatic disease of the lumbar spine. *A*, Sagittal T1-weighted SE image. Note the decreased signal intensity of the L2 vertebral body with deformity and compression fracture. There is encroachment on the spinal canal. The mottled appearance of the remaining vertebral bodies is also consistent with marrow infiltration by tumor. *B*, Sagittal T2-weighted SE image through the lumbar spine. The mottled high signal intensity of the L2 vertebral body is consistent with an infiltrative process.

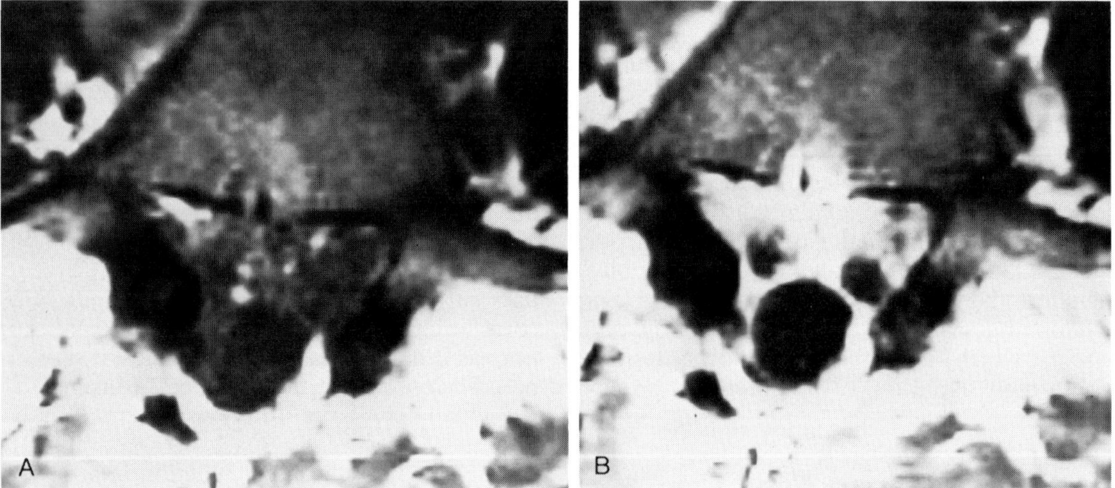

Figure 6–20. Epidural fibrosis. *A*, Axial T1-weighted SE image through the L5 vertebral body. There is evidence of a posterior laminectomy and an abnormal soft tissue signal anterior and lateral to the thecal sac obliterating the normal epidural fat signal. *B*, Axial T1-weighted SE image after administration of gadolinium-DTPA at the L5 level. The region of aberrant soft tissue noted in *A* is now seen to enhance. The exiting dural root sleeves are now appreciated surrounded by the enhancing epidural fibrosis.

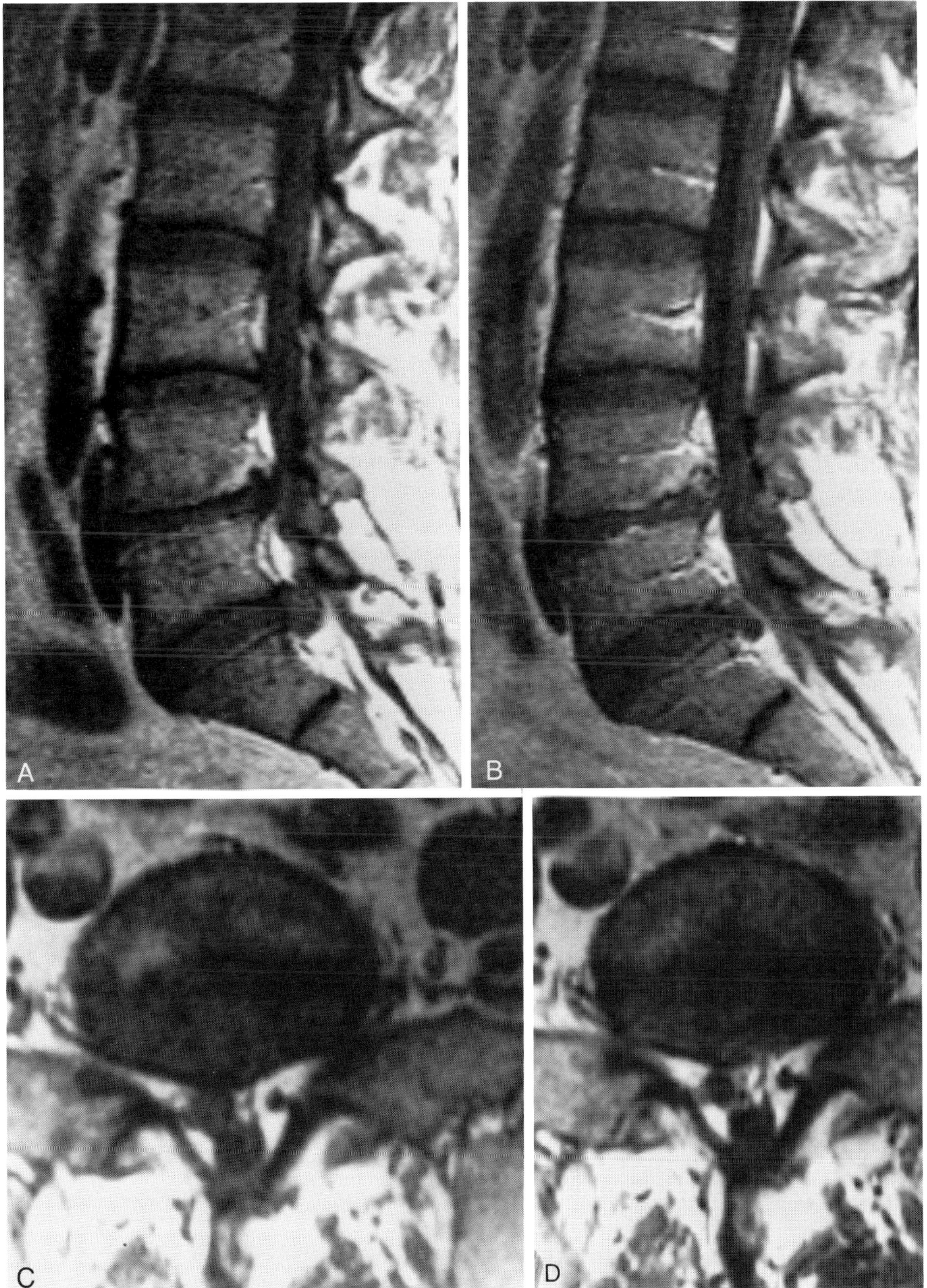

Figure 6–21. Recurrent disc herniation. Sagittal T1-weighted SE images before *(A)* and after *(B)* gadolinium administration. Axial T1-weighted SE images before *(C)* and after *(D)* gadolinium administration through the L5–S1 level. An aberrant soft tissue mass consistent with a disc herniation is noted posterior to the L5–S1 disc *(A)*. After gadolinium *(B)* the central portion of this mass does not enhance while the periphery does. *C* demonstrates an aberrant soft tissue mass representing the disc herniation at the L5–S1 level to the right midline. *D*, After gadolinium there is peripheral enhancement, but the central core of the disc herniation does not enhance.

secondary to diffusion of contrast material from adjacent scar tissue (Fig. 6–21).[18]

In both the operated and nonoperated spine, enhancement may be noted within some degenerated discs and is presumably secondary to the ingrowth of granulation tissue. This may occur in a linear or rarely a diffuse pattern. Probably by the same mechanism, enhancement is also seen with Type I vertebral body changes. Annular tears are another sequela of the degenerative process, which may show enhancement based on the presence of granulation tissue, a component of the healing process.[19] Along these same lines, enhancement has been demonstrated surrounding herniated discs in the unoperated spine in over 50 per cent of patients, and may represent a significant portion of the mass. Histologically, these areas of enhancement again seem to be related to granulation tissue.[16] Its presence is not surprising because one would expect the body to respond to tissue disruption by attempted healing.

It must be emphasized that MRI represents a tool for morphologic and biochemical analysis and also that all morphologic changes do not produce symptoms. In a study by Boden and associates, herniated disc disease was identified in 20 per cent of patients under the age of 60 in an asymptomatic population who underwent MRI.[4] In the subgroup aged 60 years or older, abnormal lumbar MRI scans were identified in 50 per cent; 36 per cent had herniated disc disease and 21 per cent spine stenosis. There was degeneration or bulging of a disc in at least one lumbar level in 35 per cent of individuals between 20 and 39 years of age and in all but one of those 60 to 80 years old. Thus, the jump from the identification of an anatomic derangement to that of a symptom complex must be made with caution.[4] The management of a patient with a spinal disorder must begin and end with a thorough clinical assessment, imaging being an intermediate test that must be integrated into, rather than isolated from, that assessment. MRI offers clear advantages over other conventional imaging techniques such as myelography and CT. MRI is noninvasive, produces no ionizing radiation, provides orthogonal imaging of the spine, directly visualizes neural structures, and images the entire lumbar spine up to the thoracolumbar junction. Because of these advantages, the authors regard MRI as the preferable imaging technique for lumbar disc herniation. Since bony compression is often a significant component of spinal stenosis, CT, particularly when combined with a water-soluble contrast agent, may provide additional information through its ability to better distinguish bony compression from soft tissue compression. In addition, the myelogram provides the surgeon with a comforting "road map" to which he may refer during decompressive surgery. Nevertheless, the authors also consider MRI the preferred test for imaging neural compression in spinal stenosis, and believe that myelography and CT should be reserved for instances in which MRI is inconclusive or unavailable.

References

1. Aguila, L. A., Piraino, D. W., Modic, M. T., et al.: The intranuclear cleft of the intervertebral disk: magnetic resonance imaging. Radiology *155*:155–158, 1985.
2. Aoki, J., Yamamoto, I., Kitamura, N., et al.: End plate of the discovertebral joint: degenerative change in the elderly adult. Radiology *164*:411–414, 1987.
3. Berns, D. H., Blaser, S. I., Ross, J. S., et al.: MR imaging with gadolinium-DTPA in leptomeningeal spread of lymphoma. J. Comput. Assist. Tomogr. *12*:499–500, 1988.
4. Boden, S. D., Davis, D. O., Dina, T. S., et al.: Abnormal magnetic resonance scans of the lumbar spine in asymptomatic subjects. J. Bone Joint Surg. *72A*:403–408, 1990.
5. deRoos, A., Kressel, H., Spritzer, C., and Dalinka, M.: MR imaging of marrow changes adjacent to end plates in degenerative lumbar disk disease. A.J.R. *149*:531–534, 1987.
6. Hendrick, R. E.: Image contrast and noise. *In* Stark, D. D., and Bradley, W. G. (eds.): Magnetic Resonance Imaging. St. Louis, C.V. Mosby Co., 1988, pp. 66–83.
7. Hueftle, M. G., Modic, M. T., Ross, J. S., et al.: Lumbar spine: postoperative MR imaging with gadolinium-DTPA. Radiology *167*:817–824, 1988.
8. Masaryk, T. J., Boumphrey, F., Modic, M. T., et al.: Effects of chemonucleolysis demonstrated by MR imaging. J. Comput. Assist. Tomogr. *10*:917–923, 1986.
9. Masaryk, T. J., Ros, J. S., Modic, M. T., et al.: High resolution MR imaging of sequestered lumbar intervertebral disks. A.J.N.R. *9*:351–358, 1988.
10. Modic, M. T., Feiglin, D. H., Piraino, D. W., et al.: Vertebral osteomyelitis: assessment using MR. Radiology *157*:157–166, 1985.
11. Modic, M. T., Steinberg, P. M., Ross, J. S., et al.: Degenerative disk disease: assessment of changes in vertebral body marrow with MR imaging. Radiology *166*:193–199, 1988.
12. Modic, M. T., Masaryk, T. J., Boumphrey, F., et al.: Lumbar herniated disc disease and canal stenosis: prospective evaluation by surface coil MR, CT and myelography. A.J.N.R. *7*:709–717, 1986.

13. Modic, M. T., Masaryk, T. J., Mulopulos, G. P., et al.: Cervical radiculopathy: prospective evaluation with surface coil MR imaging, CT with metrizamide and metrizamide myelography. Radiology *161*:753–759, 1986.
14. Modic, M. T., Masaryk, T. J., Ross, J. S., et al.: Cervical radiculopathy: value of oblique MR imaging. Radiology *163*:227–231, 1987.
15. Ross, J. S., Perez-Reyes, N., Masaryk, T. J., et al.: Thoracic disk herniation: MR imaging. Radiology *165*:511–515, 1987.
16. Ross, J. S., Modic, M. T., Masaryk, T. J., et al.: Assessment of extradural degenerative disease with gadolinium-DTPA enhanced MR imaging: correlation with surgical and pathological findings. A.J.N.R. *10*:1243–1249, 1989.
17. Ross, J. S., Modic, M. T., Masaryk, T. J., et al.: Gd-DTPA in the postoperative spine: update. Abstract 898. Presented at the R.S.N.A., Chicago, IL, November 26–December 1, 1989.
18. Ross, J. S., Delamarter, R., Hueftle, M. G., et al.: Gadolinium-DTPA enhanced MR imaging of the postoperative lumbar spine: time course and mechanism of enhancement. A.J.N.R. *10*:37–46, 1989.
19. Ross, J. S., Modic, M. T., and Masaryk, T. J.: Tears of the anulus fibrosus: assessment of gadolinium-DTPA enhanced MR imaging. A.J.N.R. *10*:1251–1254, 1989.
20. Schlesinger, S. D., Elkin, C., Pinto, R. S., and Firooznia, H.: Lumbar and cervical osseous erosions secondary to herniated disks. Comparison of CT and MR imaging. Abstract 89. Presented at the R.S.N.A., Chicago, IL, November 26–December 1, 1989.
21. Sharif, H., Clark, D. C., Aabed, M., et al.: Granulomatous spinal infections: MR imaging. Radiology *177*:101–107, 1990.
22. Smith, A., Weinstein, M., Mizushima, A., et al.: Tuberculous spondylitis: characteristics of vertebral osteomyelitis. A.J.N.R. *10*:619–625, 1989.
23. Stimac, G. K., Porter, B. A., Olsen, D. L., et al.: Gadolinium-DTPA enhanced MR imaging of spinal neoplasms. Preliminary investigation in comparison with unenhanced spin echo and STIR sequences. A.J.N.R. *9*:839–846, 1988.
24. Sze, G., Kro, L. G., Zimmerman, R. D., and Deck, M. D. F.: Intramedullary disease of the spine: diagnosis using gadolinium-DTPA enhanced MR imaging. A.J.N.R. *9*:847–858, 1988.
25. Sze, G., Abramson, A., Krol, G., et al.: Gadolinium-DTPA in the evaluation of intradural extramedullary spinal disease. A.J.N.R. *9*:153–163, 1988.
26. Sze, G., Krol, G., Zimmerman, R. G., and Deck, M. D. F.: Malignant extradural spinal tumors: MR imaging with gadolinium-DTPA. Radiology *167*:217–223, 1988.
27. Wehrli, F. W.: Principles of magnetic resonance. *In* Stark, D. D., and Bradley, W. G. (eds.): Magnetic Resonance Imaging. St. Louis, C.V. Mosby Co., 1988, pp. 3–24.
28. Yu, S., Haughton, V. M., Sether, L. A., et al.: Criteria for classifying normal and degenerated lumbar intervertebral disks. Radiology *170*:523–526, 1989.

CHAPTER

7

ELECTRODIAGNOSIS

Asa J. Wilbourn, M.D.
Michael J. Aminoff, M.D.

THE ELECTROMYOGRAPHIC EXAMINATION

Asa J. Wilbourn, M.D.

This discussion focuses on the electrodiagnostic procedure most often used in assessing patients with known or suspected lesions of the anterior horn cells within the spinal cord, and of the motor and sensory spinal roots: electromyography (EMG) or the electromyographic (EMG) examination. Unlike another electrodiagnostic technique (somatosensory and motor evoked potentials) discussed later, the EMG examination assesses primarily the peripheral, rather than the central, nervous system.

The basic EMG examination is composed of two distinct but complementary techniques: the nerve conduction studies (NCS) and the needle electrode examination (NEE). In a strict sense, the term "EMG examination" applies only to the NEE, which came into clinical use in the mid–1940s; however, most electromyographers prefer to use the term to describe the entire study, including the NCS, which were introduced a decade later. (In this chapter, "EMG" is used in this all-inclusive fashion.) In addition to the NCS and NEE, a number of other electrophysiologic studies may be performed during the EMG examination (Table 7–1). These are a heterogeneous group of procedures, mostly variations of the NCS, which have limited application. Only two are pertinent to this discussion: H responses and F waves.[16, 18]

Like every other laboratory diagnostic procedure, the EMG examination has both limitations and benefits. A major limitation is that it is assesses only the large, heavily myelinated peripheral nerve fibers. Thus, it does not evaluate any unmyelinated or lightly myelinated fibers, including pain fibers. This is not as severe a handicap as may initially appear, however, because nerve lesions rarely compromise only small fibers. Instead, they affect solely large fibers (e.g., in neurapraxia) or a combination of both large and small fibers.[16] Another practical limitation is that the techniques used in performing the EMG examination, particularly the NCS, are not standardized from one EMG laboratory to another. Hence, studies performed in different laboratories frequently are dissimilar enough to make comparisons of results difficult. The major benefit of the EMG examination is that it is the best single laboratory diagnostic procedure available for assessing both the peripheral segments of some sensory nerves and the "motor unit": the anterior horn cell, and all the muscle fibers it innervates via its axon and the terminal divisions of the latter. The EMG examination can provide objective evidence of a lesion affecting this limited portion of the peripheral neuromuscular system when the clinical examination results are normal or equivocal (because the abnormality is so mild) or unreliable

Table 7–1. VARIOUS COMPONENTS OF THE EMG EXAMINATION

"Basic" Studies
Nerve conduction studies
Motor
Sensory
Mixed
Needle electrode examination
"Special" Studies
H responses
F waves
Palmar conduction studies
Repetitive stimulation studies
Blink reflex
Single-fiber EMG

(because of a coexisting upper motor neuron lesion or incomplete voluntary effort, due to hysteria or malingering, pain on activation, and so forth).[16, 17]

Both the basic components of the EMG examination, the NCS and the NEE, have specific advantages and limitations. Fortunately, the values of one often offset the disadvantages of the other. Because they complement each other so well, both customarily are performed in every patient, although in many disorders only one of the two is of significant positive value (e.g., as will be noted, with single radiculopathies typically only the NEE is abnormal). Most of these attributes in regard to nerve fiber lesions are determined by the type of pathophysiology produced at the lesion site.

PATHOPHYSIOLOGY OF FOCAL NERVE LESIONS

The large myelinated nerve fibers are very limited in their pathophysiologic responses to the enormous variety of traumatic agents that can affect them. Regardless of etiology, most focal neurogenic lesions, including those at the root level, result in axon loss, focal demyelination, or a combination of the two; focal demyelination in turn causes either conduction slowing or conduction block at the lesion site, depending on its severity.[6, 18] A fundamental distinction between focal axon loss lesions and focal demyelinating ones is that only the latter actually remain focal; i.e., a focal demyelinating lesion does not materially affect the nerve segments proximal or distal to it. In contrast, a focal axon loss lesion always causes wallerian degeneration along the entire nerve segment distal to it, and usually some retrograde degeneration along the segment proximal to it as well. The fact that focal demyelinating lesions remain localized while "focal" axon loss lesions do not explains why only axon loss lesions at the root level can affect motor NCS performed on peripheral nerve fibers derived from the involved root.

With both demyelinating conduction block lesions and axon loss lesions, nerve impulse transmission is stopped at the lesion site, rather than merely slowed. Hence, these two processes often produce similar clinical deficits whenever they affect sufficient motor and sensory fibers. These are manifested, respectively, as muscle weakness and loss of large fiber modalities: position and vibratory sense. In addition, with axon loss lesions, two other clinical findings may be evident: muscle atrophy and, because of associated small fiber loss, impairment of pain and temperature appreciation.[5, 11, 15, 18] In contrast to demyelinating conduction block and axon loss lesions, demyelinating conduction slowing lesions produce few, if any, clinical symptoms. Because all the nerve impulses ultimately reach their destination, albeit at a slightly later time than they should, neither clinical weakness nor a fixed sensory deficit is associated with them.[15, 18] Pertinent to this is the fact that neurapraxia, the mildest type of lesion Seddon described in his classification of nerve injuries in the 1940s, is usually attributable to demyelinating conduction block; conduction slowing is not included in any clinical classification of focal nerve lesions since it is more a pathophysiologic than a clinical entity.[4, 13]

Axon loss and demyelination (and the two subdivisions of the latter) have quite different effects on the NCS and the NEE. These will be discussed, but first the various components of the EMG examination will be described.

NERVE CONDUCTION STUDIES (NCS)

During the NCS portion of the EMG examination the electrical responses evoked in muscle and nerve by nerve stimulation are recorded and analyzed. Very valuable information concerning the number of functioning nerve fibers, and the speed of conduction along those fibers, is obtained during the NCS. Both motor and sensory NCS are performed, their end points being, respectively, a compound muscle action potential (CMAP) and a sensory nerve action potential (SNAP). For technical reasons, the motor and sensory components of a mixed nerve are studied individually, rather than simultaneously, yielding two separate studies.[1, 6] In North America, most electromyographers prefer to use surface, rather than needle, recording electrodes for both stimulating and recording. The use of surface recording electrodes for motor NCS provides major benefits.

When a motor NCS is performed, recording electrodes are affixed over a muscle and its tendon; the nerve supplying it is then stimulated. For the "routine" motor NCS (Table 7–2) a small muscle of the hand or foot serves as the recorded muscle, while its nerve is stimulated at two points along its course (e.g., elbow and wrist; knee and ankle). Four parameters in all can then be assessed: the distal and proximal amplitudes, which are the heights of the evoked responses obtained on distal and proximal stimulation, respectively, measured from baseline to negative peak and reported in millivolts (mV); also the distal and proximal latencies, which are the time intervals between the shock artifacts and the onset of the CMAPs, for distal and proximal stimulation, reported in milliseconds (msec) (Fig. 7–1). Generally, only two of these four measurements are reported directly: the distal amplitude and the distal latency. The proximal amplitude is mentioned if it is considerably different than the distal one, while the proximal latency is used to determine the motor conduction velocity (CV), to be discussed.[1, 6, 18]

For sensory NCS, a sensory nerve, or the sensory component of a mixed nerve, is stimulated at one point, and the SNAP produced is recorded at some set distance along the nerve fibers, either proximal or distal to that site (usually distal). Generally, only two parameters are measured during the sensory NCS: the amplitude, which is the height of the response, measured from baseline to negative peak and reported in microvolts (μV); and the peak latency, which is the time interval between the shock artifact and the negative peak of the response, reported in msec (Fig. 7–2).[1, 6, 18] Thus, the rate of conduction for the sensory fibers is being determined for most of the conducting fibers, rather than for the fastest conducting ones, as it is for the motor fibers. This is done because the onset of the sensory response is sometimes difficult to determine with certainty. Several sensory NCS can be performed (Table 7–2). A limiting factor regarding the lower extremity sensory NCS is that they cannot be elicited bilaterally in many patients over age 60.[15, 17]

Of the various NCS results, the amplitudes (when surface recording electrodes are used) are by far the most informative with most focal neurogenic lesions, since they reflect the *number* of nerve fibers capable of conducting impulses from the stimulation to the recording sites. They are affected by pathologic processes causing focal demyelinating conduction block

Table 7–2. NERVE CONDUCTION STUDIES

Motor	Sensory
Upper Extremity	
MEDIAN: THENAR (C8, T1)	MEDIAN: INDEX (C6 and/or C7)
ULNAR: HYPOTHENAR (C8, T1)	ULNAR: FIFTH (C8)
Ulnar: first dorsal interosseus (C8, T1)	Median: thumb (C6)
Radial: extensor forearm (C6, C7)	Median: middle (C7)
Axillary: deltoid (C5, C6)	Radial: thumb base (C6 and/or C7)
Musculocutaneous: biceps (C5, C6)	Ulnar: dorsum of hand (C8)
	Lateral antebrachial cutaneous: forearm (C6)
	Medial antebrachial cutaneous: forearm (T1)
Lower Extremity	
PERONEAL: EXTENSOR DIGITORUM BREVIS (L5, S1)	SURAL: LATERAL ANKLE (S1)
POSTERIOR TIBIAL: ABDUCTOR HALLUCIS (S1, S2)	Super peroneal sensory: ankle dorsum (L5)
Peroneal: tibialis anterior (L4, L5)	*Saphenous: medial ankle (L4)
Posterior tibial: abductor digiti quinti pedis (S1, S2)	*Lateral cutaneous nerve of thigh: lateral thigh (L4)
Femoral: quadriceps (L2–L4)	

This table lists most nerve conduction studies performed. On each line, the nerve is listed first, followed by the recording point and then, in parentheses, the root innervation (motor) or derivation (sensory). The "basic" studies for each extremity are listed first in capital letters; the "uncommon" studies are listed below them, in lower case.

* Studies technically difficult to perform.

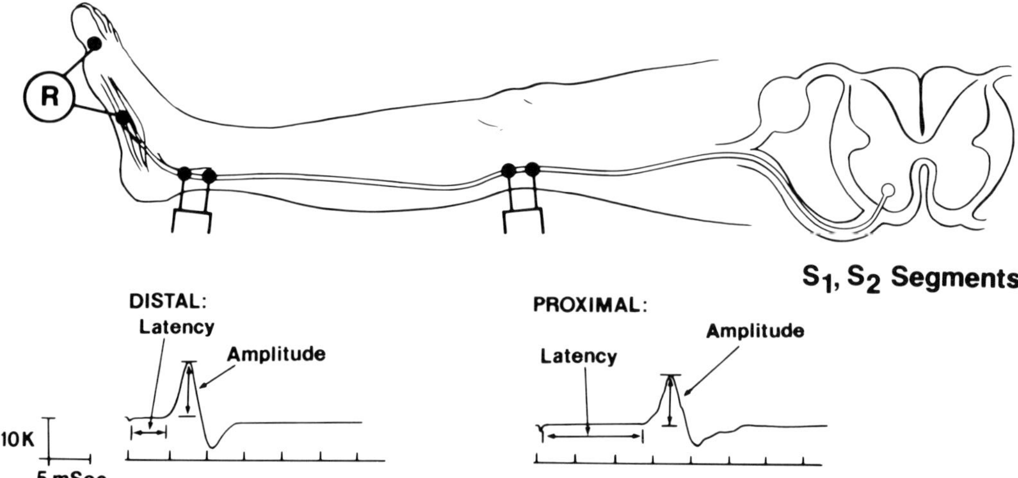

Figure 7–1. Tibial motor nerve conduction study. The distal amplitude and distal latency are reported, along with ankle-to-knee conduction velocity (obtained by substracting the distal latency from the proximal latency and dividing the result into the distance between the two stimulation points).

and by those causing axon loss. Demyelinating conduction block lesions alter the recorded amplitudes only when they are situated between the stimulation and recording points; those located proximal to the most proximal stimulation point (e.g., at the root level) cannot be detected on the NCS. Axon loss lesions, in contrast to demyelinating conduction block lesions, can affect the NCS amplitudes if they are sited anywhere along the peripheral neuraxis, from the cell bodies of origin of the peripheral nerve fibers distally. However, the degree of amplitude diminution seen is extremely variable, depending on the number of individual large nerve fibers that degenerate; it can range from none to very severe, i.e., an unelicitable response. In general, at least a moderate number of sensory axons must be affected before the SNAP amplitudes enter the abnormally low range, and even more motor axons must be lost before the CMAP amplitudes become definitely abnormal.[6, 18]

The cell bodies for the motor axons are situated within the anterior horns of the spinal cord. The sensory cell bodies, however, are within the dorsal root ganglia (DRG), which lie quite distally along the sensory (dorsal) roots, very near where the latter join with the ventral roots to form the mixed spinal nerves, at or within the intervertebral foramina (Fig. 7–3*A*).[17] Although this anatomic arrangement has relatively little clinical significance, it plays a major role in EMG localization because it permits the electromyographer to localize severe, proximal axon loss lesions to either the spinal cord and roots ("preganglionic") or to

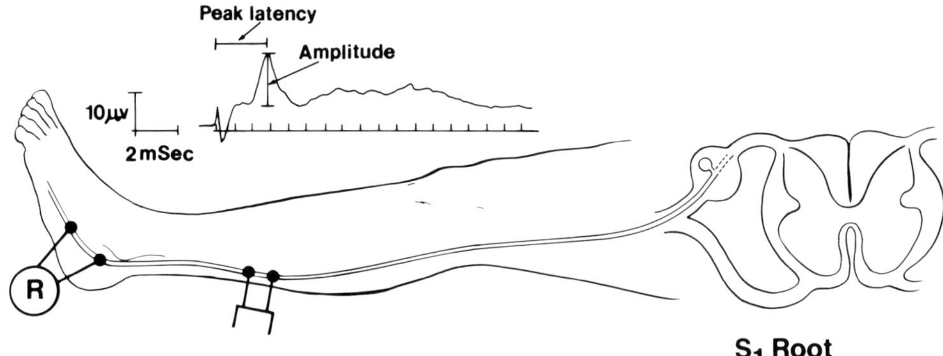

Figure 7–2. Sural (sensory) nerve conduction study. Generally, the nerve is stimulated at only one point for sensory conduction studies and the latency is measured to the peak of the response ("peak latency") rather than to the onset, as is done for motor conduction studies.

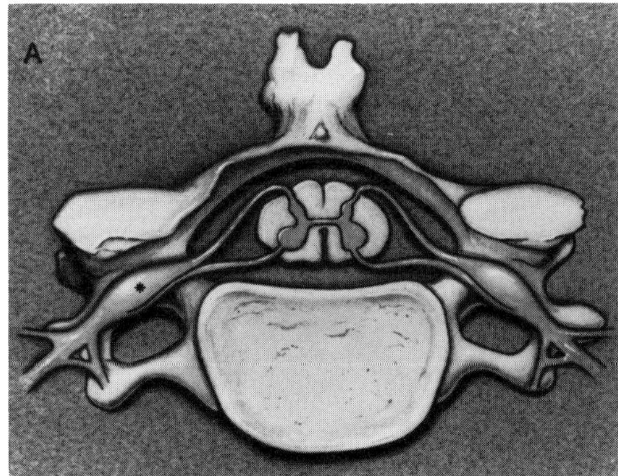

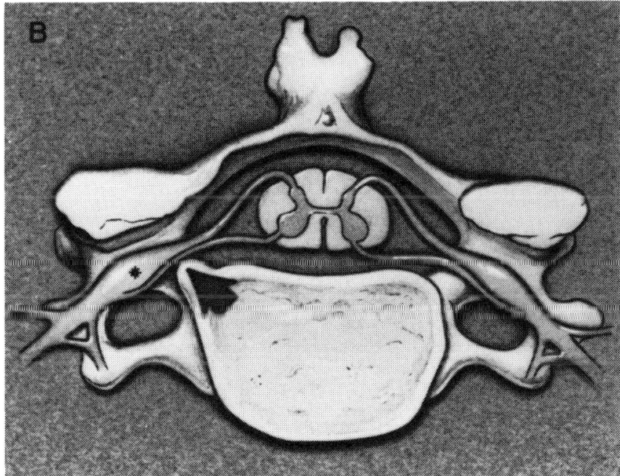

Figure 7–3. *A,* Cross section of the spinal cord, spinal roots, and surrounding structures, showing the location of the dorsal root ganglion (asterisk). *B,* Same as *A,* except the typical site of root compression with disc protrusion is shown; note that the sensory root is compromised proximal to the dorsal root ganglion (asterisk).

the plexuses or more distally ("postganglionic") (Fig. 7–3*B*). Since axon loss lesions within the intraspinal canal, e.g., myelopathies and radiculopathies, compromise the sensory root fibers *proximal* to their cell bodies in the DRG, instead of at or distal to them, they do not affect the sensory NCS amplitudes. The sensory fiber degeneration that results progresses centrally, rather than peripherally, leaving the peripheral sensory fibers intact; this occurs regardless of lesion severity and regardless of the degree of clinical sensory loss found in the appropriate dermatomal distribution. In contrast, axon loss lesions located within the plexuses or more peripherally cause sensory fibers to degenerate from that point distally, resulting in low amplitude or unelicitable SNAPs.[1, 2, 5, 6] A noteworthy anatomic point is that the sensory fibers composing the cauda equina are "preganglionic"; they are the central projections of DRG located at or within the foramina (Fig. 7–4).

Both the latencies (distal and peak) and the CVs are rate measurements. The distal/peak latencies report only the time required for impulse transmission between the (distal) stimulation site and the recording site. Therefore, they are affected almost solely by lesions causing demyelinating focal slowing (or, much less commonly, axon narrowing), situated between those two points.[6, 18] For practical purposes, the only focal neurogenic lesion encountered with any frequency that produces abnormally prolonged distal/peak latencies is carpal tunnel syndrome. The CV, unlike the distal/peak latency measurements, links the distance traversed by a nerve impulse to the time required for its transmission. CVs are calculated along a segment of nerve between two stimulation points. First, the distal latency is subtracted from the proximal latency, to obtain the time of impulse transmission, in milliseconds, between the two stimulation points. This differ-

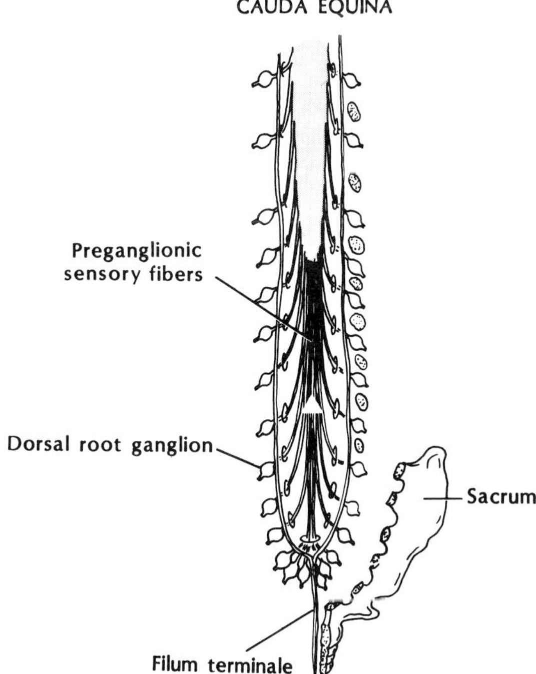

Figure 7–4. Diagrammatic coronal view of the lower spinal cord, cauda equina, and surrounding structures. Note that the sensory fibers composing the cauda equina are "preganglionic," since the dorsal root ganglia are at the foramina. Hence, an axon loss lesion of the cauda equina (shown as △) has no effect on the lower extremity sensory responses, regardless of severity.

ence is then divided into the distance (in centimeters) between those two points, as determined by surface measurements, yielding a CV, which is the speed of transmission over the fastest conducting motor fibers, reported in meters per second (m/sec). Expressing conduction rates in this manner allows those determined along nerves of markedly dissimilar length, e.g., forearm segments of the median nerve of a child and that of a professional basketball player, to be directly compared with one another. The CV, similar to the distal/peak latencies, is altered primarily by demyelinating focal slowing lesions occurring along the nerve between the two stimulation points.[1, 6, 18] For practical purposes, the only focal neurogenic lesions diagnosed with any frequency by the motor CV are some ulnar neuropathies at the elbow. (Many lesions along that segment, it should be noted, produce solely axon loss, or demyelinating conduction block, without accompanying slowing.)

Unlike the NCS amplitudes, neither the latencies nor the CVs reflect the number of axons conducting impulses, except that at least a few have to be conducting (i.e., the amplitudes cannot be zero) for them to be determined. The marked insensitivity of these NCS parameters toward detection of axon degeneration makes them of very limited value in the assessment of most focal peripheral nerve lesions, with the exceptions already noted. They rarely are affected by any acute nerve lesion, particularly one that produces clinical weakness, since the latter implies that significant axon loss or demyelinating conduction block is present, and not just some conduction slowing.[11]

LATE RESPONSES (H RESPONSES, F WAVES)

The H response is a monosynaptic reflex first described in 1918 by Hoffmann.[17] In normal adults, H responses can be obtained consistently only by stimulating the tibial nerve in the popliteal fossa, while recording from the gastrocnemius-soleus muscle group (Fig. 7–5). Thus, in regard to root assessment, only the motor and sensory fibers of the S1 root are evaluated by the H-response study.[3, 12, 15] This is a major limitation, as is the fact that H responses (1) frequently are absent bilaterally in patients over the age of 60 years, in patients

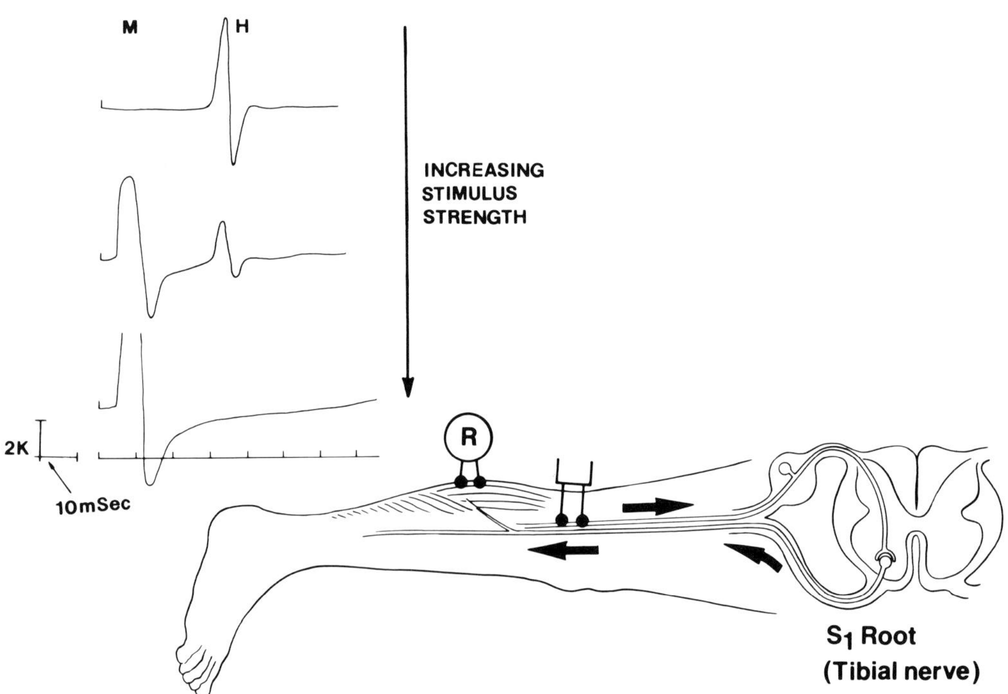

Figure 7–5. The H reflex. Note that the H response is obtained with submaximal stimulation and disappears as the stimulus strength increases; in contrast, the direct (M) response is maximal with supramaximal stimulation.

with polyneuropathies, and in those who have had lumbar laminectomies; (2) if abnormal, do not localize to the S1 root, since the fibers could be involved at other areas along their pathway (e.g., S1 cord segment, sacral plexus, sciatic nerve, proximal tibial nerve); (3) once abnormal, often remain so indefinitely.[15, 18] In spite of these limiting and confusing factors, the H response is very helpful for assessing a lower extremity, particularly when a lumbosacral radiculopathy is questioned. In part because it permits assessment of the "preganglionic" component of the S1 sensory root fibers, the H response is seldom normal with an S1 root lesion; much more often, it is of low amplitude or unelicitable. The H response has a high correlation with the Achilles tendon reflex.[15, 17]

F waves were first described by Magladery and McDougall in 1950.[17] Like H responses, they are late responses. F waves result when, owing to motor nerve stimulation, some of the impulses passing antidromically up the motor axon cause some of the motor neurons in the anterior horn to fire; the nerve impulses that travel back down the motor axons produce submaximal muscle activation, which is recorded, several milliseconds after the direct (M) wave, as F waves. Hence, F waves result from recurrent discharge after antidromic stimulation of a spinal motor neuron. Unlike H responses, F waves are not reflexes, since they traverse motor fibers exclusively; moreover, they can be elicited during any of the standard motor NCS. Unfortunately, F waves have proved a great disappointment to many electromyographers, in spite of the initial enthusiastic claims made for them. Regarding root lesions, unless there is exceptionally severe involvement of the motor fibers, normal F waves generally can still be elicited, partly because they travel over any intact fibers that are still functioning.[17]

NEEDLE ELECTRODE EXAMINATION (NEE)

The NEE is the oldest portion of the EMG examination. Unlike the NCS, it assesses only motor fibers, not sensory; also, for the most part it detects only axon loss, rather than focal demyelination. Nonetheless, it is a formidable component of the EMG examination because it is more sensitive than the NCS and late responses to motor axon loss, and it permits far more motor nerve fibers to be evaluated than do the NCS.[16] During the NEE a recording needle electrode is inserted into various muscles, and the electrical activity being generated in them, either spontaneously or volitionally, is assessed, both visually (via an oscilloscope screen) and aurally (via a loudspeaker). In contrast to the NCS, nerve stimulation is not performed during the NEE.[1, 17]

The NEE of each muscle can be divided into several phases, during each of which specific data are sought, including information about the integrity of the motor neuron (cell body and axon) supplying the muscle being evaluated.

During the "insertion" phase, the electrical activity resulting from needle movement is assessed. Normally, each such insertion injures a few muscle fibers, which generate a small burst of electrical activity called "insertional activity." Sometimes abnormal insertional activity is seen, such as "insertional positive sharp waves," which can be found in denervated muscle a few days before spontaneous fibrillation potentials appear.

During the "at rest" phase, electrical silence ordinarily prevails. However, with many disorders of the neuromuscular system, various types of "spontaneous activity" appear. Only two of these are germane to this discussion: fibrillation potentials and fasciculation potentials.

Fibrillation potentials are spontaneous, usually regularly firing, action potentials of individual muscle fibers. Fibrillation potentials have two different forms, depending on whether the tip of the recording needle is merely near the fibrillating muscle fiber, yielding the "biphasic spike" form of fibrillation potential (the "fibrillation potential" of older terminology), or whether it has actually injured it, producing the "positive sharp wave" form of fibrillation potential. Fibrillation potentials are somewhat nonspecific in that they can be seen with both myopathic and neuropathic processes. When caused by the latter, they are not seen at the onset of motor axon loss. Instead, their appearance is delayed anywhere from 14 to 35 days (stated average time: 21 days). Once established, they persist until the denervated muscle fibers generating them either (1) reinnervate or (2) degenerate for lack of a nerve supply; this usually occurs 1½ to 2 years after denervation. Fibrillation potentials are the primary means the electromyographer has of detecting motor axon loss. They are also very sensitive indicators of this process, since the loss of a single motor axon can result in up to hundreds of individual muscle fibers fibrillating within a given muscle, depending on the innervation ratio (the number of muscle fibers innervated by a motor axon). Thus, fibrillation potentials found on NEE can demonstrate motor axon loss that is far too minimal to have produced either clinical muscle weakness or muscle atrophy.[1, 15, 17]

Fasciculation potentials are spontaneous action potentials of entire motor units. They are indicative of motor unit "irritation," rather than denervation, because only intact motor units can generate them. Fasciculation potentials play a very small role in electrodiagnosis compared with fibrillation potentials. They are encountered far less often, being restricted essentially to certain anterior horn cell disorders, a few chronic entrapment mononeuropathies, some peripheral polyneuropathies, and (most often) the syndrome of "generalized benign fasciculations." They are found in a myotomal distribution so infrequently with radiculopathies that they are of no material value in the diagnosis of the latter.[1, 17]

During the "MUP activation" phase of the NEE, the muscle being assessed is voluntarily activated by the patient, and motor unit potentials (MUPs) are generated. A MUP is the summated electrical activity caused by the near-synchronous activation of the muscle fibers in a muscle that are controlled by a single anterior horn cell. MUPs are evaluated in regard to their firing characteristics and configuration.[1, 15, 17]

A "neurogenic MUP firing pattern" is seen whenever a substantial number of motor units in the muscle cannot be activated on maximal effort, because of either conduction block or axon loss. The MUPs that can fire are noted to do so in decreased numbers at a moderately rapid to rapid rate; the fewer the number of MUPs, the weaker the muscle is clinically. The rapid rate of firing of the still-functioning MUPs is important because, like fibrillation potentials, it is unequivocal evidence of a lower motor neuron lesion. Conversely, if the muscle were weak because of a upper motor neuron lesion, or incomplete voluntary effort (hysteria, malingering, pain on activation), the MUPs would fire in equally decreased numbers, but at a slow to moderate rate. A neurogenic MUP firing pattern, unlike all the other NEE changes seen with neuropathic lesions, is present from the onset of the lesion. However, it can be recognized only when conduction is blocked or lost along a substantial number of the motor axons innervating the muscle being examined. For this reason, it is of relatively little value with single radiculopathies, in which only a minority of the motor fibers are involved as a rule.[17]

A "chronic neurogenic MUP change" is an alteration in the external configuration of the MUP. The MUP increases in duration, and with some proximal chronic lesions (e.g., remote poliomyelitis, cervical spondylosis) increases in amplitude as well (generally, MUPs more than 5 mV in amplitude are considered abnormal). Chronic neurogenic MUP changes develop several months (a minimum of four to six months, hence their title "chronic") after a rather substantial axon loss lesion. Usually they are due to many of the denervated muscle fibers in the muscle being adopted, via collateral sprouting, by the surviving motor axons supplying it. Each functioning motor axon thus controls a significantly greater number of muscle fibers in the muscle than normal. Consequently when activated, it generates a larger MUP. Chronic neurogenic MUP changes, once developed, can persist indefinitely. With many remote, proximal neurogenic lesions, such as radiculopathies and particularly poliomyelitis, they are the sole electrical residual found in the entire EMG examination.[15, 17]

"Polyphasic" MUPs

Sometimes the internal configuration of MUPs is altered, so that they have five or more phases instead of the normal four or less. The MUPs with this configuration change are called "polyphasic"; they can be seen in several different circumstances, only some of which are abnormal. Three of these are pertinent in regard to neurogenic lesions. First, up to 10 per cent of the MUPs in any normal muscle may be polyphasic. Second, chronic neurogenic MUPs are almost always polyphasic in appearance; i.e., their internal as well as their external configuration is changed. Third, when reinnervation is in progress, either because of collateral sprouting or proximodistal regeneration of the axon, highly polyphasic MUPs characteristically are observed. Initially they are low in amplitude and markedly increased in duration as well, primarily because of abnormally slow conduction along the terminal fibers of recently regenerated axons.[1, 15, 17] Some electromyographers attempt to diagnose motor nerve fiber lesions, particularly radiculopathies, by finding an excess of polyphasic MUPs alone in a myotome distribution, without associated fibrillation potentials and without other MUP changes.[7, 8, 14] They believe that, for various reasons, all speculative, these MUP changes can be seen from the moment of injury. This practice, unfortunately, frequently results in false-positive EMG studies, because determining that an excess number (more than 10 per cent) of polyphasic MUPs is present in a muscle is a highly subjective task, and one easily influenced by examiner bias. Consequently, all too often the EMG diagnosis parrots the clinical impression, even when the latter ultimately proves to be erroneous. For this reason, many (probably most) electromyographers require more definite NEE abnormalities to be present for diagnosis.[1, 9, 17]

VALUE OF EMG IN DIAGNOSING RADICULOPATHIES

Widely divergent opinions are held by clinicians regarding the usefulness of the EMG examination in assessing patients with intraspinal canal lesions, especially radiculopathies. At one pole are those who consider that it rarely, if ever, is of appreciable value; at the other extreme are those who proclaim it to be a highly sensitive, almost indispensable, procedure. As is often the case in these situations, the actual value of the study appears to lie somewhere in between these markedly disparate views. In deference to its critics, I believe certain of its limitations should be conceded. First, the value of EMG in assessing radiculopathies has declined over the past two decades, relative to neuroimaging studies; it no longer is justified to consider EMG as sensitive as radiography (specifically, myelography) for detecting root lesions, as was reported by several investigators 20 to 30 years ago.[15] The reason is simple. Radiologists have added a number of procedures to their armamentarium—water-soluble dyes, computed tomography (CT), magnetic resonance imaging (MRI)—but electromyographers have continued to employ as their prime diagnostic procedure the NEE, which, although used to diagnose radiculopathies for over 40 years, has definite disadvantages. Second, EMG in many respects is ill suited for assessing lesions within the intraspinal canal, particularly those that are limited in their distribution and severity, such as, typically, most single compressive radiculopathies. These are discussed below. Third, some claims regarding the overall value of EMG in diagnosing radiculopathies are exaggerated. Realistically, the EMG study probably is definitely abnormal in only about half the patients with radiculopathies. However, it often is not appreciated that the value of EMG in assessing possible radiculopathies is highly variable, depending on a number of factors. In many patients it is of little benefit, as its critics contend; in many others it is very helpful, as its proponents claim. The two determining factors in this regard, which allow its value to be predicted with reasonable accuracy for any particular patient, are (1) the presence or absence of motor, as well as sensory, symptoms; and (2) the duration of the symptoms. As a general rule, EMG is most likely to be of benefit in diagnosing single radiculopathies when clinical weakness is present and when the lesion is of relatively recent onset. In such patients, motor axon loss is likely to have occurred and electrical evidence of it is still likely to be present; consequently the diagnostic yield is very respectable, approaching approximately 90 per cent. Conversely, EMG is least likely to provide helpful information in patients with chronic, static radiculopathies, who have pain as their sole symptom and normal results on neurologic examination. In these patients, motor axon loss may not have occurred and, even if it has, all traces of it are likely to have disappeared. As a result, the EMG diagnostic yield is low, probably less than 20 per cent, and even when some abnormalities are present they frequently are not diagnostic. Consequently, physicians who send only the latter type of patient to the EMG laboratory for evaluation are very likely to find the procedure unhelpful, just as they would conclude that lumbar laminectomies are of limited value if they referred for surgery only those patients who had already undergone several failed back operations.

EMG Examination With Single Radiculopathies

For a variety of reasons (Table 7–3) the motor NCS with single radiculopathies typically are normal. Only occasionally is motor root compromise exceptionally severe, causing so much axon loss that the CMAP recorded from one of the muscles supplied by that root becomes abnormally low. The sensory NCS are almost always normal with radiculopathies, because the sensory root compression is occurring proximal to the DRG. The H responses are abnormal with most S1 radiculopathies but unaffected by all other root lesions. The F waves, as noted, are seldom helpful with compressive radiculopathies.

Since the NCS and the late responses generally are normal with isolated radiculopathies (except the H response with S1 lesions), the NEE becomes the sole portion of the EMG examination of benefit in detecting these disorders. The EMG diagnosis therefore depends on finding abnormalities in a root, or myotome, distribution on NEE. A myotome is composed of all the muscles that receive innervation from a single spinal cord segment or root. Contiguous myotomes (e.g., L5 and S1) overlap to varying degrees; consequently, since almost all muscles receive innervation from more than one root, all are in more than one myotome.[15, 17]

Unfortunately, many unavoidable limitations, anatomic and pathophysiologic, are encountered when only the NEE can be used to detect focal neurogenic lesions, especially when those lesions are situated very proximally. These limiting circumstances ensure that false-negative results occur, regardless of the skill of the electromyographer and the extensiveness of the examination. First, the root compression may be causing focal demyelination, rather than axon loss, along the motor fibers at the lesion site. The NEE in such patients typically is normal or, at most, nondiagnostic; a prominent conduction block may cause a neurogenic MUP firing pattern to be seen in one or two of the muscles, which will be clinically weak as well, but these electrical changes are rarely found in sufficient muscles of the myotome for definite diagnosis. Second, the root compression may be causing axon loss, but only along the sensory root fibers, not the motor. Obviously, in such patients the NEE, and thus the EMG examination, will be completely normal (unless the S1 sensory root is affected, which could produce an abnormal H response). Of particular note is that sensory NCS performed on fibers of the affected dermatome are unrevealing, because the lesion characteristically is proximal to the DRG. This probably explains why some patients with radiculopathies of recent onset, particularly those manifested solely as pain, have completely normal EMG results.

Table 7–3. REASONS WHY MOTOR AND SENSORY NCS RESPONSES ARE NOT AFFECTED BY THE TYPICAL SINGLE COMPRESSIVE RADICULOPATHY

Motor NCS

Recorded muscle not innervated by involved root

Recorded muscle innervated by involved root:

1. but pathophysiology is focal demyelination.
2. and pathophysiology is axon loss but:
   a. only minority of motor fibers degenerate
   b. recorded muscle also innervated by another, uninvolved root (law of multisegmental innervation)

Sensory NCS

Lesion proximal to dorsal root ganglion (i.e., "preganglionic"); peripheral sensory fibers do not degenerate if pathophysiology is axon loss

It is obvious from the above that, if root compression is to alter the NEE materially, at least some motor fibers must be killed and undergo degeneration, thereby producing evidence of denervation—fibrillation potentials and/or chronic neurogenic MUP changes (depending on the activity and duration of the lesion)—in a myotomal distribution. To determine whether this is occurring, a number of muscles must be assessed. Theoretically, abnormalities should be found in the distribution of both the posterior primary ramus (paraspinal muscles) and the anterior primary ramus (various limb muscles) of the affected root. Regarding the latter, the changes should be found in at least two (preferably more) limb muscles innervated by the same root but by different peripheral nerves. Also, muscles not innervated by the affected root but by roots contiguous to it should be normal.[15, 17] Thus, with a C7 cervical radiculopathy, fibrillation potentials could be found in various C7-innervated limb muscles, such as the triceps and anconeus (radial innervated) and the pronator teres and flexor carpi radialis (median innervated), but not in muscles of the same limb that do not receive innervation from the C7 root, such as those innervated by the C6 root (biceps, brachioradialis, deltoideus) or the C8 root (extensor indicis proprius, first dorsal interosseus, flexor pollicis longus); fibrillation potentials could also be seen in the low cervical paraspinal muscles. Similarly, with a lumbosacral radiculopathy affecting the L5 root, fibrillation potentials could be found in several peroneal-innervated muscles (tibialis anterior, extensor hallucis, extensor digitorum brevis), some tibial-innervated muscles (tibialis posterior, flexor digitorum longus), and various proximal L5-innervated muscles (semitendinosus, gluteus medius, tensor fasciae latae), as well as the low lumbar–high sacral paraspinal muscles, but not in muscles innervated by the L2–L4 roots (vastus lateralis, adductor magnus) or the S1–S2 roots (medial gastrocnemius, abductor hallucis, short head of biceps femoris).

Unfortunately, the "classic" EMG presentation of a single radiculopathy, with fibrillation potentials found throughout the myotome, is encountered with about the same frequency as are "classic" clinical presentations of various disorders: far less often than one would wish. This is because the NEE findings are adversely influenced by a number of factors, such as regional anatomy, the severity of motor axon loss at the root level, and the timing of the EMG study in relationship to the onset of the lesion. These additional limiting factors will now be briefly discussed. First, the myotome may be composed of relatively few muscles, too few for adequate NEE assessment. With suspected thoracic radiculopathies, for example, only the paraspinal and abdominal muscles are evaluated routinely (most electromyographers avoid examining the intercostal muscles for fear of inadvertently entering the pleural space). Similarly, with possible upper lumbar (L2, L3) radiculopathies, only the paraspinal muscles, iliacus, quadriceps, and thigh adductors could show abnormalities, at most. Second, in many instances of root compression, a relatively small number of motor fibers undergo axon loss. As a result, NEE abnormalities may be restricted to only one or a few muscles innervated by the affected root, rather than appearing throughout the myotome. This can prove very misleading, even though the EMG results are abnormal. To use an L2, L3 radiculopathy as an example: the abnormalities may be limited to the limb muscles, the paraspinal muscles being normal, and thus the findings would be identical to those seen with a lumbar plexopathy. Alternatively, the changes may be restricted to a few muscles that share peripheral nerve as well as root innervation, such as the vastus lateralis and rectus femoris, rendering the findings identical to those seen with a femoral neuropathy. Third, the need for fibrillation potentials to be found in a myotomal distribution in order to diagnose a radiculopathy places significant time limitations on the study. There is a time frame, of relatively limited duration, during which the EMG examination is likely to be revealing. Results from studies performed before or after that period are often false-negative.[15,17]

The initial false-negative period encompasses the first two to three weeks after the onset of motor root axon loss, during which time fibrillation potentials will not have appeared in the partially denervated muscles, or will have developed in only some of them (beginning proximally and extending progressively more distal in the limb).[1,17] As a result, results of NEEs performed earlier than three or more weeks following the onset of a radiculopathy are very likely to be false-negative or indeterminant, even if subsequently they would be positive for a root lesion. This is a major limitation. In our impatient society, both the patient and the referring physician chafe at having to wait at least three weeks after onset of symptoms before a diagnostic study can be performed. However, this physiologic limitation cannot be circumvented, and physicians who consistently obtain EMG examinations with suspected radiculopathies earlier than three weeks after onset often obtain unreliable results of no benefit.[15,17]

The second false-negative period begins several months after the onset of a static radiculopathy and is due to the NEE abnormalities (if present) having gradually resolved, owing to progressive muscle reinnervation. The myotomal muscles with most single radiculopathies are only partially denervated at most, because each muscle is receiving innervation from a contiguous, nonaffected root, and because only some of the fibers supplying it from the affected root have degenerated. Consequently, collateral sprouting occurs from the intact motor nerve fibers supplying the muscle. As the denervated muscle fibers are reinnervated by these collateral sprouts, they cease to fibrillate. Collateral sprouting is more efficient proximally, since all the components of the sprouts must be produced within the anterior horn cell and transported distally. Thus, after the onset of a root lesion, unless progressively more motor root fibers are compressed and degenerate, any myotomal fibrillation potentials present tend to disappear from the myotome as time passes. This typically occurs in a centrifugal fashion: initially from the paraspinal muscles, then from the proximal limb muscles, and finally from the distal limb muscles. As a result, several months after the onset of static root compression, fibrillation potentials may be found on NEE in only a few of the more distal limb muscles innervated by that root, if at all, even when the root compression persists (Fig. 7–6). This is why NEEs with chronic cervical radiculopathies of more than six months' duration, and lumbosacral radiculopathies that have lasted more than 12 to 18 months, are often unrevealing. It is noteworthy that this process is not contingent upon relieving the pressure on the root fibers. Consequently, any sensory symptoms caused by comcomitant sensory root compression can continued unabated as the NEE is "normalizing with time."[15, 17]

For all the above reasons, when the "classic" EMG presentation of a radiculopathy is encountered, with fibrillation potentials found in most or all of the muscles composing the myotome, the root lesions usually are of relatively recent onset (three weeks to three months in duration), and motor root axon loss typically has been substantial. When other circumstances prevail, fibrillation potentials usually are found in only some, if any, of the muscles of the myotome; typically, these are the more distal muscles. As a corollary of this, the concept that the EMG diagnosis of a radiculopathy requires that fibrillation potentials be found throughout the myotome, or in any particular myotomal muscle, including the paraspinals, is untenable. With radiculopathies, fibrillation potentials generally are important only if they are present; their absence in any muscle does not exclude the existence of a neurogenic lesion.

Some limited information regarding the duration of the lesion can be ascertained from the NEE findings. When fibrillation potentials are seen in both the proximal and distal muscles of a myotome, unaccompanied by chronic neurogenic MUP changes, an acute radiculopathy is probably present. In contrast, when only chronic neurogenic MUP changes are noted, often limited to some of the more distal

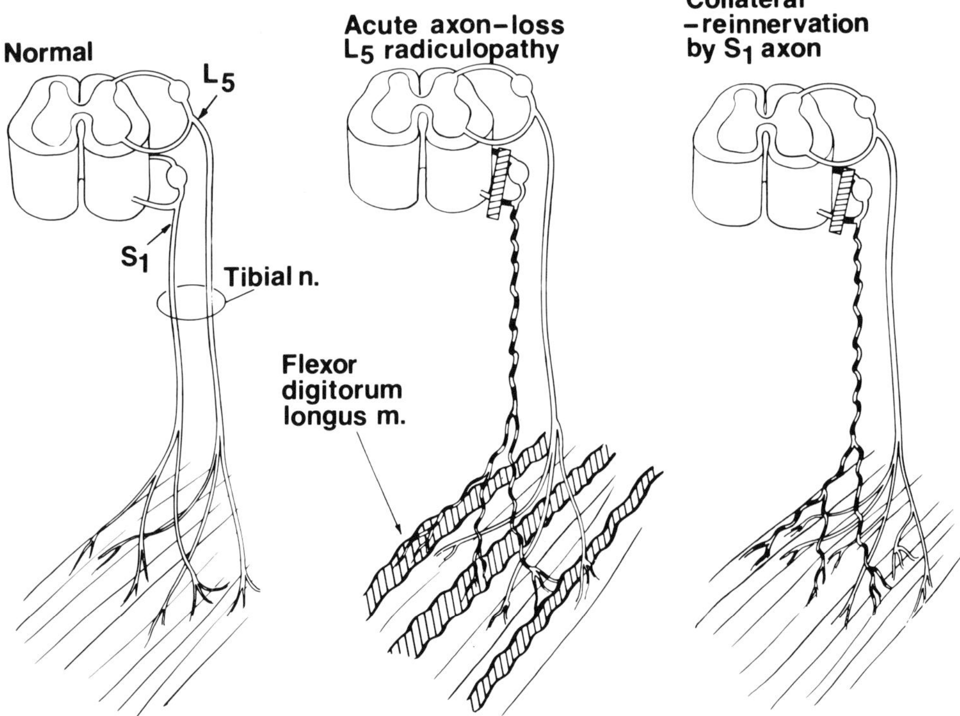

Figure 7–6. This shows how the needle electrode examination abnormalities with a static radiculopathy can resolve with the passage of time, even when the root compression persists: the muscle fibers initially denervated by the root lesion are reinnervated, via collateral sprouting, by other motor axons supplying the muscle.

muscles, the radiculopathy is likely to be both static in nature and remote in time. Finally, when both fibrillation potentials and chronic neurogenic MUP changes are found in a myotome distribution, either a chronic progressive radiculopathy is present or an acute radiculopathy has been superimposed on a chronic one.[17]

Two other disadvantages of EMG in the diagnosis of radiculopathies must be mentioned; both concern a positive study (e.g., NEE abnormalities in a root distribution). First, the etiology of the changes cannot be determined, since root compromise due to any number of causes—e.g., disc bulging, disc herniation, neoplasm encroachment, arachnoiditis, ischemic infarction—produces essentially the same EMG presentation, varying only in severity. Second, a positive EMG study pinpoints the root involved, rather than the site (i.e., the disc space) where it is involved. This limitation has far more significance in the lumbosacral region than in the cervical one. A disc herniation at the L4 level, for example, can affect the L4, L5, or S1 roots, depending on its direction and extent.[15, 17]

Despite all the limitations listed above, the EMG can play a useful role in assessing patients with suspected radiculopathy, for several reasons. First, although false-negative results are inherent in the procedure and unavoidable, false-positive results are rare when experienced electromyographers perform the studies, since most are due to examiner error or misinterpretation and thus avoidable. Consequently, the EMG examination seldom introduces misleading elements in the assessment of these patients. Second, as already noted, EMG can demonstrate findings consistent with a radiculopathy when the clinical examination is normal, unsatisfactory, or confusing for various reasons. Third, EMG is the only laboratory procedure available that directly assesses the root's physiologic integrity; hence, in contrast to the various neuroimaging techniques, it can reveal evidence of root dysfunction from causes other than compression, e.g., nerve fiber infarction, which often is responsible for lumbosacral root syndromes in patients with diabetes mellitus. Consequently, it can show abnormalities when every other diagnostic procedure is unrevealing. Also, incidental imaging abnormalities are common, especially in elderly patients, and EMG can often demonstrate which changes have clinical significance. Finally, EMG can be very helpful in distinguishing radiculopathies from other neurogenic lesions with which they can be confused clinically, and vice versa (Table 7–4).[15, 17] The results of a study reported several years ago are pertinent in this regard. Among 309 patients referred to the EMG laboratory over a six-month period for lumbosacral radiculopathy, 44 per cent were found to have definite or equivocal changes consistent with that diagnosis, while in 11 per cent the symptoms were found to have some other definite cause. These other entities ranged from upper motor neuron lesions (causing footdrop mistakenly attributed to L5 radiculopathies) to generalized myopathies (causing anterior thigh weakness erroneously thought to be due to bilateral L2–L4 radiculopathies).[15] The fact that the EMG examination so often can readily differentiate radiculopathies from other lesions with which they can be clinically confused, such as motor neuron disease, peripheral polyneuropathy, and various plexus and peripheral nerve lesions, is one of its most important attributes; by doing so, it can both prevent unnecessary laminectomies and identify patients who may benefit from surgery. Some examples of the former: (1) a patient with shoulder pain and shoulder girdle weakness, scheduled for a cervical laminectomy to relieve presumed severe C6 root compression, is shown to have neuralgic amyotrophy on EMG; (2) a patient with prominent thumb and index finger pain and paresthesias, clinically considered to have a C7 radiculopathy, has severe carpal tunnel syndrome on EMG; (3) in a patient with foot pain, foot weakness, and absent ankle jerk, scheduled for S1 root decompression, EMG reveals a tibial nerve lesion in or near the popliteal fossa (most likely a tumor); (4) a patient with back pain and bilateral foot numbness, thought to have bilateral S1 root involvement, has a severe peripheral polyneuropathy demonstrated on EMG. Even seasoned clinicians can benefit from EMG, since diagnostic errors are inevitable otherwise, at least occasionally. This statement in no way impugns the skills of the clinician, because the clinical neurologic examination, for all its good points, is an imperfect diagnostic procedure. Every ancillary neurodiagnostic technique, including EMG, was developed because of the inability of the clinical neurologic examination alone to provide all the information necessary for correct diagnosis and localization.[15]

Table 7–4. ENTITIES COMMONLY CONFUSED WITH COMPRESSIVE RADICULOPATHIES (AND VICE VERSA)

Roots	Process
Cervical	
C5, C6	Upper trunk brachial plexopathy
	Acute brachial neuropathy (neuralgic amyotrophy)
	Rotator cuff tear
	Various mononeuropathies: axillary, musculocutaneous, spinal accessory
	Motor neuron disease
	Myopathy
C6, C7	Carpal tunnel syndrome
C8, T1	Lower trunk brachial plexopathy
	Ulnar neuropathy
	Motor neuron disease
Thoracic	
T6–L2	Diabetic thoracic radiculopathy (diabetic polyradiculopathy)
Lumbosacral	
L2–L4	Diabetic amyotrophy (diabetic polyradiculopathy)
	Lumbar plexopathy
	Femoral neuropathy
	Myopathy
L5	Diabetic polyradiculopathy
	Sacral plexopathy
	Sciatic neuropathy
	Peroneal neuropathy
	Motor neuron disease
S1, S2	Sacral plexopathy
	Sciatic neuropathy
	Tibial neuropathy
	Plantar neuropathy
Bilateral (L5)	Polyneuropathy
S1, S2	

EMG With Multiple Radiculopathies

A major difference between single and multiple radiculopathies, from the EMG point of view, is that with the latter the NEE is no longer almost the sole diagnostic procedure of value; the NCS becomes informative in a positive way. This is because contiguous roots are involved with most multiple radiculopathies, and the amount of axon loss affecting each root is substantial. Consequently, the CMAPs recorded on motor NCS from muscles innervated by the involved roots frequently are abnormally low in amplitude, while the sensory NCS assessing the same roots remain normal, since the lesions are proximal to the DRG. The combination of low-amplitude or unelicitable motor CMAPs associated with normal-amplitude SNAPs is almost pathognomonic of an intraspinal canal lesion.

Cervical Root Avulsions. These lesions differ from the typical single compressive radiculopathy mainly in the degree of axon loss present. Because the entire motor supply from one or both cervical roots innervating a particular muscle has been disrupted, that muscle is severely or totally denervated. Hence, if it is used as a recorded muscle during motor NCS, the CMAP is of very low amplitude or unelicitable. Similarly, during NEE, fibrillation potentials are abundant while voluntary MUPs are sparse or absent. In contrast, the sensory NCS responses derived from the same roots are unaffected, because the sensory roots are avulsed proximal to the DRG. Thus, with C8 and T1 root avulsions, the median and ulnar CMAPs, recording hand muscles, are very abnormal, while the ulnar and medial antebrachial cutaneous SNAPs are normal. (The median SNAP, recording index finger, is also normal, but this is inconsequential since the fibers it assesses are derived from the C6 and/or C7 DRG). A similar dissociation of motor and sensory NCS responses is seen with C5–C6 root avulsions, although, because these roots are not assessed adequately by the "routine" upper extremity NCS, "uncommon" NCS must be performed, e.g., musculocutaneous motor, recording biceps; axillary motor, recording deltoid; median sensory, recording thumb; lateral antebrachial cutaneous, recording forearm (Table 7–2).

Total avulsion lesions of an upper extremity, involving roots C5 to T1, yield a characteristic EMG presentation: all the motor NCS responses, routine and "uncommon," are unelicitable, whereas all the sensory NCS responses are completely normal. Abundant fibrillation potentials and total loss of voluntary MUPs is found throughout the limb, and fibrillation potentials are usually prominent in the midcervical to upper thoracic paraspinal muscles also. The fact that the various SNAPs are normal virtually excludes the possibility of the lesion affecting the brachial plexus, rather than the roots. Conversely, the EMG localization becomes much less precise if the sensory, as well as the motor, NCS responses are unelicitable. The fact that the SNAPs are abnormal indicates involvement of the sensory fibers at or distal to the DRG, presumably at the plexus level, but does not exclude concomitant root avulsion; abundant paraspinal fibrillation potentials would suggest the latter.

Cauda Equina Lesions. Multiple lumbosacral radiculopathies are encountered rather frequently in the EMG laboratory; typically the involvement is bilateral but it often is asymmetric. Most cauda equina lesions are attributable to midline lumbar disc protrusion or lumbar canal stenosis. The S1 and S2 roots, being the more medial of the roots supplying the lower extremities, characteristically are affected. In many patients more extensive lumbosacral root involvement is seen, a particularly frequent combination being bilateral S1–S2 root compromise accompanied by unilateral or bilateral L5 root involvement. The most common electrophysiologic findings are low-amplitude or unelicitable tibial motor NCS responses, recording abductor hallucis muscles (S1–S2 myotomes) (due to the axon loss being rather severe, and affecting both roots supplying the recorded muscle); normal sural response(s) (fibers derived from the S1 DRG); bilaterally absent H responses; and fibrillation potentials and MUP loss in the S1 and S2-innervated muscles, particularly those distal to the knees (e.g., medial and lateral gastrocnemius, abductor hallucis, abductor digiti quinti pedis). When the L5 roots are also involved, the peroneal motor CMAPs may also be of low amplitude or unelicitable, and fibrillation potentials and MUP loss may be found in the L5 myotomes, especially more distally (e.g., tibialis anterior, tibialis posterior, peroneus longus, extensor hallucis, and extensor digitorum brevis). The superficial peroneal sensory NCS, which assesses fibers derived from the L5 DRG, would be normal. Because the lesions are of several months' duration in most patients, fibrillation potentials are often accompanied and sometimes overshadowed by chronic neurogenic MUP changes. Low lumbar–high sacral paraspinal fibrillation potentials are usually found bilaterally with more acute lesions but are often undetectable with chronic lesions. Cauda equina lesions involving all the lumbosacral roots supplying the lower extremities (L2–S2) are rare. When present, severe axonal degeneration is the rule and consequently the EMG picture becomes rather characteristic: very-low-amplitude or unelicitable CMAPs bilaterally, normal SNAPs bilaterally, absent H responses, and abundant denervation in both lower extremities on NEE, although sometimes, especially with L2–L4 involvement, asymmetric. A misleading factor in assessing many of these patients is the fact that they are over the age of 60 years, and their lower extremity SNAP responses and H responses often are unelicitable bilaterally secondary to age alone.[15]

LUMBAR CANAL STENOSIS

The EMG findings with lumbar canal stenosis are extremely variable, depending on the degree of axon loss (as opposed to temporary ischemia) affecting the lumbosacral motor roots. At the one extreme is a severe cauda equina lesion, producing the electrical presentation described above. These patients characteristically have a fixed clinical deficit, usually severe in degree. At the opposite end of the spectrum are patients who experience only intermittent and short-lived symptoms in whom the EMG results often are completely normal. In between these two extremes are a number of different EMG patterns: a single radiculopathy, typically S1 and sometimes found, rather surprisingly, in the less symptomatic or asymptomatic limb; unilateral or bilateral absent H responses alone; and NEE changes restricted to one or two limb muscles (most commonly muscles innervated by the S1–S2 roots). Thus, lumbar canal stenosis has no single characteristic EMG presentation.[15, 17]

FOCAL SPINAL CORD LESIONS

The EMG findings with focal myelopathies are diverse, depending predominantly on whether the anterior horn cells or their exiting fibers have been compromised. If only the descending tracts of the spinal cord are affected, the only abnormality found on EMG is in the MUP firing pattern, restricted to muscles receiving innervation from spinal cord segments caudal to the lesion; i.e., the MUPs in those muscles fire in decreased numbers at a slow to moderate rate, if at all. In contrast, if the anterior horn cells or their axons are affected, the EMG findings are those of a focal intraspinal canal lesion, characteristically bilateral but often somewhat asymmetric. The location of the lesion along the spinal cord is also a major determinant of the value of the EMG examination. For example, in our experience the EMG results with focal intra- and extramedullary tumors were very informative when the lesions were affecting the lumbosacral segments; the findings were those of a lumbar intraspinal canal lesion, often indistinguishable from a cauda equina lesion. In contrast, EMG was of little benefit when the neoplasms were affecting the upper cervical segments (C1–C4), because that region of the spinal cord cannot be assessed satisfactorily.[10] Conversely, the EMG results have been severely abnormal in many patients with syringomyelia. In most of them the lower cervical–upper thoracic cord segments were involved. Consequently, in both upper extremities the ulnar and median motor CMAPs were low in amplitude or unelicitable, while the ulnar SNAPs were normal. Since the lesions were long-standing and slowly progressive, NEE of the C8–T1 innervated muscles bilaterally typically revealed prominent MUP loss, with striking chronic neurogenic MUP changes, but often sparse fibrillation potentials. Of note is that the etiology of the intermedullary lesion, as of a single radiculopathy, cannot be determined by EMG. However, some educated guesses can be made, depending on the activity (amount of fibrillation potentials) and chronicity (amount and degree of chronic neurogenic MUP change) of the lesion, and the distribution of the abnormalities as determined by the NEE.

POSTLAMINECTOMY EMG

The specific diagnostic benefit derived from EMG studies performed after neck and back surgery varies considerably, depending mainly on the time elapsed since operation and the reason for referral. Overall, however, such studies are of limited value. In the immediate postoperative period (the first 10 to 14 days after surgery) they can reveal preexisting abnormalities, because any NEE changes seen during that period (with the exception of a neurogenic MUP firing pattern) are due to a lesion that predated the operation. In the fairly early postoperative period (three weeks to three to four months), EMG can be of substantial help in those relatively rare instances when it shows evidence of a hitherto unsuspected lesion, i.e., a lesion other than the one for which surgery was performed, such as a plexopathy, a mononeuropathy, motor neuron disease, or a different radiculopathy. It is also of considerable benefit in assessing patients with weakness, postoperative or otherwise, partly because a normal motor amplitude recorded from a weak muscle seven or more days after onset virtually excludes motor axon loss as the cause; the remaining possibilities, depending on the circumstances, are a proximal conduction block (neurapraxia), an upper motor neuron lesion, or hysteria or malingering. Thus, in patients with lower motor neuron paresis secondary to root compression, e.g. footdrop, EMG studies allow early, accurate prognostication. Also, in the rare patients who develop nonorganic weakness postoperatively, EMG can prove that the symptoms are not the result of an axon loss lesion. However, EMG cannot answer the question most often asked by the referring physicians when patients are sent to the EMG laboratory during this period: "Was the root adequately decompressed?" Unfortunately, most EMG abnormalities caused by radiculopathy do not simply disappear when root compression is relieved. The only exceptions are those due to conduction block at the root level, which can resolve rapidly after successful root decompression. Thus, with an S1 radiculopathy, a preoperatively unelicitable H response could reappear in the postoperative period (obviously, the results of a preoperative EMG examination would have to be available for this to be demonstrated). Similarly, on NEE, if conduction block had been prominent along motor root fibers, a neurogenic MUP firing pattern could disappear rapidly after decompression. However, the NEE findings most often used to diagnose radiculopathies, fibrillation potentials and/or chronic neurogenic MUP changes in a myotome distribution, do *not* resolve promptly after successful surgery. Instead, they slowly regress in a proximodistal direction, over many months, just as they do if the root impingement persists in a static (i.e., nonprogressive) manner. Consequently, EMG performed two to three months postoperatively usually show little change from those obtained before surgery. Even studies performed four to six months (upper extremity) or six to 12 months (lower extremity) after surgery can be difficult to interpret, although the amount of fibrillation potentials seen, and their distribution in the myotome, provide some clues. Fibrillation potentials that are present in abundant numbers in proximal as well as distal myotomal muscles are indicative of an active radiculopathy, either ongoing (secondary to failed surgery) or recurrent. In general, the more time that has elapsed between surgery and EMG examination, the more likely are any abnormalities seen to be caused by a progressive or "new" lesion.[15]

RECOMMENDATIONS REGARDING EMG EXAMINATION REQUESTS

Taking some of the limitations noted above into consideration, some guidelines for EMG examination can be formulated to ensure that maximal benefit is obtained from the procedure. First, the study should not be performed until at least three weeks after the onset of symptoms (in acute conditions) or after symptoms have changed appreciably (in chronic conditions). This is to allow fibrillation potentials to develop fully in any muscles that are partially denervated by the root compromise. Second, with suspected radiculopathies the examination should be performed as soon as feasible after three to five weeks' duration of symptoms, because the EMG has such a frustrating propensity to normalize with time. To be avoided is the practice of obtaining EMG studies only after lengthy periods of observation. During these waiting periods, the ratio of positive to negative EMG results can change considerably, and for the worse. Third, to ensure that electromyographers direct their attention appropriately, the specific root believed to be compromised should be indicated, rather than the suspected disc space. Fourth, a repeat EMG should not be ordered if an earlier comprehensive study was unrevealing and if the patient's symptoms have not changed significantly in the interim. In fact, because of the tendency of the EMG examination to normalize with time, any repeat EMG examinations performed in static conditions are more likely to be unhelpful than the initial ones. In this context a practice to be avoided is periodically repeating EMG examinations (often along with all other studies) in patients with long-standing but static pain. (Obviously, if the symptoms have changed since the previous study, a repeat EMG is very much indicated.) Fifth, postlaminectomy studies performed early in the recovery period to determine whether root decompression has been successful generally are of no benefit and should be avoided. Sixth, EMG should be performed in patients with suspected radiculopathies to find electrical evidence of such a lesion or of some other lesion that could explain the symptomatology; they should not be requested with the goal of "ruling out" a radiculopathy. EMG has no exclusionary value regarding radiculopathies because false-negative results are inherent in it. This fact is particularly important when EMG studies are requested for patients with normal neurologic examinations who have long-standing pain in the neck and arm or back and leg. Some physicians essentially limit such requests to this type of patient, who commonly gravitates to tertiary referral centers. Unfortunately, the diagnostic yield in this particular patient group is the lowest experienced among all those with single radiculopathies. Consequently, a normal EMG examination definitely does not exclude the possibility of a radiculopathy being present in such a patient.[15]

References

1. Aminoff, M. J.: Electromyography in Clinical Practice, 2nd ed. New York, Churchill Livingstone, 1987.
2. Bonney, G., and Gilliatt, R. W.: Sensory nerve conduction after traction lesions of the brachial plexus. Proc. R. Soc. Med. *51*:365–368, 1958.
3. Braddom, R. I., and Johnson, E. W.: Standardization of "H" reflex and diagnostic use in S1 radiculopathy. Arch. Phys. Med. Rehabil. *55*:161–164, 1974.
4. Gilliatt, R. W.: Acute compression block. *In* Sumner, A. J. (ed.): The Physiology of Peripheral Nerve Disease. Philadelphia, W. B. Saunders Co., 1980, pp. 287–315.
5. Gilliatt, R. W.: Physical injury to peripheral nerves: physiologic and electrodiagnostic aspects. Mayo Clin. Proc. *56*:361–370, 1981.

6. Hammer, K.: Nerve Conduction Studies. Springfield, IL, Charles C Thomas, 1982.
7. Johnson, E. W.: Electrodiagnosis of radiculopathy. *In* Johnson, E. W. (ed.): Practical Electromyography. 2nd ed. Baltimore, Williams & Wilkins Co., 1988, pp. 229–245.
8. LaJoie, W. V.: Introduction to clinical electromyography. Instructional Course, American Academy of Orthopedic Surgery, *21:*23–41, 1971.
9. Lambert, E.: Electromyography and electrical stimulation of peripheral nerves and muscles. *In* Youmans, J. R. (ed.): Neurological Surgery. Philadelphia, W. B. Saunders Co., 1971, pp. 358–367.
10. Madalin, K., and Wilbourn, A. J.: The value of electrodiagnostic studies with primary intraspinal canal neoplasm. Muscle Nerve *11:*976–977, 1988.
11. McDonald, W. I.: Physiological consequences of demyelination. *In* Sumner, A. J. (ed.): The Physiology of Peripheral Nerve Disease. Philadelphia, W. B. Saunders Co., 1980, pp. 265–286.
12. Schuchmann, J.: H-reflex latency in radiculopathy. Arch. Phys. Med. Rehabil. *59:*185–187, 1978.
13. Seddon, H.: A classification of nerve injuries. Br. Med. J. *2:*237–241, 1942.
14. Waylonis, G. W.: Electromyographic findings in chronic cervical radicular syndromes. Arch. Phys. Med. Rehabil. *49:*407–412, 1968.
15. Wilbourn, A. J.: The value and limitations of electromyographic examination in the diagnosis of lumbosacral radiculopathy. *In* Hardy, R. W. (ed.): Lumber Disc Disease. New York, Raven Press, 1982, pp. 65–109.
16. Wilbourn, A. J.: How can electromyography help you? Postgrad. Med.*73:*187–195, 1983.
17. Wilbourn, A. J., and Aminoff, M. J.: AAEE minimonograph 32: The electrophysiologic examination in patients with radiculopathies. Muscle Nerve *11:*1099–1114, 1988.
18. Wilbourn, A.: Nerve conduction studies in axonopathies and demyelinating neuropathies. *In* Syllabus: 1989 AAEE Course A: Fundamentals of Electrodiagnosis. American Association of Electromyography and Electrodiagnosis, Rochester, MN, 1989, pp. 7–20.

SOMATOSENSORY AND MOTOR EVOKED POTENTIALS

Michael J. Aminoff, M.D.

Somatosensory evoked potentials (SEPs) may be used to evaluate the function of both central and peripheral somatosensory pathways.[2, 3] They are usually elicited for clinical purposes by an electrical stimulus applied to a mixed or cutaneous nerve, or less commonly to the skin in the territory of an individual nerve or nerve root. Electrical stimulation of peripheral nerve excites particularly the large, fast-conducting Group Ia and Group II afferent fibers. The stimuli are selected to be of short duration (200 μs), with a repetition rate of 3 or 5 Hz and an intensity slightly above motor threshold (so that a small muscle twitch is produced when a mixed nerve is stimulated) or two or three times above sensory threshold. Any accessible nerve can be stimulated, including the median or ulnar nerve at the wrist, the peroneal nerve at the knee, and the posterior tibial nerve at the ankle. Responses are recorded with either surface or needle electrodes from a more proximal portion of the nerve and over the spine and scalp. There is no unanimity concerning the optimal recording montage, although guidelines have been published by the American Electroencephalographic Society.[1]

The size of the cerebral response elicited by a single sensory stimulus is small compared with the ongoing activity of the brain (i.e., the electroencephalogram [EEG]), but the response occurs at a fixed time after the stimulus, in contrast to background electrocerebral activity and any noncerebral artifacts. The use of simple computers permits the response of interest to be extracted from background activity by averaging after repeated stimuli. Individual stimuli trigger the analysis sweep of the computer: the responses, which occur at the same time in relation to sweep onset, are summed and enhanced as the stimulus is repeated, whereas activity having a random relationship to sweep onset cancels out. The quality of the recording and the amount of background noise govern the number of trials that need to be averaged, but usually between 500 and 2000 trials are averaged for responses derived from stimulation of the upper limbs, and between 1000 and 4000 responses to stimulation of the lower limbs. At least two averages are always obtained to ensure the replicability of the findings.

Responses are characterized by their polarity (i.e., positivity or negativity at the active electrode with respect to the reference point) and normal mean latency. In the SEPs derived by stimulation of a nerve in the arm, it is generally possible to recognize an Erb's point potential, an N13/P13–14 in recordings made between the neck and the midfrontal region of the scalp (FZ), and a P13–14 and N20 in the recording made between the contralateral "hand" area of scalp and an inactive reference site (Fig. 7–7). Other early components have also been described but are not present consistently in normal subjects. The N20 is probably generated in the somatosensory cortex. It is followed by a number of different peaks, depending on the site of recording over the scalp, and these probably have distinct cortical generators. When a nerve in the lower extremity is stimulated, potentials can generally be recorded over the cauda equina and spine. In addition, conspicuous P27 and N35 peaks can be identified over the vertex of the scalp with stimulation of the peroneal nerve at the knee, and P37 (sometimes designated P40) and N45 components are found when the posterior tibial nerve is stimulated at the ankle (Fig. 7–8).

In evaluating the response, the latency of individual components and the interval between different components (the intercomponent latency) are determined and related to height or limb length. The presence or absence of individual components of the response is also noted. Alterations in amplitude and morphology of the response are also evaluated, although these are less reliable for determining abnormality.

PLEXUS INJURIES

It may be difficult to determine clinically whether patients with traumatic brachial plexopathy have a postganglionic lesion rather than preganglionic rupture of nerve roots. This distinction is important, however, with regard to management and prognosis. For this reason, SEPs (obtained by stimulation of nerve trunks in the affected arm) have been used to clarify the site of the lesion in patients with unilateral

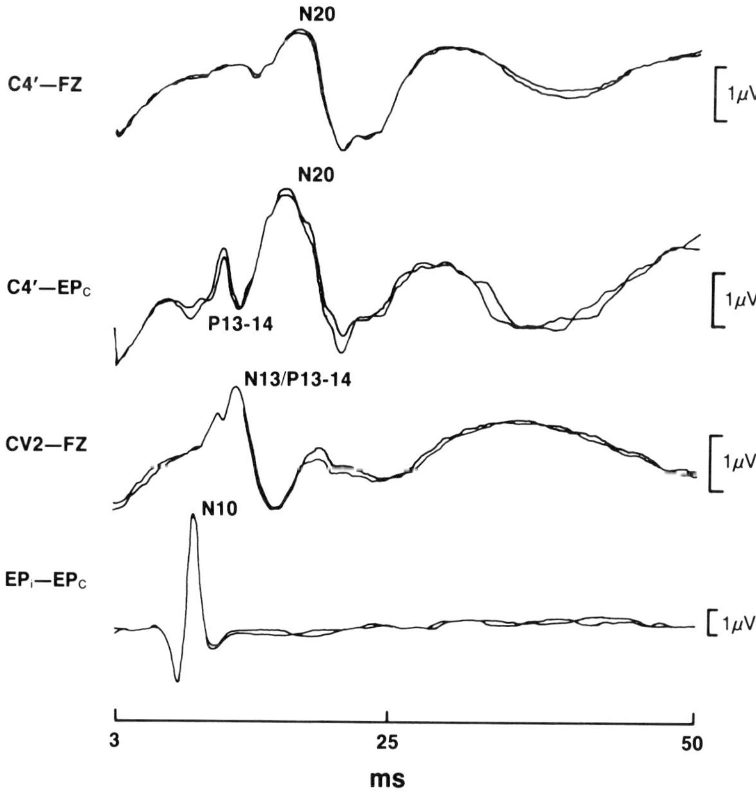

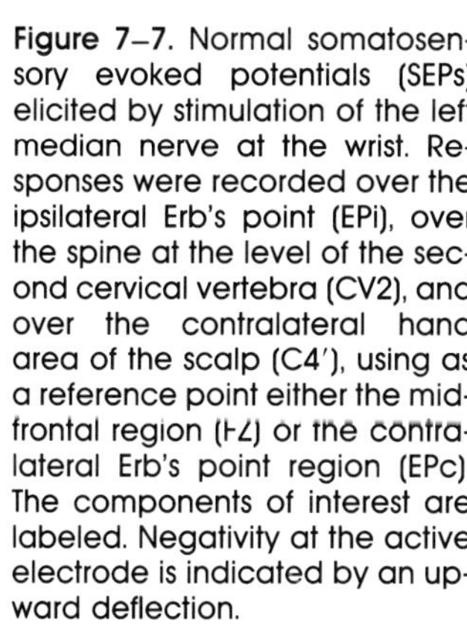
Figure 7–7. Normal somatosensory evoked potentials (SEPs) elicited by stimulation of the left median nerve at the wrist. Responses were recorded over the ipsilateral Erb's point (EPi), over the spine at the level of the second cervical vertebra (CV2), and over the contralateral hand area of the scalp (C4′), using as a reference point either the midfrontal region (FZ) or the contralateral Erb's point region (EPc). The components of interest are labeled. Negativity at the active electrode is indicated by an upward deflection.

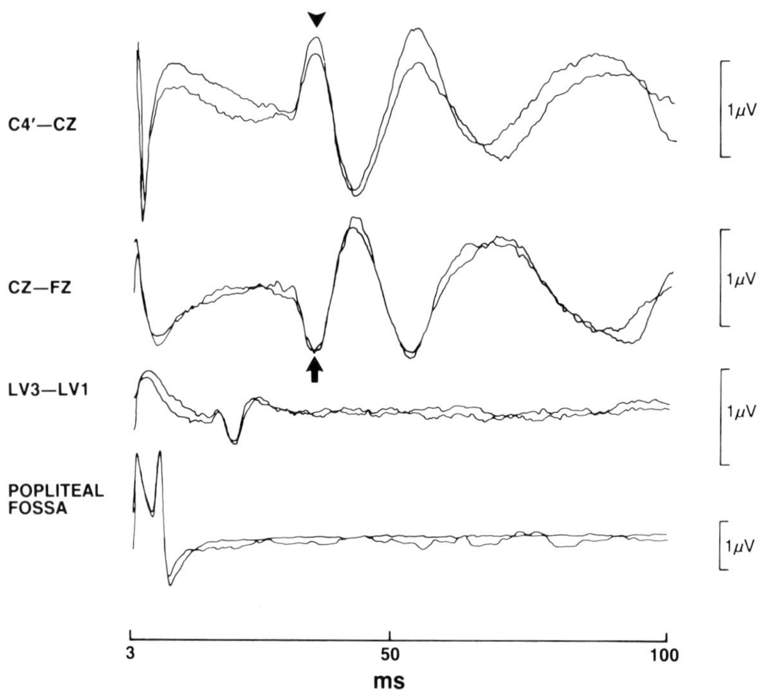

Figure 7–8. SEPs elicited by tibial nerve stimulation at the left ankle in a normal subject. The peripheral volley is recorded over the nerve at the popliteal fossa. The cauda equina response is recorded over the spine between the third and first lumbar vertebrae (LV3 and LV1). Over the scalp a positivity is recorded (*arrow*) at the vertex (CZ) with reference to the midfrontal region (FZ), and a corresponding negativity between C4′ and the vertex (CZ) (*arrowhead*). Negativity at the active electrode is indicated by an upward deflection.

injuries of the brachial plexus. Their use in this regard is based on the belief that the N9 peak recorded at Erb's point depends on the integrity of postganglionic fibers in the arm and is attenuated by damage to these fibers, whereas attenuation of the N13–P13 component reflects the total extent of pre- and postganglionic damage. Thus, a postganglionic lesion is said to have occurred if the N9 component is reduced to the same extent as or more than the N13–P13 component, whereas a preganglionic or combined lesion is diagnosed if the N9 peak is less attenuated. Although the technique has been held to be useful, critical evaluation of the published data suggests a more limited role. For example, Jones and colleagues[17] compared the sites of lesions determined at operation and electrophysiologically, and found that in only half of their 16 patients were they able to localize the lesion correctly by the SEP findings; in three patients the site of the lesion as determined electrophysiologically differed markedly from the findings at surgery.

If SEPs are to be used to localize the lesion to a particular segment within the plexus itself, it may be necessary to record the SEPs obtained by stimulating a number of different nerves in turn.[32] Even then, misleading information may be obtained if there are multiple lesions, because the findings may reflect merely the most distal of these lesions.

Despite these limitations, SEPs may occasionally be helpful in the evaluation of traumatic plexopathies.[6] For example, in one of our patients with attenuated peripheral sensory nerve action potentials, the presence of small SEPs over the Erb's point region, but without any response over the cervical spine or scalp, suggested the possibility of multiple root avulsions in addition to more peripheral pathology, and this was subsequently confirmed radiologically and at surgery. Further, the SEPs may be helpful when the extent of functional continuity in the plexus is unclear. Finally, intraoperative stimulation of specific nerve roots, with recording of responses over the scalp, may help to indicate functional continuity of nerve fibers when this is not clinically evident.

In patients with neurogenic or classic thoracic outlet syndrome, SEP studies may show abnormalities,[34] but results of other, more conventional, electrophysiologic studies (such as electromyography) are also abnormal.[6] In patients with the non-neurogenic variety of thoracic outlet syndrome, findings from SEPs obtained by stimulation of median, ulnar, and radial nerves are normal, as are those from other electrophysiologic studies.[6]

RADICULOPATHIES

SEP studies are the only easy, noninvasive electrophysiologic technique for evaluating function in sensory fibers of the nerve roots, but there are a number of theoretical limitations to their use. First, any slowing of conduction velocity (CV) over a small segment of the nerve fibers traversing a particular nerve root may be masked by the long distance from the point of peripheral stimulation to the site at which responses are generated. Second, focal conduction block in some fibers in the nerve root may not be detected because conduction is normal in the remaining fibers. Third, SEPs vary so much in size between individuals and between sides in the same individual that only loss of responses can be regarded as abnormal. Fourth, abnormal SEP results do not suggest either the age or nature of the underlying lesion and provide only limited information concerning the site of the lesion proximal to the nerve plexus. Accordingly, it is not surprising that in patients with isolated compressive lumbosacral root lesions, the peroneal-derived SEP result has always been normal in our experience.[4, 5] Some authors have claimed a high incidence of abnormalities but have not provided sufficient details to permit independent review of these claims.

In cervical spondylosis, patients with subjective complaints, such as pain and paresthesias, but with no objective neurologic signs, generally have normal median, ulnar, or radial SEPs. When radicular signs are present, the SEP results may be abnormal, regardless of whether there is an accompanying myelopathy.[13, 15, 33] However, an abnormal SEP finding is generally accompanied by abnormalities on needle electromyography, so that little is gained by the additional electrophysiologic study.

Cutaneous Nerve Stimulation

Instead of stimulating a multisegmental nerve trunk, a cutaneous nerve, which is segmentally more specific, can be stimulated in order to elicit SEPs. Using this technique, Eisen and colleagues[12] reported that 57 per cent of 28 patients with suspected root lesions had abnormal scalp-recorded SEPs, but the diagnostic yield by needle electromyography was greater (75 per cent). The most common SEP abnormality was a reduction in amplitude or alteration in morphology; latency abnormalities were uncommon. Subsequently, Perlik and associates[25] used a similar technique to study 27 patients with low back pain, unilateral radicular symptoms, and abnormal CT scans. In 21 patients there were scalp-recorded SEP abnormalities; only six of these showed other electrophysiologic changes and they also had clinical abnormalities. The findings from this study therefore suggest that SEPs elicited from cutaneous nerves may be very sensitive to compressive radiculopathies, but clearly further verification of this is required from others. In this regard, Seyal and associates[28] were unable to confirm the high yield of scalp-recorded SEPs in patients with compressive lumbosacral radiculopathy, although they did find it useful to record SEPs at the lumbar root entry zone after stimulation of segmentally specific cutaneous nerves in the legs. This latter approach may ultimately be more fruitful in evaluating patients with radiculopathies.

Dermatomal Stimulation

Another approach to increase the specificity of SEP studies has been to record the response over the scalp to stimulation in the cutaneous territory of individual nerve roots. Such dermatomally elicited SEPs have been used to investigate patients with isolated compressive root lesions. Early reports of a high diagnostic yield in lumbosacral root entrapment syndromes are of questionable validity, because of an absence of data from normal subjects and the use of apparently arbitrary criteria for abnormality.[27] The studies by Aminoff and colleagues[4, 5] showed that in only about 25 per cent of patients with clinically unequivocal L5 or S1 compressive root lesions did the SEP findings permit the diagnosis to be confirmed. By contrast, needle electromyography had the greatest yield, showing signs of denervation in a myotomal pattern in 75 per cent. Katifi and Sedgwick[18] claimed a much higher diagnostic yield for dermatomal SEPs, using a technique similar to that of Aminoff and associates, and indeed the normal results obtained by the two groups were remarkably similar. However, evaluation of this study is difficult because patients had widespread disease and more generous criteria for electrophysiologic abnormality were employed, complicating the interpretation of the electrophysiologic findings. The operative findings were regarded as the "gold standard" permitting a definitive diagnosis, and inspection of the data of Katifi and Sedgwick reveals that dermatomal SEPs indicated abnormalities of 12 roots that were not involved at operation, and in only four of their 21 patients were the operative findings accurately and completely predicted by the SEP studies.

In a more recent study, dermatomal SEPs were held to be useful in the evaluation of patients with cervical radiculopathy.[19] Of 24 patients with radiologically verified cervical disc prolapse, 16 (67 per cent) showed abnormal findings on needle electromyography. Only 13 of the patients underwent dermatomal SEP studies and in 11 the results were abnormal. However in six the abnormality was at the wrong level, and in three of these six patients this was the sole SEP abnormality. Therefore, dermatomal SEP studies appear to have a very limited role in the diagnosis of cervical root lesions.

Magnetic Stimulation

One new approach to the electrophysiologic diagnosis of radiculopathies by SEP studies merits consideration. The spinal roots and the proximal and distal portions of the peripheral nerves can be stimulated magnetically, and cerebral responses recorded over the scalp. In patients with radiculopathy, initial studies suggest that the response is delayed,[30] but this needs to be established more clearly.

DYSFUNCTION OF CENTRAL NERVOUS SYSTEM

SEPs have been used to detect lesions involving the central somatosensory pathways in the spinal cord or brain (Figs. 7–9, 7–10). They may also provide a guide to the location of the lesion. However, the findings are never pathognomonic of specific diseases. An abnormal SEP result may be important in indicating that vague sensory complaints have an organic

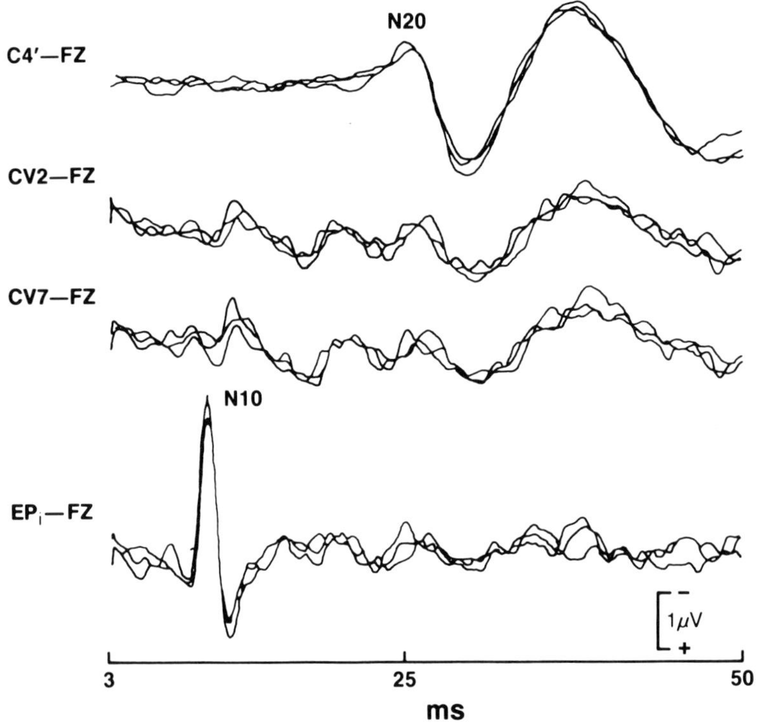

Figure 7–9. SEPs elicited in a patient with a foramen magnum lesion after median nerve stimulation at the right wrist. The potential recorded over the Erb's point region is well formed and of normal latency, but there is a poorly defined response over the lower (CV7) and upper (CV2) cervical spine, and the N20 response over the scalp has a latency of 26 ms, which is grossly prolonged.

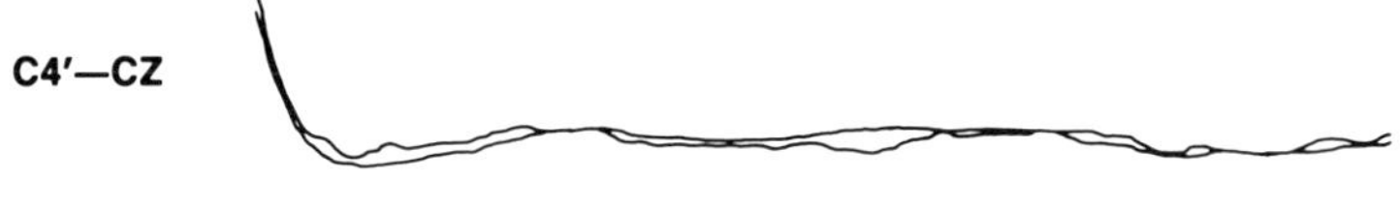

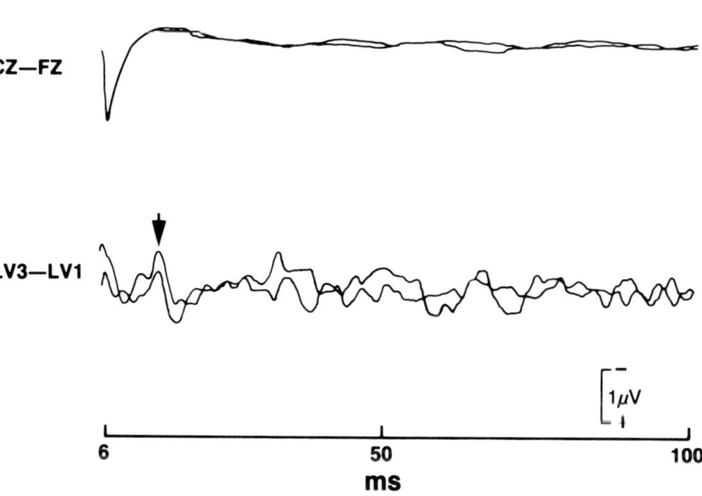

Figure 7–10. SEPs elicited by peroneal nerve stimulation at the left knee in a patient with a mild cervical spondylotic myelopathy. A reproducible potential is present over the lumbar spine (*arrow*), but there is no response over the scalp.

basis, but a normal SEP does not indicate that sensory complaints are of nonorganic origin.

With intrinsic cord lesions such as syringomyelia, SEPs elicited from nerves in the upper limbs may be attenuated or absent over the cervical spine, and central conduction time (i.e., the interval between the responses recorded over spine and scalp) may be prolonged.[7]

SEPs have been used to evaluate patients with spinal injuries. It was initially hoped that the presence or absence of a response over the scalp after stimulation of a nerve below the level of the lesion would provide some guide to the completeness of the lesion. However, it often is not possible to record any scalp response in the acute stage following a spinal injury, irrespective of whether the lesion is partial or complete. A preserved SEP, or the early return of a response after spinal injury, would however indicate an incomplete lesion and therefore imply a better prognosis for recovery than otherwise.[11]

Noel and Desmedt[23] found in patients with a cervical compressive myelopathy that the SEP result obtained by sural nerve stimulation was often more abnormal than that obtained by stimulation of a digital nerve in the upper limb. Such a finding suggests that the recording of sural-derived SEPs (or of SEPs derived by stimulation of other nerves in the legs) in patients who show no clinical evidence of cord involvement may help in determining which patients with cervical spondylosis are at particular risk of developing a spondylotic myelopathy (Fig. 7–10). Veilleux and Daube[31] found that ulnar-derived SEPs may also be particularly helpful in this regard. In cervical spondylotic myelopathy, Perlik and Fisher[24] found that the tibial-derived SEP was abnormal in all of 13 patients, and Yu and Jones[35] reported that such abnormalities were strongly correlated with ipsilateral posterior column signs, and that the SEP was a more sensitive means of detecting sensory pathway involvement than clinical examination. Of particular importance, Yu and Jones found that the correlation of SEP and radiologic findings was poor; SEPs were abnormal in six of eight patients with clinical myelopathy but no radiologic evidence of posterior cord compression, perhaps because an impairment of blood supply was partly responsible for the myelopathy.

It has been suggested that the SEP abnormalities found in cervical spondylotic myelopathy are occasionally helpful in distinguishing this disorder from amyotrophic lateral sclerosis, when this is a diagnostic consideration.

However, SEP abnormalities have been reported in the latter disorder, especially when elicited by stimulation of nerves in the legs.[8,26]

SEP results may be abnormal in patients with spinal disease that does not relate to an acquired structural abnormality or require surgical treatment. For example, SEPs are commonly abnormal in patients with multiple sclerosis or hereditary spinocerebellar degenerations.[11] The findings do not distinguish between different spinal disorders, or, for example, between compressive and ischemic spondylotic myelopathies. The SEP findings are helpful only in revealing an abnormality and perhaps also—if a number of different nerves are stimulated—in localizing the lesion. If an expanded recording montage is used, it may be possible to resolve the N14 peak that is recorded between electrodes placed on the neck and forehead into several individual components. This enhances the ability to detect and localize cervical cord lesions on the basis of the median-derived SEP.[14,21]

Noninvasive magnetic stimulation of spinal nerves or nerve roots has been used to elicit SEPs, and in patients with myelopathy these cerebral responses may be delayed.[30] This approach is being further evaluated, and definition of its role in the functional localization of spinal lesions studied.

MOTOR RESPONSES TO ELECTRICAL OR MAGNETIC STIMULATION OVER SPINE

Marsden and associates[20] showed that motor responses elicited by percutaneous electrical stimulation over the cervical or lumbar vertebral column can be recorded from muscles of the upper and lower limbs, respectively. This results mainly from excitation of the proximal portion of the motor roots.[22] Tabaraud and associates[29] investigated the use of such motor evoked responses in the diagnosis of radiculopathy, recording bilaterally from the tibialis anterior and soleus muscles after lumbar spinal stimulation in 25 control subjects and 45 patients with unilateral L5 or S1 root pain due to radiologically demonstrated disc protrusions. Among the patients with radiculopathy, the motor evoked response latency was prolonged on the symptomatic side by more than three standard deviations of the mean interside latency difference in normal subjects in 72 per cent of those with an L5 lesion and 66 per cent of those with an S1 lesion. Abnormalities were found in patients who had no signs of root disease, as well as in those with objective neurologic deficits.

Chokroverty and associates[9] used magnetic lumbar stimulation to evaluate patients with lumbosacral root lesions. A magnetic coil placed over the central sacral region produced pulsed magnetic fields that generated electric currents, activating impulses in nerve roots. They reported prolonged latencies and decreased amplitudes of the evoked motor potentials recorded from muscles supplied by the affected roots. They have used a somewhat similar technique to evaluate patients with cervical radiculopathy.[10] The role of the technique in the management of patients with root lesions remains to be established.

In some patients with cervical spondylotic myelopathy, quite marked slowing of conduction has been found in central motor pathways when magnetic stimulation was applied to the head and then just lateral to the cervical spine while motor responses were recorded from a muscle in the hand.[16] Such slowed conduction in central motor pathways has also been found in patients with multiple sclerosis and certain other neurologic disorders, and the role of this technique in the detection and differential diagnosis of spinal disorders awaits delineation.

References

1. American Electroencephalographic Society: Guidelines for clinical evoked potential studies. J. Clin. Neurophysiol. *1:*3–53, 1984.
2. Aminoff, M. J.: Use of somatosensory evoked potentials to evaluate the peripheral nervous system. J. Clin. Neurophysiol. *4:*135–144, 1987.
3. Aminoff, M. J.: The use of somatosensory evoked potentials in the evaluation of the central nervous system. Neurol. Clin. *6:*809–823, 1988.
4. Aminoff, M. J., Goodin, D. S., Barbaro, N. M., et al.: Dermatomal somatosensory evoked potentials in unilateral lumbosacral radiculopathy. Ann. Neurol. *17:*171–176, 1985.
5. Aminoff, M. J., Goodin, D. S., Parry, G. J., et al.: Electrophysiologic evaluation of lumbosacral radiculopathies: electromyography, late responses and somatosensory evoked potentials. Neurology *35:*1514–1518, 1985.
6. Aminoff, M. J., Olney, R. K., Parry, G. J., and Raskin, N. H.: Relative utility of different electrophysiologic techniques in the evaluation of brachial plexopathies. Neurology *38:*546–550, 1988.
7. Anderson, N. E., Frith, R. W., and Synek, V. M.:

Somatosensory evoked potentials in syringomyelia. J. Neurol. Neurosurg. Psychiatry *49:*1407–1410, 1986.
8. Bosch, E. P., Yamada, T., and Kimura, J.: Somatosensory evoked potentials in motor neuron disease. Muscle Nerve *8:*556–562, 1985.
9. Chokroverty, S., Sachdeo, R., and Duvoisin, R. C.: Magnetic stimulation of the lumbosacral roots: a new diagnostic technique. Neurology *38*(Suppl. 1):387, 1988.
10. Chokroverty, S., and DiLullo, J.: Magnetic stimulation of the human cervical vertebral column. Neurology *39* (Suppl. 1):394, 1989.
11. Eisen, A., and Aminoff, M. J.: Somatosensory evoked potentials. *In* Aminoff, M. J. (ed.): Electrodiagnosis in Clinical Neurology. 2nd ed. New York, Churchill Livingstone, 1986, pp. 535–573.
12. Eisen, A., Hoirch, M., and Moll, A.: Evaluation of radiculopathies by segmental stimulation and somatosensory evoked potentials. Can. J. Neurol. Sci. *10:*178–182, 1983.
13. El Negamy, E., and Sedgwick, E. M.: Delayed cervical somatosensory potentials in cervical spondylosis. J. Neurol. Neurosurg. Psychiatry *42:*238–241, 1979.
14. Emerson, R. G., and Pedley, T. A.: Effect of cervical spinal cord lesions on early components of the median nerve somatosensory evoked potential. Neurology *36:*20–26, 1986.
15. Ganes, T.: Somatosensory conduction times and peripheral, cervical and cortical evoked potentials in patients with cervical spondylosis. J. Neurol. Neurosurg. Psychiatry *43:*683–689, 1980.
16. Jarratt, J. A.: Magnetic stimulation for motor conduction. *In* Syllabus, International Symposium on New Concepts in Electrodiagnosis, A.A.E.E., 1986, pp. 27–33.
17. Jones, S. J., Wynn Parry, C. B., and Landi, A.: Diagnosis of brachial plexus traction lesions by sensory nerve action potentials and somatosensory evoked potentials. Injury *12:*376–382, 1981.
18. Katifi, H. A., and Sedgwick, E. M.: Evaluation of the dermatomal somatosensory evoked potential in the diagnosis of lumbosacral root compression. J. Neurol. Neurosurg. Psychiatry *50:*1204–1210, 1987.
19. Leblhuber, F., Reisecker, F., Boehm-Jurkovic, H., et al.: Diagnostic value of different electrophysiologic tests in cervical disc prolapse. Neurology *38:*1879–1881, 1988.
20. Marsden, C. D., Merton, P. A., and Morton, H. B.: Percutaneous stimulation of spinal cord and brain: pyramidal tract conduction velocities in man. J. Physiol. (Lond.) 328:6P, 1982.
21. Mauguiere, F., and Ibanez, V.: The dissociation of early SEP components in lesions of the cervicomedullary junction: a cue for routine interpretation of abnormal cervical responses to median nerve stimulation. Electroencephalogr. Clin. Neurophysiol. *62:*406–420, 1985.
22. Mills, K. R., and Murray, N. M. F.: Electrical stimulation over the human vertebral column: which neural elements are excited? Electroencephalogr. Clin. Neurophysiol. *63:*582–589, 1986.
23. Noel, P., and Desmedt, J. E.: Cerebral and far-field somatosensory evoked potentials in neurological disorders involving the cervical spinal cord, brainstem, thalamus and cortex. Prog. Clin. Neurophysiol. *7:*205–230, 1980.
24. Perlik, S. J., and Fisher, M. A.: Somatosensory evoked response evaluation of cervical spondylytic myelopathy. Muscle Nerve *10:*481–489, 1987.
25. Perlik, S., Fisher, M. A., Patel, D. V., and Slack, C.: On the usefulness of somatosensory evoked responses for the evaluation of lower back pain. Arch. Neurol. *43:*907–913, 1986.
26. Radtke, R. A., Erwin, A., and Erwin, C. W.: Abnormal sensory evoked potentials in amyotrophic lateral sclerosis. Neurology *36:*796–801, 1986.
27. Scarff, T. B., Dallmann, D. E., Toleikis, J. R., and Bunch, W. H.: Dermatomal somatosensory evoked potentials in the diagnosis of lumbar root entrapment. Surg. Forum *32:*489–491, 1981.
28. Seyal, M., Sandhu, L. S., and Mack, Y. P.: Spinal segmental somatosensory evoked potentials in lumbosacral radiculopathies. Neurology *39:*801–805, 1989.
29. Tabaraud, F., Hugon, J., Chazot, F., et al.: Motor evoked responses after lumbar spinal stimulation in patients with L5 or S1 radicular involvement. Electroencephalogr. Clin. Neurophysiol. *72:*334–339, 1989.
30. Tsuji, S., Murai, Y., and Yarita, M.: Somatosensory potentials evoked by magnetic stimulation of lumbar roots, cauda equina, and leg nerves. Ann. Neurol. *24:*568–573, 1988.
31. Veilleux, M., and Daube, J. R.: The value of ulnar somatosensory evoked potentials (SEPs) in cervical myelopathy. Electroencephalogr. Clin. Neurophysiol. *68:*415–423, 1987.
32. Yiannikas, C., Shahani, B. T., and Young, R. R.: The investigation of traumatic lesions of the brachial plexus by electromyography and short latency somatosensory potentials evoked by stimulation of multiple peripheral nerves. J. Neurol. Neurosurg. Psychiatry *46:*1014–1022, 1983.
33. Yiannikas, C., Shahani, B. T., and Young, R. R.: Short-latency somatosensory-evoked potentials from radial, median, ulnar, and peroneal nerve stimulation in the assessment of cervical spondylosis. Arch. Neurol. *43:*1264–1271, 1986.
34. Yiannikas, C., and Walsh, J. C.: Somatosensory evoked responses in the diagnosis of thoracic outlet syndrome. J. Neurol. Neurosurg. Psychiatry *46:*234–240, 1983.
35. Yu, Y. L., and Jones, S. J.: Somatosensory evoked potentials in cervical spondylosis. Brain *108:*273–300, 1985.

CHAPTER

8

PATHOPHYSIOLOGY OF THE INTERVERTEBRAL DISC AND ADJACENT NEURAL STRUCTURES*

Björn Rydevik, M.D., Ph.D.
Sten Holm, Ph.D.

One of the most expensive and incapacitating medical and social problems of our times, especially in industrialized countries, is low back pain.[12, 65, 119, 189–192, 254] Considering the magnitude of the problem, there are surprisingly few attempts made to approach low back pain from a multidisciplinary social, mechanical, and metabolic point of view. This may be due to the enormous complexity of the problem, including connective tissue biochemistry and metabolism, message transport in nerve fibers, and translation in the cortex of the brain with compounding psychologic contribution.[5, 58, 189, 196, 197]

In most patients the cause of the symptoms remains virtually unknown, although some relevant clues have been discovered over the last few years. Some factors that are thought to either induce, or potentially affect, low back pain can be seen in Figure 8–1. Pathoanatomic conditions that can occur in the spinal motion segment, and are generally accepted as related to the symptoms of low back disorders and pain, include disc herniations, fractures, infections, spinal stenosis, spondyloarthropathies, and spondylolisthesis. For acute low back pain, however, only in about 2 to 4 per cent of cases can an adequate clear diagnosis be made, whereas this increases to 30 per cent if the pain lasts for three months.[189, 193]

In many patients low back pain conditions are thought to be related to changes in the intervertebral disc, either directly through disc herniation or indirectly, as degenerative discs may lead to the development of atypical stresses on other spinal structures.[98, 116, 134, 296] It has also been suggested that intradiscal pathology and disruption without disc herniation may play an important role in nonspecific low back pain disorders.[294]

Most tissue components of the motion segment are innervated with sensory nerve endings, and therefore are potential sources of pain in cases of tissue injury to any of these structures. Interestingly, the nucleus pulposus of the discs, the main culprit in sciatica and

*Acknowledgments: This review is in part based on work supported by the Swedish Medical Research Council (project no. 8685).

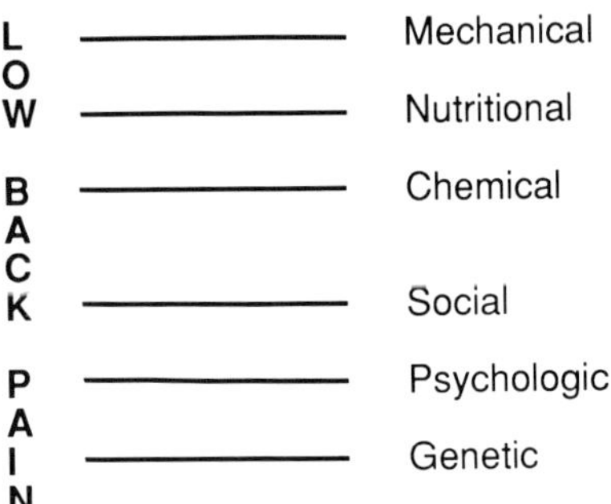

Figure 8–1. Factors that may initiate or potentiate low back pain.

one of the best studied, evaluated, diagnosed and treated conditions of the spine, seems to be the only structure that is devoid of sensory innervation. A herniated nucleus pulposus can cause pain, however, by affecting nearby neural structures, for example, both in the posterior longitudinal ligament and the nerve root, rather than through intrinsic pain receptors.

In this chapter the structure, function, and pathophysiologic mechanisms of the intervertebral disc and adjacent neural structures are discussed, along with the mechanisms of interaction between disc and nerve tissue.

THE INTERVERTEBRAL DISC

Tissue Structure and Function

Much previous work related to the etiology of low back pain has concentrated on the morphology of healthy and degenerated intervertebral discs (Fig. 8–2).[9, 180, 252] The mechanical behavior of the disc has been the subject of numerous investigations,[65, 254, 309, 311] and it now seems to be generally accepted that the normal function of the disc depends on its ability to maintain hydration under load. How the observed biochemical changes affect hydration and hence load transmission through the disc has been a matter of controversy.[200, 234] Additional biochemical changes with age and degeneration have also been evaluated and attempts made to correlate these changes with pain.[4, 43, 81, 99, 181, 196, 200]

Another area of speculation has been the pathophysiologic mechanisms related to nutrition of the intervertebral disc. Some authors have postulated that nutritional deficiencies could lead to disc degeneration.[109, 111, 112, 114, 188, 189, 195, 216, 287, 289] This is possible since disc tissue is not inactive but has a low, but significant, rate of turnover.[44, 109, 151, 288, 289]

The adult lumbar discs are large (occupying about 35 per cent of the volume of the spine) and avascular.[252, 287] Because of this it is unclear how nutrients enter and metabolites leave these structures. Although metabolic activity is slow, it is present and requires a flow of substrates to maintain its viability. Because of the absence of blood supply to the discs, studies have been performed to determine whether diffusion alone can supply nutrients to the cells in various parts of the discs to sustain them adequately in a healthy functional state.[109, 116, 130, 172, 195] Mechanisms other than pure diffusion have been postulated for nutrient transport, e.g., pumping of fluid in and out of the disc under changes in load[109, 188] and slow flow of

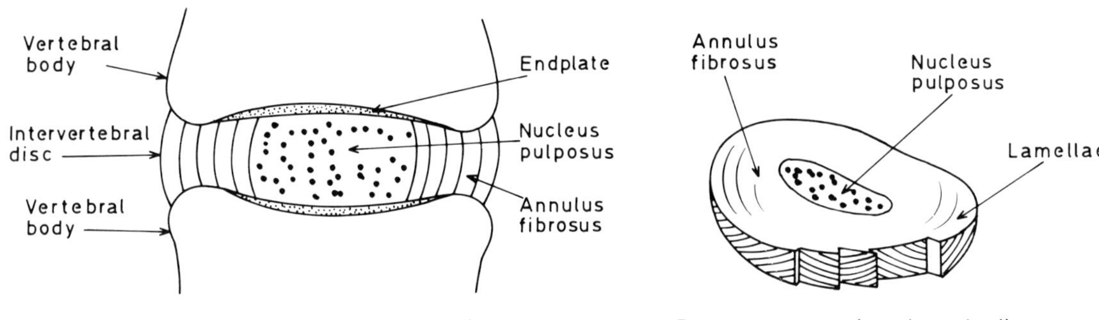

Figure 8–2. Schematic view of the spine and the different regions in the intervertebral disc. Included is also the arrangement of the annulus lamellae, showing alternating direction of collagen bundles. (From Schultz, A. B.: Mechanics of the human spine: invited feature article. Appl. Mech. Rev. *27*:1487–1497, 1974. By permission of "Applied Mechanics Reviews," a publication of ASME.)

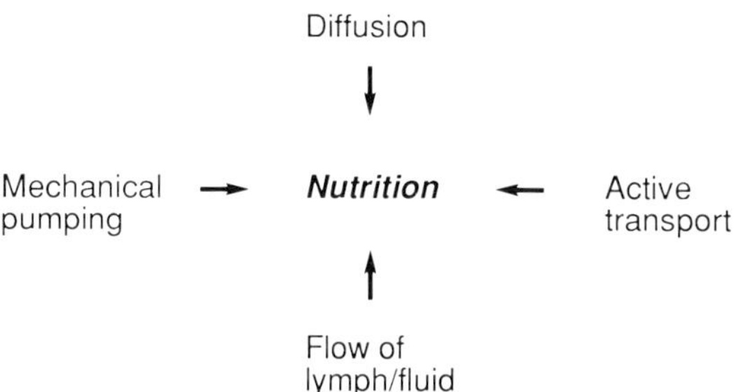

Figure 8–3. Potential nutritional mechanisms that can supply the intervertebral disc with nutrients.

lymph or other nutrient fluid through the disc (Fig. 8–3).[61]

The normal existence, and the metabolic capacity, of the disc depend on a supply of nutrients from, as well as disposal of waste products into, surrounding fluids. Only a few quantitative studies have been published on solute transport in disc tissue.[109, 112, 114, 172, 221, 287] Urban[287] and Urban and Maroudas[292, 293] describe factors (i.e., diffusion coefficient, partition coefficient, swelling pressure, and hydraulic permeability) that control swelling and fluid flow in the intervertebral disc, as well as the transport properties of various solutes.

The intervertebral disc is a specialized connective tissue designed to provide strength, mobility, and resistance to strain. For its normal function it must possess elastic properties. A normal disc allows the spine to move in various directions and to resist axial load (Fig. 8–4). The matrix of the intervertebral disc is able to fulfill these requirements through its very specialized collagen network and its highly concentrated proteoglycan-water gel. Any changes in the structure, and hence the mechanical efficiency, of the disc are likely to interfere with such functions, which are essential for the equalization and absorption of the various stresses placed on the vertebral column.[201]

The proteoglycan gel of the nucleus, with its high swelling pressure and ability to maintain hydration under large external loads, resists compression, while the specialized weave of the collagen network acts in tension to restrain the proteoglycan and yet allow bending and torsion of the disc. The mechanical properties of the disc are therefore dependent on the interplay of these two components. In addition, although the disc has a relatively low cell density, cells are present and necessary for the continued renewal and replacement of the proteoglycans. Nutrition of these cells is essential for maintenance of the integrity of the disc matrix. Inadequate nutrition or accumulation of waste products could be one of the causes of disc degeneration. Since the intervertebral discs are large, avascular structures, it has been questioned whether diffusion alone can adequately supply nutrients to the cells throughout the disc. Mechanisms of nutritional transport other than diffusion, e.g., fluid pumping, have been estimated to contribute to approximately 5 to 10 per cent of the total solute transport.[109] Any disturbance in transport, nutritional supply or composition, or highly activated enzy-

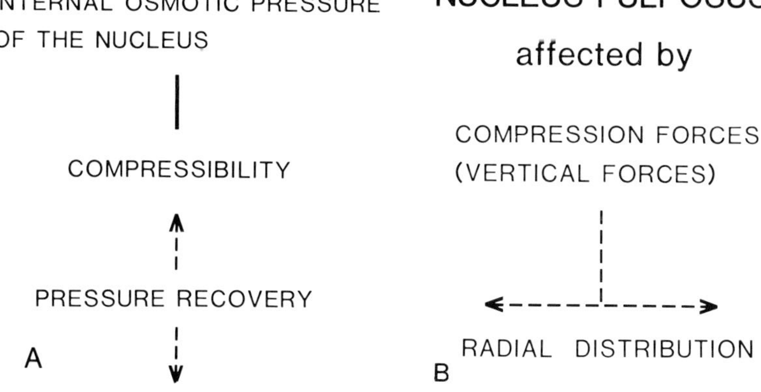

Figure 8–4. Mechanical factors affecting *(A)* the annulus and *(B)* the nucleus. The diagrams indicate how the forces are distributed.

matic degradation may lead to mechanical dysfunction of the entire lumbar motion segment.

The intervertebral disc structure consists of three main parts: the outer annulus fibrosus, the inner gelatinous nucleus pulposus, and the cartilaginous end plates, which are interposed between the bony vertebral bodies and the disc material.

The annulus fibrosus is organised into lamellae of coarse collagen fibrils. These run obliquely to each other in alternating layers, which surround the nucleus pulposus. It has a banded appearance resulting from the intricate arrangement of these fibrous lamellae (see Fig. 8–2). The annulus is less hydrated than the nucleus, and the changes that occur with age are not as apparent. The distinction between annulus and nucleus, while pronounced in young individuals, is not sharply defined in adults. In the junctional area there is a gradual change from the more fibrous annulus to the more gelatinous nucleus.

The nucleus pulposus occupies about 30 to 60 per cent of the disc volume. Its composition and appearance changes markedly throughout life. Nuclei in young discs are highly hydrated (80 to 88 per cent water). In adults the hydration decreases markedly and, as the tissues become firmer and lose translucency, the boundary between nucleus and annulus becomes more difficult to distinguish. The nucleus lies slightly posterior to the center of the disc, but it is equidistant from the anterior margin of the disc. In flexion and extension

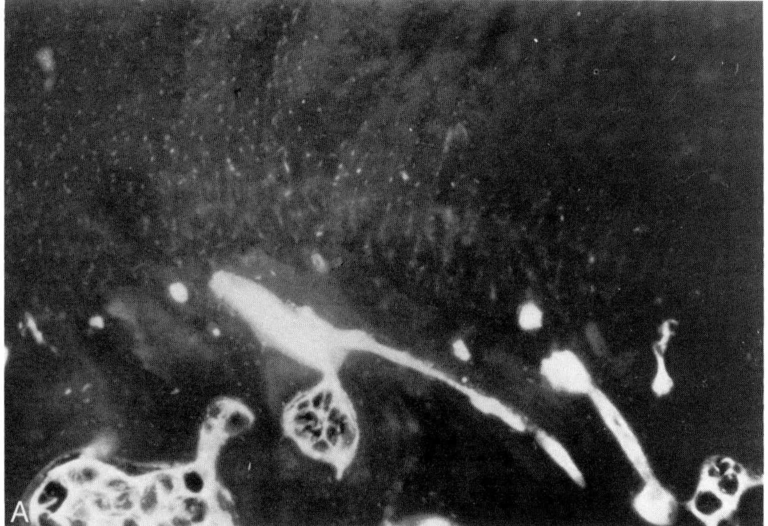

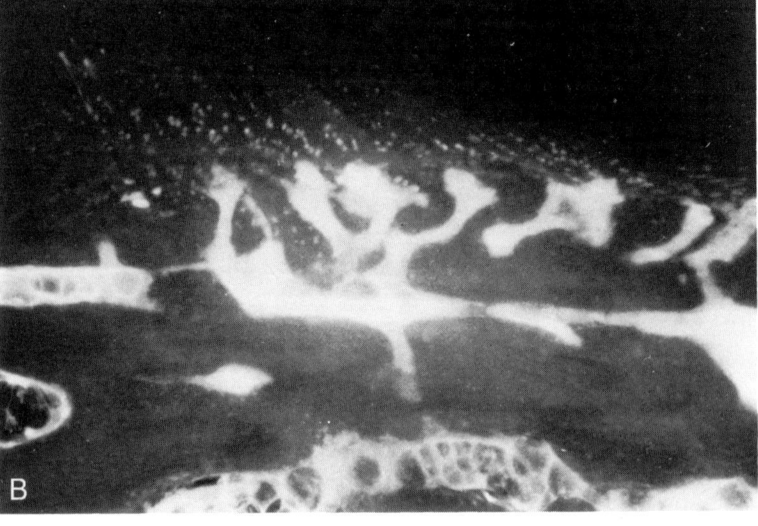

Figure 8–5. The bone-disc interface in *(A)* the region of the inner annulus fibrosus and *(B)* the area of the nucleus-annulus interface. Tetracycline was injected intravenously and the discs were excised. After histologic preparation, disc slices were viewed in a fluorescence microscope.

	SAGITTAL SECTION	
	ANTERIOR	POSTERIOR
OUTER ANNULUS FIBROSUS	17.2 ± 3.7	25.8 ± 4.1
INNER ANNULUS FIBROSUS	38.7 ± 6.4	43.5 ± 7.3
NUCLEUS PULPOSUS	83.6 ± 4.2	84.9 ± 5.0

Figure 8–6. Blood vessel contacts (percentage and S.D.) close to the canine intervertebral disc.

the undegenerated nucleus tissue displaces backward and forward with these movements of the spine.

The vertebral end plates, consisting of layers of hyaline cartilage, are attached to the cranial and caudal aspects of the disc.[51] They serve to anchor the disc fibers and act as a barrier between the vascular spongiosa of the vertebral body and the avascular disc. There are numerous pits and perforations in the adult end plate that may serve as channels for fluid and chemical interchange between the spongiosa and the disc.[201, 231] Furthermore, the end plates serve as a major transport route into the disc, and mediate solutes to and waste products from the blood vessels (Fig. 8–5). The blood vessels, which are present in the vertebral bodies as well as within the epidural space, are essential for the nutrition of the avascular disc. The size of the contact area of the blood vessels, with the bony end plate and the periphery of the discs, governs the transport rates of various solutes. For adequate disc nutrition a very large and efficient capillary contact area is essential (Fig. 8–6).[109]

The intrinsic stability of the motion segment, and thus of the whole spine, is due mainly to the intervertebral discs and the ligaments associated with them. The extrinsic stability is related to the paraspinal and trunk muscles. The anterior and posterior longitudinal ligaments consist of dense fibrous connective tissue in close union with the annulus fibrosus. The former is attached to the vertebral end plates. The posterior longitudinal ligament is thinner than the anterior and consists of a series of fanlike bands that span across the posterolateral aspects of each disc and are not attached very firmly to it (Fig. 8–7). The posterior vertebral arches support the interspinous and supraspinous ligaments and the ligamenta flava. The articular facets restrict anteroposterior gliding and rotation movements, but they have only a small part to play in the distribution of stress applied to that segment of the spine. Furthermore, the axis of bending does not pass through the center of the vertebral body and the disc, but passes through the center of the nucleus pulposus.[201]

Matrix of the Disc

The matrix of the intervertebral disc is very similar in composition to that of articular cartilage. It consists principally of collagen fibers embedded in a proteoglycan-water gel. Contained within this matrix are cells, which are actively maintaining and repairing it. Because of the low cellularity, the properties of the disc depend chiefly on the constituents of the matrix. The relative proportions of the latter vary with position in the disc and with age.

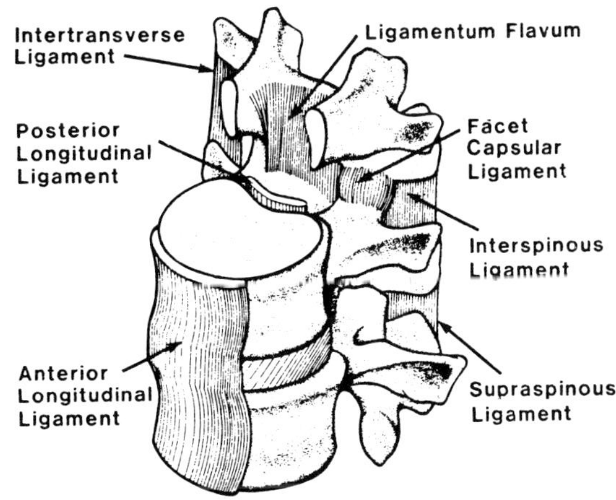

Figure 8–7. The motion segment (the disc and two adjacent intervertebral bodies) with its stabilizing ligaments. (From Bogduk, N., Windsor, M., and Inglis, A.: The innervation of the cervical intervertebral discs. Spine *13*:2–8, 1988.)

Proteoglycans. Proteoglycans are a family of macromolecules that consist of a central protein core attached to glycosaminoglycan (GAG) side chains (Fig. 8–8). The proteoglycans of the disc, like those of articular cartilage, are heterogeneous and polydisperse.[4, 28, 269, 270] In articular cartilage most proteoglycans exist as aggregates formed by the interaction of a single chain of hyaluronic acid with many proteoglycan molecules.[93] Although there is a considerable amount of hyaluronate in the human disc compared with cartilage (about 4 per cent of the total GAG in the disc is hyaluronate, compared with less than 1 per cent in articular cartilage),[92] only about 5 to 10 per cent of disc proteoglycan is aggregated.[57] Hence, disc proteoglycans are of smaller size than those in other cartilaginous tissues. This is probably why a large proportion of the proteoglycans can easily be extracted with dilute salts.[4, 57, 81] Adams and Muir[4] suggested that the portion of the proteoglycans that cannot be extracted is closely associated with the collagen fibrils, and increases with age.

The GAG side chains in the disc consist predominantly of chondroitin-6-sulfate (CS) and keratan sulfate (KS).[278] Both glycosaminoglycans, i.e., CS and KS, contain charged acidic groups (SO_3^- and COO^-), which give the matrix a net negative charge. CS has two negative charges per disaccharide unit, whereas KS has only one. There may also be some disulfated or nonsulfated disaccharides in the polymer.[151] However, in the case of articular cartilage, the correlation between the directly measured fixed charge density and the concentration of GAG determined by chemical analysis indicates that these cannot constitute more than a very small fraction of the total GAG.[171]

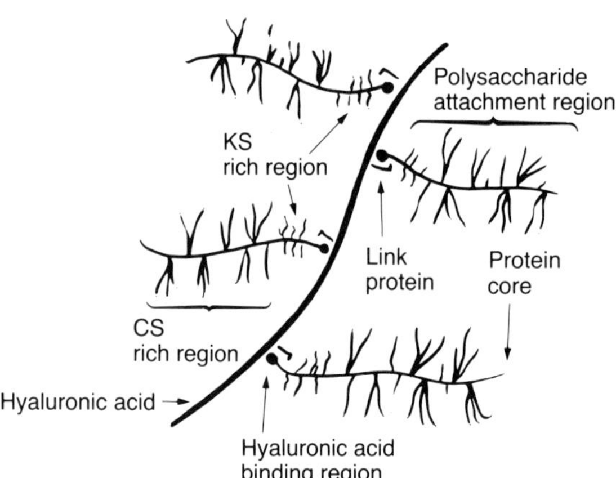

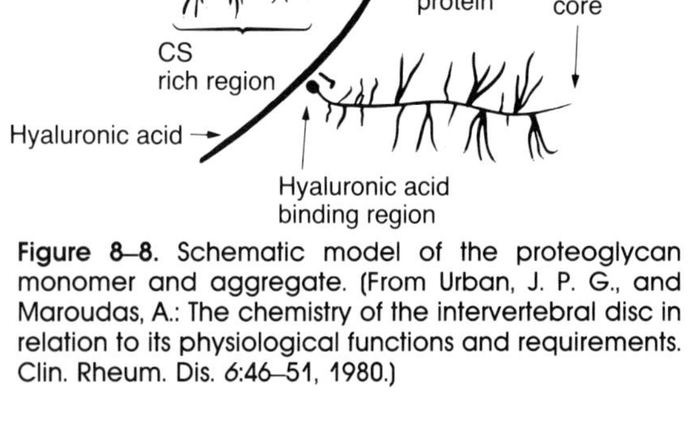

Figure 8–8. Schematic model of the proteoglycan monomer and aggregate. (From Urban, J. P. G., and Maroudas, A.: The chemistry of the intervertebral disc in relation to its physiological functions and requirements. Clin. Rheum. Dis. *6*:46–51, 1980.)

	Dog (3 yrs)	Pig (3 yrs)	Man (30 yrs)
Outer annulus (ant)	350	500	900
Inner annulus (ant)	420	700	1050
Nucleus	750	900	1350
Inner annulus (post)	630	800	1170
Outer annulus (post)	510	630	990

Figure 8–9. Turnover time in days (i.e., the time necessary to totally replace the proteoglycan molecules) in various areas of the intervertebral disc of different species. For a 30-year-old man, a replacement of a proteoglycan molecule in the nucleus pulposus takes more than three years!

The ratio of CS to KS varies across the disc and also changes with age and with degeneration. In general the proportion of KS rises with age. Therefore, the charge density does not increase as fast as the proportion of total GAG in the tissue. Furthermore, the turnover time (time for total replacement of the proteoglycan molecule) also changes with age and position within the tissue (Fig. 8–9).[8, 74, 75]

The GAGs, because they are charged and flexible, develop a large "swelling pressure" in the matrix, which enables the disc to resist compressive loads. It is the fixed charge density itself, rather than the proteoglycan concentration, that determines solute equilibrium in the tissue, and therefore properties such as the swelling pressure of the disc.

Collagen. Collagen is a fibrous protein of great tensile strength. The organization and size of its fibers vary widely from tissue to tissue. The constituent molecular type is also specific for each tissue. In the disc there is a gradation of collagen type from nucleus to annulus. In the outer annulus the collagen belongs mostly to Type 1,[59] the type present in tissues such as dermis, bone, and tendon.[11] In the inner part of the annulus Type II collagen predominates.[11, 60] Only Type II is found in a healthy nucleus pulposus, and Type II collagen is characteristic of articular cartilage.[11]

In the disc, as in cartilage, the collagen fibrils are embedded in a proteoglycan-water gel. The difficulty of extracting the final fraction of proteoglycan from the tissue[94] has been interpreted as implying a close association between collagen and some portion of the proteoglycans.[4] The nature of that association is not known, but entanglement and interpenetration, as well as electrostatic interactions, have been suggested. However, since the polymeric cartilage collagen has been found to have no net charge at physiologic pH,[171] the latter explanation for the association seems unlikely.

The organization of collagen fibrils in the disc is highly specialized. The three-dimensional collagen framework has been described by Inoue,[125] Takeda,[280] and Inoue and Takeda[126] (Fig. 8–10). In the annulus, collagen is arranged in 15 to 20 concentric lamellae[278] made up of parallel bundles, 10 to 50 microns in size. Each bundle is composed of fine fibrils, reported by Takeda[280] and Inoue and Takeda[126] as 0.1 to 0.2 microns in diameter, but by Szirmai[278] as finer than this. These lamellae are visible to the naked eye and vary from 200 to 400 microns in width, the outer lamellae being the thickest. The lamellae in the posterior aspect of the disc are not as wide as in the rest of the tissue.[280] The fiber bundles of each lamella run obliquely between the adjacent vertebral bodies and are firmly anchored either to them or to the cartilaginous end plate.[103, 278] The resulting angle formed between the fiber bundles of the lamellae and the vertebral bodies varies between 40 and 70 degrees, the direction of the fibers alternating in neighboring lamellae.[278] Naylor[200] showed how the angle changes with the position in the annulus.

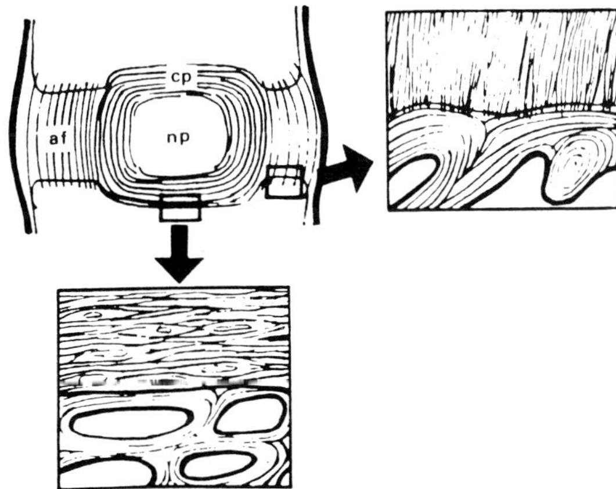

Figure 8–10. Schematic representation of the collagen framework of the intervertebral disc and interconnection of the nucleus pulposus (np), annulus fibrosus (af), and cartilage end plate (cp). (From Inoue, H.: Three dimensional observation of collagen framework of intervertebral discs in rats, dogs and humans. Arch. Histol. Jpn. *36*:39–56, 1973.)

In the nucleus the collagen fibrils are about 500 Å in diameter and are much finer than in the annulus. They are arranged in an irregular meshwork. The nucleus fibers are not connected to the cartilaginous end plate.[280] However, at the boundary with the annulus these fibrils merge with those of the inner concentric lamellae.

The arrangement of the collagen network in the disc has an important influence on how load is distributed. Since the lamellae are only loosely interconnected, the angle between the fiber bundles of the adjacent lamellae is changeable.[278] Thus, even though the collagen molecule itself is only slightly extensible, the fact that the lamellae can move separately gives the total structure considerable extensibility, especially in the vertical direction.[66] The annulus is able to bulge outward under evenly applied pressure because of the gel-like nucleus. When, with age, the nucleus loses its gel-like character, it is no longer able to act hydrostatically and comes to act more like a viscoelastic solid. Compressive stresses are then no longer evenly distributed to the end plates and annulus. High local stresses in the annulus may then occur and lead to its eventual degeneration.[103]

Noncollagenous Proteins. In addition to collagen and proteoglycan, the disc contains a considerable fraction of noncollagenous proteins, glycoproteins, and other uncharacterized material. The biologic function of these substances is not yet understood.[73, 91]

Cells. The disc has a low cell density. The mean figure for cells in a human disc is 5800 cells/mm^3,[172] whereas for the canine intervertebral disc the mean figure is in the region of 17,000 to 18,000 cells/mm^3. The cell density is not uniformly distributed throughout the tissue but higher at the periphery of the annulus and close to the end plates (Fig. 8–11).[112, 116, 172]

The cells are different in shape and are separated from each other by intervening matrix. Cells do, however, occur in groups in the tissue, especially along the lamellae. In the nucleus pulposus the cells are rounded,

Figure 8–11. Cell density profiles across the intervertebral disc. The density profile for the human disc is very flat, whereas for animals the profiles tend to decrease very close to the vertebral end plate, where a flood-layer is generally seen. (From Holm, S. and Urban, J.: The intervertebral disc: factors contributing to its nutrition and matrix turnover. *In* Helminen, H. J., Kiviranta, I., Tammi, M., et al. (eds.): Joint Loading. Chapter 8, Bristol, Wright, 1987, pp. 187–226).

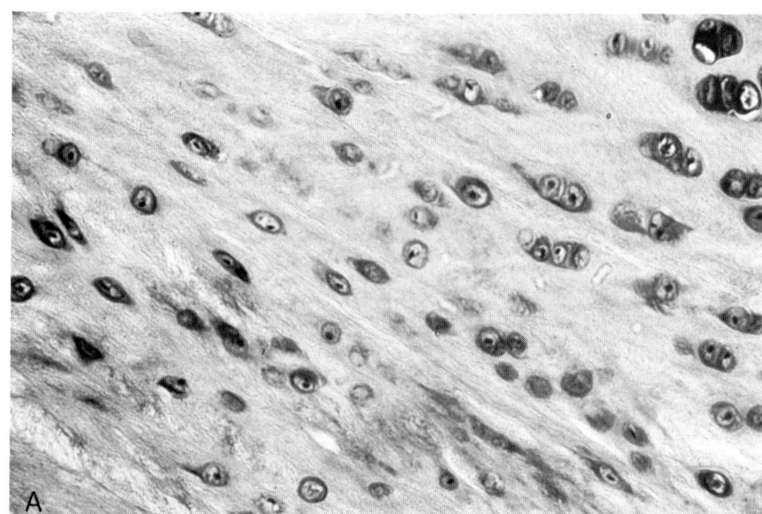

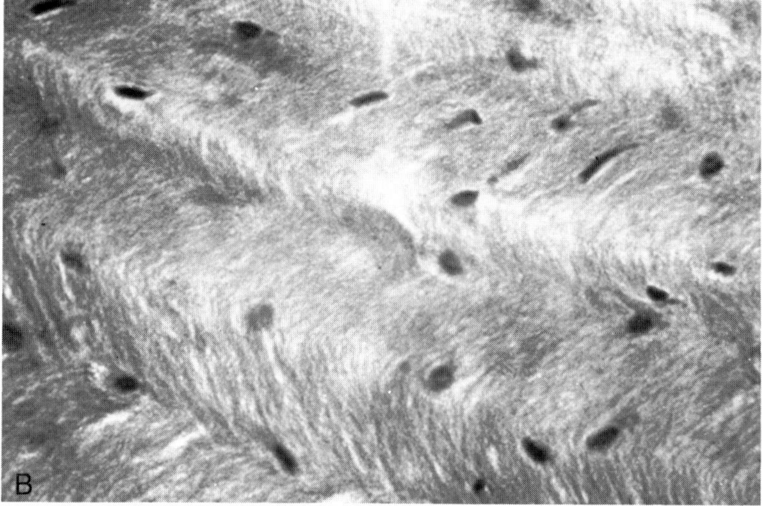

Figure 8–12. Human disc cells (30-year-old man). *A*, Rounded cells in the nucleus pulposus. *B*, Elongated cells in the annulus fibrosus.

whereas in the annulus cells are more cigar shaped (Fig. 8–12).[172, 201]

These observations suggest that there is possibly a functional relationship between the shape of the cells and the degree of fibril orientation. Thus, in the annulus cells the fibrils concentrate at the end of the cells where newly produced fibrils occur. They are oriented parallel to the existing ones. In the nucleus, however, the fibrils are randomly oriented among the pyknotic cells.[201, 233]

Water. Water containing dissolved solutes is the main constituent of the disc; it occupies 65 to 90 per cent of the tissue volume, depending on age and region (Table 8–1). Since the cell density is low, most of this water is extracellular. Some of it is associated with the collagen fibers as intrafibrillar water, but the proportion of the native collagen of the disc is not known. In articular cartilage intrafibrillar water is freely exchangeable.[169] However, it is not known whether it is accessible to larger molecules such as immunoglobulins, or to the proteoglycan molecules themselves.[171] If it were inaccessible to the proteoglycans, this would result in a considerable osmotic pressure difference between extra- and intrafibrillar fluid regions.[171]

Relative Proportions of Matrix Constituents. The proportions of matrix constituents vary considerably with position in the tissue and also with age. The composition of the disc changes markedly throughout life. It can be seen that the water content of the nucleus, very high in juveniles, decreases rapidly to approach that of the annulus in mature adults.

Table 8–1. WATER CONTENT (PERCENTAGE) IN THE ANNULUS AND NUCLEUS OF PORCINE, CANINE, AND HUMAN DISCS OF VARIOUS AGES

	Nucleus Pulposus	Inner Annulus	Outer Annulus
Pig			
Young	88	76	70
Adult	76	70	65
Old	70	65	61
Dog			
Young	85	75	73
Adult	80	69	65
Old	75	65	60
Man			
Young	81	70	68
Adult	70	65	58
Old	60	57	53

The water content of the annulus, however, stays fairly steady throughout life (Table 8–1). The fraction of hexosamine in the total dry weight of disc tissue also decreases with age,[81, 86] while the collagen content increases in both the nucleus[4, 87] and annulus.[4] The nonextractable portion of the matrix also increases with age,[4, 81, 87] as does the KS:CS ratio.

The changes that occur with age are such that, over time, in many respects the composition of the nucleus seems to approach that of the annulus. The nucleus becomes less hydrated. The water content drops from over 85 per cent in preadolescence to about 70 to 75 per cent in middle age.[81] The fixed charge density of the nucleus falls from about 0.3 to about 0.1 mEq per ml[291] over the same period. However, with age the ratio of keratan to chondroitin sulfate in the nucleus increases to well above the level found in the annulus.[4, 86] This increase could result from a shortening of the protein core with age; the molecular weight of the proteoglycans from the nucleus has been found to decrease with age.[28, 32]

Very little information is available on how the composition of the disc changes with the anatomic level in the spine. Adams and Muir[4] found some variations in a mature spine (44 years) but none of significance in younger spines (16 and 8 years). In a mature spine the fraction of collagen on a dry weight basis increases considerably between T12–L1 and L5–S1.

Nutrition: Transport and Metabolism

For an understanding of disc nutrition, the factors that control transfer of solutes into the disc must be quantified. With regard to the area of contact, previous studies[24, 88, 109, 195] have indicated the existence of two routes into the disc, via the periphery of the annulus and through the disc bone interface (Fig. 8–13). However, only a few attempts have been made to quantify the relative importance of the two routes.[109, 130, 172, 287, 289]

The metabolism of the disc is predominantly anaerobic, since the proportion of glucose being converted to carbon dioxide is no more than 2 to 5 per cent of the total glucose consumed, even at a high oxygen concentration.[109] Moreover, oxygen consumption per cell

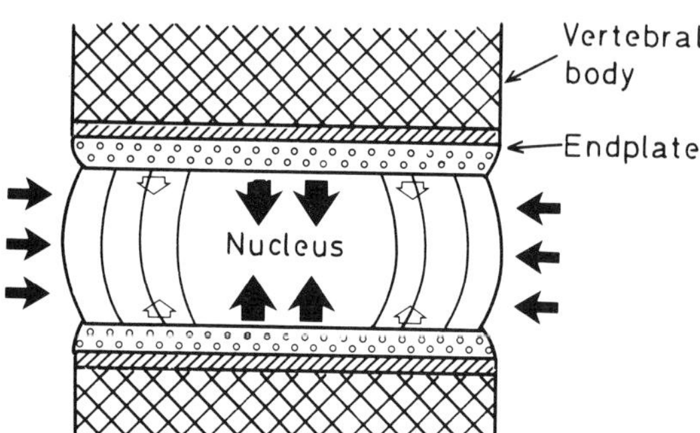

Figure 8–13. Schematic representation of the nutritional routes into the intervertebral disc system. (From Holm, S., Maroudas, A., Urban, J. P. G., et al.: Nutrition of the intervertebral disc. Connect. Tissue Res. *8*:101–119, 1981.)

is comparable with that of other avascular tissues, such as cornea, stroma, and articular cartilage.[109] However, it is only about one twentieth of the oxygen consumption per cell of tissues such as liver or kidney. The rate of production of lactic acid is relatively high. This is consistent with the finding of Diamant and colleagues that the pH in the center of the disc is considerably lower than the normal pH 7 level.[48]

Holm and associates[109] showed that the oxygen consumption per cell is similar in all regions of the disc. However, because of differences in cell density, this leads to a far lower oxygen consumption per gram of tissue in the nucleus than in the outer annulus. Because the disc is a large avascular tissue, and the nutrients can reach the cells only by passive diffusion from the peripheral blood vessels, there are large gradients in the concentration of oxygen and other metabolites (Fig. 8–14). The oxygen tension in the center of the nucleus is very low, being only about 2 to 5 mm Hg.[109] It has been shown that only at a very low oxygen tension (in the range of 0 to 4 mm Hg) does oxygen consumption show strong dependence on oxygen concentration (Table 8–2).[109] Therefore, differences in oxygen content across the disc probably have only a small influence on the basic metabolism of disc cells, but they may play a part in controlling matrix production.[141, 166]

Transport Properties

Diffusion. Diffusion can be thought of as the motion of solute molecules in response to a driving force provided by the gradient in chemical potential. In dilute solutions, where no interactions between solutes occur and where the behavior of solutes is close to ideal, diffusion can be described by Fick's first law, with solute flux proportional to the concentration gradient (Fig. 8–15).

The solute diffusivity is constant throughout a given disc system when considering low solute concentrations, or for systems in which the gradient in concentration is equal to the gradient in chemical potential. For diffusion of electrolytes through an electric field, which could be the case in a charged matrix or in a mixture of other ionic solutes, the chemical

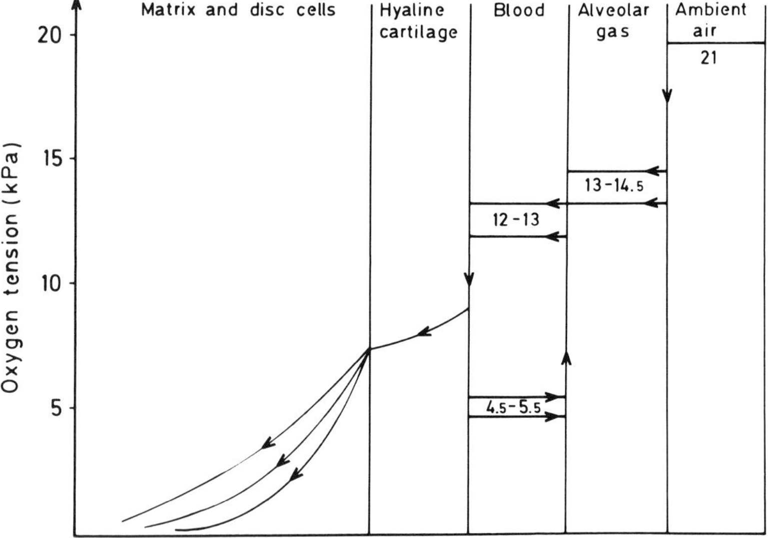

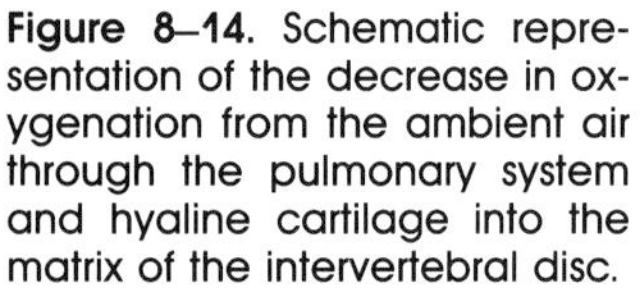
Figure 8–14. Schematic representation of the decrease in oxygenation from the ambient air through the pulmonary system and hyaline cartilage into the matrix of the intervertebral disc.

Table 8–2. RATES OF GLYCOLYSIS IN THE NUCLEUS PULPOSUS OBTAINED AFTER INCUBATION AT VARIOUS OXYGEN TENSION LEVELS, INCLUDING ALSO VARIOUS OXYEN CONSUMPTION RATES OBTAINED IN A GILSON RESPIROMETER

Oxygen Tension (kPa)	Oxygen Uptake (μmol/g/hr)	Glucose Uptake (μmol/g/hr)	Lactic Acid Production (μmol/g/hr)	Carbon Dioxide Production (μmol/g/hr)
0.3	0.039	3.3	6.4	0.042
0.9	0.10	3.3	6.4	0.075
1.8	0.13	2.9	6.0	0.13
3.9	0.165	2.7	5.1	0.13
9.8	0.18	2.3	4.5	0.17
19.9	0.19	2.3	4.6	0.17

From Holm, S., Maroudas, A., Urban, J. P. G., et al.: Nutrition of the intervertebral disc. Connect. Tissue Res. *8*:101–119, 1981.

potential is dependent on the field as well as the solute concentration. Diffusion under these conditions can be described by the Nernst-Planck equation.[97] A limitation of this equation, however, is that it does not take into account solute-solute or solvent-solute interactions, unless these alter the electric field gradient. However, a convertive term can be added to include the effect of solvent flow on solute transport.

TRANSPORT WITHIN THE DISC

$$\frac{\partial \bar{m}}{\partial t} = \frac{1}{\varrho}\frac{\partial J}{\partial x} + \frac{R}{S}\bar{m}$$

FICK'S LAW $\quad \frac{J}{\varrho} = -\bar{D}\frac{\partial \bar{m}}{\partial x}$

↓

$$\frac{\partial \bar{m}}{\partial t} = \bar{D}\frac{\partial^2 \bar{m}}{\partial x^2} + \frac{R}{S}\bar{m}$$

BOUNDARY CONDITIONS

$$\frac{\partial \bar{m}(A)}{\partial t} = \bar{D}\frac{\partial^2 \bar{m}(A)}{\partial x^2} + \frac{R}{S}\bar{m}(A)$$

R = Reaction rate

S = Total amount of non-tracer A

↑

energy demands
cell density
cell distribution
age/position/dimensions
blood vessels

Figure 8–15. Theoretical equations describing the transport of solutes within the disc and the boundary conditions, which must be evaluated in the calculations. (From Urban, J. P. G.: Fluid and solute transport in the intervertebral disc. Ph.D. Thesis, London University, 1977. Reproduced with kind permission from the author.)

Diffusion in a two-component system can be described in terms of a single diffusion coefficient. The diffusion coefficients, based on different reference systems, can be related to the "mutual"-diffusion coefficient based on constant volume.[35] When a system remains at constant composition, except for the interchange of radioactive isotopes, the process is described by the "self"-diffusion coefficient. In this case the "driving force" for diffusion is specific activity[97] and diffusion will continue until the system is at uniform specific activity.

In the disc charged solutes present an equilibrium concentration gradient, which has to be taken into account when tracer diffusion is considered.[287] The diffusion coefficient of a solute in a gel matrix is generally lower than that for the same solute in free solution, for several reasons. Helfferich[97] summarized these as follows:

1. Part of the tissue is occupied by the matrix so that the effective area for diffusion is less than that in free solution, and the diffusion paths are longer.
2. Frictional effects can retard molecules, which are moving through pores of similar diameter to their own.
3. Interaction with fixed groups may slow down counter-ion diffusion.

The diffusion coefficient characterizes the rate at which a solute moves by molecule diffusion: the larger the value of the diffusion coefficient, the faster is the rate of diffusion. The diffusion coefficient varies considerably with the size of the solute, and also in various solutions. Solutes diffuse more slowly in the disc than in a free solution. This is due to the presence of solutes within the tissue, which act as obstacles and lead to an increased tortuosity: the solute has to move through a longer path to cover a given distance than it would in free solution. The diffusion coefficient of small solutes in the disc, whether the solutes are charged or not, have values equal to about 40 to 60 per cent of their value in water.[221, 287, 288] Tortuosity increases with the concentration of solute in the matrix. Thus, solute diffusion coefficients in the annulus are lower than those in the more highly hydrated nucleus.[287] For large solutes the diffusion coefficient should be even further reduced, because, in addition to tortuosity, frictional effects also tend to retard the motion of these molecules within the matrix. In the degenerated tissue, with a decreased water content, the diffusional transport properties are accordingly reduced in comparison with normal highly hydrated tissue.

Partition Coefficient. The partition coefficient (or distribution coefficient) (Fig. 8–16) is defined as the ratio between the concentration in the tissue and the concentration in the external solution. Solute distribution depends on both charge and size.[109, 287]

Large solutes are sterically excluded by the macromolecules of the matrix. Anions are practically excluded by the fixed negative charges of the glycosaminoglycan groups, while cations, conversely, are preferentially taken up. Ions are distributed between the matrix of the disc and an external equilibrating solution in accordance with the Gibbs-Donnan equilibrium relationship.

Swelling of Disc Tissue. The matrix of the disc consists of two major structural components, collagen and proteoglycans. The proteo-

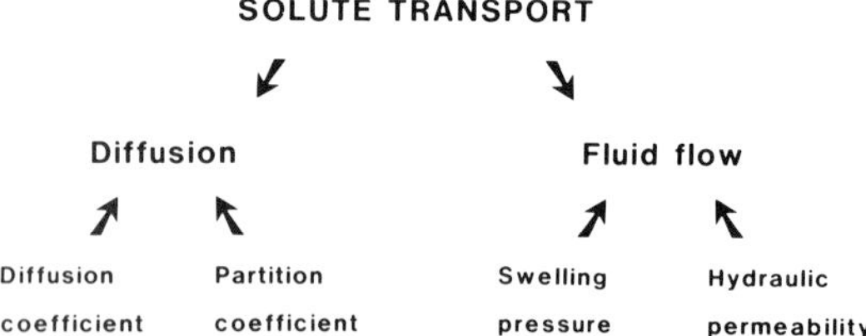

Figure 8–16. Solute transport into the avascular intervertebral disc is predominantly a function of diffusion and fluid flow, which in turn are dependent on more basic physicochemical parameters.

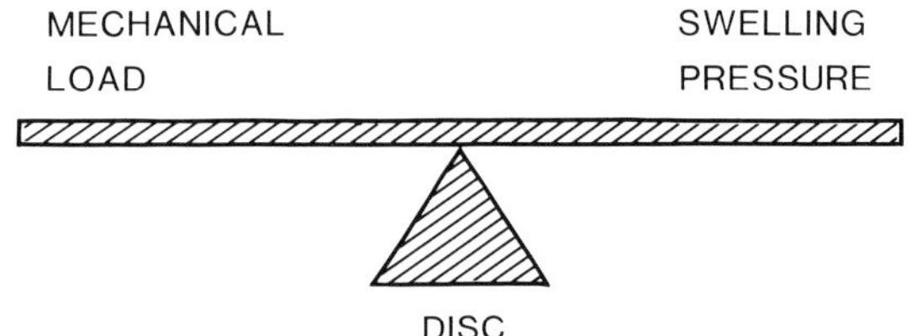

Figure 8–17. The intervertebral disc must at steady stage balance all applied mechanical loads via the swelling pressure created by the proteoglycans in the tissue. When the load exceeds the swelling pressure, fluid is lost from the disc. At rest, there is usually a re-imbibition of fluid back to equilibrium.

glycan solution has a high osmotic pressure and tends to imbibe water and inflate the specialized network of collagen fibers. The turgor of the disc is thus maintained, even under high compressive loads. The proteoglycans are also responsible for the very fine effective "pore size" of the tissue, thereby providing a high resistance to fluid flow and influencing the partition and transport of solutes. Both the osmotic pressure and the "pore size" of the proteoglycan solution are strongly concentration dependent. The behavior of the disc is therefore dictated to a large extent by its proteoglycan content.

The discs are known to possess a high osmotic pressure, which enables them to support physiologic loads of several atmospheres (Fig. 8–17).[170, 171, 291] This high osmotic pressure is generally attributed to the proteoglycan component. It arises partly from an ionic contribution in accordance with the Gibbs-Donnan equilibrium, and partly from a contribution by the polymeric nature of the proteoglycan molecules. Collagen adds little to the osmotic pressure of the tissue as such. At physiologic hydrations, the tension in the collagen network opposes the swelling tendency of the proteoglycans. The net swelling pressure (P_s) can be defined as the pressure that, when applied to tissue in contact with solution, is just sufficient to stop the tissue from losing or gaining water (Fig. 8–18).[170] If the proteoglycan swelling tendency is P_g and the resisting force of the collagen network is E, then at equilibrium

$$P_s = P_g - E = P_{Don} + P_{Poly} - E$$

where P_{Don} is the Donnan swelling pressure. The latter results from the excess of positive ions in the tissue due to the fixed charges of

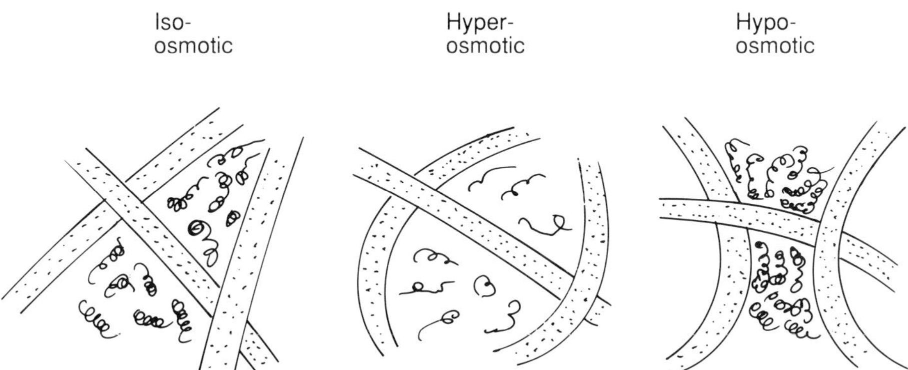

Figure 8–18. Schematic representation of a normal (iso-osmotic), swollen (hyperosmotic), and shrunken (hypo-osmotic) collagen-proteoglycan matrix in the intervertebral disc. Changes in the osmotic pressure and/or mechanical properties may result in increased swelling after imbibition of fluid, thus changing concentration gradients and transport properties of the tissue.

the glycosaminoglycan groups. P_{Poly}, the colloid swelling pressure, is derived from an entropic contribution resulting from the configurational possibilities of the polymer chains. The magnitude of both P_{Don} and P_{Poly} depends on the GAG concentration.

At physiologic hydration, the values of both P_{Don} and P_{Poly} lie in the range of 1.5 to 2.5 atmospheres for the nucleus, as well as the annulus.[287] These results are similar to those found in articular cartilage.[170]

The collagen resisting force (E) at physiologic hydrations is about 2 atmospheres in the annulus and about 1 atmosphere in the nucleus. The swelling pressure, which balances the original hydration, ranges from about 2 to 5 atmospheres.[287] The pressure exerted on the lumbar discs in vivo is of this magnitude.[194] Decreased hydration would lead to a less flexible structure and increased risk of, for example, disc rupture.

Hydraulic Permeability. The rate of solute transport depends on the number of blood vessel contacts with the disc, since solutes have to be transported to and from the avascular disc by blood vessels surrounding it. It has been found from in vivo work[24, 88, 288] and from in vivo studies on excised disc plugs[195] that there are two distinguishable nutritional routes into the disc: one from the blood vessels surrounding the outer region of the annulus, and the other from the blood vessels in the vertebral bodies. The outer portion of the bone end plate is virtually impermeable. In effect, only about one third of the end plate area, mainly in the region of the nucleus and the annulus, has blood vessels penetrating close to the interface with the disc. On the other hand, the periphery of the annulus is highly vascularized and completely permeable. Although the permeable area is the same for all solutes, the relative proportion of a particular solute that diffuses into the disc through each route depends on its partition coefficient at the disc interface. For uncharged solutes, such as glucose or oxygen, there will be little selectivity, and approximately equal amounts of solutes will travel by each pathway (see Fig. 8–13). For a negatively charged solute, such as the sulfate ion, because of the great exclusion force exerted by the highly charged nucleus, diffusion through the end plates is less efficient. On the other hand, for a positively charged solute such as calcium, penetration through the end plates is much greater than through the periphery of the annulus fibrosus.[288]

Nachemson and colleagues[195] found that in a significant proportion of the adult human discs studied, the permeability of the end plates was much reduced. There was a strong correlation between end plate closure and disc degeneration. Brown and Tsaltas[26] found that the end plate permeability of rabbit discs decreased with age. Since the cells in the nucleus and in the annulus are dependent on these routes both for supply of nutrients and for removal of waste products, closure of the end plate may be expected to lead to nutritional deficiencies, as well as to a build-up of metabolic end products. Thus, changes in end plate permeability could be a path to disc degeneration.

The hydraulic permeability for tissues such as articular cartilage and corneal stroma is higher than in the disc at similar hydration, although the swelling-pressure curves are markedly different.[287] At a hydration of 70 per cent, corneal stroma has a swelling pressure of 0.6 atmospheres, articular cartilage one to six atmospheres, and discs (annulus fibrosus) one to six atmospheres. Both hydraulic permeability and swelling pressure are functions of the composition of the tissue. Since at normal hydrations flow occurs chiefly through the proteoglycan-water gel, the concentration of the proteoglycans governs the permeability.

Fluid Flow. From studies on articular cartilage[135, 170, 171] and the intervertebral disc,[287] it is clear that fluid flow plays an important role in determining the load-bearing behavior of connective tissue (see Fig. 8–16).

Tests of load deformation have shown the pattern of behavior of discs under additional compressive loads.[89, 168] As the load is applied, there is a rapid initial deformation, due almost entirely to bulging of the disc. When the load is removed, the disc returns to its original height. If the load is maintained after this initial elastic response, the disc continues to deform, but at a considerably reduced rate owing to loss of fluid. The fluid, squeezed out when load is applied to the disc and reabsorbed when load is removed, carries solutes with it.

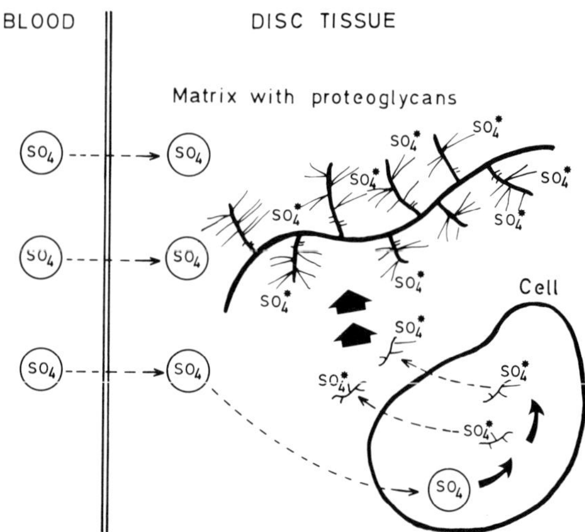

Figure 8–19. Incorporation of sulfate by the cells forming proteoglycan fragments and finally aggregation, thus creating a large proteoglycan molecule.

Metabolism

A major function of the cells is to synthesize proteoglycans. This helps ensure that the water-binding capacity is adequate. In order to do so, the metabolic reactions involve synthesis of proteoglycan fragments. Sulfate ion plays an important role in these processes (Fig. 8–19).[263]

The energy requirements for this synthesis are partially fulfilled by the anaerobic breakdown of glucose to lactic acid by the disc tissue. This process seems to follow the same pathways as that in other tissues, namely, the glycolytic sequence of reactions described in the Embden-Meyerhof process. Enzymes act catalytically by combining with their specific substrates, which place them in a functional state and capable of undergoing the specific chemical reactions. Thus, in series a large number of separate activated enzyme reactions occur. These reactions are linked in a chain through which, for example, in this particular case, glucose is converted into lactic acid.[109, 152, 167]

Certain other substances, besides the specific enzymes and their substrates, are essential for the breakdown of glucose to lactic acid. These are coenzymes such as adenosine triphosphate (ATP) and diphosphopyridine nucleotide (DPN). ATP is the coenzyme of phosphorylation and DPN is involved with oxidations and reductions.[272]

Coenzymes might be considered a type of substrate, since they are chemically changed in the reaction, but they differ from the substrates of metabolism in that they are constantly regenerated. DPN is involved in many different reactions, including glycolysis. The latter describes the breakdown of one molecule of glucose to two molecules of lactic acid. The oxidation-reduction system of DPN may be written:

$$DPN^+ + 2H^+ + 2E \rightarrow DPNH + H^+$$

One equivalent of acid (i.e., H^+) is formed during the reduction of DPN.

The second coenzyme of glycolysis, ATP, takes part in four reactions in the glycolytic breakdown of glucose. The overall reaction of glucose breakdown is

$$C_6H_{12}O_6 + 2H_3PO_4 + 2ADP \rightarrow 2C_3H_6O_3 + 2ATP + 2H_2O$$

For each molecule of glucose, combined with two molecules of ADP and two of inorganic phosphate, two molecules of lactic acid are produced and two molecules of ATP are formed.[109]

Oxidative Metabolism of Carbohydrate. When glucose is converted to lactic acid in the disc tissue cells, by way of the glycolytic cycle, oxygen is not used. However, a small but significant amount of oxygen is consumed by the disc. Therefore, pathways of oxidation must be considered (Table 8–2).[314]

The Cytochrome System. The ultimate choice of an acceptor in respiration is molecular oxygen. The direct reduction of molecular oxygen in most tissues occurs through the cytochrome system. Electrons are transferred from the substrate, usually by the use of coenzymes and flavoproteins to cytochrome C. This reduced cytochrome C is then reoxidized by means of the enzyme cytochrome oxidase and oxygen:

$$\text{reduced cytochrome C} + 0.5\ O_2 \rightarrow \text{cytochrome C} + H_2O.$$

The hydrogen (electrons) of the metabolite is passed from coenzyme to coenzyme until it reduces oxygen and is removed as water. The respiration of cells and tissues is accompanied by the incorporation of inorganic phosphate into ADP to form ATP. Oxidation therefore results in an increase of the available energy within the tissue, in the form of high-energy phosphate.[267, 272]

The Citric Acid Cycle of Oxidation. Under anaerobic conditions the pyruvic acid that arises from the glycolytic breakdown of glucose is reduced to lactic acid. This is the end product.[215] However, under aerobic conditions the pyruvic acid is oxidized, step by step, to carbon dioxide and water in a series of reactions known as the citric acid, or Krebs, cycle. The overall reaction is represented by the following formula, although there are many intermediate steps:

$$\text{Acetyl } C_OA + 3NAD^+ + FAD + GDP + P_i + H_2O \rightarrow 2CO_2 + 3NADH + FADH_2 + GTP + 2H^+ + C_OA$$

The substances that enter the cycle are acetyl coenzyme A and water. Molecular oxygen does not participate directly in the citric acid cycle. However, the cycle operates only under aerobic conditions, because NAD^+ and FAD can be regenerated in the mitochondrion only by electron transfer to molecular oxygen. Glycolysis has both an aerobic and an anaerobic mode, whereas the citric acid cycle is strictly aerobic. Glycolysis can proceed under anaerobic conditions because NAD^+ is regenerated in the conversion of pyruvate to lactate.[272]

Oxidation of pyruvate through the citric acid cycle is certainly the main pathway in many animal tissues, not only for the oxidation of carbohydrates, but also for fatty acids and amino acids. In the intervertebral disc, however, the use of the citric acid cycle seems to be in the range of a small percentage of the total metabolic process.

However, there are other routes whereby glucose can be directly oxidized. Of these the best understood is the "hexosemonophosphate shunt." The significance of this pathway of oxidation in the disc has not been evaluated.

Pathophysiologic Mechanisms

Despite the clinical importance of lumbar intervertebral disc degeneration, no well-supported concept of its pathogenesis has emerged. The nucleus pulposus is the functional center of the disc, and when it loses its plasticity, and hence its load-bearing capacity, minor movements and loading may cause mechanical effects on the annulus, with the occasional result of annular ruptures and disc herniations.[180] Hirsch[102] hypothesized that disc herniation is a manifestation of disc degeneration. No ruptures occur in an annulus without the nucleus showing advanced structural changes.[103–105]

The most widely accepted reason for disc degeneration is an insufficient nutritional state of the disc tissue. Interestingly, blood vessels disappear from the disc at about the ages of 18 to 20 years. At the same age the first signs of degeneration can be seen.[228, 285] Reduced permeability of the vertebral end plate in connection with disc degeneration and age changes of the disc[26, 195] are associated with impaired transport of solutes and waste products. The latter causes accumulation of lactate and other end products, and hence lowers the pH. This in turn may activate matrix-degrading enzymes (Fig. 8–20).[109] All these processes occur at

AGE - DEGENERATION

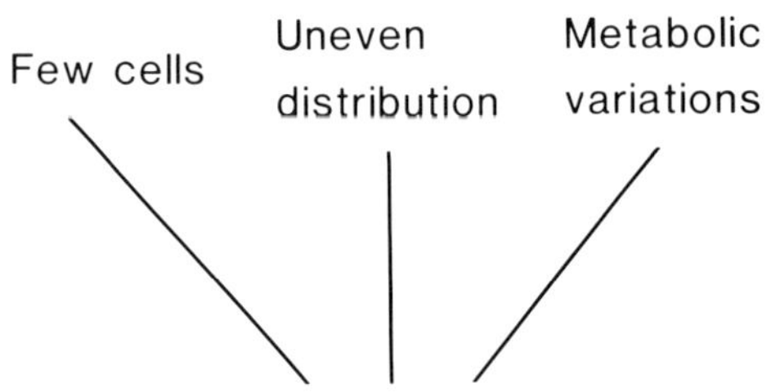

NUTRITIONAL DEFICIENCY

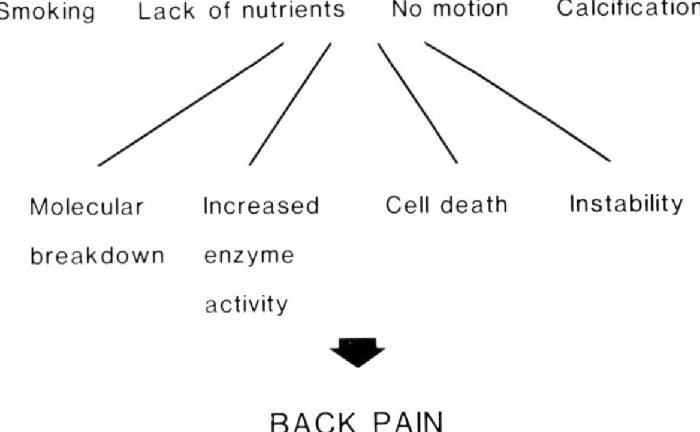

BACK PAIN

Figure 8–20. By age and degenerative processes, a nutritional deficiency occurs. Several other factors can potentiate this process, and the final result can be back pain in combination with other spinal disorders.

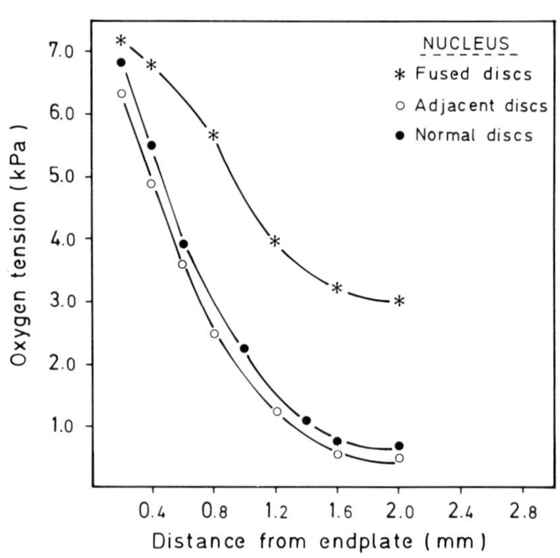

Figure 8–21. Oxygen tension profiles in the nucleus pulposus in fused spine, measured in vivo by thin needle electrodes. In the central area of the fused disc a roughly fivefold increase of oxygen tension was noted as compared with the normal and adjacent discs. Close to the vertebral end plate, the different discs exhibited oxygen tensions of a similar order of magnitude. (From Holm, S., and Nachemson, A.: Nutrition changes in the canine intervertebral disc after spinal fusion. Clin. Orthop. *169*:243–258, 1982.)

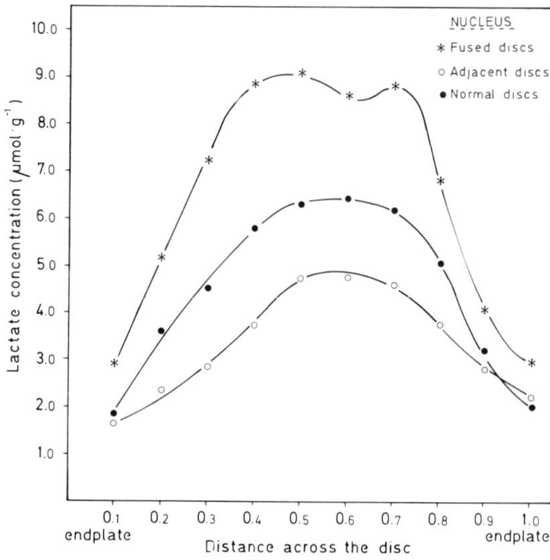

Figure 8–22. Lactate concentration profiles across the nucleus pulposus (end plate and end plate section) for normal discs and discs being fused for eight months. In the central nucleus of the fused disc, the lactate concentration increased significantly both in respect to the normal disc and to the adjacent discs ($p < 0.01$). The concentration profile decreased toward the end plates. (From Holm, S., and Nachemson, A.: Nutrition changes in the canine intervertebral disc after spinal fusion. Clin. Orthop. *169*:243–258, 1982.)

similar times, after age 20 to 25. Interestingly, radiographic changes suggesting degenerated discs are rarely seen below this age, and low back pain complaints manifest themselves increasingly from this age over the next two decades of life.

Models of Changes in Nutrition and Morphology

Fusion of Motion Segment. Fusion immobilizes the fused segment and changes mechanical stresses in both the fused and the adjacent discs.[110, 282] Holm and Nachemson[110] reported significant changes in several solutes (sulfate, glucose, oxygen) necessary for disc cell metabolism. The concentration of these solutes fell with time in the fused segments after fusion was achieved (Fig. 8–21). Consistent with the concentration fall in the fused segments, the activity in the adjacent discs increased. These changes suggest that metabolic activity is possibly triggered by spinal motion. There is also a large increase of lactic acid accumulation in the nucleus of the fused discs (Fig. 8–22). Perhaps this occurs because in the fused area

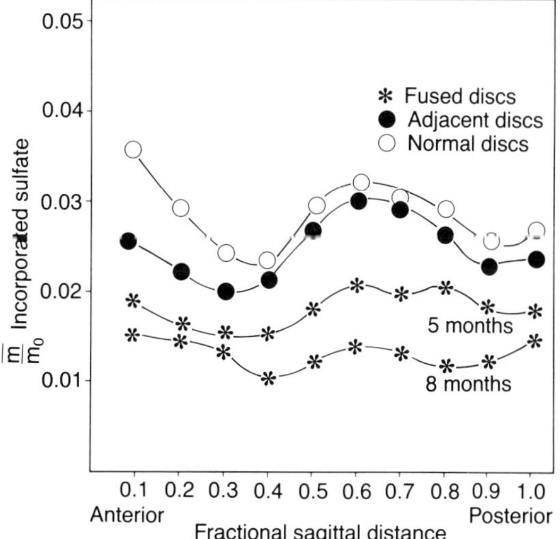

Figure 8–23. Incorporation of radioactive sulfate in both normal and fused intervertebral discs. The adjacent discs correspond to and should be compared with the disc being fused for eight months. In the anterior part of the annulus of the adjacent discs the incorporation was significantly increased in comparison with the normal discs ($p < 0.05$), whereas in other parts of the tissue the difference was not significant although it was higher. (From Holm, S., and Nachemson, A.: Nutrition changes in the canine intervertebral disc after spinal fusion. Clin. Orthop. *169*:243–258, 1982.)

the blood supply to the end plate of the disc is gradually reduced, thus partially closing one route for movement of solutes out of the tissue and allowing the concentration of metabolic products to build up.[109] Again, it is of specific interest to note that in the discs adjacent to the fused segments, which presumably also undergo abnormal mechanical stress, the changes are seen in the opposite direction to those seen in the fused segments, and are more like those observed in the discs of trained (i.e., physically conditioned) subjects (Fig. 8–23).

Exercise. There is no direct experimental evidence of the effect of exercise on proteoglycan synthesis rates in the disc. Animal studies performed by Holm and Nachemson[111] did not examine the proteoglycan composition of the disc as such, but rather evaluated the total production rate. The changes found in the thoracolumbar region, especially, were in direct contrast to those found in the discs of the fused segments (Fig. 8–24). In the former an increase in the transport rate of solutes was found and a greater consumption rate by the cells.[110, 111] The results indicate that various kinds of exercise improve nutritional properties (Fig. 8–25), while fusion results in a diminution of blood vessel capillary efficiency. Exercise does affect capillary growth in other tissues.[123] It is, however, difficult to judge what kind of training modes are beneficial for disc metabolism. At present it is impossible to differentiate sufficiently between various regimens, but results suggest that moderate exercising programs, as well as lateral bending, may be beneficial for transport properties (Table 8–3).

In tests in which there is an overload of stress involved, the rate of degenerative processes may increase. In studies using bipedal mice and rats, as well as those using rats on a treadmill exercising regimen, degenerative changes are created, especially in the nucleus.[101, 115, 317] Explanations for this have suggested the possibility of an increasing thickness of a calcified layer between the disc and the vertebral body, and also that the nutritional route through the end plate could be interrupted by increasing calcification and that this cessation of nutritional supply may lead to the observed disorders of the disc.

In all experimental, as well as clinical, models, when load is applied to the disc system, fluid is squeezed out of the tissue, thus resulting in a creep pattern. Urban[287] calculated that during a normal walking cycle, when the applied pressure is increased by about 15 per cent for one second, approximately 0.005 per cent of disc fluid is lost. During the day the applied pressures vary between 0.6 and 0.8 MN/m^2, depending on activity. The disc then loses about 10 per cent of its height as a result of viscoelastic creep during a 16-hour day. Because swelling is faster than creep, disc height can recover during the eight-hour night resting period, when the pressure on the disc returns to about 0.2 MN/m^2. Creep, occurring in all the discs of the spine, is probably re-

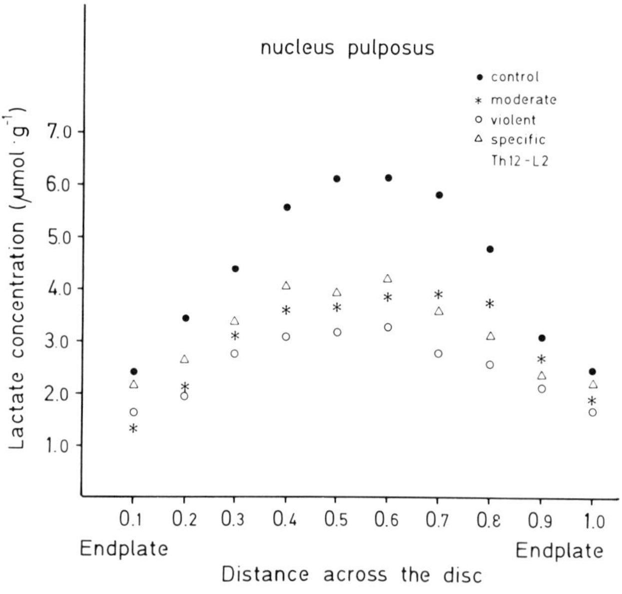

Figure 8–24. Lactate concentration profiles across the nucleus of thoracolumbar discs. The control animals were kept in cages, whereas three other groups of animals were exposed to either moderate, violent, or specific exercise. (From Holm, S., and Nachemson, A.: Variations in the nutrition of the canine intervertebral disc induced by motion. Spine *8*:866–874, 1983.)

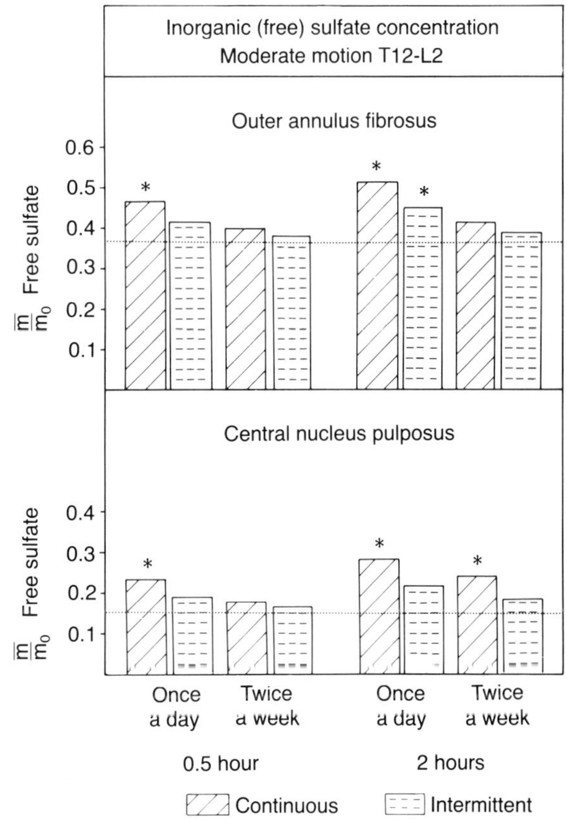

Figure 8–25. Exercise procedures of the canine spine, showing inorganic sulfate transport. Significant levels ($p < 0.05$) are indicated by a star. The exercising regimens are either continuous or intermittent (5-min exercise + 5-min rest, etc.) and the speed was moderate (jogging pace). (From Holm, S., and Nachemson, A.: Variations in the nutrition of the canine intervertebral disc induced by motion. Spine *8*:866–874, 1983.)

sponsible for the fact that the average person is about 1 to 3 per cent shorter at the end of the day than in the morning.

The magnitude of creep in the disc can be appreciated from the experimental observation of Kazarian,[131] who showed, as expected, that the creep rate depends on load applied and the grade of disc degeneration. The higher the load, or the greater the degree of degeneration, the faster is the creep rate. For a load of 10 kg the loss in height in 120 minutes was found to be 0.031 cm in a normal thoracic disc and 0.048 cm in a degenerative disc (Grade 3).[131]

Prolapse. End plate lesions (Schmorl's nodes), annular tears, and fissures in relation to biochemical changes for the prolapsed disc have been discussed by Taylor and Akeson.[281] The glycosaminoglycan content of prolapsed discs has been found to be lower, and the collagen content higher, than that of a normal comparable disc.[43, 181, 225] The water content of prolapsed discs is also lower than that of normal discs.[43] Whether the changes occurring are a result of proteoglycan loss or collagen increase after herniation, or whether prolapse follows changes in tissue biochemistry, is not known.

Table 8–3. TRANSPORT OF RADIOACTIVE SULFATE AND METHYLGLUCOSE INTO THE INTERVERTEBRAL DISCS

Disc Level	Outer Annulus Fibrosus *Sulfate*	Outer Annulus Fibrosus *Methylglucose*	Central Nucleus Pulposus *Sulfate*	Central Nucleus Pulposus *Methylglucose*
T12–L2	+19.5*	+30.4	+29.5**	+35.6
L3–L6	+13.2	+19.1	+17.0*	+22.4
L7	+ 5.1	+ 8.8	+10.4	+14.7

A daily halfhour program including continuous moderate exercise was used. Results are presented as a percentage from the results obtained in the control group. Positive (+) signs mean an increased rate of concentration. The levels of significance are indicated by stars (* = $p<0.05$, and ** = $p<0.01$).

From Holm, S., and Nachemson, A.: Variations in the nutrition of the canine intervertebral disc induced by motion. Spine *8*:866–874, 1983.

Scoliosis. Scoliosis often develops during the adolescent growth phase of life and is frequently idiopathic. However, scoliosis may also occur secondary to inherited connective tissue disorders such as Ehlers-Danlos syndrome and Marfan's syndrome. Changes in the biochemistry of discs, in cases of idiopathic scoliosis, as compared with normal controls, have been found by Ghosh,[76] Pedrini,[221] and Parsons[220] and their colleagues. In general, the findings show a decrease in glycosaminoglycan content of scoliotic discs and a proportional increase in collagen content. These changes in composition may result from alterations in the loading pattern on the spine because of the scoliosis.

Vibration. Epidemiologic studies have demonstrated an increasing incidence of back pain in subjects exposed to vibration.[227, 251, 258, 259] The intervertebral discs occupy about one third of the lumbar spine, and one of their major functions is to act like shock absorbers, equalizing and distributing applied loads. Normally, during lifetime, discs are subjected to forces acting variously in compression, distraction, torsion, shear, and vibration. Little is known about how the different forces influence the disc, its nutrition, and the synthesis rates of the cells. It is the cells and their nutritional support system that enable the largest avascular structure in the body to function in a physiologically acceptable manner. Although the cells are inhomogeneously distributed and sparse, they nevertheless must continue to produce collagen and proteoglycan macromolecules, in order to maintain specific mechanical properties of the discs. Vibration is known to have deleterious effects on different microvascular systems in the body. Therefore, there are reasons to assume that vibration may also affect the nutrition of the avascular lumbar intervertebral discs, which are critically dependent on highly efficient microcirculation close to the vertebral end plate and the periphery of the annulus fibrosus (Figs. 8–26, 8–27).[90, 114]

Permeable fraction of the porcine vertebral endplate (nucleus pulposus)	6 months %	1.5 yrs %	3 yrs %
Normal	85	78	65
Diabetic	73	65	50
Smoke exposed	50	43	30
Applied axial vibrations	62	55	45
Malnutrition	81	70	61

Figure 8–26. Permeable fraction of glucose of the porcine end plate in the nucleus region of the L4–L5 disc. The animals were of various ages and were exposed to induced diabetes (six months), smoke exposure (three hours), axial vibrations (six hours), and malnutrition (six months).

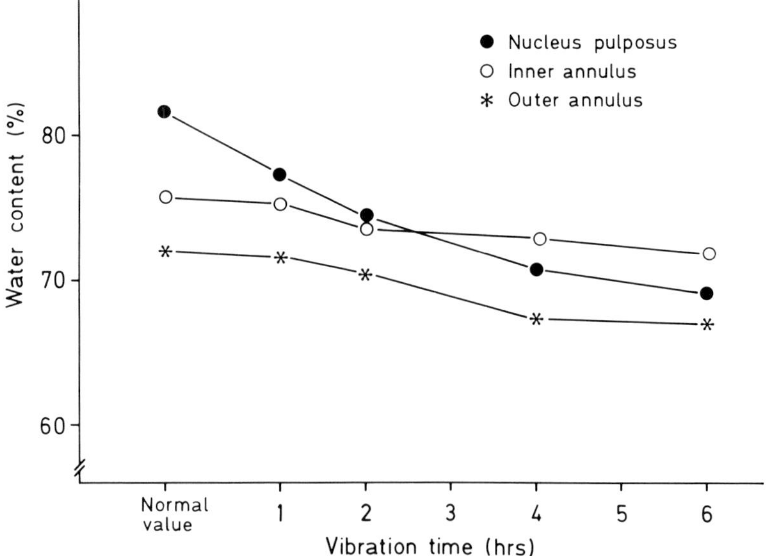

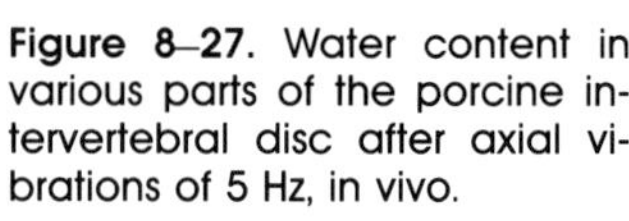

Figure 8–27. Water content in various parts of the porcine intervertebral disc after axial vibrations of 5 Hz, in vivo.

Smoking. The efficiency of solute delivery from the capillaries, the capacity of the avascular disc bed, and the dimensions of the disc systems are factors of specific importance. This is particularly true in the case of the large human discs in which the balance between nutrient utilization and supply is precarious. Any loss in blood vessel contact or reduction in blood flow at the periphery of the disc could lead to nutritional deficiencies and a build-up of waste products.[109, 112, 113, 117]

Several factors may be of potential risk in developing blockage of capillaries or acting directly on capillary walls, inducing constriction and consequently affecting blood flow. One such risk factor is cigarette smoking. Smoking is also regarded as a potential risk factor for initiating low back pain.[64, 134] The epidemiologic studies implicating smoking with low back pain unfortunately evaluated only the symptoms of low back pain and not any structural changes. Therefore, the conclusions of these studies are controversial and not conclusive.

Cigarette smoking has clearly been shown to affect the circulatory system outside the intervertebral disc, as well as cellular uptake rates and metabolite production within the disc (Figs. 8–26, 8–28). By reducing the transport of substrate into the disc and waste products out of the system, the inevitable consequence over a long period is deficient nutrition, leading to degenerative metabolic processes, disc dehydration, instability, and probably low back pain.

Diabetes. As mentioned above, the microcirculatory system outside the disc is critical for the supply of relevant nutrients, as well as disposal of waste products from the disc. Any disturbance in the capillary network may lead to problems for the centrally located cells and inevitably lead to degenerative processes in the tissue. One risk factor that may change the arterial transport properties outside the disc system is diabetes. Diabetes often leads to acceleration of atherosclerosis and consequently may induce impairment of circulation. It has been shown that experimentally induced diabetes causes a significant negative process in the intervertebral disc.[107] From the studies of experimentally induced diabetes, one can conclude that the circulatory system outside the disc supplies nutrients to the avascular structures, and cannot undergo any significant negative changes and continue to meet the

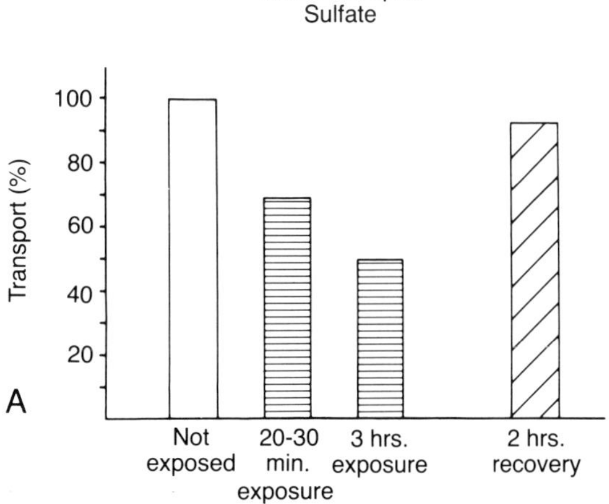

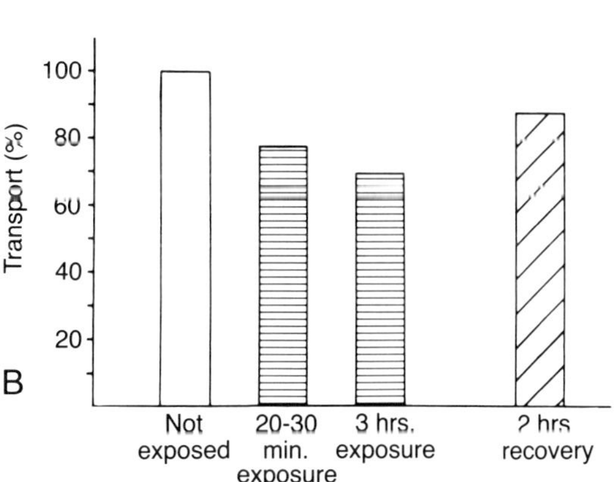

Figure 8–28. Solute transport (*A*, sulfate and *B*, methylglucose) into the porcine disc after various times of acute exposure of cigarette smoke. Included are also normal transport rates and the situation after two hours of recovery. (From Holm, S., and Nachemson, A.: Immediate effects of cigarette smoke on nutrition of the intervertebral disc of the pig. Orthop. Trans. *8*:380, 1984.)

metabolic requirements of the disc tissue cells (see Fig. 8–26). Consequently, a reduction in the blood flow and nutritional exchange area close to the intervertebral disc may lead to a breakdown of the disc tissue.

Experimental Disc Degeneration. Most observations of the degenerative process of the disc are made on whole discs, which have been obtained as surgical or postmortem specimens at a specific time point of tissue during degeneration. Therefore, neither sequential changes, nor changes occurring in specific areas, have been assessed. A few different models of experimental disc degeneration have, however, been developed. Bercovici and Paraschivesco injected hyaluronidase into the disc.[14] Intradiscal injection of chymopapain has also been used to induce experimental disc degeneration.[22] The clinical use of intradiscal injection of chymopapain to treat disc herniation and sciatica is well known.[25, 177, 198] Lindblom produced degeneration in the discs of rat tails by tying them up in the shape of a U and maintained the position for several weeks.[146] The most frequent method to produce experimental disc degeneration, however, is the model described by Lipson and Muir[149, 150] which was used as early as 1951 by Smith and Walmsley.[261] An injury is made surgically to the disc of the rabbit by incision with a knife in the ventral part of the annulus. In most previous studies using this model, only morphology and histology were examined. Lipson and Muir, however, also examined the proteoglycan changes in the disc of the rabbit during the healing and the degeneration process. They observed that the annulus healed by scar tissue within three to four weeks after surgery. All other parts of the disc, except the posterior part of the annulus, started to disorganize and degenerate progressively. In six months the disc had the "crabmeat" appearance seen in advanced human disc degeneration.

The chemical changes seen in this model include decrease of water and total proteoglycan (uronic acid) contents on the first day after the operation, followed by a rapid return to the normal state on the fourth day, after which the contents of water and proteoglycans of the discs were progressively lost. The contents of uronic acid also decreased rapidly in the first week and continued to decrease slowly thereafter. However, the size of the proteoglycan monomers did not change with degeneration. In the new aggregates there was an initial fall for three weeks, after which time they were restored. After six weeks, however, the proportions of the aggregates began to decline progressively. The early events in the proteoglycan metabolism appear to be an attempt by the tissue to repair the defect.[148]

Disc Degeneration versus Aging

In most cases no specific, identifiable cause for disc degeneration can be demonstrated; i.e., the condition may be called idiopathic disc degeneration. The word "idiopathic" means "of unknown causation"[52] and with regard to disc degeneration, this term relates to the widespread appearance of degenerated discs in the population (Fig. 8–29). There are conflicting data regarding the possible role of such degenerated discs in the occurrence of low back pain.[67, 148, 180] Intervertebral disc degeneration is often demonstrated in adults with low back pain,[132] but a direct causal relationship between the existence of disc degeneration and low back pain has not definitively been proved.[67, 124, 164] However, herniation of the intervertebral disc with compression of the nearby spinal nerve root is a condition in which there seems to be a direct relation between changes in the disc and the occurrence of pain, in this instance sciatic pain, although details in the pathophysiologic mechanisms behind such nerve root pain are incompletely understood.[85, 133, 182, 235, 242, 245, 303] It has also been extensively debated whether disc degeneration is primarily a disease process or a phenomenon more related to physiologic aging.[67, 148] In discussing this matter, it should be considered that the intervertebral disc has a basic, well-defined reaction pattern in terms of a sequence of degenerative changes, regardless of the cause of these alterations.[108, 148] Specific causes have been discussed above, but for most cases of disc degeneration it may not be possible to establish any particular etiology, just as for low back pain itself.

NEURAL STRUCTURES

Morphologic and Physiologic Aspects

Innervation of Motion Segment

Local tissue innervation has been shown to exist in most tissues in the motion segment, except in the nucleus pulposus.[19, 77, 102, 136, 199, 222, 260, 318] The terminal innervation of various tissues is derived from the sinuvertebral nerve (often called the nerve of Luschka), which branches from the first part of the spinal nerve and/or from the dorsal root ganglion.[216] The sinuvertebral nerve passes in the upper part of the intervertebral foramen toward the posterior longitudinal ligament. Each nerve divides into cranially and caudally coursing branches that innervate the various tissues in the spinal motion segment.[216] It may be of clinical significance that each nerve seems to innervate at

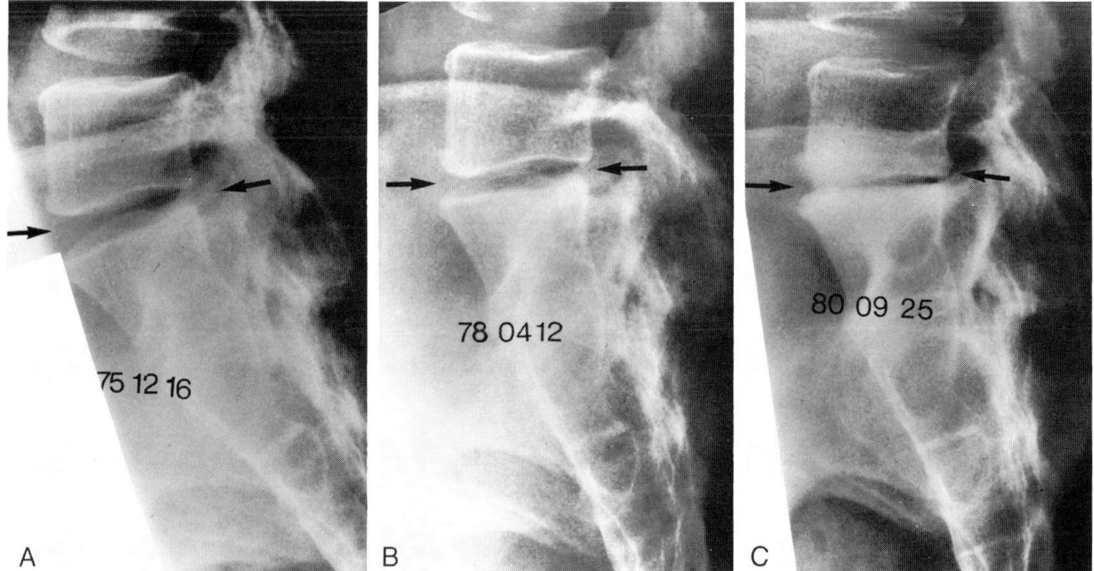

Figure 8–29. *A* to *C,* Lateral radiographs of the lumbosacral junction in the same individual during a period of five years, showing the gradual loss of disc height of the L5–S1 disc *(arrows).* There was no known cause for the reduction of disc height, i.e., this is a case of idiopathic disc degeneration.

least two intervertebral discs and that there can be contralateral neural overlap as well as multisegmental distribution of branches of the sinuvertebral nerve.[136, 216] Such neuroanatomic characteristics of the motion segment may explain the often diffuse localization of pain in the lumbar spine.

The posterior longitudinal ligament is richly innervated,[102, 216, 308] but there is some disagreement in the literature regarding the innervation of the annulus fibrosus. Some studies have shown it to be without innervation,[217, 222, 271] while others indicate that at least the outer parts of the annulus fibrosus have nerve endings.[19, 20, 165, 318]

In recent years interest has been directed to the existence of certain neuropeptide-containing nerve fibers in various tissues of the motion segment.[33, 137] Such studies, based on the use of immunohistochemical techniques, indicate not only the anatomic location of various neurons, but also some biochemical characteristics of the nerve fibers. This may relate to normal and pathologic nerve function, including pain production in various tissue injury situations.

Spinal Nerve Roots

The spinal nerve roots constitute the anatomic connection between the central and peripheral nervous systems. The anatomy of the nerve roots is complex, as they pass through the spine in close relation to structures such as the intervertebral discs and the vertebrae. In the subarachnoid space in the lumbar spine, the dorsal and ventral nerve roots form the cauda equina. At the level of each intervertebral foramen, a pair of ventral and dorsal nerve roots join to gradually form the spinal nerve. Also in this region is the dorsal root ganglion.[31, 95, 242, 301] The neural structures, close to the intervertebral disc in the region of the intervertebral foramen, may be called "the nerve root complex."[230, 242, 308] The general arrangement and relation between spinal nerve roots, spinal nerve, and peripheral nerves is depicted in Figure 8–30 and described in further detail in Chapter 4.

Microscopic Anatomy. The nerve roots in the spinal canal are covered by a thin, relatively permeable root sheath.[7] The nerve roots are in the cerebrospinal fluid (CSF), enclosed by arachnoid membrane and dura. The spinal nerve roots receive their blood supply from vessels approaching along the peripheral nerve components, as well as proximally from the spinal cord.[218, 219, 226] The microvasculature of spinal nerve roots seems to be less well developed than that of peripheral nerves. However, spinal nerve roots also derive some portion of

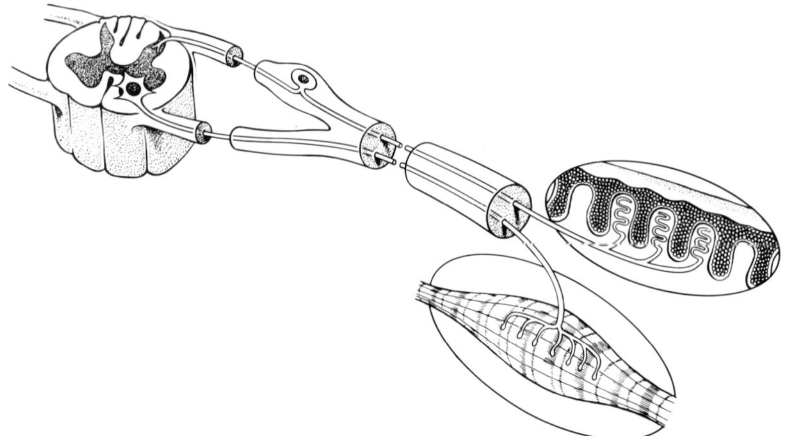

Figure 8–30. Schematic drawing of a segment of the spinal cord, the motor (ventral) and sensory (dorsal) nerve roots, the dorsal root ganglion, the spinal nerve, and the peripheral nerve with the target organs for the innervation. (From Lundborg, G.: Nerve regeneration and repair—a review. Acta Orthop. Scand. *58*:145–169, 1987. © 1987 Munksgaard International Publishers Ltd., Copenhagen, Denmark.)

their nutrition through diffusion from the CSF.[246] The nutritional mechanisms of spinal nerve roots are less well understood than those of the intervertebral disc.

As mentioned above, the nerve roots are covered by specific connective tissue sheaths. The root sheath covering the nerve roots in the cauda equina is very thin and permeable to certain substances.[175, 268] The spinal dura, on the other hand, is a relatively thick, efficient diffusion barrier.[7] The subarachnoid space usually ends at about the level of the dorsal root ganglion (Fig. 8–31). At, or just distal to, the dorsal root ganglion, the dura gradually forms the epineurium of the peripheral nerve. Some of the basement membrane substance, which originates from the root sheath, and the tissue layer between the spinal dura and the arachnoid gradually form the perineurium, which surrounds each fascicle in the peripheral nerves.[7, 175] The spinal nerve gradually becomes a peripheral nerve.

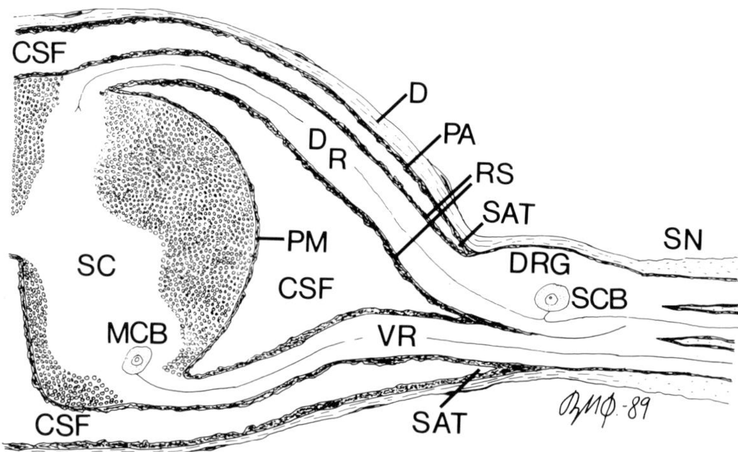

Figure 8–31. Cross section of a segment of the spinal cord (SC), ventral nerve root (VR), and dorsal nerve root (DR). The cell bodies of the motor axons (MCB), which run in the ventral nerve root, are in the anterior horn of the gray matter of the spinal cord. The cell bodies of the sensory axons (SCB), which run in the dorsal nerve root, are in the dorsal root ganglion (DRG). The ventral and dorsal nerve roots blend just caudal to the dorsal root ganglion to form the spinal nerve (SN). The spinal cord is covered with the pia mater (PM). This sheath continues on the spinal nerve roots as the root sheath (RS). The root sheath reflects to the pia-arachnoid (PA) at the subarachnoid triangle (SAT). Together with the dura (D), the pia-arachnoid forms the spinal dura. The spinal cord and nerve roots are floating freely in the cerebrospinal fluid (CSF) in the subarachnoid space. (From Olmarker, K.: Spinal nerve root compression. Experimental studies on effects of acute, graded compression on nerve root nutrition and function, with an *in vivo* compression model of the porcine cauda equina. Doctoral Thesis, University of Göteborg, 1990. Reproduced with kind permission from the author.)

The nerve fibers, both in spinal nerve roots and in peripheral nerves, are of two principally different kinds, myelinated and unmyelinated (Fig. 8–32). In both types of nerve fibers the main component is a central axon. Each nerve fiber constitutes a long cellular process from a nerve cell body lying in the dorsal root ganglion (sensory neurons) or in the anterior horn of the spinal cord (motor neurons). The nerve fibers have varying diameters. The large-diameter fibers are usually myelinated. In these types of fibers, Schwann cells have formed myelin sheaths that surround the axon. The myelin sheath is a multilayered structure made up of lipid and protein components. In unmyelinated nerve fibers, which usually are of smaller diameter, one Schwann cell surrounds several axons. In the myelinated nerve fibers, the Schwann cells are longitudinally arranged near the surface of the axon. The Schwann cells come into close contact with each other at the nodes of Ranvier, where the oxidative activity in the nerve fibers is concentrated.[232] At the nodes of Ranvier, cellular processes from the Schwann cells interdigitate and thereby form a space that permits various extracellular ions to reach the axon, while the myelin sheaths between the nodes of Ranvier insulate the axon. The diameter of the myelinated nerve fibers is usually 5 to 20 microns. The conduction velocity within this group of nerve fibers has been shown to be proportional to the nerve fiber diameter.[69] The rapid conduction velocity in the myelinated, large-diameter nerve fibers, compared with the thinner unmyelinated nerve fibers, is partly due to the fact that the impulse propagation in myelinated fibers is saltatory. This means that the action potential jumps from one node of Ranvier to the next, which results in a higher conduction velocity than occurs with continuous impulse propagation along unmyelinated axons. Large-diameter nerve fibers are more susceptible to compression than thinner nerve fibers, a difference that may be due to more deformation of large fibers than of thin fibers at a given pressure.[40, 70, 162, 244]

The sensory nerve cell bodies are found in the dorsal root ganglion (DRG), usually close to or in the intervertebral foramen.[31, 95] It has been suggested that the small-diameter (less than 20 microns) sensory nerve cell bodies are involved in the transmission of pain impulses, the medium-sized nerve cell bodies in transmission of impulses from viscera, and the large-diameter (over 100 microns) sensory nerve cell bodies in temperature, tactile, and proprioceptive impulses.[283] In dorsal root ganglion cells certain neuropeptides, such as substance P and vasoactive intestinal peptide (VIP), are also produced. Such neuropeptides have been implicated in low back pain disorders.[305–307] Each sensory nerve cell body has two axons: one approaches the nerve cell body via the peripheral nerve and one projects from the nerve cell body toward the spinal cord in the dorsal nerve root.

Neural Function and Axonal Transport. Each nerve fiber has two basic functions. These are the propagation of electrical impulses and the intra-axonal or axonal transport of various substances, such as proteins and organelles. Both impulse propagation and axonal transport are energy-dependent processes. The propagation of impulses along the axons is based on the action potential, which is an all-or-none phenomenon. It is elicited in the axon once its resting membrane potential is changed enough to initiate this process. The fact that the impulse propagation is energy dependent means that this process may be blocked by, for example, local ischemia of a nerve or nerve root. The action potential that can be recorded from a peripheral nerve or a nerve root is called a compound nerve action potential. It represents the summation of the action potentials in the individual nerve fibers during the recording procedure.

Because of the specific anatomic configuration of neurons, with very long processes (the axons) extending from nerve cell bodies, there is a need for efficient communication systems between the various parts of the nerve cells. The length:diameter ratio of an axon is remarkable in that the axonal length may be 10,000 to 15,000 times greater than the diameter of the nerve cell bodies. Most of the proteins and other substances that are needed for the structural and functional integrity of the neuron are synthesized in the nerve cell body. Such substances are transported from the nerve cell body out to the periphery, and also in the opposite direction, through axonal transport systems. Axonal transport from the nerve cell body to the periphery is called anterograde axonal transport; the process in the opposite direction is called retrograde axonal transport. Two main components of anterograde axonal transport have been identified.[17, 23, 53, 82, 178] Slow anterograde axonal transport takes place at velocities of about 1 to 6 mm per day, and with this phase cyto-

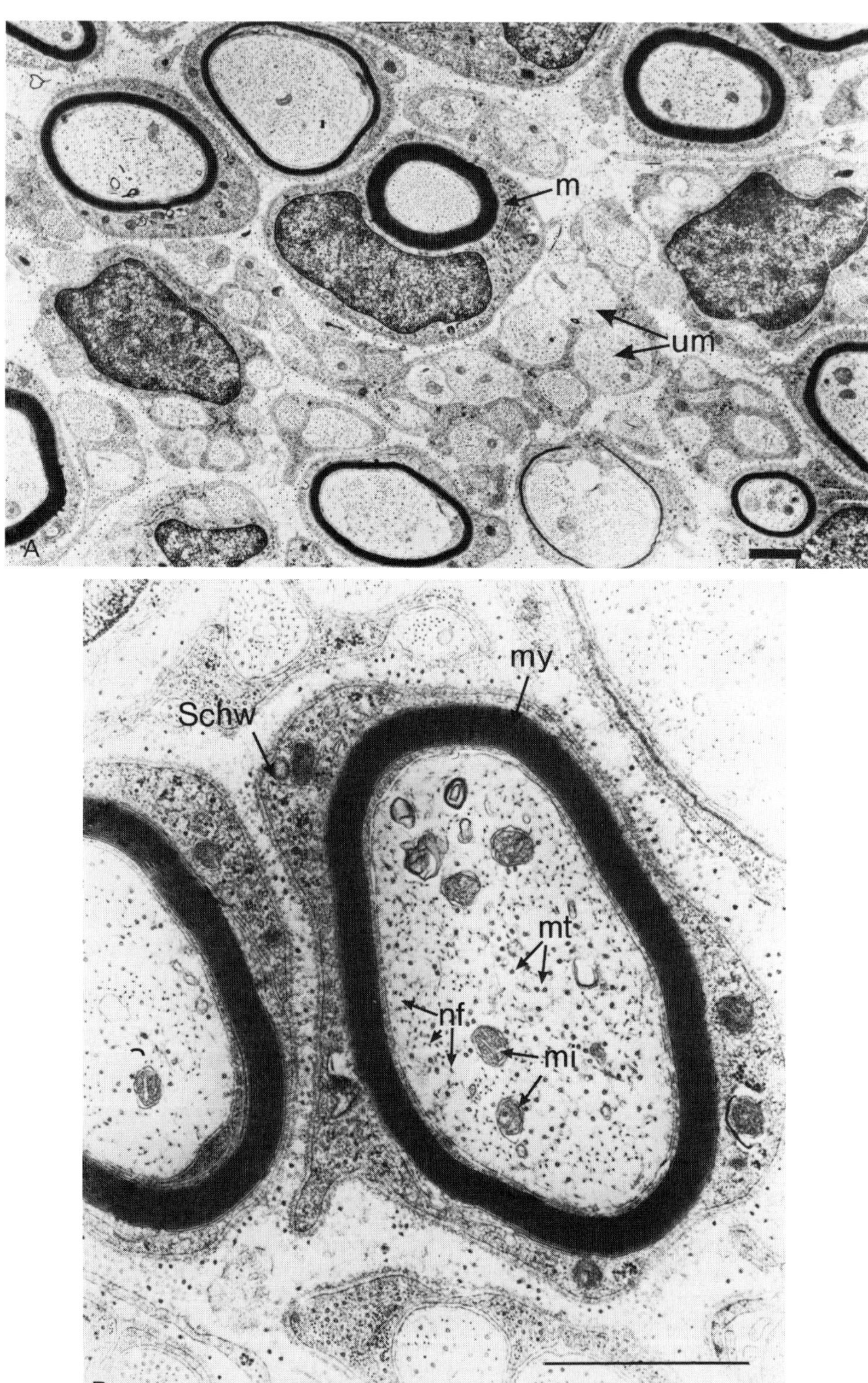

Figure 8–32. *A,* Electron micrograph showing myelinated (m) and unmyelinated (um) nerve fibers (bar gauge = 1 u). *B,* Electron micrograph showing myelinated fibers containing Schwann cell cytoplasm (Schw), myelin (my), mitochondrium (mi), microtubule (mt), and neurofilament (nf) (bar gauge = 1 μ). (From Lundborg, G., Rydevik, B., Manthorpe, M., et al.: Peripheral nerve: the physiology of injury and repair. *In* Woo, S. L.-Y., and Buckwalter, J. A. (eds.): Injury and Repair of the Musculoskeletal Soft Tissues. Symposium. Park Ridge, IL, American Academy of Orthopaedic Surgeons, 1988.)

skeletal elements such as microtubules and microfilaments are transported. Fast anterograde axonal transport takes place at speeds up to about 400 mm per day and involves transport of various enzymes, glycoproteins, lipids, and transmitter substance vesicles.[41, 142, 204, 310] Retrograde axonal transport systems with transportation of material at speeds from about 1 to 300 mm per day have also been identified in many neuronal systems.[15, 16, 138, 139, 155] The exact functions and physiologic significance of axonal transport in normal and pathologic conditions are not fully understood. Axonal transport systems may be impaired in various pathologic conditions such as ischemia, compression, and axonal degeneration and regeneration.[38, 39, 42, 145, 238] The importance of interaction between the nerve cell body and the axon is illustrated by the response pattern of the nerve cell body following nerve injury, including the chromatolytic reaction. This reaction in the nerve cell body may be based on interruption of the retrograde axonal transport systems.

The axonal transport systems, as well as impulse propagation, require a local energy supply along the axon in order to maintain normal function. Anoxia and ischemia, as shown both in vitro and in vivo, may block fast and slow anterograde axonal transport as well as retrograde axonal transport.[38, 145, 238] Although both axonal transport and impulse propagation are dependent on a continuous supply of energy, these two processes are not based on exactly the same cellular mechanisms. This is illustrated by the fact that axonal transport can be maintained over a nerve segment, which does not conduct impulses after inhibition of the excitability of the nerve membrane by a blocking substance such as procaine.[203, 253]

Blood Supply. The vascular supply to the spinal cord and the spinal nerve roots was first described during the latter part of the 19th century.[1, 2, 54, 55, 129] Later, further details of the vascular supply of the spinal cord and spinal nerve root were clarified.[3, 34, 37, 46, 50, 63, 78, 100, 143, 144, 273, 297] Parke and colleagues performed extensive investigations on the vascular supply of lumbosacral spinal nerve roots in the human lumbar spine.[218, 219] The spinal nerve roots, including the dorsal root ganglia, receive their blood supply both from arteries that enter the spinal nerves lateral to the intervertebral foramen and from centrally located arteries coursing caudally from the spinal cord.[37, 49, 218, 219] Thus, unlike peripheral nerves, the spinal roots in the cauda equina are not supplied by regional, segmental arteries. The blood vessels, running in the nerve roots from cranial and caudal directions, approach each other in a region of "relative hypovascularity" (Fig. 8–

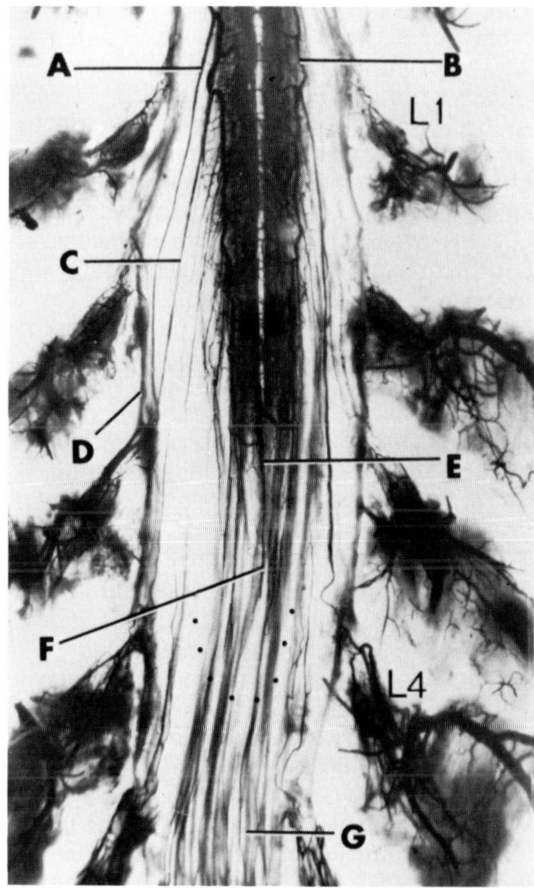

Figure 8–33. Microangiographic representation of the blood supply to the human fetal spinal cord, cauda equina nerve roots, and dorsal root ganglia. The conus medullaris terminates opposite the third lumbar ganglion. Below this point, the content of the lumbar canal consists only of the lumbosacral nerve roots. The last dorsal medullary artery is seen following the right fourth lumbar nerve root, and all other vessels inferior to this are true radicular arteries. The distal radicular vessels in the lower part of the cauda equina (G) are shown ascending toward the proximal descending vessels. The area of relative hypovascularity is obvious between these two sets of vessels and is marked as a U-shaped area *(dots)* around the termination of the conus, which is approximately one segment lower than in the adult. A, Small dorsal medullary artery of the third lumbar level; B, right dorsolateral spinal artery; C, ventral medullary artery from the third lumbar level; D, strip of lateral dura left to preserve relationships; E, anterior spinal artery, terminating in the filum termnale (F). (From Parke, W. W., Gammell, K., and Rothman, R. H.: Arterial vascularization of the cauda equina. J. Bone Joint Surg. *63A*:53–62, 1981.)

33).[218, 219] This region of the cauda equina may represent a site of the spinal nerve roots that is vulnerable to, for example, compression.

The arteries in the spinal nerve root are mainly in the outer layers of the root sheath. However, arterial vessels may also be found deeper in the nerve root tissue between, or within, the fascicles.[219] Arterial coils and vascular loops may compensate for elongation of the nerve roots and their vessels during spinal motion.[219, 226] Endoneurial capillaries usually run parallel to the axons. The general arrangement of the spinal nerve root venous system is similar to that of the arteries. However, large veins often have a deep course in the nerve roots in a spiral manner.[219] Several of the anatomic characteristics of human spinal nerve root blood supply have also been found in nerve roots of porcine cauda equina.[209, 215]

Nutrition Via Cerbrospinal Fluid. The nerve fibers of spinal nerve roots, as well as those of peripheral nerves, depend on a continuous and adequate supply of nutrients in order to maintain normal function.[156, 158, 276] The vascular supply to the spinal nerve roots seems to be less well developed than to peripheral nerves.[219, 226] One may therefore speculate that additional nutritional support systems should be necessary in this region of the spinal nerve roots. Using radioisotope techniques, Rydevik and associates[246] showed that the spinal nerve roots in the subarachnoid space derive a significant portion of their nutrition via diffusion from the surrounding CSF. This means that the intrathecal parts of the spinal nerve roots have dual nutritional pathways: (1) via the intraneural microvessels and (2) via diffusion from the CSF (Fig. 8–34). The significance of these characteristics for spinal nerve root nutrition in normal and pathologic situations is not fully understood.

Dorsal Root Ganglion: Blood Supply and Nutrition. The blood supply of the dorsal root ganglia differs from other parts of the nerve roots in that the ganglia have a very rich microvascular supply.[10, 219] Furthermore, the blood vessels in the dorsal root ganglia are more permeable than the intraneural blood vessels at other levels of the nerve roots.[212] These specific anatomic characteristics in terms of the rich vascular blood supply, as well as the higher vascular permeability of the microvasculature in the dorsal root ganglia, probably reflect the high level of metabolic and nutritional demand of the ganglion cells. The nerve cell bodies are responsible for the synthesis of several essential substances for the whole neuron, e.g., proteins, which are needed for the maintenance of the structural and functional integrity of the sensory neurons. The dorsal root ganglion has been implicated in various low back pain disorders, at least as related to changes in neuropeptide dynamics.[305–307]

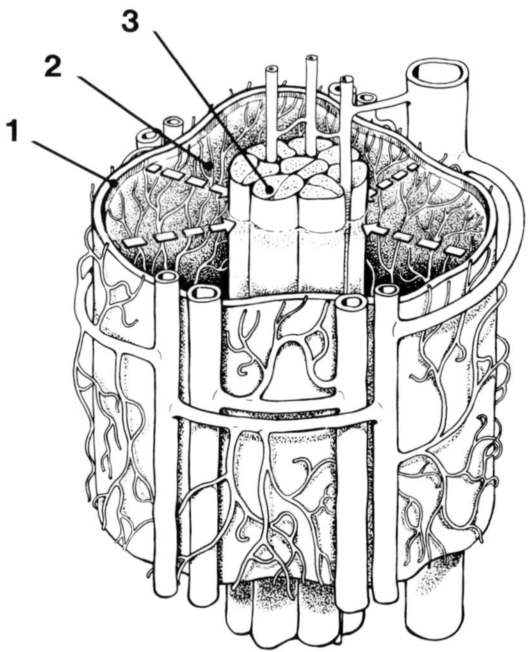

Figure 8–34. Schematic drawing of a segment of the spinal canal, indicating the dual nutritional system to the spinal nerve roots. The results indicate that nutrients seem to be transported from the vasculature in the membranes surrounding the spinal canal via diffusion through the cerebrospinal fluid *(arrows)*, but also directly to the nerve root tissue via the intraneural vasculature. 1, Dura and arachnoid; 2, cerebrospinal fluid; 3, nerve roots. (From Rydevik, B., Holm, S., Brown, M.D., and Lundborg, G.: Diffusion from the cerebrospinal fluid as a nutritional pathway for spinal nerve roots. Acta Orthop. Scand. *138*:247–248, 1990. © 1990 Munksgaard International Publishers Ltd., Copenhagen, Denmark.)

Pathophysiologic Mechanisms

The spinal nerve roots are generally well protected from external trauma by the bony elements of the vertebral column. However, since nerve roots do not possess the same amount and organization of protective connective tissue layers as peripheral nerves, the roots seem to be susceptible to mechanical deformation by intraspinal disorders such as disc herniation, spinal stenosis, and other degenerative conditions.[242] In addition, it has been suggested that nerve roots may be affected by various chemical substances from degenerated invertebral discs and/or facet joints.[242, 304]

Mechanical Deformation of Nerve Roots

General Aspects of Nerve Compression. Compression of peripheral nerves or spinal nerve roots can induce clinical symptoms such as numbness, pain, and muscle weakness.[158, 276] The pathophysiologic basis for the various functional changes has been investigated extensively.[13, 62, 84, 156, 179, 238–240]

When a nerve or nerve root is compressed, there are both "direct" mechanical effects on the nerve fibers and "indirect" effects via impairment of the blood supply to the nerve tissue. It has been shown that a nerve can function if exposed to high pressures in a compression chamber, provided that there is an adequate concentration of oxygen.[84] However, nerve function rapidly deteriorates if oxygen is removed, even at normal pressure levels. This led to the conclusion that ischemia is more important for changes in nerve conduction than the actual pressure level.[84] However, this finding was based on experiments performed in vitro on isolated nerve specimens. Other studies have shown that local compression of a nerve in vivo may induce changes and that the pressure level is of major significance for both structural and functional changes.[13, 62, 202, 239]

Local compression of a nerve may induce direct mechanical effects on the nerve fibers, such as deformation of the nodes of Ranvier and invagination of the paranodal myelin sheaths.[56, 202, 239] However, such effects have been seen only after compression at considerably high pressure levels.[202] Changes induced by compression at lower pressure levels (i.e., less than about 200 mm Hg) are more likely to be due to impairment of the nutritional supply to the nerve tissue than to direct structural injury to the nerve fibers.

Compression-induced Neurophysiologic Changes. The critical pressure limits for the occurrence of various changes induced in nerve roots during compression have been analyzed in an in vivo compression model of the porcine cauda equina (Fig. 8–35).[205, 209] Graded compression of the nerve roots in the porcine cauda equina is achieved by an inflatable balloon system. With such an experimental approach, the effects of graded compression on basic physiologic events in the nerve roots such as blood flow, nutritional supply, and nerve conduction have been analyzed.[206, 208, 210, 247] Vital microscopy of the nerve roots has shown that compression at very low pressure levels (5 to 10 mm Hg) induces acute changes in the intraneural microcirculation in terms of reduced venular blood flow.[206] Blood flow in the capillaries in the nerve roots seems to be dependent on an efficient venular blood flow. Retrograde stasis in capillaries, due to venular congestion, has previously been suggested to be an important pathophysiologic mechanism in nerve compression syndromes.[275] Experimental observations indicate that a corresponding mechanism might be of significance in spinal nerve root compression, i.e., that low-pressure compression may affect venular blood flow, thereby creating retrograde stasis in capillaries with impaired nutrition of the nerve fibers in the nerve roots. Total ischemia of the compressed nerve root segments is induced at

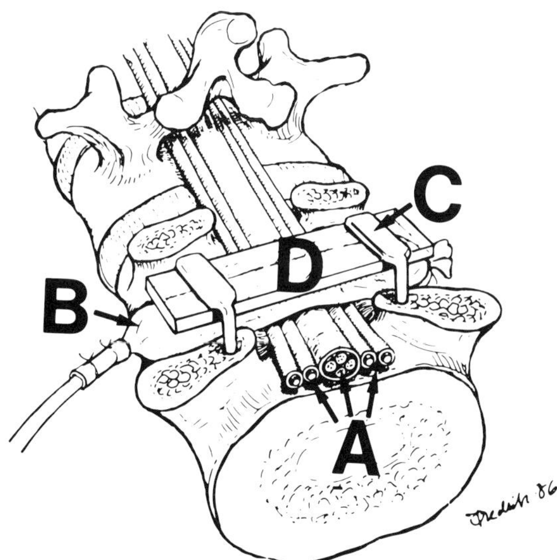

Figure 8–35. Schematic drawing of an experimental model for nerve root compression. The cauda equina (A) is compressed by an inflatable balloon *(B)*, which is fixed to the spine by two L-shaped pins (C) and a Plexiglas plate (D). (From Olmarker, K., Rydevik, B., and Holm, S.: Edema formation in spinal nerve roots induced by experimental, graded compression. An experimental study on the pig cauda equina with special reference to differences in effects between rapid and slow onset of compression. Spine *14*:569–573, 1989.)

pressure levels close to mean arterial blood pressure. Experimental compression of the porcine cauda equina at two levels may induce ischemia not only at the locations of compression but also in the nerve root segments between the compression sites.[279]

Nutrients may be transported to the nerve roots through intrinsic blood vessels and via diffusion from the surrounding CSF.[246] The nerve roots thus seem to have dual nutritional pathways, and theoretically impairment of one of these two pathways might, at least partly, be compensated for by the remaining nutritional route. However, studies performed on the effects of compression on transport of intravenously injected ^{3}H-labeled methylglucose to the nerve roots, which reflects the contribution from the blood vessels in the nerve roots and from the CSF, have indicated that even very low-pressure compression may impair the overall nutritional transport to the nerve roots.[208] Compression at 10 mm Hg, for instance, induced an acute reduction of the transport of methylglucose to the nerve roots to about 70 to 80 per cent of normal values.[208]

The blood vessels in the nerve roots, like all other blood vessels in the body, react to mechanical injury by increased permeability, resulting in edema formation. Experimentally, intraneural edema formation has been induced in spinal nerve roots by compression at 50 mm Hg for two minutes.[207] Edema in the nerve root tissue may increase endoneurial fluid pressure.[153, 160, 183, 242, 243] Such increased pressure may lead to impairment of intraneural blood flow.[154, 184–186] Intraneural edema may persist for some time after removal of a compressive agent, and this edema may negatively affect nerve roots for a longer time than the compression itself. Long-standing intraneural edema appears to lead to fibrosis formation in the nerve tissue,[236, 237] which may contribute to the slow recovery seen in some patients with nerve compression disorders. Endoneurial vessels of nerve roots, and in particular the dorsal root ganglia, are more permeable to plasma proteins than the endoneurial vessels of peripheral nerves.[10, 127, 212] This means that there is no effective blood-nerve barrier in nerve roots. These characteristics may add to the tendency toward edema formation in nerve roots. The nerve roots also are devoid of perineurium, which in peripheral nerves is known to act as a diffusion barrier to macromolecules.[213, 214] Since the nerve roots lack perineurium, the nerve fibers in the roots may be relatively freely exposed to substances not only in the bloodstream, but also in the subarachnoid space.

Electrophysiologic analyses of the effects of compression on nerve root function have indicated that there is an acute pressure threshold for the occurrence of changes in spinal nerve root conduction. This occurs between 50 and 75 mm Hg (Fig. 8–36*A*, *B*).[223, 247] Compression at higher pressure levels (100 to 200 mm Hg) demonstrates that impulse conduction in motor nerve roots recovers more rapidly and more completely than in the sensory roots after release of pressure (Fig. 8–36*C*, *D*). Thus, local compression of the cauda equina may injure sensory nerve roots more than motor nerve roots. Systemic hypotension may increase the susceptibility of the nerve roots of the cauda equina to compression.[68] Double- or multiple-level compression causes more pronounced changes in motor nerve conduction than single-level compression at corresponding pressure levels.[211]

Biomechanics of Nerve Root Deformation. Mechanical deformation of nerve roots basically affects all the tissue components of the roots: the nerve fibers, connective tissue elements, and blood vessels. A discussion of nerve root biomechanics should take into account the fact that nerve roots are complex structures in which each tissue component has distinct mechanical properties. Data on peripheral nerve biomechanics cannot be directly applied to spinal nerve root biomechanics owing to anatomic differences between these two components of the nervous system.[242, 249]

Within certain limits the spinal nerve roots may adapt to mechanical deformation without functional changes. However, if the applied force and the resulting deformation exceed certain limits, structural and functional changes may occur. The nerve roots in the subarachnoid space lack epineurium and perineurium, but under tensile loading they exhibit both elasticity and tensile strength.[277] The ultimate load for human ventral spinal nerve roots from the cauda equina is between 2 and 22 N; for dorsal nerve roots the corresponding value is between 5 and 33 N.[276, 277] The length of the nerve roots from the spinal cord to the foramina in the human lumbosacral spine varies from about 60 mm at the L1 level to about 170 mm at the S1 level.[274] The mechanical properties of human spinal nerve roots differ

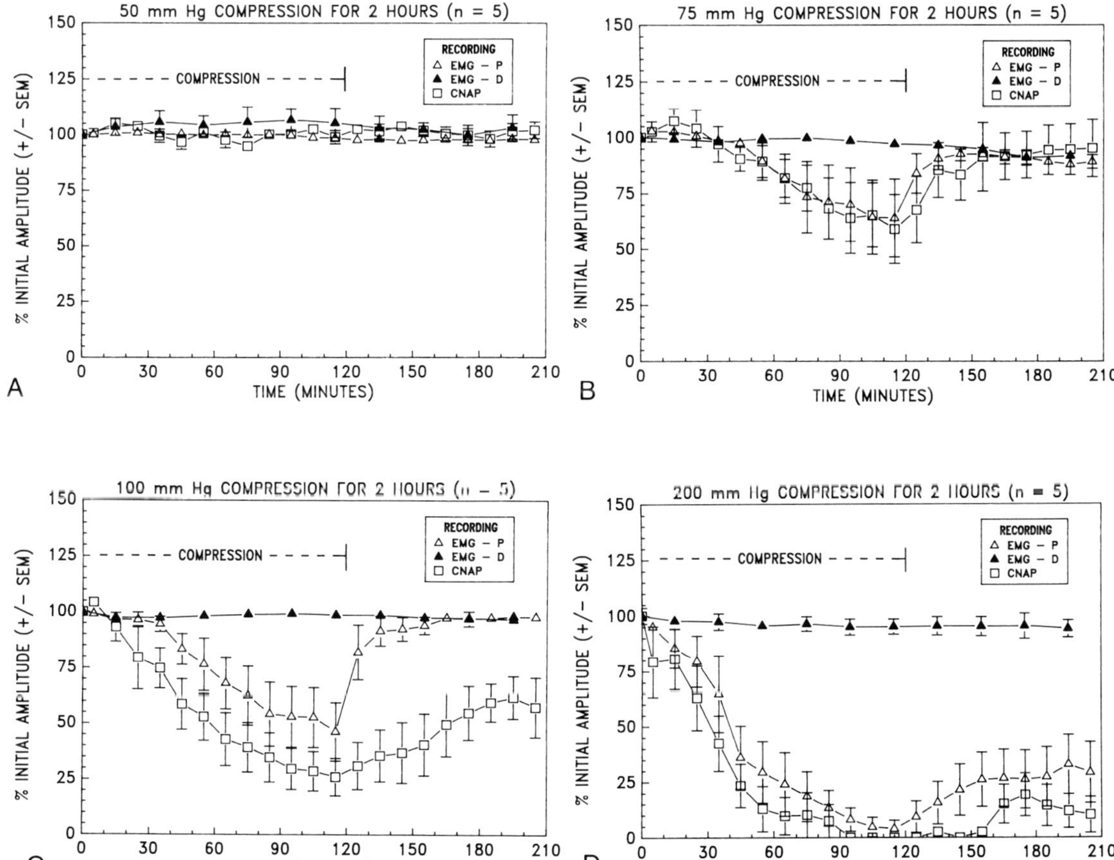

Figure 8–36. *A* to *D,* Diagrams showing the effects of nerve root compression at 50, 75, 100, and 200 mm Hg for two hours including 90 minutes' recovery. EMG-P, Amplitude of tail muscle EMG after stimulation of the cauda equina through the screws in the sacral lamina, proximal to the compression. EMG-D, Amplitude of tail muscle EMG after stimulation of the cauda equina through a retractable electrode distal to the compression. CNAP, Compound nerve action potential recorded from screws in the sacral lamina after stimulation of nerves in the tail through needle electrodes. Note that there were no effects of 50 mm Hg for two hours. During compression at 75 mm Hg for two hours, there was partial impairment of both afferent and efferent conduction. After compression at 100 mm Hg, there was a differential recovery with complete recovery of EMG amplitude to baseline, but only patial recovery of compound nerve action potential. Compression at 200 mg Hg induced corresponding, but more pronounced, changes (From Rydevik, B. L., Pedowitz, R. A., Hargens, A. R., et al.: Effects of acute, graded compression on spinal nerve root function and structure. An experimental study of the pig cauda equina. Spine 1991 (in press) and from Garfin, S. R., Cohen, M. S., Massie, J. B., et al.: Nerve-roots of the cauda equina. The effects of hypotension and acute grade compression on function. J. Bone Joint Surg. *72A*:1185–1192, 1990.)

for a given nerve root in its location in the spinal canal compared with the tissue in the lateral intervertebral foramen region. For example, for the S1 nerve root the ultimate load for the intrathecal portion is 13 N, and for the foraminal portion about 73 N. Corresponding differences between intrathecal and foraminal components have also been verified for the L5 nerve roots. Thus, the ultimate load values for the foraminal nerve root segments are about five times higher than for the intrathecal portion of the same nerve root under tensile loading. However, if one takes into account the larger cross-sectional area of the nerve root in the intervertebral foramen, compared with that in the subarachnoid space, the ultimate tensile stress values are more comparable in the two locations. The ultimate strain under tensile loading is 13 to 19 per cent for the human nerve root at the L5–S1 level.[248]

The nerve roots in the spine are not static structures; they move relative to surrounding tissues (e.g., vertebrae and discs) with spinal motion. Furthermore, the nerve roots may adapt to such motion by their elasticity. To allow for the relative motion of nerve roots in, for example, the intervertebral foramen, there must be a gliding capacity of the spinal nerve roots. It has been found that during straight leg raising the nerve roots move approximately 2 to 5 mm at the level of the intervertebral foramina.[79] Chronic irritation with subsequent fibrosis in and around the nerve roots may impair this gliding mechanism (see below).

The effects of compression on spinal nerve roots are related not only to pressure level and duration of compression, but also to the onset rate of compression. It has thus been found that a rapid onset rate (0.05 to 0.1 sec) causes much more tissue changes than a slow onset rate (20 sec) when compared at corresponding pressure levels. A rapid onset rate induced

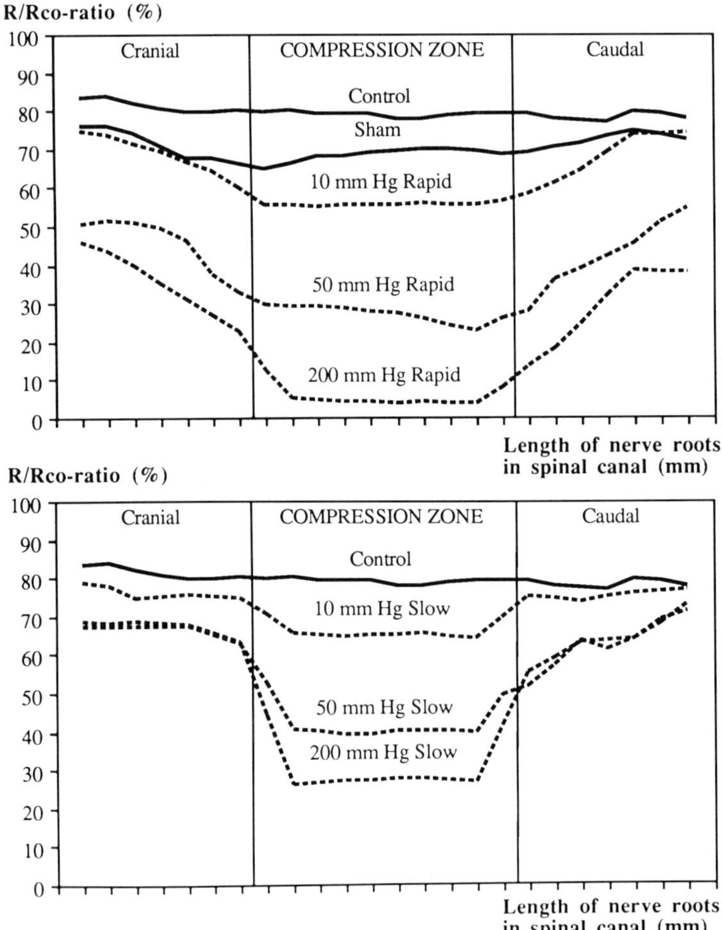

Figure 8–37. Diagrams showing the effects of graded compression on the nutritional supply of the spinal nerve roots of the pig cauda equina. Average R/Rco ratio (the concentration of the tracer in the nerve roots as related to blood concentration) for control, sham-compression, and compression at rapid onset rate *(top)*, and control and slow onset rate *(bottom)*. (From Olmarker, K., Rydevik, B., Hansson, T., and Holm, S.: Compression-induced changes of the nutritional supply to the porcine cauda equina. J. Spinal Dis. *3*:25–29, 1990.)

more pronounced changes than a slow onset rate in terms of edema formation in the nerve roots, impairment of nutritional transport (Fig. 8–37), and changes in impulse conduction (Fig. 8–38).[206, 208, 209]

Chronic Nerve Root Injury. A series of changes in nerve roots such as alterations in intraneural blood flow, microvascular permeability, axonal transport, nutritional supply, and impulse propagation may take place as a result of mechanical effects on the nerve root. Significant changes in certain of these physiologic functions, e.g., intraneural blood flow, axonal transport (Fig. 8–39), and nutritional supply, are induced at low pressure levels of compression. If such compression is prolonged, there may be secondary alterations leading to functional changes, which, under certain conditions, may include nerve root pain. For example, mechanical compression may induce edema formation, which in turn may lead to fibroblast invasion and fibrosis formation in the nerve tissue.[236, 237, 242] Long-standing impairment of the nutritional supply to a compressed nerve root or nerve roots may lead not only to deficient nutrition of the nerve fibers, but also to accumulation of waste products. Waste products may include various acid components that, under certain circumstances, may alter the local ionic and homeostatic balance in the nerve roots, leading to pain production. Watanabe and Parke[302] described the neuropathologic changes in nerve roots of the cauda equina in a case of spinal stenosis. Various kinds of structural nerve fiber reactions were found, along with thickening of the meningeal membranes. Such fibrotic changes might lead to impairment of nerve root nutrition by altered diffusion from the CSF.[246]

Chronic fibrosis formation in and around the nerve root may also significantly impair the gliding capacity of the nerve root complex in the intervertebral foramina. If nerve roots in this manner are restricted in their motion, "microstretching injuries" in the nerve roots may occur. Such tissue reactions may further potentiate the injury.

The nerve fibers react to injury by either local demyelination or, if more severe damage is induced, axonal degeneration. Nerve segments with demyelinated nerve fibers are probably susceptible to further mechanical deformation, and again, perhaps, involved in the etiology of pain production (see also below).

Spinal Stenosis and Disc Herniation. Spinal nerve roots may be subjected to mechanical compression in spinal stenosis and disc herniation. Spinal stenosis is usually a slowly developing process where the nerve roots are circumferentially compressed at a slow rate. In a dorsolateral disc herniation, the situation is different: there will be local compression, leading to some flattening of the nerve root, but also intraneural tension, since the nerve root normally adheres to the surrounding tissues above and below the intervertebral disc.[264, 265] The contact force between a simulated disc herniation in cadavers and the overlying deformed nerve root has been measured by Spencer and associates.[266] Taking the area of contact into account, they assumed a contact pressure of approximately 400 mm Hg. With reduced disc height the contact force and pressure between the experimental disc herniation and the nerve root was reduced owing to slackening of the nerve root. These authors suggested that their findings may in part explain the relief of sciatic pain following chemonucleolysis and, after time, as disc degeneration progresses, with reduced disc height.

Experimental studies on human cadaver spines, involving constriction of the dural sac and the cauda equina with a round clamp, have indicated that the minimal measured cross-sectional area for the cauda equina, including the dural sac at the L3 level, is 77 ± 13 mm^2.[233] During gradual constriction of the dural sac, pressure starts to increase among the nerve roots at or just below this "critical" cross-sectional area. For the L3 level, this value is about 45 per cent of the normal cross-sectional area of the dural sac. In order to induce an acute pressure increase to 50 mm Hg among the nerve roots, the cross-sectional area of the cauda equina has to be further constricted to an area of 63 ± 13 mm^2 (about 37 per cent of the normal dural sac size at this level). The corresponding degree of acute constriction needed to induce a pressure elevation to 100 mm Hg is 57 ± 11 mm^2 (corresponding to 33 per cent of the normal dural sac size at this level).[257] These data indicate that constriction of the cauda equina in the human lumbar spine down to a cross-sectional area of the dural sac less than approximately 75 mm^2 is likely to lead to increased pressure in the dural sac and compression of the cauda equina, which may affect nerve root physiology. The values reported for critical areas of the dural sac correlate well to the cross-sectional area of

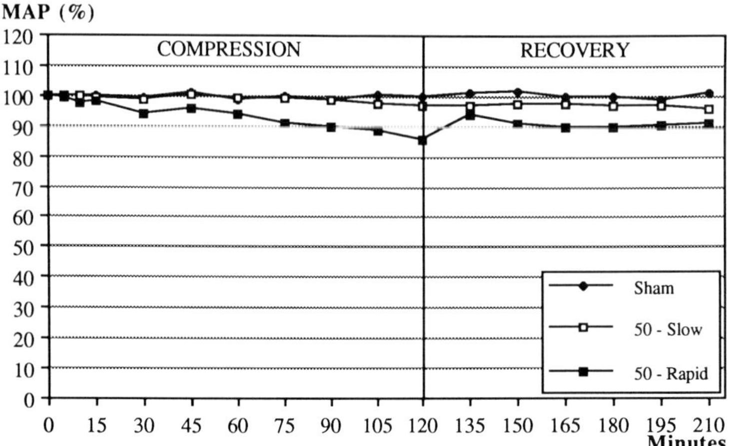

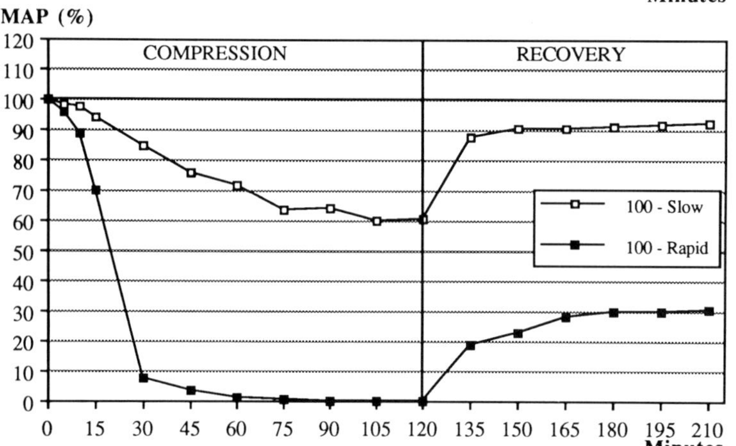

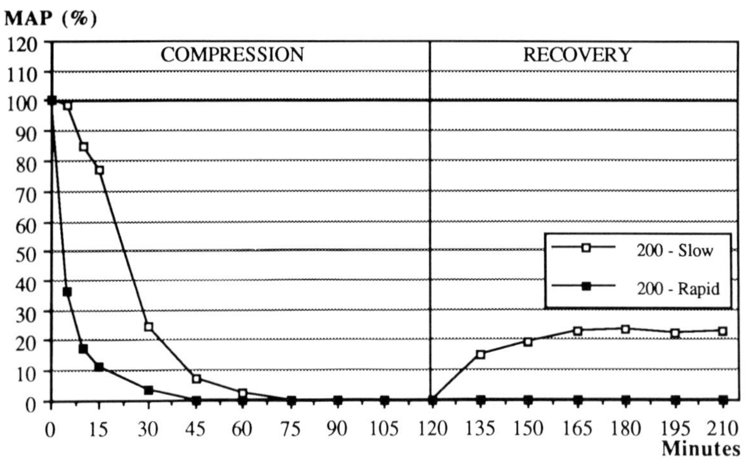

Figure 8–38. Data from experimental graded compression of the pig cauda equina. Average amplitude of MAP (muscle action potential), representing conduction of the fastest conducting motor nerve fibers, expressed in percentage of baseline value. The diagrams show the results of two hours of compression and 1.5 hours of recovery for sham-compression and for rapid and slow onset of compression at 50, 100, and 200 mm Hg. Note that there are more pronounced effects of rapid onset of compression than of slow onset of compression, particularly at 100 mm Hg compression in this model. (From Olmarker, K., Holm, S., and Rydevik, B.: Importance of compression onset rate for the degree of impairment of impulse propagation in experimental compression injury of the porcine cauda equina. Spine *15*:416–419, 1990.)

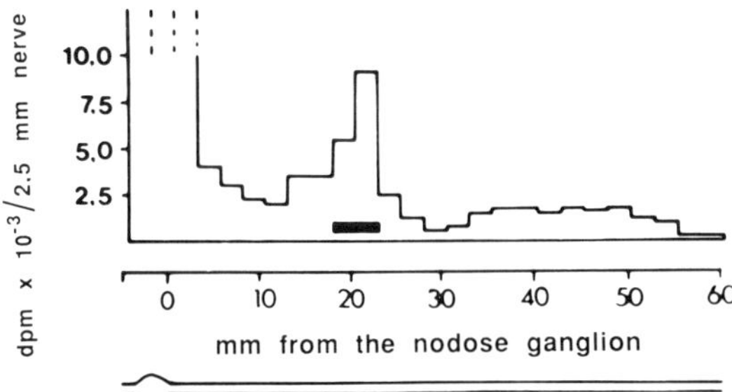

Figure 8–39. Diagram that illustrates a block of axonal transport induced by compression. The rabbit vagus nerve is compressed by means of a small inflatable cuff. The cuff is applied around the nerve, which thereby is compressed at controlled pressure. Radioactively labeled amino acid (^{3}H-leucine) is injected into the nodose ganglion of the nerve. These amino acids are then incorporated into the proteins, which are synthesized in the ganglion, and then transported down the axon at a speed of about 400 mm per 24 hours. The nerve is shown schematically beneath the horizontal axis; the amount of radioactivity along the nerve is shown on the vertical axis. The site of compression is indicated by the black bar. The compression has in this nerve induced an accumulation of axonally transported proteins, seen as a peak at the site of compression. Such impairment of axonal transport has been found to occur when pressure as low as 30 mm Hg is applied to the nerve. (From Rydevik, B., Brown, M. D., and Lundborg, G.: Pathoanatomy and pathophysiology of nerve root compression. Spine 9:7–15, 1984.)

the dural sac in patients with symptoms of central spinal stenosis (90 ± 35 mm^2).[256] It should be noted that there are considerable variations in the size of the spinal canal with not only flexion and extension, but also axial load. Such size variations of the spinal canal may explain the posture dependency of symptoms in patients with central spinal stenosis.

Delamarter and colleagues studied the effects of prolonged compression of the cauda equina by a constriction band of nylon in beagle dogs.[45] The cauda equina was acutely constricted circumferentially down to 75, 50, or 25 per cent of the normal cross-sectional area. The effects of such constriction were analyzed for up to three months of constriction, and it was found that with constriction to 75 per cent of the normal value there were no neurologic deficits, but with constriction to 50 or 25 per cent of the normal value there was both motor and sensory impairment, as well as structural damage to the nerve roots. These observations correlate with the studies on the human lumbar spine by Schönström and associates,[255, 257] in which pressure changes among the nerve roots were first induced when the cross-sectional area of the dural sac was reduced to about 45 per cent of the initial normal value. In the dog model neurologic improvement was seen, even in cases of very severe constriction, when decompression was performed three months after the onset of compression.[45]

Dorsal Root Ganglion Reactions. The possible role of the dorsal root ganglion in low back pain and sciatica was first alluded to by Lindblom and Rexed in 1948.[147] These investigators performed cadaver dissections and found that compression of the dorsal root ganglion was often induced as a result of dorsolateral lumbar disc herniation. In some specimens, hypertrophied facet joints were found also to cause nerve root deformation. The microscopic appearance of the ganglia showed gross alterations of the internal structure with, for example, an increase in the amount of connective tissue. Howe and colleagues[121] noted that compression of a normal dorsal root ganglion may induce a neurophysiologic response consistent with pain production. In this regard the ganglion seems to be different from other parts of the nerve root complex in that nerve roots are normally not sensitive to mechanical stimulation in terms of pain production (see also below).

The vascular supply to the dorsal root ganglion can be affected by mechanical compression; edema formation may be easily induced in the ganglion. Edema in the ganglion can lead to a significant increase in pressure in this structure.[243] Such pressure elevation may in turn affect the nutritional supply to the cells in the ganglion.

Arachnoiditis

Spinal arachnoiditis may develop after spine surgery and after myelography with certain agents, and may be related to various long-standing disease conditions in the spine. Both mechanical and chemical factors may be implicated in the pathogenic mechanisms behind arachnoiditis. The pathology of arachnoiditis is characterized by thickening and opacity of the arachnoid membrane, which generally becomes adherent to the dura, nerve roots, or pia.[30] The subarachnoid space may become obliterated by connective tissue components, rendering nerve roots compressed, ischemic, or both. These pathologic changes do not seem to respond to corticosteroid or radiation therapy, and surgical intervention with decompression or division of connective tissue adhesions confers no certain benefit.[96] Holm and associates[118] experimentally analyzed arachnoiditis from a nutritional, histologic, and radiologic point of view. It was found that even with relatively mild arachnoiditis seen radiologically, there was significant impairment of the nutritional supply to the nerve roots. This reduced nutrition appears to be based on certain structural changes at the microscopic level in terms of arachnoidal cell proliferation and collagen production within the root sheaths. These findings indicate that pronounced changes in nerve root nutrition may occur before radiologic changes become apparent.

INTERACTION BETWEEN DISC AND NERVE TISSUE

It is well known that the occurrence of degenerative changes in the intervertebral discs is sometimes associated with back pain, with or without nerve root involvement. Some possible pathophysiologic mechanisms behind such spinal pain syndromes are discussed below, with special reference to nerve root involvement associated with degenerative disc disease conditions.

Mechanical and Chemical Effects

In association with conditions such as disc herniation and spinal stenosis, nerve roots may be subjected to mechanical deformation, leading to a series of intraneural tissue reactions, the severity of which are dependent on, for example, the magnitude of the deforming forces and the time factors involved. Compression may lead to impairment of nerve root blood flow.[206, 319] Mechanical compression may also induce increased permeability of the nerve root microvessels, leading to formation of edema in the nerve root tissue.[207] Subsequently, fibrosis may develop in and around nerve roots.[122] There are also reasons to believe that nerve root compression may cause impairment of axonal transport.[38, 39, 238, 242] It has been suggested that nerve root compression at the level of, for example, the cervical spine or the lumbar spine may lead to axonal transport blockage at the level of compression, resulting in distal depletion of axonally transported material such as proteins, which are essential for the maintenance of normal integrity of the peripheral nerve fibers.[286] It has also been proposed that such a mechanism leads to increased susceptibility to compression of the distally located nerve fibers, thereby providing a pathophysiologic mechanism for the so-called "double-crush syndrome."[286] This condition is characterized by simultaneously occurring compression of a nerve root and its corresponding peripheral nerve. Thus, mechanical nerve root compression by, for example, herniated disc material may lead to changes in biochemical properties of the nerve fibers, with certain clinical implications in terms of enhanced susceptibility to additional nerve compression.

Acute compression of a normal peripheral nerve does not usually cause pain, but rather numbness, paresthesias, motor weakness, and related symptoms and signs.[158] This phenomenon is seen in situations such as when the peroneal nerve is compressed in a person sitting with crossed legs. Experimental human investigations in vivo with compression of the median nerve in the carpal tunnel indicate that compression-induced numbness is caused by ischemia, not just mechanical nerve fiber deformation.[159] Compression of normal spinal nerve roots seems to induce corresponding changes in sensory and motor functions, without associated pain.[140, 163, 262] These observations were obtained by subjecting nerve roots to mechanical deformation during lumbar spine surgery under local anesthesia, or by postoperatively causing mechanical deformation of nerve roots by (for example) inflatable balloons placed close to the nerve root at the time of surgery. If the nerve root in question had been compressed by a herniated disc, i.e., if the root was irritated, even minimal mechanical deformation resulted in reproduction of the sciatic pain. Observations during laminectomy and disc excision, performed under epidural anesthesia, indicate that the nerve root close to the disc herniation is very sensitive to mechanical deformation.[27, 71, 83] It was noted that, although all tissues in the lumbar spine were well anesthetized, even careful retraction of the irritated nerve root induced radiating leg pain. The observations in humans regarding the increased mechanosensitivity of irritated nerve roots in terms of pain production correlate well with experimental findings on the neurophysiologic response of normal and irritated peripheral nerves and nerve roots in animals.[47, 121] Therefore, it seems reasonable to assume that nerve root irritation is a significant factor that has to be present for mechanical nerve root deformation to induce radiating pain. However, it should be noted that the dorsal root ganglion has been found to be mechanosensitive and that deformation even of a normal ganglion, without irritation, may induce corresponding pain production.[120, 121] It has also been shown that neurons of the dorsal root ganglia become spontaneously active as a result of a lesion to their peripheral processes, i.e., to the spinal or peripheral nerve.[29, 300]

At the site of mechanical compression, there may also be structural nerve fiber reactions, including myelin changes and axonal membrane alterations,[202, 239, 242] contributing to various kinds of functional changes such as motor weakness, sensory disturbances, and sometimes pain. Injured nerve fibers appear to react with ectopic impulse generation.[29, 47, 80, 298, 299] Clinical observations support findings that spontaneous ectopic activity from sites of axonal injury in the spine, or in the periphery, may be associated with pain and paresthesias. Factors such as local hypoxia, with or without compression, of an abnormal segment of a nerve or nerve root may induce or enhance ectopic impulse generation.[29, 47]

The causes and histologic characteristics of both intra- and extraneural irritation and fibrosis have been the subject of extensive debate.[122, 128, 235, 242, 264] From the discussion above, it is clear that mechanical factors such as compression and traction of spinal nerve roots may induce a series of tissue reactions, leading to a state of irritation or inflammation of the nerve roots. The exact nature and the functional consequences of such nerve root irritation are not fully known, but there is reason to believe that the histologic characteristics include, for example, edema, fibrosis, and demyelination.[242]

It has been proposed that not only mechanical but also biochemical factors may be involved in the production of such nerve root irritation. Breakdown products from a degenerating nucleus pulposus may come into contact with the nerve root, inducing a "chemical radiculitis."[173, 174] Furthermore, a degenerated intervertebral disc may create an intradiscal acidic local environment, which may contribute to adhesion formation around the nerve root that courses close to the disc.[187] It has also been suggested that autoimmune mechanisms may be involved in the tissue reactions seen in and around nerve roots in association with disc degeneration.[18, 72] However, no experimental or clinical studies are available to provide conclusive evidence that such biochemical interactive mechanisms between intervertebral disc and nerve root exist. Conflicting, experimentally obtained evidence is reported in the literature in this regard; application of normal, nondegenerated, autologous nucleus pulposus to a rabbit tibial nerve did not increase or otherwise alter the severity of controlled compression injury of the nerve,[241] but homogenized, autologous nucleus pulposus induced local tissue inflammation when injected epidurally in dogs.[176] If such biochemical mechanisms exist, it should be important to identify them and analyze their role in neural irritation. Better understanding in this area might allow the development of new and improved forms of treatment for at least some conditions of nerve root involvement in degenerative disc disease.

Clinical Considerations

In most cases of acute low back pain, the exact mechanism behind the pain is unclear; in these instances the condition may be called idiopathic low back pain.[312] As stated above, all tissues in the lumbar spine, except in the nucleus pulposus, seem to be supplied with sensory innervation, thereby being potential sources of pain in case of injury to these tissues. The natural history of low back pain is generally very favorable, with a rapid remission of symptoms within the first weeks after onset of pain.[189, 191, 193] Although the cause of back pain in most cases is unclear, there are reasons to believe that at least some low back pain conditions may be based on tissue injury in the lumbar spine, e.g., in the outer annulus fibrosus, ligaments, joints, and muscles. Such tissue injuries are likely to heal, at least in part, within a few weeks, a period consistent with the natural history of low back pain. There is a positive effect of motion on tissues that may cause back pain, including the disc.[6, 21, 111, 193, 250, 284, 295, 315, 316] Recently developed rehabilitation programs for low back pain, with early initiated, gradually increasing physical activity, are in part based on such knowledge of the beneficial response of injured tissues to controlled motion.[191, 193]

The tissue reactions that occur in spinal nerve roots in association with, for example, disc herniation, obviously have a complex background, involving mechanical and possibly also biochemical factors. The symptoms induced by nerve root compression may show a wide range of variability, including sensory changes, muscle weakness, and sometimes pain. However, spinal nerve root compression has been shown to exist also in asymptomatic individuals.[106, 313]

The functional changes in spinal nerve roots, induced by (for example) compression by a herniated intervertebral disc, may be of two different kinds: (1) loss of nerve function, clinically seen as sensory deficits or muscle weakness; and (2) hyperexcitability of the nerve tissue (Fig. 8–40). The hyperexcitability, which clinically is likely to be related to nerve root pain, seems to be based on ectopic impulse generation.[47, 229, 298] The two different kinds of functional changes (loss of nerve function and hyperexcitability) can be present simultaneously in a given nerve root. This means that an involved nerve root may show, for example, decreased conduction velocity or block of impulse propagation at the site of injury, although this injury site is hypersensitive to further mechanical deformation. Clinically, loss of nerve function can be analyzed by examination of sensory nerve conduction and electromyography. However, such objective neurophysiologic measurements may not necessarily correlate with the amount of nerve root pain experienced by the patient. The neurophysiologic examination merely provides information on whether a nerve root is affected or not, and may allow some degree of quantification of such involvement.

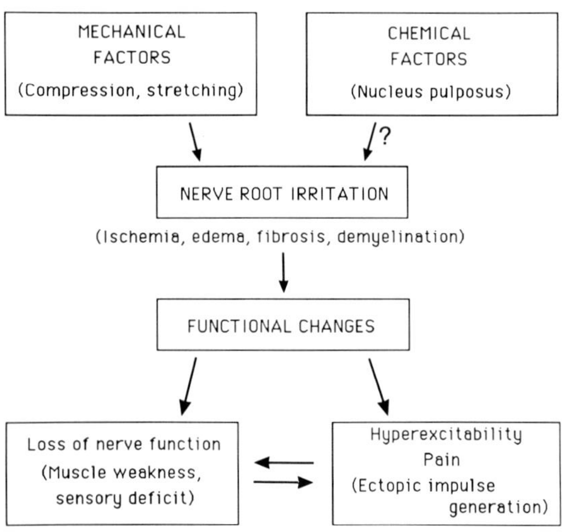

Figure 8–40. Proposed sequence of events leading to nerve root involvement in connection with disc herniation (i.e., sciatica). Mechanical, and possibly chemical, factors may lead to nerve root irritation, which in turn may induce various functional changes. Note that loss of nerve function is distinct from hyperexcitability, although these two kinds of functional changes may exist simultaneously in an injured nerve root segment. (Modified from Rydevik, B., and Garfin, S. R.: Spinal nerve root compression. *In* Szabo, R. (ed.): Nerve Compression Syndromes. Diagnosis and Treatment. Thorofare, NJ, Slack, 1989, pp. 247–261.)

CONCLUSION

The intervertebral discs play a crucial role in both normal function of the spine and in various pathologic conditions such as spinal disease and trauma. Normal structure and function of the discs is dependent on an adequate supply of nutrients. The discs, which in the adult state are avascular, receive their nutrition by diffusion through the end plates of the vertebral bodies and through the annulus fibrosus. Interference with these transport mechanisms may lead to degenerative changes in the discs. Biochemical and biomechanical alterations in the nucleus pulposus, which is devoid of sensory innervation, may lead to back pain owing to secondary (acute and chronic) effects of the nucleus pulposus on surrounding tissues. Thus, changes in the normal structure and function of the intervertebral discs may, via mechanical and possibly also biochemical mechanisms, affect adjacent neural structures, in terms of involvement of local sensory nervous system components in the motion segment, as well as the spinal nerve roots. Such pathophysiologic events can lead to various clinical symptoms, including back and nerve root pain.

References

1. Adamkiewicz, A.: Die Blutgefässe des menschlichen Rückenmarkes. I. Die Gefässe der Rückenmarkssubstanz. Sitzungsb. Akad. Wissensch. Wien. Math.-Naturw. *84*:469–502, 1881.
2. Adamkiewicz, A.: Die Blutgefässe des menschlichen Rückenmarkes. II. Die Gefässe der Rückenmark-

soberfläcke. Sitzungsb. Akad. Wissensch. Wien. Math.-Naturw. *85*:101–130, 1882.

3. Adams, H. D., and van Geertruyden, H. H.: Neurologic complications of aortic surgery. Ann. Surg. *144*:574–610, 1956.
4. Adams, P., and Muir, H.: Qualitative changes with age of proteoglycans of human lumbar disks. Ann. Rheum. Dis. *35*:289–296, 1976.
5. Akeson, W. H., and Murphy, R. W.: Editorial comment: low back pain. Clin. Orthop. *129*:2–3, 1977.
6. Akeson, W. H., Amiel, D., Abel, M. F., et al.: Effects of immobilization on joints. Clin. Orthop. *219*:28–37, 1987.
7. Andres, K. H.: Über die Feinstruktur der Arachnoidea und Dura mater von Mammalia. Z. Zellforsch. *79*:272–295, 1967.
8. Antonopolous, C. A.: Glycosaminoglycans of human nucleus pulposus. Identification and variation in their concentration with age. Acta Univ. Lund *11*:3–7, 1965.
9. Armstrong, J. R.: Lumbar Disc Lesions. Edinburgh, Livingstone, 1965.
10. Arvidsson, B.: Distribution of intravenously injected protein tracers in peripheral ganglia of adult mice. Exp. Neurol. *63*:388–410, 1979.
11. Bailey, A. J., and Robins, S. P.: Current topics in biosynthesis, structure and function of collagen. Sci. Prog. *63*:419–444, 1976.
12. Benn, R. T., and Wood, P. H. N.: Pain in the back Rheumatol. Rehabil. *14*:121–128, 1975.
13. Bentley, F. H., and Schlapp, W.: The effects of pressure on conduction in peripheral nerve. J. Physiol. *102*:72–82, 1943.
14. Bercovici, S., and Paraschivesco, E.: Recherche experimentale sur la discopathie vertebrale degenerative. Rev. Rhum. *25*:487–499, 1959.
15. Bisby, M. A.: Orthograde and retrograde axonal transport of labeled protein in motoneurons. Exp. Neurol. *50*:628–640, 1976.
16. Bisby, M. A.: Retrograde axonal transport. *In* Hertz, L., Fedoroff, S., and Hertz, L. (eds.): Advances in Cellular Neurobiology. Vol. 1. New York, Academic Press, 1980, pp. 69–117.
17. Black, M. M., and Lasek, R. J.: Slow components of axonal transport: two cytoskeletal networks. J. Cell. Biol. *86*:616–623, 1980.
18. Bobechko, W. P., and Hirsch, C.: Auto-immune response to nucleus pulposus in the rabbit. J. Bone Joint Surg. *47B*:574–580, 1965.
19. Bogduk, N., Tynan, W., and Wilson, A. S.: The nerve supply to the human lumbar intervertebral discs. J. Anat. *132*:39–56, 1981.
20. Bogduk, N., Windsor, M., and Inglis, A.: The innervation of the cervical intervertebral discs. Spine *13*:2–8, 1988.
21. Bortz, W. M.: The disuse syndrome. West. J. Med. *141*:691–694, 1984.
22. Bradford, D. S., Oegema, T. R., Jr., Cooper, K. M., et al.: Chymopapain, chemonucleolysis and pulposus regeneration. A biochemical and biomechanical study. Spine *9*:135–147, 1984.
23. Brady, S. T., and Lasek, R. J.: The slow components of axonal transport movements, compositions and organization. *In* Weiss, D. G. (ed.): Axoplasmic Transport. Berlin, Springer-Verlag, 1982, pp. 206–217.
24. Brodin, H.: Paths of nutrition in articular cartilage and intervertebral discs. Acta Orthop. Scand. *24*:177–180, 1955.
25. Brown, M. D.: Intradiscal Therapy—Chymopapain or Collagenase. Chicago, Year Book, 1983.
26. Brown, M. D., and Tsaltas, T. T.: Studies on the permeability of the intervertebral disc during skeletal maturation. Spine *1*:240–244, 1976.
27. Brown, M. D., Gepstein, R., and Pallares, V.: Somatosensory evoked potentials during epidural anaesthesia. 32nd Annual Meeting of the Orthopaedic Research Society (Trans.), New Orleans, February, 1986.
28. Buckwalter, J. A., Pedrini-Mille, A., Pedrini, V., and Tudisco, C.: Proteoglycans of human infant intervertebral disc. Electron microscopic and biochemical studies. J. Bone Joint Surg. *67A*:284–294, 1985.
29. Burchiel, K. J.: Effects of electrical and mechanical stimulation on two foci of spontaneous activity which develop in primary afferent neurons after peripheral axotomy. Pain *18*:249–265, 1984.
30. Burton, C. V.: Lumbosacral arachnoiditis. Spine *3*:24–30, 1978.
31. Cohen, M. S., Wall, E. J., Brown, R. B., et al.: Cauda equina anatomy. Part II: Extrathecal nerve roots and dorsal root ganglia. Spine *15*:1248–1251, 1990.
32. Comper, W. D., and Preston, B. N.: Model connective tissue systems: a study of polyion mobile ion and of excluded-volume interactions of proteoglycans. Biochem. J. *143*:1–9, 1974.
33. Coppes, M. H., Marani, E., Thomeer, R. T. W. M., and Oudega, M.: Innervation of annulus fibrosus in low back pain. Lancet *336*:189–190, 1990.
34. Corbin, J. L.: Anatome et Pathologie Arterielles de la Moelle. Paris, Masson & Cie, 1961.
35. Crank, J.: The Mathematics of Diffusion. Oxford, Oxford University Press, 1975.
36. Crock, H. V., and Yoshizawa, H.: The blood supply of the lumbar vertebral column. Clin. Orthop. *115*:6–21, 1976.
37. Crock, H. V., and Yoshizawa, H.: The Blood Supply of the Vertebral Column and Spinal Cord in Man. New York, Springer-Verlag, 1977.
38. Dahlin, L. B., Rydevik, B., McLean, W. G., and Sjöstrand, J.: Changes in fast axonal transport during experimental nerve compression at low pressures. Exp. Neurol. *84*:29–36, 1984.
39. Dahlin, L. B., and McLean, W. G.: Effects of graded experimental compression on slow and fast axonal transport in rabbit vagus nerve. J. Neurol. Sci. *72*:19–30, 1986.
40. Dahlin, L. B., Shyu, B. C., Danielsen, N., and Andersson, S. A.: Effects of nerve compression or ischemia on conduction properties of myelinated and non-myelinated nerve fibers. An experimental study in rabbit common peroneal nerve. Acta Physiol. Scand. *136*:97–105, 1989.
41. Dahlström, A.: Axoplasmic transport (with particular respect to adrenergic neurons). Philos. Trans. R. Soc. Lond. (Biol.) *261*:325–358, 1971.
42. Danielsen, N., Lundborg, G., and Frizell, M.: Nerve repair and axonal transport: distribution of axonally transported proteins during maturation period in regenerating rabbit hypoglossal nerve. J. Neurol. Sci. *73*:269–277, 1986.

43. Davidson, E. A., and Woodhall, B.: Biochemical alterations in herniated intervertebral disks. J. Biol. Chem. *234*:2951–2954, 1959.
44. Davidson, E., and Small, W.: Metabolism in vivo of connective tissue mucopolysaccharides. Chondroitin sulphate C and keratan sulphate of nucleus pulposus. Biochim. Biophys. Acta *69*:445–452, 1963.
45. Delamarter, R. B., Bohlman, H. H., Dodge, L. D., and Biro, C.: Experimental lumbar spinal stenosis: analysis of the cortical evoked potentials, microvasculature and histopathology. J. Bone Joint Surg. *72A*:110–120, 1990.
46. Desproges-Gotteron, R.: Contribution à l'étude de la sciatique paralysante. Thesis No. 342, Paris, 1955.
47. Devor, M.: The pathophysiology of damaged peripheral nerves. *In* Wall, P. D., and Melzack, R. (eds.): Textbook of Pain. 2nd ed. Edinburgh, Churchill Livingstone, 1989, pp. 63–81.
48. Diamant, B., Karlsson, J., and Nachemson, A.: Correlation between lactate levels and pH in discs of patients with lumbar rhizopathies. Experientia *24*:1195–1196, 1968.
49. Dommisse, G. F.: Morphological aspects of the lumbar spine and lumbosacral region. Orthop. Clin. North Am. *6*:163–175, 1975.
50. Dommisse, G. F.: Arteries and veins of the lumbar nerve roots. Clin. Orthop. *115*:22–29, 1976.
51. Donnish, E. W., and Trapp, W.: The cartilage endplates of the human vertebral column (some considerations of postnatal development). Anat. Rec. *169*:705–716, 1971.
52. Dorland's Illustrated Medical Dictionary. 27th ed. Philadelphia, W. B. Saunders Co., 1988.
53. Droz, B.: Synthetic machinery and axoplasmic transport: maintenance of neuronal connectivity. *In* Tower, D. B. (ed.): The Nervous System. Vol. 1. The Basic Neurosciences. New York, Raven Press, 1975, pp. 111–127.
54. Duret, H.: Note sur les artères nourriciéres et sur les vaisseaux capillaires de la moelle épinère. Progr. Med. *1*:284, 1873.
55. Duret, H.: Conclusion d'un mémoire sur la circulation bulbaire. Arch. Physiol. Norm. Pathol. *50*:88–89, 1873.
56. Edwards, D. J., and Cattell, M. K.: Further observations on decrement in nerve conduction. Am. J. Physiol. *87*:359–367, 1928.
57. Emes, J. H., and Pearce, R. H.: The proteoglycans of human intervertebral discs. Biochem. J. *145*:549–556, 1975.
58. Evans, W., Jobe, W., and Seibert, C.: A cross-sectional prevalence study of lumbar spine degeneration in a working population. Spine *14*:60–64, 1989.
59. Eyre, D. R., and Muir, H.: Types I and II collagens in intervertebral disc. Biochem. J. *157*:267–270, 1976.
60. Eyre, D. R., and Muir, H.: Quantitative analysis of types I and II collagens in human intervertebral discs at various ages. Biochim. Biophys. Acta *492*:29–42, 1977.
61. Finneson, B. E.: Low Back Pain. Philadelphia, J. B. Lippincott Co., 1973.
62. Fowler, R. J., Danta, G., and Gilliatt, R. W.: Recovery of nerve conduction after a pneumatic tourniquet: observations on the hind-limb of the baboon. J. Neurol. Neurosurg. Psychiatry *35*:638–647, 1972.
63. Fried, L. C., and Doppman, J.: The arterial supply to the lumbosacral spinal cord in the monkey. A comparison with man. Anat. Rec. *178*:41–48, 1958.
64. Frymoyer, J. W., Pope, M. H., Clements, J. H., et al.: Risk factors in low-back pain: an epidemiological study. J. Bone Joint Surg. *65A*:213–218, 1983.
65. Frymoyer, J. W., and Gordon, S. L.: New Perspectives on Low Back Pain. American Academy of Orthopaedic Surgeons, 1989.
66. Galante, J. O.: Tensile properties of the human lumbar annulus fibrosus. Acta Orthop. Scand. (Suppl.) 100, 1967.
67. Garfin, S. R., and Herkowitz, H. N.: Disc disease—does it exist? *In* Weinstein, J. N., and Wiesel, S. W. (eds.): The Lumbar Spine. Philadelphia, W. B. Saunders Co., 1990, pp. 369–380.
68. Garfin, S. R., Cohen, M. S., Massie, J. B., et al.: Nerve-roots of the cauda equina. The effects of hypotension and acute graded compression on function. J. Bone Joint Surg. *72A*:1185–1192, 1990.
69. Gasser, H. S.: Conduction in nerves in relation to fiber types. Proc. Assoc. Res. Nerv. Ment. Dis. *15*:35–59, 1935.
70. Gasser, H. S., and Erlanger, J.: The role of fiber size in the establishment of a nerve block by pressure and cocain. Am. J. Physiol. *88*:581–591, 1929.
71. Gepstein, R., and Brown, M. D.: Somatosensory-evoked potentials in lumbar nerve root decompression. Clin. Orthop. *245*:69–71, 1989.
72. Gertzbein, S. D., Tile, M., Gross, A., et al.: Autoimmunity in degenerative disc disease of the lumbar spine. Orthop. Clin. North Am. *6*:67–73, 1975.
73. Ghosh, P., Taylor, T. K. F., Braund, K. G., and Larsen, L. H.: The collagenous and non-collagenous protein of the canine intervertebral disc and their variation with age, spinal level and breed. Gerontology *22*:124–132, 1976.
74. Ghosh, P., Taylor, T. K. F., and Braund, K. G.: Variation of the glycosaminoglycans of the canine intervertebral disc with ageing. I. Chondrodystrophoid breed. Gerontology *23*:87–98, 1977.
75. Ghosh, P., Taylor, T. K. F., and Braund, K. G.: Variation of the glycosaminoglycans of the intervertebral disc with ageing. II. Non-chondrodystrophoid breed. Gerontology *23*:99–109, 1977.
76. Ghosh, P., Bushell, G. R., Taylor, T. K. F., and Sutherland, J. M.: The influence of spinal curvature on collagen distribution across the normal and scoliotic disc. Trans. Am. Orthop. Res. Soc., 24th Annual Meeting, 1978.
77. Giles, L. G. F., and Taylor, J. R.: Innervation of lumbar zygapophyseal joint synovial folds. Acta Orthop. Scand. *58*:43–46, 1987.
78. Gillilan, L. A.: The arterial blood supply of the human spinal cord. J. Comp. Neurol. *110*:75–103, 1958.
79. Goddard, M. D., and Reede, J. D.: Movements induced by straight leg raising in the lumbo-sacral roots, nerves and plexus, and in the intrapelvic section of the sciatic nerve. J. Neurol. Neurosurg. Psychiatry *28*:12–18, 1965.

80. Govrin-Lippman, R., and Devor, M.: Ongoing activity in severed nerves: source and variation with time. Brain Res. *159*:406–410, 1978.
81. Gower, W. E., and Pedrini, V.: Age related variations in protein-polysaccharides from human nucleus pulposus, annulus fibrosus, and costal cartilage. J. Bone Joint Surg. *51A*:1154–1162, 1969.
82. Grafstein, B., and Forman, D. S.: Intracellular transport in neurons. Physiol. Rev. *60*:1167–1283, 1980.
83. Greenbarg, P. E., Brown, M. D., Pallares, V. S., et al.: Epidural anesthesia for lumbar spine surgery. J. Spinal Dis. *1*:139–143, 1988.
84. Grundfest, H.: Effects of hydrostatic pressure upon the excitability, the recovery, and the potential sequence of frog nerve. Cold Spring Harb. Symp. Quant. Biol. *4*:179–187, 1936.
85. Hakelius, A.: Prognosis in sciatica: a clinical follow-up of surgical and non-surgical treatment. Acta Orthop. Scand. (Suppl.) 129, 1970.
86. Hallen, A.: Hexosamine and ester sulphate content of the human nucleus pulposus at different ages. Acta Chem. Scand. *12*:1869–1872, 1958.
87. Hallen, A.: The collagen and ground substance of human disc at different ages. Acta Chem. Scand. *16*:705–709, 1962.
88. Hansen, H. J., and Ullberg, S.: Uptake of ^{35}S in the intervertebral disc after injection of ^{35}S sulphate. An autoradiographic study. Acta Orthop. Scand. *30*:84–90, 1961.
89. Hansson, T., Keller, T., and Spengler, D.: Mechanical behavior of the human lumbar spine. II: Fatigue strength during dynamic compressive loading. J. Orthop. Res. *5*:479–487, 1987.
90. Hansson, T., and Holm, S.: Clinical implications of vibration-induced changes in the lumbar spine. Orthop. Clin. North Am. *22*:247–254, 1991.
91. Happey, F.: A biophysical study of the human intervertebral disc. *In* Jayson, M. I. V. (ed.): The Lumbar Spine and Back Pain. London, Pitman Medical, 1976, pp. 293–316.
92. Hardingham, T. E.: The role of link protein in the structure of articular cartilage proteoglycans aggregates. Biochem. J. *177*:237–247, 1979.
93. Hardingham, T. E., and Muir, H.: The specific of hyaluronic acid with cartilage proteoglycans. Biochim. Biophys. Acta *279*:401–405, 1972.
94. Hascall, V. C., and Sajdera, S. W.: Physical properties and polydispersity of proteoglycan from bovine nasal cartilage. J. Biol. Chem. *245*:4920–4930, 1970.
95. Hasue, M., Kunogi, J., Konno, S., and Kikuchi, S.: Classification by position of dorsal root ganglia in the lumbosacral region. Spine *14*:1261–1264, 1989.
96. Haughton, V. M., Ho, K. C., Larson, S. J., et al.: Comparison of arachnoiditis produced by meglumine iocarmate and metrizamide myelography in an animal model. A. J. R. *131*:129–132, 1978.
97. Helfferich, F.: Ion Exchange. New York, McGraw-Hill Book Co., 1962.
98. Heiliövaara, M.: Occupation and risk of herniated lumbar intervertebral disc or sciatica leading to hospitalization. J. Chronic Dis. *3*:259–264, 1987.
99. Hendry, N. G. C.: Hydration of the nucleus pulposus and its relation to intervertebral disc derangement. J. Bone Joint Surg. *40B*:132–144, 1958.
100. Herren, R. Y., and Alexander, L.: Sulcal and intrinsic blood vessels of human spinal cord. Arch. Neurol. Psychiat. *41*:678–687, 1939.
101. Higuchi, M., Abe, K., and Kaneda, K.: Changes in the nucleus pulposus of the intervertebral disc in bipedal mice. Clin. Orthop. *175*:251–257, 1983.
102. Hirsch, C.: Studies on the mechanism of low back pain. Acta Orthop. Scand. *20*:261–274, 1951.
103. Hirsch, C., and Schajowicz, F.: Studies on the structural changes in the lumbar annulus fibrosus. Acta Orthop. Scand. *22*:184–192, 1952.
104. Hirsch, C., and Schajowicz, S.: Studies on structural changes in the lumbar annulus fibrosus. Acta Orthop. Scand. *22*:184–231, 1953.
105. Hirsch, C., and Nachemson, A.: New observations on mechanical behaviour of lumbar discs. Acta Orthop. Scand. *23*:254–283, 1954.
106. Hitselberger, W. E., and Witten, R. M.: Abnormal myelograms in asymptomatic patients. J. Neurosurg. *28*:204–206, 1968.
107. Holm, S.: Does diabetes induce degenerative processes in the lumbar intervertebral disc? Kyoto, Japan, Proceedings of the International Society for the Study of the Lumbar Spine, 1989.
108. Holm, S. H.: Nutrition of the intervertebral disc. *In* Weinstein, J. N., and Wiesel, S. W. (eds.): The Lumbar Spine. Philadelphia, W. B. Saunders Co., 1990, pp. 244–260.
109. Holm, S., Maroudas, A., Urban, J. P. G., et al.: Nutrition of the intervertebral disc. Connect. Tissue Res. *8*:101–119, 1981.
110. Holm, S., and Nachemson, A.: Nutrition changes in the canine intervertebral disc after spinal fusion. Clin. Orthop. *169*:243–258, 1982.
111. Holm, S., and Nachemson, A.: Variations in the nutrition of the canine intervertebral disc induced by motion. Spine *8*:866–874, 1983.
112. Holm, S., and Nachemson, A.: Cellularity of the lumbar intervertebral disc and its relevance to nutrition. Orthop. Trans. *7*:457–458, 1983.
113. Holm, S., and Nachemson, A.: Immediate effects of cigarette smoke on nutrition of the intervertebral disc of the pig. Orthop. Trans. *8*:380, 1984.
114. Holm, S., and Nachemson, A.: Nutrition of the intervertebral disc: effects induced by vibrations. Orthop. Trans. *9*:451, 1985.
115. Holm, S., and Rosenqvist, A.-L.: Morphological and nutritional changes in the intervertebral disc after spinal motion. Scand. J. Rheumatol. (Suppl.) *60*:A117, 1986.
116. Holm, S., and Urban, J.: The intervertebral disc: factors contributing to its nutrition and matrix turnover. *In* Helminen, H. J., Kiviranta, I., Tammi, M., et al. (eds.): Joint Loading. Bristol, Wright, 1987, pp. 187–226.
117. Holm, S., and Nachemson, A.: Nutrition of the intervertebral disc: acute effects of cigarette smoking. An experimental animal study. Upsala J. Med. Sci. *93*:91–99, 1988.
118. Holm, S., Rydevik, B., Nordborg, C., et al.: Experimental spinal arachnoiditis: a nutritional, radiographic and histologic investigation. Submitted to Spine, 1991.
119. Horal, J.: The clinical appearance of low back disorders in the city of Gothenburg, Sweden. Acta Orthop. Scand. (Suppl.) 118, 1969.
120. Howe, J. F., Calvin, W. H., and Losser, J. D.: Impulses reflected from dorsal root ganglia and from focal nerve injuries. Brain Res. *116*:139–144, 1976.
121. Howe, J. F., Loeser, J. D., and Calvin, W. H.:

Mechanosensitivity of dorsal root ganglia and chronically injured axons: a physiological basis for the radicular pain of nerve root compression. Pain *3*:25–41, 1977.
122. Hoyland, J. A., Freemont, A. J., and Jayson, M. I. V.: Intervertebral foramen venous obstruction. A cause of periradicular fibrosis? Spine *14*:558–568, 1989.
123. Hudlicka, O., and Tyler K. R.: The effect of long-term high-frequency stimulation on capillary density and fiber types in rabbit fast muscles. J. Physiol. (Lond.) *353*:435–445, 1984.
124. Hult, L.: Cervical, dorsal and lumbar spine syndromes. Acta Orthop. Scand. *17* (Suppl.):65–73, 1954.
125. Inoue, H.: Three dimensional observation of collagen framework of intervertebral discs in rats, dogs and humans. Arch. Histol. Jpn. *36*:39–56, 1973.
126. Inoue, H., and Takeda, T.: Three dimensional observations of collagen framework of lumbar intervertebral discs. Acta Orthop. Scand. *46*:949–956, 1975.
127. Jacobs, J. M., Macfarlande, R. M., and Cavanagh, J. B.: Vascular leakage in the dorsal root ganglia of the rat studied with horseradish peroxidase. J. Neurol. Sci. *29*:95–107, 1976.
128. Jayson, M. I. V., Keegan, A. L., Million, R., and Tomlinson, I.: A fibrinolytic defect in chronic back pain syndromes. Lancet *24*:1186–1187, 1984.
129. Kadyi, H.: Über die Blutgefässe des menschlichen Rückenmarkes. Anat. Anz. *1*:304–314, 1886 (cited by Gillilan, 1958).
130. Katz, M. M., Hargens, A. R., and Garfin, S. R.: Intervertebral disc nutrition. Diffusion versus convection. Clin. Orthop. *210*:243–245, 1986.
131. Kazarian, L. E.: Creep characteristics of the human spinal column. Orthop. Clin. North Am. *6*:3–18, 1975.
132. Kellgren, J. H., and Lawrence, J. S.: Osteoarthrosis and disc degeneration in an urban population. Ann. Rheum. Dis. *17*:388–397, 1958.
133. Kelsey, J. L.: An epidemiological study of the relationship between occupation and acute herniated lumbar intervertebral discs. Int. J. Epidemiol. *4*:197–205, 1976.
134. Kelsey, J. L., Githens, P. B., and O'Connor, T.: Acute prolapsed lumbar intervertebral disc. An epidemiologic study with special reference to driving automobiles and cigarette smoking. Spine *9*:608–613, 1984.
135. Kempson, G. E., Muir, H., and Pollard, C.: The tensile properties of the cartilage of human femoral condyles related to the content of collagen and glycosaminoglycans. Biochim. Biophys. Acta *297*:456–472, 1973.
136. Kimmel, D. L.: Innervation of spinal dura mater and dura mater of the posterior cranial fossa. Neurology *11*:800–809, 1961.
137. Korkala, O., Grönblad, M., Liesi, P., and Karaharju, E.: Immunohistochemical demonstration of nociceptors in the ligamentous structures of the lumbar spine. Spine *10*:156–157, 1985.
138. Kristensson, K., and Sjöstrand, J.: Retrograde transport of protein tracer in the rabbit hypoglossal nerve during regeneration. Brain Res. *45*:175–181, 1972.
139. Kristensson, K., and Olsson, Y.: Retrograde transport of horseradish peroxidase in transected axons. 3. Entry into injured axons and subsequent localization in perikaryon. Brain Res. *115*:201–213, 1976.
140. Kuslich, S. D., and Ulstrom, C. L.: The origin of low back pain and sciatica: a microsurgical investigation. *In* Williams, R. W., McCulloch, J. A., and Young, P. H. (eds.): Microsurgery of the Lumbar Spine. Rockville, MD, Aspen Publishers, 1990, pp. 1–7.
141. Lane, J. M., Brighton, C. T., and Menkowitz, B. J.: Anaerobic and aerobic metabolism in articular cartilage. J. Rheumatol. *4*:334–342, 1977.
142. Lasek, R. J.: Protein transport in neurons. Int. Rev. Neurobiol. *13*:289–324, 1970.
143. Lazorthes, G., Gouazé, A., Bastide, G., et al.: La vascularisation artérielle du renflement lombaire. Étude des variations et des suppléances. Rev. Neurol. *114*:109–122, 1966.
144. Lazorthes, G., Gouazé, A., Zadeh, J. O., et al.: Arterial vascularization of the spinal cord. Recent studies of the anatomic substitution pathways. J. Neurosurg. *35*:253–262, 1971.
145. Leone, J., and Ochs, S.: Anoxic block and recovery of axoplasmic transport and electrical excitability of nerve. J. Neurobiol. *9*:229–245, 1978.
146. Lindblom, K.: Experimental ruptures of intervertebral discs in rat tails. J. Bone Joint Surg. *34A*:123–128, 1952.
147. Lindblom, K., and Rexed, B.: Spinal nerve injury in dorso-lateral protrusions of lumbar disks. J. Neurosurg. *5*:413–432, 1948.
148. Lipson, S. J.: Aging versus degeneration of the intervertebral disc. *In* Weinstein, J. N., and Wiesel, S. W. (eds.): The Lumbar Spine. Philadelphia, W. B. Saunders Co., 1990, pp. 261–265.
149. Lipson, S. J., and Muir, H.: Vertebral osteophyte formation in experimental disc degeneration. Arthritis Rheum. *23*:319–324, 1980.
150. Lipson, S. J., and Muir, H.: Proteoglycans in experimental intervertebral disc degeneration. Spine *6*:194–210, 1981.
151. Lohmander, S., Antonopoulos, C. A., and Friberg, U.: Chemical and metabolic heterogeneity of chondroitin sulphate and keratan sulphate in guinea pig cartilage and nucleus pulposus. Biochim. Biophys. Acta *304*:430–448, 1973.
152. Longmuir, J. S.: Respiration rate of rat liver cells at low oxygen concentration. Biochem. J. *65*:378–382, 1957.
153. Low, P. A., and Dyck, P. J.: Increased endoneurial fluid pressure in experimental lead neuropathy. Nature *269*:427–428, 1977.
154. Low, P. A., Dyck, P. J., and Schmelzer, J. D.: Chronic elevation of endoneurial fluid pressure is associated with low-grade fiber pathology. Muscle Nerve *5*:162–165, 1982.
155. Lubinska, L.: On axoplasmic flow. Int. Rev. Neurobiol. *17*:241–296, 1975.
156. Lundborg, G.: Structure and function of the intraneural microvessels as related to trauma, edema formation, and nerve function. J. Bone Joint Surg. *57A*:938–948, 1975.
157. Lundborg, G.: Nerve regeneration and repair—a review. Acta Orthop. Scand. *58*:145–169, 1987.
158. Lundborg, G.: Nerve Injury and Repair. Edinburgh, Churchill Livingstone, 1988.

159. Lundborg, G., Gelberman, R. H., Minteer-Convery, M., et al.: Median nerve compression in the carpal tunnel—functional response to experimentally induced controlled pressure. J. Hand Surg. *7*:252–259, 1982.
160. Lundborg, G., Myers, R., and Powell, H.: Nerve compression injury and increased endoneurial fluid pressure: a "miniature compartment syndrome." J. Neurol. Neurosurg. Psychiatry *46*:1119–1124, 1983.
161. Lundborg, G., Rydevik, B., Manthorpe, M., et al.: Peripheral nerve: the physiology of injury and repair. *In* Woo, S. L. Y., and Buckwalter, J. A. (eds.): Injury and Repair of the Musculoskeletal Soft Tissues. American Academy of Orthopaedic Surgeons Symposium. Parke Ridge, IL, American Academy of Orthopaedic Surgeons, 1988.
162. MacGregor, R. J., Sharpless, S. K., and Luttges, M. W.: A pressure vessel model for nerve compression. J. Neurol. Sci. *24*:299–304, 1975.
163. Macnab, I.: The mechanism of spondylogenic pain. *In* Hirsch, C., and Zotterman, Y. (eds.): Cervical Pain. New York, Pergamon Press, 1972, pp. 89–95.
164. Magora, A., and Schwartz, A.: Relation between the low back pain syndrome and x-ray findings. I. Degenerative osteoarthritis. Scand. J. Rehabil. Med. *8*:115–125, 1976.
165. Malinsky, J.: The ontogenetic development of nerve terminations in the intervertebral discs of man. Acta Anat. *38*:96–113, 1959.
166. Marcus, R. E.: The effect of low oxygen concentration on growth, glycolysis and sulphate incorporation by articular chondrocytes in monolayer culture. Arthritis Rheum. *16*:646–656, 1973.
167. Marcus, R. E., and Srivastava, V. M. L.: Effect of low oxygen tensions on glucose-metabolizing enzymes in cultured articular chondrocytes. Proc. Soc. Exp. Biol. Med. *143*:488–491, 1973.
168. Markolf, K. L., and Morris, J. M.: The structural components of the intervertebral disc. J. Bone Joint Surg. *56A*:675–685, 1974.
169. Maroudas, A.: Distribution and diffusion of solutes in articular cartilage. Biophys. J. *10*:365–379, 1970.
170. Maroudas, A.: Glycosaminoglycan turnover in articular cartilage. Philos. Trans. R. Soc. Lond. *271*:292–313, 1975.
171. Maroudas, A.: Physico-chemical properties of articular cartilage. *In* Freeman, M. A. R. (ed.): Adult Articular Cartilage. 2nd ed. London, Pitman Medical, 1979.
172. Maroudas, A., Stockwell, R. A., Nachemson, A., and Urban, J.: Factors involved in the nutrition of the human lumbar intervertebral disc: cellularity and diffusion of glucose in vitro. J. Anat. *120*:113–130, 1975.
173. Marshall, L. L., and Trethewie, E. R.: Chemical irritation of nerve-root in disc prolapse. Lancet *2*:320, 1973.
174. Marshall, L. L., Trethewie, E. R., and Curtain, C. C.: Chemical radiculitis: a clinical, physiological and immunological study. Clin. Orthop. *129*:61–67, 1977.
175. McCabe, J. S., and Low, F. N.: The subarachnoid angle: an area of transition in peripheral nerve. Anat. Rec. *164*:15–34, 1969.
176. McCarron, R. F., Wimpee, M. W., Hudkins, P. G., et al.: The inflammatory effect of nucleus pulposus: a possible element in the pathogenesis of low back pain. Spine *12*:760–764, 1987.
177. McCollough, J. A., and Macnab, I.: Sciatica and Chymopapain. Baltimore, Williams & Wilkins Co., 1983.
178. McLean, W. G., McKay, A. L., and Sjöstrand, J.: Electrophoretic analysis of axonally transported proteins in rabbit vagus nerve. J. Neurobiol. *14*:227–236, 1983.
179. Meek, W. J., and Leaper, W. E.: The effect of pressure on conductivity of nerve and muscle. Am. J. Physiol. *27*:308–322, 1911.
180. Miller, J. A. A., Schmatz, C., and Schultz, A. B.: Lumbar disc degeneration: correlation with age, sex and spine level in 600 autopsy specimens. Spine *13*:173–178, 1988.
181. Mitchell, P. E. G., Hendry, N. G. C., and Billewicz, W. Z.: The chemical background of intervertebral disc prolapse. J. Bone Joint Surg. *43B*:141–151, 1961.
182. Mixter, W. J., and Barr, J. S.: Rupture of the intervertebral disc with involvement of the spinal canal. N. Engl. J. Med. *211*:210–215, 1934.
183. Myers, R. R., and Powell, H. C.: Endoneurial fluid pressure in peripheral neuropathies. *In* Hargens, A. R. (ed.): Tissue Fluid Pressure and Composition. Baltimore, William & Wilkins Co., 1981, pp. 193–207
184. Myers, R. R., Mizisin, A. P., Powell, H. C., and Lampert, P. W.: Reduced nerve blood flow in hexachlorophene neuropathy. Relationship to elevated endoneurial fluid pressure. J. Neuropathol. Exp. Neurol. *41*:391–399, 1982.
185. Myers, R. R., and Powell, H. C.: Galactose neuropathy: impact of chronic endoneurial edema on nerve blood flow. Ann. Neurol. *16*:587–594, 1984.
186. Myers, R. R., Murakami, H., and Powell, H. C.: Reduced nerve blood flow in edematous neuropathies: a biomechanical mechanism. Microvasc. Res. *32*:145–151, 1986.
187. Nachemson, A.: Intradiscal measurements of pH in patients with lumbar rhizopathies. Acta Orthop. Scand. *40*:23–42, 1969.
188. Nachemson, A.: Towards a better understanding of low-back pain: a review of the mechanics of the lumbar disc. Rheumatol. Rehabil. *14*:129–143, 1975.
189. Nachemson, A.: The lumbar spine. An orthopaedic challenge. Spine *1*:59–71, 1976.
190. Nachemson, A.: The natural course of low back pain. *In* White, A. A., and Gordon, S. L. (eds.): Symposium on Idiopathic Low Back Pain. St. Louis, C. V. Mosby Co., 1982, pp. 46–51.
191. Nachemson, A.: Work for all. For those with low back pain as well. Clin. Orthop. *179*:77–85, 1983.
192. Nachemson, A.: Prevention of chronic back pain. The orthopaedic challenge for the 80's. Bull. Hosp. Joint Dis. Orth. Inst. *44*:1–15, 1984.
193. Nachemson, A.: The future of low back pain. *In:* Weinstein, J. N., and Wiesel, S. W. (eds.): The Lumbar Spine. Philadelphia, W. B. Saunders Co., 1990, pp. 56–70.
194. Nachemson, A., and Elfström, G.: Intravital dynamic pressure measurements in lumbar discs. A study of common movements, maneuvers and exercises. Scand. J. Rehabil. Med. *2* (Suppl. 1):1–40, 1970.
195. Nachemson, A., Lewin, T., Maroudas, A., and

Freeman, M. A. R.: In vitro diffusion of dye through the end-plates and the annulus fibrosus of human lumbar intervertebral discs. Acta Orthop. Scand. *41*:589–607, 1970.

196. Nachemson, A., Schultz, A. B., and Berkson, M. H.: Mechanical properties of human spine motion segments. Influence of age, sex, disc level and degeneration. Spine *4*:1–8, 1979.
197. Nachemson, A. L., and Andersson, G. B. J.: Classification of low-back pain. Scand. J. Work Environ. Health *8*:134–136, 1982.
198. Nachemson, A., and Rydevik, B.: Chemonucleolysis for sciatica—a critical review. Acta Orthop. Scand. *59*:5–62, 1988.
199. Nade, S. M. L., Bell, E., and Wyke, B. D.: The innervation of the lumbar spinal joints and its significance. J. Bone Joint Surg. *62B*:255–261, 1980.
200. Naylor, A.: The biophysical and biochemical aspects of intervertebral disc herniation and degeneration. Ann. R. Coll. Surg. Engl. *31*:91–114, 1962.
201. Naylor, A.: The structure and function of the intervertebral disc. Orthopaedics (Oxford) *3*:7–22, 1970.
202. Ochoa, J., Fowler, T. J., and Gilliatt, R. W.: Anatomical changes in peripheral nerves compressed by a pneumatic tourniquet. J. Anat. *113*:433–455, 1972.
203. Ochs, S.: Systems of material transport in nerve fibers (axoplasmic transport) related to nerve function and trophic control. Ann. N. Y. Acad. Sci. *228*:202–223, 1974.
204. Ochs, S.: Axoplasmic transport. *In* Tower, D. (ed.): The Nervous System. Vol. 1. The Basic Neurosciences. New York, Raven Press, 1975, pp. 137–146.
205. Olmarker, K.: Spinal nerve root compression. Experimental studies on effects of acute, graded compression on nerve root nutrition and function, with an *in vivo* compression model of the porcine cauda equina. Doctoral Thesis, University of Göteborg, Sweden, 1990.
206. Olmarker, K., Rydevik, B., Holm, S., and Bagge, U.: Effects of experimental, graded compression on blood flow in spinal nerve roots. A vital microscopic study on the porcine cauda equina. J. Orthop. Res. 7:817–823, 1989.
207. Olmarker, K., Rydevik, B., and Holm, S.: Edema formation in spinal nerve roots induced by experimental, graded compression. An experimental study on the pig cauda equina with special reference to differences in effects between rapid and slow onset of compression. Spine *14*:569–573, 1989.
208. Olmarker, K., Rydevik, B., Hansson, T., and Holm, S.: Compression-induced changes of the nutritional supply to the porcine cauda equina. J. Spinal Dis. *3*:25–29, 1990.
209. Olmarker, K., Holm, S., Rosenqvist, A.-L., and Rydevik, B.: Experimental nerve root compression. A model of acute, graded compression of the porcine cauda equina, and an analysis of neural and vascular anatomy. Spine *16*:61–69, 1991.
210. Olmarker, K., Holm, S., and Rydevik, B.: Importance of compression onset rate for the degree of impairment of impulse propagation in experimental compression injury of the porcine cauda equina. Spine *15*:416–419, 1990.
211. Olmarker, K., Holm, S., and Rydevik, B.: Cauda equina compression at single versus multiple levels. An experimental study on the porcine cauda equina with analyses of impairment of nerve impulse conduction properties. Clin. Orthop. 1991 (in press).
212. Olsson, Y.: The involvement of vasa nervorum in diseases of peripheral nerves. *In* Vinken, P. S., and Bruyn, G. W. (eds.): Handbook of Clinical Neurology. Vol. 12. Vascular Diseases of the Nervous System. New York, Elsevier, 1972, pp. 644–664.
213. Olsson, Y., and Kristensson, K.: Permeability of blood vessels and sheath in the peripheral nervous system to exogenous proteins. Acta Neuropathol. *5* (Suppl.):61–69, 1971.
214. Olsson, Y., and Kristensson, K.: The perineurium as a diffusion barrier to protein tracers following trauma to nerves. Acta Neuropathol. *23*:105–111, 1973.
215. Oshino, N., Sugano, T., and Oshino, R., et al.: Mitochondrial function under hypoxic conditions: the steady states of cytochrome alpha+ alpha3 and their relation to mitochondrial energy states. Biochim. Biophys. Acta *368*:298–310, 1974.
216. Parke, W. W.: Applied anatomy of the spine. *In* Rothman, R. H., and Simeone, F. (eds.): The Spine. 2nd ed. Vol. 1. Philadelphia, W. B. Saunders Co., 1982, pp. 18–51.
217. Parke, W. W.: The innervation of connective tissues of the spinal motion segment. Presented at the International Symposium on Percutaneous Lumbar Discectomy. Philadelphia, PA, November 1987.
218. Parke, W. W., Gammell, K., and Rothman, R. H.: Arterial vascularization of the cauda equina. J. Bone Joint Surg. *63A*:53–62, 1981.
219. Parke, W. W., and Watanabe, R.: The intrinsic vasculature of the lumbosacral spinal nerve roots. 1985 Volvo Award in Basic Science. Spine *10*:508–515, 1985.
220. Parsons, D. B., Brennan, M. B., Glimcher, M. J., and Hall, J.: Scoliosis: collagen defect in the intervertebral disc. Trans. Orthop. Res. Soc. *7*:52, 1982.
221. Paulson, S., and Sylven, B.: Biophysical and physiological investigations on cartilage and other mesenchymal tissues. III. The diffusion rate of various substances in normal bovine nucleus pulposus. Biochim. Biophys. Acta. *7*:207–213, 1951.
222. Pedersen, H. E., Blunck, C. F. J., and Gardner, E.: Anatomy of lumbosacral rami and meningeal branches of spinal nerves. J. Bone Joint Surg. *38A*:377–391, 1956.
223. Pedowitz, R. A., Garfin, S. R., Massie, J. B., et al.: Effects of magnitude and duration of compression on spinal nerve root conduction. Spine 1991 (in press).
224. Pedrini, V. A., Ponseti, I. V., and Dohrman, S. C.: Glycosaminoglycans of intervertebral discs in idiopathic scoliosis. J. Lab. Clin. Med. *82*:938–950, 1973.
225. Pedrini-Mille, A., Pedrini, V. A., Tudicio, C., et al.: Proteoglycans of human scoliotic intervertebral disc. J. Bone Joint Surg. *65A*:815–823, 1983.
226. Petterson, C. Å. V., and Olsson, Y.: Blood supply of spinal nerve roots. An experimental study in the rat. Acta Neuropathol. *78*:455–461, 1989.
227. Pope, M. H., Wilder, D. G., and Frymoyer, J. W.:

Vibration as an aetiological factor of low back pain. *In* Engineering Aspects of the Spine. Mech. Eng. Publ. No. 1980–2, 1980.

228. Putschar, W.: Comparative disc pathology. Lab. Invest. *8*:1259–1263, 1959.

229. Rasminsky, M.: Ectopic generation of impulses in pathological nerve fibers. *In* Jewett, D. L., and McCarroll, H. R. (eds.): Nerve Repair and Regeneration—Its Clinical and Experimental Basis. St. Louis, C. V. Mosby Co., 1980, pp. 178–185.

230. Rauschning, W.: Normal and pathologic anatomy of the lumbar root canals. Spine *12*:1008–1019, 1987.

231. Roberts, S., Menage, J., and Urban, J. P. G.: Biochemical and structural properties of the cartilage endplate and its relation to the intervertebral disc. Spine *14*:166–174, 1989.

232. Romanul, F. C. A., and Cohen, R. B.: A histochemical study of oxidative enzymes in the sciatic nerve of the rabbit. Am. J. Pathol. *35*:713–720, 1959.

233. Rosenqvist, A.-L., and Holm, S.: Morphological and nutritional changes in the vertebral endplate of the rat induced by exercise. Submitted to Spine, 1990.

234. Rothman, R. H., and Simeone, F. A.: The Spine. 2nd ed. Philadelphia, W. B. Saunders Co., 1982.

235. Rydevik, B. L.: Etiology of sciatica. *In* The Lumbar Spine. Weinstein, J. N., and Wiesel, S. W. (eds.): Philadelphia, W. B. Saunders Co., 1990, pp. 132–140.

236. Rydevik, B., Brånemark, P.-I., Nordborg, C., et al.: Effects of chymopapain on nerve tissue. An experimental study on the structure and function of peripheral nerve tissue in rabbits after local application of chymopapain. Spine *1*:137–148, 1976.

237. Rydevik, B., Lundborg, G., and Nordborg, C.: Intraneural tissue reactions induced by internal neurolysis. Scand. J. Plast. Reconstr. Surg. *10*:3–8, 1976.

238. Rydevik, B., McLean, W. G., Sjöstrand, J., and Lundborg, G.: Blockage of axonal transport induced by acute, graded compression of the rabbit vagus nerve. J. Neurol. Neurosurg. Psychiatry *43*:690–698, 1980.

239. Rydevik, B., and Nordborg, C.: Changes in nerve function and nerve fibre structure induced by acute, graded compression. J. Neurol. Neurosurg. Psychiatry *43*:1070–1082, 1980.

240. Rydevik, B., Lundborg, G., and Bagge, U.: Effects of graded compression on intraneural blood flow. An in vivo study on rabbit tibial nerve. J. Hand Surg. *6*:3–12, 1981.

241. Rydevik, B., Brown, M. D., Ehira, T., et al.: Effects of graded compression and nucleus pulposus on nerve tissue: an experimental study in rabbits. Acta Orthop. Scand. *54*:670–671, 1983.

242. Rydevik, B., Brown, M. D., and Lundborg, G.: Pathoanatomy and pathophysiology of nerve root compression (invited paper). Spine *9*:7–15, 1984.

243. Rydevik, B. L., Myers, R. R., and Powell, H. C.: Pressure increase in the dorsal root ganglion following mechanical compression. Closed compartment syndrome in nerve roots. Spine *14*:574–576, 1989.

244. Rydevik, B., Lundborg, G., and Skalak, R.: Biomechanics of peripheral nerves. *In* Nordin, M., and Frankel, V. H. (eds.): Basic Biomechanics of the Musculoskeletal System. Philadelphia, Lea & Febiger, 1989, pp. 75–87.

245. Rydevik, B., and Garfin, S. R.: Spinal nerve root compression. *In* Szabo, R. (ed.): Nerve Compression Syndromes. Diagnosis and Treatment. Thorofare, NJ, Slack, 1989, pp. 247–261.

246. Rydevik, B., Holm, S., Brown, M. D., and Lundborg, G.: Diffusion from the cerebrospinal fluid as a nutritional pathway for spinal nerve roots. Acta Physiol. Scand. *138*:247–248, 1990.

247. Rydevik, B. L., Pedowitz, R. A., Hargens, A. R., et al.: Effects of acute, graded compression on spinal nerve root function and structure. An experimental study of the pig cauda equina. Spine *16*:487–493, 1991.

248. Rydevik, B. L., Kwan, M. K., Myers, R. R., et al.: Biomechanical analyses of human lumbosacral spinal nerve roots. Submitted to Spine, 1991.

249. Rydevik, B. L., Kwan, M. K., Myers, R. R., et al.: An in vitro mechanical and histological study of acute stretching on rabbit tibial nerve. J. Orthop. Res. *8*:694–701, 1990.

250. Salter, R. B.: Regeneration of articular cartilage through continuous passive motion—past, present and future. *In* Straub, L. R., and Wilson, P. D., Jr. (eds.): Clinical Trends in Orthopaedics. New York, Thieme-Stratton, pp. 101–107, 1982.

251. Sandover, J.: Dynamic loading as a possible source of low back pain disorders. Spine *8*:652–658, 1983.

252. Schmorl, G., and Junghanns, H.: The Human Spine in Health and Disease. New York, Grune & Stratton, 1971.

253. Schnapp, B. J., and Reese, T. S.: New developments in understanding rapid axonal transport. Trends Neurosci. *9*:155–162, 1986.

254. Schultz, A. B.: Mechanics of the human spine: invited feature article. Appl. Mech. Rev. *27*:1487–1497, 1974.

255. Schönström, N., Bolender, N. F., Spengler, D. M., et al.: Pressure changes within the cauda equina following constriction of the dural sac: an in vitro experimental study. Spine *9*:604–607, 1984.

256. Schönström, N., Bolender, N., and Spengler, D.: The pathomorphology of spinal stenosis as seen on CT scans of the lumbar spine. Spine *10*:806–811, 1985.

257. Schönström, N., and Hansson, T.: Pressure changes following constriction of the cauda equina. An experimental study in situ. Spine *13*:385–388, 1988.

258. Seidel, H., and Heide, R.: Long-term effects of whole body vibration: a critical survey of the literature. Int. Arch. Occup. Environ. Health *58*:1–26, 1986.

259. Seidel, H., Bluethner, R., and Hinz, B.: Effects of sinusoidal whole body vibration on the lumbar spine: the stress-strain relationship. Int. Arch. Occup. Environ. Health *57*:207–223, 1986.

260. Shinohara, H.: A study on lumbar disc lesions: significance of histology of free nerve endings in lumbar discs. J. Jpn. Orthop. Assoc. *44*:553–570, 1970.

261. Smith, J. W. and Walmsley, R.: Experimental incisions of the intervertebral disc. J. Bone Joint Surg. *33B*:612–625, 1951.

262. Smyth, M. J., and Wright, V.: Sciatica and the intervertebral disc. An experimental study. J. Bone Joint Surg. *41A*:1401–1418, 1958.

263. Souter, W. A., and Taylor, T. K. F.: Sulphated acid mucopolysaccharide metabolism in the rabbit in-

tervertebral disc. J. Bone Joint Surg. *52B*:371–384, 1970.

264. Spencer, D. L.: Mechanisms of nerve root compression due to a herniated disc. *In* Weinstein, J. N., and Wiesel, S. W. (eds.): The Lumbar Spine. Philadelphia, W. B. Saunders Co., 1990, pp. 141–145.
265. Spencer, D. L., Irwin, G. S., and Miller, J. A.: Anatomy and significance of fixation of the lumbosacral nerve roots in sciatica. Spine *8*:672–679, 1983.
266. Spencer, D. L., Miller, J. A., and Bertolini, J. E.: The effects of intervertebral disc space narrowing on the contact force between the nerve root and a simulated disc protrusion. Spine *9*:422–426, 1984.
267. Starlinger, H., and Lübbers, D. W.: Polarographic measurements of the oxygen pressure performed simultaneously with optical measurements of the redox state of the respiratory chain in suspensions of mitochondria under steady-state conditions at low oxygen tensions. Pflügers Arch *341*:15–22, 1973.
268. Steer, J. M.: Some observations on the fine structure of rat dorsal spinal nerve roots. J. Anat. *109*:467–485, 1971.
269. Stevens, R. L., Ewans, R. J. F., Revell, P. A., and Muir, H.: Proteoglycans of the intervertebral disc. Biochem. J. *179*:561–572, 1979.
270. Stevens, R. L., Dondi, P., and Muir, H.: Proteoglycans of the intervertebral disc. Biochem. J. *179*:573–578, 1979.
271. Stilwell, D. L., Jr.: The nerve supply of the vertebral column and its associated structures in the monkey. Anat. Rec. *125*:139–169, 1956.
272. Stryer, L.: Biochemistry. San Francisco, W. H. Freeman & Co., 1975.
273. Suh, T. H., and Alexander, L.: Vascular system of the human spinal cord. Arch. Neurol. Psychiat. *41*:659–677, 1939.
274. Sunderland, S.: Avulsion of nerve roots. *In* Vinken, P. J., and Bruyn, G. W. (eds.): Handbook of Clinical Neurology. Vol. 25. Injuries of the Spine and Spinal Cord. New York, Elsevier, 1975, pp. 393–435.
275. Sunderland, S.: The nerve lesion in the carpal tunnel syndrome. J. Neurol. Neurosurg. Psychiatry *39*:615–626, 1976.
276. Sunderland, S.: Nerves and Nerve Injuries. 2nd ed. Edinburgh, Churchill Livingstone, 1978.
277. Sunderland, S., and Bradley, K. C.: Stress-strain phenomena in human spinal nerve roots. Brain *84*:120–124, 1961.
278. Szirmai, J. A.: Structure of the intervertebral disc. *In* Balazs, E. A. (ed.): Chemistry and Molecular Biology of the Intracellular Matrix. New York, Academic Press, 1970, pp. 1279–1308.
279. Takahashi, K., Olmarker, K., Rydevik, B., and Holm, S.: Analyses of intraneural blood flow at double level cauda equina compression in the pig. Transactions, Orthopaedic Research Society, Annual Meeting, Anaheim, CA, March 1991.
280. Takeda, T.: Three-dimensional observation of collagen framework of human lumbar discs. J. Jpn. Orthop. Assoc. *49*:45–57, 1975.
281. Taylor, T. K., and Akeson, W. H.: Intervertebral disc prolapse: a review of morphologic and biochemic knowledge concerning the nature of prolapse. Clin. Orthop. *76*:54–79, 1971.
282. Taylor, T. K. F., Ghosh, P., Braund, K. G., et al.: The effect of spinal fusion on intervertebral disc composition: an experimental study. J. Surg. Res. *21*:91–104, 1976.
283. Tennyson, V. M., and Gershon, M. D.: Light and electron microscopy of dorsal root, sympathetic, and enteric ganglia. *In* Dyck, P. J., Thomas, P. K., Lambert, E. H., and Bunge, R. (eds.): Peripheral Neuropathy. 2nd ed. Vol. 1. Philadelphia, W. B. Saunders Co., 1984, pp. 121–155.
284. Tipton, C. M., Vailas, A. C., and Mattehs, R. D.: Experimental studies on the influences of physical activity on ligaments, tendons and joints: a brief review. Acta Med. Scand. *711* (Suppl.):157–168, 1985.
285. Twomey, L., and Taylor, J.: Age changes in lumbar intervertebral disc. Acta Orthop. Scand. *56*:496–499, 1985.
286. Upton, R. M., and McComas, A. J.: The double-crush in nerve entrapment syndromes. Lancet *2*:359–362, 1973.
287. Urban, J. P. G.: Fluid and solute transport in the intervertebral disc. Ph.D. Thesis, London University, 1977.
288. Urban, J., Holm, S., Maroudas, A., and Nachemson, A.: Nutrition of the intervertebral disc. An in vivo study of solute transport. Clin. Orthop. *129*:101–114, 1977.
289. Urban, J. P. G., Holm, S., and Maroudas, A.: Diffusion of small solutes in the intervertebral disc; an in vivo study. Biorheology *15*:202–223, 1978.
290. Urban, J. P. G., and Maroudas, A.: Measurement of fixed charge density in the intervertebral disc. Biochim. Biophys. Acta *586*:166–178, 1979.
291. Urban, J. P. G., Maroudas, A., Bayliss, M. T., and Dillon, J.: Swelling pressures of proteoglycans at the concentrations found in cartilaginous tissues. Biorheology *16*:447–464, 1979.
292. Urban, J. P. G., and Maroudas, A.: The chemistry of the intervertebral disc in relation to its physiological functions and requirements. Clin. Rheum. Dis. *6*:46–51, 1980.
293. Urban, J. P. G., and Maroudas, A.: Swelling of the intervertebral disc in vivo. Connect. Tissue Res. *9*:1–10, 1981.
294. Vanharanta, H., Guyet, R. D., Ohnmeiss, D. D., et al.: Disc deterioration in low-back syndromes. Spine *13*:1349–1351, 1988.
295. Videman, T.: Connective tissue and immobilization. Key factors in musculoskeletal degeneration? Clin. Orthop. *221*:26–32, 1987.
296. Videman, T., Nurminen, T., Tola, S., et al.: Low back pain in nurses and some loading factors of work. Spine *9*:400–404, 1984.
297. Viraswami, V.: A study of the blood supply of the nerve roots in man and the rabbit with an experimental analysis of the collateral circulation following ligature of the arteries. Thesis, London, 1963.
298. Wall, P. D., and Gutnick, M.: Properties of afferent nerve impulses originating from a neuroma. Nature *248*:740–743, 1974.
299. Wall, P. D., Waxman, S., and Basbaum, A. I.: Ongoing activity in peripheral nerve: injury discharge. Exp. Neurol. *45*:576–589, 1974.
300. Wall, P. D., and Devor, M.: Sensory afferent impulses originate from dorsal root ganglia as well as from the periphery in normal and nerve injured rats. Pain *17*:321–339, 1983.

301. Wall, E. J., Cohen, M. S., Massie, J. M., et al.: Cauda equina anatomy. Part I: Intrathecal nerve root organisation. Spine *15*:1244–1247, 1990.
302. Watanabe, R., and Parke, W. W.: Vascular and neural pathology of lumbosacral spinal stenosis. J. Neurosurg. *65*:64–70, 1986.
303. Weber, H.: Lumbar disc herniation: a controlled, prospective study with ten years of observation. Spine *8*:131–140, 1983.
304. Wehling, P., Bandara, G., and Evans, C. H.: Synovial cytokines impair the function of the sciatic nerve in rats: a possible element in the pathophysiology of radicular syndromes. Neuro-Orthop. *7*:55–59, 1990.
305. Weinstein, J.: Mechanisms of spinal pain: the dorsal root ganglion and its role as a mediator of low back pain. Spine *11*:999–1001, 1986.
306. Weinstein, J. N., Pope, M., and Schmidt, R.: The effects of low frequency vibration on dorsal root ganglion substance "P." Neuro-Orthop. *4*:24–30, 1987.
307. Weinstein, J. N., Pope, M., Schmidt, R., et al.: Neuropharmacological effects of vibration: an animal model. Spine *13*:521–525, 1988.
308. Weinstein, J., LaMotte, R., Rydevik, B., et al.: Nerve. *In* Frymoyer, J. W., and Gordon, S. L. (eds.): New Perspectives on Low Back Pain. Park Ridge, IL, American Academy of Orthopaedic Surgeons, 1989.
309. Weinstein, J. N., and Wiesel, S. W.: The Lumbar Spine. Philadelphia, W. B. Saunders Co., 1990.
310. Weiss, D. G.: General properties of axoplasmic transport. *In* Weiss, D. G. (ed.): Axoplasmic Transport. Berlin, Springer-Verlag, 1982, pp. 1–14.
311. White, A. A., and Panjabi, M. M.: Clinical Biomechanics of the Spine. Philadelphia, J. B. Lippincott Co., 1978.
312. White, A. A., and Gordon, S. L.: Symposium on Idiopathic Low Back Pain. St. Louis, C. V. Mosby Co., 1982.
313. Wiesel, S. W., Tsourmas, N., Feffer, H. L., et al.: A study of computer-assisted tomography. 1. The incidence of positive CAT scans in an asymptomatic group of patients. Spine *9*:549–551, 1984.
314. Wilson, D. F., Erecinska, M., Drown, C., and Silver, J. A.: The oxygen dependence of cellular energy metabolism. Arch. Biochem. Biophys. *195*:485–493, 1979.
315. Woo, S. L.-Y., Gelberman, R. H., Cobb, N. G., et al.: The importance of controlled passive mobilization on flexor tendon healing. A biomechanical study. Acta Orthop. Scand. *52*:615–622, 1981.
316. Woo, S. L.-Y., and Buckwalter, J. A.: Injury and repair of the musculoskeletal soft tissues. Symposium. Park Ridge, IL, American Academy of Orthopaedic Surgeons, 1988.
317. Yamada, K.: The dynamics of experimental posture. Experimental study of intervertebral disc herniation in bipedal animals. J. Exp. Med. *8*:350–361, 1962.
318. Yoshizawa, H., O'Brien, J. P., Smith, W. T., et al.: Neuropathology of intervertebral disc removed for low back pain. J. Pathol. *132*:95–104, 1980.
319. Yoshizawa, H., Kobayashi, S., and Kubota, K.: Effects of compression on intraradicular blood flow in dog. Spine *14*:1220–1225, 1989.

SECTION 2

THE CHILD'S SPINE

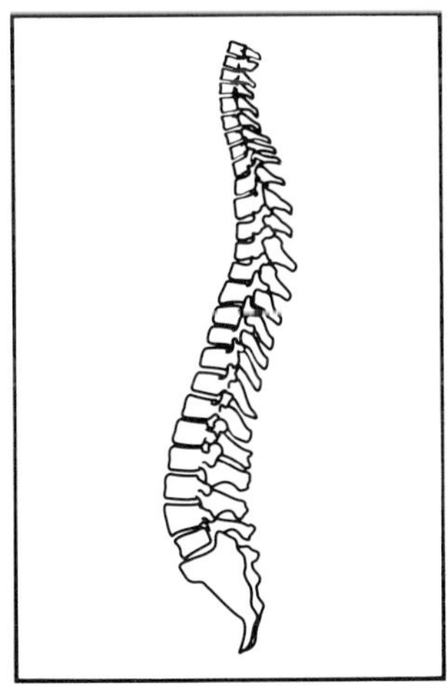

CHAPTER 9

BACK PAIN IN CHILDREN AND ADOLESCENTS

William H. Dillin, M.D.
Robert G. Watkins, M.D.

Sherlock Holmes is the most famous detective in literature. It is not surprising that the creator of this legend of deductive reasoning was a physician, Sir Arthur Conan Doyle. While Holmes confronted the diverse and nefarious elements of criminal behavior, he remained steadfast in his pursuit by following a system of evaluation that allowed him to interpret the information he received. Perhaps the greatest witness to the "process" of Holmes is the continued popularity of the detective in the context of the changed face of science. We still marvel at his thinking. Doyle expressed it this way: "It is an old maxim of mine that when you have eliminated the impossible, whatever remains, however improbable, must be the truth."[1] Even in the context of emotionally adverse conclusion, logic prevails. Most clinicians confronting a pediatric patient with back pain are naturally inclined to be conservative, to treat the symptom with temporizing measures and wait. But is this logical? When confronted with the probable, wouldn't Holmes have followed the leads to their inevitable conclusion rather than loiter? Are there probabilities in the pediatric age group that suggest we should pursue rather than tarry? Are these patients little adults with back pain, or is their pathologic potential somehow different during growth from that experienced by mature adults?

In a study performed by Hensinger involving 100 pediatric patients with back pain, only 15 per cent failed to have a condition discoverable by diagnosis.[2] This suggests a very high yield of conclusions derived from evaluation of the symptom of pediatric back pain. A similar study of King demonstrated that in 63 per cent of patients under the age of 19 with back pain there is a specified, definable diagnosis.[3] We can conclude that evaluating pediatric back pain will surrender specific results.

Why not allow the benign natural histories of adult back pain to prevail and treat accord-

Table 9–1. POSSIBLE DIAGNOSES OF BACK PAIN IN CHILDREN

Mechanical Disorders	**Inflammatory Processes**
Postural problems	Disc space infection
Muscular disorders	Discitis
"Overuse syndromes"	Disc space calcification
Herniated nucleus pulposus	Vertebral osteomyelitis
"Ruptured disc"	Collagen vascular disorders
Developmental Abnormalities	Sacroiliac joint infections
Spondylolysis/ spondylolisthesis	**Neoplastic Diseases**
Scheuermann's disease	Spinal canal
Thoracic kyphosis	Vertebral column
Lumbar spine	Muscle
	Conversion reaction

Table 9–2. POSSIBLE DIAGNOSES OF BACK PAIN IN CHILDREN BY AGE

Up to 10 Years	10 Years and Over
Infections	Spondylolysis/spondylolisthesis
Tumor	Scheuermann's disease
Column	Herniated nucleus pulposus
Cord	Overuse syndrome
Vertebral osteomyelitis	Tumors

ingly? While it is true that many of the factors in back pain in adults are difficult to discover, the pathologic conditions that produce the symptoms are assumed to be related to degeneration of the tissue (muscle, ligament, disc, bone).[3] But these degenerative processes are the unlikely cause of pediatric back pain.[4] Table 9–1 are the probable diagnoses for the symptom of back pain in the pediatric age group.[5] Clearly, the other diagnoses need to be considered and discovered because the consequences are different and so are the natural histories.

King further suggested that the probabilities of specific diagnoses may be further subdivided in relation to patients over and under 10 years of age (Table 9–2).[5]

References

1. Bartlett J.: Familiar Quotations. Secaucus, N.J., Carol Publishing Group, 1983.
2. Hensinger, R. M.: Back pain in children. *In* Bradford, D. S., and Hensinger, R. M. (eds.): The Pediatric Spine. New York, Thieme, 1985, pp. 41–60.
3. King, H.: Evaluating the child with back pain. Pediat. Clin. North Am. *33:* 1489–1493; 1986.
4. Dillin, W. H.: Conservative management of acute back pain and sciatica. Semin. Spine Surg. *1:*18–27, 1989.
5. King, H.: Back pain in children. Pediatr. Clin. North Am. *31:* 1083–1094, 1984.
6. Bunnell, W. P.: Back pain in children. Orthop. Clin. North Am. 13: 587–604, 1982.

HISTORY

As in all areas of clinical medicine, the history is the most important aspect of clinical information.

Chief Complaint. The chief complaint is expressed by patients as their primary concern. In the spine, this area may be amplified by obtaining details of the pattern of possible referral: referral to the iliac crests, tailbone, flank, trochanteric areas, anterior thigh, posterior thigh, lateral thigh, and groin; knee pain; anterior, lateral, and posterior calf pain; and foot pain. The authors usually review the pain diagram at this time as a pictorial representation of the chief complaint and ask about abdominal pain. How bad is the pain on a scale of 1 to 10?

In the pediatric population, a child may not be able to furnish a coherent history suggestive of specific pathologic conditions, and the parents may have to be interviewed to seek regression in signs of developmental milestones, failure to achieve the developmental milestones, or the more subtle issues related to gait disturbances.

Onset. The pain complaint needs to be identified in terms of temporal factors: acute, subacute, or insidious onset. If this is not the first episode of pain or if chronic pain has worsened, this chronology requires clarification. It is important to elicit the interval between episodes, the number of episodes, the start of the last episode, and the variation in intensities of the episodes.

Course. A detailed chronologic history is obtained. All previous diagnostic efforts are assessed: bone scan, x-rays, myelography, plain computed tomography (CT), contract CT, magnetic resonance imaging (MRI) of spine, MRI or CT of pelvis, electromyography (EMG) and nerve conduction velocity. If these tests have been done, dates, physicians, and hospitals are inquired about. A history is obtained of the patient's previous visits to anyone who treated their back and the information obtained as a result of those visits. Specific details of conservative treatments are sought along with their effect on the symptoms: manipulation, physical therapy modalities, back exercises, traction, therapeutic injections, anti-inflammatory agents, pain medications, muscle relaxants. If the history reveals previous spinal surgery, details of the symptoms before surgery, the effect of the operation on the symptoms, and the pain-free interval is sought. The surgical and hospital records are obtained. Finally, patients are asked if the symptoms are worsening, improving, or plateaued and exactly how much and what kind of medicine they are taking.

Medical History. Back pain may be of non-spinal origin or influenced by factors that are nonspinal. The medical history is important. Details to be requested include current medications, allergies, previous nonspinal operations, family history of spinal and nonspinal diseases, previous medical diagnoses, previous extensive medical evaluation (inpatient or outpatient), new nonspinal symptoms, symptoms related to depression or psychiatric illness and any recent travel.

Relationship to Activity. A critical concept is the development of information that points to a mechanical or nonmechanical history of symptoms. Specific activities are detailed to assess whether pain is worse, better, or unchanged and whether radiation of pain is induced. Most important is the question regarding a position for pain relief or whether the pain is unrelated to position or activity. Patients should be asked if they are surrendering activities to accommodate pain and if their activities changed (increased intensity of sport or a new sport undertaken) before the symptoms appeared. Information related to Valsalva maneuvers: coughing or sneezing, straining to go to the bathroom, and the effect on pain is requested.

The activities of daily life are inventoried. sitting, walking, standing, running, lifting, bending. Specifically, does sitting aggravate symptoms or relieve them? If the patient is old enough, inquire about the effects of driving. If there is intolerance of sitting, how long can the patient sit comfortably? Is there stiffness after sitting? Walking history will reveal whether surfaces are a factor and whether ascending or descending stairs is relevant. If pain is caused during walking, the distances should be quantitated, and what the patient does to obtain relief documented. Are the symptoms relieved by lying down or are they aggravated by lying on the stomach, the back, or a particular side? Does the simple act of standing cause pain and does the patient have a sensation of listing? Symptoms related to the effects of lifting, twisting, reaching and rotating, bending forward with rotation, bending backward, and bending forward alone should be reviewed. Finally, pain should be analyzed with reference to the day-night cycle. Is there a history of night pain, waking from sleep, stiffness on arising, and progressive improvement or deterioration during the day?

Neurologic Effects. It is important to conceptualize back pain as a potential neurologic symptom, and thus details involving the whole neurologic system are relevant. Blurred vision, double vision, syncope, dizziness, headaches, hearing loss, fine motor and gross motor incoordination, Lhermitte's phenomenon, and gait disturbances provide a screen of possible underlying neurologic disease. Details of bowel and bladder habits as well as progressive changes in the feet, are sought. Further information is elicited on arm pain, weakness, and sensory loss and whether the hands are numb and clumsy. Any numbness over the back and thorax is questioned. Specific information is obtained on lower extremity atrophy, numbness, tingling dysthesia, and developing muscle weakness. Is pain present over the cervical or thoracic spine besides the lumbar involvement?

Chronic Inflammatory Factors. Inquire about pain in other joints, its relationship to menstrual periods, and the effects of the weather.

Physical Examination. This begins with inspection. Identification of the normal sagittal plane curves is made from the side. Is there normal cervical lordosis, thoracic kyphosis, and lumbar lordosis? Is the sacrum verticalized or exaggerated? The skin should be surveyed for evidence of cutaneous changes: hairy patches, subcutaneous lesions, pigmentation changes, multiple lipomas, café au lait spots, dermal sinus, angioma, and surgical scars. Palpation should include the cervical, thoracic, and lumbosacral bony prominences and adjacent soft tissues. The cervical range of motion is recorded and evidence of torticollis sought. Does the patient have a list? The forward bending test allows comparison of the symmetry of both sides of the spine. Is a rib hump present? Is scoliosis visible? Is a paraspinous muscle hump present? If prominence on one side is suggested, a level may be utilized to quantitate the difference. Observe from the side the degree of thoracic kyphosis. Returning the patient to the neutral standing position, a plumb line dropped from the C7 spinous process can demonstrate decompensation if it does not strike between the gluteal folds, and its lateralization can be quantified. Shoulder level should be assessed and differences measured with a level. General flexibility of the thoracolumbar spine is measured by having the patient forward flex, extend, lateral bend, and axially rotate to the left and right. Assess the patient for an active list with flexion, and any reversal of lumbar lordosis. Pain at specific range of motion and in a specific direction is recorded. With the patient sitting, the patellar and Achilles reflexes are assessed, sensory testing made for soft touch and pinprick, temperatures assessed in the lower extremities, and thigh and calf circumferences recorded. A sitting root test is performed. With the patient supine, the straight leg raising (SLR) test is performed as well as full hip range of motion and a Fabere test. The iliopsoas muscles, hip abductors and adductors, quadrilaterals, extensor hallucis longus muscle, and peroneii and posterior tibial muscles are graded for strength on resistive testing. Leg lengths are measured from the anterosuperior iliac spine to the medium malleolus bilaterally. Gaenslen's test is performed on either side of the examining table with the patient supine. With the patient prone, a reverse SLR test is performed, and hamstring strength assessed. Finally, with the patient standing, a Romberg test, tandem walk, rapid alternative movements, and object recognition tests are performed. Anterior tibial and gastrocnemius muscle strength is determined by heel and toe walking, respectively, and the patient's gait is observed.

Other joints are assessed for flexibility and examined meticulously if complaints are present. Chest wall deformities and secondary sexual characteristics are recorded (e.g., breast, hair, and scrotal development).

Laboratory Evaluation. The degree of laboratory evaluation depends on clinical suspicion. Many different studies may be useful, such as complete blood count and sedimentation rate for infection, urinalysis for urinary tract infection, and rheumatoid factor and HLA-B27 if arthritis is suspected. Further chemical panels may be indicated under appropriate clinical circumstances, especially in screening for medical causes of low back pain.

Summary. The purpose of gathering clinical information is the formulation of potential diagnoses. Not all patients who manifest clinical problems can express the symptoms or be examined with unequivocal accuracy. Table 9–3 lists observable and historical facts that may lead the clinician to suspect intraspinal pathology.[1]

Table 9–3. CLINICAL FINDINGS SUGGESTIVE OF INTRASPINAL PATHOLOGY

Dorsal Cutaneous Abnormalities
Hypertrichosis
Dimples
Pigmented nevi
Hemangioma
Dermoid cyst
Dermal sinus
Lipoma
Neurologic Abnormalities
Gait disturbance
Muscle atrophy
Sensory impairment
Bowel or bladder changes
Spinal Anomalies
Congenital scoliosis
Spinal dysraphism
Increased interpedicular distance
Left thoracic scoliosis
Orthopedic Deformities
Cavovarus feet
Clubfoot
Sprengels deformity
Intestinal Anomalies
Neurenteric cysts
Intestinal duplication

Reference

History

1. Sutterlin, C., Grogan, D., and Ogden, J.: Diagnosis of developmental pathology of the neuraxis by magnetic resonance imaging. J. Pediatr. Orthop 7:291–297, 1987.

X-RAY EVALUATION

Since we have concluded that evaluation is necessary for pediatric patients with low back pain, a question arises concerning the type of radiographic studies that may be appropriate. What constitutes sufficient evaluation? The general principles for use of radiologic tests center around securing a diagnosis, and then using the information to determine treatment. Thus, natural histories, pathophysiologies, and treatments impact on decision making and must be known for the physician to comprehend when to stop further testing. In addition, false-positive and false-negative test results for each radiologic technique in relationship to each specific pathology need to be defined. These clinical correlations are continually refined with the emerging diagnostic technologies. However, no test is perfect and no test replaces clinical understanding.

Plain X-rays

The plain x-ray is the traditional first test for assessing pediatric low back pain. Two views are initially selected, anteroposterior (AP) and lateral. What information can be gleaned from plain x-rays? On the AP view, the alignment of the spinous processes, rotation of the pedicles, integrity of the transverse processes, and, importantly, the interpedicular distance and erosion of the pedicles should be reviewed. It is always important to assess the paravertebral soft tissues and intrapelvic tissues if the gonads are not shielded. On the lateral x-ray, the vertebral body structure and alignment, apophyses, end plates, and bone density can be estimated. In addition, the sagittal curve of the lumbar spine, the height of the disc spaces, and the presence of calcification can be considered. There should be a careful inventory on both films of architectural defects and components that are absent, distorted, or unsegmented.

Oblique x-rays profile the pars interarticularis and neural foramen. Some authors advocate routine oblique x-rays because spondylolysis was demonstrated only on oblique views in 20 per cent of patients. Other authors suggest that lateral deviation and rotation of a spinous process on the AP view is associated with pars interarticularis defects, especially with spondylolisthesis.

If the clinical examination suggests that an x-ray is appropriate for evaluation of scoliosis or kyphosis, standing lateral and standing AP x-rays may be indicated. Bending films to assess curve flexibility in scoliosis are usually not recommended unless the information is required for treatment, but hyperextension films to assess kyphosis flexibility has been recommended in Scheuermann's disease and some other kyphoses as a form of pretreatment evaluation.

Flexion-extension radiographs are usually necessary only if radiographic changes in alignment (angulation or translation) are important for clinical decision making.

Bone Scans

Bone scans are a valuable adjunct in the assessment of pediatric back pain. Many diagnoses in this age group fall in the detection range of the bone scan. Although destructive bony lesions may be the final consequence of vertebral osteomyelitis, the bone scan may be positive before the radiographic picture has evolved. Despite being a sensitive test, a normal bone scan does not exclude infection. The value of the bone scan in bone lesions such as the aneurysmal bone cyst and osteoid osteoma has been demonstrated, and its role in the evaluation of primary bone tumors is a critical feature. But perhaps the most common use of the bone scan is in the definition of stress reactions in bone and spondylolysis in the very active athletic population under 20. Bone scans have been correlated with the radiologic defects of spondylolysis, but the correlation is not perfect. In some individuals positive bone scans and normal x-rays are indicative of an acute ongoing stress reaction in bone; in others with radiographically evident spondylolysis there may be a negative bone scan indicating a process that has been completed in the past.

Some authors have suggested that a positive scan in the absence of radiographic findings is an indication for bracing and represents an incipient fracture. Occasionally, other anatomic areas may present with pathologic stress reactions simulating another cause of low back pain, and this is frequently detectable on bone scintography; stress reaction of the sacroiliac joint is an example.

Computed Tomography (CT)

Perhaps the greatest advantage of CT is in the sagittal, coronal, and axial reconstruction of bony detail. CT can be used to visualize the herniated intervertebral disc, the "limbus vertebra," and the ring apophysis lesion. It is helpful in identifying the pars interarticularis fracture as an acute event or unhealed defect, and also useful in detecting the healing and healed pars fracture. Occasional fractures of the posterior elements or transverse process fractures, diagnosable on plain x-ray, are discovered on CT during a back pain evaluation. CT is invaluable for evaluating the aneurysmal bone cyst, osteoid osteoma, and osteoblastoma. Reports of soft tissue identification of adipose tissue in the filum terminale as an indication of possible spinal cord tethering have also been exhibited on CT. CT remains a valuable tool for bone definition, but more frequently MRI and contrast-enhanced CT and myelography have supplanted CT for soft tissue definition.

Direct sagittal contrast-enhanced CTD has been used for dorsal ventral plane evaluation of diverse pediatric lesions: "lipoma and dysraphism, lipomyelomeningocele, lipomyelocystocele, lumbosacral agenesis with cord regression, capillary hemangioma, and vertebral osteomyelitis."[22] Combinations of myelography and contrast-enhanced CT have been invaluable in the diagnosis of the intraspinal causative anomalies presenting as scoliosis, leg weakness, and foot deformity. Contrast-enhanced CT and lumbar myelography retain a role in the evaluation of intraspinal pathology, including disc herniation in the pediatric patient.

Magnetic Resonance Imaging (MRI)

The clinical utility of MRI in conjunction with its noninvasive attributes has prompted some authors to propose it as the procedure of choice in the evaluation of pediatric intraspinal pathology. In a few small series comparing MRI with metrizamide myelography and CT in pediatric spinal cord disorders, MRI was found equally as effective as these procedures in delineating the pathology. MRI has been effective in outlining skip lesions and extension along the longitudinal axis of the spinal cord. It is also valuable in detecting a wide variety of pediatric spinal disorders, not only as a definitive test but as an initial screen for undiagnosed variations in potential pathologies. One retrospective study analyzed broad categories of spinal dysraphism, scoliosis, and neoplasia, comparing MRI with myelography and CT and confirming many of the diagnoses obtained from these modalities at surgery.[28] The authors concluded that MRI was the indicated procedure in pediatric spinal evaluation with the notable exceptions of severe scoliosis, metastatic tumor seeding, and a thin dorsal neural placode.

MRI has become increasingly popular in the search for occult spinal dysraphism because its noninvasive technique may allow the discovery of unexpressed pathology before the onset of neurologic consequences. In a group of patients studied with MRI because of the presence of scoliosis and/or an evolving neurologic pattern, MRI defined the anatomic factors of dysraphism clearly and provided "more information than myelography or CT."[29] The evaluation of the tethered cord has gained further proponents for MRI, with the additional recommendation that ultrasonograph is useful for patients under 1 year of age. Sonography has been used intraoperatively in patients with spinal dysraphism and syringohydromyelia, and clinically in infants and postoperative patients in whom a bony aperture exists, but more recently, MRI been used to image pulsatile cord motion to provide a dynamic interpretation of potential tethering. "With MRI imaging alone, it is possible to either localize and characterize the anatomic alterations associated with dysraphism, or to exclude the presence of surgically remedial spinal dysraphism as a cause of patients' symptomatology."[34]

MRI has become useful in evaluating suspected correctable etiologies in childhood scoliosis, in identifying conditions amenable to treatment before addressing the issue of scoliosis, and in identifying the lesions in which change in spinal alignment might precipitate neurologic catastrophe.

MRI has developed its advocates in the analysis of acute and chronic musculoskeletal infection and in differentiating soft tissue from bony infection. It was recommended as the study of initial choice in the evaluation of spine infection, and was found to be superior to myelography and CT in the following lesions: epidural abscess without meningitis, myelitis, osteomyelitis, and disc space infection. It was helpful in distinguishing tumor and infection, but required adjunctive assistance in the form of myelography and CT in the presence of epidural abscess combined with meningitis.[24, 29, 35–37]

The solid central nervous system (CNS) tumors of childhood have been analyzed by MRI. The focus of more recent investigations using gadolinium-DTPA–enhanced MRI in addition to conventional MRI has several presumed advantages: (1) tumor localization and delineation apart from edema, (2) in areas of enhanced biologic neoplastic behavior, (3) in distinguishing reactive biology from malignant, and (4) in potentially differentiating quiescent from dynamic pathology.[40]

While no test is unassailably accurate, a dualism of pathologic structure and development can at times obscure the talents of the most astute clinician. Diagnostic tests can supplement the judgment of the physician who understands the spectrum of developmental biologic potentials. The biology may be progressive and cause symptoms or the child may be progressing in growth, the pathology staid, and the conflict productive of symptoms. It is difficult to discriminate between the unusual features of a common problem and the common features of the unusual in the best of circumstances. Adults have difficulty in communicating their symptoms, but the difficulty is even more obvious in children. In addition, the dormant lesion may exist, hiding the final manifestations of its effects, but diagnosable by suspicion and the appropriate diagnostic tests.

References

X-ray Evaluation

1. Libson, E., Bloon, R., Dinari, G., et al.: Oblique lumbar spine radiographs: importance in young patients. Radiology *151:* 89–90, 1984.
2. Ravichandran, G.: A radiologic sign in spondylolisthesis. A.J.R. *134:* 113–117, 1980.
3. Moriossy, R.: Clinical and radiologic evaluation of spinal disease. *In* Bradford, D. S., and Hensinger, R. M. (eds.): The Pediatric Spine. New York, Thieme, 1985.
4. Bolivar, R., Kohl, S., and Pickering, L.: Vertebral osteomyelitis in children: report of four cases. Pediatrics *62:* 549–553, 1978.
5. Epremian B. E., and Perez, L. A.: Imaging strategy in osteomyelitis. Clin. Nucl. Med. *2:*218, 1977.
6. Gelfand, M. J., and Silbertstein, E. B.: Radionuclide imaging: use in diagnosis of osteomyelitis in children. J.A.M.A, *237:*245–247, 1977.
7. Hudson, T.: Scintigraphy of aneurysmal bone cysts. A.J.R. *142:* 761–765, 1984.
8. Helms, C., Hattner, R., and Vogler, J.: Osteoid osteoma: radionuclide diagnosis. Radiology *151:* 779–784, 1984.
9. Winter, P. F., Johnson, P. M., and Hilal, S. R.: Scintigraphic detection of osteoid osteoma. Radiology *122:*177–178, 1977.
10. Heyman, S., and Treves, S.: Scintigraphy in pediatric bone tumors. *In* Jaffe, N. (ed.): Bone Tumors in Children. Littleton, MA, Wright-Publishing Sciences Group, 1979, pp. 79–96.
11. Simon, M. A., and Kirchner, P. T.: Scintigraphic evaluation of primary bone tumors. J. Bone Joint Surg. *62A:*758–764, 1989.
12. Papanicolaou, N., Wilkinson, R., Emans, J.: Bone scintigraphy and radiology in young athletes with low back pain. A.J.R. *145:*1039–1044, 1985.
13. Gelfand, M., Strife, J., and Kereiakes, J.: Radionuclide bone imaging in spondylolysis of the lumbar spine in children. Radiology *140:*191–195, 1981.
14. Van Der Oever, M., Merrick, M., and Scott, J. H. S.: Bone scintigraphy in symptomatic spondylolysis. J. Bone Joint Surg. *69B:*453–456, 1987.
15. Marymont, J., Lynch, M., and Henning, C.: Exercise-related stress reaction of the sacroiliac joint. Am. J. Sports Med. *4:*320–323, 1986.
16. Fitz, C.: Diagnostic imaging in children with spinal disorders. Pediatr. Clin. North Am. *32:*1537–1558, 1985.
17. Rothman, S.: Computed tomography of the spine in older children and teenagers. Clin. Sports Med. *5:*247–270, 1986.
18. Haney, P., Gellad, F., and Swartz, J.: Aneurysmal bone cyst of the spine: CT appearance. CT *7:*319–322, 1983.
19. Gamba, J., Martinez, S., Apple, J., et al.: Computed tomography of axial skeletal osteoid osteomas. A.J.R.: *142:*769–772, 1984.
20. Wang, A., Lipson, S., and Haykal, M.: Computed tomography of aneurysmal bone cyst of the L1 vertebral body. J. Comput. Assist. Tomogr. *8:*1186–1189, 1984.
21. McClendon, R., Oakes, W., and Heinz, E.: Adipose tissue in the filbum terminale: a computed tomographic finding that may indicate tethering of the spinal cord. Neurosurgery *22:*873–876, 1988.
22. Altman, N., Harwood-Nash, D., and Fitz, C.: Evaluation of the infant spine by direct sagittal computed tomography. A.J.N.R. *6:*65–69, 1985.
23. Tadmor, R., Ravid, M., and Findler, G.: Importance of early radiologic diagnosis of congenital anomalies of the spine. Surg. Neurol. *23:*493–501, 1985.
24. Bale, J., Bell, W., and Dunn, V.: Magnetic resonance imaging of the spine in children. Arch. Neurol. *43:*1253–1256, 1986.
25. Duthey M., and Lund, G.: MR imaging of the spine in children. Eur. J. Radiol. *8:*188–195, 1988.
26. Sutterlin, C., Grogan, D., and Ogden, J.: Diagnosis of developmental pathology of the neuraxis by magnetic resonance imaging. J. Pediatr. Orthop. *7:*291–297, 1987.
27. Packer, R., Zimmerman, R., Sutton, L., et al.: Magnetic resonance imaging of spinal cord disease of childhood. Pediatrics *78:*251–256, 1986.
28. Davis, P., Hoffman, J., Jr., and Ball, T.: Spinal abnormalities in pediatric patients: MR imaging findings compared with clinical, myelographic, and surgical findings. Radiology *166:*629–685, 1989.
29. Szalay, E., Roach, J., and Smith, H.: Magnetic resonance imaging of the spinal cord in spinal dysraphisms. J. Pediatr. Orthop. *7:*541–545, 1987.
30. Hall, W., Albright, A. L., and Brunberg, J.: Diagnosis of tethered cords by magnetic resonance imaging. Surg. Neurol. *30:*60–64, 1988.
31. Quencer, R., Motalvo, B., Naidich, T., et al.: Intraoperative sonography in spinal dysraphism and syringohydromyelia. A.J.R. *148:*1005–1013, 1987.
32. Raghavendra, B., and Epstein, F.: Sonography of the spine and spinal cord. Radiol. Clin. North Am. *13:*91–104, 1985.
33. Levy, L., DiChiro, G., and McCullough, D. C.: Fixed spinal cord: diagnosis with MR imaging. Radiology *169:*773–778, 1988.
34. Brunberg, J. A., Latchaw, R., Kanal, E., et al.: Magnetic resonance imaging of spinal dysraphism. Radiol. Clin. North Am. *26:*181–204, 1988.
35. Nokes, S., Murtagh, F. R., Jones, J. D., III, et al.: Childhood scoliosis: MR imaging. Radiology *164:*791–797, 1987.
36. Modic, M., Pflanze, W., and Feiglin, D. H.: Magnetic resonance imaging of musculoskeletal infections. Radiol. Clin. North Am. *24:*247–258, 1986.
37. Post, M. J., Quencer, R. M., Montalvo, B. M., et al.: Spinal infection: evaluation with MR imaging and intraoperative US. Radiology *169:*765–771, 1988.
38. Kucharczyk, W., Brant-Zawadzki, M., and Sobel, D.:

Central nervous system tumors in children: detection by magnetic resonance imaging. Radiology *155*:131–136, 1985.

39. Stimac, G. K., Porter, B., Olson, D., et al.: Gadolinium-DTPA–enhanced MR imaging of spinal neoplasms: preliminary investigation and comparison with unenhanced spin-echo and STIR sequences. A.J.R. *151*:1185–1192, 1988.
40. Sze, G., Krol G., Zimmerman, R., and Deck, M.D.: Intramedullary disease of the spine: diagnosis using gadolinium-DTPA–enhanced MR imaging. A.J.R. *151*:1193–1204, 1988.

LUMBAR DISC HERNIATION

Lumbar disc herniation does occur in childhood and adolescence. The incidence in these age groups is not clearly defined, but estimates of surgical case series reveal a 2 per cent or less operative rate compared with other age groups.[1] The presenting complaints usually concentrate on leg pain with typical sciatic distribution.[1, 2] In adolescents, the painful hamstring that does not improve may represent sciatica. Back pain is an initial feature but is often outweighed by the degree of leg pain (Fig. 9–1).[1, 2]

Many authors have proposed that lumbar disc herniations in children are essentially different from those in adults, stressing the mechanical nature as opposed to the neurologic findings.[3] However, in one series comparing adults and children, the incidence of reflex loss and sensory alteration was greater in adults but muscle weakness was the same.[2] Other authors have flatly stated that disc herniations are "difficult to diagnose because of the paucity of neurologic abnormalities."[4] Whether there is an appreciable difference between adults and children with regard to neurologic deficits or not, the mechanical signs of disturbance are salient features of the childhood and adolescent disc herniation. The array of abnormal mechanics includes loss of lumbar lordosis, scoliosis, muscle spasm, gait abnormalities, and SLR test results.[1–7] Perhaps the most important clinical feature of adolescent disc herniation is seen in the SLR test. In one series multiple other diagnoses were considered in lieu of disc herniation, including spinal cord tumor, juvenile rheumatoid arthritis, hip disease, low back strain, infection, hematoma, psychosomatic gout, poliomyelitis, and leg length discrepancy.[1] Whether neurologic disorders are present, lumbar disc herniation should be strongly considered when mechanical signs as demonstrated by the SLR test are defined on physical examination (Fig. 9–2).

The conservative treatment of childhood and adolescent disc herniation consists of bed rest, activity restriction, and anti-inflammatory medications. In one series conservative treatment was ineffective in 60 per cent, and others have cited its failure to resolve symptoms.[3, 5, 7]

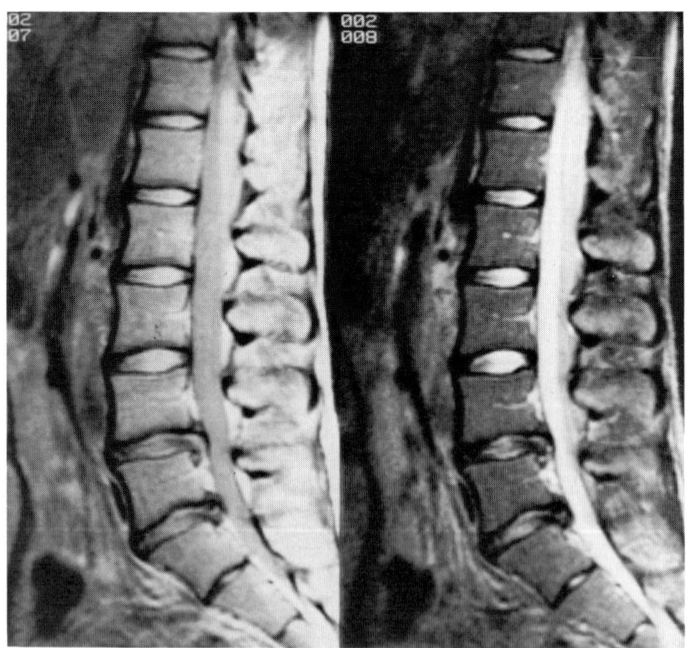

Figure 9–1. MRI scan in a 16-year-old with degenerative disc disease at L4–L5 and L5–S1 and apparent herniations at each of these levels.

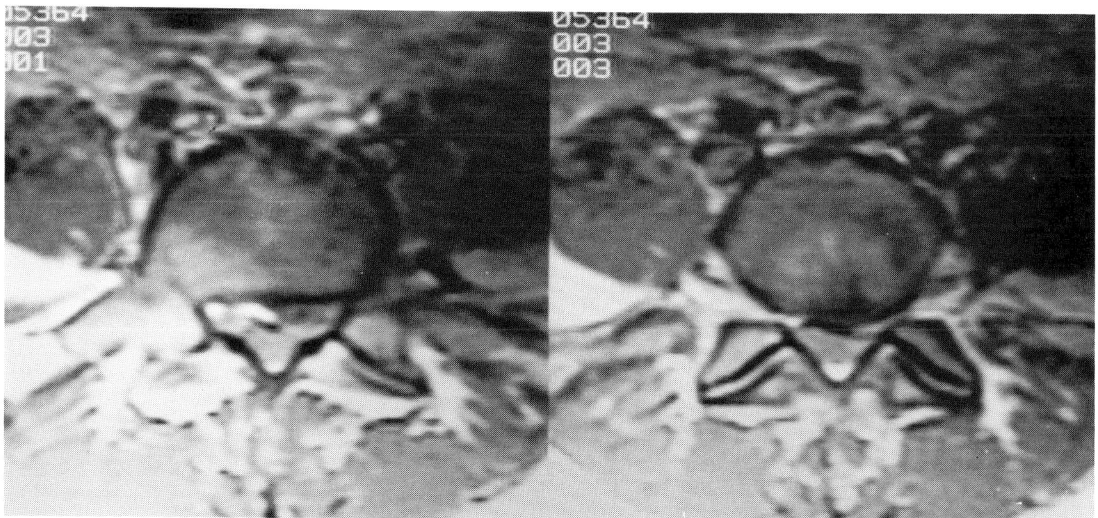

Figure 9–2. MRI scan in a 16-year-old with left L5–S1 disc herniation and no neurologic deficits, but a positive left-sided straight leg raising (SLR) test and a contralateral cross SLR test.

Most series depict the role of trauma as a causative agent in disc herniation.[1-7] Is lumbar disc herniation a symptom of early degenerative disc disease or is trauma a de novo insult to a normal structure (disc) that fails mechanically?

The association of structural abnormalities in individuals with adolescent and childhood disc herniation has been noted.[1,2,4] Spina bifida occulta, sacralization of L5 and six lumbar vertebrae, constituted 30 per cent of structural abnormalities in one series.[2] In another series, transitional vertebrae were demonstrated with elevated frequency.[4]

The preoperative evaluation should include diagnostic tests to confirm and localize the pathology. Before the advent of MRI scan myelography was recommended as the procedure of choice.[1-7] Others proposed EMG and CT to establish the pathologic condition.[4] MRI is emerging as perhaps the initial and very possibly a sufficient diagnostic entity in the evaluation of possible disc herniation.

Most series cite universally good results in the surgical management of lumbar disc herniation in the adolescent and child.[1-7] Interlaminal laminectomy without fusion has been recommended as the procedure of choice and variations of that surgical theme have been prescribed.[1-7] Spinal fusion in addition to discectomy did not produce a better result than discectomy alone.[1] The recurrence rate at the operative level was 6.1 per cent and 12.1 per cent at another level in a group followed for an average of 19 years. In this same group none of the patients who had a poor result had undergone spinal fusion.[?] The role of fusion remains unclear.

References

Lumbar Disc Herniation

1. Bradford, D. S., and Garcia, A.: Lumbar intervertebral disk herniations in children and adolescents. Orthop. Clin. North Am. *2*:583–592, 1971.
2. DeOrio, J., and Bianco, A.: Lumbar disc excision in children and adolescents. J. Bone Joint Surg. *64A*:991, 1982.
3. Garrido, E., Humphreys, R. P., Hendrick, E. B., and Hoffman, H. J.: Lumbar disc disease in children. Neurosurgery *2*:22–26, 1978.
4. Epstein, J. A., Epstein, N., and Marc, J.: Lumbar intervertebral disk herniation in teenage children: recognition and management of associated anomalies. Spine *9*:427–431, 1984.
5. Kurihara, A., and Kataoka, O.: Lumbar disc herniation in children and adolescents. Spine *5*:443–451, 1989.
6. Russwurm, H., and Bjerkreim, I.: Lumbar intervertebral disc herniation in the young. Acta Orthop. Scand. *40*:148–163, 1978.
7. Kamel, M., and Rosman, M.: Disc protrusion in the growing child. Clin. Orthop. *185*:46–52, 1984.

SLIPPED VERTEBRAL APOPHYSIS

The differential diagnosis of the symptomatic herniated lumbar disc may contain pathologic variants inducing the same clinical signs and symptoms. In the series of Garrido and colleagues three of 38 patients operated on for sciatica were discovered to have a "posteriorly dislocated epiphysis."[1] Some authors have contested that this is the spinal equivalent of the slipped capital femoral epiphysis. The pathologic specimens consisted of bone and cartilage fragments. Proposals for etiologic mechanisms have included trauma and the additive mechanical stress on a posterior vertebral margin secondary to bordering anomalies. Some authors have suggested that this clinicopathologic group represents "a posterior variant of marginal cartilaginous nodes." Scheuermann's disease was considered to be present in 50 per cent of patients in one series.[3] The mechanism proposed for posterior marginal node is the intrusion of disc material in a fashion that displaces the posterior ring apophysis from the vertebra and thus ultimately increases the mechanical vulnerability of this area to further herniation and displacement with the development of symptoms (Figs. 9–3, 9–4).

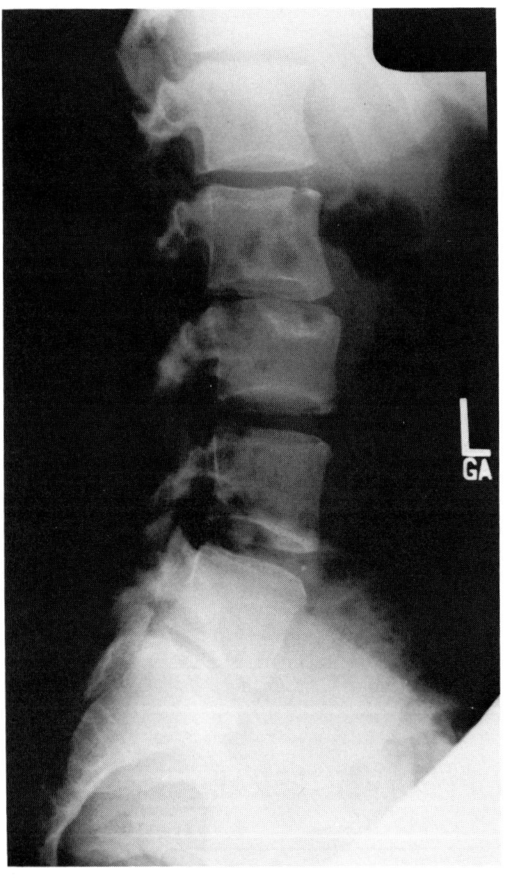

Figure 9–3. Lateral x-ray film of a 17-year-old pole vaulter with acute back pain. Note the end plate depression at L3.

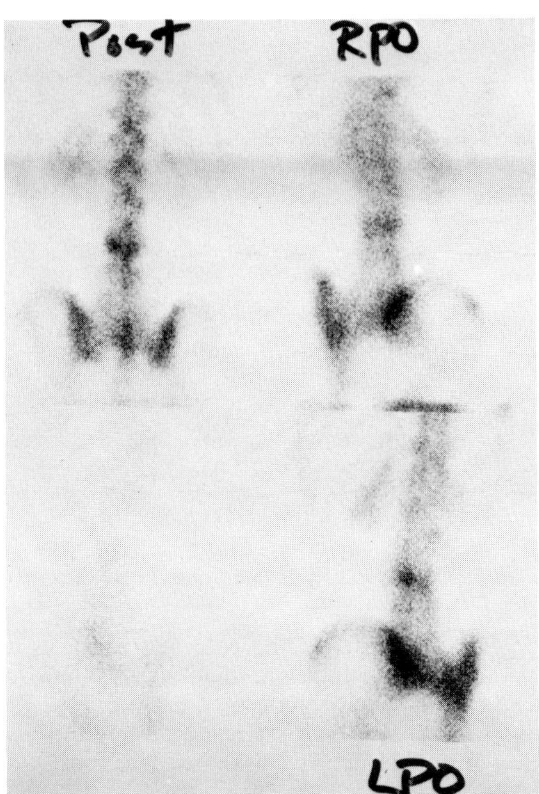

Figure 9–4. A positive bone scan in the patient shown in Figure 9–3 consistent with end plate compression fracture.

The lateral lumbar spine film demonstrates two factors: bone protruding into the spinal canal and posteroinferior marginal defect. The anteroposterior x-ray is less helpful. CT is definitive and provides additional information regarding the accompanying disc material. The inferior margin of the L4 vertebra appears to be the most common site of origin of a slipped apophysis. The indications for surgery are the same as for "pure disc herniation." Surgical considerations should include excision of both the herniated disc and the slipped apophysis.

References

Slipped Vertebral Apophysis

1. Garrido, E., Humphreys, R. P., Hendrick, E. B., and Hoffman, H. J.: Lumbar disc disease in children. Neurosurgery *2*:22–26, 1978.

2. Callahan, D., Pack, L., Brean, R., et al.: Intervertebral disc impingement syndrome in a child. Spine *11*:402–404, 1986.
3. Laredo, J. D., Bard, M., Chretien, J., and Kahn, M. F.: Lumbar posterior marginal intraosseous cartilaginous node. Skeletal Radiol. *15*:201–208, 1986.
4. Pettersson, H., Harwood-Nash, D. C., Fitz, C. R., et al.: The CT appearance of avulsion of the posterior vertebral apophysis. A case report. Neuroradiology *21*:145–147, 1981.

DISCITIS

Discitis is an inflammatory state of the intervertebral disc of presumed infectious etiology, but antecedent infection of extraspinal origin is uncommonly discovered in the history.

The presentation of discitis may be variable. In one series patients were categorized into those who had difficulty walking or standing, those who had abdominal pain, and those who had back pain or an abnormal spinal posture.[3]

Difficulty in walking or standing is more common in the younger age group with discitis (mean age 22 months) than in the older. The differential diagnosis of limb pain (Table 9–4) is extensive and involves a spectrum of biologic processes invoking different etiologies. It is not surprising that the time to diagnose the condition after presentation may be prolonged. Examination of the extremities is usually performed under such circumstances, but examination of the lumbar spine is mandatory. In one clinical series the diagnosis of discitis was not considered because many consulting physicians did not perform a spinal examination.[3]

Abdominal pain is another potential source of pain referral from discitis. The average age is usually older (7.8 years mean), and although the complaints draw an abdominal focus, the

Table 9–4. DIFFERENTIAL DIAGNOSIS OF LIMB PAIN IN CHILDHOOD

- **Organic Conditions**
  - Traumatic
    - Stress fracture
    - Myohematoma
    - Myositis ossificans
  - Orthopedic
    - Chondromalacia patellae
    - Osteochondritis dissecans
    - Osgood-Schlatter disease
    - Slipped capital femoral epiphysis
    - Legg-Calvé-Perthes disease
    - Hypermobility syndromes
  - Collagen Vascular
    - Juvenile rheumatoid arthritis
    - Systemic lupus erythematosus
    - Dermatomyositis
    - Mixed connective tissue disease
    - Henoch-Schönlein purpura
    - Familial Mediterranean fever
    - Palindromic rheumatism
    - Rheumatic fever
    - Inflammatory bowel disease
  - Infectious
    - Bacterial
      - Osteomyelitis
      - Discitis
      - Septic arthritis
      - Pyogenic myositis
    - Viral
      - "Toxic synovitis"
      - "Transient" synovitis
      - Rubella vaccination
      - Viral myositis
- **Neoplastic Disorders**
  - Leukemia
  - Lymphoma
  - Neuroblastoma
  - Histiocytosis X
  - Bony tumors
    - Osteogenic sarcoma
    - Ewing's sarcoma
    - Chondrosarcoma
  - Soft tissue tumors
    - Rhabdomyosarcoma
    - Fibrosarcoma
    - Synovial cell sarcoma
- **Hematologic Disorders**
  - Sickle cell anemia
  - Hemophilia
- **Endocrine Disorders**
  - Hypercortisolism
  - Hyperparathyroidism
  - Hypothyroidism
  - Osteoporosis
  - Myopathies
- **Nutritional Disorders**
  - Scurvy (vitamin C)
  - Rickets (vitamin D)
  - Hypervitaminosis A
  - Hypercholesterolemia
- **Miscellaneous Disorders**
  - Storage disease
    - Mucopolysaccharidoses
    - Recurrent arthralgias/myalgias associated with streptococcal and other infections
- **Syndromes of Unknown Origin**
  - Fibromyalgia
  - Growing pains
- **Psychosomatic Disorders**
  - Hysteria/conversion reactions
  - Reflex neurovascular dystrophy
  - School phobia

physical examination does not elicit localized findings consistent with intra-abdominal pathology. These patients usually undergo a thorough diagnostic search for potential abdominal conditions before the spine examination. Frequently, spasm, tenderness, postural rigidity, and hamstring tightness are found upon examination. Most patients present with back pain or an abnormal spinal posture.

Despite the spectrum of complaints in discitis, certain constant feaures are discoverable on physical examination in most patients: back spasm and rigid posturing, tenderness, abnormal postures with lordosis exaggerated, or scoliosis when standing or sitting. An SLR test may be elicited.

Consistent objective data that may stimulate the consideration of the diagnosis of discitis are low-grade fever, an elevated sedimentation rate, and disc space narrowing on plain x-ray examination. Early in the biologic permeation of discitis, the plain x-rays may be normal, but within two to four weeks disc space narrowing at the affected level is present, and with progression blurring of end plate margins may occur. In retrospect, subtle disc space narrowing was often present on lumbar x-rays interpreted as normal or on other investigative studies, such as intravenous pyelography.[3]

Advocates of radioisotopic scanning to evaluate back pain in children point to the potential early diagnosis of discitis on scan. In one series the scan was positive in patients with normal x-rays, and the diagnosis of discitis was established before radiographic alteration was noted.[3] The child may present while the radiologic changes of disc space narrowing on the normal x-ray are in transition, so that the static representation of this dynamic state is obscured. The value of the dynamic aspect of radionuclide scintigraphy has been established.

The pathophysiology of disc space infection in children has been presumed to be due to numerous vascular channels into the disc. This vascular access to the disc diminishes with maturity. Microangiographic studies suggest that the pathology of bone infection requires bone infarction due to septic emboli, and that children have relative protection from a rich arcade of intraosseous anastomoses, whereas in adults the metaphyseal vessels are end arteries, and septic emboli often result in the bone infarction.[8] The authors concluded that the clinical and radiologic aspects of childhood discitis are explainable on the basis of "intermetaphyseal anastomoses which allow septic thrombosis to spread to transequatorial metaphyses, without affecting the intervening equatorial zones."[8]

The differentiation between discitis and vertebral osteomyelitis is important. Discitis is considered a self-limited process, but vertebral osteomyelitis can lead to deformity and potential neurologic sequelae. Sequential radiographic changes may facilitiate the discrimination between osteomyelitis and discitis. Disc space narrowing, adjacent end plate changes, and autofusion of contiguous vertebra favor discitis, while destruction of vertebral body architecture favors osteomyelitis.

However, vertebral osteomyelitis may not allow an indolent analysis of sequential radiographs and retrospective diagnosis. Witness the fulminant course of *Salmonella* vertebral osteomyelitis and subsequent epidural abscess formation in the presence of normal initial x-rays.

The criteria for the diagnosis of osteomyelitis are typical radiographic changes, bacteriologic identification, and biopsy changes consistent with the process. In a report on four children with vertebral osteomyelitis, all presented with abdominal pain rather than back pain, staphylococcus was the causative agent, and half did not show initial x-ray abnormalities.[13] Clinical suspicion may warrant additional diagnostic evaluation to include radionuclide imaging, computerized tomography, and MRI scanning to detect the difference between discitis and vertebral osteomyelitis.

Besides vertebral osteomyelitis and subsequent conditions such as epidural or paravertebral abscesses, meningitis must be considered as a diagnostic possibility in children who refuse to walk or present with back stiffness or pain. The clinical findings in meningitis that are common irrespective of etiology are fever, lethargy, neck and back stiffness, Kernig's sign, and Bradzinski's sign. Lumbar puncture and cerebrospinal fluid (CSF) examination is the cornerstone of diagnosis for bacterial meningitis. Since the clinical presentation may be highly variable in terms of age and source, clinical awareness of the possibility must be considered in the evaluation of the child or adolescent with back pain or stiffness, fever, or refusal to walk or stand, in order to prevent potentially devastating sequelae.

The treatment of discitis involves bed rest and immobilization. Some authors have advocated casts for immobilization. The natural history of discitis is clinical improvement in six weeks to two months and resolution of laboratory abnormalities. The standard recommendation for the treatment of discitis does not include the use of antibiotics, about which dissenting opinions have been recorded. Criteria for antibiotic usage in discitis have included failure of the disease process to follow the natural history, pain and immobilization, positive cultures, continuous elevation of sedimentation rate, radiographically noted progression of disease, and systemic sepsis.

Aspiration or biopsy is not usually recommended. In clinical series the recovered organism has usually been *S. aureus*. Criteria for aspiration or biopsy of the disc space include failure to improve, a more septic course, radiographic evidence of progression, and recurrent symptoms.

References

Discitis

1. Spiegel, P., Kengla, K., and Isaacson, A.: Intervertebral disc-space inflammation in children. J. Bone Joint Surg. *54A:* 284–296, 1972.
2. Smith, T. K.: Diskitis in children. *In* Bradford D. S., and Hensinger, R. M. (eds.): The Pediatric Spine. New York, Thieme, 1985, pp. 63–67.
3. Wenger, D. R., Bobechko, W. P., and Gilday, D. L.: The spectrum of intervertebral disc-space infection in children. J. Bone Joint Surg. *60A:*100–108, 1978.
4. Bowyer, S. L., and Hollister, J. R.: Limb pain in childhood. Pediatr. Clin. North Am. *31:*1053–1080, 1984.
5. Rocco, H. D., and Eyring, E. J.: Intervertebral disk infection in children. Am. J. Dis. Child. *123:*448–451, 1972.
6. Grünebaum, M., Horodniceanu, C., Mukamel, M., et al.: The imaging diagnosis of non-pyogenic discitis in children. Pediatr. Radiol. *12:*123–127, 1982.
7. Peterson, H. A.: Disk-space infection in children. Instr. Course Lect. *32:*50–60, 1983.
8. Ratcliffe, J. F.: Anatomic basis for the pathogenesis and radiologic features of vertebral osteomyelitis and its differentiation from childhood discitis. Acta Radiol. Diagn. *26:*137–143, 1985.
9. Collert, S.: Osteomyelitis of the spine. Acta Orthop. Scand. *48:*282–290, 1977.
10. Ambramovitz, J., Batson, R. A., and Yablon, J. S.: Vertebral osteomyelitis. Spine *11:*418–420, 1986.
11. Eismont, F. J., Bohlmann, H. M., Goldberg, V. M., et al.: Pyogenic and fungal vertebral osteomyelitis with paralysis. J. Bone Joint Surg. *65A:*19–29, 1983.
12. Gardner, R.: Salmonella vertebral osteomyelitis and epidural abscess in a child with sickle cell disease. Pediatr. Emerg. Care *1:*87–89, 1985.
13. Bolivar, R., Kohl, S., and Pickering, L. K.: Vertebral osteomyelitis in children: report of four cases. Pediatrics *62:*549–553, 1978.
14. Fernandez-Ullsa, M., Vasavada, P. J., Hanslits, M. L., et al.: Diagnosis of vertebral osteomyelitis: clinical, radiological and scintigraphic features. Orthopedics *8:*1144–1150, 1985.
15. Whelan, M. A., Schonfeld, S., Post, J. D., et al.: Computed tomography of nontuberculous spinal infection. J. Comput. Assist. Tomogr. *9:*280–287, 1985.
16. Post, J. D., Quencer, R. M., Montalvo, B. M., et al.: Spinal infection: evaluation with MR imaging and intraoperative US. Radiology *169:*765–771, 1988.
17. Modic, M. T., Pflanze, W., Feiglin, D. H., et al.: Magnetic resonance imaging of musculoskeletal infections. Radiol. Clin. North Am. *24:*247–258, 1986.
18. Francke, E.: The many causes of meningitis. Postgrad. Med. *82:*175–178, 181–183, 187–188, 1987.
19. Gururaj, V. J., Russo, R. M., Allen, J. E., et al.: To tap or not to tap, and what are the best indicators for performing a lumbar puncture in an outpatient child? Clin. Pediatr. *12:*488, 1973.
20. Strampfer, J. J., Domenico, P. and Cunha, B. A.: Laboratory aids in the diagnosis of bacterial meningitis. Heart Lung *17:*605–607, 1988.
21. Wallace, S. J.: Meningitis: diagnosis and treatment. Public Health *102:*447–454, 1988.
22. Scoles, P. V., and Quinn, T. P.: Intervertebral discitis in children and adolescents. Clin. Orthop. *162:*31–36, 1982.
23. Boston, H. C., Bianco, A., and Rhodes, K. H.: Disk space infections in children. Clin. North Am. *6:*953–963, 1975.

SPONDYLOLYSIS AND SPONDYLOLISTHESIS

Spondylolysis and spondylolisthesis are important diagnostic entities in childhood back pain. Their natural history has been defined. At age 6 there is a 4.4 per cent incidence, increasing to 6 per cent at adult ages.[1] It is unusual for children to present with spondylolysis before age 5 and unusual for young children to present with severe spondylolisthesis (Grades III or IV). When symptoms appear, the complaints cluster around the growth spurt of adolescence. The risk of progression after adolescence is rare, but progression has been estimated to occur in about 15 per cent during adolescence. Since symptoms cannot be exclusively correlated with the degree of slip, and high-degree slips may generate deformity, the question arises as to the appropriate monitoring of patients with spondylolysis or spondylolisthesis, especially during the adolescent growth years (Fig. 9–5).

Although spondylolisthesis has been classified into five pathologic versions, this discussion will focus on the most common entity to arouse clinical suspicion in childhood and adolescence: the Type 2 isthmic lesion. A cornerstone of thought regarding the isthmic type is that it is derived from a stress fracture. These stress concentrations may be a biomechanical consequence of shear on the pars interarticularis, especially with extension. In addition, contributing pathomechanics of rotational forces in conjunction with lordosis may accentuate stresses in the pars. From an epidemiologic aspect, children and adolescents exposed to repeated biomechanical challenge duplicating proposed mechanisms of stress concentrations in the pars have a significantly higher incidence of spondylolysis than expected. The concept of repetitive microtrauma with concentration of these stresses in the pars has become increasingly recognized, and there is additional confirmation of the increased incidence of spondylolysis in the adolescent athlete, and of the biomechanical coercion of certain sports such as gymnastics, and weight lifting. Spondylolysis in a sense represents a spectrum from incipient stress fracture (stress reaction), healing stress fracture, to the point of persistent radiographic defect. Since symptoms may precede any radiographic abnormality and spondylolysis may exist as a radiographically defined but asymptomatic lesion, the search for the cause of back pain in teenage athletes is pursued with the idea of early detection in the symptomatic patient and the exclusion of other causes. Mechanical pain in the athlete may be derived from diverse sources: the sacroiliac joint, muscle strains, iliac apophysitis, ligament sprains, interspinous bursitis, anterior ring epiphyseal growth plate injury (Scheuermann's variants), degenerative disc disease, and disc herniation fractures of the posterior element other than the pars (pedicles and articular, transverse, and spinous processes). Although it is convenient to describe mechanical causes of back complaints in a teenager or child athlete, other pathologies such as tumors and infection may occur and need to be excluded. The bone scan is an invaluable diagnostic tool for evaluating back pain because of its sensitivity and dynamic format. A normal bone scan does not preclude spondylolysis, and perhaps a more common diagnosis is "spondylogenic back pain" associated with "hyperlordotic posturing of the lumbar spine, tight hip flexors, and frequently relatively tight hamstrings and lumbodorsal fascia."[12]

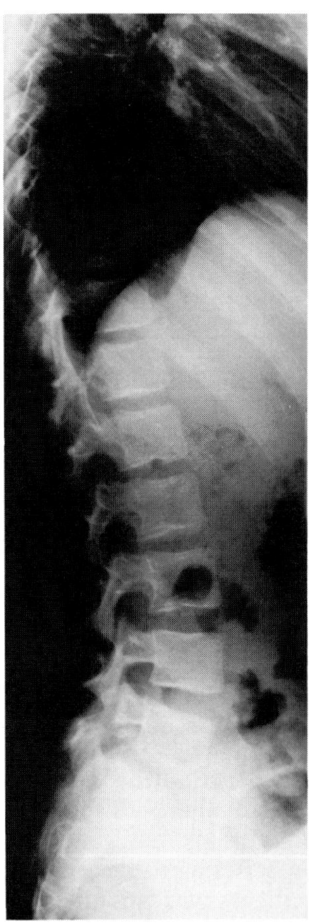

Figure 9–5. A gymnast with Grade I, Type II isthmic spondylolisthesis.

Children may present with back pain, back pain and associated radicular pain, or "poor posture." Back pain is usually activity related and relieved by rest or limitation of activities. Pain may radiate into the posterior thighs but rarely below the knee. For the lower-grade slips (I or II) the most common findings on physical examination are hamstring tightness (53 per cent), increased lordosis (25 per cent), mild scoliosis (21 per cent), muscle spasm (14 per cent), and no abnormalities (21 per cent).[3] High-grade slips (III, IV, spondyloptosis) associated with lumbosacral kyphosis and a vertebral sacrum may present with a portrait of "flattening of the buttocks, malrotated pelvis, lordosis extending into the thoracic spine and inability to stand straight with the knees fully extended."[2] The patient may not be able to assume flexion of the hips in the presence of a straight leg. The pelvic waddle may be related to hamstring tightness and lumbosacral kyphosis demonstrable as the gait pattern of spondylolisthesis.

The spectrum of neurologic involvement runs from rare to more common with higher-grade slips. In patients with idiopathic scoliosis the incidence of spondylolysis was 6.2 per cent.[28] Scoliosis in association with spondylolisthesis is usually compensatory rather than structural. In one study, "patients with a higher degree of lumbosacral kyphosis and more severe slipping also had a statistically higher degree of lumbar scoliosis."[39] Although spondylolysis is most common at the lumbosacral junction, it can occur at higher levels, L1 to L3.

Unilateral spondylolysis is thought to occur in 20 per cent of all patients with this disease. Some authors have associated this with "hyperplasia of the vertebral body and neural arch."[32] Sherman described contralateral hypertrophy of the pedicle and sclerosis in association with unilateral spondylolysis.[44]

A standing lateral x-ray may be sufficient to demonstrate the slip of spondylolisthesis, but in spondylolysis (especially the unilateral variety) oblique x-rays may be necessary to demonstrate the break in the pars interarticularis, represented as a defect in the neck of the "Scottie dog of La Chapele."[33] Some authors say that indirect signs of spondylolysis are observable on the frontal view as an offset in a line drawn through the spinous processes and hyperostosis in a contralateral pedicle and pars. Amato and colleagues demonstrated lamina fragmentation on the anteroposterior or up-angled view in 14.2 per cent of cases of spondylolysis.[35] In addition to patients with clear-cut spondylolysis on x-ray, a subgroup of "dysplastic types" exist in which the pars is attenuated and appears to resemble a greyhound on the oblique view.

The role of the bone scan cannot be overemphasized in the detection of spondylolysis before x-ray identification (stress reaction, stress fracture) and in establishing the probability of recent onset in those with an established defect.

CT is useful in the detection of spondylolysis as an acute event or unhealed defect, and in differentiating a "hot spot" on bone scan in the differential diagnosis with osteoid osteoma.

Treatment options for spondylolysis and spondylolisthesis include observation, rest, restriction of activity, exercise, bracing, and surgery. Brace treatment in symptomatic spondylolysis has its advocates. Micheli showed that 32 per cent healed and 88 per cent were able eventually to resume pain-free activity levels after bracing, even if healing did not occur.[24] Bell and colleagues used an antilordotic brace in the treatment of Grades I and II spondylolisthesis during the "adolescent growth time" and demonstrated no increases in slip percentage and ultimate resolution of pain symptoms.[3] Patients with more than a 50 per cent slip or children or adolescents who have intractable leg or back pain with lesser slips are generally recommended to have fusion operations.[5, 6, 10, 39, 40]

Although the natural history is considered benign in spondylolysis and spondylolisthesis, regular evaluation of the child or adolescent with back pain should be performed to detect any progression.[11, 39]

Micheli recommended abdominal exercises, pelvic tilts, and hamstring stretching in the population of symptomatic spondylolysis patients who are braced.[24] In addition to trunk exercise and lower extremity stretching, Micheli noted that some children had sufficient spondylogenic back pain for short-term bracing to be recommended in the absence of radiographically verifiable defects.[24]

A study of 255 patients followed for 20 years or more depicted a relatively small risk of slipping and no correlation with degree of slip or onset of age.[41] At follow-up, the risk of low back symptoms correlated with "greater than 25 per cent slipping, low lumbar index in L5 spondylolysis, spondylolysis at L4 level, and early disc degeneration."[41]

Risk factors associated with slipping and symptoms are listed in Table 9–5.[10]

Table 9–5. RISK FACTORS ASSOCIATED WITH SLIPPING

Clinical	Radiologic
Adolescent growth	Dysplastic slip
Female gender	Domed sacrum: trapezoidal L5 >50% slip
History of back pain	Slip angle >40–50%
	Increased-motion dynamic views

References

Spondylolysis and Spondylolisthesis

1. Fredrickson, B. E., Baker, D., McHolick, W. J., et al.: The natural history of spondylolysis and spondylolisthesis. J. Bone Joint Surg. *66A:*699–707, 1984.
2. Hensinger, R. M.: Back pain in children. *In* Bradford, D. S., and Hensinger, R. M. (eds.): Spine. New York, Thieme, 1985, pp. 41–63.
3. Bell, D. F., Ehrlich, M. G., and Zaleske, D.: Brace treatment for symptomatic spondylolisthesis. Clin. Orthop. *236:*192–198, 1988.
4. LaFond, G.: Surgical treatment of spondylolisthesis. Clin. Orthop. *22:*175, 1962.
5. Boxall, D., Bradford, D. S., Winter, R. B., et al.: Management of severe spondylolisthesis in children and adolescents. J. Bone Joint Surg. *61A:*479, 1979.
6. Hensinger, R. M., Lang, J. R., and MacEwen, G. D.: Surgical management of the spondylolisthesis in children and adolescents. Spine *1:*207, 1976.
7. Blackburne, J. S., and Velikas, E. P.: Spondylolisthesis in children and adolescents. J. Bone Joint Surg. *59B:*490, 1977.
8. Vebostad, A.: Spondylolisthesis. A review of 71 patients. Acta Orthop. Scand. *45:*715,1974.
9. Lusskin, R.: Pain patterns in spondylolisthesis—a correlation of symptoms, local pathology, and therapy. Clin. Orthop. *40:*123, 1965.
10. Bradford, D. S.: Spondylolysis and spondylolisthesis in children and adolescents: current concepts on management. *In* Bradford, D. S., and Hensinger, R. M. (eds.): The Pediatric Spine. New York Thieme, 1985, pp. 403–425.
11. Winter, R. B.: The natural history of spondylolysis and spondylolisthesis (letter). J. Bone Joint Surg. *67A:*823, 1985.
12. Wiltse, L. L., Newman, P. M., and MacNab, I.: Classification of spondylolysis and spondylolisthesis. Clin. Orthop. *117:*23–29, 1976.
13. Wiltse, L. L., Widell, E. M., and Jackson, D. W.: Fatigue fracture: the basic lesion in isthmic spondylolisthesis. J. Bone Joint Surg. *57A:*17–22, 1975.
14. Kenz, J., and Troup, J. D. G.: The structure of the pars interarticularis of the lower lumbar vertebrae and its relation to the etiology of spondylolysis. J. Bone Joint Surg. *55B:*735–741, 1973.
15. Neithard, F. B.: Scheuermann's disease and spondylolysis. Orthop. Trans. *7:*103, 1983.
16. Jackson, D. W., Wiltse, L. L., and Cirincione, R. J.: Spondylolysis in the female gymnast. Clin. Orthop. *117:*68, 1976.
17. Ichikawa, N., Ohara, Y., Morishita, T., et al.: An etiological study on spondylolysis from a biomechanical aspect. Br. J. Sports Med. *16:*135–141, 1982.
18. Commandre, F. A., Taillan, B., Gagnerie, F., et al.: Spondylolysis and spondylolisthesis in young athletes: 28 cases. J. Sports Med. Phys. Fitness *28:*104–107, 1988.
19. Kono, S., Hayashi, N., Kashahara, G., et al.: A study on the etiology of spondylolysis with reference to athletic activities. J. Jpn. Orthop Assoc. *49:*125, 1975.
20. Rossi, F.: Spondylolysis, spondylolisthesis and sports. J. Sports Med. Phys. Fitness *18:*317–340, 1978.
21. Papanicolaou, N., Wilkinson, R. H., Emans, J. B., et al.: Bone scintigraphy and radiography in young athletes with low back pain. A.J.R. *145:*1039–1044, 1985.
22. Marymont, J., Lynch, M., and Henning, C. E.: Exercise-related stress reaction of the sacroiliac joint. Am. J. Sports Med. *14:*320–323, 1986.
23. Keene, J. S., and Drummond, D. S.: Mechanical back pain in the athlete. Compr. Ther. *11:*7–14, 1985.
24. Micheli, L. L.: Back injuries in gymnastics. Clin. Sports Med. *4:*85–93, 1985.
25. Micheli, L. L.: Low back pain in the adolescent: differential diagnosis. Am. J. Sports Med. *7:*362, 1979.
26. Newman, P. H.: A clinical syndrome associated with severe lumbosacral subluxation. J. Bone Joint Surg. *47B:*472, 1965.
27. Turner, R. H., and Bianco, A. J., Jr.: Spondylolysis and spondylolisthesis in children and teenagers. J. Bone Joint Surg. *53A:*1298, 1971.
28. Fisk, J. R., Moe, J. H., and Winter, R. B.: Scoliosis, spondylolysis, and spondylolisthesis: their relationship as reviewed in 539 patients. Spine *3:*234–245, 1978.
29. Seitsalo, S., Osterman, K., and Poussa, M.: Scoliosis associated with lumbar spondylolisthesis. Spine *13:*899–904, 1988.
30. Lowe, J., Libson, E., and Ziv, I.: Spondylolysis in the upper lumbar spine. J. Bone Joint Surg. *69B:*582–586, 1987.
31. Wiltse, L. L.: Spondylolisthesis in children. Clin. Orthop. *21:*156–163, 1961.
32. Porter, R. W., and Park, W.: Unilateral spondylolysis. J. Bone Joint Surg. *64B:*344–348, 1982.
33. Sherman, F. C., Wilkinson, R. M., and Hall, J. E.: Reactive sclerosis of a pedicle and spondylolysis in the lumbar spine. J. Bone Joint Surg. *59A:*49–54, 1977.
34. Commandre, F. A., Gagnerie, G., and Zakarian, M.: The child. The spine and sport. J. Sports Med. Phys. Fitness *28:*11–19, 1988.
35. Amato M., Totty, W. G., and Giluda, L. A.: Spondylolysis of the lumbar spine: demonstration of defects and laminal fragmentation. Radiology *153:*627–629, 1984.
36. Gelfand, M. J., Strife, J. L., and Kereiakes, J. G.: Radionuclide bone imaging in spondylolysis of the lumbar spine in children. Radiology *140:*191–195, 1981.
37. Van Den Oever, M., Merrick, M. V., and Scott, J. H.: Bone scintigraphy in symptomatic spondylolysis. J. Bone Joint Surg. *69B:*453–456, 1987.
38. Rothman, S.: Computed tomography of the spine in older children and teenagers. Clin. Sports Med. *5:*247–270, 1986.
39. Seitsalo, S., Osterman, K., and Poussa, M.: Spondylolisthesis in children under 12 years of age: long-term results of 56 patients treated conservatively or operatively. J. Pediatr. Orthop. *8:*516–521, 1988.
40. Pizzutillo, P. D., Mirenda, W., and MacEwen, G. D.: Posterolateral fusion for spondylolisthesis in adolescence. J. Pediatr. Orthop. *6:*311–316, 1986.
41. Saraste, M.: Long-term clinical and radiological follow-up of spondylolysis and spondylolisthesis. J. Pediatr. Orthop. *7:*631–638, 1987.

SCHEUERMANN'S DISEASE

Scheuermann's disease is associated with radiographic criteria: end plate irregularities, disc space narrowing, three or more contiguous vertebrae wedged greater than 5 degrees, Schmorl's node formation, and kyphosis.[1–3] Patients with Scheuermann's disease are more likely to seek medical attention for deformity than for back pain, and some authors have stated that the lumbar and thoracolumbar involvement of Scheuermann's is often associated with low back symptoms as opposed to the more clinically silent thoracic form. Decision making in patients with Scheuermann's kyphosis has been well documented, heralding the value of the Milwaukee brace and the criteria for surgery.[5] Surgery was recommended for "kyphosis of more than 60 degrees that was increasing and was not controlled by the brace."[5]

The relationship between Scheuermann's disease and back pain has some variations in the scientific literature (Fig. 9–6). Stoddard and Osborn selected 853 people at random and compared these with 925 symptomatic low back pain patients.[7] They demonstrated Scheuermann's disease in 42.6 per cent of the symptomatic and 13.1 per cent of the control group.[7] They also described spondylolysis prevalence in Scheuermann's as compared with the prevalence in control groups, and raised the specter of future back symptoms with the finding of typical Scheuermann's disease and an accelerated presence of spondylolysis. Other authors cited the issue of "underdiagnosis" of lumbar and thoracolumbar Scheuermann's as a cause of back pain. Fisk and associates evaluated over 500 17- and 18-year-olds, discovering a 56.3 per cent incidence of Scheuermann's in males compared with 30.3 per cent in females.[9] These authors further concluded that the problem was universal, with no relationship to significant physical activity, but was associated, by inference, with "prolonged static high intradiscal pressures associated with too much sitting on our behinds."[9] Still other reports have linked physical activity in association with juvenile kyphosis and the striking incidence among males at adolescent ages.[10–12]

Greene and colleagues reported adolescents with mechanical back pain and many of the constellation of abnormalities characteristic of Scheuermann's disease located at the thoracolumbar junction.[4] In over 75 per cent of this group, trauma or significant activity was implicated with symptoms. Spondylolysis or spondylolisthesis was discovered in 32 per cent. Ogilvie and Sherman documented a 50 per cent incidence of spondylolysis in patients with Scheuermann's kyphosis and increased lumbar lordosis.[13] In support of traumatic etiology for back pain and vertebral body changes similar to Scheuermann's disease in the lumbar spine, Blumenthal and associates categorized such a group of adolescent athletes exposed to axial spinal stresses and labeled them as "atypical Scheuermann's."[14] The biomechanical theory supporting changes of the end plate and vertebral body in adolescence concentrates on the concept of the relative weakness of the end plate compared with the disc under axial load, and the concept that loads imposed on the preflexed spine can predispose to the mechan-

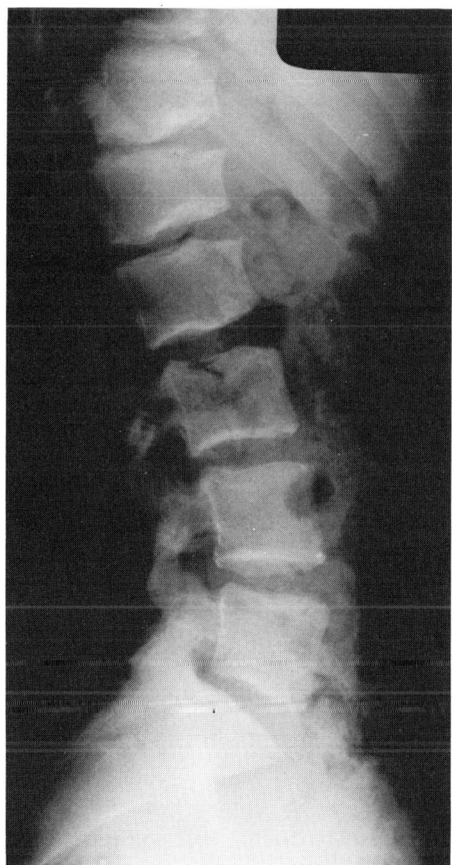

Figure 9–6. A 15-year-old with vertebral end plate changes consistent with dorsolumbar Scheuermann's disease and chronic low-grade back pain.

ical failure of the end plate and potential implosion of nuclear material. The events would lead to a spectrum of spinal abnormalities: localized abnormalities of a nonprogressive nature and progressive fixed kyphosis on the other end.[4] The pathology of "atypical Scheuermann's" thus might differ from the "osteochondroses, juvenilis Scheuermann's" in which some researchers have concluded "that a disturbance of collagen or ground substance biosynthesis is of importance."[17]

Patients with "atypical Scheuermann's" and dorsolumbar Scheuermann's may present with back pain and relatively high symptoms (thoracolumbar junction). Pain usually increases with activity and is relieved by rest. Pain may be accentuated with flexion. Treatment consists of anti-inflammatory medications, restriction of activity, guided therapy to return to activity level, and bracing if kyphosis progresses or mechanical pain does not subside.

Vertebral body changes secondary to overload of the immature skeleton may be a cause of adolescent back pain and need to be considered in a differential diagnosis of pediatric back pain. Classical juvenile kyphosis with Scheuermann's end plate changes may be associated with back pain, but a careful evaluation should be made of other potential causes of low back pain such as spondylolysis and spondylolisthesis. Typical thoracolumbar involvement meeting the classic criteria of Scheuermann's can cause low back pain in the adolescent.

References

Scheuermann's Disease

1. Hensinger, R. M.: Back pain in children. *In* Bradford, D. S., and Hensinger, R. M. (eds.): The Pediatric Spine. New York, Thieme, 1985, pp. 41–60.
2. Bradford, D. S.: Vertebral osteochondrosis. Clin. Orthop. *158*:83–90, 1981.
3. Grünebaum, M., Horodniceanu, C., Mukamel, M., et al.: The imaging diagnosis of non-pyogenic discitis in children. Pediatr. Radiol. *12*:123–127, 1982.
4. Greene, T. L., Hensinger, R. M., and Hunter, L. Y.: Back pain and vertebral changes simulating Scheuermann's disease. J. Pediatr. Orthop. *5*:1–7, 1985.
5. Wilcox, P. G., and Spencer, C. W.: Dorsolumbar kyphosis or Scheuermann's disease. Clin. Sports Med. *5*:343–351, 1986.
6. Sachs, B., Bradford, D., and Winter, R.: Scheuermann's kyphosis. J. Bone Joint Surg. *69A*:50–57, 1987.
7. Stoddard, A., and Osborn, J. F.: Scheuermann's disease or spinal osteochondrosis. J. Bone Joint Surg. *61B*:56–58, 1979.
8. Lings, S., and Mikkelsen, L.: Scheuermann's disease with low localization. Scand. J. Rehabil. Med. *14*:77–79, 1982.
9. Fisk, J. W., Baigent, M. L., Hill, P. D.: Scheuermann's disease. Am. J. Phys. Med. *63*:18–30, 1984.
10. Scheuermann, V. H.: Kyphosis dorsalis juvenilis. Z. Orthop. Chir. *41*:305–317, 1921.
11. Wassmann, K.: Kyphosis juvenilis Scheuermann–an occupational disorder. Acta Orthop. Scand. *21*:65–74, 1946.
12. Micheli, L. J.: Low back pain in the adolescent: differential diagnosis. Am. J. Sports Med. *7*:362–364, 1977.
13. Ogilvie, J., and Sherman, J.: Spondylolysis in Scheuermann's disease. Spine *12*:251–253, 1987.
14. Blumenthal, S. L., Roach, J., and Henning, J. A.: Lumbar Scheuermann's—a clinical series and classification. Spine *12*:929–932, 1987.
15. Jayson, M. I., Herbert, C. M., and Barks, J. S.: Intervertebral discs: nuclear morphology and bursting pressures. Ann. Rheum. Dis. *32*:308–315, 1973.
16. Roaf, R.: A study of the mechanics of spinal injuries. J. Bone Joint Surg. *42B*:810–823, 1960.
17. Aufdermann, M., and Spycher, M.: Pathogenesis of osteochondrosis juvenilis Scheuermann. J. Orthop. Res. *4*:452–457, 1986.

SCOLIOSIS

Scoliosis is usually a clinically silent process in terms of pain, and if undetected can lead to severe deformity. The focus of the last decade in spinal deformity has been the study of the natural history of idiopathic scoliosis, the role of screening techniques, the effectiveness of nonsurgical management, the analysis of curve progression risk, and the dramatic alteration in the concepts of internal fixation.[1–14] School screening has been used to identify patients who should be treated before curves progress to the range of surgical necessity.[1–4] This is precisely the point: scoliosis is painless and progression has to be identified visually, not by sophisticated pain inventory.

What is to be expected in the profile of idiopathic scoliosis: right-sided thoracic curve, left lumbar curve, positive family history? Any child or adolescent who does not fit this profile needs to be considered for further evaluation. Any child or adolescent who has back pain and scoliosis must be evaluated diagnostically to determine the associative cause of back pain in conjunction with scoliosis or the identification of the pathology that is generating a painful curve. Additional clues to the potentially serious underlying pathology are an unusually rapid alteration in the magnitude of a curve or the identification of neurologic signs and symptoms. We have already alluded to the statistical association of spondylolysis and spondylolisthesis with scoliosis and the frequent presentation of "sciatic scoliosis" in adolescents with herniated discs, and the potential for discitis or other infectious processes to present with deformed skeletal structure. However, there are still other pathologic conditions that may stimulate curvature and cause pain.

Citron and colleagues' review of intramedullary cord tumors presenting as scoliosis scrutinized the importance of diagnostic evaluation of painful scoliosis.[15] They pointed out that the only objective sign may be spinal curvature and that the identification of occult intraspinal tumor may prevent inappropriate scoliosis surgery and enhance the quality of results for tumor surgery.[15] Of the patients in this series 66 per cent had spinal pain. Careful search of plain x-rays may yield erosive bony changes or pedicle splaying, but there are pitfalls to these objective parameters. What constitutes normal interpedicular distance may coincide with the pathologic range in children, severe deformity may make the assessment difficult, and lesions of the cervical spine may be responsible for an observed curve lower in the spine.[15]

Osteoid osteoma and osteoblastoma may induce a scoliosis that is initially postural, but may promote structural characteristics with time.[16, 17] Kirwan and colleagues demonstrated that the size of the induced curve and the degree of rotational deformity was directly related to age of symptom onset and duration. The results of surgery were tied to the issue of time and skeletal maturity, and spontaneous curve resolution was the stated goal after surgical excision of the lesion.[16, 17]

Congenital scoliosis may be associated with occult intraspinal anomalies. From a conceptual perspective, it is easy to visualize that any intimate disturbance in the structural housing of the neurologic elements could be associated with maldevelopment of that same neurologic constitution.[18]

In one clinical series, over 50 per cent of intraspinal anomalies consisted of diastematomyelia, the remainder being distributed among various other conditions such as dermoid, lipoma, neurenteric cyst, tethered cord, and lateral meningocele.[19] Gillespie and colleagues localized specific anomalies to a cluster of spinal regions (Table 9–6), and also identified the most common clinical presentations: neurologic abnormalities such as food deformity or scoliosis without concurrent neurologic findings.[19]

Table 9–6. Intraspinal Anomalies in Congenital Scoliosis

Lower Level in Spine	Higher Level in Spine
Diastematomyelia	Dermoid
Lipoma of cauda equina	Neurenteric cyst
Tethered cord	
Orthopedic Presentation	**Neurologic Presentation**
Unilateral foot deformity	Pain and stiff back
Short leg	Onset of weakness
	Bladder disturbance
	Long tract signs

McMaster reviewed 251 cases of congenital scoliosis, exposing an 18 per cent occurrence of intraspinal abnormality.[18] Diastematomyelia was by far the most common diagnosis. "Other less common anomalies, occurring alone or in association with a diastematomyelia, were: neurenteric, epidermoid, and dermoid cysts; teratoma; lipofibroma; absence of nerve roots; fibrous bands; and a tight filum terminale." McMaster concluded that the incidence of congenital scoliosis with intraspinal anomaly is at least 20 per cent or higher; in this series, 33 per cent presented with skin changes on the back or lower limb and/or bladder neurologic dysfunction.[18] The remainder were evaluated for scoliosis. Various midline skin changes connected with the most common intraspinal anomaly associated with congenital scoliosis (diastematomyelia) are: "hairy tuft, dermal dimple, hemangioma, skin sinus, nevus, lipoma, and pilonidal sinus."[20] The congenital scoliosis itself requires an exclusion of occult intraspinal process before any anticipated surgical correction to avoid making neurologic deficits worse or precipitating them.[21] Careful evaluation of patients with congenital scoliosis is also warranted because of the high incidence of nonspinal anomalies of various organ systems.[22]

Plain radiographs cannot be used to exclude the intraspinal anomalies because the structural distortion of the spine from scoliosis may obscure those entities suggested by x-ray films.[18] It is necessary to investigate with myelography, CT, and/or MRI. Of intraspinal anomalies, 74 per cent manifested cutaneous changes, although midline cutaneous findings are not pathognomonic. Only 17 per cent of patients in McMaster's series had normal lower extremities with an intraspinal anomaly.[18]

Some authors have speculated that the tethered cord is more common than the various entities making up spinal dysraphism, although they present in similar fashions.[23]

References

Scoliosis

1. Bunnell, W. P.: The natural history of idiopathic scoliosis. Clin. Orthop. *229:*20–25, 1988.
2. Lonstein, J. E.: Natural history and school screening for scoliosis. Orthop. Clin. North Am. *19:*227–237, 1988.
3. Rinsky, L. A., and Gamble, J. G.: Adolescent idiopathic scoliosis. West. J. Med. *148:*182–190, 1988.
4. McCarthy, R. E.: Prevention of the complications of scoliosis by early detection. Clin. Orthop. *222:*73–78, 1987.
5. Lonstein, J. E.: Comparison of symposium papers on natural history of idiopathic scoliosis. Spine *11:*807, 1986.
6. Mellencamp, D. D., and Blount, W. P.: Late results revisited. Spine *11:*805–806, 1986.
7. McCullough, N. C.: Nonoperative treatment of idiopathic scoliosis using surface electrical stimulation. Spine *11:*802–804, 1986.
8. Emans, J. B., Kaelin, A., and Bancel, P.: Boston bracing system for idiopathic scoliosis. Spine *11:*792–801, 1986.
9. Winter, R. B., Lonstein, J. E., and Drogt, J.: The effectiveness of bracing in the nonoperative treatment of idiopathic scoliosis. Spine *11:*790–791, 1986.
10. Ascani, E., Bartolozzi, P., and Logroscino, C. A.: Natural history of untreated idiopathic scoliosis after skeletal maturity. Spine *11:*784–789, 1986.
11. Weinstein, S. L., and Ponseti, I. V.: Curve progression in idiopathic scoliosis. J. Bone Joint Surg. *65A:*447–455, 1983.
12. Weinstein, S. L., Zavala, D. C., and Ponseti, I. V.: Idiopathic scoliosis. J. Bone Joint Surg. *63A:*702–711, 1981.
13. Weinstein, S. L.: Idiopathic scoliosis: naural history. Spine *11:*780–783, 1986.
14. Bunnell, W. P.: Natural history of idiopathic scoliosis before skeletal maturity. Spine *11:*773–776, 1986.
15. Citron, N., Edgar, M. A., Sheehy, J., et al.: Intramedullary spinal cord tumors presenting as scoliosis. J. Bone Joint Surg. *66B:*513–517, 1984.
16. Ransford, A. O., Pozo, J. L., Hutton, P. A., et al.: The behavior pattern of the scoliosis associated with osteoid osteoma or osteoblastoma of the spine. J. Bone Joint Surg. *66B:*16–20, 1984.
17. Kirwan, E. O., Hutton, P. A., Pozo, J. L. and Ransford, A. O.: Osteoid osteoma and benign osteoblastoma of the spine. J. Bone Joint Surg. *66B:*21–26, 1984.
18. McMaster, M. J.: Occult intraspinal anomalies and congenital scoliosis. J. Bone Joint Surg. *66A:*588–601, 1984.
19. Gillespie, R., Faithfull, D. K., Roth, A., et al.: Intraspinal anomalies in congenital scoliosis. Clin. Orthop. *93:*103–109, 1973.
20. Eid, K., Hochberg, J., and Saunders, D. E.: Skin abnormalities of the back in diastematomyelia. Plast. Reconstr. Surg. *63:*534–539, 1979.
21. Winter, R. B., Haven, J. J., and Moe, J. H, et al.: Diastematomyelia and congenital spine deformities. J. Bone Joint Surg. *56A:*27–39, 1974.
22. Bernard, T. N., Jr., Burke, S. W., Johnston, C. E. III, and Roberts, J. M.: Congenital spine deformities. Orthopedics *8:*777–783, 1985.
23. Hoffman, M. J., Hendrick, E. B., and Humphreys, R. P.: The tethered spinal cord: its protean manifestations, diagnosis and surgical correction. Childs Brain *2:*145–155, 1976.

BONE TUMORS

Bone tumors, whether malignant or benign, primary or metastatic, may present clinically in a similar fashion. The unholy triad of pain, deformity, and neurologic deficit may be encountered together or as separate existences, and may represent a benign local process or a devastatingly destructive malignancy. Back pain in children and adolescents, whether it is activity related or accentuated at night, should raise the specter of tumor. It is an absolute consideration in persistent back pain.

In addition to careful history taking and vigorous physical assessment, the clinician has two major allies: first, that the diagnosis of tumor has been considered and second, that the bone scan is available. The latter represents the single best screening test for childhood tumors that involve the skeleton.[1] Plain x-ray, tomography, CT, myelography, and MRI play an important role in the definition of tumor pathology. Criteria for staging musculoskeletal neoplasms have been defined by Enneking, and treatment considerations addressed.[2] The natural histories reflecting the biologic behavior of these disparate lesions, and the definition of results by treatment option, are the basis for management and decision making.

Benign Lesions

Osteoid Osteoma and Osteoblastoma. Osteoid osteoma and osteoblastoma are benign lesions presenting usually between the ages of 10 and 20 (osteoblastoma slightly later). Males are affected more frequently and osteoid osteoma has been called the most common cause of painful scoliosis.[2] The most common position of the tumors is in the posterior elements, especially in the lumbar spine, and when they are localized in the lumbar or thoracolumbar area, 86 per cent of patients demonstrate scoliosis.[3]

Increased pain with activity and at night have been recorded in 95 per cent of patients, 29 per cent had pain sufficient to awaken from sleep and 90 per cent reported relief with aspirin; 27 per cent of osteoblastomas in the spine and 6.5 per cent of osteoid osteomas were associated with "definite neurological abnormalities."[2]

The average time from symptom onset to diagnosis was 28 months.[3] Bone scan reduced the time before diagnosis by 66 per cent. No false-negative bone scans have been recognized, and multiple series have depicted the sensitivity of bone scan for these tumors.[3, 5–11]

Treatment consists of complete excision of the tumor. Since the spontaneous resolution of the deformity is related to the duration of symptoms, failure to identify the cause of painful scoliosis may lead to permanent structural deformity and progression even after tumor excision.[2] In one series, 15 months appeared to be a critical junction for the scoliosis prognosis.[3]

A bone scan is mandatory in the evaluation of painful scoliosis.[3–11]

Eosinophilic Granuloma. Eosinophilic granuloma is usually discovered in patients between the ages of 5 and 10 years, and when it involves the spine produces "vertebral plana," considered a classic spinal manifestation of the biology.[12] The lesion may be single or multiple and has an excellent prognosis even with partial restoration of vertebral structure.[13] The value of the bone scan is not as apparent with eosinophilic granuloma as with other pediatric back pain etiologies, and scans may be positive (hot) or negative (cold).[12, 14] Conventional radiography is an important mainstay in diagnosis.[12, 14]

Aneurysmal Bone Cyst. Aneurysmal bone cyst may present with spinal involvement and may precipitate a neurologic sign or back pain.[15, 23] In one series all patients had posterior element involvement, and in patients in whom the vertebral body showed involvement the pedicle was also implicated.[13] Since the lesion is expansible, it may involve contiguous structures and has to be considered in the broad differential diagnosis of expansile lesions of the vertebrae (osteochondroma, osteoblastoma, giant cell tumor, hemangioma, eosinophilic granuloma, fibrous dysplasia, chordoma, metastasis, angiosarcoma, osteosarcoma, chondrosarcoma, and lymphoma).[17] Treatment of choice is resection (partial or complete) or curettage.[15, 16, 19, 21–23] Radiation is controversial but may be necessary to control growth in surgically inaccessible areas.[15, 16, 19, 21–23]

Giant Cell Tumor. Giant cell tumor is not a common tumor of the spine, but when present may present as an expansile lesion similar to aneurysmal bone cyst.[25] The sacrum can become involved in giant cell tumor and was noted in 33 of 407 cases.[26] In inaccessible areas the traditional treatments of curettage and bone grafting may yield to embolization and even adjunctive radiation, despite the risks of complicating sarcomas.[24] Surgical aggression with the resection of lesions and reconstruction has become more expansively applied in the spine, particularly focusing on the greater technical capacity to deal with sacral tumors.[27]

Hemangioma. Hemangioma is a "vascular hamartoma," and when it rarely presents with symptoms under the age of 20, pain is the dominant theme. Some authors have suggested radiation therapy under these circumstances.[28] Surgery is rarely indicated for neurologic signs, but when it is contemplated preoperative embolization with subsequent lesion excision and spinal reconstruction is recommended.[28]

Osteochondroma. The treatment of symptomatic osteochondroma consists of surgical excision, although this entity is rarely symptomatic in childhood.[28]

Malignant Lesions

The presentation of malignant lesions may include pain, deformity, and neurologic deficit. The pathologic consequences of primary origin tumors from bone or its marrow may mean the alteration of pain-sensitive structures and thus the risk during physiologic load of pathologic fracture, or the development of symptoms from tumor insinuation.

In a Mayo Clinic series of osteosarcoma of the spine, the median survival rate was ten months.[29] All patients presented with pain and 70 per cent with neurologic complaints or physical dysfunction. Treatment spanned the spectrum from laminectomy to laminectomy, plus radiation, and a few patients had adjunctive chemotherapy.[29]

Other primary tumors of marrow origin are non-Hodgkin's lymphoma and leukemia, and Ewing's sarcoma.[30] The latter is a malignant round cell tumor of bone with an extremely poor prognosis. It must be considered when spinal osteolysis and destruction is encountered in the pediatric group.[31, 32]

Metastatic skeletal lesions in the pediatric age group have been analyzed, and while skeletal metastasis from primary bone tumors is more common, symptoms derived from skeletal embarrassment of extraosseous origin tumors may be the initial symptom of occult neoplasm.[33] Observers have noted the paradox that metastases to bone are more common in young children.[33] The manifestations of tumor biology may cover the spectrum of malevolent consequences: restriction of use of involved segments, soft tissue masses, pathologic fracture, and neurologic catastrophe.[33] The most common pathologic fracture was vertebral compression, and of these, 50 per cent presented with cord compression. Leeson and Makley revealed that all possibilities of bony abnormality may be encountered, and frequently the clinician's conceptual framework and clinical history are the cornerstones to accurate assessment. Since 79 per cent of patients exhibited spinal metastasis in the Leeson and Makley series, spinal pain clearly mandates careful evaluation and at least consideration of malignant possibility.[33] Neuroblastoma was by far the most common tumor, producing skeletal metastases with an average of three bones involved, with the spine entangled in 81 per cent.[33] There are no pathognomonic radiographic findings. Other potential sources are rhabdomyosarcoma (the most common pediatric soft tissue malignancy), Wilms' tumor, retinoblastoma, and medulloblastoma. Survival time for tumors presenting with pathologic fractures is poor.[33]

References

Bone Tumors

1. Gilday, D. L., Ash, J. M., and Reilly, B.: Radionuclide skeletal survey for pediatric neoplasms. Radiology *123:*399–406, 1977.
2. Enneking, W. F.: A system for staging musculoskeletal neoplasms. Clin. Orthop. *204:*9–24, 1986.
3. Pettise, K., Klassen, R.: Osteoid-osteoma and osteoblastoma of the spine. J. Bone Joint Surg. *68A:*354–361, 1986.
4. Swee, R. G., McLeod, R. A., Beabout, J. W.: Osteoid osteoma. Detection, diagnosis and localization. Radiology *130:*117–123, 1979.
5. Ransford, A. O., Pozo, J. L., Hutton, A. N., et al.: The behavior problem of the scoliosis associated with osteoid osteoma or osteoblastoma of the spine. J. Bone Joint Surg. *66B:*16–20, 1984.
6. Myles, S. T., and McCrae, M. E.: Benign osteoblastoma of the spine in childhood. J. Neurosurg. *68:*884–888, 1988.
7. Kirwan, E., Huton, P. A., Pozo, J. L, et al.: Osteoid osteoma and benign osteoblastoma of the spine. J. Bone Joint Surg. *66B:*20–26, 1984.
8. Azouz, E. M., Kozlowski, K., and Marton, D.: Osteoid osteoma and osteoblastoma of the spine in children. Pediatr. Radiol. *16:*25–31, 1986.
9. Healey, J. M., and Ghelman, B.: Osteoid osteoma and osteoblastoma. Clin. Orthop. *204:*76–86, 1986.
10. Haibach, M., Farrell, C., and Gaines, R. W.: Osteoid osteoma of the spine: surgically correctable cause of painful scoliosis. Can. Med. Assoc. J. *135:*895–898, 1986.
11. Preston, P. G.: Case of the month. A painful scoliosis. Br. J. Radiol. *59:*1233–1235, 1986.
12. MacKenzie, W. G., and Morton, K. S.: Eosinophilic granuloma of bone. Can. J. Surg. *31:*264–267, 1988.
13. Hensinger, R. M.: Back pain in children. *In* Bradford, D. S., and Hensinger, R. M. (eds.): The Pediatric spine. New York, Thieme, 1985, pp. 41–60.
14. Crone-Muzebrock, W., and Brassow, F.: A comparison of radiographic and bone scan findings in histiocytosis X. Skeletal Radiol. *9:*170–173, 1983.
15. Capama, R., Albisinni, V., and Picci, P.: Aneurysmal bone cyst of the spine. J. Bone Joint Surg. *67B:*527–531, 185.
16. Lifeso, R. M., and Younge, D.: Aneurysmal bone cysts of the spine. Int. Orthop. *8:*281–285, 1985.
17. Kunar, R., Guinto, F., and Madewell, J. E.: Expansile bone lesions of the vertebra. Radiographics *8:*749–769, 1988.
18. Morton, K. S.: Aneurysmal bone cyst: A review of 26 cases. Can. J. Surg. *29:*110–115, 1986.
19. Cole, W. G.: Treatment of aneurysmal bone cysts in childhood. J. Pediatr. Orthop. *6:*326–329, 1986.
20. Daffner, R. H., Linetsky, L., and Zabkar, J. H.: Case report 433: aneurysmal bone cyst of TB. Skeletal Radiol. *16:*428–432, 1989.
21. Worlock, P., and Clifford, P.: Aneurysmal bone cyst of the sacrum. J. R. Coll. Surg. Edinb. *30:*196–199, 1985.
22. Nicastro, J. F., and Leatherman, K. D.: Two-stage resection and spinal stabilization for aneurysmal bone cyst. Clin. Orthop. *180:*173–178, 1983.
23. Schaffer, L., Kranzler, L. I., and Sigueira, E. B.: Aneurysmal bone cyst of the spine. A case report. Spine *10:*389–393, 1985.
24. Walker, D. R., Rankin, R. N., and Anderson, C.: Giant-cell tumor of the sacrum in a child. Can. J. Surg. *31:*47–49, 1988.
25. Savini, R., Gherlinzoni, F., Morandi, M., et al.: Surgical treatment of giant-cell tumor of the spine. J. Bone Joint Surg. *65A:*1283–1289, 1983.
26. Dahlin, D. C.: Caldwell lecture. Giant cell tumor of bone: highlights of 407 cases. A.J.R. *144:*955–960, 1985.

27. Sung. M. W., Shu, W. P., and Wang, H. M.: Surgical treatment of primary tumors of the sacrum. Clin. Orthop. *215*:91–98, 1987.
28. Savani, R., Giunti, A., and Boriani, S.: Benign and malignant spinal tumors. *In* Bradford, D. S., and Hensinger, R. M. (eds.): The Pediatric Spine. New York, Thieme, 1985, pp. 131–154.
29. Shives, T. C., Dahlin, D. C., Sim, F. H., et al.: Osteosarcoma of the spine. J. Bone Joint Surg. *68A*:660–668, 1986.
30. Variend, S.: Small cell tumors in childhood: A review. J. Pathol. *145*:1–25, 1985.
31. Wilkins, R. M., Pritchard, D. J., and Burgert, E. M.: Ewing's sarcoma of bone. Cancer *58*:2551–2555, 1986.
32. Meyers, P. A.: Malignant bone tumors in children: Ewing's sarcoma. Hematol. Oncol. Clin. North Am. *1*:667–673, 1982.
33. Leeson, M. C., Makley, J. T., and Carter, J. R.: Metastatic skeletal disease in the pediatric population. J. Pediatr. Orthop. *5*:261–267, 1985.

SPINAL CORD TUMORS

How do spinal cord tumors present? One would naturally suspect that the sequelae of intraspinal tumor would be neurologic deficit. But is this true, especially early in the process?

Ker and Jones' review of 32 primary tumors of the cauda equina catalogued the complaints: low back pain (31 per cent), back pain and sciatica (34 per cent), sudden onset of pain (20 per cent), night pain (25 per cent), no neurologic abnormalities (66 per cent), and intermittent pain (30 per cent).[1] "The average delay in diagnosis was 39 months," instigating the quote attributed to Allen: "the stage of onset is the stage of errors."[1]

Seljeskog expressed it this way: "All too frequently the child presents with signs and symptoms that are non-neurologic."[2] He enumerated the historical factors: pain, change in functional abilities (walking, running, regression in toilet training), and back stiffness.[2] He specified the physical attributes: motor weakness, spinal deformity, reflex changes, muscle atrophy, and midline defects (cutaneous changes such as lipoma, dermal sinus, hair patch, and angioma).[2]

Hydrocephalus or increased intracranial pressure may be a result of CSF tumor seeding, and conversely an intraspinal tumor may point suspicion toward the head.[2]

Epstein and Wisoff, discussing intramedullary tumors of the spinal cord, emphasized the variability of clinical symptoms: the sway of improvement and deterioration and the onset of symptoms in occasional cases with minor trauma, presumably to the compromise of "peritumoral edema."[3] The salient point is that intraspinal tumors are not necessarily linear and progressive but may wax and wane, and thus intermittency cannot be used to exclude their presence. Gait disturbance is the communal deployment of spinal cord dysfunction ("late walker," refusal to walk, altered stride), and perhaps the subtle emergence of weakness.[3] Spinal pain is present in 70 per cent, radicular pain in 10 per cent, and dysesthesias in 10 per cent; bladder dysfunction is rare.

Kumar and associates described three patients who illustrate the complexity of diagnosis of intraspinal tumors.[4] In all three the symptoms were referable to the hip, and radiographic changes consistent with hip pathology were identified. All three patients exhibited concomitant scoliosis, leading to the suggestion that in patients with uncommon hip disorders and associated postural deformities (torticollis, scoliosis), intraspinal tumor should be considered.

Abdominal pain has been associated with intraspinal tumor.[5]

Intramedullary Tumors. The most common tumors are astrocytoma and ependymoma (Fig. 9–7). Syringomyelia and hydromyelia are in the differential diagnosis, but syringomyelia usually has an earlier associated event, and hydromyelia is associated with posterior fossa abnormalities.[2]

Astrocytoma of the spinal cord presented with pain (62.5 per cent), gait disturbance (43.7 per cent), numbness (18.8 per cent), and sphincter dysfunction (18.8 per cent).[6] Neurologic findings were a Babinski response (50 per cent), posterior column dysfunction (40 per cent), and paraparesis (37.5 per cent). Postlaminectomy spinal deformity was viewed as a significant residual of treatment, and the necessity of close observation for deformity progression was emphasized.[6] The distribution of the astrocytoma may be from "the cervicomedullary junction to the conus medullaris" or may exist more focally, spanning fewer spinal segments.[3] MRI is excellent and gadolinium-enhanced MRI may prove even more definitive; 24-hour delayed CT scans are sometimes necessary for tumor definition.[3]

Ependymoma of the spinal cord and cauda equina has been extensively reviewed by Vijavakumar and colleagues. An interesting point is that although treatment failures are

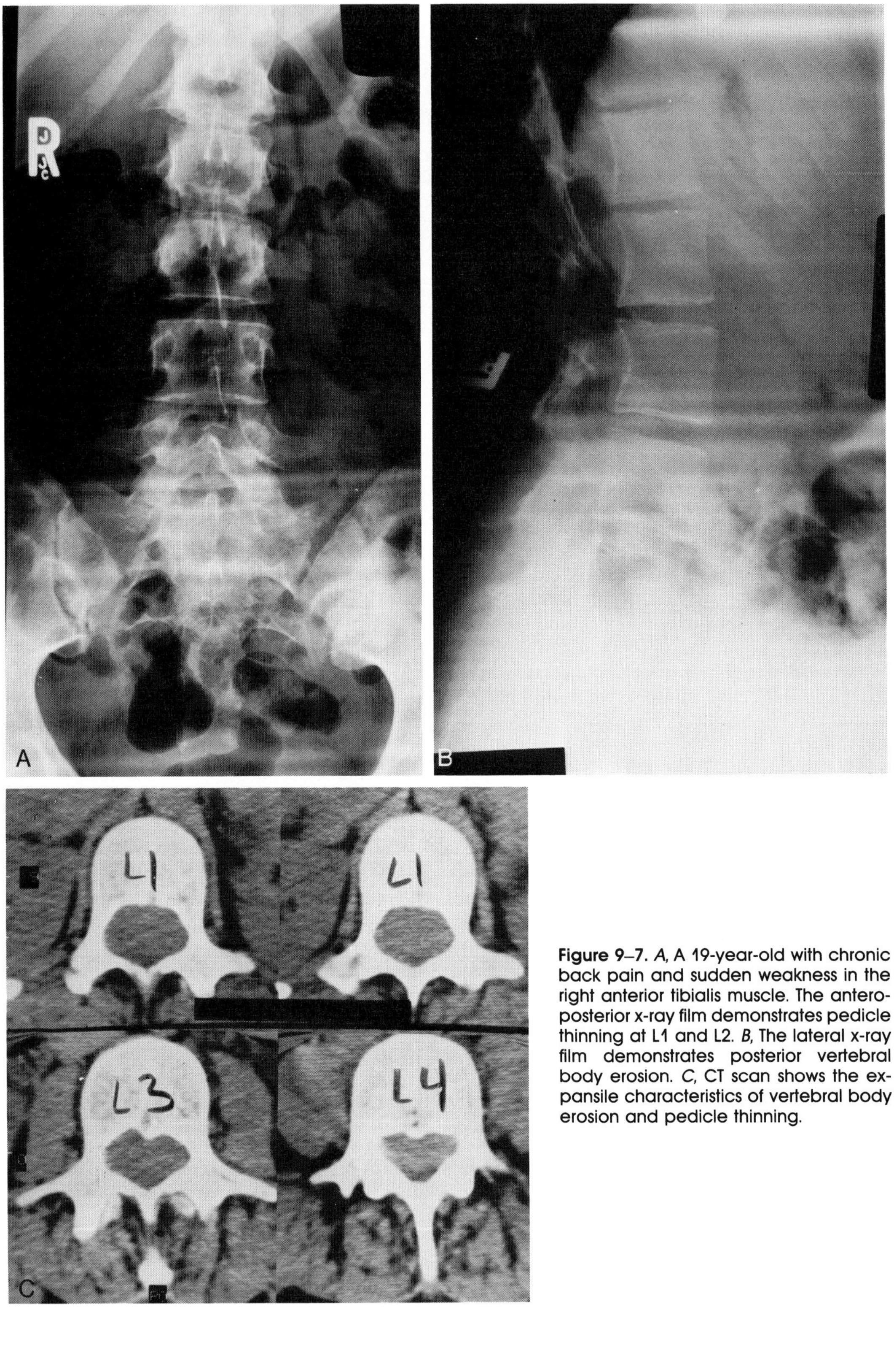

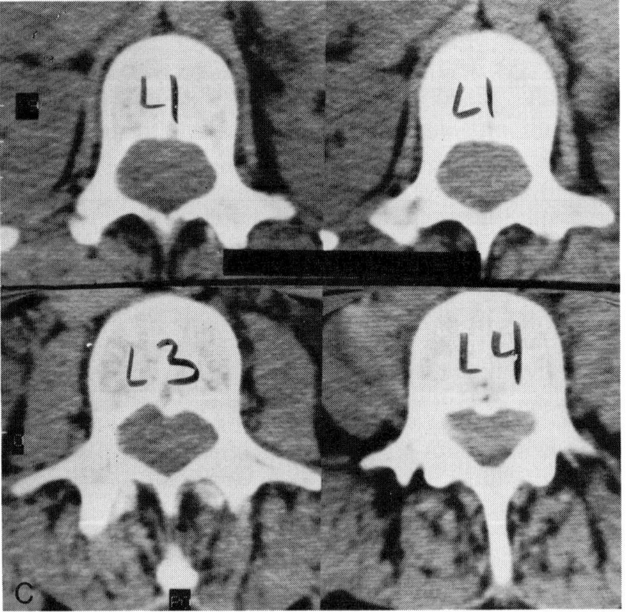

Figure 9–7. *A*, A 19-year-old with chronic back pain and sudden weakness in the right anterior tibialis muscle. The anteroposterior x-ray film demonstrates pedicle thinning at L1 and L2. *B*, The lateral x-ray film demonstrates posterior vertebral body erosion. *C*, CT scan shows the expansile characteristics of vertebral body erosion and pedicle thinning.

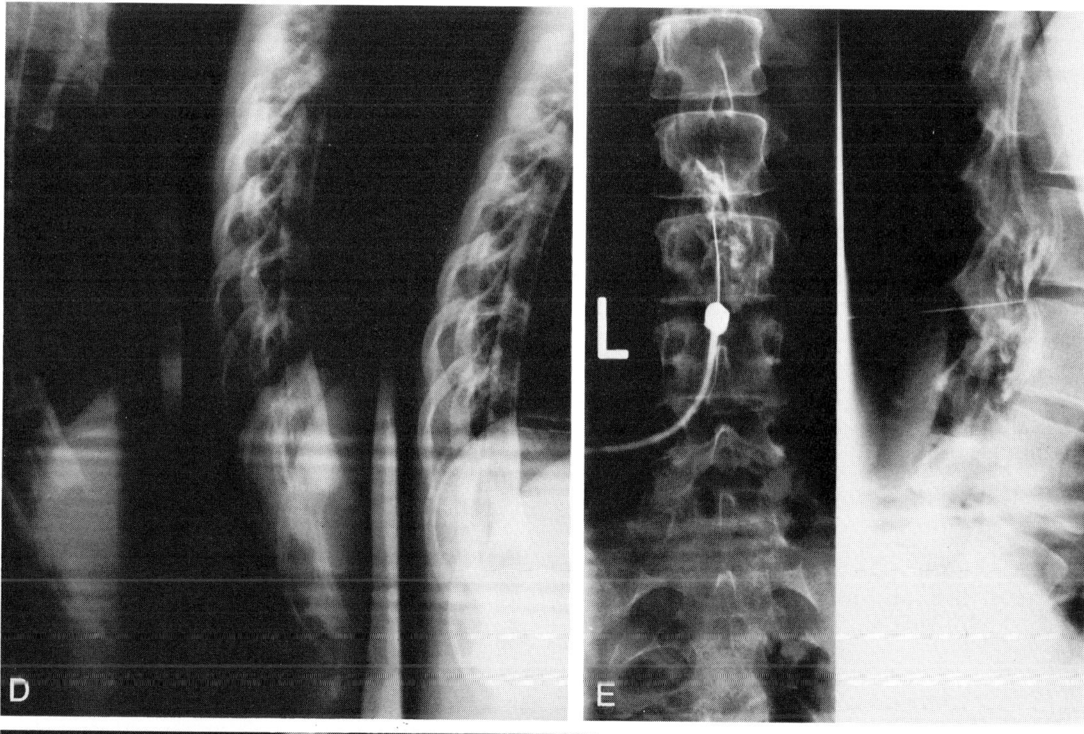

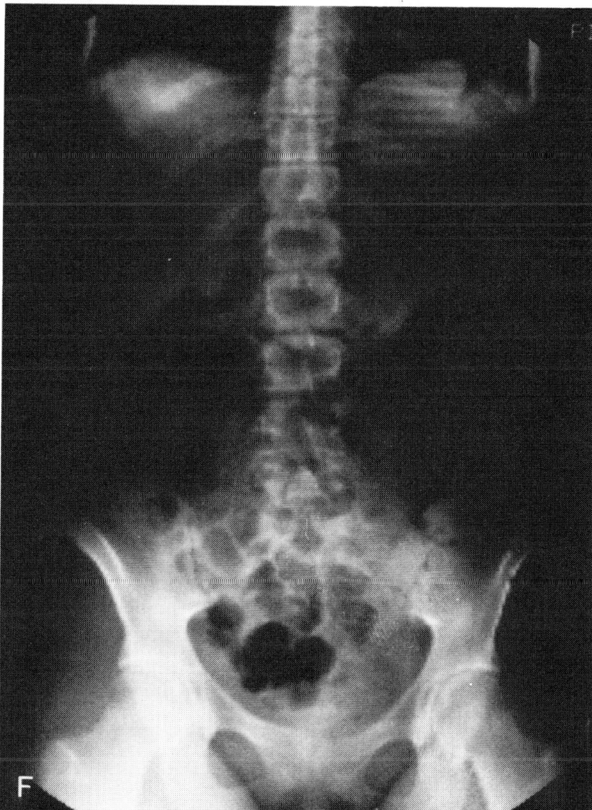

Figure 9–7 *Continued D*, Anteroposterior and lateral myelograms show ependymoma. *E*, The lateral myelogram shows complete block at the thoracolumbar junction with dye introduced via a C1–C2 puncture. *F*, Scout CT scan shows a block at the T12–L1 level.

presumably local recurrences of ependymoma of the cauda equina, metastases have been reported, and the risk of dissemination within the CNS is stated at approximately 7 per cent. The ependymoma is most commonly located at the caudal area.[7]

Other intraspinal tumors have been recognized as lesions such as intramedullary lipomas.

Intradural Extramedullary Tumors. Developmental tumors are frequently in the lumbar spine and may demonstrate radiologic bony anomalies (spina bifida occulta) or cutaneous midline changes; examples include epidermoid and dermoid tumors, lipoma, and teratoma.[2] Many of these tumors ultimately represent the common development of spinal cord tethering, which is probably the risk of neurologic progression.[8]

Nerve sheath tumors such as the neurofibromas and neuronomas, schwannomas, and neurofibromas are rarer in the pediatric group, as is spinal meningioma.[2] When present, nerve sheath tumors and meningiomas occurred between the ages of 10 and 15 years and the common complaint was pain.[3] Multiple neurofibromatosis is associated with incidence in adolescence.[3]

CSF Metastasis. Medulloblastoma and ependymoma of intracranial origin may metastasize to involve spinal cord neurologic structures, the so-called "drop metastases." This seeding may expand the cord via attached tumor or adhere to the cauda equina.[9] Water-soluble myelography was used to demonstrate the metastases in one series.[9] Perhaps contrast-enhanced MRI may be fruitful in this area? There is a case report of spinal intramedullary spread of medulloblastoma diagnosed via MRI.[10]

Spinal Cord Disease in Systemic Cancer. In children with known systemic cancer, complaints referable to the spine or neurologic symptoms should be investigated. In one series the average delay was two weeks from symptom onset to diagnosis.[11] The initial signs and symptoms were back pain (80 per cent), weakness (67 per cent), sphincter dysfunction (57 per cent), and sensory abnormality (14 per cent) and the accuracy of diagnostic modalities for cord compression was myelography 100 per cent, bone scan 54 per cent, plain x-ray 35 per cent, CT 100 per cent, and MRI 100 per cent. "Other nonmetastatic etiologies that must be considered included infectious or radiation-related transverse myelopathy, spinal cord stroke, intradural or extradural hematoma and extradural abscess."[11]

References

Spinal Cord Tumors

1. Ker, N. B., and Jones, C. B.: Tumors of the cauda equina. The problem of differential diagnosis. J. Bone Joint Surg. *67B:*358–362, 1985.
2. Seljeskog, E. L.: Pediatric intraspinal tumors. *In* Bradford, D. S., and Hensinger, R. M. (eds.): The Pediatric Spine. New York, Thieme, 1985, pp. 155–166.
3. Epstein, F. J., and Wisoff, J. H.: Intramedullary tumors of the spinal cord. *In* McLaurin, R. L., Schut, L., Venes, J. L., and Epstein, F. (eds.): Pediatric Neurosurgery. Surgery of the Developing Nervous System. 2nd ed. Philadelphia, W. B. Saunders Co., 1989, pp. 428–442.
4. Kumar, S. J., Marks, H. G., Ghiragossian, J. D., et al.: Intraspinal tumors in children presenting primarily with hip symptoms: a report of three cases. J. Pediatr. Orthop. *8:*529–531, 1988.
5. Eeg-Olofsson, O., Carlsson, E., and Jeppsson, S.: Recurrent abdominal pains as the first symptom of a spinal cord tumor. Acta Paediatr. Scand. *70:*595–597, 1981.
6. Reimer, R., and Onofrio, B. M.: Astrocytomas of the spinal cord in children and adolescents. J. Neurosurg. *63:*669–675, 1985.
7. Vijavakumar, S., Estes, M., Hardy, R., et al.: Ependymoma of the spinal cord and cauda equina: a review. Clev. Clin. Med. *55:*163–170, 1988.
8. Pierre-Kahn, A., Lacombe, J., Pichon, J., et al.: Intraspinal lipomas with spina bifida. J. Neurosurg. *65:*756–761, 1986.
9. Stanley, P., Senac, M., and Segall, M. D.: Intraspinal seeding from intracranial tumors in children. A. J. R. *144:*157–161, 1985.
10. Barnwell, S. L., and Edwards, M. S.: Spinal intramedullary spread of medulloblastoma. J. Neurosurg. *65:*253–255, 1986.
11. Lewis, D. W., Packer, R. J., Raney, B., et al.: Incidence, presentation and outcome of spinal cord disease in children with systemic cancer. Pediatrics *78:*438–443, 1986.

CHILDHOOD ARTHRITIS

Chronic arthritis of childhood is noted in a variety of groups: "systemic-onset disease (20 per cent), rheumatoid factor–negative polyarthritis (25 per cent), rheumatoid factor–positive polyarthritis (5 per cent), pauciarthritis associated with antinuclear antibodies and chronic iridocyclitis (30–35 per cent), and pauciarthritis associated with sacroilitis and HLA-B27 (10–15 per cent)."[1]

Table 9–7. Conditions That Can Mimic JRA

Infectious Diseases
Septic arthritis
Osteomyelitis
Virus-related arthritis
Childhood Malignancies
Leukemia
Neuroblastoma
Others
Noninflammatory Conditions of Bones and Joints
Limb pains ("growing pains")
Psychogenic rheumatism
Musculoskeletal trauma
Miscellaneous orthopedic conditions (slipped capital femoral epiphysis, Osgood-Schlatter disease, chondromalacia patellae, discitis, Scheuermann's disease, avascular necrosis, etc.)
Genetic and congenital syndromes
Rheumatic Diseases
Systemic lupus erythematosus
Rheumatic fever
Dermatomyositis
Vasculitis syndromes
Scleroderma
Mixed connective tissue disease

The differential diagnoses cover broad categories, but particular attention needs to be paid to infectious and neoplastic conditions. Since there are no pathognomonic tests for childhood arthritis, part of the establishment of the diagnosis is the exclusion of other possibilities.[1]

The spectrum of changes encountered in the lumbar spine associated with childhood arthritis include the ravages of spondylitis, apophyseal joint ankylosis, scoliosis, and compression fractures.[2] Patients with arthritis and scoliosis may complain of back stiffness and pain. Differential growth may be a factor in scoliosis. Some suggest that scoliosis is present in 15 to 20 per cent, with the overall incidence of thoracic and lumbar occurrence 5 per cent in childhood arthritis.[2]

In juvenile ankylosing spondylitis most present with peripheral joint involvement rather than spinal complaints.[3] Only 25 per cent have demonstrated sacroiliac joint changes within one year of peripheral joint involvement.[3]

Schaller stressed the importance of excluding "the potentially treatable diseases such as septic arthritis, osteomyelitis or malignancy."[4] Consequently, peripheral blood smears, joint aspirate Gram stain, culture, cell count, and bone scan need to be considered. Sedimentation rates, HLA-B27, rheumatoid factor, antinuclear antibody, and urinalysis may be adjunctive tests.[4] Careful scrutiny of the x-rays may reveal other conditions mimicking arthritis.

Clearly, in a child with back pain, a history of other joint involvement should be sought.

An important diagnostic dilemma is posed by the sacroiliac joint. Symptoms originating from this joint may be due not only to trauma but to infection and arthritis. Physical findings associated with sepsis sacroiliac joint involvement include local tenderness, iliac wing compression resulting in symptoms, Gaenslen's test, Fabere test, SLR test, and inability to stand on the ipsilateral leg. Since the symptoms of sacroiliac joint involvement have a wide range of presentation, clinical suspicion is an important factor in its discovery.

The bone scan may not always be positive and should be supplemented with tests of sedimentation and pelvic x-rays. Aspiration of the joint is important in sacroiliac joint infection, as well as CT to demonstrate any contiguous abscess.[5] Ankylosing spondylitis and Type II pauciarticular chronic juvenile rheumatoid arthritis may involve the sacroiliac joint.[5]

References

Childhood Arthritis

1. Schaller, J. G.: Chronic arthritis in children. Juvenile rheumatoid arthritis. Clin. Orthop. *182:*79–89, 1984.
2. Jones, E. T.: Involvement in childhood arthritis. *In* Bradford, D. S., and Hensinger, R. M. (eds.): New York, Thieme, 1985, pp. 80–87.
3. Calabro, J. J.: Clinical aspects of juvenile and adult ankylosing spondylitis. J. Rheumatol. *22*(Suppl 2):104–109, 1983.
4. Schaller, J. G.: Arthritis in children. Pediatr. Clin. North Am. 1565–1580, 1986.
5. Reilly, J. P., Gross, R. H., and Emans, J. B.: Disorders of the sacroiliac joint in children. J. Bone Joint Surg. *70A:*31–40, 1988.

MISCELLANEOUS CONDITIONS

It is not possible to catalog every clinical possibility in pediatric back pain, and many etiologies may not fit into specific groupings.

Extraspinal disease has been alluded to. Before relegating the occult source of patient complaint to the trash heap of psychogenic factors, we must consider whether our perspective has been too narrow. Disease exists outside the confines of our specialties, and it is entirely possible that viscerogenic etiologies may indeed be the culprit. The unusual does occur. We do not need to define it more precisely, only to consider its possibility. We practice at a specific point in time. Perhaps the diagnosis has not been contemplated. Perhaps the disease process is too immature to permit detection. Perhaps our devices are too insensitive to recognize. Although the incidence and probability of disease are our guideposts, there are always those singular moments when the clinical assumes the cloak of a Sherlock Holmes, and doggedly pursues to a satisfactory conclusion "the brilliant diagnosis."

Intervertebral disc calcification in chlidren is usually found in the cervical rather than the lumbar spine, can be associated with systemic inflammation (fever, increased sedimentation rate, increased white blood cell count), may be symptomatic (pain and stiffness), and may be associated with herniation. Most children are treated expectantly. The cause is unknown.[1-3]

Symptomatic congenital spinal stenosis, in the absence of achondroplasia, is rarely demonstrated clinically below the age of 20.[4] The variability of presentation depends on the most symptomatic levels of structure (local versus global). Achondroplasia may be associated with decreased interpediculate distance, thickened and reduced pedicles and inferior facets, diminished anteroposterior diameter, and decreased cross-sectional and nerve root canal areas.[6] These factors may conspire to produce nerve root compression, transverse myelopathy (acute or chronic), or intermittent claudication.[6] Eisenstein stated that congential stenosis existed if "anteroposterior diameter was less than 15 mm and transverse diameter less than 20 mm."[7, 8] Symptoms may include leg pain on walking and standing, numbness, weakness in the lower extremities, and sphincter dysfunction. Achondroplasia may produce kyphosis at the thoracolumbar junction and neurologic sequelae.[6]

A rare form of osteoporosis occurring in the prepubertal child with no associated identifiable genetic predisposition may be responsible for kyphosis, and compression fractures and has been reported in association with scoliosis.[9, 10] The condition is self-limiting, although residual deformity may not resolve.[9, 10] It should be differentiated from osteogenesis imperfecta.[9]

Back pain has been reported, with a high incidence in cystic fibrosis, independent of thoracic kyphosis, but related to postural abnormalities or vertebral wedging.[11, 12]

Storage diseases may weaken the bone and predispose to pathologic fracture as in Gaucher's disease.[13] The vertebrae may be osteopenic and depict vertebral body "beaking."[14]

Bone infarction from sickle cell disease may cause back pain and can be differentiated from osteomyelitis by Tc-99m MDP bone scanning followed by Ga 67 citrate scintigraphy in doubtful cases.[15]

Tuberculosis does exist. It may cause significant deformity (kyphosis) and subsequent neurologic sequelae if unrecognized. Skin tests, sedimentation rate tests, and careful radiologic scrutiny may reveal "haziness and loss of trabecular pattern in the vertebral body, and there is an adjacent fusiform paravertebral shadow."[16] Antitubercular medicines, bracing, and possibly surgery are the clinical mainstays of treatment.

References

Miscellaneous Conditions

1. Sonnabend, D. H., Taylor, T. K. F., and Chapman, G. K.: Intervertebral disc calcification syndromes in children. J. Bone Joint Surg. *64B:*25–31, 1982.
2. McGregor, J. C., and Butler, P.: Disc calcification in childhood: computed tomographic and magnetic resonance imaging appearances. Br. J. Radiol. *59:*180–182, 1986.
3. Hatfield, K. D.: Disc calcification in childhood—a case report with CT findings. Australas. Radiol. *31:*397–399, 1987.
4. Dauser, R. C., and Chandler, W. F.: Symptomatic congenital spinal stenosis in a child. Neurosurgery *11:*61–63, 1982.
5. Dharker, S. R., Raman, P. T., Mathai, K. V., et al.: Congenital stenosis of the lumbar canal. Neurology India *26:*1–6, 1978.
6. Holder, J. C., FitzRandolph, R. L., and Flanigan, S.: The spectrum of spinal stenosis. Curr. Probl. Diagn. Radiol. *14:*1–33, 1985.
7. Eisenstein, S.: The morphometry and pathological anatomy of the lumbar spine in South African Negroes and Caucasoids with special reference to spinal stenosis. J. Bone Joint Surg. *59B:*173, 1977.
8. Eisenstein, S.: Measurements of the lumbar spinal canal in two racial groups. Clin. Orthop. *115:*42, 1976.
9. Jones, E. T., and Hensinger, R. M.: Spinal deformity in idiopathic juvenile osteoporosis. Spine *6:*1–4, 1981.

10. Bartal, E., and Gage, J. R.: Idiopathic juvenile osteoporosis and scoliosis. J. Pediatr. Orthop. *2:*295–298, 1982.
11. Rose, J., Gamble, J., Schultz, A., et al.: Back pain and spinal deformity in cystic fibrosis. Am. J. Dis. Child. *141:*1313–1316, 1987.
12. Denton, J. R., Tietjen, R., and Gaerlan, P. F.: Thoracic kyphosis in cystic fibrosis. Clin. Orthop. *155:*71–74, 1981.
13. Katz, K., Cohen, I. J., Ziv, N., et al.: Fractures in children who have Gaucher disease. J. Bone Joint Surg. *69A:*1361–1370, 1987.
14. Stowens, D. W., Teitelbaum, S. L., Kahn, A. J., et al.: Skeletal complications of Gaucher's disease. Medicine *64:*310–322, 1985.
15. Koren, A., Garty, I., and Katzuni, E.: Bone infarction in children with sickle cell disease: early diagnosis and differentiation from osteomyelitis. Eur. J. Pediatr. *142:*93–97, 1984.
16. Hensinger, R. M.: Back pain in children. *In* Bradford, D. S., and Hensinger, R. M. (eds.): The Pediatric Spine. New York, Thieme, 1985, pp. 41–60.

CONCLUSION

The evils are several. On the one hand, the clinician must decide when testing is appropriate and what period is reasonable for observation or nonspecific treatment. We have sought to emphasize the interval between onset of symptoms and the final diagnosis in specific causes of pediatric back pain. This represents observation, not criticism. The individual patient is a challenge, and although we cannot, in blanket fashion, test everybody, our threshold for discovery must be lower for the child than for the adult—the incidence of pathologies is different. There is a plethora of pathology, but as Sherlock Holmes demonstrated, knowledge and observation form the rational basis for discovery.

CHAPTER

10

CONGENITAL ANOMALIES OF THE CERVICAL SPINE

Robert N. Hensinger, M.D.

Congenital anomalies of the cervical spine occur infrequently and receive little attention when pathologic conditions of the spine are considered. However, these spinal abnormalities have great impact on afflicted individuals, and physicians who deal with problems of the spine should be familiar with their diagnosis and management. These structural defects originate early in fetal development, and when discovered in childhood appear to be static and unchanging. This appearance is deceptive, as with further growth many may prove to be capable of dramatic change and progressive deformity, and may be life-threatening, particularly in the cervical spine. Many anomalies are not discovered until a complication occurs. Anomalies of the occipitocervical junction often remain undetected until late childhood or adolescence, and some remain hidden well into adult life.

Other anomalies of the spine, although recognized in early life, may not become clinically significant until adulthood. During the growing years, a delicate balance is struck between the congenitally distorted bony elements of the vertebral column and the neurologic elements. Later, in adult life, factors such as aging or intercurrent trauma may alter this relationship. The patient with an os odontoideum may gradually develop laxity of the supporting structures after countless flexion-extension movements of the neck or, after a seemingly trivial injury, may develop serious instability of the atlantoaxial joint and spinal cord compression. Those afflicted with the Klippel-Feil syndrome may gradually develop symptoms of degenerative arthritis at the hypermobile articulations adjacent to the cervical synostosis.

Diagnosis and assessment of these congenital spinal conditions are hampered by the difficulties encountered during roentgenographic evaluation. In the normal child, the pattern of vertebral growth and ossification has wide variation and often is not complete until late in the second decade. Fixed bony deformities often prevent proper positioning for standard views. Nonstandard views and oblique projections add to diagnostic confusion and hinder complete assessment of the patient. Laminagraphy, cineradiography, myelography, and arteriography are helpful at times in the evaluation of these conditions and should be available to the physician engaged in treating the more complex problems.

This chapter is especially concerned with the treatment of these spinal anomalies. Too often a policy of observation is adopted, whereas more vigorous management could control, ameliorate, and even on occasion correct the deformity. Sufficient information is available about the natural history of these anomalies, and attention must now be directed to the results of treatment. Operative stabilization of the patient with chronic atlantoaxial instability may prevent a neurologic disaster.

Physicians who treat these children must be concerned with their total care. It is tempting to focus attention on the problems of the spine to the exclusion of all others, but it is imperative to be aware of the high incidence of associated anomalies with vertebral malformations. Recognition of a vertebral abnormality should stimulate a thorough and intensive search for associated anomalies. Poor management of these related problems, particularly urinary complications, may nullify a well planned and executed orthopedic program. Particular emphasis is placed on related anomalies of the central nervous system (CNS), which may be subtle in their manifestation yet have great impact on the patient's social and educational adjustment to life. A hearing deficit may be unrecognized until well into the school years. Mirror motions of the upper extremities may limit effective two-handed activity, such as playing a piano or climbing a ladder. These and other learning disabilities can be an important part of the condition and yet may not be appreciated by the physician, teacher, or parent. Early recognition and appropriate treatment of these problems can substantially contribute to the general well-being of the child.

BASILAR IMPRESSION

Basilar impression (or invagination) is a deformity of the bones of the base of the skull at the margin of the foramen magnum. The floor of the skull appears to be indented by the upper cervical spine, and therefore the tip of the odontoid is more cephalad, sometimes protruding into the opening of the foramen magnum, and it may encroach upon the brain stem. This increases the risk of neurologic damage from injury, circulatory embarrassment, or impairment of cerebrospinal fluid (CSF) flow. Chamberlain in 1939[3] first called attention to the clinical significance of this anomaly with this vivid description:

The changes shown by the roentgenogram give the impression of softening of the base of the skull and moulding through the force of gravity. It is as though the weight of the head has caused the ears to approach the shoulders, while the cervical spine, refusing to be shortened, has pushed the floor of the posterior fossa upward into the brain space.

The terms "platybasia" and "basilar impression" are often used as synonyms but are not related anatomically or pathologically. Platybasia has no clinical significance; it is merely an anthropologic term used to denote flattening of the angle formed by the intersection of the plane of the anterior fossa with the plane of the clivus. Basilar impression, which is invagination in the region of the foramen magnum, does have clinical significance. Patients with symptomatic basilar impression are seldom found to have an associated platybasia.

There are two types of basilar impression: (1) primary, a congenital abnormality often associated with other vertebral defects such as atlanto-occipital fusion, hypoplasia of the atlas, bifid posterior arch of the atlas, odontoid abnormalities, and Klippel-Feil syndrome; and (2) secondary, a developmental condition usually attributed to softening of the osseous structures at the base of the skull, with the deformity developing later in life. This is occasionally seen in conditions such as osteomalacia, rickets, Paget's disease,[5] osteogenesis imperfecta, renal osteodystrophy, rheumatoid arthritis, neurofibromatosis, and ankylosing spondylitis.

Roentgenographic Features

Basilar impression is difficult to assess roentgenographically, and many measurement schemes have been proposed. Those most commonly referred to are Chamberlain's,[3] McGregor's,[12] and McRae's lines in the lateral roentgenogram (Fig. 10–1), and in the anteroposterior projection, Fischgold-Metzger's line. Chamberlain's line[3] (a line drawn from the dorsal marginal hard palate to the posterior lip of the foramen magnum) is seldom used because the posterior lip of the foramen magnum (opisthion) is difficult to define on a standard roentgenogram (Fig. 10–2*A*) and is often itself invaginated in basilar impressions. McGregor's[12] (a line drawn from the upper surface of the posterior edge of the hard palate to the most caudal point of the occipital curve of the skull) is easier to identify (Figs. 10–1, 10–2) and therefore preferable. The position of the tip of the odontoid is measured in relation to this baseline, and a distance of 4.5 mm above McGregor's line is considered to be on the extreme edge of normality.[12] However,

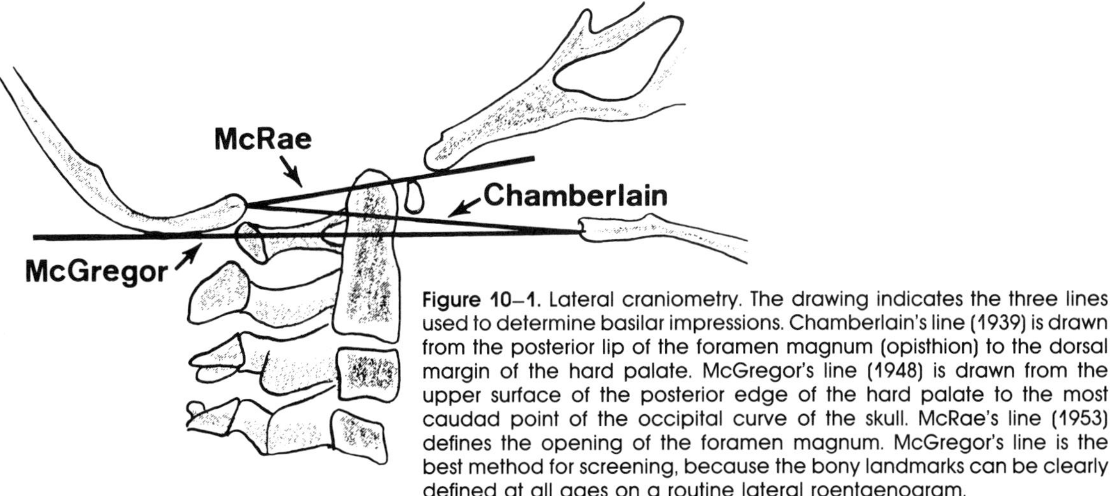

Figure 10–1. Lateral craniometry. The drawing indicates the three lines used to determine basilar impressions. Chamberlain's line (1939) is drawn from the posterior lip of the foramen magnum (opisthion) to the dorsal margin of the hard palate. McGregor's line (1948) is drawn from the upper surface of the posterior edge of the hard palate to the most caudad point of the occipital curve of the skull. McRae's line (1953) defines the opening of the foramen magnum. McGregor's line is the best method for screening, because the bony landmarks can be clearly defined at all ages on a routine lateral roentgenogram.

the study of normal variations by Hinck and associates[9] demonstrated a wide range of normality, as well as difference between males and females. McRae's line defines the opening of the foramen magnum and is derived from his observation that if the tip of the odontoid lies below the opening of the foramen magnum, the patient will probably be asymptomatic. McRae's line is an accurate guide in the clinical assessment of patients with basilar impression.

A criticism of the lateral lines (McGregor's and Chamberlain's) is that the hard palate is not actually a part of the skull and may be

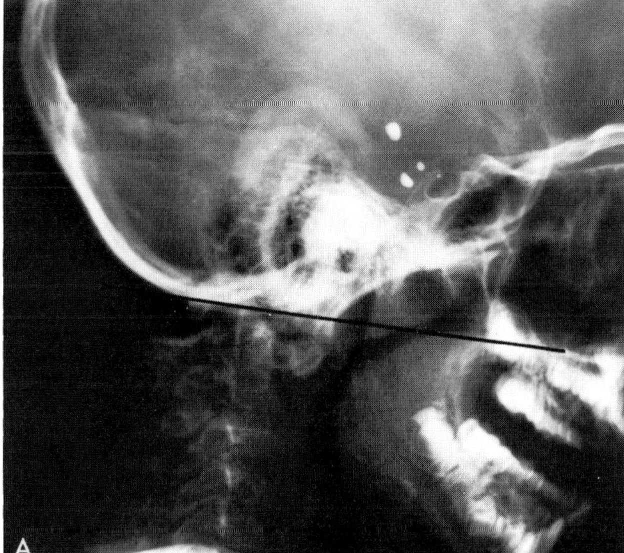

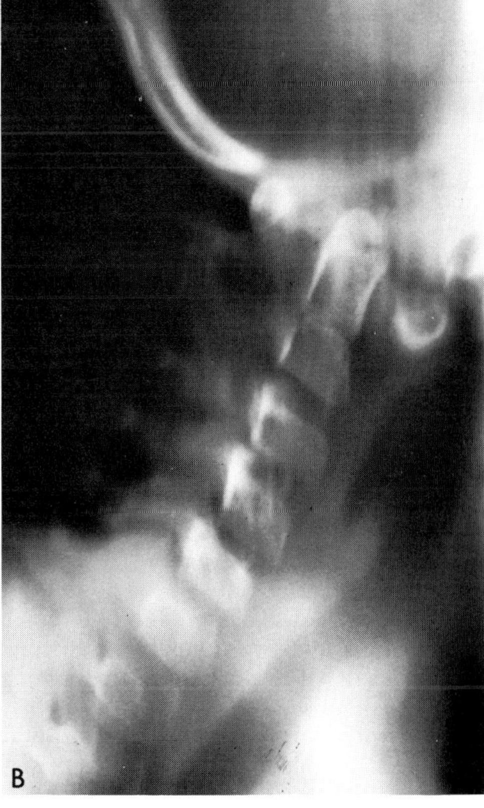

Figure 10–2. A 6-year-old female with a history of an unusual gait and a recent episode of unconsciousness after mild head trauma. *A*, Routine lateral roentgenogram suggests that the odontoid is displaced proximally into the opening of the foramen magnum. McGregor's line has been drawn from the most caudal portion of the occiput to the hard palate. The tip of the odontoid is more than 5 mm above this line, indicating basilar impression. *B*, Lateral laminagram demonstrates subluxation of C1 and C2 and that the tip of the odontoid is above the opening of the foramen magnum (McRae's line).

distorted by an abnormal facial configuration or a highly arched palate, quite independent of a craniovertebral anomaly. In addition, the patient may have an abnormally long or short odontoid or an abnormality of the axis or occipital facets, which can diminish the value of the measurements. With the development of computed tomographic (CT) reconstructions and magnetic resonance imaging (MRI), it is now possible to view the relationship at the occipitocervical junction in much greater detail.[10, 11] Reports indicate that these techniques are largely replacing the older tomography techniques, particularly the anteroposterior measurement of Fischgold and Metzger,[6] which was previously the most accurate method. However, the lateral reference lines are still important for screening.

In summary, McGregor's line is the best method for routine screening, because the landmarks can be clearly defined at all ages on a routine lateral roentgenogram. More detailed techniques (CT and MRI) are generally reserved for patients in whom the routine examination or clinical findings may suggest an occipitocervical anomaly.[10, 11] McRae's line is a helpful guide in assessing the clinical significance of basilar impression.

Clinical Features

Patients with basilar impression frequently have a deformity of the skull or neck (a short neck in 78 per cent, asymmetry of the face or skull or torticollis in 68 per cent.[4] These physical findings are often noted in patients without basilar impression (Klippel-Feil syndrome, occipitalization) and are not considered pathognomonic.

The symptoms (or lack of them) even in severe basilar impression are difficult to explain.[4] Basilar impression is frequently associated with anomalous neurologic conditions such as the Arnold-Chiari malformation[4] and syringomyelia, which can further cloud the clinical picture. Symptoms are generally due to crowding of the neural structures at the level of the foramen magnum, particularly the medulla oblongata. There is an unusually high incidence of basilar impression in northeast Brazil, and the work of De Barros and colleagues[4] has been helpful in delineating the symptoms and signs. Patients who were symptomatic with pure basilar impression had the dominant complaints of motor and sensory disturbances, and 85 per cent had weakness and paresthesia of the limbs. In contrast, patients who were symptomatic with pure Arnold-Chiari malformation were more likely to have cerebellar and vestibular disturbances (unsteadiness of gait, dizziness, and nystagmus). In both conditions, there may be impingement of the lower cranial nerves as they emerge from the medulla oblongata, particularly the trigeminal (V), glossopharyngeal (IX), vagus (X), and hypoglossal (XII).[4] Headache and pain in the nape of the neck, in the distribution of the greater occipital nerve, is a common finding.[4]

Posterior encroachment may cause blockage of the aqueduct of Silvius, and the presenting symptoms may be from increased intercranial pressure or hydrocephalus.[4, 12] Compression of the cerebellum with vestibular involvement or herniation of the cerebellar tonsils (the Arnold-Chiari malformation) is a frequent finding,[4] leading to vertical or lateral nystagmus in 65 per cent of cases. These symptoms may be due not to direct pressure from the posterior rim of the foramen magnum, but rather to a thickened band of dura not visible on plain roentgenograms; this has prompted several authors to recommend routine myelographic evaluation. If this situation is unrecognized, bony decompression alone (without opening the dura) will be unsuccessful in obtaining remission of symptoms or halting progression of the neurologic injury.[4]

There is a high incidence of vertebral artery anomalies in basilar impression, atlanto-occipital fusion, and absence of the C1 facet.[2] In addition, the vertebral arteries may be compressed as they pass through the crowded foramen magnum, causing symptoms suggestive of vertebral artery insufficiency such as dizziness, seizures, mental deterioration, and syncope.[2, 12] These symptoms may occur alone or in combination with those of spinal cord compression.[2, 4, 8, 12] Michie and Clark[13] and Bachs and associates[1] theorized that one explanation for the frequent association of syringomyelia or syringobulbia and basilar impression is that the vertebral arteries and the anterior spinal artery are compromised in the region of the foramen magnum, with subsequent degeneration of the spinal cord and medulla. Unfortunately, arteriographic studies are not available to confirm this interesting thesis. Children with occipitocervical anomalies may be more susceptible to vertebral artery injury and brain stem ischemia, particularly those who undergo skull traction for correction of scoliosis. Even moderate amounts of traction (less than 15 lbs) that normally would be well tolerated may compromise these abnormal vessels. Careful roentgenographic evaluation of the occipitocervical junction should precede any use of skull traction, even if only minimal traction forces are planned.

Although this condition is congenital, many patients do not develop symptoms until the second or third decade of life.[4] This may be due to a gradually increasing instability from ligamentous laxity caused by aging, similar to the delayed myelopathies reported after atlantoaxial dislocations or the increasing instability of C1 and C2 in patients with odontoid agenesis.[7] These persons often develop premature cervical osteoarthritis, as found in the family studies of Gunderson and colleagues.[8] Chamberlain[3] and others theorized that the young developing brain may be more tolerant to compressive effects, later proving deleterious to older tissues. Similarly, arteriosclerotic changes in the vertebral arteries may make these vessels more susceptible to minor constrictions. The symptoms frequently occur in older patients in whom a congenital anomaly would not ordinarily be considered. Patients with this malformation have been mistakenly diagnosed as having multiple sclerosis, posterior fossa tumors, amyotrophic lateral sclerosis, or traumatic injury. It is therefore important to survey this area whenever such a diagnosis is considered and whenever this malformation is in any way suspected.

Treatment

Treatment depends on the cause of the symptoms, often requiring the combined talents of the orthopedist, neurosurgeon, neurologist, and radiologist. It is possible to have a severe basilar impression without neurologic symptoms, and a search for associated conditions must be conducted. If the symptoms are predominantly due to anterior impingement from a hypermobile odontoid, stabilization of the occipitocervical junction, in extension,[14] may be required. If the odontoid cannot be reduced, an anterior excision can be considered, preceded by stabilization in extension. Posterior impingement usually requires suboccipital craniectomy and decompression of the posterior ring of C1 and possibly C2, coupled with posterior stabilization. Most authors suggest opening the dura to look for a tight posterior dural band.[4] These are generalizations regarding treatment, and appropriate references should be consulted in the evaluation of individual patients.

References

Basilar Impression

1. Bachs, A., Barraquer-Bordas, L., Barraquer-Ferre, L., et al.: Delayed myelopathy following atlantoaxial dislocations by separated odontoid process. Brain *78:*537, 1955.
2. Bernini, F., Elefante, R., Smaltino, F., and Tedeschi, G.: Angiographic study on the vertebral artery in cases of deformities of the occipitocervical joint. Am. J. Roentgenol. Radium Ther. Nucl. Med. *107:*526, 1969.
3. Chamberlain, W. E.: Basilar impression (platybasia): a bizarre developmental anomaly of the occipital bone and upper cervical spine with striking and misleading neurologic manifestations. Yale J. Biol. Med. *11:*487, 1939.
4. De Barros, M. C., Farias, W., Ataide, L., and Lins, S.: Basilar impression and Arnold-Chiari malformation: a study of 66 cases. J. Neurol. Neurosurg. Psychiatry *1:*596, 1968.
5. Epstein, B. S., and Epstein, J. A.: The association of cerebellar tonsillar herniation with basilar impression incident to Paget's disease. Am. J. Roentgenol. Radium Ther. Nucl. Med. *107:*535, 1969.
6. Fischgold, H., and Metzger, J.: Étude radiotomographique de l'impression basilaire. Rev. Rhum. Mal. Osteoartic. *19:*261, 1952.
7. Fromm, G. H., and Pitner, S. E.: Late progressive quadriparesis due to odontoid agenesis. Arch. Neurol. *9:*291, 1963.
8. Gunderson, C. H., Greenspan, R. H., Glaser, G. H., and Lubs, H. A.: Klippel-Feil syndrome: genetic and clinical reevaluation of cervical fusion. Medicine *46:*491–511, 1967.
9. Hinck, V. C., Hopkins, C. E., and Savara, B. S.: Diagnostic criteria of basilar impression. Radiology *76:*572, 1961.
10. Kulkarni, M. V., Williams, J. C., Yeakley, J. W., et al.: Magnetic resonance imaging in the diagnosis of the cranio-cervical manifestations of the mucopolysaccharidoses. Magn. Res. Imaging *5:*317, 1987.
11. McAfee, P. C., Bohlman, H. H., Han, J. S., and Salvagno, R. T.: Comparison of nuclear magnetic resonance imaging and computed tomography in the diagnosis of upper cervical spinal cord compression. Spine *11:*295, 1986.
12. McGregor, M.: The significance of certain measurements of the skull in the diagnosis of basilar impression. Br. J. Radiol. *21:*171, 1948.
13. Michie, I., and Clark, M.: Neurological syndromes associated with cervical and craniocervical anomalies. Arch. Neurol. *18:*241, 1968.
14. Whitesides, T. E., Jr., and Pendleton, E. B.: Lateral approach to the upper cervical spine for treatment of upper cervical-occipital-cervical disorders. J. Bone Joint Surg. *57A:*1025, 1975.

ATLANTOAXIAL INSTABILITY

The clinical significance of a bony anomaly in the region of the atlantoaxial joint is primarily related to its influence on the stability of this articulation. The precipitating factor may be an abnormal odontoid, atlanto-occipital fusion, or laxity of the transverse atlantal ligament, but the end result is narrowing of the spinal canal and impingement on the neural elements. It is important not to lose sight of this basic problem, but frequently it becomes obscure in roentgenographic detail, conflicting reports, and unusual clinical symptoms and signs. Therefore, it is important to review atlantoaxial instability before a detailed discussion of the individual anomalies that may be contributory.

Pathomechanics

The articulation between the first and second cervical vertebrae is the most mobile part of the vertebral column and normally has the least stability of any of the vertebral articulations. The normal cervical spine permits about 90 degrees of rotatory motion. Fifty per cent of this motion occurs in the atlantoaxial joint. Considerable shifting from side to side (lateral slide) also occurs as a component of this rotatory motion. Flexion and extension are permitted to a limited degree (normally about 10 degrees of extension and 5 degrees of forward flexion), and more than 10 degrees of flexion indicates subluxation.[20] The odontoid acts as a bony buttress to prevent hyperextension, but the remainder of the normal range of motion is maintained and is solely dependent on the integrity of the surrounding ligaments and capsular structures.

The articulation between the condyles of the skull and the atlas (the atlanto-occipital joint) normally allows only a few degrees of flexion-extension, a slight nodding motion of the head. In rotation, the atlas and head turn as a unit. The articulation between the axis and the third cervical vertebra permits some flexion-extension but is similarly restricted in rotation. Thus, the atlantoaxial joint is extremely mobile but structurally weak and is located between two relatively fixed points, the atlanto-occipital and C2–C3 joints.

Motion of the atlantoaxial articulation is usually accentuated in patients with bony anomalies of the occipitocervical junction. An excellent example is the patient with atlanto-occipital fusion, who is frequently found to have compensatory hypermobility of the atlantoaxial joint. If this same patient has an associated synostosis of C2–C3, it is reasonable to expect that this additional stress on the atlantoaxial articulation may eventually lead to significant instability.[34] This assumption has clinical support, in that 60 per cent of patients with symptomatic atlanto-occipital fusion have associated fusion of C2–C3.[22]

Nonetheless, it is unusual for patients to become symptomatic before the third decade. What accounts for this delay? We must assume that at least initially a delicate balance is struck between the hypermobile articulation and the adjacent spinal cord. Motion is maintained without neurologic compromise. This relationship must be altered before symptoms develop. In the symptomatic patient, trauma is an immediate suspect, but statistically it is not often associated or is of a minor nature. More likely, the degenerative changes of aging cause the lower cervical articulations to become more rigid. This gradual restriction of motion below places an increased demand on the ligaments and capsular structures of the atlantoaxial articulation with the development of instability.[14] With aging, the CNS itself becomes less tolerant of intermittent compression, and its ability to recover is diminished. There is evidence to suggest that intermittent compression is more harmful or irritating to the spinal cord than static, constant compression.[31] Arteriosclerosis and loss of elasticity from aging affect the vertebral arteries, making them more sensitive to compression at the foramen magnum.[24]

As a consequence, the symptomatic patient often presents with a puzzling clinical picture. Only a few patients present initially with a history of head or neck trauma, neck pain, torticollis, quadriparesis, or signs of high spinal cord compression, any of which would facilitate the diagnosis. A changing, intermittent pattern of symptoms is more typical than the localized pattern suggested by the roentgenograms alone. Many are mistakenly diagnosed as having a diffuse demyelinating disease such as multiple sclerosis or amyotrophic lateral sclerosis.

In patients with basilar impression or atlanto-occipital fusion, the clinical findings suggest that the major damage is occurring anteriorly from the odontoid. The symptoms and signs of pyramidal tract irritation, muscle weakness and wasting, ataxia, spasticity, hyperreflexia, and pathologic reflexes are commonly found.[1, 22] Autopsy findings consistently demonstrate that the brain stem is indented by the abnormal odontoid.[1, 23] Other less common complaints include diplegia, tinnitus, earaches, dysphasia, and poor phonation, all of which are due to cranial nerve or bulbar irritation from direct pressure of the odontoid on the medulla. If the primary area of impingement is posterior from the rim of the foramen magnum, the dural band, or the posterior ring of the atlas (typical of odontoid anomalies), there will be symptoms referable to the posterior columns with alterations in deep pain and vibratory responses and proprioception. If there is also an associated cerebellar herniation, nystagmus, ataxia, and incoordination may be observed. Symptoms referable to vertebral artery compression—dizziness, seizures, mental deterioration, and syncope—may occur alone or in combination with those of spinal cord compression.[14]

In children the presenting symptoms may be quite subtle and nonspecific. Perovic and colleagues reported that in most of their patients, the only presenting symptom was generalized weakness manifested as lack of physical endurance, a history of frequent falling, or the child's asking to be carried.[26] Pyramidal tract signs appeared later, and posterior column signs and sphincter disturbances were less frequently encountered.[26] Similarly, in achondroplasia, retardation of motor skills and increasing hydrocephalus may be the only clinical manifestation of impending quadriparesis due to basilar stenosis.

Atlantoaxial instability is commonly associated with other anomalies of the spine, many of which lead to scoliosis. Patients with congenital scoliosis, Down syndrome, spondyloepiphyseal dysplasia, osteogenesis imperfecta, and neurofibromatosis are all capable of having significant atlantoaxial instability, which may be unrecognized. Radiologic surveys, particularly flexion-extension views of C1–C2 articulation, should be obtained before administration of general anesthesia or preliminary spinal traction in the management of the scoliosis.

Roentgenographic Features

The atlas-dens interval (ADI) is the space seen on the lateral roentgenogram between the anterior aspect of the dens and the posterior aspect of the anterior ring of the atlas (Fig. 10–3). In children the ADI should be no greater than 4.0 mm,[20] particularly in flexion where the greatest distance can be noted. The upper limit of normal in adults is less than 3 mm. Occasionally the space between the odontoid and the ring of C1 forms a "V" shape in flexion; in this situation the ADI is measured at the midportion of the odontoid. A subtle increase in the ADI in the neutral position may indicate disruption of the transverse atlantal ligament. This is a valuable aid in evaluation of acute injury, when standard flexion-extension views would be potentially hazardous.[18, 20] Fielding noted that the shift of C1–C2

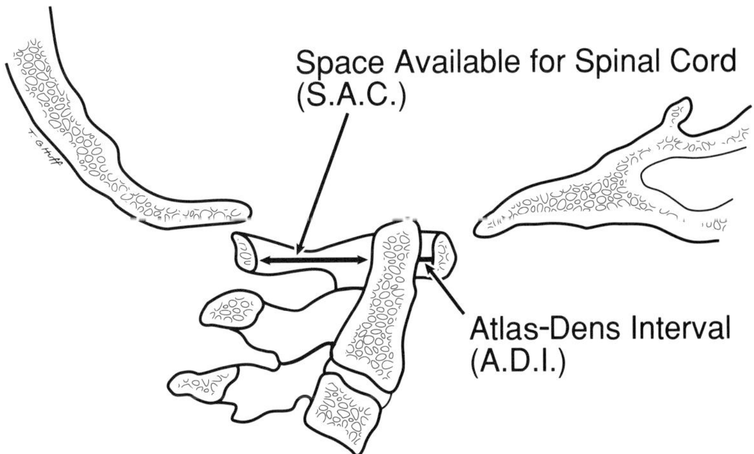

Figure 10–3. Atlantoaxial joint demonstrating the normal atlas-dens interval (ADI) and the normal space available for the spinal cord (SAC), the distance between the posterior aspect of the odontoid, and the nearest posterior structure.

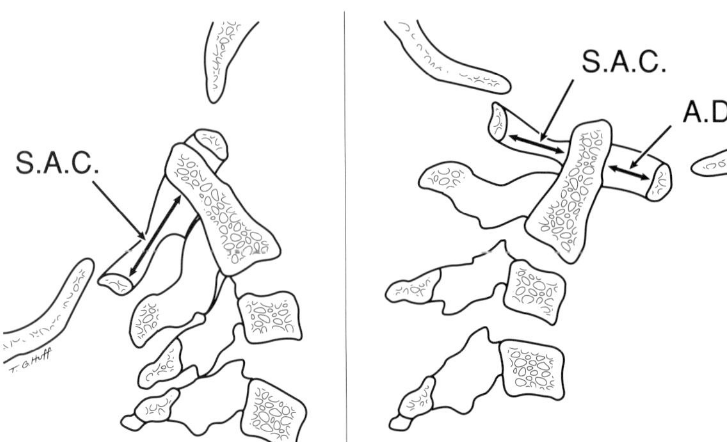

Figure 10–4. Atlantoaxial instability with intact odontoid. *A*, Flexion—forward sliding of the atlas with increased ADI and decreased SAC. *B*, Extension—the ADI and SAC return to normal as the intact odontoid provides a bony block to subluxation in hyperextension.

does not exceed 3 mm in adults if the transverse ligament is intact.[5] The transverse ligament ruptures within the range of 5 mm.[7] Unfortunately, similar data are not available for children.

The ADI is of limited value in evaluating chronic atlantoaxial instability due to congenital anomalies, rheumatoid arthritis, or Down syndrome. In these conditions the odontoid is frequently found to be hypermobile with a widened ADI, particularly in flexion (Fig. 10–4), but not all are symptomatic nor do all require surgical stabilization.[2] In this situation, attention should be directed to the amount of space available for the spinal cord (SAC). This is accomplished by measuring the distance from the posterior aspect of the odontoid or axis to the nearest posterior structure (the foramen magnum or posterior ring of the atlas). This measurement is particularly helpful in evaluating a patient with nonunion of the odontoid or os odontoideum, as in both conditions the ADI may be normal, yet in flexion or extension there may be considerable reduction in the space available for the spinal cord (Fig. 10–5).[16] Lateral flexion-extension views should be conducted voluntarily by the patient, particularly those with a neurologic deficit (Fig. 10–6). Most symptomatic patients exhibit significant instability.

Patients with a normal odontoid process and an attenuated or ruptured transverse atlantal ligament are particularly at risk; with anterior shift of the atlas over the axis, the spinal cord is easily damaged by direct impingement against the intact odontoid process,[16, 28] such as in atlanto-occipital fusion. The situation is less dangerous if the odontoid process is absent or fractured and is carried forward with the atlas (os odontoideum).[6] In a large series of patients with os odontoideum reported by Fielding and associates, the average displace-

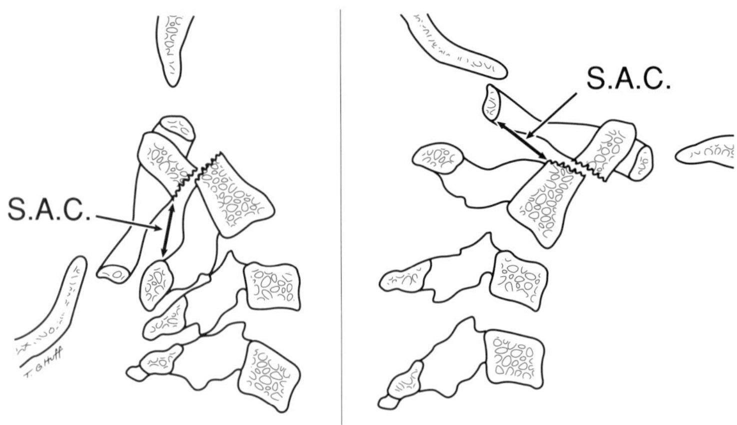

Figure 10–5. Atlantoaxial instability with os odontoideum, absent odontoid, or traumatic nonunion. *A*, Flexion—forward sliding of the atlas with reduction of SAC but no change in ADI. *B*, Extension—posterior subluxation with reduction in SAC and no change in ADI.

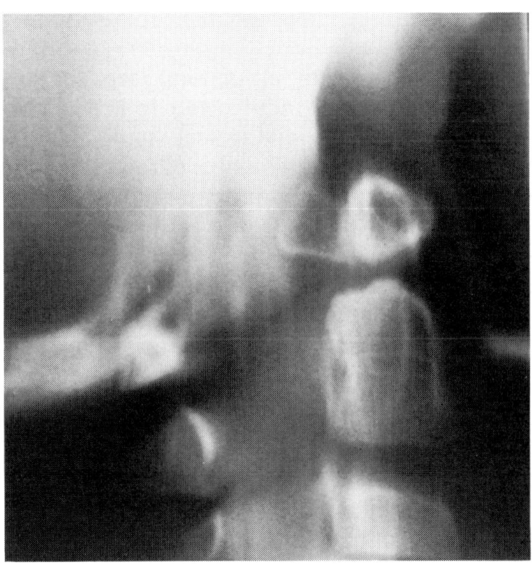

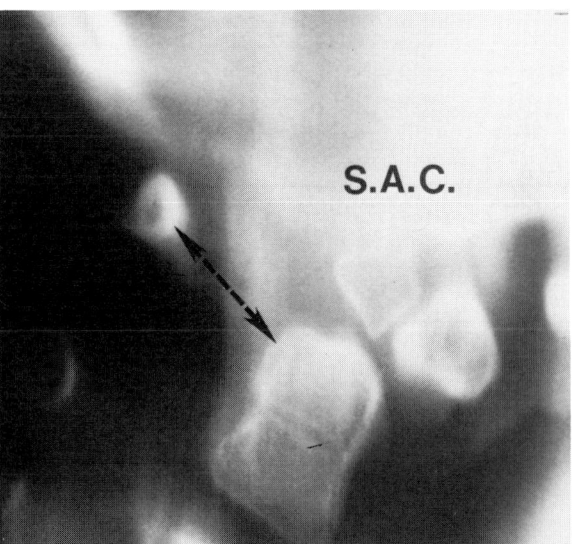

Figure 10–6. Lateral flexion-extension roentgenograph of an os odontoideum. *A*, Extension. *B*, Flexion. The odontoid ossicle is fixed to the anterior ring of the atlas and moves with it in flexion and extension and lateral slide. The SAC decreases with flexion and the ossicle moves into the spinal canal with extension.

ment was 1 cm, mostly either anterior or posterior, but some were unstable in all directions.[6]

In patients with multiple anomalies, the usual roentgenographic views are not always reliable in confirming the presence or absence of an odontoid.[26] Similarly, in patients with abnormal bone, such as those with Morquio's syndrome or spondyloepiphyseal dysplasia, the odontoid may be present but dysplastic, blending with the surrounding abnormal bone, and cannot be differentiated. In these situations, adequate visualization can be obtained by using lateral laminagraphic techniques (Fig. 10–2). When the exact cut at the level of the odontoid is determined, it is repeated in flexion-extension to ascertain the stability of the atlantoaxial articulation. Extension views should not be ignored. Many patients have been found to have significant posterior subluxation.[6, 12] Dynamic (flexion-extension) CT scans have been used to demonstrate this area, particularly with lateral reconstruction, and may well replace the laminagraphic technique.[28] Early reports of the use of MRI demonstrate direct vision of the neurologic structures and in many cases the site of bony impingement.[21]

Steel[32] called attention to the checkrein effect of the alar ligaments and how they form the second line of defense after disruption of the transverse atlantal ligament (Fig. 10–7). This secondary stability no doubt plays an important role in patients with chronic atlantoaxial instability.[8] Steel's anatomic studies provided a simple rule that is helpful to physicians evaluating this area. He defined the "rule of thirds" in that the area of the vertebral canal at the first cervical vertebra can be divided into one third "space," which represents a safe zone in which displacement can occur without neurologic impingement and is roughly equivalent to the transverse diameter of the odontoid (usually 1 cm).[32] In chronic atlantoaxial instability, it is of prime importance to recognize when the patient has exceeded the "safe zone" of Steel and enters the area of impending spinal cord compression. At this point the second line of defense, the alar ligaments, has failed and there is no longer a margin of safety (Fig. 10–7).[7] Experimentally, Fielding and associates[7] found that after rupture of the transverse ligament the alar ligaments are usually inadequate to prevent further displacement of C1–C2 when a force similar to that which ruptured the transverse ligament is applied. Although the alar ligaments appear thick and strong, they stretch with relative ease and permit significant displacement.

McRae[22] was first to call attention to the relationship of neurologic symptoms and the

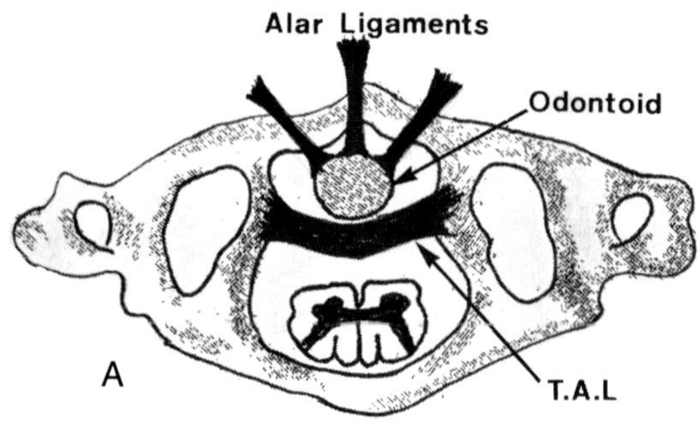

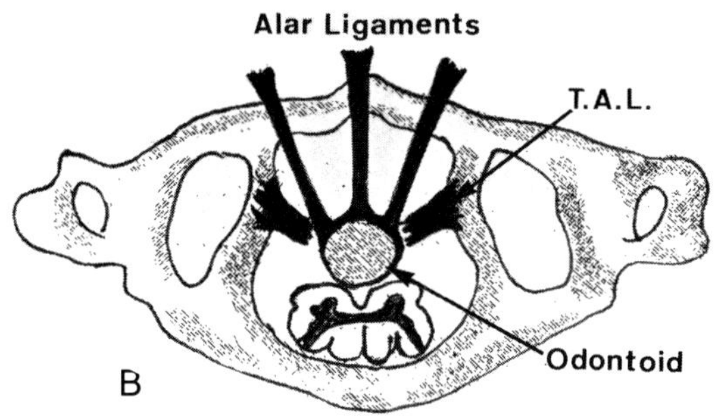

Figure 10–7. Atlantoaxial joint as viewed from above. *A*, Normal. *B*, Disruption of transverse atlantal ligament (TAL): odontoid occupies the "safe zone of Steel." The intact alar ligaments (second line of defense) prevent spinal cord compression.

sagittal diameter of the spinal canal (SAC [space available for cord]) (see Fig. 10–3). He noted that in his patients with atlanto-occipital fusion, those with less than 10 mm of available space behind the odontoid or atlas were always symptomatic. However, with the availability of more clinical data, this measurement has been more specifically defined. Greenberg,[14] after an extensive review of the literature, determined that in adults spinal cord compression always occurs if the sagittal diameter of the cervical canal behind the dens is 14 mm or less. Cord compression is possible between 15 and 17 mm and never occurs if the distance is 18 mm or more. However, variations in patient size and the presence or absence of soft tissue elements will affect the clinical significance of the measurement. Myelography has demonstrated in some patients a ventral impingement due to a thick wad of radiolucent soft tissue posterior to the dysplastic odontoid and the body of the axis.[26]

Information on normal variations in sagittal and transverse diameter of the cervical spine has been collected for infants, children, and young adults.[15, 18, 25] As might be expected, these measurements in general are smaller than those found in adults and follow a predictable growth curve. Clinical significance is determined by means of two parameters: (1) comparison of the absolute diameter to the known norms for that vertebral level and age and (2) comparison of successive vertebral levels within the same individual. Variations in the latter are more sensitive in determining an abnormality involving a single vertebra, because there is good correlation between adjacent levels in the same child. These measurements should be readily available when evaluating the growing spine for both pathologic narrowing and expansion.[5] The transparencies developed by Haworth and Keillor[15] are particularly helpful in this regard and provide an efficient screening test for assessing the transverse diameter of the spinal canal in the growing child. The sagittal diameter of the cervical canal is largest at C1 and gradually narrows in size until C5–C7. The appearance is similar to a funnel, and enlargement in the outline suggests an intraspinal mass, even if the absolute measurements do not exceed the upper limits of normal.[5]

In children there are several normal variations in cervical spine mobility that can be alarming to physicians who are aware of them. Cattell and Filtzer[3] called attention to the frequent (20 per cent) finding of overriding of the anterior arch of the atlas on the odontoid with extension of the neck. This is due to normal elasticity of ligaments and diminishes with growth; it is not present after age 7 years. Pseudosubluxation of 3 mm of C2 on C3 can be found in more than one half of the children under age 8 years (Fig. 10–8).[3, 9] Less frequently, hypermobility occurs at the C3–C4 interspace. Recognition becomes particularly important when evaluating a young child who has the Klippel-Feil syndrome or has undergone recent trauma.

In children the normal pattern of ossification of the cervical spine can pose problems in roentgenographic interpretation. At birth the odontoid is separated from the body of the axis by a wide cartilaginous band, which represents the vestigial disc space, referred to as the neurocentral synchondrosis (see "Anomalies of Odontoid"). On the lateral radiograph, this lucent line is similar in appearance to an epiphyseal growth plate. This may be confused

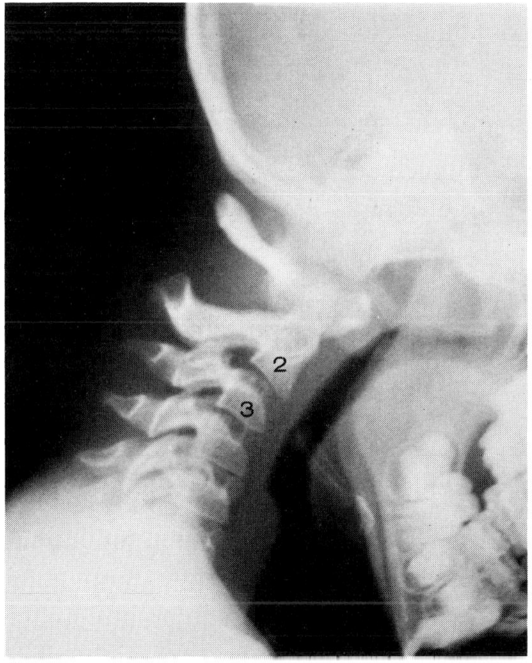

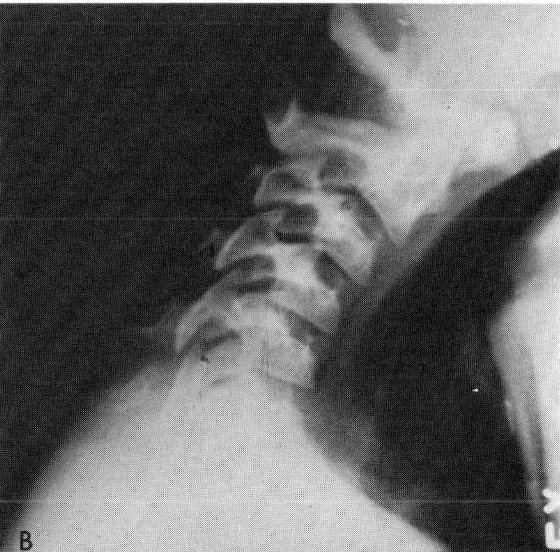

Figure 10–8. *A*, Pseudosubluxation of C2 on C3 in a child at age 5 years. *B*, Same patient at age 10. Flexion view of the cervical spine demonstrating normal motion without pseudosubluxation. This normal variation can be found in more than half of children under the age of 8 years.

with the jointlike articulation between the odontoid and the body of the atlas found in os odontoideum. This is present in nearly all children at age 3 and absent in most by age 6. Consequently, the diagnosis of os odontoideum in children must be confirmed by demonstrating motion between the odontoid and the body of the axis. Atlantoaxial fusion may be difficult to diagnose in the young child, as a significant portion of the ring of C1 is unossified at birth. There is usually a 5- to 9-mm gap posteriorly, which ossifies by age 4.[34] The anterior arch of the atlas is not visible in 80 per cent of infants, and the entire ring may not be completely ossified until age 10.[34]

Myelographic evaluation can be of great help in defining an area of constriction. In this regard, gas or a water-soluble contrast agent (metrizamide) myelography should be used in preference to oil contrast media (Fig. 10–9).[10, 22, 26, 29] CT in conjunction with metrizamide myelography is particularly helpful in evaluating children with rotational deformities or compromise of the neural canal in the upper cervical spine.[10, 28, 29] Similarly, MRI allows a more complete and accurate examination of the soft tissues and brain stem, and assists in identifying the area of direct impingement in those with occipitocervical anomalies.[71] Vertebral arteriography is helpful in evaluating patients who exhibit symptoms of transient brain stem ischemia. If cerebellar herniation (Arnold-Chiari malformation) is suspected, arteriography combined with myelography can demonstrate the anomaly (Fig. 10–10).[29]

Treatment

In general, effective treatment can be provided only if the exact cause of symptoms has been determined. This must be accomplished by a careful correlation of the clinical and radiologic findings. Before surgical intervention, reduction of the atlantoaxial articulation should be achieved by either positioning or traction.[8, 9] Operative reduction should never be attempted, as it is associated with increased morbidity and mortality rates.[30, 35] The patient should be maintained in the reduced position preoperatively until spinal cord edema and local irritation resolve. This is usually accompanied by improvement of the neurologic

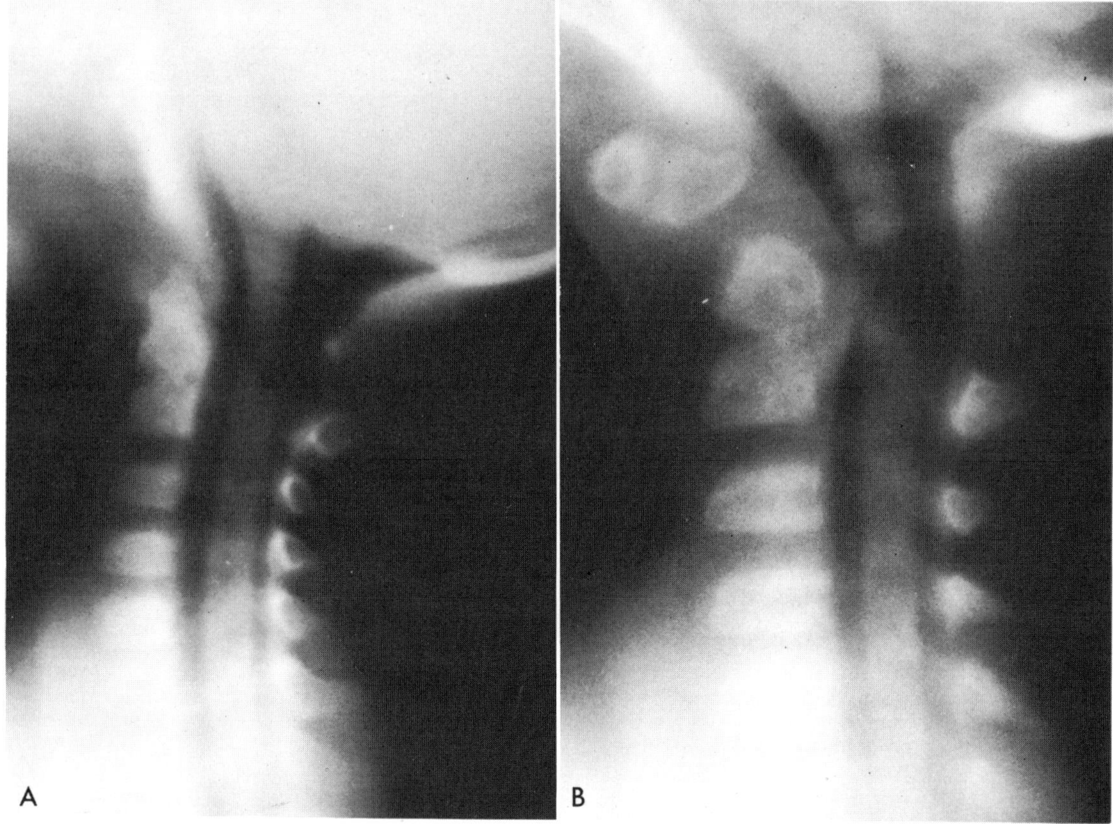

Figure 10–9. Normal gas myelogram-polytomograms. *A,* A 3-year-old dwarf with slightly abnormal odontoid, no atlantoaxial instability, and no neurologic signs or symptoms. *B,* Atlantoaxial instability without cord compression and myelopathy. A 7-year-old dwarf with a congenitally detached odontoid that dislocates forward with the anterior arch of the atlas. The posterior ring of the atlas is absent, and therefore posterior impingement of the spinal cord against the axis is avoided. (Roentgenograms courtesy of Steven E. Kopits, M.D., Division of Orthopaedics, Johns Hopkins University; and Milos Perovic, M.D., Department of Radiology, University of Connecticut.)

status and often remission of symptoms. If neurologic symptoms are unchanged with reduction and rest, the physician should carefully seek other causes.

Too little attention has been paid in the past to occult respiratory dysfunction in these patients.[13, 19] Many have an unrecognized decrease in vital capacity and chronic alveolar hypoventilation as a result of the neurologic injury to the brain stem. Similarly, the gag and cough reflexes are often depressed[13] and the patient may not be able to clear pulmonary secretion adequately in the postoperative period. Periods of apnea and respiratory distress, either during surgery or in the immediate postoperative period, have frequently resulted in death or have required prolonged respiratory support. Preoperative pulmonary evaluation can be of help in limiting the severity of respiratory complications. If pulmonary function is significantly reduced or if the gag and cough reflexes are depressed, consideration should be given to preoperative tracheostomy.[13] Equipment for mechanical respiratory support must be immediately available during the postoperative period.

Laxity of Transverse Atlantal Ligament

This is a diagnosis of exclusion suggested by the clinical occurrence of chronic atlantoaxial dislocation without a predisposing cause.[22] There is no history of trauma, congenital anomaly, infection, or rheumatoid arthritis to account for the radiologic finding. Most pa-

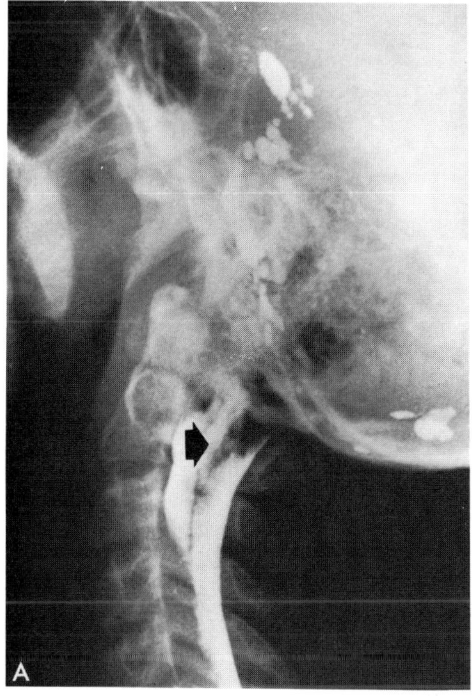

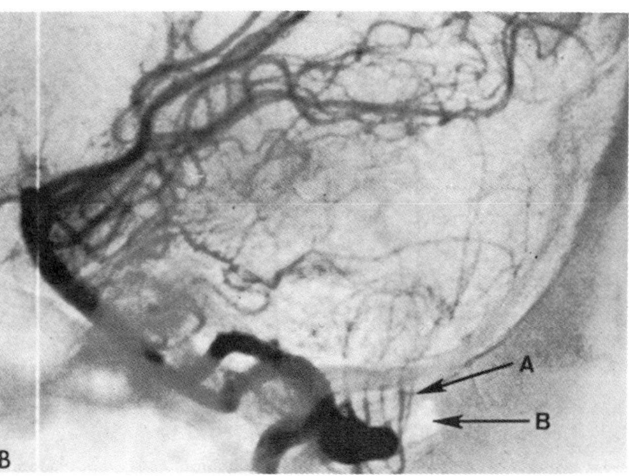

Figure 10–10. A 12-year-old with nystagmus and cerebellar ataxia. *A*, Myelogram demonstrates the Arnold-Chiari malformation with herniation of the cerebellar tonsils through the foramen magnum. The arrow indicates the distal migration of the tonsils. *B*, Same patient. Vertebral arteriography demonstrates inferior cerebellar vessels looping down to the spinal canal. A *(arrow)*, inferior cerebellar vessels. B *(arrow)*, posterior ring of atlas. (Roentgenograms courtesy of Frank Lee, M.D., Department of Radiology, Jefferson Medical College, Philadelphia, Pennsylvania.)

tients discovered have the typical symptoms of atlantoaxial instability and require surgical stabilization.

Laxity of the transverse atlantal ligament is unusually common in patients with Down syndrome, the reported incidence being 15 per cent (Fig. 10–11).[2, 27] The lesion may be found in all age groups, with no age preponderance.[2] It appears that these patients have rupture or attenuation of the transverse atlantal ligament with encroachment of the "safe zone of Steel" (Fig. 10–7), but at least initially they are protected by checkrein action of the alar ligaments from spinal cord compression (Fig. 10–11). In other words, many have excessive motion, but relatively few are symptomatic and most are discovered only by radiologic survey.[4] If roentgenograms of the upper cervical spine indicate an atlas-dens interval of more than 5 mm, instability is considered to be present. Usually, if the symptoms are present, instability of greater than 7 mm or even 10 mm is found.

Unfortunately, complete data are still not available regarding the best way to manage this problem.[2, 4, 27] We still know very little about the natural history despite roentgenographic examination of hundreds of children.[4] Studies have indicated that some children become progressively looser with time; others who manifest small degrees of instability can, on occasion, become stable.[2] Currently, roentgenographic examination on a routine basis is recommended for children with Down syndrome, particularly those who will be competing in athletics.[27] Certainly, any child with Down syndrome who has a musculoskeletal complaint, such as subluxing patella, dislocating hips, or unsteady gait, should be investigated. With our present knowledge, prophylactic stabilization does not appear to be indicated, but more clinical information is required. Those who have minor degrees of hypermobility or instability should be followed with flexion-extension x-rays on a regular basis. They should not engage in contact sports, somersaults, trampoline exercises, or similar activities that favor neck flexion,[27] and the potential risks should be discussed with the parents. Any child who has neck symptoms due to instability or a history of neurologic problems should be stabilized.[2]

Occipital Atlantal Instability

This is a rare condition often due to trauma or, less commonly, congenital abnormalities.[11]

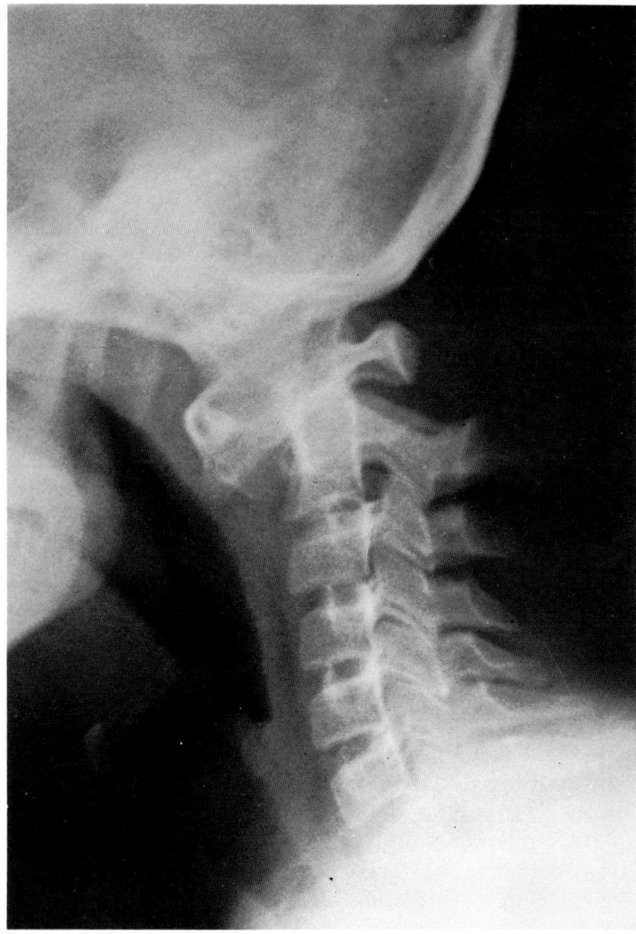

Figure 10–11. An 11-year-old with Down syndrome and gross atlantoaxial instability. The patient's gait was clumsy. Physical examination revealed poor coordination of the extremities. There was no other evidence of motor or sensory impairment or pathologic reflexes. The patient had no symptoms referable to the cervical spine two years after surgical stabilization.

Previously, most patients did not survive this injury, but with improved resuscitatory measures the problem has been reported more frequently. Clinical and neurologic manifestations include cardiorespiratory arrest, motor weakness, quadriplegia, torticollis, pain in the neck, vertigo, and projectile vomiting.[11] Surgical stabilization is usually necessary. Anomalies of the upper cervical spine can also lead to this condition and it has been reported in association with Down syndrome.

References

Alantoaxial Instability

1. Bharucha, E. P., and Dastur, H. M.: Craniovertebral anomalies (a report on 40 cases). Brain *87*:469, 1964.
2. Burke, S. W., French, H. G., Roberts, J. M., et al.: Chronic atlanto-axial instability in Down syndrome. J. Bone Joint Surg. *67A*:1356, 1985.
3. Cattell, H. S., and Filtzer, D. L.: Pseudosubluxation and other normal variations in the cervical spine in children. J. Bone Joint Surg. *47A*:1295, 1965.
4. Davidson, R. G.: Atlantoaxial instability in individuals with Down's syndrome: a fresh look at the evidence. Pediatrics *81*:857, 1988.
5. Dolan, K. D.: Expanding lesions of the cervical spinal canal. Radiol. Clin. North Am. *15*:203, 1977.
6. Fielding, J. W., Hensinger, R. N., and Hawkins, R. J.: Os odontoideum. J. Bone Joint Surg. *62A*:376, 1980.
7. Fielding, J. W., Cochran, G. V., Lawsing, J. F., III, and Hohl, M.: Tears of the transverse ligament of the atlas. J. Bone Joint Surg. *56A*:1683, 1974.
8. Fielding, J. W., Hawkins, R. J., and Ratzan, S. A.: Spine fusion for atlanto-axial instability. J. Bone Joint Surg. *58A*:400, 1976.
9. Garber, J. N.: Abnormalities of the atlas and axis vertebrae, congenital and traumatic. J. Bone Joint Surg. *46A*:1782, 1964.
10. Geehr, R. B., Rothman, S. L. G., and Kier, E. L.: The role of computed tomography in the evaluation of upper cervical spine pathology. Comput. Tomogr. *2*:79, 1978.
11. Georgopoulos, G., Pizzutillo, P. D., and Lee, M. S.: Occipito-atlantal instability in children. A report of

five cases and review of the literature. J. Bone Joint Surg. *69A:*429, 1987.
12. Giannestras, N. J., Mayfield, F. H., Provencio, F. P., and Maurer, J.: Congenital absence of the odontoid process. A case report. J. Bone Joint Surg. *46A:*839, 1964.
13. Grantham, S. A., Dick, H. M., Thompson, R. C., Jr., and Stinchfield, F. E.: Occipito-cervical arthrodesis. Indications, technic and results. Clin. Orthop. *65:*118, 1969.
14. Greenberg, A. D.: Atlantoaxial dislocations. Brain *91:*655, 1968.
15. Haworth, J. B., and Keillor, G. W.: Use of transparencies in evaluating the width of the spinal canal in infants, children and adults. Radiology *79:*109, 1962.
16. Hensinger, R. N.: Osseous anomalies of the craniovertebral junction. Spine *111:*323, 1986.
17. Hinck, V. C., and Hopkins, C. E.: Measurement of the atlantodental interval in the adult. Am. J. Roentgenol. *84:*945, 1960.
18. Hinck, V. C., Hopkins, C. E., and Savara, B. S.: Sagittal diameter of the cervical spinal canal in children. Radiology *79:*97, 1962.
19. Krieger, A. J., Rosomoff, H. L., Kuperman, A. S., and Zingesser, L. H.: Occult respiratory dysfunction in a craniovertebral anomaly. J. Neurosurg. *31:*15, 1969.
20. Locke, G. R., Gardner, J. I., and Van Epps, E. F.: Atlas dens interval (ADI) in children: a survey based on 200 normal cervical spines. Am. J. Roentgenol. *97:*135, 1966.
21. McAfee, P. C., Bohlman, H. H., Han, J. S., and Salvagno, R. T.: Comparison of nuclear magnetic resonance imaging and computed tomography in the diagnosis of upper cervical spinal cord compression. Spine *11:*295, 1986.
22. McRae, D. L.: Bony abnormalities in the region of the foramen magnum: correlation of the anatomic and neurologic findings. Acta Radiol. *40:*335, 1953.
23. McRae, D. L.: The significance of abnormalities of the cervical spine. Am. J. Roentgenol. *84:*3, 1960.
24. Nagashima, C.: Atlanto-axial dislocation due to agenesis of the os odontoideum or odontoid. J. Neurosurg. *33:*270, 1970.
25. Naik, D. R.: Cervical spinal canal in normal infants. Clin. Radiol. *21:*323, 1970.
26. Perovic, N. M., Kopits, S. E., and Thompson, R. C.: Radiologic evaluation of the spinal cord in congenital atlanto-axial dislocations. Radiology *109:*713, 1973.
27. Pueschel, S. M., and Scola, F. H.: Atlantoaxial instability in individuals with Down's syndrome: epidemiologic, radiographic, and clinical studies. Pediatrics *80:*555, 1987.
28. Roach, J. W., Duncan, D., Wenger, D. R., and Maravilla, A.: Atlanto-axial instability and spinal cord compression in children. Diagnosis by computerized tomography. J. Bone Joint Surg. *66A:*708, 1984.
29. Resjo, M., Harwood-Nash, D. C., and Fitz, C. R.: Normal cord in infants and children examined with computed tomographic metrizamide myelography. Radiology *130:*691, 1979.
30. Sinh, G., and Pandya, S. K.: Treatment of congenital atlanto-axial dislocations. Proc. Aust. Assoc. Neurol. *5:*507, 1968.
31. Spillane, J. D., Pallis, C., and Jones, A. M.: Developmental abnormalities in the region of the foramen magnum. Brain *80:*11, 1957.
32. Steel, H. H.: Anatomical and mechanical considerations of the atlanto-axial articulations. J. Bone Joint Surg. *50:*1481, 1968.
33. Sullivan, C. R., Bruwer, A. J., and Harris, L. E.: Hypermobility of the cervical spine in children. A pitfall in the diagnosis of cervical dislocation. Am. J. Surg. *95:*636, 1958.
34. von Torklus, D., and Gehle, W.: The Upper Cervical Spine. New York, Grune & Stratton, 1972.
35. Wadia, N. H.: Myelopathy complicating congenital atlanto-axial dislocation (a study of 28 cases). Brain *90:*449, 1967.

ATLANTO-OCCIPITAL FUSION (OCCIPITALIZATION, OCCIPITOCERVICAL SYNOSTOSIS, ASSIMILATION OF ATLAS)

This condition is characterized by a partial or complete congenital union between the atlas and the base of the occiput (Fig. 10–12). It ranges from total incorporation of the atlas into the occipital bone to a bony or even fibrous band uniting one small area of the atlas to the occiput. Basilar impression is commonly associated with occipitocervical synostosis; other associated anomalies include Klippel-Feil syndrome, occipital vertebrae, and condylar hypoplasia.[16]

Occipitocervical synostosis, basilar impression, and odontoid anomalies are the most common developmental malformations of the occipitocervical junction. Incidence ranges from 1.4 to 2.5 per 1000 children, both sexes being equally affected.[9, 16]

Clinical Features

Most patients have an appearance much like that in the Klippel-Feil syndrome, with a short broad neck, a low hairline, torticollis, a high scapula, and restricted neck movements.[3, 11, 15] The skull may be deformed and shaped like a "tower." Kyphosis and scoliosis are frequent occurrences. Other associated anomalies occasionally seen include dwarfism, funnel chest, pes cavus, syndactylies, jaw anomalies, cleft palate, congenital ear deformities, hypospadias, and sometimes genitourinary tract defects.

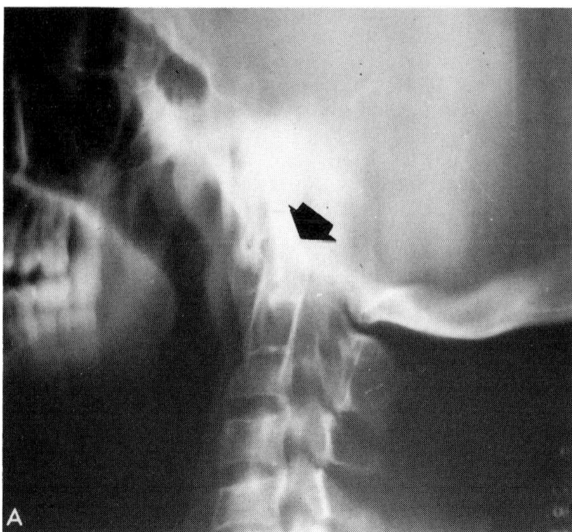

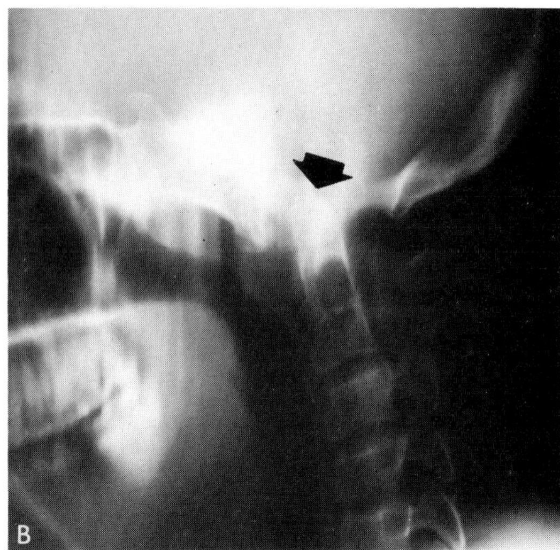

Figure 10–12. A 22-year-old with symptomatic atlanto-occipital fusion and hypermobile odontoid. Lateral laminagraphic views in *A*, extension; *B*, flexion. The odontoid extends well into the opening of the foramen magnum (McRae's line), and with flexion the odontoid moves posteriorly with impingement of the brain stem. (Roentgenograms courtesy of Donald L. McRae, M.D., Department of Radiology, University of Toronto, Canada. Reproduced by permission from Am. J. Roentgenol. 84:3–25, 1960.)

Neurologic symptoms do not usually occur until the third or fourth decade but can present during childhood. They progress in a slow, unrelenting manner and may be initiated by traumatic or inflammatory processes. It is rare that symptoms begin dramatically, but they have been reported even as a cause of instant death.[8] It is difficult to explain why neurologic problems develop so late and progress so slowly in these patients. It may be that the frequently associated atlantoaxial instability progresses with age and the resultant added demands placed upon it, producing gradual spinal cord or vertebral artery compromise.

McRae and Barnum[11] suggested that the key to development of neurologic manifestations lies with the odontoid and its position—an indication of the degree of actual or relative basilar impression. If the odontoid lies below the foramen magnum, the patient is usually asymptomatic.[10] However, with the decrease in vertical height of the atlas, the odontoid may project well into the foramen magnum, producing brain stem pressure, a fact well documented by autopsy.[3, 12]

Anterior compression of the brain stem from the backward-projecting odontoid is most common (Fig. 10–12). This produces a variety of findings, depending on the location and the degree of pressure. Pyramidal tract signs and symptoms (spasticity, hyperreflexia, muscle weakness and wasting, and gait disturbances) are most common, but cranial nerve involvement (diplopia, tinnitus, dysphagia, and auditory disturbances) may be seen less often. Compression from the posterior lip of the foramen magnum or the constricting band of dura may disturb the posterior columns, resulting in loss of proprioception, vibration, and tactile discrimination. Nystagmus, a common occurrence, is probably due to posterior cerebellar compression.

Vascular disturbances from vertebral artery involvement may occasionally result in syncope, seizures, vertigo, and unsteady gait, among other signs and symptoms of brain stem ischemia.

Disturbed mechanics of the cervical spine may result in a dull aching pain in the posterior occiput and neck with episodic neck stiffness and torticollis. Tenderness noted in the area of the posterior scalp may be due to irritation of the greater occipital nerve.

The following most common signs and symptoms occur, in decreasing order of frequency: pain in the occiput and neck, vertigo, unsteady gait, paresis of the limbs, paresthesias, speech disturbances, hoarseness, double vision, syncope, auditory noise or disturbance, and interference with swallowing. All these may be manifestations of underlying atlantoaxial instability, which, as an isolated lesion, may produce neck pain, headaches, and neurologic deficits from cord or root irritation and, rarely, sudden death.[7, 17]

Roentgenographic Features

Standard roentgenograms of this area can be difficult to interpret. Tomography, CT, and MRI may be necessary to clarify the pathologic condition (Fig. 10–12). Most commonly the anterior arch of the atlas is assimilated into the occiput, usually in association with a hypoplastic posterior arch. The condition may range from total incorporation of the atlas into the occipital bone to a bony or even fibrous band uniting one small area of the atlas to the occiput. Laminagrams are often necessary to demonstrate bony continuity of the anterior arch of the atlas with the occiput. Posterior fusion is not usually evident, as this portion of the ring may be represented only by a short bony fringe on the edge of the foramen magnum. Despite its innocuous radiologic appearance, this fringe is frequently directed downward and inward, can compromise the spinal canal posteriorly, and has been found to create a groove in the spinal cord. It is usually assumed that the assimilated atlas is fused symmetrically to the occipital opening, but several autopsy specimens have demonstrated a posterior positioning of the atlas.[11] This in effect pushes the odontoid posteriorly, narrowing the spinal canal and the space available for the spinal cord.

Ossification of the atlas proceeds from paired centers—one for each of the lateral masses. These progress posteriorly into the neural arches, which are fully ossified at birth except for a gap of 5 to 9 mm posteriorly that closes by the fourth year. The anterior arch of the atlas is not visible in 80 per cent of neonates. This area most commonly ossifies from a single center, which appears during the first year of life and fuses to the remainder of the atlas by the third year.[1, 4, 7, 16]

There is varying loss of height of the atlas, allowing the odontoid to project upward into the foramen magnum and creating a "relative" basilar impression (Fig. 10–12).[18] The position of the odontoid relative to the foramen magnum was described under "Basilar Impression." McRae[11, 12] measured the distance from the posterior aspect of the odontoid to either the posterior arch of the atlas or the posterior lip of the foramen magnum (SAC), which was closer. He stated that a neurologic deficit would be present if this distance was less than 19 mm. This distance should be determined in flexion, because this position most dramatically reduces the space available for the cord.

Flexion-extension stress films (Fig. 10–12) often show posterior displacement of the odontoid from the anterior arch of the atlas of as much as 12 mm.[11] Associated atlantoaxial instability has been reported to develop eventually in 50 per cent of patients.[16] This is determined by measuring the distance from the anterior border of the odontoid to the posterior aspect of the anterior arch of the atlas. A distance greater than 4 mm in young children who probably have considerable cartilage present and 3 mm in older children and adults is considered pathologic.[1, 4, 6] The odontoid itself often has an abnormal shape and direction; it frequently is longer, and its angle with the body of the axis is directed more posteriorly.[11, 17]

McRae[10] was first to note the frequent occurrence of congenital fusion of C2–C3 (70 per cent) in patients with atlanto-occipital fusion (Fig. 10–13). This suggests that greater demands are placed on the atlantoaxial articulation, particularly in flexion and extension when the joints above and below are fused.[3, 11] von Torklus and Gehle noted that approximately 50 per cent of patients develop late onset of atlantoaxial instability and the resultant potential for compromise of the spinal cord.[16]

Another commonly associated abnormality is the presence of a constricting band of dura posteriorly. This has been found to create a groove in the spinal cord and may be the primary cause of symptoms. The band cannot be visualized on routine roentgenograms, nor does it correlate with the presence or absence of the posterior bony fringe of the atlas. Consequently, CT and MRI should be an integral part of the evaluation. Water-soluble contrast material (metrizamide) along or in conjunction with CT can visualize the spinal canal and its contents. A properly performed study will yield valuable information regarding the presence of a dural band, tonsillar herniation, and the size, shape, and position of the spinal cord in the spinal canal.[2, 15]

Treatment

Management of this fortunately uncommon problem may be hazardous. Unlike anomalies

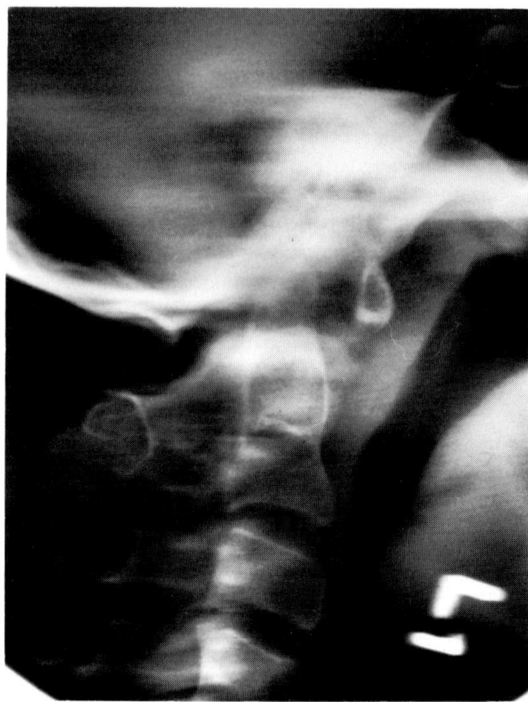

Figure 10–13. A 23-year-old male with the Klippel-Feil syndrome, ataxic gait, hyperreflexia, and a history of several episodes of unconsciousness. Lateral laminagraphic view of the cervical spine and base of the skull demonstrates a C2–C3 fusion and fusion of the ring of C1 to the opening of the foramen magnum (occipitalization). The odontoid is hypermobile. Patients with this pattern of fusion are at great risk. With aging, the odontoid may become hypermobile, and the space available for the spinal cord posteriorly may be compromised.

of the odontoid, surgical intervention carries a much higher risk of morbidity and mortality.[3, 13, 17]

Nonoperative methods such as cervical collars, braces, plaster, and traction should be attempted initially in some of these patients. These methods are often helpful in patients with persistent complaints of head and neck pain, and are particularly helpful if symptoms follow minor trauma or infection. If neurologic deficits are present, immobilization may achieve only temporary relief. Patients presenting with evidence of a compromised situation in the upper cervical area must take precautions not to expose themselves to undue trauma.

With anterior spinal cord signs and symptoms due to an unstable atlantoaxial complex, an occiput to C2 fusion is suggested with preliminary traction to attempt reduction, if necessary. If reduction is possible and there are no neurologic signs, surgical intervention carries an improved prognosis.[3, 7, 17] Operative reduction should be avoided, because this has frequently resulted in death.[14, 17] No satisfactory solution for the unreducible odontoid has been determined; the reader is referred to the reports of Bharucha and Dastur,[3] Greenberg,[7] and Wadia.[17]

Posterior signs and symptoms and myelographic evidence of bony or dural compression, depending on the degree of neurologic involvement, may be indications for a posterior decompression and stabilization of the occiput to C2. Results of this vary from complete remission of symptoms to increased neurologic deficits and even death.[3, 13, 18]

Anomalies of Ring of C1

Dubousset called attention to a previously unrecognized problem with the ring of C1, the hemiatlas.[5] Although there had been an occasional case report, he presented the first large study to review the problem in depth. He reported 17 patients in whom he was able to document absence of the facet of C1, which led to a severe and progressive torticollis in young children (Fig. 10–14). Initially, the deformity is flexible and can be passively corrected. As the child ages, the torticollis becomes more severe and eventually fixed. Radiographic diagnosis using tomography or CT have been helpful in identifying this deformity. Use of traction to align the head and neck at the time of the study assists in highlighting the problem. If the patient is passively correctable, a single posterior fusion, occiput to C2, is performed. A halo cast is applied postoperatively to maintain the head in a satisfactory alignment until the fusion is complete. Although the time at which this becomes a fixed deformity was not defined, Dubousset reported good results in teenagers. This can also accompany the Klippel-Feil syndrome with anomalies of the lower cervical spine as well. Dubousset found an increased incidence of anomalies of the vertebral vessels in these children and suggested arteriographic evaluation before the use of traction or surgical intervention, which could further compromise a precarious blood supply to the midbrain and spinal cord.[5]

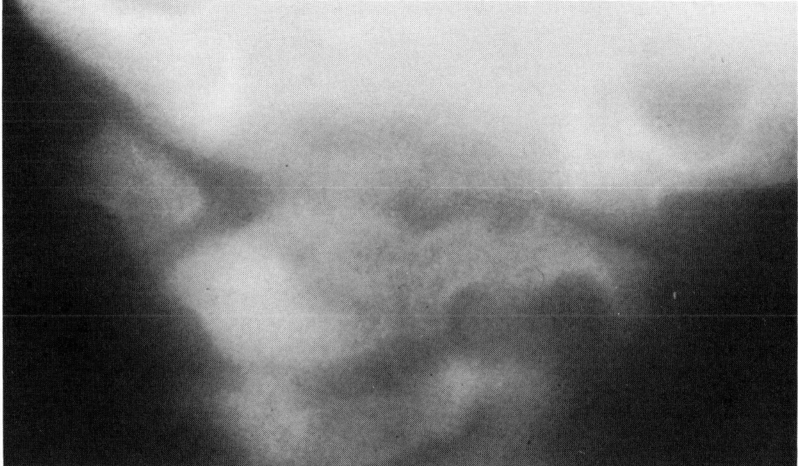

Figure 10–14. Absence of the C1 facet in a 5-year-old with severe and progressive torticollis. Laminagraph demonstrates a hemiatlas, with complete absence of the left portion of the C1 ring. (Roentgenogram courtesy of Luther C. Fisher III, M.D., Department of Orthopaedics, University of Mississippi Medical Center.)

References

Atlanto-occipital Fusion

1. Bailey, D. K.: The normal cervical spine in infants and children. Radiology *59:*712, 1962.
2. Baird, P. A., Robinson, G. C., and Buckler, W. St J.: Klippel-Feil syndrome. Am. J. Dis. Child. *113:*546, 1967.
3. Bharucha, E. P., and Dastur, H. M.: Craniovertebral anomalies (a report on 40 cases). Brain *87:*469, 1964.
4. Caffey, J.: Paediatric X-ray Diagnosis. Chicago, Year Book Medical Publishers, 1967.
5. Dubousett, J.: Torticollis in children caused by congenital anomalies of the atlas. J. Bone Joint Surg. *68A:*178, 1986.
6. Fielding, J. W.: The cervical spine in the child. Curr. Pract. Orthop. Surg. *5:*31, 1973.
7. Greenberg, A. D.: Atlantoaxial dislocations. Brain *91:*644, 1968.
8. Hadley, L. A.: The Spine. Springfield, IL, Charles C Thomas, 1956.
9. Macalister, A.: Notes on the development and variations of the atlas. J. Anat. Physiol. *27:*519, 1983.
10. McRae, D. L.: Bony abnormalities in the region of the foramen magnum: correction of the anatomic and neurologic findings. Acta Radiol. *40:*335, 1953.
11. McRae, D. L., and Barnum, A. S.: Occipitalization of the atlas. Am. J. Roentgenol. Radium Ther. Nucl. Med. *70:*23, 1953.
12. McRae, D. L.: The significance of abnormalities of the cervical spine. Am. J. Roentgenol. Radium Ther. Nucl. Med. *84:*3, 1960.
13. Nicholson, J. S., and Sherk, H. H.: Anomalies of the occipitocervical articulation. J. Bone Joint Surg. *50A:*295, 1968.
14. Sinh, G., and Pandya, S. K.: Treatment of congenital atlantoaxial dislocations. Proc. Aust. Assoc. Neurol. *5:*507, 1968.
15. Spillane, J. D., Pallis, C., and Jones, A. M.: Developmental abnormalities in the region of the foramen magnum. Brain *80:*11, 1957.
16. von Torklus, D., and Gehle, W.: The Upper Cervical Spine. New York. Grune & Stratton, 1972.
17. Wadia, N. H.: Myelopathy complicating congenital atlantoaxial dislocation (a study of 28 cases). Brain *90:*449, 1967.
18. Wilkinson, M.: Cervical Spondylosis. 2nd ed. Philadelphia, W. B. Saunders Co., 1971.

ANOMALIES OF ODONTOID (DENS)

Congenital anomalies of the odontoid can lead to an unstable atlantoaxial complex, with potential neurologic sequelae and even death due to spinal cord pressure.[25] Several gradations or variations of anomalies of the odontoid exist, ranging from aplasia (complete absence) to hypoplasia (partial absence) and to os odontoideum (Fig. 10–15).

Aplasia or agenesis of the odontoid is a complete absence of development. Hypoplasia is a partially developed odontoid, ranging in size from a short, stubby, peglike projection to an odontoid of almost normal size. Os odontoideum is an anomaly in which the odontoid process is divided by a wide transverse gap, leaving the apical segment without support from the base.[33] Distinguishing aplasia or hypoplasia from os odontoideum is of limited importance, because they usually lead to atlantoaxial instability, and clinical signs, symptoms, and treatment are identical. The only distinctive features are roentgenographic.

Incidence

The frequency of these anomalies is unknown, and like many anomalies that may be asymptomatic, they are probably more com-

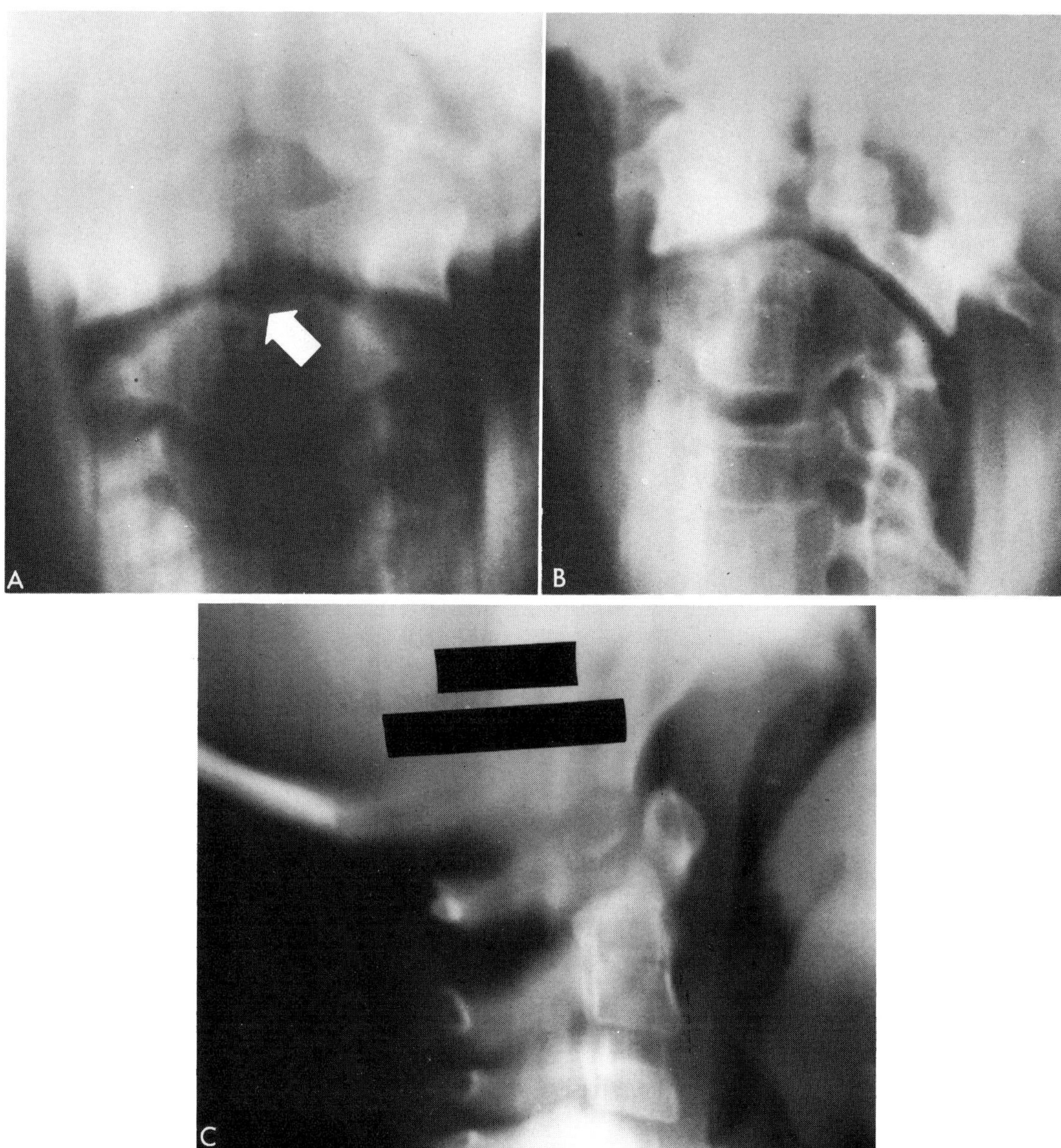

Figure 10–15. *A*, Agenesis of the odontoid (open-mouth laminagraphic view). Note the slight depression between the superior articular facets of the axis *(arrow)*. A short bony remnant in this position is termed odontoid hypoplasia. *B*, Os odontoideum (open-mouth laminagraphic view). The os odontoideum is an oval or round ossicle, usually approximately half the normal size of the odontoid, with a smooth cortical border of uniform thickness. There is a jointlike articulation between the os odontoideum and the body of the axis, which appears radiologically as a wide radiolucent gap and usually extends above the level of the superior facets. *C*, Lateral roentgenogram of an os odontoideum. The odontoid ossicle is fixed to the anterior ring of the atlas, and moves with it in flexion and extension and lateral slide. There is usually a short bony remnant projecting superiorly from the body of C2.

mon than is recognized. They are often incidental findings or are seen in patients sustaining trauma or symptoms sufficient to require roentgenographic investigation.

In our experience, aplasia is extremely rare. McRae[31] noted that there was no proved case of odontoid aplasia at the Montreal Neurological Institute up to 1960. Many previous reports have confused aplasia for hypoplasia, and probably, as previously emphasized, aplasia has been a misnomer, because it almost never describes an associated absence of the portion below the articular facets that contributes to the body of the axis. Hypoplasia and os odontoideum are infrequently reported and can be considered rare.[19, 23, 34, 41, 50] With more recent awareness, however, these lesions are being recognized more commonly than previous literature might indicate—especially os odontoideum.[15] In a large series reported by Wollin, the average age of diagnosis was 30 years,[50] but in a later series it was 18.9 years, suggesting earlier recognition.[15] An increasing number of children with these anomalies are being discovered.

In such conditions as Down syndrome, Morquio's syndrome, Klippel-Feil syndrome, and some skeletal dysplasias, odontoid anomalies in association with ligamentous laxity producing atlantoaxial instability are much more common than in the general population.[4, 7, 8, 24, 25, 32, 44, 45] Associated regional malformations may occur, but unlike many congenital cervical anomalies, they are rare.[3, 25, 41]

Development of Odontoid

The body of the odontoid is derived from the mesenchyme of the first cervical sclerotome and is actually the centrum of the first cervical vertebra, which, during development, becomes separated from the atlas to fuse with the remainder of the axis.[27, 42, 44] The apex of the odontoid process is derived from the mesenchyme of the most caudad occipital sclerotome or proatlas. Ossification of these two segments of the odontoid then proceeds along separate lines.

Between the first and fifth prenatal months the dens begins to ossify from two centers, one on each side of the midline. By the time of birth they have fused into a single mass.[2, 5, 12] Occasionally the right and left halves of the odontoid are not fused at birth and a longitudinal midline cleft may be seen. At birth the tip of the odontoid has not ossified, is V-shaped, and is known as a dens bicornis (Fig. 10–16). A separate ossification center within the V, known as a "summit ossification center" or ossiculum terminale, usually appears at age 3 years and fuses with the remainder of the dens by age 12.[2, 5, 39] Cattell and Filtzer[6] found an ossiculum terminale in 26 per cent of 70 normal children aged 5 to 11 years.

An ossiculum terminale may never appear or may occasionally fail to fuse with the dens; it is then called an ossiculum terminale persistens. It is occasionally discernible as either a cyst or an area of increased density. These developmental anomalies are of little clinical significance.[10, 25] Sherk and Nicholson,[44] however, reported a rare case of quadriplegia and death in a Down syndrome child that was directly attributable to atlantoaxial instability secondary to an ossiculum terminale. This is the only such report; the ossiculum terminale usually is firmly bound to the main body of the dens by cartilage and consequently is seldom the source of instability.

At birth the dens is separated from the body of the axis by a cartilaginous band (Fig. 10–16) that represents the epiphyseal growth plate. This plate does not run across the base of the dens at the level of the superior articular facets of the axis, but lies well below this level within the body of the axis (Fig. 10–16*B*). Therefore, the part of the odontoid below the articular facets contributes to the body of the axis. On the open-mouth view, the odontoid fits like a "cork in a bottle," lying sandwiched between the neural arches (Fig. 10–16*B*). This epiphyseal line is present in almost all children by age 3 years and 50 per cent of children by age 4, but absent in most by age 6.[6, 12] It rarely persists into adolescence and adult life. If present, it is not seen at the base of the dens where a fracture would be anticipated, but lies well below the level of the superior articular facets within the body of the axis. In the young child the unossified portions of the odontoid may give the false impression of odontoid hypoplasia. Similarly, one may erroneously conclude that the child has C1–C2 instability, as the anterior arch of the atlas commonly may slide upward and actually may protrude beyond the ossified portion of the odontoid[6] on the lateral extension roentgenogram (Fig. 10–17).

The blood supply to the odontoid is from

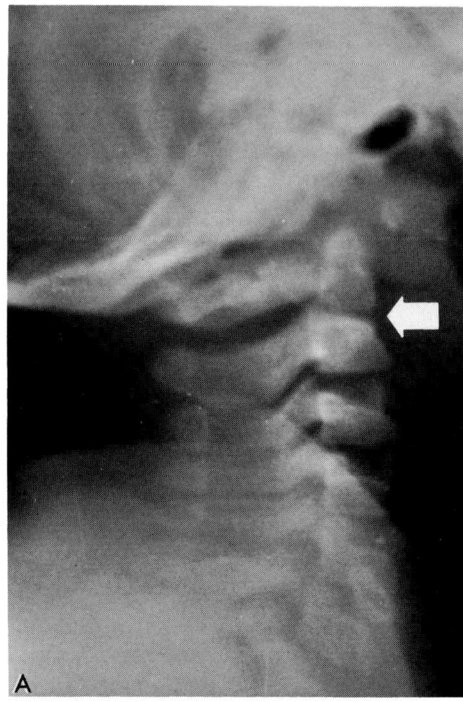

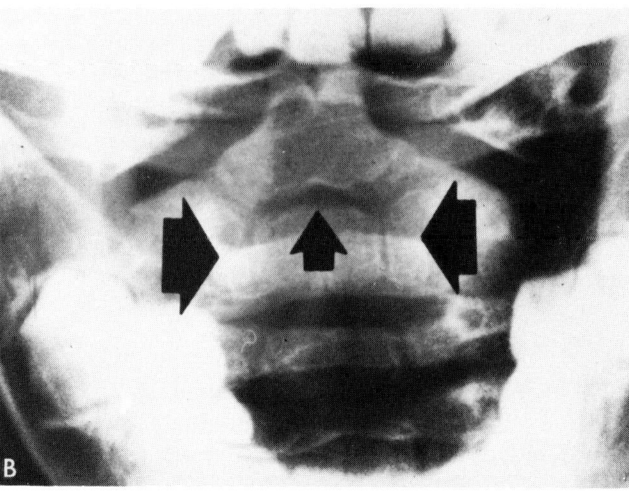

Figure 10–16. *A,* A 6-month-old infant. The odontoid is normally formed and recognizable on routine roentgenograms at birth but is separated from the body of the axis by a broad cartilaginous band *(arrow),* similar in appearance to an epiphyseal plate. It represents the vestigial disc space and is referred to as the neurocentral synchondrosis. *B,* The neurocentral synchondrosis is not at the anatomic base of the dens, at the level of the superior articular facets of the axis. This open-mouth view demonstrates that the embryologic base of the odontoid is below the articular facets and contributes a substantial portion to the body of the axis. The odontoid appears to fit like a cork in a bottle, lying sandwiched between the neural arches. This radiolucent line is present in nearly all children at age 3 years and in 50 per cent by age 4; it is absent in most by age 6.

two sources. The vertebral arteries provide both an anterior and a posterior ascending artery that arise at the level of C3 and pass ventral and dorsal to the body of the axis and the odontoid, anastomosing in an apical arcade in the region of the alar ligaments. These arteries supply small penetrating branches to the body of the axis and the odontoid. Lateral to the apex of the odontoid, the anterior ascending arteries and apical arcade receive anastomotic derivatives from the carotids by way of the base of the skull and the alar ligaments. This curious arrangement of the blood supply is necessary because of the embryologic development and anatomic function of the odontoid. The transient neurocentral synchondrosis between the odontoid and the axis prevents the development of any significant vascular channels between the two structures. The body of the odontoid is surrounded entirely by synovial joint cavities, and its fixed position relative to the rotation of the atlas precludes vascularization by direct branches from the vertebral arteries at the C1 segmental level.

Etiology and Pathogenesis

A congenital etiology for the os odontoideum has been assumed, and two theories have been advanced: (1) failure of fusion of the apex or ossiculum terminale to the odontoid—this is unlikely, because the fragment is too small and never approximates the size of the os odontoideum; (2) failure of fusion of the odontoid to the axis—this too is doubtful, as one would expect a crater or depression of C2, since a substantial portion of C2 is derived from the odontoid, and this has not been reported. Rather, there is more often an associated short, stubby projection or hypoplastic odontoid remnant in the area of the odontoid base.[33, 50] Hypoplasia and os odontoideum can be acquired secondary to trauma or, rarely, infection.[1, 11, 13, 15, 30, 39, 50] Several cases of "os odontoideum" that developed several years after trauma when a normal odontoid was initially present have been reported (Fig. 10–17).[11, 13, 15, 17] Most patients have a significant episode of trauma before the diagnosis of os odontoideum.[15]

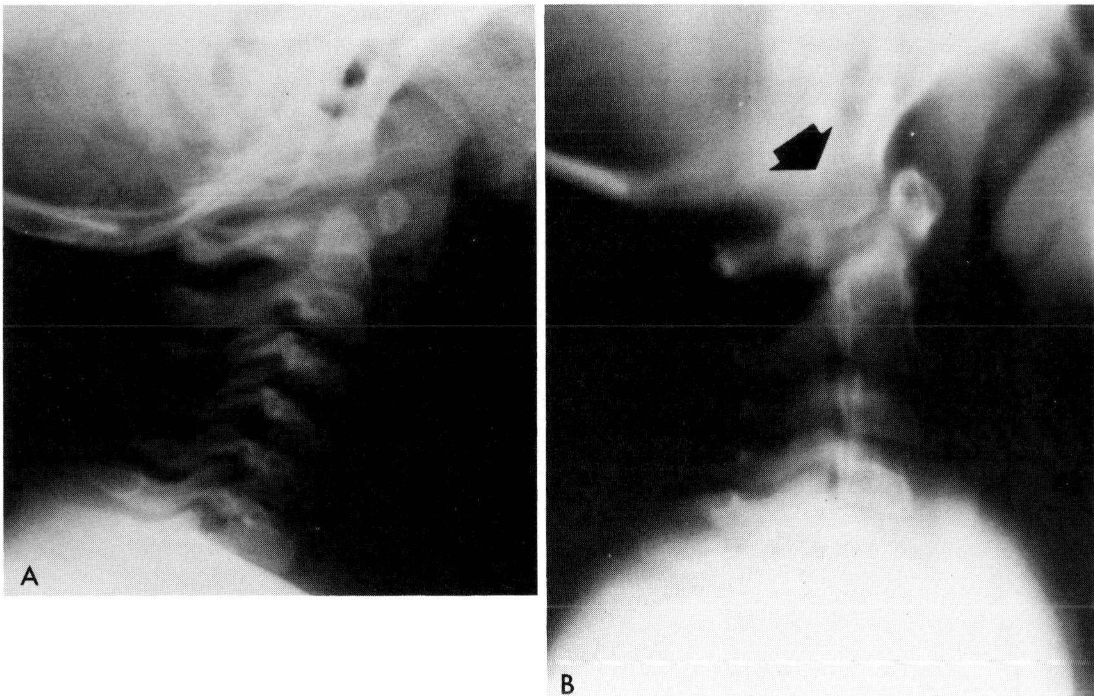

Figure 10–17. *A*, A 5-year-old male who at age 2 years fell from a couch. Lateral roentgenogram demonstrates a normal-appearing odontoid and cervical spine. He complained of pain in the neck and occiput and presented with torticollis. Symptoms and signs gradually resolved over one month. *B*, The child was asymptomatic until age 5, when over a period of six months he developed increasing neck pain and stiffness without neurologic complaints or findings. Roentgenograms revealed an os odontoideum and 7 mm of flexion-extension motion. The patient subsequently underwent C1–C2 stabilization.

Fielding and associates suggested that the great weight of evidence favors an unrecognized fracture in the region of the base of the odontoid as the most common cause, and less often a congenital origin.[15] They postulated that after fracture of the odontoid there may be only slight separation of the fragments, but with time contracture of the alar ligaments, which attach to the tip of the odontoid, exert a distraction force that pulls the fragment away from the base and closer to their origin at the occiput (Fig. 10–18). The blood supply to the odontoid is precarious, because it passes up along the sides of the odontoid, is easily traumatized, and contributes to poor fracture healing or callus formation that may retard retraction of the fragment. The position of the odontoid adjacent to the ring of C1 is maintained by the intact transverse atlantal ligament. The blood supply to the fragment is maintained by the proximal arterial arcade, from the carotid to the alar ligaments, and may be sufficient to maintain only a portion of the odontoid. Similarly, the blood supply to the proximal portion of the odontoid can be interrupted by excessive traction on these ligaments.[15]

It is probable that both congenital and posttraumatic forms of hypoplasia and os odontoideum exist. It is thought that failure of fusion of the apex of the odontoid (derived from the proatlas) to the main body of the atlas (derived from the first cervical sclerotome) results in the congenital form of os odontoideum.

The free ossicle of the os odontoideum usually appears fixed to the anterior arch of the atlas and moves with it in flexion and extension (see Fig. 10–6). Instability can reduce the SAC but not the ADI.[26] The instability may be predominantly anterior or posterior or grossly unstable in all directions.[14, 15] In a group of patients requiring surgery, the average displacement was 11.0 mm.

There is controversy regarding the presence of associated bony anomalies in the area of the hypoplastic dens or os odontoideum. In

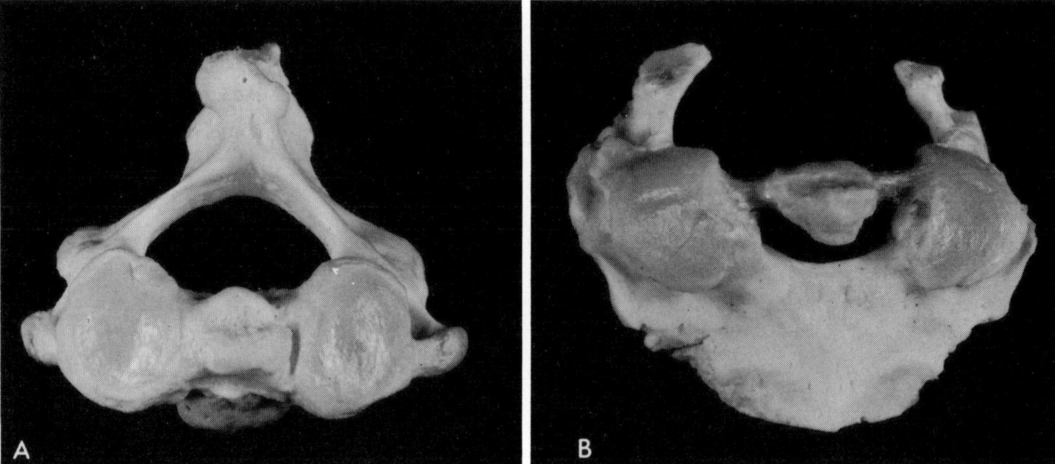

Figure 10–18. *A,* Anatomic specimen of an os odontoideum from a 17-year-old male with multiple congenital anomalies who died from renal disease. The previous bony attachment of the odontoid to the axis was rough and blunted. There was a fibrocartilate pseudarthrosis between the os odontoideum and C2. *B,* The occiput and occipital joints, with the os odontoideum suspended between the facets. The transverse ligament was intact but loosened during the preparation of the specimen. The alar ligaments remain attached to the tip of the os odontoideum. They are shortened and appear to have pulled the residual odontoid tip closer to their origin on the occiput. The os odontoideum was firmly attached by soft tissue to the occiput and ring of C1 and moved freely with these structures on C2. The foramen magnum is incomplete posteriorly. The posterior ring of C1 (not pictured) was intact and otherwise normal in its appearance. The spinal cord was narrowed and attenuated at the level of C1.

our experience, these changes are occasionally present, but with improved awareness they will undoubtedly be found more often. The posterior arch of C1 may be hypoplastic while the anterior arch is hypertrophied.[19, 21] If the posterior ring of C1 is narrow and there is abnormal anterior displacement of C1, there is less available space for the cord, and hence an increased danger of neurologic sequelae.

Clinical Features

Patients may present clinically with no symptoms, local neck symptoms, transitory episodes of paresis after trauma, or frank myelopathy secondary to cord compression.[25, 48] Minor trauma is commonly associated with the onset of symptoms, often of sufficient degree to warrant radiologic evaluation of the cervical spine. Symptoms may be mechanical, owing to local irritation of the atlantoaxial articulation, such as neck pain, torticollis, or headache. Neurologic symptoms are due to C1–C2 displacement and spinal cord compression. An important factor differentiating os odontoideum from other anomalies of the occipitovertebral junction is that these patients seldom have symptoms referable to cranial nerves,[34] as the area of the spinal cord impingement is below the foramen magnum.

If the clinical manifestations are limited to neck pain and torticollis (local joint irritation) without neurologic involvement (40 per cent of cases),[23] the prognosis is excellent.[15, 29, 34, 40] Similarly, patients who exhibit only transient weakness of the extremities and dysesthesia after trauma usually have complete return of function. However, those in whom there is an insidious onset and slowly progressive neurologic impairment have a greater potential for permanent deficit.[3, 15] Sudden death has been reported.[41] Damage may be mixed, with involvement of both the anterior and posterior spinal cord structures. Weakness and ataxia are more common complaints than is sensory loss. However, spasticity, increased deep tendon reflexes, clonus, loss of proprioception, and sphincter disturbances in various combinations have all been described.

A few patients may have symptoms and signs of cerebral and brain stem ischemia, seizures, mental deterioration, syncope, vertigo, and visual disturbances.[14, 16, 40, 42] In these patients there typically is a paucity of cervical spinal cord signs and symptoms, and it is presumed that they are experiencing vertebral artery compression at the foramen magnum or just below it. Thus, the diagnosis can be confusing, and many patients are misdiagnosed or thought to have progressive neurologic illness. Whenever a diagnosis of Friedreich's ataxia, multiple sclerosis, or other unexplained neurologic complaints is encountered, survey of the occipitocervical junction is suggested.

Roentgenographic Features

Recommended roentgenographic views are open-mouth, anteroposterior, and lateral, in addition to tomography, flexion-extension or CT reconstructions.[4] Tomograms are of value because plain films do not always show the anomaly or the extent of motion (Figs. 10–6, 10–19).

Cineradiography has been valuable for understanding odontoid anomalies, particularly those that cause atlantoaxial instability, but owing to high radiation exposure it has been largely replaced by CT in flexion and extension and CT reconstruction.[28, 38] Most children with these lesions have a predominance of either anterior or posterior instability, but these can exist together. Myelography is seldom necessary, because the pathology is usually obvious.

Normal Variations

At birth the normal odontoid can be visualized in the lateral view with its epiphyseal plate (see Fig. 10–16). A mistaken impression of hypoplasia may be given by a lateral extension roentgenogram, because the anterior arch of the atlas may slide upward and actually protrude beyond the ossified tip of the dens, especially in very young patients.

Agenesis or Hypoplasia of Odontoid

This extremely rare anomaly may be recognized from birth onward and is best seen in the open-mouth view, sometimes difficult to obtain in infancy (see Fig. 10–15). The diagnostic feature is the absence of the basilar portion of the odontoid, which normally dips down into and contributes to the body of the axis. This basilar portion is well below the level of the superior articular facets of the axis. The lateral view is of little help in distinguishing this anomaly from hypoplasia.

The most common form of hypoplasia presents with a short, stubby peg of odontoid projecting just above the lateral facet articulations (see Fig. 10–15). Tomography is necessary to confirm whether an os odontoideum is present in addition to the hypoplasia.

In patients with multiple anomalies, the usual roentgenographic views are not always reliable in confirming the presence or absence of an odontoid. Similarly, in patients with abnormal bone, such as in Morquio's syndrome and spondyloepiphyseal dysplasia,[25] the odontoid may be present but dysplastic, blending with the surrounding abnormal bone, and cannot be differentiated (Fig. 10–19*A*). In these situations, good results have been obtained by using lateral laminagraphic techniques (Fig. 10–19*B, C*). When the exact cut at the level of the odontoid is determined, it is repeated in flexion and extension to ascertain the stability of the atlantoaxial articulation. The extension view should not be ignored. Many patients have been found with significant posterior subluxation.[15, 19] Giannestras and associates reported a youngster who became quadriparetic from prolonged hyperextension while lying prone watching television.[19]

Os Odontoideum

In os odontoideum, there is a jointlike articulation between the odontoid and the body of the axis, which appears radiologically as a wide radiolucent gap (see Fig. 10–15*B, C*). This gap may be confused with the normal neurocentral synchondrosis (see Fig. 10–16) before age 5 years. Therefore, in children the diagnosis of os odontoideum is confirmed by demonstrating motion between the odontoid and the body of the axis. In adults the diagnosis of os odontoideum is suggested by observing a radiolucent defect between the dens and the body of the axis. However, the radiologic appearance of the condition may be similar to a traumatic nonunion, and frequently they cannot be differentiated.[30, 50] In os odontoideum the gap between the free ossicle and the axis usually extends above the level of the superior facets and is wide with a smooth edge. The ossicle is usually approximately one half the normal size of the odontoid and is round or oval in shape, and the cortex is of uniform thickness. In traumatic nonunion the gap between the fragments is characteristically narrow and irregular

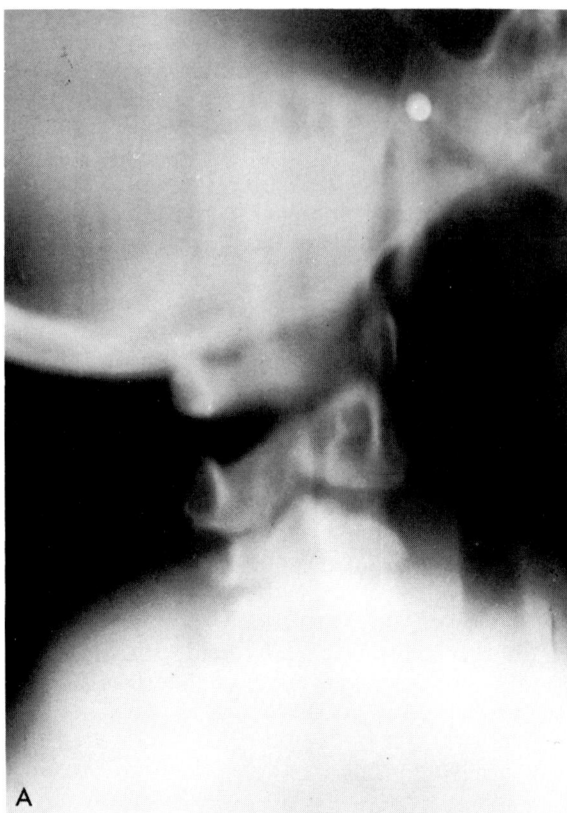

Figure 10–19. *A*, A 7-year-old with the diagnosis of spondyloepiphyseal dysplasia. *A*, The patient was discovered to have an absent odontoid. Lateral laminagraphic views demonstrate a stable atlantoaxial articulation in *B*, extension, and *C*, flexion. The patient is neurologically normal.

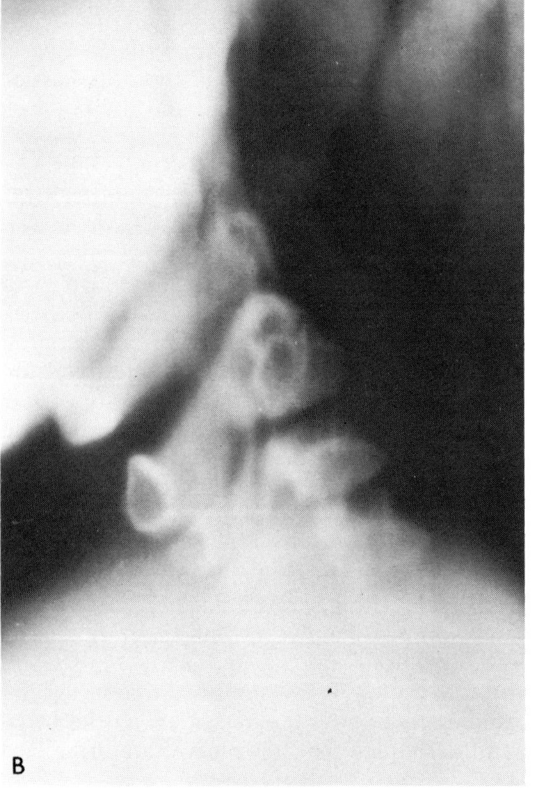

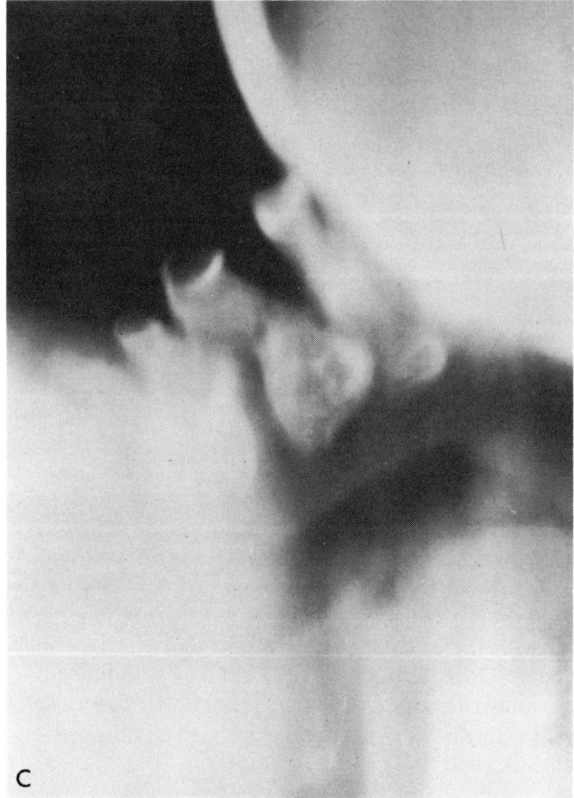

and frequently extends into the body of the axis below the level of the superior facets of the axis. The bone fragments appear to "match" and there is no marginal cortex at the level of the fracture or the rounded-off appearance found with os odontoideum.[39] Laminagrams may be helpful in determining these subtle differences. The odontoid ossicle is fixed firmly to the anterior ring of the atlas and moves with it in flexion, extension, and lateral slide. The anterior portion of the atlas is usually hypertrophied and the posterior portion of the ring may be hypoplastic or absent.[15, 34]

Recommended roentgenographic views are the open-mouth and lateral flexion-extension views. Lateral laminagrams or CT reconstructions are indicated when routine views are not satisfactory in demonstrating the anomaly. Lateral flexion-extension stress views should be conducted voluntarily by patients, particularly those with a neurologic deficit. The degree of anteroposterior displacement of the atlas on the axis should be documented (Fig. 10–20). The os odontoideum will move with the ring of C1, and consequently measurements of its relationship to C1 are of little value. Measurements can be made using a line projected superiorly from the posterior border of the body of the axis to a line projected inferiorly from the posterior border of the anterior arch of the atlas. Measurements greater than 3 mm should be considered pathologic. Most symptomatic patients exhibit significant instability.[15] In a large series reported

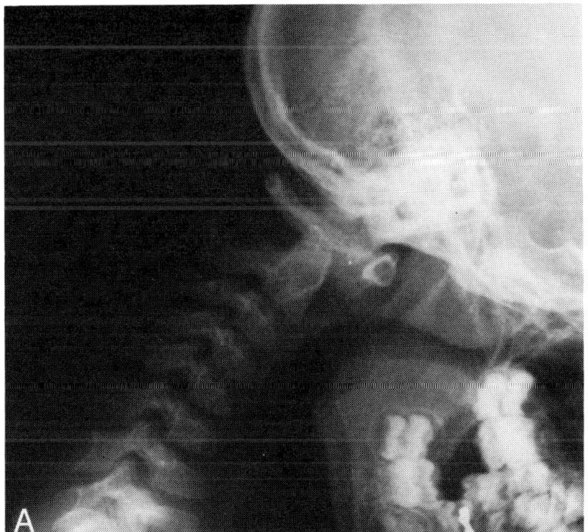

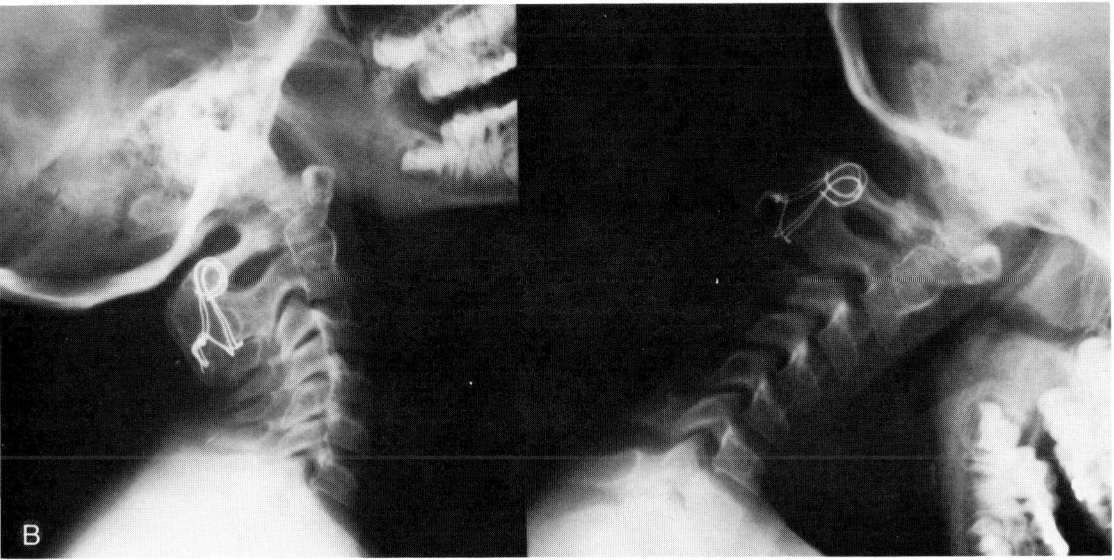

Figure 10–20. A 7-year-old had a one-year history of peculiar posturing and stiffness of the neck. *A,* Flexion roentgenograms demonstrated an os odontoideum, and subluxation of C1–C2. The degree of anteroposterior displacement of the atlas on the axis should be documented. The os odontoideum will move with the ring of C1, and consequently measurements of its relationship to C1 are of little value. Measurements can be made using a line projected inferiorly from the posterior border of the anterior arch of the atlas. *B, C,* Extension and flexion roentgenograms after posterior stabilization. Reduction must be accomplished before surgery, and if wire stabilization is selected, care must be taken to avoid further flexion of the neck during surgery.

by Fielding and associates, the average was 1 cm; most were either anterior or posterior, but some were unstable in all directions.[15] Posteriorly, the lumen of the spinal canal or the SAC should be determined (see Figs. 10–5, 10–6).

Treatment

Patients with congenital anomalies of the odontoid lead a precarious existence. The concern is that a trivial insult superimposed on an already weakened and compromised structure may be catastrophic. It is our experience that patients with these problems either have or develop gross atlantoaxial instability, and with it the possibility of progressive myelopathies, or even death.

Patients with local symptoms or transient myelopathies may expect recovery, at least temporarily.[29, 34, 40] Cervical traction or immobilization may be helpful in such circumstances. Surgical stabilization is indicated if there is neurologic involvement (even if transient), if there is instability of 10 mm or more in flexion and extension, if there is progressive instability, or if there are persistent neck complaints associated with atlantoaxial instability.

Considerable controversy exists over the role of prophylactic stabilization in asymptomatic patients with instability.[18, 20, 29, 34] The safety of stability, and with it the ability to lead a normal active life, must cause one to weigh the possible complications of surgery against the catastrophic dangers of instability with secondary cord pressure. In the pediatric age group, it may be difficult or impossible to curtail activity, even in the presence of marked instability.[14, 15, 43] If possible, reduction of the atlantoaxial articulation must be accomplished before surgery either by careful positioning of the patient or by skull traction. Open reduction during surgery is discouraged, as it has proved extremely hazardous and may result in respiratory distress, apnea, or death.[18] Ideally the patient should be maintained in the reduced position one to two weeks before surgery to allow recovery of neurologic function and to lessen spinal cord irritation. When fusion is undertaken, regardless of the indication, preoperative halo traction is often required to achieve reduction, which may have to be continued during surgery and postoperatively until transfer to a suitable immobilization device.[22, 34]

The suggested method of stabilization is posterior cervical fusion of C1–C2, employing wire fixation and an iliac bone graft (Fig. 10–20). This is not without risk, as slight flexion is often required to pass the wire beneath the posterior ring of the atlas, and it can have tragic results.[34] In the patient with a marginally functioning neurologic status, it may be wiser to perform an occiput to C2 arthrodesis and plan to maintain immobilization in extension during the postoperative period.[34] In this regard, the halo-cast is helpful. Incomplete development of the posterior ring of C1 is uncommon but is reported to occur with increased frequency in patients with os odontoideum.[15] The completeness of the C1 arch should be evaluated preoperatively, as a large gap may preclude wire fixation. If wire fixation is employed, excessive tightening of the wire should be avoided. The articulation is frequently unstable in both flexion and extension, and posterior dislocations may occur owing to overcorrection, with disastrous results.

Patients in whom the C1–C2 dislocation is unreducible after an adequate trial of traction pose a difficult management problem.[9] In this situation, posterior decompression by laminectomy has been associated with increased morbidity and mortality.[34] In addition, posterior decompression alone may potentiate C1–C2 instability, and if performed must be accompanied by occiput to C2 arthrodesis.[9, 15] For patients with no neurologic deficit, a simple in situ posterior fusion is the least hazardous procedure. If reduction of the C1–C2 dislocation is considered necessary or if the clinical situation precludes posterior stabilization, an anterior approach should be considered.[21, 49] The lateral retropharyngeal approach described by Whitesides and McDonald has provided anterior exposure of the C1–C2 articulation adequate to perform decompression, reduction, and stabilization.[49] This route is preferred to the transoral or mandibular and tongue-splitting approaches, which are associated with an increased incidence of infection.[49]

A common clinical problem is differentiation between a fractured odontoid and os odontoideum. Discovery is usually made after trauma in both conditions, and an accurate diagnosis may not be possible by roentgenographic techniques alone. In this situation a period of immobilization (skull traction or cast) is recommended. Overdistraction, particularly in children, should be avoided, because it can lead to os odontoideum.[15] If the lesion represents an acute fracture, healing usually occurs. If a congenital or traumatic nonunion is present, surgical stabilization will be necessary if atlantoaxial instability is demonstrated.

Summary

Anomalous development of the odontoid is uncommon, and its clinical significance lies in its potential to produce serious neurologic sequelae due to atlantoaxial instability. Although there are several recognized variations (aplasia, hypoplasia, and os odontoideum), clinically they share the same signs and symptoms, and treatment is identical. Symptoms are usually due to instability of the atlantoaxial joint, with compression of the spinal cord anteriorly against the axis or posteriorly from the ring of the atlas. Patients may present with no symptoms, persistent neck complaints, or transient or permanent neurologic deficits or may die suddenly. Symptoms from cranial nerve irritation seldom occur, but symptoms of cerebral and brain stem ischemia are occasionally noted owing to compression of the vertebral arteries in the area of the atlas.

If the condition is suspected, the diagnosis can usually be confirmed on lateral flexion-extension roentgenograms. Special techniques are often required, particularly lateral flexion-extension laminagrams. Flexion-extension stress roentgenograms are often necessary to determine the presence and degree of atlantoaxial instability.

The role of prophylactic surgical stabilization is not yet established. If marked instability is demonstrated or if there are clinical findings of neurologic compromise, there is general agreement that surgical fusion should be performed. Operative reduction should be avoided, and preoperative correction by traction or positioning is preferred. Posterior surgical stabilization of the first and second cervical vertebrae is sufficient, if this can be accomplished without further flexing the head. In this situation, occiput to C2 stabilization is recommended to avoid all possibility of further neurologic trauma during the procedure.

References

Anomalies of Odontoid

1. Ahlback, I., and Collert, S.: Destruction of the odontoid process due to axial pyogenic spondylitis. Acta Radiol. [Diagn.] (Stockh.) *10:*394, 1970.
2. Bailey, D. K.: The normal cervical spine in infants and children. Radiology *59:*712, 1962.
3. Basset, F. H., and Goldner, J. L.: Aplasia of the odontoid process. Proc. A.A.O.S. *50A:*833, 1968.
4. Burke, S. W., French, H. G., Roberts, J. M., et al.: Chronic atlanto-axial instability in Down syndrome. J. Bone Joint Surg. *67A:*1356, 1985.
5. Caffey, J.: Pediatric X-ray Diagnosis. Chicago, Year Book Medical Publishers, 1967.
6. Cattell, J. S., and Filtzer, D. L.: Pseudosubluxation and other normal variations in the cervical spine in children. J. Bone Joint Surg. *47A:*1295, 1965.
7. Curtis, B. H., Blank, S., and Fisher, R. L.: Atlantoaxial dislocation in Down's syndrome. J.A.M.A. *205:*464, 1968.
8. Dzenitis, A. J.: Spontaneous atlantoaxial dislocation in a mongoloid child with spinal cord compression. Case report. J. Neurosurg. *25:*458, 1966.
9. Dyck, P.: Os odontoideum in children: neurological manifestations and surgical management. Neurosurgery *2:*93, 1978.
10. Evarts, C. M., and Lonsdale, D.: Ossiculum terminale—an anomaly of the odontoid process: report of a case of atlantoaxial dislocation with cord compression. Cleve. Clin. Q. *37:*73, 1970.
11. Fielding, J. W.: Disappearance of the central portion of the odontoid process. J. Bone Joint Surg. *47A:*1228, 1965.
12. Fielding, J. W.: The cervical spine in the child. Curr. Pract. Orthop. Surg. *5:*31, 1973.
13. Fielding, J. W., and Griffin, P. O.: Os odontoideum: an acquired lesion. J. Bone Joint Surg. *56A:*187, 1974.
14. Fielding, J. W., Hawkins, R. J., and Ratzan, S.: Fusion for atlantoaxial instability. J. Bone Joint Surg. *58A:*400, 1976.
15. Fielding, J. W., Hensinger, R. N., and Hawkins, R. J.: Os odontoideum. J. Bone Joint Surg. *62A:*376, 1980.
16. Ford, F. K.: Syncope, vertigo, and disturbances of vision resulting from intermittent obstruction of the vertebral arteries due to a defect in the odontoid process and excessive mobility of the axis. Bull. John Hopkins Hosp. *91:*168, 1952.
17. Freiberger, R. H., Wilson, P. D., Jr., and Nicholas, J. A.: Acquired absence of the odontoid process. J. Bone Joint Surg. *47A:*1231, 1965.
18. Garber, J. N.: Abnormalities of the atlas and axis vertebrae. J. Bone Joint Surg. *46A:*17892, 1964.
19. Giannestras, J. J., Mayfield, F. H., Provencio, F. P., and Maurer, J.: Congenital absence of the odontoid process. J. Bone Joint Surg. *46A:*839, 1964.
20. Gillman, C. L.: Congenital absence of the odontoid process of the axis: report of a case. J. Bone Joint Surg. *41A:*340, 1959.
21. Greenberg, A. D.: Atlantoaxial dislocations. Brain *91:*644, 1968.
22. Greenberg, A. D., Scovillo, W. B., and Davey, L. M.: Transoral decompression of atlantoaxial dislocation due to odontoid hypoplasia: report of two cases. J. Neurosurg. *28:*266, 1968.
23. Gwinn, J. L., and Smith, J. L.: Acquired and congenital absence of the odontoid process. Am. J. Roentgenol. Radium Ther. Nucl. Med. *88:*424, 1962.
24. Hensinger, R. N., Lang, J. R., and MacEwen, G. D.: The Klippel-Feil syndrome: a constellation of related anomalies. J. Bone Joint Surg. *56A:*1246, 1974.

25. Hensinger, R. N.: Osseous anomalies of the craniovertebral junction. Spine *11*:323, 1986.
26. Locke, G. R., Gardner, J. I., and Van Epps, E. F.: Atlas-dens interval (ADI) in children: a survey based on 200 normal cervical spines. Am. J. Roentgenol. *97*:135, 1966.
27. Macalister, A.: Notes on the development and variations of the atlas. J. Anat. Physiol. *27*:519, 1982.
28. McAfee, P. C., Bohlman, H. H., Han, J. S., and Salvagno, R. T.: Comparison of nuclear magnetic resonance imaging and computed tomography in the diagnosis of upper cervical spinal cord compression. Spine *11*:295, 1986.
29. McKeever, F. M.: Atlantoaxial instability. Surg. Clin. North Am. *48*:1375, 1968.
30. McRae, D. L.: Bony abnormalities in the region of the foramen magnum: correlation of the anatomic and neurologic findings. Acta Radiol. *40*:335, 1953.
31. McRae, D. L.: The significance of abnormalities of the cervical spine. Am. J. Roentgenol. Radium Ther. Nucl. Med. *84*:3, 1960.
32. Martel, W., and Fishler, J. M.: Observation of the spine in mongoloidism. Am. J. Roentgenol. Radium Ther. Nucl. Med. *97*:630, 1966.
33. Michaels, L., Prevost, M. J., and Crong, D. F.: Pathological changes in a case of os odontoideum (separate odontoid process). J. Bone Joint Surg. *51A*:965, 1969.
34. Minderhoud, J. M., Braakman, R., and Penning, L.: Os odontoideum: clinical, radiological, and therapeutic aspects. J. Neurol. Sci. *89*:521, 1969.
35. Pizzutillo, P. D., Woods, M. W., and Nicholson, L.: Risk factors in Klippel-Feil syndrome. Orthop. Trans. *11*:473, 1987.
36. Pueschel, S. M., and Scola, F. H.: Atlantoaxial instability in individuals with Down's syndrome: epidemiologic, radiographic, and clinical studies. Pediatrics *80*:555, 1987.
37. Ramenofsky, M. L., Buyse, M., Goldberg, M. J., and Leape, L.: Gastroesophageal reflux and torticollis. J. Bone Joint Surg. *60A*:1140, 1975.
38. Roach, J. W., Duncan, D., Wenger, D. R., et al.: Atlanto-axial instability and spinal cord compression in children. Diagnosis by computerized tomography. J. Bone Joint Surg. *66A*:708, 1984.
39. Rothman, R. H., and Simeone, F. A.: The Spine. Philadelphia, W. B. Saunders Co., 1982, 2nd ed.
40. Rowland, L. P., Shapiro, J. H., and Jacobson, H. G.: Neurological syndromes associated with congenital absence of the odontoid process. Arch. Neurol. Psychiatr. *80*:286, 1958.
41. Schiller, F., and Nieda, I.: Malformations of the odontoid process. Report of a case and clinical survey. Calif. Med. *86*:394, 1957.
42. Shapiro, R., Youngsberg, A. S., and Rothman, S. L. G.: The differential diagnosis of traumatic lesions of the occipito-atlanto-axial segment. Radiol. Clin. North Am. *3*:505, 1971.
43. Shepard, C. N.: Familial hypoplasia of the odontoid process. J. Bone Joint Surg. *48A*:1224, 1966.
44. Sherk, H. H., and Nicholson, J. L.: Ossiculum terminale and mongolism. J. Bone Joint Surg. *51A*:957, 1969.
45. Spitzer, R., Rabinowitch, J. Y., and Wybar, K. C.: Study of the abnormalities of the skull, teeth and lenses in mongolism. Can. Med. Assoc. J. *84*:567, 1961.
46. Stratford, J.: Myelopathy caused by atlantoaxial dislocation. J. Neurosurg. *14*:97, 1957.
47. Swischuk, L. E., Hayden, C. K., and Sarwar, M.: The posteriorly tilted dens. A normal variation mimicking a fractured dens. Pediatr. Radiol. *8*:27, 1979.
48. Wadia, N. H.: Myelopathy complicating congenital atlantoaxial dislocation (a study of 28 cases). Brain *90*:449, 1967.
49. Whitesides, T. E., and McDonald, A. P.: Lateral retropharyngeal approach to the upper cervical spine. Orthop. Clin. North Am. *9*:1115, 1978.
50. Wollin, D. G.: The os odontoideum: separate odontoid process. J. Bone Joint Surg. *45A*:1459, 1963.

KLIPPEL-FEIL SYNDROME (CONGENITAL SYNOSTOSIS OF CERVICAL VERTEBRAE, BREVICOLLIS)

In 1912 Klippel and Feil[20] published the first complete description of the clinical aspects and pathology of this condition. Their attention was attracted to a patient with the unusual clinical findings of marked shortening of the neck, a low posterior hairline, and severe restriction of neck motion. The patient died, and at the postmortem they discovered a complete fusion of the cervical vertebrae. Subsequently, Feil was able to collect 13 additional examples and published a thesis in 1919[10] that included his findings from this larger group and a review of the literature. The term "Klippel-Feil syndrome" in its present usage refers to all patients with congenital fusion of the cervical vertebrae, whether it involves two segments, congenital block vertebrae (Fig. 10–21), or the entire cervical spine (Fig. 10–22). Feil originally suggested a system of classification based on the extent and type of the cervical fusion. However, with the exception of the area of genetics,[9, 13] this classification has not proved clinically useful. Instead, as additional patients were discovered and roentgenographic techniques improved, it became apparent that certain anomalies of the occipitocervical junction (see "Basilar Impression," "Atlanto-occipital Fusion," and "Anomalies of Odontoid") should be considered separately from the original syndrome. Although these conditions occur commonly in conjunction with fusion of the lower cervical vertebrae, their significance is dependent on how they influence the atlantoaxial joint. Their prognostic and therapeutic implications are distinctly

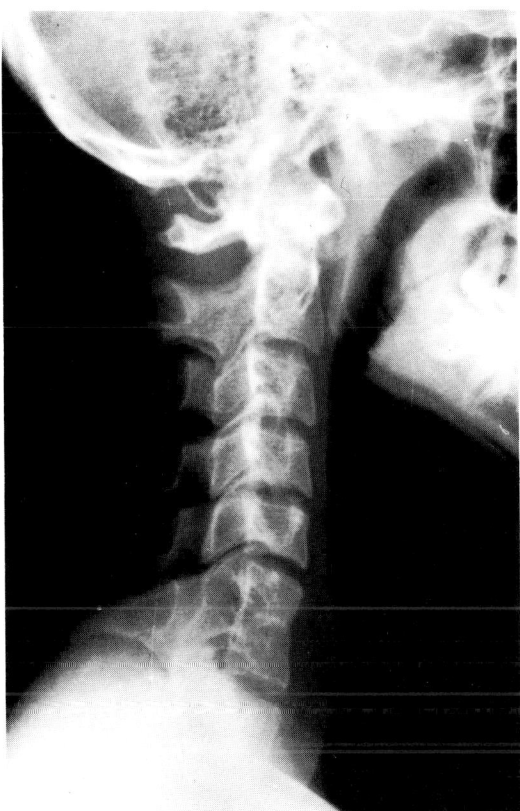

Figure 10–21. Congenital block vertebrae C6–C7. Symptoms are directly related to the number and level of involved vertebrae; thus, this represents the most benign form of the Klippel-Feil syndrome.

different, and they occur with sufficient frequency to warrant individual analysis.

Congenital cervical fusion is the result of failure of normal segmentation of the cervical somites during the third to eighth weeks of life. With the exception of a few patients in whom this condition is inherited,[13, 14] the etiology is as yet undetermined. It is important to note that the effect of this embryologic abnormality is not limited to the cervical spine: the entire fetus may be adversely affected. Patients with the Klippel-Feil syndrome, even those with minor cervical lesions, may have other less apparent or even occult defects in the genitourinary,[16, 24, 36] nervous,[3, 4] and cardiopulmonary systems,[2, 28, 32] and even hearing impairment.[16, 25, 34, 40] Many of these "hidden" abnormalities may be more detrimental to the patient's general well-being than the obvious deformity of the neck. In the review by Hensinger and associates,[16] a high incidence of related congenital anomalies was found (Table 10–1), emphasizing that all patients with the Klippel-Feil syndrome should be thoroughly investigated.

Clinical Features

The classical clinical description of the syndrome is a triad—low posterior hairline, short neck, and limitation of neck motion—but fewer than one half of the patients have all three signs (Figs. 10–23, 10–24).[16] The presence of these signs is directly related to the degree of cervical spine involvement. Clinically, the most consistent finding is limitation of neck motion.[13] However, if fewer than three vertebrae are fused or if only the lower cervical

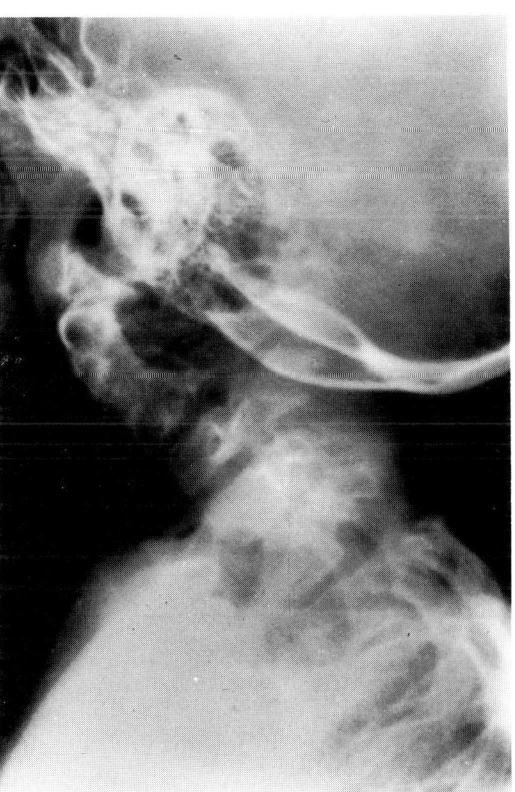

Figure 10–22. A 12-year-old female with the Klippel-Feil syndrome and iniencephaly: enlarged foramen magnum and absent posterior laminae. Note the fixed hyperextension and the long segment of cervical fusion (C2–C6) and an abnormal occipitocervical articulation. This pattern could be viewed as a more elaborate variation of the C2–C3 pattern of McRae. Flexion-extension and rotational forces are concentrated in the area of the abnormal occipitocervical junction. These patients may be at risk of developing instability with aging.

Table 10–1. ABNORMALITIES ASSOCIATED WITH THE KLIPPEL-FEIL SYNDROME

Common	Percentage
Scoliosis	60
Renal abnormalities	35
Sprengel's deformity	30
Deafness	30
Synkinesis	20
Congenital heart disease	14
Less Common	
Ptosis	
Duane's contracture	
Lateral rectus palsy	
Facial nerve palsy	
Syndactyly	
Hypoplastic thumb	
Upper extremity hypoplasia	

segments are fused, the patient generally has no detectable limitation.[13] In addition, many patients with marked cervical involvement are able to compensate with hypermobility at the unfused joints and to maintain a deceptively good range of motion.[16] Several of our patients have 90 degrees of flexion-extension, occurring at the only open interspace (Fig. 10–25). Generally, flexion-extension is better preserved than rotation or lateral bend. Rarely, patients have no detectable motion and fixed hyperextension of the neck; this is usually associated with iniencephaly (absence of the posterior cervical laminae and an enlarged foramen magnum) (see Fig. 10–22).[38]

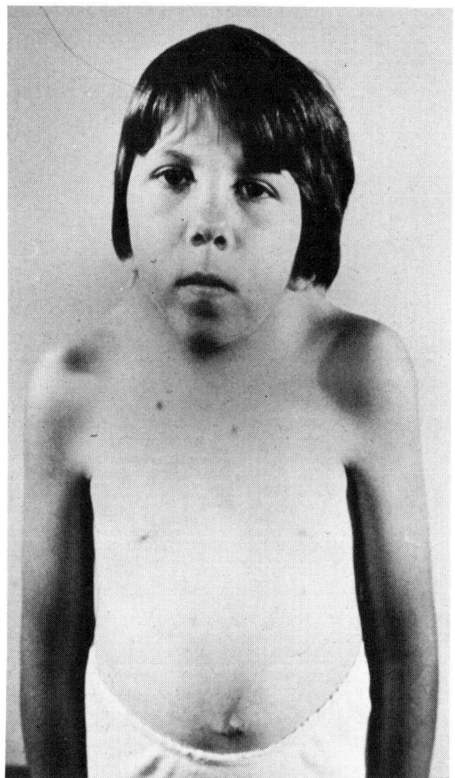

Figure 10–23. A 9-year-old with the Klippel-Feil syndrome, demonstrating short neck with a tendency to webbing, mild torticollis, and asymmetry of eye level. The patient clinically has marked restriction of neck motion, impaired hearing, and mirror motions (synkinesia) of the upper extremities.

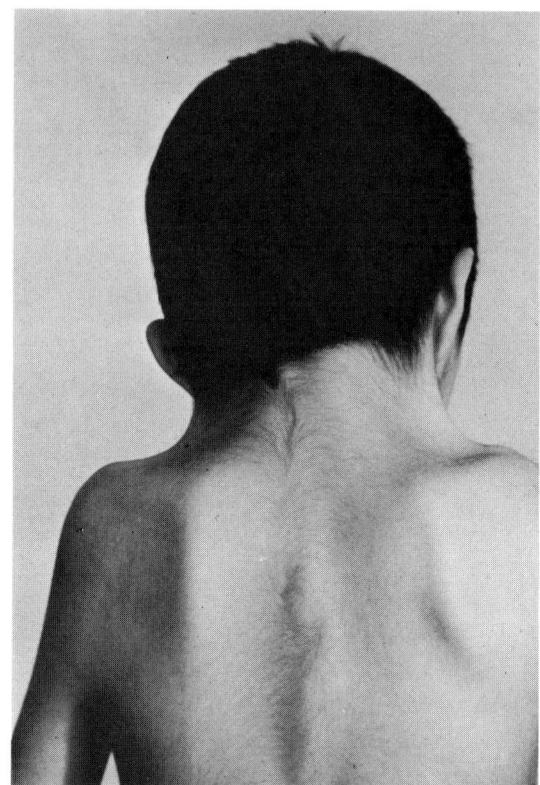

Figure 10–24. Extreme form of webbing of the neck, pterygium colli. Note the low posterior hairline.

Shortening of the neck, unless extreme, is a subtle finding. Similarly, the low posterior hairline is not constant (see Figs. 10–23, 10–24). Less than 20 per cent of patients with the Klippel-Feil syndrome have obvious facial asymmetry, torticollis, or webbing of the neck.[13, 16] When extreme, webbing of the neck is called "pterygium colli" and consists of large skin folds extending from the mastoid to the acromion (see Fig. 10–24).[12] The underlying muscles may be involved, but surgical release generally does not result in improved neck motion.

Sprengel's deformity occurs in 25 to 35 per

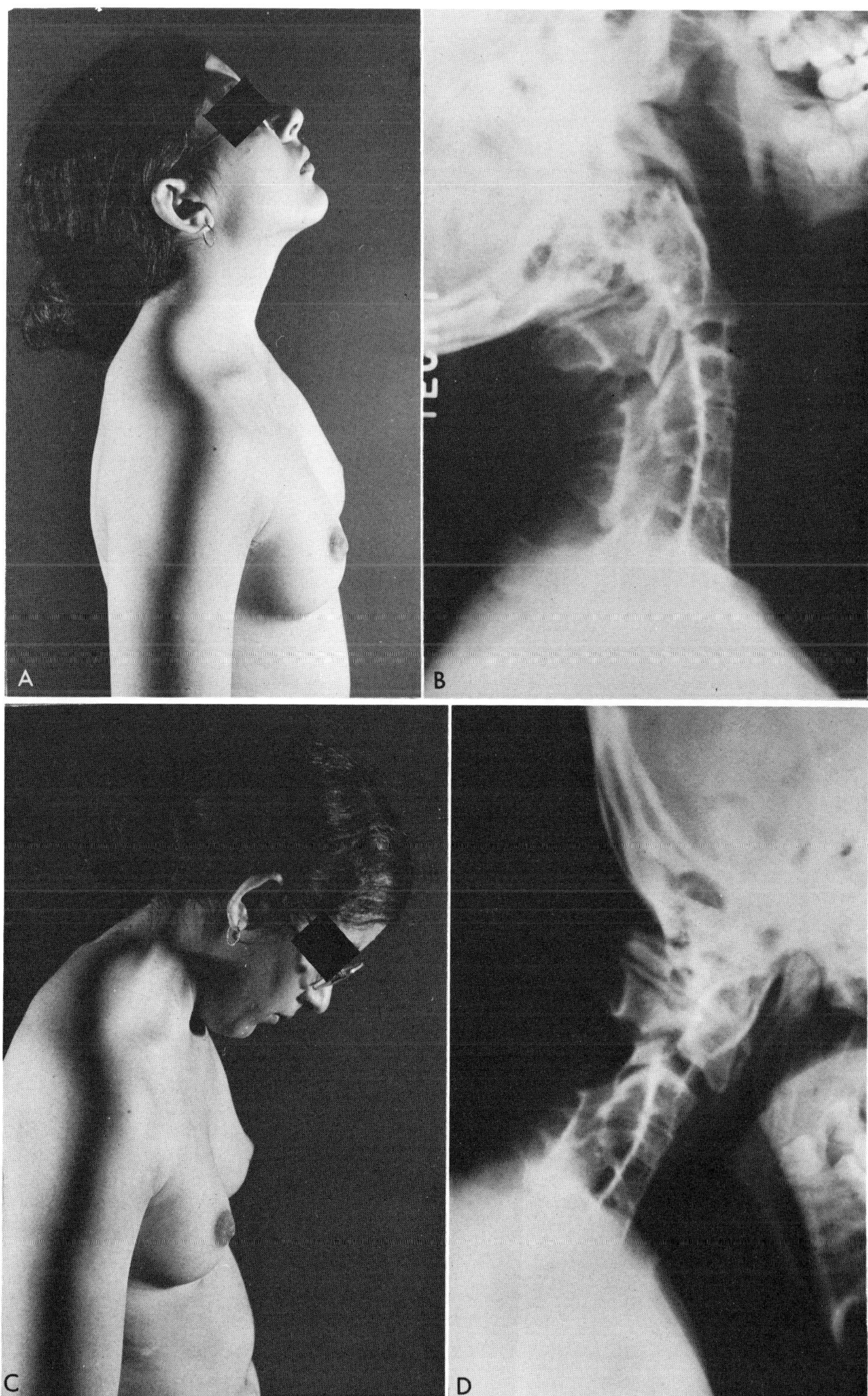

Figure 10–25. An 18-year-old female with the Klippel-Feil syndrome demonstrating flexion-extension of the cervical spine, both clinically *(A, C)* and radiologically *(B, D)*. Most of the neck motion is occurring at the C3–C4 disc space. Clinically the patient is able to maintain an adequate range (90 degrees) of flexion-extension. At present she is asymptomatic, but with aging this hypermobile articulation may become unstable.

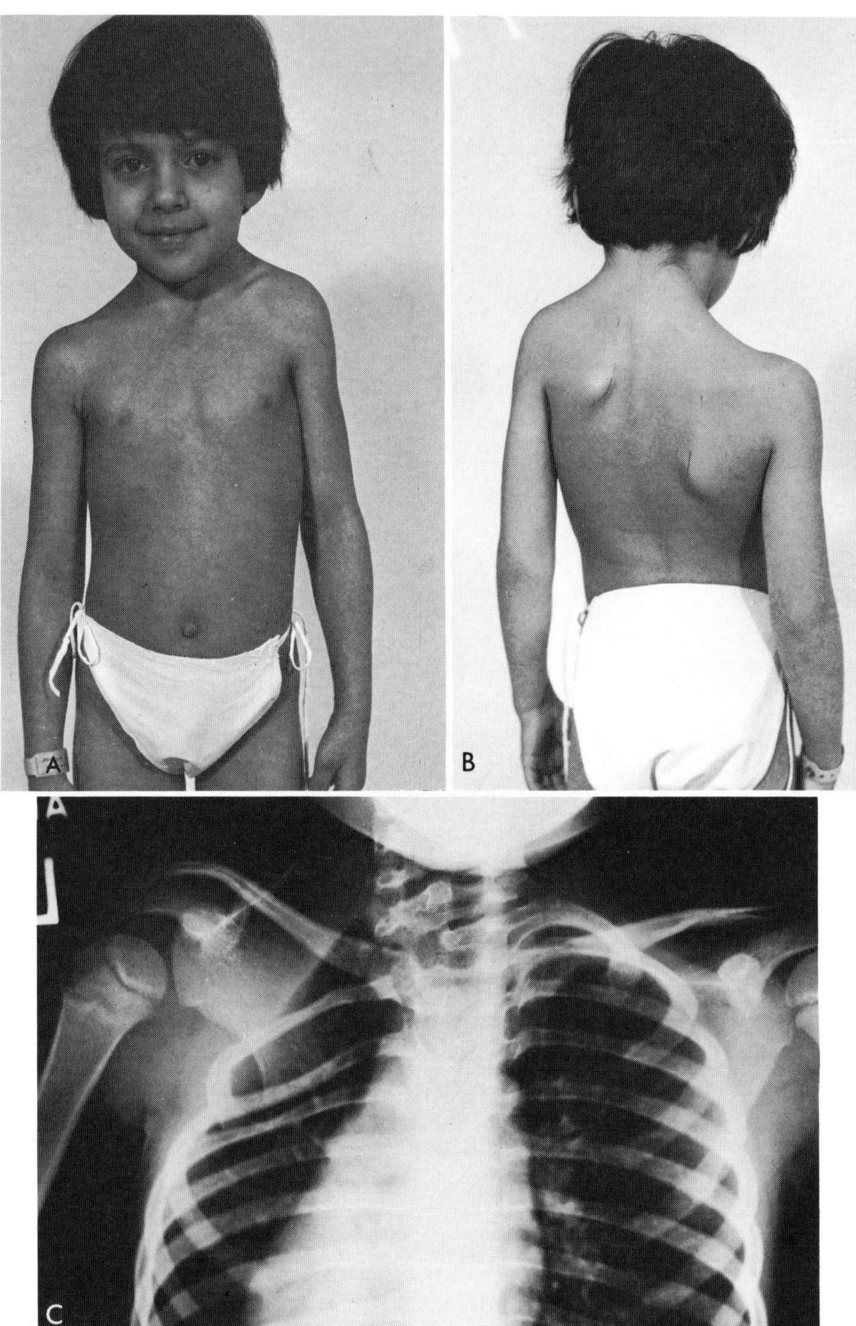

Figure 10–26. A 6-year-old with the Klippel-Feil syndrome and Sprengel's deformity on the left. *A*, Frontal view. *B*, Posterior view. *C*, Roentgenographic appearance demonstrating the posterior vertebral anomalies of the cervical spine and the high-riding left scapula. Patient subsequently had a left scapuloplasty.

cent unilaterally or bilaterally (Fig. 10–26).[9, 13, 16, 24, 39] At the third week of gestation, the scapula develops from mesodermal tissue high in the neck at the level of C4. It descends into the thoracic position by the eighth week, or approximately at the same time that the Klippel-Feil lesion is thought to occur.[9, 13] Therefore, it is logical to expect a significant relation between these two anomalies. Occasionally, there is a bony bridge between the cervical spine and scapula, an omovertebral bone. Its removal may permit an increase in neck and shoulder motion.

Probably for the same embryologic reasons, other clinical findings are occasionally found (Table 10–1): ptosis of the eye, Duane's contracture (contracture of the lateral rectus muscle),[13] lateral rectus palsy, facial nerve palsy, and a cleft or high-arched palate. Abnormalities of the upper extremities include syndactyly, hypoplastic thumb, supernumerary digits, and hypoplasia of the upper extremity. Abnormalities of the lower extremities are infrequent.

Symptoms

With the exception of the anomalies that involve the atlantoaxial joint, there are no symptoms that can be directly attributed to the fused cervical vertebrae. All symptoms commonly associated with the Klippel-Feil syndrome originate at the open segments where the remaining free articulations may become compensatorily hypermobile. Owing to the increased demands placed on these joints or in response to trauma, this hypermobility can lead to frank instability or early degenerative arthritis.[39] Symptoms may then arise from two sources: (1) mechanical symptoms due to irritation of the joint and (2) neurologic symptoms due to root irritation or spinal cord compression. Patients with a short-segment fusion are less likely to develop symptoms,[13] because the loss of motion is adequately compensated by the remaining free segments. Patients with synostosis of the lower cervical spine are at less risk, because the limitation is minimal and can be adequately compensated by the more normally mobile joints above. Most patients who develop symptoms are in the second or third decade of life,[13] suggesting that the instability is in part a function of time with increasing ligament laxity.

Neurologic symptoms are generally localized to the head, neck, and upper extremities and result from direct irritation or impingement of the cervical nerve roots with radicular symptoms in the upper extremities.[27] The symptoms can usually be localized to the hypermobile joints adjacent to the fused segments. There may be constriction and narrowing of the nerve root at the foramen from osteophytic spurring.[27] If joint instability is progressive or if there is appropriate trauma, the spinal cord may be involved to varying degrees, from mild spasticity, hyperreflexia, and muscular weakness to sudden complete quadriplegia after minor trauma.[11, 13, 17, 39]

Roentgenographic Features

In the severely involved child, an adequate roentgenographic evaluation can be difficult. Fixed bony deformities frequently prevent proper positioning, and overlapping shadows from the mandible, occiput, or foramen magnum may obscure the upper vertebrae (Fig. 10–27).

In this situation, flexion-extension laminagraphic views help provide the information necessary to assess stability. Another technique that has gained wide acceptance in the diagnosis of cervical instability is CT.[37] This technique coupled with flexion-extension of the cervical spine can delineate more precisely the presence or absence of spinal cord compression. This can be further enhanced by a contrast myelography. With MRI, the relationship between the bony elements and neurologic structures can be viewed directly in flexion and extension to show the origin of neural compression.[23] This is particularly helpful for patients who have abnormal bone such as in Morquio's disease.[22] With these techniques, the space available for the spinal cord can be measured directly rather than inferred by use of the atlas-dens interval.[23] Knowledge of the normal variations in cervical spine mobility, particularly in children, is important in evaluating patients with the Klippel-Feil syndrome.[6, 41] Pseudosubluxation of C2 on C3 with flexion can be observed in 45 per cent of normal children under 8 years of age (see Fig. 10–8).[6] Marked angulation at a single interspace during flexion, rather than a uniform arc of vertebral motion, can be observed in normal children (16 per cent)[7] and may be misinterpreted as vertebral fusion below.

Fusion of cervical vertebrae is the hallmark of the Klippel-Feil syndrome. This may be simply synostosis of two bodies (congenital

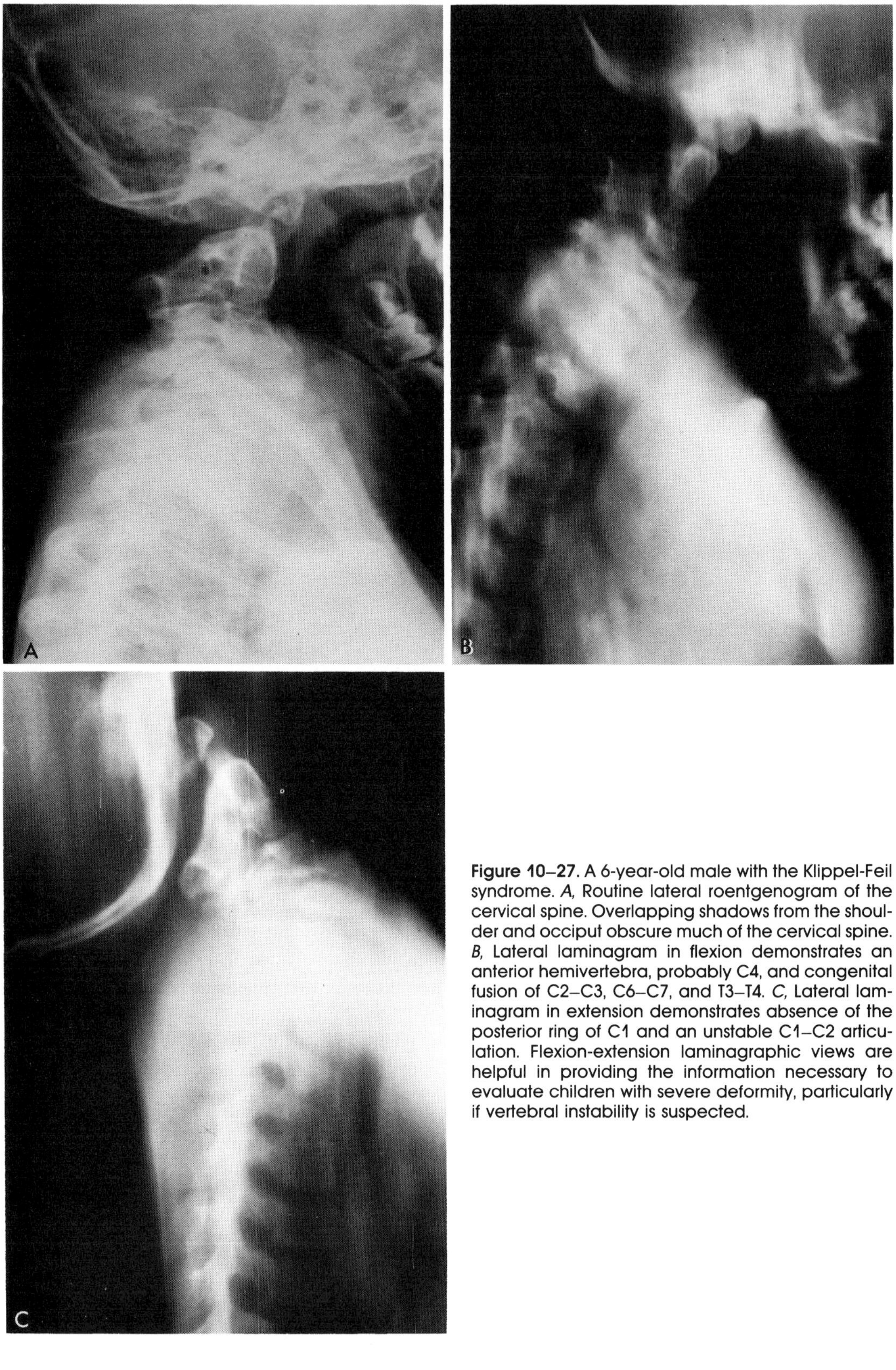

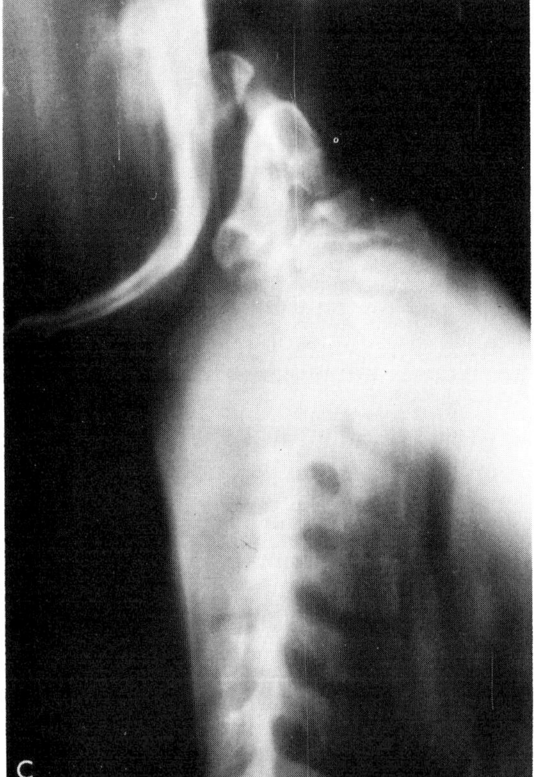

Figure 10–27. A 6-year-old male with the Klippel-Feil syndrome. *A*, Routine lateral roentgenogram of the cervical spine. Overlapping shadows from the shoulder and occiput obscure much of the cervical spine. *B*, Lateral laminagram in flexion demonstrates an anterior hemivertebra, probably C4, and congenital fusion of C2–C3, C6–C7, and T3–T4. *C*, Lateral laminagram in extension demonstrates absence of the posterior ring of C1 and an unstable C1–C2 articulation. Flexion-extension laminagraphic views are helpful in providing the information necessary to evaluate children with severe deformity, particularly if vertebral instability is suspected.

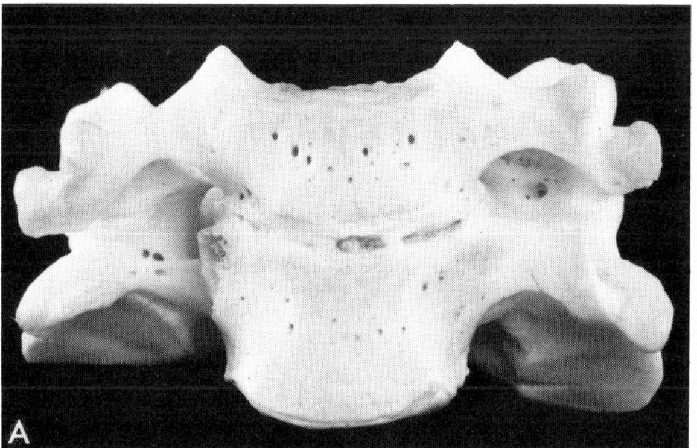

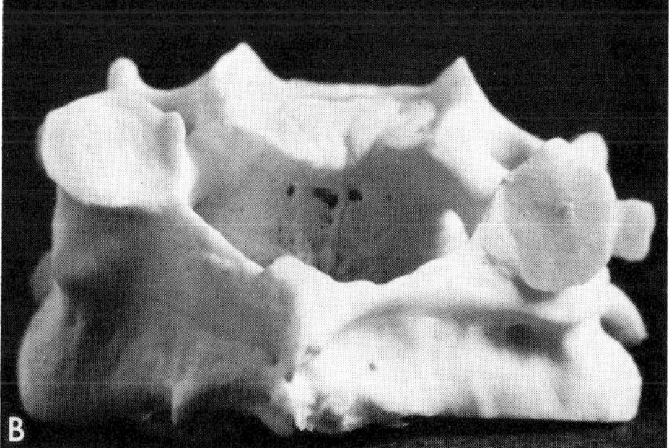

Figure 10–28. Postmortem specimen of a congenital block vertebra of C3–C4. *A,* Anterior view. *B,* Posterior view. The specimen demonstrates complete fusion, but remnants of the cartilaginous vertebral end plates can still be seen.

block vertebrae) (Figs. 10–21, 10–28) or massive fusion of vertebrae, which was found in Klippel and Feil's first patient (see Fig. 10–22).[20]

Aside from vertebral fusion, flattening and widening of the involved vertebral bodies and absent disc spaces are the most common findings. Hypoplasia of the disc space or remnants of it can often be seen (Fig. 10–28). In the young child, narrowing of the cervical disc space cannot always be appreciated, because the ossification of the vertebral body is in-

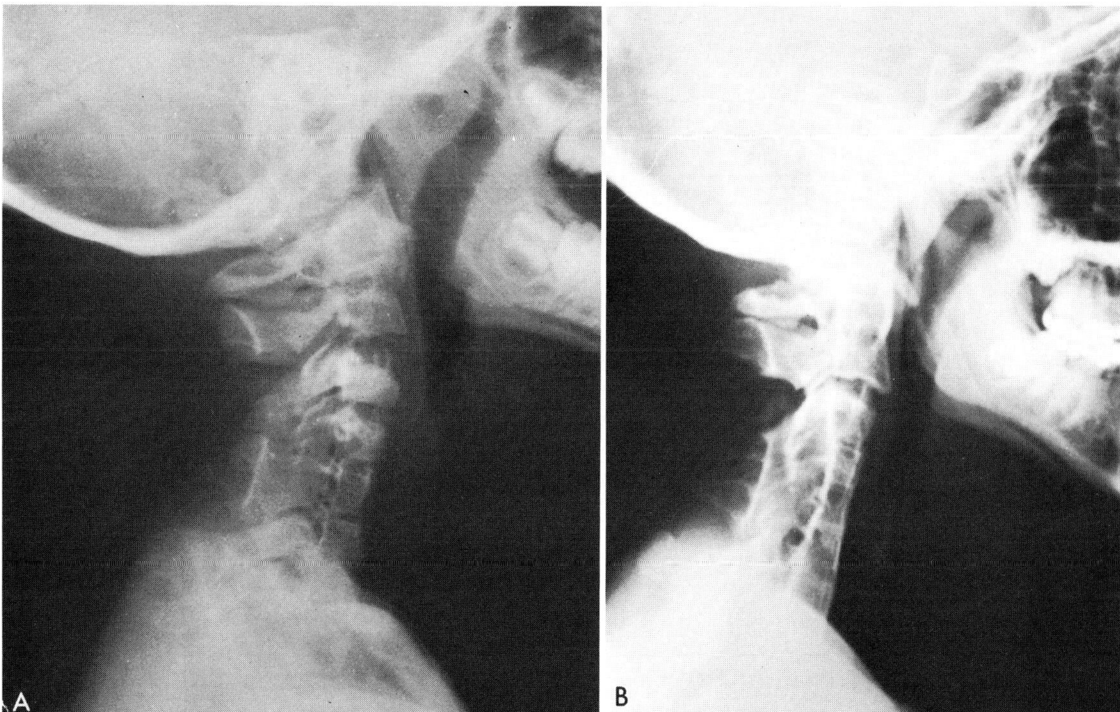

Figure 10–29. *A,* An 8-year-old demonstrating posterior fusion of the laminae and spinous process but incomplete fusion of the vertebral bodies anteriorly. *B,* Same patient at age 19, now demonstrating complete fusion of the vertebral bodies C2–C3 and C4–C7. In children, narrowing of the cervical disc spaces cannot always be appreciated, as ossification of vertebral bodies is not completed until adolescence. The unossified cartilage end plates can give a false impression of a normal disc space.

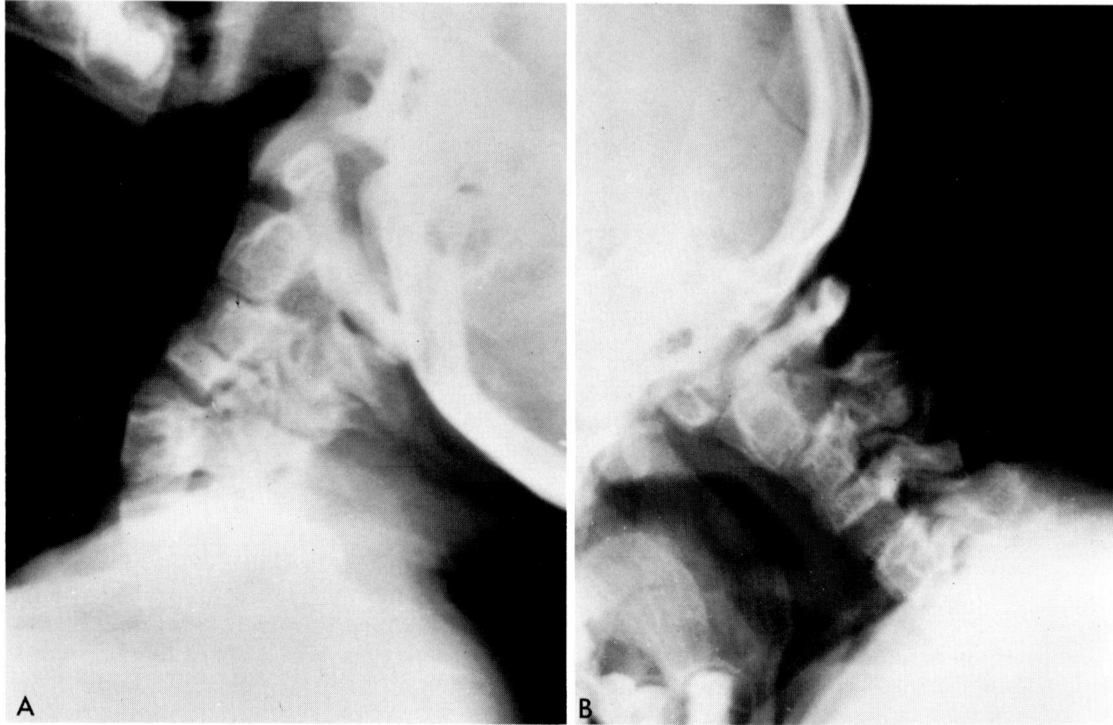

Figure 10–30. A 3-year-old with the Klippel-Feil syndrome and congenital scoliosis. Lateral flexion-extension roentgenograms of the cervical spine *(A, B)* demonstrate that neck motion occurs predominantly between C4 and C5. Flexion-extension views are helpful in determining the type and extent of congenital fusion in young children.

complete and the unossified end plates may give the false impression of a normal disc space (Fig. 10–29). However, with continued growth, the ossification of the vertebral bodies is completed and the fusion becomes obvious. If fusion is suspected in a child, it may be confirmed by flexion-extension views (Fig. 10–30). Juvenile rheumatoid arthritis (Fig. 10–31) rheumatoid spondylitis, and infection can mimic the roentgenographic findings, but usually the clinical history and physical examination indicate the correct diagnosis.

Hemivertebrae are common (Fig. 10–32); they occurred in 74 per cent of patients in the review of Gray and associates,[13] and the incidence increases with the number of segments fused. Posterior element fusion usually parallels that of the vertebral bodies. In the young child, particular attention should be paid to the laminae, because fusion posteriorly is often more apparent than anteriorly in early life (Fig. 10–33).[16]

The sagittal and transverse diameters of the spinal canal are usually normal. Narrowing of the spinal canal, if it occurs, is usually seen in adult life and is due to degenerative changes (osteoarthritic spurs) or hypermobility.[18, 34] Enlargement of the cervical canal is uncommon, and if found may indicate conditions such as syringomyelia, hydromyelia, or the Arnold-Chiari malformation.[31, 42] The intervertebral foramina are usually smooth in contour, but are frequently smaller than normal and oval rather than circular in shape (Fig. 10–34). Posterior spina bifida is common (45 per cent), but anterior spina bifida is rare. Rarely, there is complete absence of the posterior elements. This is usually accompanied by enlargement of the foramen magnum and fixed hyperextension of the neck, referred to as iniencephaly (see Fig. 10–22).[38]

All these defects may extend into the upper thoracic spine, particularly in severely involved patients. A disturbance of the upper thoracic spine on a routine chest roentgenogram may be the first clue to an unrecognized cervical synostosis. With a high thoracic congenital scoliosis, the roentgenographic evaluation should routinely include lateral views of the cervical spine.

Patterns of Cervical Motion. One can gain insight into the problem of instability by reviewing the lateral flexion-extension films of the Klippel-Feil patient. The type or pattern of cervical motion depends on the location and extent of the fused cervical vertebrae. Those with fusion of the lower cervical vertebrae or with more than two disc spaces between fused segments seem to be at low risk for serious problems.

Pizzutillo and colleagues[35] reviewed the patients from the Alfred I. DuPont Institute and those reported in the literature to determine the long-term problems found in the Klippel-Feil syndrome. In their classification, they noted that those who have upper segment instability were more likely to be younger and to have neurological problems. Conversely, degenerative changes were more common in the older patient with low segment hypermobility. This finding emphasizes the importance of screening the upper cervical spine in the young child for instability. There are three high-risk patterns of cervical spinal motion that potentially have a poor prognosis, from either early instability or late degenerative osteoarthritis.

Pattern 1 is fusion of C2 and C3 with occipitalization of the atlas (see Fig. 10–12). Complications associated with this pattern were first reported by McRae in 1953[26] and they received substantial support in the literature.[27] Flexion-extension is concentrated in the area of C1 and C2. With aging, an odontoid can become hypermobile, narrowing the spinal canal and compromising the spinal cord and brain stem.

Pattern 2 is a long fusion with an abnormal occipitocervical junction (see Fig. 10–22). This is similar to the C2–C3 fusion of McRae and could be reviewed as a more elaborate variation. The force of flexion-extension and rotation is concentrated in the area of the abnormal

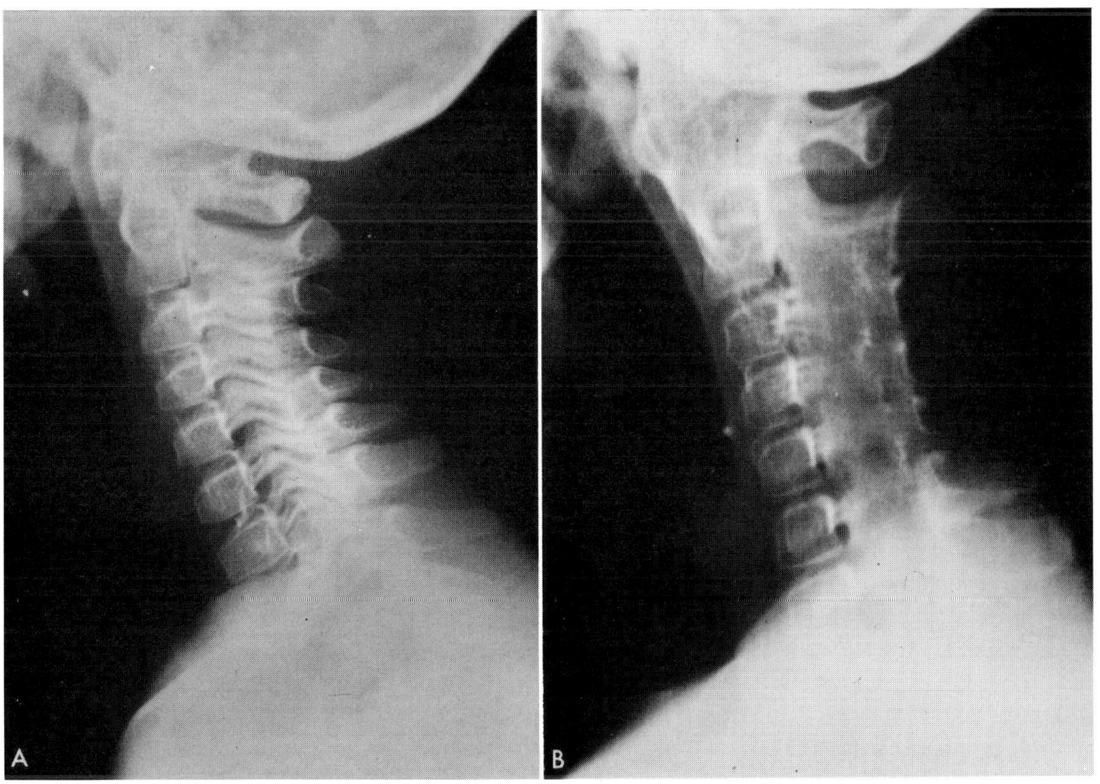

Figure 10–31. Juvenile rheumatoid arthritis. *A,* Roentgenographic appearance of the cervical spine, age 5, at the onset of the rheumatoid process. *B,* Same patient at age 10 with complete fusion of the laminae posteriorly and severely restricted neck motion. We would expect that with further growth these vertebral bodies will subsequently fuse.

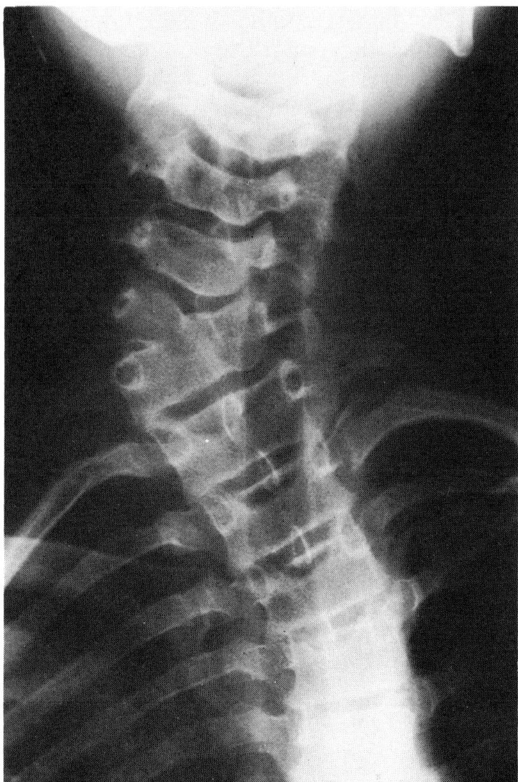

Figure 10–32. A 14-year-old with cervical hemivertebrae. Hemivertebrae are common in the Klippel-Feil syndrome but usually are found in the dorsal or lumbar vertebral segments.

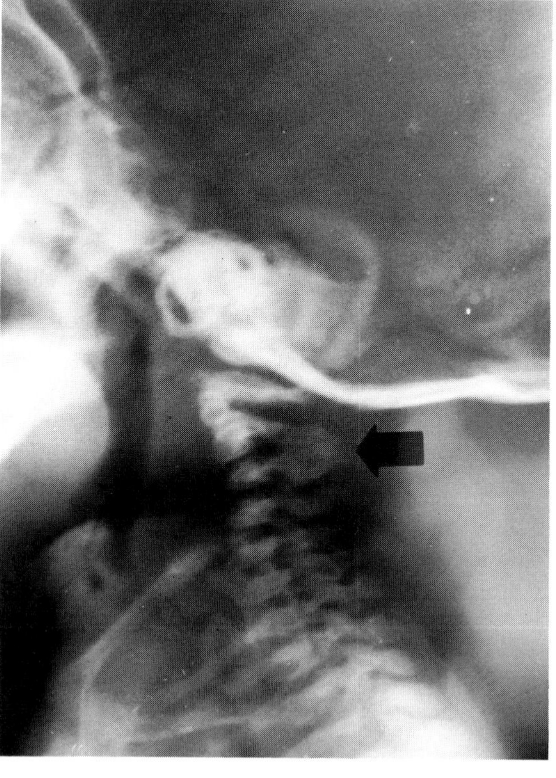

Figure 10–33. A 3-month-old with the Klippel-Feil syndrome. The roentgenograms demonstrate posterior fusion of the laminae of C2–C3 *(arrow)*. In young children, particular attention should be paid to the laminae, because fusion posteriorly is often more apparent than anteriorly in early life.

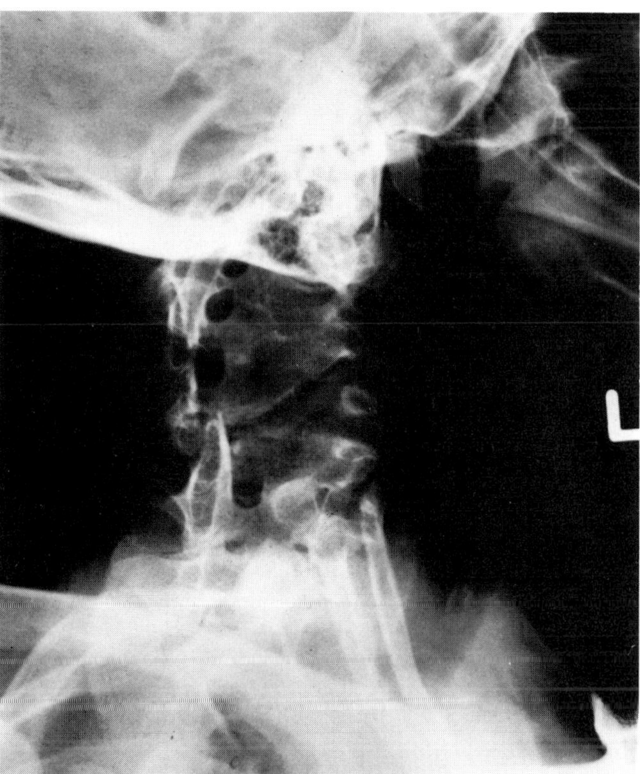

Figure 10–34. Oblique view of the cervical spine demonstrating the smooth contour of the intervertebral foramina, which are frequently smaller than normal and oval rather than circular in shape.

odontoid or poorly developed ring of C1, which cannot withstand the wear and tear of aging. It is important to differentiate this pattern from the patient with a long fusion and a normal C1–C2 articulation (Fig. 10–35), which is usually compatible with a normal life expectancy.

Pattern 3 is a single open interspace between two fused segments (Fig. 10–36). In this situation, cervical spine motion is concentrated at the single open articulation. In some patients, this hypermobility may lead to frank instability or degenerative osteoarthritis (Fig. 10–37).[13, 27, 39] This pattern can be easily recognized, because the cervical spine appears to angle or hinge at the open segment.

Associated Conditions

(Table 10–1)

Scoliosis is the most frequent anomaly found in association with the syndrome.[16, 24] Sixty per cent of these patients have a significant degree of scoliosis (greater than 15 degrees by the Cobb method).[16] Most of these require treatment and should be followed through the growth years. The roentgenographic examinations should include lateral views of the spine, because increasing kyphosis may make the need for treatment of the scoliosis more urgent. If the deformity is recognized early, many children can be successfully controlled with standard spinal orthotics such as the Milwaukee brace. At present, most of these patients have required posterior spinal stabilization, partly owing to late recognition.[4, 11, 16, 24]

Two types of scoliosis can be identified: congenital scoliosis due to vertebral anomalies and differential growth patterns (Fig. 10–38) and compensatory scoliosis below the area of vertebral involvement. In our series, congenital scoliosis is the most common (55 per cent), and in more than one half of the children the curvature was progressive and required treatment.[16] Most (75 per cent) required posterior spinal fusion to arrest an increasing deformity, and the remainder were controlled with a brace or cast.[16] Of interest is the frequent occurrence of progressive scoliosis in the normal-appearing vertebrae below the primary congenital curve. If only the congenitally involved seg-

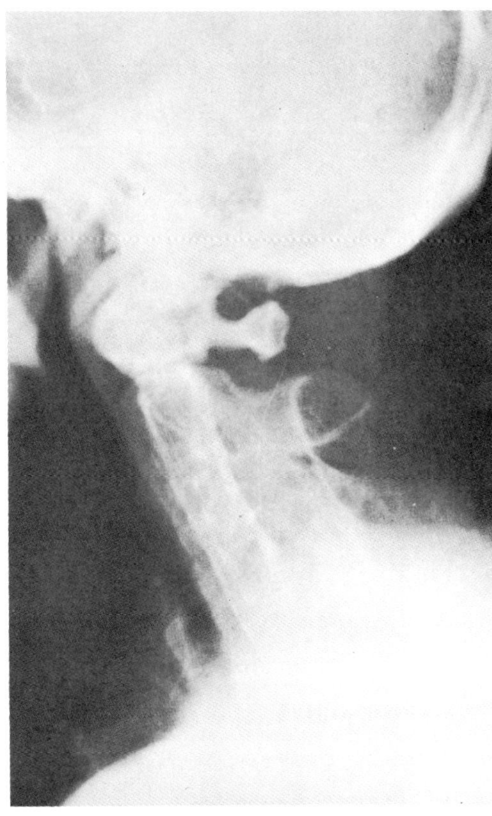

Figure 10–35. A 45-year-old male with the Klippel-Feil syndrome. The patient has complete fusion of C2–C7. Flexion-extension occurs only at the atlantoaxial articulation. There are no symptoms referable to the neck, despite two previous serious falls. This pattern appears to be relatively safe, because the normal occipitocervical junction serves as a protection from late instability.

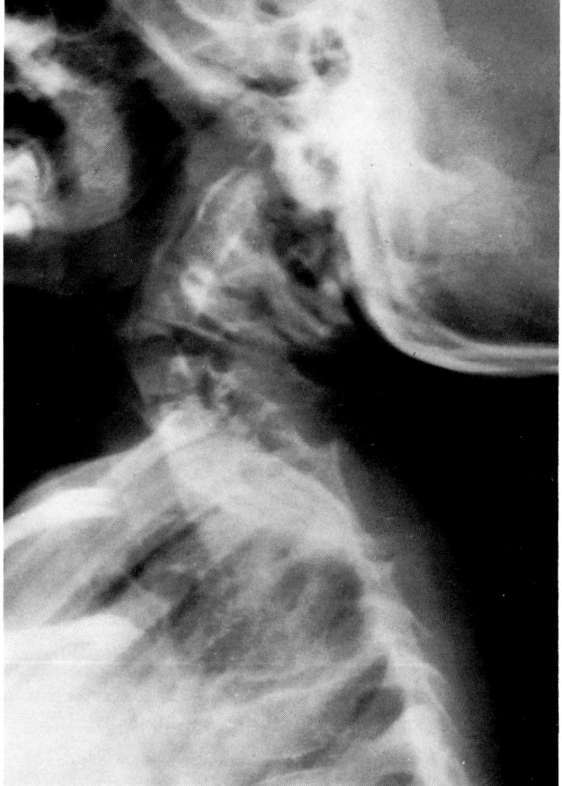

Figure 10–36. Open interspace between two fused segments. A 7-year-old with the Klippel-Feil syndrome has flexion-extension motion of the neck occurring primarily at one interspace. The cervical spine appears to angle or hinge at this point. This is a worrisome pattern, because wear and tear of aging may lead to early degenerative change or instability and narrowing of the spinal cord.

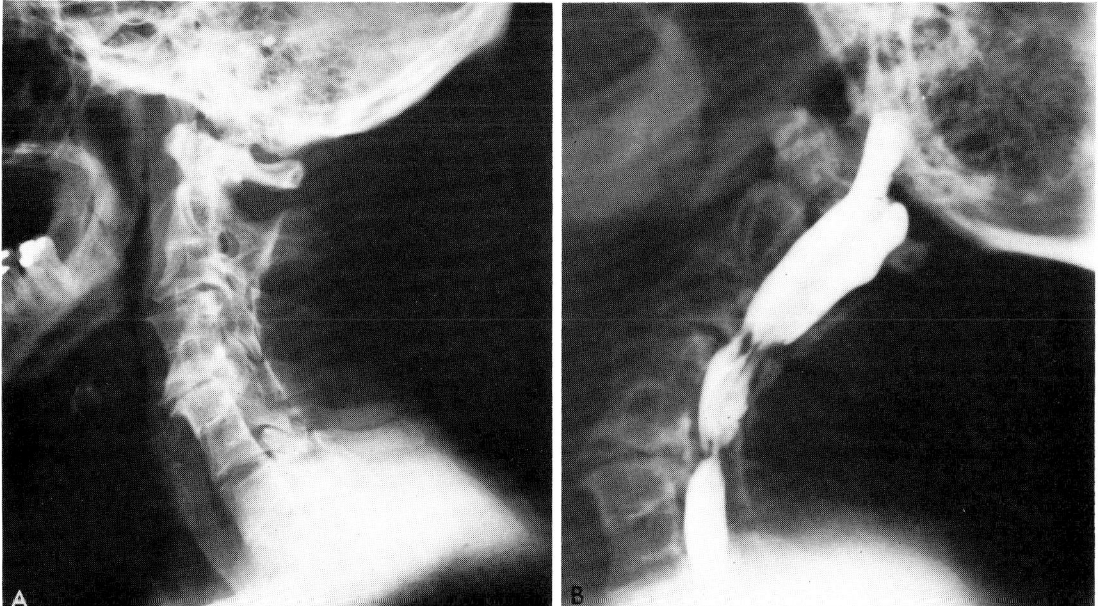

Figure 10–37. A 54-year-old male with a four-month history of persistent neck pain with radiation into the upper extremities. He had no history of neck complaints but a long history of occipital headaches. He recently noted paresthesias in the upper and lower extremities. Neurologic examination and EMG were within normal limits. *A*, Lateral roentgenogram of the cervical spine, demonstrating congenital fusion between C2–C3, C4–C5, and C6–C7. Note marked changes of degenerative osteoarthritis with large osteophyte formation at the open interspace of C3–C4 and C5–C6. *B*, Myelogram during extension of the cervical spine demonstrates narrowing of the spinal canal due to the large osteoarthritic spurs at C3–C4 and C5–C6. He subsequently underwent spine stabilization with relief of neck complaints.

ments are examined in follow-up, an increasing compensatory scoliosis in the lower vertebrae may not be recognized and its significance may not be appreciated until serious deformity results. When surgical intervention is required, the same principles apply as used in congenital scoliosis. When spinal fusion is performed, the orthopedist should carefully consider the overall alignment of the patient's spine. The temptation to achieve maximal radiologic correction of the mobile segments must be tempered by careful consideration of the congenitally fixed segments. Failure to observe this principle may result in an unbalanced spine; the patient will have traded one deformity for another that may be even worse than the original.

Documented progression of scoliosis, whether in the congenitally distorted elements or in the compensatory curve below, demands immediate and appropriate treatment to prevent serious additional deformity. Progressive scoliosis in the thoracic spine may seriously compromise pulmonary function.[2, 16] More subtle occult abnormalities can lead to respiratory difficulty in some Klippel-Feil patients. Abnormal rib spacing, congenital fusion of the ribs, and deformed costovertebral joints may inhibit full expansion of the rib cage during respiration.[1] Although not causing an angular deformity, fusion of the thoracic vertebrae may decrease the size of the thoracic cage. The spondylothoracic dwarf may represent a severe form of this problem, leading to early respiratory death.[30] Also, Krieger and associates[21] reported on the relationship of occult respiratory dysfunction and craniovertebral anomalies. They noted that in addition to the obvious problems of bony impingement or traction upon the brain stem, these patients may have subtle hydrocephalus, which may adversely affect respiratory function.

This information has particular application when cervical distraction devices are contemplated in the treatment of scoliosis (halofemoral or halopelvic traction). When considering the use of such devices, the physician should be aware that children with the Klippel-Feil syndrome may be more susceptible to

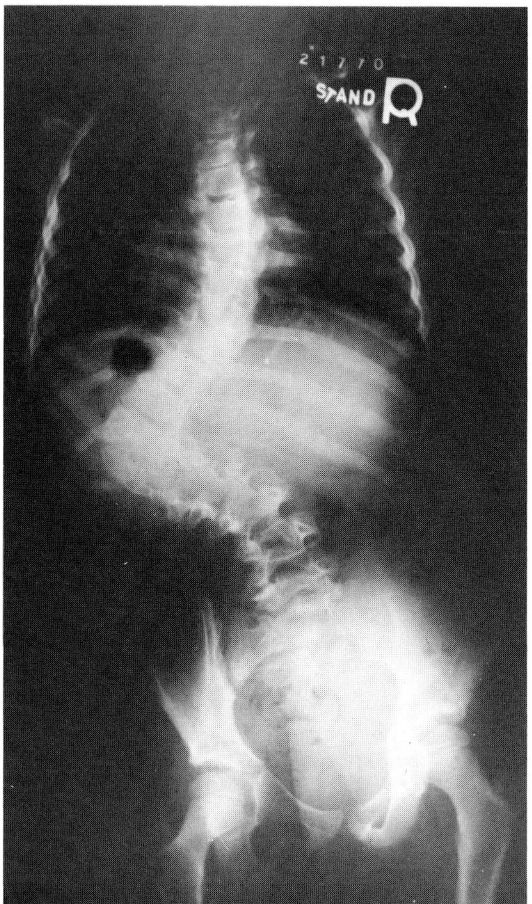

Figure 10–38. An 8-year-old with the Klippel-Feil syndrome and deafness. The severe kyphoscoliosis subsequently required spine correction and stabilization.

neurologic or vascular injury and that the presence of cervical anomalies may preclude the use of cervical distraction.[16]

Renal Abnormalities. Over one third of the children with the Klippel-Feil syndrome can be expected to have a significant urinary tract anomaly. These anomalies are often asymptomatic in the young. Previously, we have recommended that such anomalies be evaluated with intravenous pyelography (Fig. 10–39).[16] However, it has been found that ultrasonography offers a noninvasive way to screen adequately for the anomalies associated with the Klippel-Feil syndrome.[7] The pronephros, the embryologic tissue destined to become the genitourinary tract, develops between the seventh and 14th somites, in the same region and at the same time as the cervical spine,[1, 29] quite similar to the scapulae in Sprengel's deformity. The most frequent abnormality is unilateral absence of a kidney. Other abnormalities include a double collecting system, renal ectopia, a horseshoe kidney, and hydronephrosis from ureteropelvic obstruction. Two of 50 patients in our series developed severe pyelonephritis in the remaining kidney, requiring renal transplantation.[16] Indeed, in Klippel and Feil's original case report, the patient died from nephritis.[20]

Cardiovascular Abnormalities. The literature notes the association of the Klippel-Feil syndrome with congenital heart disease (4.2 to 14 per cent).[11, 16, 28, 32] The most common lesion reported has been an interventricular septal defect occurring alone or in combination with other defects, such as a patent ductus arteriosus and abnormal position of the heart and aorta.

Deafness. The association of hearing impairment and even deafness in the Klippel-Feil

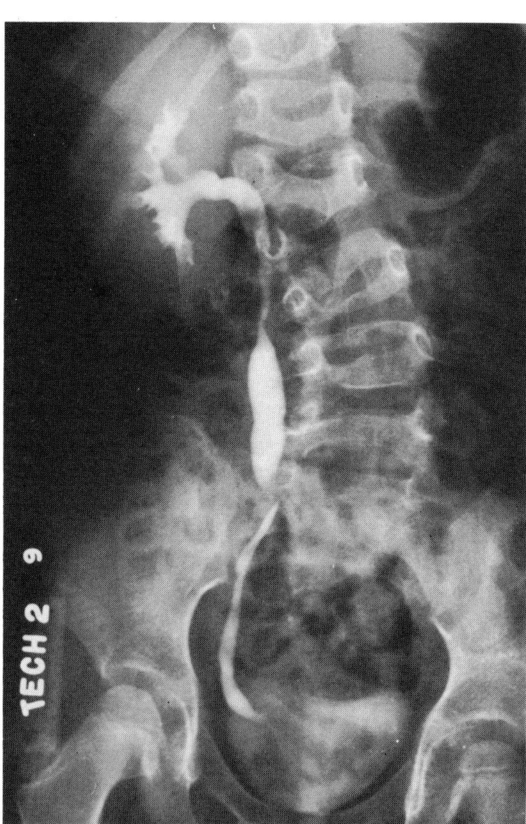

Figure 10–39. A 10-year-old patient with the Klippel-Feil syndrome. Roentgenograms demonstrate multiple vertebral anomalies, unilateral absence of the kidney, and hydroureter. Ureteral reimplantation was required for ureteral reflux and hydronephrosis.

syndrome (over 30 per cent) has been reported in the otology literature,[18, 25, 34, 40] but it is seldom mentioned in orthopedic reports.[16, 24] Other defects include absence of the auditory canal and microtia.

Jalladeau[18] is credited with the first report of deafness. Stark and Borton[40] noted that detailed audiologic data were not yet available, and the precise defect is often not known. There is no characteristic audiologic anomaly, and all types of hearing loss (conductive, sensorineural, and mixed) have been described. These patients should undergo a complete audiometric evaluation when these are discovered. The relationship between hearing loss and speech-language retardation is well documented, and early detection of hearing impairment can lessen the retardation by permitting early initiation of speech and language training.[40]

Mirror Motions (Synkinesis). Synkinesis consists of involuntary paired movements of the hands and occasionally the arms. The patient is unable to move one hand without similar reciprocal motion of the opposite hand. Mirror motion was first described by Bauman, who found it in four of six patients with the Klippel-Feil syndrome.[4] This condition has been noted to occur occasionally in normal preschool children and patients with cerebral palsy or Parkinson's disease, but most of those afflicted with this condition have the Klippel-Feil syndrome.[9] Approximately 20 per cent demonstrate mirror motions clinically.[16] Baird and associates,[3] using electromyography to examine 13 patients with the Klippel-Feil syndrome, found 10 patients with electrically detectable paired motion in the opposite extremity. This suggests that many patients may be subclinically affected and may be more clumsy at two-handed activities. Some authors have suggested it should be included as part of the syndrome.[3, 9]

The etiology of synkinesis is unknown, but it appears to be a separate congenital neurologic defect not due to bony impingement or irritation of the spinal cord.[1, 15] The examination of two autopsy specimens suggests that the clinical findings are due to inadequate or incomplete decussation of the pyramidal tracts in conjunction with a dysraphic cervical spinal cord. As a consequence, cerebral control over the upper extremities must follow less direct pathways located in the extrapyramidal system, and afflicted patients require more extensive practice to dissociate the movements of the individual extremities.

Synkinesis is most pronounced in young children, particularly those under 5 years of age. Fortunately, the condition tends to decrease with age. Occupational therapy has been helpful in teaching control over the extremities, or at least in disguising the reciprocal motion to a tolerable cosmetic level. Still, many patients may find discriminating two-handed activity difficult, such as playing the piano, typing, sewing, or ladder climbing.[33]

Treatment

The minimally involved patient with the Klippel-Feil syndrome can be expected to lead a normal active life with no or only minor restrictions or symptoms. Many severely involved patients can enjoy the same good prognosis if early and appropriate treatment is instituted when needed. This is particularly applicable in the area of associated scoliosis and renal abnormalities. Prevention of further deformity or complications can be of great benefit. The actual treatment of the Klippel-Feil syndrome is confined mostly to the area of associated conditions and is discussed under the respective headings.

At present, treatment choices for the cervical spine anomalies are quite limited. Patients with major areas of cervical synostosis or high-risk patterns of cervical spinal motion should be strongly advised to avoid activities that place stress on the cervical spine. In these, the mobile articulations are under greater mechanical demands and are less capable of protecting them against traumatic insults.

As discussed, sudden neurologic compromise or death after minor trauma has been reported in the Klippel-Feil syndrome and is usually due to disruption at the hypermobile articulation.[13, 27, 39] The role of prophylactic surgical stabilization in asymptomatic patients has not yet been defined. There is no satisfactory answer to when the risk of instability warrants further reduction of neck motion.

For symptomatic patients with mechanical problems, the usual treatment measures for degenerative osteoarthritis are applicable and include traction, a cervical collar, and analgesics. Symptoms that suggest neurologic compromise require careful consideration and evaluation by a neurologist, neurosurgeon, and orthopedist (see Fig. 10–37). The exact area of irritation must be determined before surgical intervention. Attempts should be made preoperatively to obtain reduction of the bony architecture in advance of surgical stabilization. The physician must be mindful that there are other associated abnormalities, both in the brain stem and in the spinal cord itself, that may be contributing to the symptoms.

Treatment of the cosmetic aspects of this deformity has met with limited success. Occasionally, children with the fixed torticollis posture may be improved with bracing. However, this requires long-term application and excellent patient cooperation. Surgical correction of the bony deformity by direct means such as wedge osteotomy is not recommended. Occasionally, carefully selected patients who have cervical congenital scoliosis may obtain some correction and improvement of appearance by use of the halo-cast combined with posterior cervical fusion. Bonola[5] described a method of rib resection to attain apparent increase in neck length and motion. However, this procedure is an extensive surgical experience and is a great risk to the patient. No subsequent reports have appeared in the literature.

Soft tissue procedures, Z-plasty, and muscle resection may achieve cosmetic improvement in properly selected patients.[24] It can restore a more natural contour to the shoulders and neck as well as an apparent increase in neck length. These procedures generally do not increase neck motion, and the scars may be extensive, particularly in the patient with a large skin web. If an omovertebral bone is present, its removal may permit an increase in neck and shoulder motion. The surgeon should be aware that the risk of brachial plexus injury from traction is higher in those with the Klippel-Feil syndrome, because there are likely to be anomalous origins of the cervical nerve roots in these patients. Iniencephaly and absence of the posterior cervical elements (see Fig. 10–23) may be associated with Sprengel's deformity and must be identified if surgical correction is considered.[38]

Summary

The Klippel-Feil syndrome is an uncommon condition due to congenital fusion of two or more cervical vertebrae. Most afflicted individuals are asymptomatic or have a mild restriction of neck motion. If symptoms referable to the cervical spine occur, it is usually in adult life and is due to degenerative arthritis or instability of the hypermobile articulations adjacent to the area of synostosis. Most respond to conservative treatment measures; a small percentage require judicious surgical stabilization. Cosmetic surgery is of limited benefit in treatment of the neck deformity.

The relatively good prognosis of the cervical lesion is overshadowed by the "hidden" or unrecognized associated anomalies. The high incidence of significant scoliosis, renal anomalies, deafness, neurologic malformations, Sprengel's deformity, and cardiac anomalies should be of great concern to the physician. Early recognition and treatment of these problems may be of substantial benefit, sparing the patient further deformity or serious illness.

References

Klippel-Feil Syndrome

1. Avery, L. W., and Rentfro, C. C.: The Klippel-Feil syndrome: a pathologic report. Arch. Neurol. Psychiatr. *36:*1068, 1936.
2. Baga, N., Chusid, E. L., and Miller, A.: Pulmonary disability in the Klippel-Feil syndrome. Clin. Orthop. *67:*105, 1969.
3. Baird, P. A., Robinson, G. C., and Buckler, W. St. J.: Klippel-Feil syndrome. Am. J. Dis. Child. *113:*546, 1967.
4. Bauman, G. I.: Absence of the cervical spine: Klippel-Feil syndrome. J.A.M.A. *98:*129, 1932.
5. Bonola, A.: Surgical treatment of the Klippel-Feil syndrome. J. Bone Joint Surg. *38B:*440, 1956.
6. Catell, H. S., and Filtzer, D. L.: Pseudosubluxation and other normal variations in the cervical spine in children. J. Bone Joint Surg. *47A:*1295, 1965.
7. Drvaric, D. M., Ruderman, R. J., Conrad, R. W., et al.: Congenital scoliosis and urinary tract abnormalities: are intravenous pyelograms necessary? J. Pediatr. Orthop. *7:*441, 1987.
8. Epstein, J. A., Carras, R., Epstein, B. S., and Levine, L. S.: Myelopathy in cervical spondylosis with vertebral subluxation and hyperlordosis. J. Neurosurg. *32:*421, 1970.
9. Erskine, C. A.: An analysis of the Klippel-Feil syndrome. Arch. Pathol. *41:*269, 1946.
10. Feil, A.: L'absence et la diminution des vertèbres cervicales (étude clinique et pathogenique): le syndrome de réduction numérique cervicale. Thèses de Paris, 1919.
11. Forney, W. R., Robinson, S. J., and Pascoe, D. J.: Congenital heart disease, deafness, and skeletal malformations; a new syndrome? J. Pediatr. *68:*14, 1966.
12. Frawley, J. M.: Congenital webbing. Am. J. Dis. Child. *29:*799, 1925.
13. Gray, S. W., Romaine, C. B., and Skandalakis, J. F.: Congenital fusion of the cervical vertebrae. Surg. Gynecol. Obstet. *118:*373, 1964.

14. Gunderson, C. H., Greenspan, R. H., Glaser, G. H., and Lubs, H. A.: Klippel-Feil syndrome; genetic and clinical reevaluation of cervical fusion. Medicine *46:*491, 1967.
15. Gunderson, C. H., and Solitare, G. B.: Mirror movements in patients with the Klippel-Feil syndrome: neuropathologic observations. Arch. Neurol. *18:*675, 1968.
16. Hensinger, R. N., Lang, J. R., and MacEwen, G. D.: The Klippel-Feil syndrome: a constellation of related anomalies. J. Bone Joint Surg. *56A:*1246, 1974.
17. Illingworth, R. S.: Attacks of unconsciousness in association with fused cervical vertebrae. Arch. Dis. Child. *31:*8, 1956.
18. Jalladeau, J.: Malformations congénitales associées syndrome de Klippel-Feil. Thèse de Paris, 1936.
19. Kirkham, T. H.: Cervico-oculo-acusticus syndrome with pseudopapilloedema. Arch. Dis. Child. *44:*504, 1969.
20. Klippel, M., and Feil, A.: Un cas d'absence des vertèbres cervicales avec cage thoracique remontant jusqu'a la base du crane. Nouv. Icon. Salpet. *25:*223, 1912.
21. Krieger, A. J., Rosomoff, H. L., Kuperman, A. S., and Zingesser, L. H.: Occult respiratory dysfunction in a craniovertebral anomaly. J. Neurosurg. *31:*15, 1969.
22. Kulkarni, M. V., Williams, J. C., Yeakley, J. W., et al.: Magnetic resonance imaging in the diagnosis of the cranio-cervical manifestations of the mucopolysaccharidoses. Magn. Res. Imaging *5:*317, 1987.
23. McAfee, P. C., Bohlman, H. H., Han, J. S., and Salvagno, R. T.: Comparison of nuclear magnetic resonance imaging and computed tomography in the diagnosis of upper cervical spinal cord compression. Spine *11:*295, 1986.
24. McElfresh, E., and Winter, R.: Klippel-Feil syndrome. Minn. Med. *56:*353, 1973.
25. McLay, K., and Maran, A. G.: Deafness and the Klippel-Feil syndrome. J. Laryngol. Otol. *83:*175, 1969.
26. McRae, D. L.: Bony abnormalities in the region of the foramen magnum: correlation of the anatomic and neurologic findings. Acta Radiol. *40:*335, 1953.
27. Michie, I., and Clark, J.: Neurological syndromes associated with cervical and craniocervical anomalies. Arch. Neurol. *18:*241, 1968.
28. Morrison, S. G., Perry, L. W., and Scott, L. P.: Congenital brevicollis (Klippel-Feil syndrome) and cardiovascular anomalies., Am. J. Dis. Child. *115:*614, 1968.
29. Moore, W. B., Matthews, T. J., and Rabinowitz, R.: Genitourinary anomalies associated with Klippel-Feil syndrome. J. Bone Joint Surg. *57A:*355, 1975.
30. Moseley, J. E., and Bonforte, R. J.: Spondylothoracic dysplasia—a syndrome with congenital heart disease. Am. J. Dis. Child. *102:*858, 1961.
31. Naik, D. R.: Cervical spinal canal in normal infants. Clin. Radiol. *21:*323, 1970.
32. Nora, J. J., Cohen, M., and Maxwell, G. M.: Klippel-Feil syndrome with congenital heart disease. Am. J. Dis. Child. *102:*858, 1961.
33. Notermans, S. L. H., Go, K. G., and Boonstra, S.: EMG studies of associated movements in a patient with Klippel-Feil syndrome. Psychiatr. Neurol. Neurochir. *73:*257, 1970.
34. Palant, D. I., and Carter, B. L.: Klippel-Feil syndrome and deafness. Am. J. Dis. Child. *123:*218, 1972.
35. Pizzutillo, P. D., Woods, M. W., and Nicholson, L.: Risk factors in the Klippel-Feil syndrome. Orthop. Trans. *11:*473, 1987.
36. Ramsey, J., and Bliznak, J.: Klippel-Feil syndrome with renal agenesis and other anomalies. Am. J. Roentgenol. Radium Ther. Nucl. Med. *113:*460, 1971.
37. Roach, J. W., Duncan, D., Wenger, D. R., et al.: Atlanto-axial instability and spinal cord compression in children. Diagnosis by computerized tomography. J. Bone Joint Surg. *66A:*708, 1984.
38. Sherk, H. H., Shut, L., and Chung, S.: Iniencephalic deformity of the cervical spine with Klippel-Feil anomalies and congenital elevation of the scapula. J. Bone Joint Surg. *56A:*1254, 1974.
39. Shoul, M. I., and Ritvo, M.: Clinical and roentgenological manifestations of the Klippel-Feil syndrome (congenital fusion of the cervical vertebrae, brevicollis): report of eight additional cases and review of the literature. Am. J. Roentgenol. Radium Ther. Nucl. Med. *68:*369, 1952.
40. Stark, E. W., and Borton, T. E.: Hearing loss and the Klippel-Feil syndrome. Am. J. Dis. Child. *123:*233, 1972.
41. Sullivan, R. C., Bruwer, A. J., and Harris, L.: Hypermobility of the cervical spine in children: a pitfall in the diagnosis of cervical dislocation. Am. J. Surg. *95:*636, 1958.
42. Yousefzadeh, D. K., El-Khoury, G. Y., and Smith, W. L.: Normal sagittal diameter and variation in the pediatric cervical spine. Pediatr. Radiol. *144:*319, 1982.

MUSCULAR TORTICOLLIS (WRYNECK)

This is a common condition usually discovered in the first six to eight weeks of life. The deformity is due to contracture of the sternocleidomastoid muscle, with the head tilted toward the involved side and the chin rotated toward the contralateral shoulder (Fig. 10–40*A*). If the infant is examined within the first four weeks of life, a mass or "tumor" is usually palpable in the neck (Fig. 10–41).[14] It is generally a nontender, soft enlargement that is mobile beneath the skin and attached to or located within the body of the sternocleidomastoid muscle. The mass attains maximal size within the first month of life and then gradually regresses. If the child is examined after 4 to 6 months of age, the mass is usually absent and the contracture of the sternocleidomastoid muscle and the torticollis posture are the only clinical findings (Fig. 10–42). The mass is frequently unrecognized and was undetected in

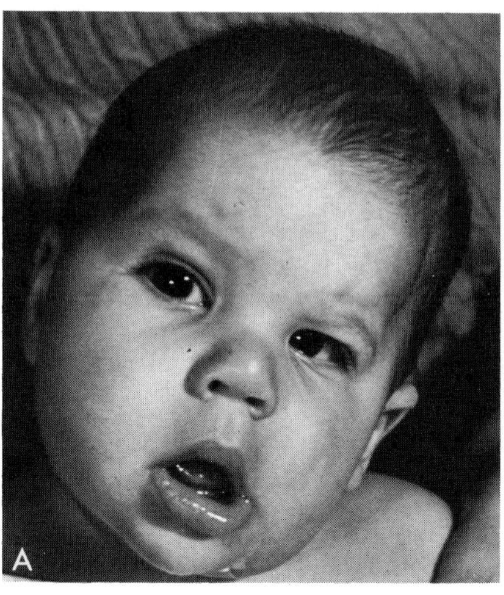

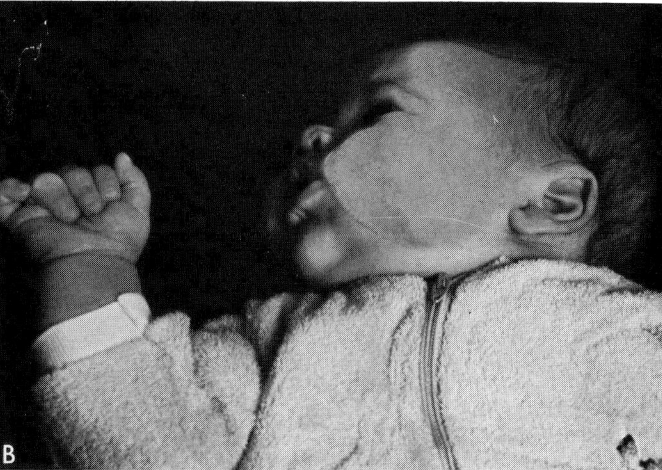

Figure 10–40. A 6-month-old with right-sided congenital muscular torticollis. *A,* Note the rotation of the skull and asymmetry and flattening of the face on the side of the contracted sternocleidomastoid. *B,* Same patient with the head resting on glass and photographed from below. Note how the face conforms to the surface. When the child sleeps, usually prone, it is more comfortable to have the affected side down, and consequently the face remodels to conform to the bed.

80 per cent of the patients of Coventry and Harris.[6]

If the condition is progressive, deformities of the face and skull can result and are usually apparent within the first year. Flattening of the face on the side of the contracted sternocleidomastoid muscle may be particularly impressive (Fig. 10–40*A*). The deformity is probably due to the position the child assumes when sleeping (Fig. 10–40*B*). In a study of children in the United States, it was found that they generally sleep prone,[1] and in this position it is more comfortable to have the affected side down. As a consequence, the face remod-

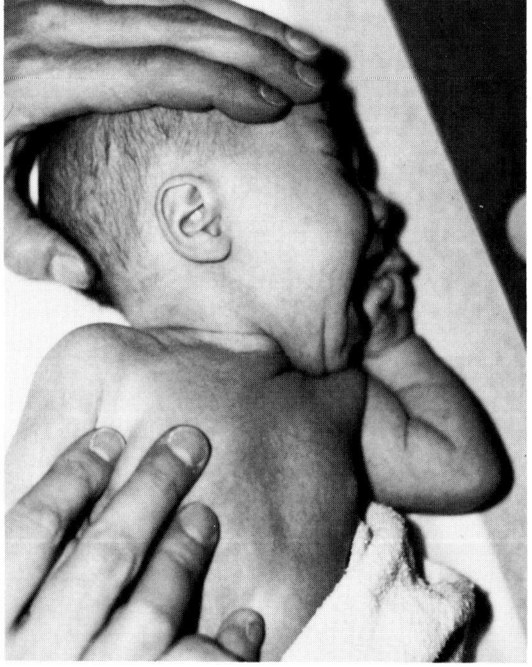

Figure 10–41. A 6-week-old with swelling in the region of the sternocleidomastoid muscle. The mass is usually soft, nontender, and mobile beneath the skin but is attached to the muscle.

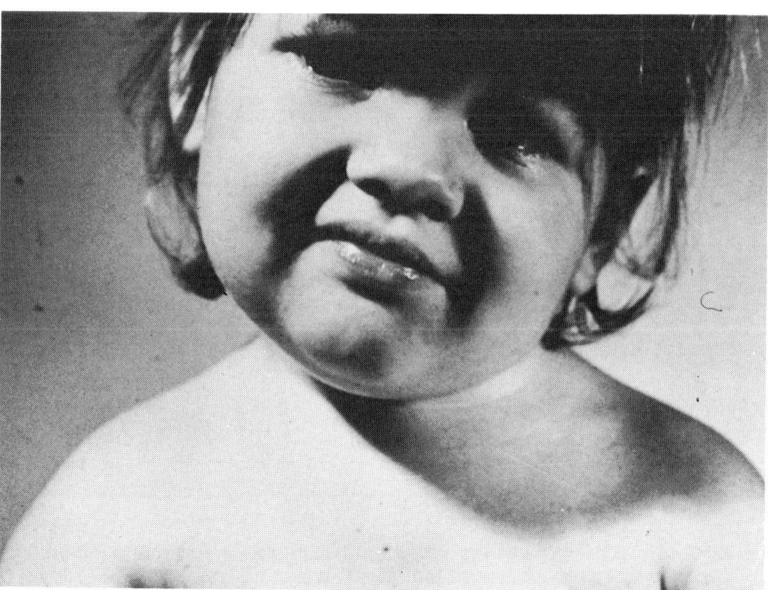

Figure 10–42. An 18-month-old with torticollis resistant to stretching exercises and requiring surgical release.

els to conform to the bed. In children who sleep supine, reverse modeling of the contralateral aspect of the skull is evident. If the condition remains untreated during the growth years, the level of the eyes and ears becomes distorted and may result in considerable cosmetic deformity.

Etiology

At present, congenital muscular torticollis is believed to be the result of local compression to the soft tissues of the neck at the time of delivery. Birth records of affected children demonstrate a preponderance of breech or difficult deliveries or primiparous births.[14, 15] However, the deformity has occurred after otherwise normal deliveries and has been reported in infants born by cesarean section.[14, 15] Microscopic examinations of resected surgical specimens and experimental work with dogs[2] suggest that the lesion is due to occlusion of the venous outflow of the sternocleidomastoid muscle. This results in edema, degeneration of muscle fibers, and eventual fibrosis of the muscle body. Coventry and Harris[6] suggested that the clinical deformity is related to the ratio of fibrosis to remaining functional muscle. If sufficient normal muscle is present, the sternocleidomastoid will stretch with growth and the child will probably not develop the torticollis posture, whereas if there is a predominance of fibrosis, there is very little elastic potential. Pathologic studies demonstrated that with time the fibrosis of the sternal head may entrap and compromise the branch of the accessory nerve to the clavicular head of the muscle (progressive denervation), leading to a late increase in the deformity.[20] There is some evidence to suggest the problem may be due to uterine crowding or "packing syndrome," as in three of four children the lesion is on the right side.[14, 15] Also, 20 per cent of children with congenital muscular torticollis have congenital dysplasia of the hip, which is believed to be due to restriction of infant movement in the tight maternal space.[13] Roentgenograms of the cervical spine should be obtained to rule out congenital anomaly of the cervical spine.

Treatment

Conservative Measures. Excellent results can be obtained with conservative measures in most patients.[3, 6, 14, 15] Ninety per cent of the patients of Coventry and Harris responded to stretching exercises alone.[6] The exercises are performed by the parent, with guidance from the physical therapist and physician. Standard maneuvers include positioning of the ear opposite the contracted muscle to the shoulder, and touching the chin to the shoulder on the affected side. It must be emphasized that when adequate stretching has been obtained in the neutral position, these maneuvers should be repeated with the head hyperextended, to

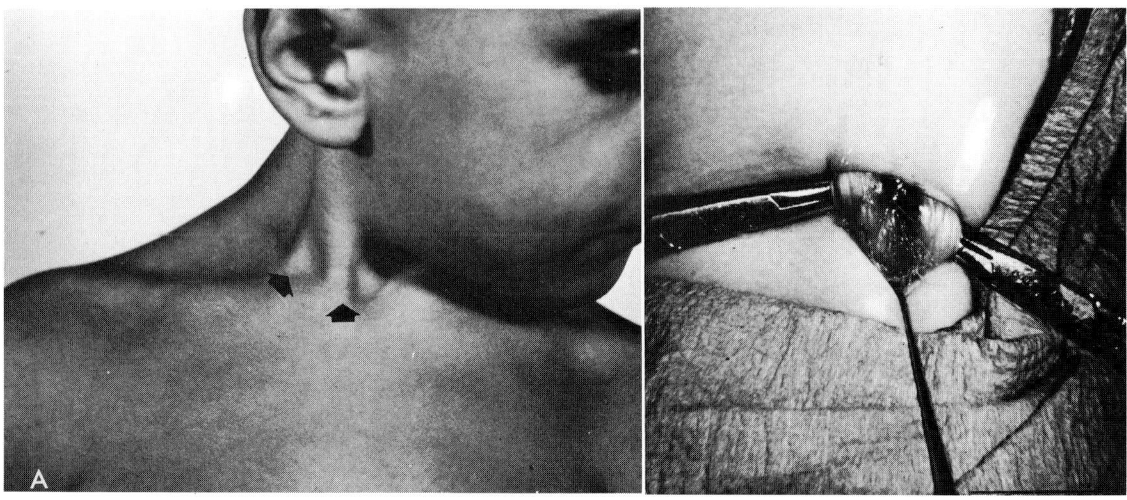

Figure 10–43. *A,* Clinical appearance of a 6-year-old with congenital muscular torticollis. Note the appearance of the two heads of the sternocleidomastoid *(arrows). B,* Operative exposure of the same patient demonstrating complete replacement with fibrous tissue of the two heads of the sternocleidomastoid.

achieve maximal stretching and prevent residual contractures. Additional measures include positioning of the crib and toys so that the neck is stretched when the infant tries to reach and grasp. The use of a "sleeping helmet" has been suggested to reduce the deformity and hasten face and skull remodeling.[5]

Surgery. If the condition persists beyond 1 year of age, nonoperative measures are rarely successful.[3] Similarly, established facial asymmetry and limitation of normal motion of more than 30 degrees usually preclude a good result, and surgical intervention will be required to prevent further facial flattening and poor cosmesis (Fig. 10–43).[3] However, a good (but not perfect) cosmetic result can be obtained in children as old as 12 years of age (Fig. 10–44).[6] Asymmetry of the skull and face will

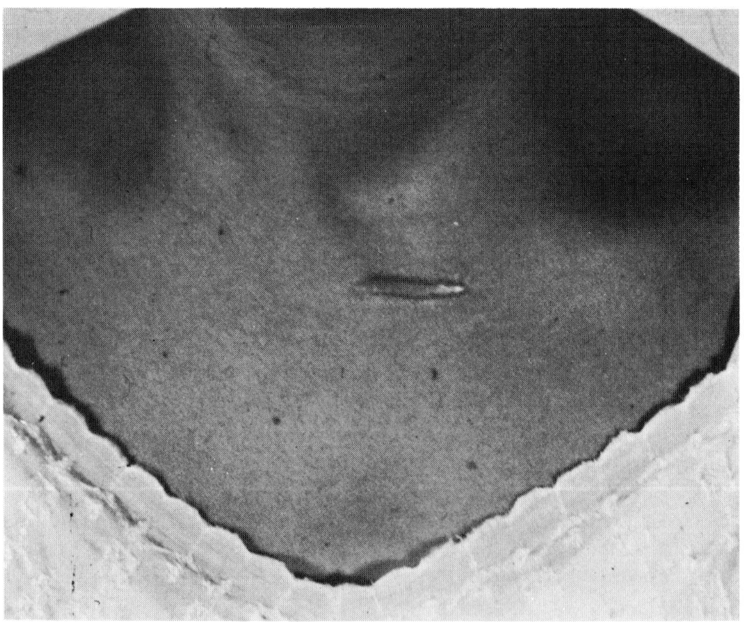

Figure 10–44. An 18-year-old after resection of a portion of the sternocleidomastoid. The incision was placed too near the clavicle and consequently spread, becoming cosmetically unacceptable.

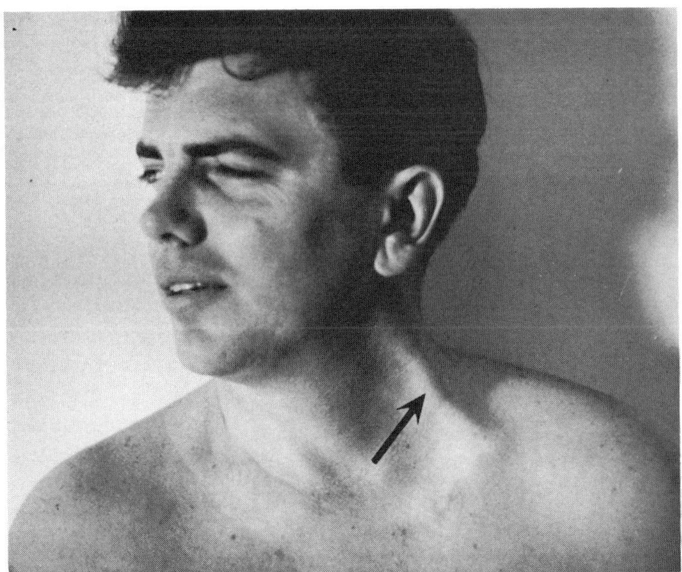

Figure 10–45. A 23-year-old male who underwent release of the sternocleidomastoid. There is a residual fascial band *(arrow)* and slight restriction of neck motion.

improve as long as adequate growth potential remains after the deforming pull of the sternocleidomastoid is removed (Fig. 10–45).[6]

Surgery consists of resection of a portion of the distal sternocleidomastoid muscle (Fig. 10–43). At least a 1-cm segment of the tendon should be removed to guard against anomalous reattachment and recurrence of the deformity. A transverse incision is made low in the neck to coincide with a normal skin fold.[22] It is important not to place the incision near or over the clavicle, because scars in this area tend to spread and are cosmetically unacceptable (Fig. 10–44).[14] Similarly, closure with a subcuticular suture is preferred.[10] The most common postoperative complaint is that of disfiguring scars.[14, 15, 22] The two heads of the sternocleidomastoid are identified, and both are sectioned (Fig. 10–43). It is important to release the investing fascia about the sternocleidomastoid, as this too is frequently contracted.[14] Rotation of the chin and head at this point generally reveal the adequacy of the surgery, and palpation of the neck demonstrates any extraneous tight bands that could lead to partial recurrence or incomplete correction (Fig. 10–45).[15] In the older child, an accessory incision is often required to section the muscle at its origin on the mastoid process. The whole muscle should not be excised, because this may lead to reverse torticollis[15] or additional deformity from asymmetry in the contour of the neck.[14]

The postoperative regimen includes passive stretching exercises performed in the same manner as those done preoperatively. They should begin as soon as the patient can tolerate manipulation of the neck. Occasionally, head traction at night is helpful, particularly with an older child. Bracing or cast correction may be necessary if the deformity has been of long duration or if the torticollic posture has become a strong habit. Results of surgery have been uniformly good, with a low incidence of complications or recurrence, and almost all patients are pleased with the results.[3, 6, 14, 15] Slight restriction of neck motion and anomalous reattachment occur frequently,[15, 22] but are generally unnoticed by the patient. If the patient is young, the facial asymmetry can be expected to resolve completely unless there is persistence of the torticollis, particularly from residual fascial bands (Fig. 10–45).[15]

Differential Diagnosis

Torticollis is a common childhood complaint. The etiology is diverse, and identifying the cause can pose a difficult diagnostic problem (Tables 10–2, 10–3).

Congenital muscular torticollis is the most common cause of wryneck posture in the infant and young child, but there are other problems that lead to this unusual posture. Head tilt and rotatory deformity of the head and neck (torticollis) usually indicates a problem at C1–C2,

Table 10–2. DIFFERENTIAL DIAGNOSIS OF TORTICOLLIS

Congenital
Occipitocervical anomalies
Basilar impressions
Atlanto-occipital fusion
Odontoid anomalies
Hemiatlas
Pterygium colli (skin web)
Congenital muscular torticollis
Klippel-Feil syndrome
Acquired
Neurogenic
Spinal cord tumors
Cerebellar tumors (posterior fossa)
Syringomyelia
Ocular dysfunction
Bulbar palsies
Traumatic (particularly C1–C2)
Subluxations
Dislocations
Fractures
Inflammatory
Cervical adenitis
Spontaneous hyperemic atlantoaxial rotatory subluxation
Tuberculosis
Typhoid
Rheumatoid arthritis
Acute calcification of a disc
Miscellaneous
Sandifer's syndrome (hiatal hernia with esophageal reflux)

whereas head tilt alone indicates a more generalized problem in the cervical spine. If the posturing of the head and neck is noted at or shortly after birth, congenital anomalies of the cervical spine should be considered. Bony anomalies of the cervical spine, particularly those that involve C1–C2, typically present as a rigid deformity, and the sternocleidomastoid muscle is *not* contracted or in spasm.

Gyorgyi[11] examined 20 cases of congenital torticollis and found the following coexisting anomalies: congenital cervical fusions, asymmetric facet joints, basilar impression, atlantoaxial dislocation, assimilation of the atlas, and deformities of the odontoid process. Interestingly, he noted that in children with congenital torticollis, 40 per cent had a history of breech presentation. Many occipitocervical malformations present with torticollis.[12, 17, 18, 24] De Barros and associates[7] noted that 68 per cent had basilar impression, most commonly unilaterally. Approximately 20 per cent of patients with the Klippel-Feil syndrome have associated torticollis.[9, 12] With asymmetric development of the occipital condyles or the facets of C1, the head tilt may result in a torticollis unless compensated for by a tilt of the lower cervical spine like that which occurs in the milder forms.[7, 8, 10]

If torticollis is noted in the weeks following delivery, the usual cause is congenital muscular torticollis. If the child is under 2 months of age, a palpable lump may be found in the sternocleidomastoid. Congenital muscular torticollis is painless, is associated with a contracted or shortened sternocleidomastoid muscle, and is unaccompanied by any bony abnormalities or neurologic deficit. Soft tissue problems are less common and include abnormal skin webs or folds (pterygium colli), which maintain the torticollis posture. Tumors in the region of the sternocleidomastoid, cystic hygroma, brachial cleft cyst, and thyroid teratoma are rare but should be considered.

Inflammatory conditions can include local irritation from cervical lymphadenitis, which may lead to the appearance of a wryneck or tilt of the head. Another less frequent cause is a retropharyngeal abscess after inflammation of the posterior pharynx or tonsillitis. Children with polyarticular juvenile rheumatoid arthritis frequently develop involvement of the cervical joints. Torticollis and limitation of cervical motion may be the only clinical signs. Spontaneous atlantoaxial rotatory subluxation may follow acute pharyngitis.[9, 19] Radiographic confirmation is difficult, and the CT methods for evaluation suggested by Phillips and Hensinger should be used.[19] Early diagnosis and reduction of the displacement is important. If it becomes

Table 10–3. TORTICOLLIS DUE TO BONY ANOMALIES

Congenital anomalies of craniocervical junction
Klippel-Feil syndrome
Atlanto-occipital synostosis (unilateral)
Basilar impression (unilateral)
Odontoid anomalies
Aplasia
Hypoplasia
Os odontoideum
Occipital vertebra
Asymmetry of occipital condyles (hypoplasia)
Acquired anomalies of craniocervical junction
Traumatic
Subluxations
Dislocations
Fractures
Inflammatory
Rheumatoid arthritis
Idiopathic
Atlantoaxial rotary displacement
Subluxation
Fixation

fixed, it poses a considerable treatment problem.[19] A rare inflammatory cause is acute calcification of a cervical disc,[16, 21] which can be visualized on routine roentgenographic study of the neck (Fig. 10–46).

Traumatic causes should always be considered and carefully excluded early in the evaluation. If unrecognized, they may have serious neurologic consequences. In general, torticollis most commonly follows injury to the C1–C2 articulation. Minor trauma can lead to spontaneous C1–C2 subluxation. Fractures or dislocation of the odontoid may not be apparent in the initial roentgenographic views (see Fig. 10–18), and consequently a high index of suspicion and careful follow-up is required.

Children with bone dysplasia, Morquio's syndrome, spondyloepiphyseal dysplasia, and Down syndrome have a high incidence of C1–C2 instability and should be evaluated routinely.

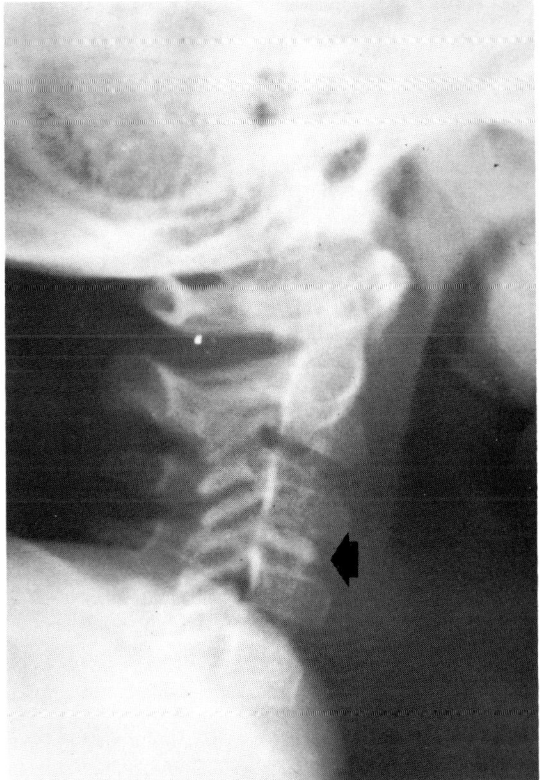

Figure 10–46. A 6-year-old female with acute onset of torticollis and neck pain but no history of trauma or recent infection. Lateral roentgenograph of the cervical spine demonstrates acute calcification of the disc between C3 and C4 *(arrow).* The child was treated conservatively with a neck collar, and there was spontaneous resolution of the torticollis and symptoms over a two-week period. The disc calcification, however, was still radiologically visible at six months after onset of symptoms but not at 12 months.

Intermittent torticollis can occur in the young child. A seizure-like disorder called "benign paroxysmal torticollis of infancy" has many neurologic causes, including drug intoxication. Similarly, Sandifer's syndrome, involving gastroesophageal reflux with sudden posturing of the trunk and torticollis, is being recognized more often, particularly in neurologically handicapped children, such as those with cerebral palsy.[23]

Neurologic disorders, particularly space-occupying lesions of the central nervous system, such as tumors of the posterior fossa or spinal column, cordoma, and syringomyelia, are often accompanied by torticollis. Generally, there are additional neurologic findings, such as long tract signs and weakness in the upper extremities. Uncommon neurologic causes include dystonia musculorum deformans and problems of hearing and vision that can result in head tilt. Although uncommon, hysterical and psychogenic etiologies exist, but these should be diagnosed only after other causes are carefully excluded.

Roentgenographic Features

All children with torticollis should be evaluated with roentgenography to exclude a bony abnormality or fracture. Roentgenographic interpretation of congenital torticollis may be difficult because of the fixed abnormal head position and the restricted motion. In those with a painful wry neck, it may be impossible to position them appropriately for a standard view of the occipitocervical junction. A helpful guide is that the atlas moves with the occiput, and if the x-ray beam is directed 90 degrees to the lateral skull, a satisfactory view of the occipitocervical junction usually results (Fig. 10–47). Flexion-extension stress films, laminagraphy, or cineradiography may be necessary to confirm atlantoaxial instability. The bony anomalies that may be present in congenital torticollis are documented under "Occipitocervical Synostosis," "Anomalies of Odontoid," "Klippel-Feil Syndrome," and "Basilar Impression."

Rotatory subluxation of C1 on C2 presents a unique problem. Plain roentgenographs seldom differentiate the position of C1 and C2 during subluxation from that in a normal child whose head is rotated, because both give the same picture. Open-mouth views have been difficult to obtain and interpret. Unfortu-

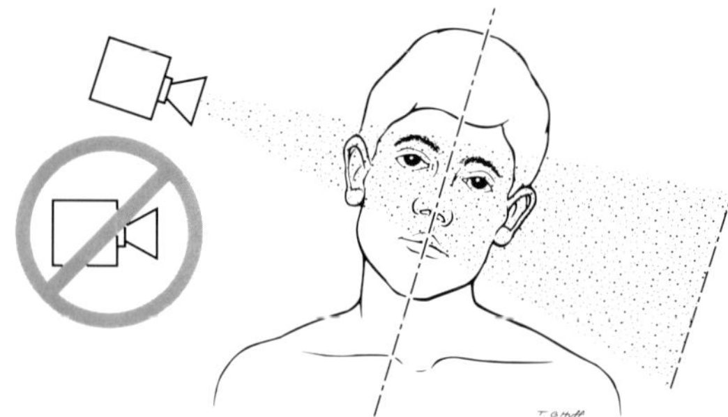

Ring of C1 stays with the Occiput

Figure 10–47. Obtaining a satisfactory radiograph may be hampered by the patient's limited ability to cooperate, fixed bony deformity, and overlapping shadows from the mandible, occiput, and foramen magnum. A helpful guide is that the atlas moves with the occiput, and if the x-ray beam is directed 90 degrees to the lateral of the skull, a satisfactory view of the occipitocervical junction usually results.

nately, lack of cooperation and decreased neck motion on the part of the child can make it impossible to obtain these special views. Fielding and Hawkins[9] recommended cineradiography, but the radiation dosage is relatively high, and again patient cooperation may be difficult to obtain owing to muscle spasm. The normal relationship between the occiput and the atlas is thought to be rarely affected in atlantoaxial rotatory subluxation. Thus, a lateral radiograph of the skull may demonstrate the relative position of the atlas and axis more clearly than a lateral radiograph of the cervical spine, in which tilting of the head will also tilt the atlas, and overlapping shadows make interpretation difficult (Fig. 10–47). Similarly, if during CT scans the child is in the torticollic position, the image may be interpreted by the radiologist as showing rotation of C1 on C2. Conversely, in the child with rotatory subluxation, the rotation of C1 on C2 may be within the range of normal, as is usually the case. Early in this condition the radiologist may contribute the finding to patient positioning.[19] This dilemma can be resolved by paying close attention to proper positioning of the patient, obtaining CT cuts at the level of C1, and then rotating the head to the right and left and demonstrating the facets to be locked in that position.[19]

References

Torticollis

1. Brackbill, Y., Douthitt, T. C., and West, H.: Psychophysiologic effects in the neonate of prone versus supine placement. J. Pediatr. *82:*82, 1973.
2. Brooks, B.: Pathologic changes in muscle as a result of disturbances of circulation. Arch. Surg. *5:*188, 1922.
3. Canale, S. T., Griffin, D. W., and Hubbard, C. N.: Congenital muscular torticollis. Long-term follow-up. J. Bone Joint Surg. *64A:*810, 1982.
4. Chandler, F. A.: Muscular torticollis. J. Bone Joint Surg. *30A:*556, 1948.
5. Clarren, S. K., Smith, D. W., and Hampton, J. W.: Helmet treatment for plagiocephaly in congenital muscular torticollis. J. Pediatr. *94:*43, 1979.
6. Coventry, M. B., and Harris, L. E.: Congenital muscular torticollis in infancy: some observations regarding treatment. J. Bone Joint Surg. *41A:*815, 1959.
7. De Barros, M. C., Farias, W., Ataide, L., and Lins, S.: Basilar impression and Arnold-Chiari malformation: a study of 66 cases. J. Neurol. Neurosurg. Psychiatr. *1:*596, 1968.
8. Dubousett, J.: Torticollis in children caused by congenital anomalies of the atlas. J. Bone Joint Surg. *68A:*178, 1986.
9. Fielding, J. W., and Hawkins, R. J.: Atlanto-axial rotatory fixation (fixed rotatory subluxation of the atlanto-axial joint). J. Bone Joint Surg. *59A:*37, 1977.
10. Gray, S. W., Romaine, C. B., and Skandalakis, J. F.: Congenital fusion of the cervical vertebrae. Surg. Gynecol. Obstet. *118:*373, 1964.
11. Gyorgyi, G.: Les changements morphologiques de la region occipitocervicale associés au torticollis. J. Radiol. Electrol. Med. Nucl. *45:*797, 1965.
12. Hensinger, R. N., Lang, J. R., and MacEwen, G. D.: The Klippel-Feil syndrome: a constellation of related anomalies. J. Bone Joint Surg. *56A:*1246, 1974.
13. Hummer, D. C., Jr., and MacEwen, G. D.: The coexistence of torticollis and congenital dysplasia of the hip. J. Bone Joint Surg. *54A:*1255, 1972.
14. Ling, C. M., and Low, Y. S.: Sternomastoid tumor and muscular torticollis. Clin. Orthop. *86:*144, 1972.
15. MacDonald, C.: Sternomastoid tumor and muscular torticollis. J. Bone Joint Surg. *51B:*432, 1969.
16. Melnick, J. C., and Silverman, F. N.: Intervertebral disk calcification in childhood. Radiology *80:*399, 1963.
17. McRae, D. L.: Bony abnormalities in the region of the foramen magnum: correction of the anatomic and neurologic findings. Acta Radiol. *40:*335, 1953.
18. McRae, D. L.: The significance of abnormalities of the cervical spine. Am. J. Roentgenol. Radium Ther. Nucl. Med. *84:*3, 1960.
19. Phillips, W. A., and Hensinger, R. N.: The management of rotatory atlanto-axial subluxation in children. J. Bone Joint Surg. *71A:*664, 1989.
20. Sarant, J. B., and Morrissy, R. T.: Idiopathic torticollis: sternocleidomastoid myopathy and accessory neuropathy. Muscle Nerve *4:*374, 1981.
21. Schechter, L. S., Smith, A., and Pearl, M.: Intervertebral disk calcification in childhood. Am. J. Dis. Child. *123:*608, 1972.
22. Staheli, L. T.: Muscular torticollis: late results of operative treatment. Surgery *69:*469, 1971.
23. Sutcliff, J.: Torsion spasms and abnormal postures in children with hiatus hernia: Sandifer's syndrome. Prog. Pediatr. Radiol. *2:*190, 1969.
24. von Torklus, D., and Gehle, W.: The Upper Cervical Spine. New York, Grune & Stratton, 1972.

CHAPTER

11

CONGENITAL ANOMALIES OF THE SPINAL CORD

Leslie Sutton, M.D.

MYELOMENINGOCELE

Myelomeningocele is the most common significant birth defect involving the spine. The condition is manifest at birth and is characterized by herniation of a malformed spinal cord through a defect in the bony canal and skin. It almost always results in permanent disability regardless of medical intervention, and often deprives the victim of "those qualities held in high esteem by our society—independence, physical powers and intelligence."[13] No consensus has been reached regarding the timing, the nature, or even the wisdom of intervention. It is hoped that informed parents and compassionate professionals working together will arrive at decisions that are individualized and appropriate for each affected newborn.

Embryology

Myelomeningocele is one of a group of neural tube defects, which also includes anencephaly, encephalocele, and craniorachischisis.[30, 31] The most severe of these are incompatible with life and occur earliest in embryogenesis.

By 18 days of development, the embryo is a flattened oval disc with all three germ layers present. A longitudinal depression, the neural groove, appears in the neural plate, which is destined to become the brain and spinal cord. By 22 days, the neural groove has deepened, and fusion of the adjacent tissue begins the transformation of the flat neural plate into a hollow neural tube. The entire process is called neurulation, which begins in the dorsal midline and simultaneously progresses in both cephalad and caudal directions. The final portions of the tube to close are the rostral opening (the anterior neuropore, at 24 days) and the caudal opening (the posterior neuropore, at 28 days). Thus, by the first month of gestation the entire process has been completed. The development of the meninges begins after closure of the posterior neuropore, as does formation of the bony laminae.[30]

Theories regarding myelomeningocele and other neural tube defects fall into two basic groups: (1) those postulating that the tube never undergoes a normal closure at a given site and (2) those postulating that it closes normally, but then reopens. The issue is of some importance, since the period of development during which potential teratogens could act is entirely different in the two cases. The traditional nonclosure theory is supported by the fact that anencephaly and myelomeningocele occur at the sites of the embryonic anterior and posterior neuropores, and also by studies of human embryos that have shown failure of neurulation at a very early stage.[29] The reopening theories have been most recently popularized by Gardner, who proposes that failure of the fourth ventricle to open results in distention of the central canal of the spinal cord with cerebrospinal fluid (CSF). The spinal cord eventually ruptures to produce the myelomeningocele.[14–16] This "hydrodynamic theory" has been criticized because it does not explain total myeloschisis, since rupture at a single point would be expected to decompress the cerebral canal and limit the abnormality. Furthermore, embryos with neural tube defects have been found at a stage before the choroid plexus has formed.[29, 45] Thus, although the hydrodynamic theory does not account for all aspects of the genesis of neural tube defects, it undoubtedly helps to explain delayed symptomatic hydrosyringomyelia, which often accompanies myelomeningocele.

Epidemiology

The etiology of myelodysplasia is unknown, and evidence exists for both environmental[59] and multifactorial genetic influences.[5] The incidence of myelomeningocele is approximately one to two per 1000 live births in the United States, but is considerably higher in the British Isles (8.7 per 1000 births in Belfast, Northern Ireland).[12] Populations migrating from areas of high or low incidence appear to retain their characteristic malformation rate.[26] The risk is higher in Caucasians and among persons of lower socioeconomic class.[26] In addition, the risk increases markedly after the birth of an affected child, to 2 to 5 per cent.[25] An interesting finding in some studies is an increased incidence in babies born during winter months.[11]

Little is known about possible environmental factors in man, but experimental work in rodents reveals a number of teratogenic agents that may induce neural tube defects, including x-rays, vitamin A excess, vitamin E and folic acid deficiency, and some chemical agents.[18] It has been difficult to prove, however, that vitamin supplements prevent myelodysplasia in humans.[27, 44] A suggestion that potato avoidance during pregnancy could prevent myelodysplasia has not been supported by further study.[43]

Prenatal Diagnosis

The use of amniocentesis to detect neural tube defects was first described by Brock and Sutcliffe in 1972.[3] Skin-covered lesions, which represent 5 to 20 per cent of all neural tube malformations, are not detected by this technique, however, and it involves an invasive procedure. Screening populations at risk has been carried out with measurement of maternal serum alpha-fetoprotein obtained at 16 to 18 weeks of gestation. An abnormal result is followed by amniocentesis. This technique has proved valuable as a screening technique, but false-positive results are noted in multiple pregnancies, in hydronephrosis, and for no apparent reason.[42] Screening ultrasonography performed on mothers at increased risk between 16 and 20 weeks of gestation has also proved valuable,[4] and it is estimated that more than 90 per cent of open neural tube defects can be positively identified by a combination of amniocentesis and ultrasonography in time for therapeutic abortion.[19, 49]

Initial Evaluation

The initial assessment of the newborn infant with a myelomeningocele begins with a detailed examination to evaluate its general well-being and to seek associated anomalies. In particular, fatal urologic or cardiac anomalies may be evident that would favor nonoperative treatment. Some infants may have abnormal facies suggesting Down syndrome, and although chromosomal studies should be obtained, these are most often normal, and the facial appearance becomes normal with age. Approximately 80 per cent of children with myelomeningocele present with hydrocephalus or develop it within the newborn period.[40] A large head circumference or bulging fontanelle suggests the need for early head ultrasonography via the fontanelle. Stridor, apnea, or bradycardia in the absence of overt intracranial hypertension suggests a symptomatic Arnold-Chiari malformation and hindbrain dysfunction, which carries a poor prognosis.[2, 7]

The myelomeningocele is then inspected using sterile gloves. If the sac is intact, it should not be ruptured. The red granular neural placode is surrounded by the pearly zona epitheliosa, which interfaces with full-thickness skin. This tissue must be excised at the time of surgery to prevent dermoid inclusion cysts from developing later in life. Most myelomeningoceles are slightly oval in shape, with the long axis oriented vertically. If the lesion is more horizontally oriented, it may be easier to close the skin defect horizontally. If the sac is ruptured, the placode will be readily visible. A vertically oriented groove within it represents the opened central canal of the spinal cord and may be dripping CSF. The spinal level of the lesion is estimated, as is its size. Associated scoliosis is noted.

The neurologic examination is difficult in neonates, and it is easy to confuse reflex motion with voluntary motor movements. Fixed contractures and foot deformity suggest paralysis of the spinal segments innervating those joints. Any movement in response to painful stimulation of the same extremity must be viewed as potentially reflexive. Crying in response to a painful stimulus suggests intact sensation at that level. Table 11–1 lists the segmental innervation of the lower extremities in man and may be used as a guide in assigning a functional level. It is more useful, however, to document function of the individual muscle groups rather than simply to record a spinal level.

Virtually all patients with myelomeningocele have abnormal bladder function, but it is difficult to assess this in the newborn period. A patulous anus lacking in sensation and a distended bladder on physical examination or ultrasonography confirm a neurogenic bladder. A full bladder may be emptied by the Credé maneuver, but a renal and bladder ultrasound examination is still necessary to evaluate the upper tracts and to assess the adequacy of emptying.

Initial Management and Treatment Options

The ethics of selecting newborn infants with severe congenital anomalies for aggressive or "conservative" management is controversial, and a thorough discussion goes beyond the scope of this book. Several reviews have been written on this topic.[20, 21, 32, 33, 36, 44, 54, 56] It is generally agreed, however, that initial evaluation and family counseling are ideally performed by a multidisciplinary team that is expert in managing children with myelomeningocele of all ages and can offer a realistic discussion regarding long-term prognosis. Evidence suggests that with broad-spectrum antibiotic coverage, surgery can be delayed for up to a week without increased risk to the infant in order to allow face-to-face discussion with both parents.[6, 56] Other authors, however, still suggest that surgery is best performed 24 to 48 hours after birth to prevent ventriculitis.[40, 51, 52] It is vital to emphasize to the family that surgical closure of the myelomeningocele is a life-saving measure but does not alter preexisting neurologic deficits.

Table 11–1. INNERVATION OF THE LEG MUSCLES

Hip flexion	L1–L3
Hip adduction	L2–L4
Knee extension	L2–L4
Ankle inversion	L4
Toe extension	L5–S1
Hip abduction	L5–S1
Hip extension	L5–S2
Knee flexion	L5–S2
Ankle plantar flexion	S1–S2

Data from Sharrard, W. J. W.: The segmental innervation of the lower limb muscles in man. Ann. R. Coll. Surg. *35*:106–122, 1964.

Pending plans for definitive care, the infant is nursed in the prone position with a sterile saline-soaked gauze dressing loosely applied to the sac or placode. Broad-spectrum antibiotics (ampicillin and cefotaxime) are begun intravenously pending discussion with the parents.

As a rule, the back is closed initially and hydrocephalus is treated with a ventriculoperitoneal shunt at a separate procedure. In patients with overt hydrocephalus and intracranial hypertension at birth, it may be advisable to perform both procedures at the same sitting, since failure to treat the hydrocephalus may allow continued leakage of CSF into the back and threaten the closure.

The goal of back closure is to seal, using multiple tissue layers, the spinal cord and subarachnoid space against entry of bacteria from the skin. At the same time, the surgeon must preserve whatever neurologic function remains, and attempt to prevent tethering of the spinal cord. The technique is generally that described by Poppen,[48] with modifications by McLone[37] and Reigel and McLone.[51]

The child is positioned in the prone position under general anesthesia. Rolls are placed under the chest and hips to allow the abdomen to hang freely and minimize epidural bleeding

(Fig. 11–1*A*). If the sac is intact, fluid is aspirated and sent for culture. The surgeon then gently attempts to approximate the base of the sac or defect vertically and then horizontally to determine which direction will produce the smallest skin defect. An elliptical incision is then made, oriented along that axis, outside the junction of the normal, full-thickness skin and the thin, pearly zona epitheliosa. Full-thickness skin forming the base of the sac

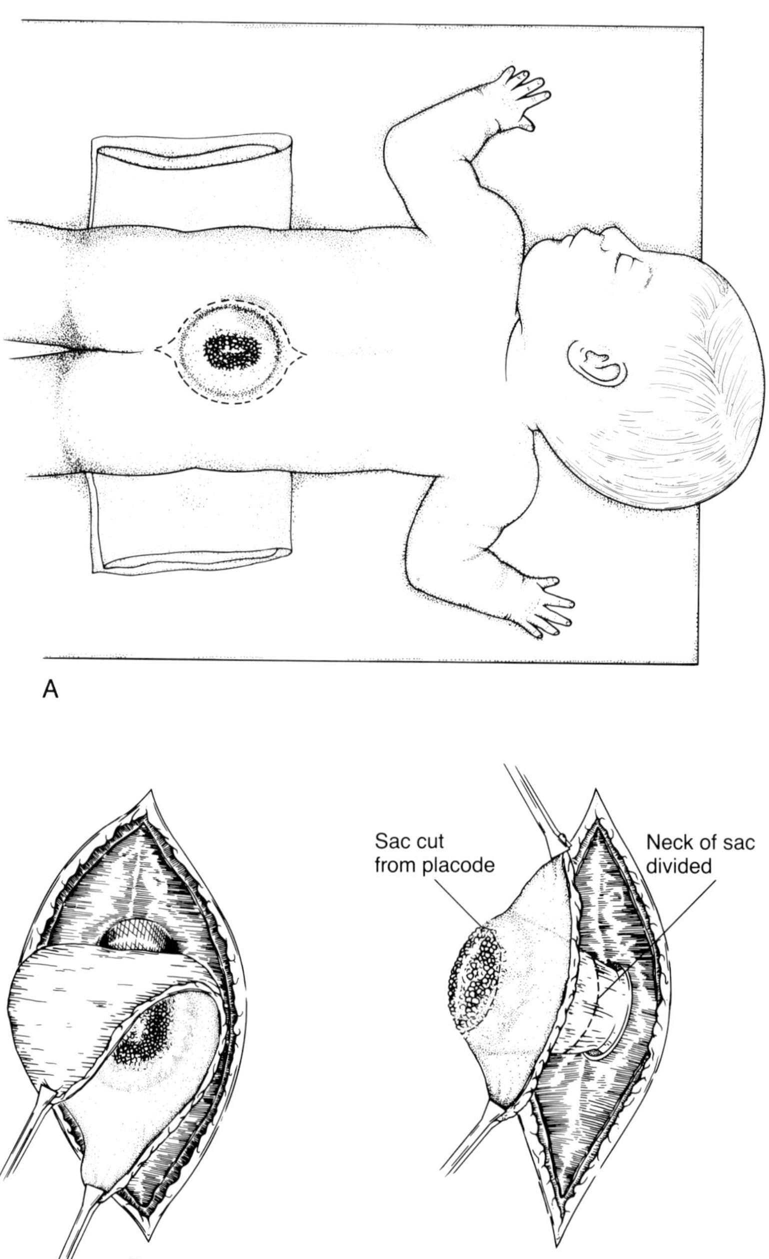

Figure 11–1. Technique for closure of a myelomeningocele (see text). *A,* The infant is placed in the prone position with towel rolls under the hips. An elliptic incision is outlined just outside the zona epitheliosa, which may be oriented on a vertical or horizontal axis. *B,* The incision is to the level of the lumbodorsal fascia. The apices of the island of skin within the incision are grasped with clamps, and the skin is undermined medially until the dural sac is seen to funnel through the fascial defect. *C,* The dural sac is first incised at its base. The skin is then excised from the placode and discarded, allowing the placode to fall into the spinal canal.

is viable and should not be excised. This incision is carried through the subcutaneous tissue until the glistening layer of everted dura or fascia is encountered. The base of the sac is then mobilized medially until it is seen to enter the fascial defect (Fig. 11–1*B*). The sac is entered by radially incising the cuff of skin surrounding the placode. This skin is then sharply excised circumferentially around the placode and discarded, care being take to avoid damaging the placode (Fig. 11–1*C*). It is important that all the zona epitheliosa be removed to prevent later development of an epidermoid tumor. At this point the placode is floating freely inside the everted dura (Fig. 11–1*D*).

In some instances it is appropriate to "reconstruct" the placode so that it fits better within the canal, and to reconstruct the tubular form of the spinal cord so that a pial surface is in contact with the dural closure. The purpose of this is to prevent retethering. This is accomplished by interrupted 6-0 sutures to approximate the pia-arachnoid–neural junction of one side with the other. The central canal is thus closed along its entire length.

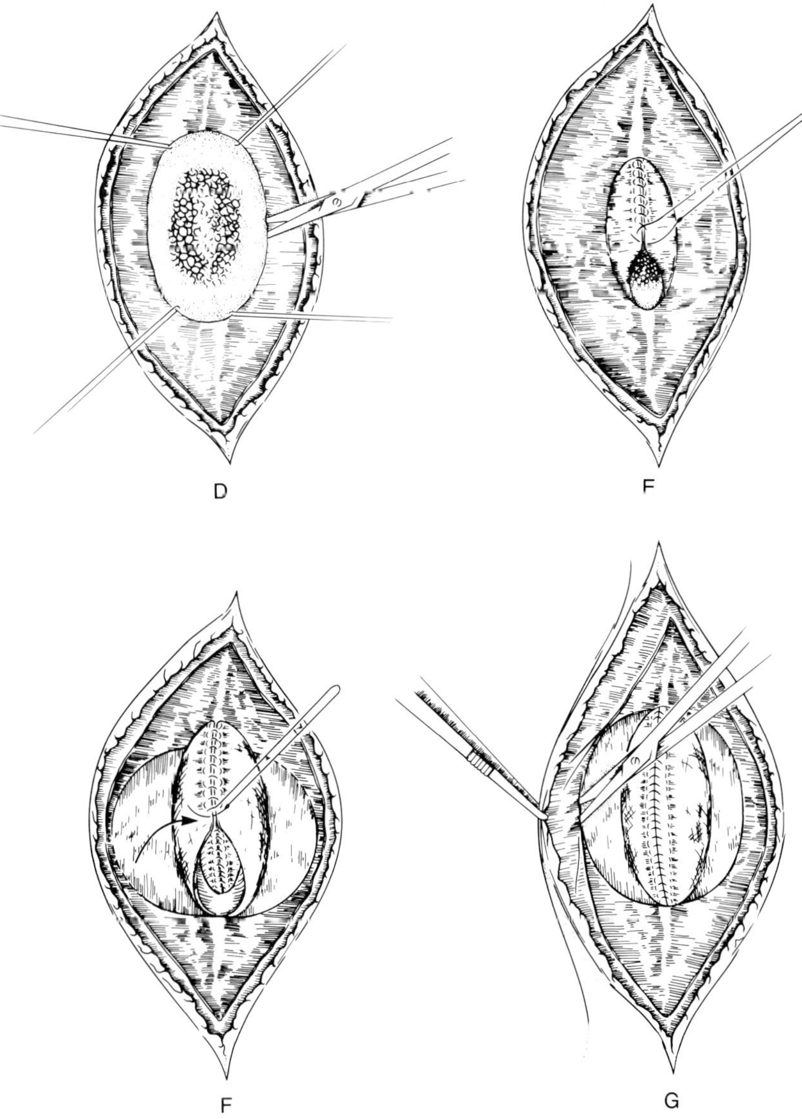

Figure 11–1 *Continued D,* The everted dura is undermined and reflected medially to envelop the placode. *E,* The dural layer is closed with nonabsorbable suture, using a running stitch. *F,* The fascia is incised to the muscle, undermined, and reflected medially to create a second layer of closure. *G,* The skin is undermined using blunt techniques to permit closure.

Attention is now directed toward the dura, which is everted and loosely attached to the underlying fascia. It is undermined bluntly and reflected medially on each side until enough has been mobilized to effect closure (Fig. 11–1*E*). The dura is very thin medially where the root sleeves exit and is easily torn. Once it is free, the dura is closed in a watertight fashion with 4-0 Nurolon.

If the dural closure is suboptimal, it is desirable also to close the fascia as a separate layer. The fascia is incised laterally in a semicircular fashion on either side, elevated from the underlying muscle, and reflected medially (Fig. 11–1*F*). It is closed with 4-0 Nurolon over the underlying dural closure. The fascia is poor at the caudal end of a lumbar myelomeningocele or with sacral lesions, and the closure may be incomplete.

Mobilization of the skin is by blunt dissection with scissors or a finger and it may be necessary to free it up all the way anteriorly to the abdomen (Fig. 11–1*G*). In most instances the closure is easiest in the midsagittal (vertical) plane, but occasionally less tension is required for a horizontal closure. A two-layer closure with vertical mattress skin sutures is preferred.

Very large lesions require special techniques. There is often an associated gibbous deformity and it is helpful to rongeur the everted lamina, which, if left in place, will produce pressure points on the skin closure. Large circular defects may be closed by means of an S-shaped skin opening, allowing the use of rotation flaps (Fig. 11–2).[34] Alternatively, a Z-rhomboid flap may be employed.[9] Lateral relaxing incisions and muscle flaps have been described but should be avoided if possible.[28, 35]

A very few infants are so severely affected that no realistic benefit can follow aggressive management. For these, antibiotics are not given and they are discharged home to the care of the parents. It is understood that if the child survives or if the parents change their minds and opt for aggressive treatment, the infant will again become a candidate for surgical intervention.

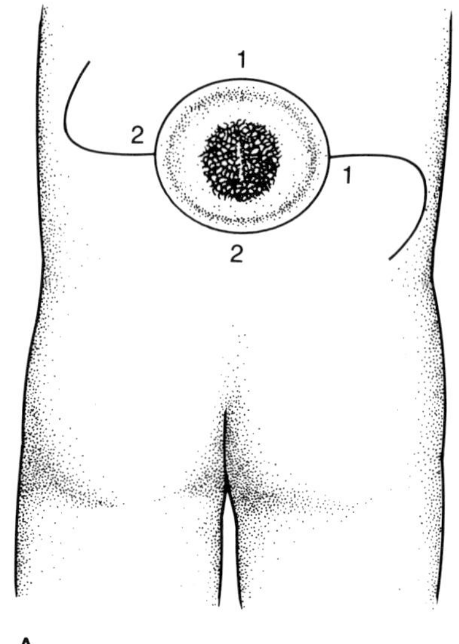

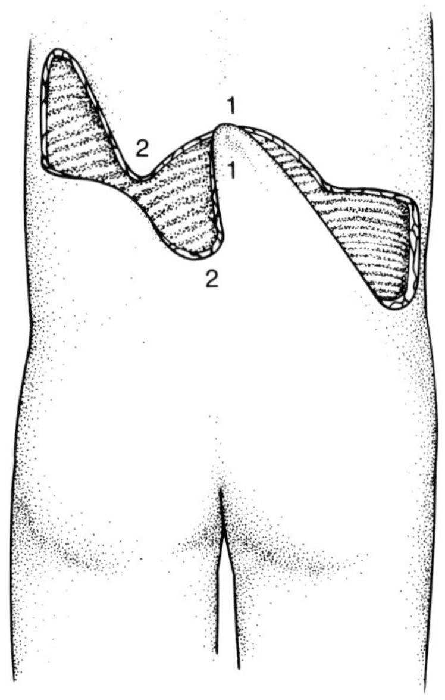

Figure 11–2. *A, B,* Z-plasty closure for large circular skin defects. A horizontal, S-shaped skin incision is used with the defect in the center. Closure is effected by approximating the points of the skin edge to the troughs of the opposing skin edge, as shown in *B.*

Late Deterioration

Myelomeningocele is a birth defect, and although there are often severe neurologic sequelae, they should remain static. Any sign of worsening in a child or adult with spina bifida should provoke an intense search for a cause, which is usually treatable. Possible reasons for neurologic deterioration include un-

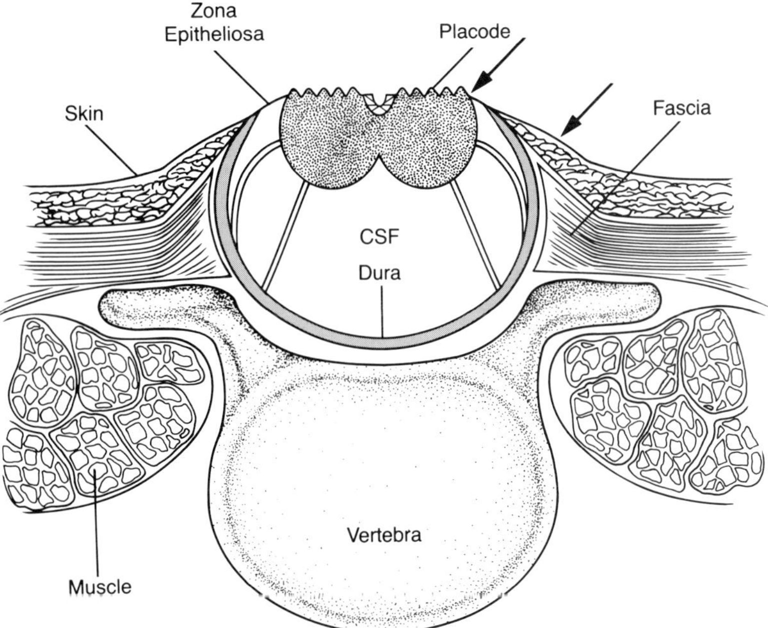

Figure 11–3. Cross-sectional anatomy of a typical myelomeningocele.

controlled hydrocephalus, Chiari malformation, hydromyelia, tethered cord syndrome, epidermoid/dermoid inclusion cyst, and reactive depression. Unfortunately, even with modern diagnostic techniques it may prove difficult to determine which of the above factors is responsible for worsening in a particular patient. This is true in part because the anatomic changes (such as Chiari malformation or tethered cord) are present in the vast majority of children with myelodysplasia, whether or not they are symptomatic.

Tethered Cord

It is now generally recognized that spinal cord tethering in patients with myelomeningocele may result in progressive loss of function similar to that seen with occult spinal dysraphism.[50] Signs and symptoms usually appear during the first decade of life and include back and leg pain, decrease in urinary control, gait difficulty and leg weakness, progressive foot deformity, and possibly scoliosis. Urinary and gait difficulties are complaints confined to patients with low-level lesions, who are already functioning quite well neurologically and clearly have the most to lose. In the more severely affected patient who may already be wheelchair bound, pain may be the only manifestation of cord tethering and may be confused with appendicitis, hernia, urinary tract infection, or traumatic arthritis associated with abnormal posture or gait. Work-up consists of magnetic resonance imaging (MRI) of the complete spine, including sagittal and axial views. This will invariably show a low-lying, dorsally displaced spinal cord and perhaps an associated diastematomyelia or hydromyelia. Unfortunately, these same findings are noted even in asymptomatic patients and their presence does not by itself indicate the need for surgery. It is important that all children with myelomeningocele be carefully followed by a specialty group, including orthopedist, pediatrician, and physical therapist, so that subtle signs of deterioration can be documented, since the decision to operate is made largely on clinical grounds.

The surgery to release a tethered spinal cord in a patient with myelomeningocele is similar to that for a lipomyelomeningocele. Patients are operated on in the prone position with rolls under the chest and hips. A vertical midline incision is used, regardless of the type of closure used for the initial myelomeningocele closure. The most caudal normal lamina above the palpable spina bifida defect is identified and removed, and the underlying normal dura is opened at this level, exposing normal (but low-lying) spinal cord. With the aid of magnification, the dorsally and laterally attached placode is carefully dissected free from adhesions, working in a caudal direction. This is best done with sharp instruments. When the spinal cord has been released, it will fall into the patulous sac of the anterior spinal canal. Any associated diastematomyelia or dermoid inclusion cyst is removed. The dura is closed primarily or with a patch graft.

As with lipomyelomeningocele, the aim of surgery is to prevent further deterioration of function, but occasionally improvement is seen, even in preexisting deficits of long-standing duration. Reigel reported improvement in bladder function in five of nine patients with recent deterioration and 77 per cent of patients with gait difficulty and motor weakness.[50] Pain almost invariably improves.

It has been suggested that spinal cord tethering may play a role in the etiology of scoliosis in patients with myelomeningocele.[50] This has been difficult to prove since there are many other reasons why children with spina bifida might develop scoliosis, including bony abnormality, Chiari malformation, or hydromyelia.[47] In patients with a minor degree of scoliosis, tethered cord release may appear to halt progression, but it is unclear what the natural history would have been without surgery. Children with severe curvature require fusion with or without an untethering procedure.

Hydromyelia

The routine availability of metrizamide spinal computed tomography (CT) and MRI has heightened awareness of this entity. Hydromyelia presumably is the result of hydrodynamic forces arising from persistent fetal or untreated hydrocephalus that force CSF down the central canal of the spinal cord.[14–16] This accounts for the frequency of symptomatic hydromyelia in patients with unshunted ventriculomegaly, or those considered to have "compensated" hydrocephalus, whose nonfunctional shunts were not revised because they lacked overt signs or symptoms of intracranial hypertension.[22]

Symptoms of hydromyelia in spina bifida differ somewhat from those in classical syringomyelia. The latter entity typically produces a dissociated sensory loss (relative loss of pain and temperature modalities with preservation of light touch), atrophy, and fasciculations primarily affecting the shoulder girdle and hands. When found in association with myelomeningocele, hydromyelia typically results in progressive bladder dysfunction, spasticity of both upper and lower extremities, quadriparesis, and generally preserved sensation. The myelomeningocele repair may become swollen and tender.[22] In part, symptoms may be due to the direct effects of the hydrocephalus stretching the cortical motor fibers. Hydromyelia may also be seen with progressive scoliosis.

Work-up consists of CT or MRI of the head followed by MRI of the entire spine to visualize the extent of the syrinx, as well as any associated Chiari malformation and tethered spinal cord. The hydromyelic cavity may be localized to a few spinal segments or extend throughout the length of the spinal cord. There may be multiple cavities and septations.

Treatment of symptomatic hydromyelia begins with a ventriculoperitoneal shunt or shunt revision if the ventricles are enlarged. If the ventricles are small, or if the hydromyelia persists without improvement in symptoms after this procedure, a shunt is placed from the hydromyelia to the pleural cavity. This is ideally done in the thoracic area but should be at the spinal level where the cavity is largest. The shunt is made to drain at a very low pressure. A follow-up MRI scan is taken when the patient is stable. Shunt failure is common.

Other procedures have been described. Terminal ventriculostomy was advocated by Gardner and colleagues for classical syringomyelia,[17] but the myelotomy tends to scar closed with time. In addition, the negative pressure provided by the pleural end of a shunt provides more decompression than simply allowing the hydromyelia to communicate with the subarachnoid space.[58] Park and associates advocated posterior fossa decompression and plugging of the obex to prevent CSF fluid from the fourth ventricle from entering the central canal in patients in whom ventriculoperitoneal shunt revisions do not alleviate symptoms.[47] This is a formidable procedure, however, and recurrent vomiting may occur from irritation or compression of the brain stem at the obex.

Chiari Malformation

The Chiari malformations are anomalies of craniovertebral function characterized by downward displacement of the cerebellar vermis, tonsils, and cervicomedullary junction into the spinal canal. Chiari described three types in 1891.[8]

Type I becomes symptomatic primarily in young adults or adolescents without myelomeningocele. The medulla and cerebellar vermis extend downward into the cervical spinal canal as a tongue of tissue plastered against the dorsal surface of the spinal cord. There may be associated hydromyelia, but hydrocephalus is rare. Symptoms include lower cranial nerve palsies, vertigo, oscillopsia, truncal ataxia, headache, or syncope in association with the Valsalva maneuver. In addition, the classical symptoms of syringomyelia, such as weakness and atrophy of the hands and dissociated sensory loss, may be seen if there is an associated cavitation of the spinal cord.

Type II nearly always occurs in association with myelomeningocele, and symptoms may be apparent in infancy, childhood, or adulthood. Anatomically, the cerebellum is small, as is the posterior fossa itself, and the foramen magnum is large. The vermis projects as a tongue of tissue into the cervical spinal canal, and the vermis tongue and fourth ventricle may extend as low as the thoracic spine (Fig. 11–4). Commonly, there is a kink in the medulla, and the cervical nerve roots are seen to project in an upward direction. Hydrocephalus is present in 90 per cent of cases.

Type II lesions typically present in infancy with inspiratory stridor due to vocal cord paralysis, weakness in feeding, bradycardia, apnea, or "blue spells." Patients are often erroneously diagnosed as suffering from croup or asthma.[2, 7, 10, 23, 23, 46, 57] In older children and adults, symptoms are similar to those seen with Type I lesions.

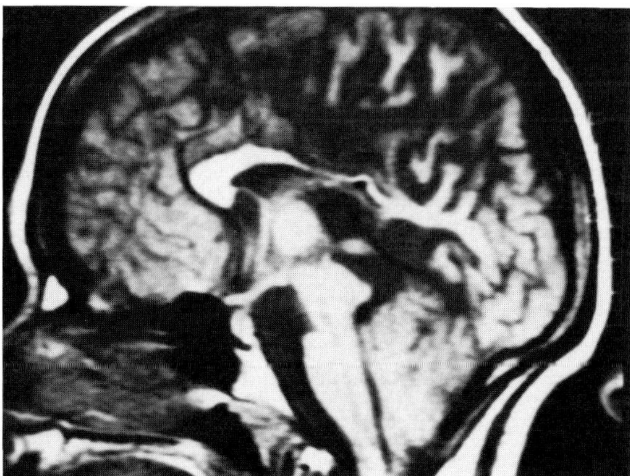

Figure 11–4. MRI scan showing a typical Chiari II malformation seen in association with myelomeningocele. The brain stem and cerebellum are fused into a "vermian pseudotumor," the posterior fossa is shallow, and the vermis protrudes into the spinal canal. The transverse sinuses and torcular are at the level of the foramen magnum.

Type III is uncommon and consists of cervical spina bifida with cerebellar hernia. It is usually fatal in the newborn period.

MRI is the procedure of choice for initial evaluation, because the lesion is readily visualized and associated abnormalities are easily excluded. Midsagittal views show the tongue of cerebellum extending below the foramen magnum in Type I lesions, and the "vermian pseudotumor," consisting of the fused brain stem and cerebellum, in Type II lesions.

Chiari Type II lesions presenting in the infant with myelomeningocele are particularly dificult to manage. Much of the symptomatology may derive from disordered brain stem nuclei, which do not improve with surgical decompression.[2, 7] If the associated hydrocephalus is under optimal control, however, consideration must be given to posterior fossa decompression and cervical laminectomy despite the dismal outlook. Patients are operated on in the prone position. A midline incision is used to expose the suboccipital bone, as well as the cervical spine down to the level of the cerebellar hernia as seen on the MRI scan, and a laminectomy is performed. The tonsillar hernia can usually be seen through the translucent dura, which is opened in the midline, beginning at the lowest point of the laminectomy and progressing upward. In this way, silver clips can be used to control bleeding from the anomalous venous sinuses that usually are in the posterior fossa. The dural opening should include the fibrous band usually present at the foramen magnum. The dura is then left open and the muscles, fascia, and skin are closed as usual. If the child does not improve and stridor and apnea persist, a frank discussion with the family is indicated. Options include tracheostomy and feeding gastrostomy and chronic ventilator therapy, if needed. Such treatment seriously lowers the quality of life, and some families may opt for conservative management.

Older children and adults with Chiari malformations who present with Type I symptoms respond to decompression more favorably, presumably because the cranial nerve nuclei are functional and symptoms are due to compression. The surgical procedure is the same as that described above.

Summary

Signs or symptoms of worsening in a patient with myelodysplasia should provoke a thorough evaluation. The importance of careful history taking and physical examination cannot be overemphasized, since radiologic studies often reveal a plethora of abnormalites, and only the astute clinician can discern which is responsible for a particular complaint. If symptoms involve only the lower extremities and sphincters, possible causes include decompensated hydrocephalus, hydromyelia, or tethered cord. If the upper extremities or brain stem are involved, possible causes include hydrocephalus, hydromyelia/hydrobulbia, and Chiari malformation. At times the clinician is forced to simply treat the various lesions serially until symptoms improve.

Outcome

Significant progress has been made in the understanding and management of myelomeningocele over the past 25 years, particularly in the widespread use of multidisciplinary teams of specialists to manage children with this condition. Among those who undergo early back closure, 92 per cent survive infancy[56] and 86 per cent are alive at 3½ to 7 years of follow-up.[39] Death is due to problems associated with the Chiari II malformation, restrictive lung disease secondary to chest deformity, shunt malfunction, and urinary sepsis. Among those who were not closed immediately, approximately half went on to die at a mean of 6 weeks of age and 50 per cent were eventually closed in one series.[56]

Approximately 75 per cent of children with myelomeningocele are ambulatory, although most require braces and crutches.[1, 39] The likelihood that a child will ambulate is related to the level of the lesion; virtually all sacral and lumbosacral patients will walk, yet only half of those with thoracic or thoracolumbar lesions achieve this skill, with the use of braces and crutches. Those with high-level lesions often can walk as young children, but fall into the wheelchair group as they get older, gain weight, or simply discover that wheelchair locomotion requires less energy than ambulation with crutches.[40]

Overall, approximately 75 per cent of surviving infants have normal intelligence (IQ greater than 80),[40, 56] although this falls to only 50 to 60 per cent of those who require shunts for hydrocephalus.[1, 55] Intelligence is also related to the level of the lesion: approximately 55 per cent of those with thoracic lesions have significant developmental delay, compared with only 25 per cent of those with lesions at lower levels.[56] The cause of mental retardation in children with myelodysplasia remains controversial. McLone and colleagues attributed it to ventriculitis,[38] but this does not account for all cases, and it is likely that in most cases forebrain dysfunction is simply part of the complex of anomalies associated with myelodysplasia (Fig. 11–4).

Although virtually all children with myelomeningocele have abnormal bladder function, urinary continence with the use of clean intermittent catheterization approaches 90 per cent in the population 5 to 9 years old.[40]

References

1. Ames, M. D., and Schut, L.: Results of treatment of 171 consecutive myelomeningoceles—1963–1968. Pediatrics *50:*466–470, 1972.
2. Bell, W. O., Charney, E. B., Bruce, D. A., et al.: Symptomatic Arnold-Chiari malformation: review of experience with 22 cases. J. Neurosurg. *66:*812–816, 1987.
3. Brock, D. J. H., and Sutcliffe. R. G.: Alpha-fetoprotein in the antenatal diagnosis of anencephaly and spina bifida. Lancet *2:*197–199, 1972.
4. Campbell, S.: Early prenatal diagnosis of neural tube defects by ultrasound. Clin. Obstet. Gynecol. *20:*351–359, 1977.
5. Carter, C. O., David, P. A., and Laurence, K. M.: A family study of major central nervous system malformations in South Wales. J. Med. Genet. *5:*81–106, 1968.
6. Charney, E. B., Weller, S. C., Sutton, L. N., et al.: Management of the newborn with myelomeningocele: time for a decision-making process. Pediatrics *75:*58–64, 1985.
7. Charney, E. B., Rorke, L. B., Sutton, L. N., and Schut, L.: Management of Chiari II complications in infants with myelomeningocele. J. Pediatr. *111:*364–371, 1987.
8. Chiari, H.: Ueber Veränderungen des Kleinhirns in Folge von Hydrocephalie des Grosshirns. Dtsch. Med. Wochenschr. *17:*1172–1175, 1891.
9. Cruz, N. I., Ariyan, S., Duncan, C. C., et al.: Repair of lumbosacral myelomeningoceles with double Z-rhomboid flaps. Technical note. J. Neurosurg. *59:*714–717, 1983.
10. Duhaime, A. C., Schut, L., and Sutton, L. N.: The Arnold-Chiari malformation. Int. Pediatr. *2:*38–42, 1987.
11. Edwards, J. H.: Congenital malformations of the central nervous system in Scotland. Br. J. Prev. Soc. Med. *12:*115, 1958.

12. Elwood, J. H., and Nevin, N. C.: Factors associated with anencephalus and spina bifida in Belfast. Br. J. Prev. Soc. Med. *27:*73–86, 1973.
13. French, B. N.: Midline fusion defects and defects in formation. *In* Youmans, J. R. (ed.): Neurological Surgery. 3rd ed. Philadelphia, W. B. Saunders Co., 1990, pp. 1081–1235.
14. Gardner, W. J.: Myelomeningocele, the result of rupture of the embryonic neural tube. Cleve. Clin. Q. *27:*88–100, 1960.
15. Gardner, W. J.: Rupture of neural tube: cause of myelomeningocele. Arch. Neurol. *4:*1–7, 1961.
16. Gardner, W. J.: Dysraphic States: From Syringomyelia to Anencephaly. Amsterdam, Excerpta Medica, 1973.
17. Gardner, W. J., Bell, H. S., Poolos, P. N., et al.: Terminal ventriculostomy for syringomyelia. J. Neurosurg. *46:*609–617, 1977.
18. Giroud, A.: Causes and morphogenesis of anencephaly. *In* Wolstenholme, G. E. W., and O'Connor, C. M. O. (eds.): Ciba Foundation Symposium on Congenital Malformations. London, Churchill, 1960, p. 1960.
19. Globus, M. S., Loughman, W. D., Epstein, C. J., et al.: Prenatal genetic diagnosis in 3000 amniocenteses. N. Engl. J. Med. *300:*157–163, 1979.
20. Gross, R. H., Cox, A., Tatyrek, R., et al.: Early management and decision making for the treatment of myelomeningocele. Pediatrics *72:*450–458, 1983.
21. Gross, R. H.: Newborns with myelodysplasia—the rest of the story. N. Engl. J. Med. *312:*1632–1633, 1985.
22. Hall, P. V., Campbell, R. L., and Kalsbeck, J. E.: Meningomyelocele and progressive hydromyelia. Progressive paresis in myelodysplasia. J. Neurosurg. *43:*457–463, 1975.
23. Hoffman, H. J., Hendrick, E. B., and Humphreys, R. P.: Manifestations and management of Arnold-Chiari malformations in patients with myelomeningocele. Childs Brain *1:*255–259, 1975.
24. Holinger, P. C.: Respiratory obstruction and apnea in infants with bilateral abductor vocal cord paralysis, meningomyelocele, hydrocephalus and Arnold-Chiari malformation. J. Pediatr. *92:*368–373, 1978.
25. Holmes, L. B., Driscoll, S. G., and Atkins, L.: Etiologic heterogeneity of neural tube defects. N. Engl. J. Med. *294:*365–369, 1976.
26. Laurence, K. M., Carter, C. O., and David, P. A.: Major central nervous system malformations in South Wales. II. Pregnancy factors, seasonal variation and social class effects. Br. J. Prev. Soc. Med. *22:*212–222, 1968.
27. Laurence, K. M.: Prevention of neural tube defects by improvement in antenatal diet and preconception folic acid supplementation. Prog. Clin. Biol. Res. *163:*383–388, 1985.
28. Lehrman, A., and Owen, M. P.: Surgical repair of large myelomeningoceles. Ann. Plast. Surg. *12:*501–507, 1984.
29. Lemire, R. J., Shepard, T. H., and Alvord, E. C.: Caudal myeloschisis (lumbosacral spina bifida cystica) in a 5 millimeter (horizon XIV) human embryo. Anat. Rec. *152:*9–16, 1965.
30. Lemire, R. J., Loeser, J. D., Leech, R. W., and Alvord, E. C.: Normal and Abnormal Development of the Human Nervous System. Hagerstown, MD, Harper & Row, 1975, pp. 54–69.
31. Lemire, R. J.: Neural tube defects: clinical correlations. Clin. Neurosurg. *30:*165–177, 1983.
32. Lorber, J.: Early results of selective treatment of spina bifida cystica. Br. Med. J. *4:*201–204, 1973.
33. Lorber, J., and Salfield, S. A. W.: Results of selective treatment of spina bifida cystica. Arch. Dis. Child. *56:*822–830, 1981.
34. Matson, D. D.: Surgical repair of myelomeningocele. J. Neurosurg. *27:*180–186, 1967.
35. McDevitt, N. B., Gillespie, R. P., Wodsey, R. E., et al.: Closure of thoracic and lumbar dysraphic defects using bilateral latissimus dorsi myocutaneous flap transfer with external gluteal fasciocutaneous flaps. Childs Brain *9:*394–399, 1982.
36. McLaughlin, J. F., Shurtleff, D. B., Lamars, J. Y., et al.: Influence of prognosis on decisions regarding the care of newborns with myelodysplasia. N. Engl. J. Med. *312:*1589–1594, 1985.
37. McLone, D. G.: Technique for closure of myelomeningocele. Childs Brain *6:*65–73, 1980.
38. McLone, D. G., Czyzewski, D., Raimondi, A. J., et al.: Central nervous system infection as a limiting factor in the intelligence of children with myelomeningocele. Pediatrics *70:*338–342, 1982.
39. McLone, D. G.: Results of treatment of children born with a myelomeningocele. Clin. Neurosurg. *30:*407–412, 1983.
40. McLone, D. G., Dias, L., Kaplan, W. E., et al.: Concepts in the management of spina bifida. Concepts Pediatr. Neurosurg. *5:*97–106, 1985.
41. McLone, D. G.: Treatment of myelomeningocele: arguments against selection. Clin. Neurosurg. *33:*359–370, 1986.
42. Milunsky, A., Apert, E., Neff, R. K., et al.: Prenatal diagnosis of neural tube defects. IV. Maternal serum alpha-fetoprotein screening. Obstet. Gynecol. *55:*60–66, 1980.
43. Nevin, N. C., and Merrett, J. D.: Potato avoidance during pregnancy in women with a previous infant with either anencephaly and/or spina bifida. Br. J. Prev. Soc. Med. *29:*111–115, 1975.
44. Nevin, N. C.: The role of periconceptual vitamin supplementation in the prevention of neural tube defects. Part B: Epidemiology, early detection and therapy and environmental factors. Prog. Clin. Biol. Res. *163:*389–396, 1985.
45. Osaka, K., Tanimura, T., Hirayama, A., et al.: Myelomeningocele before birth. J. Neurosurg. *49:*711–724, 1978.
46. Papasozomenos, S., and Roessman, V.: Respiratory distress and Arnold-Chiari malformation. Neurology *31:*97–100, 1981.
47. Park, T. S., Cail, W. S., Maggio, W. M., et al.: Progressive spasticity and scoliosis in children with myelomeningocele. Radiologic investigation and surgical treatment. J. Neurosurg. *62:*367–373, 1985.
48. Poppen, J. L.: An Atlas of Neurosurgical Techniques. Philadelphia, W. B. Saunders Co., 1960.
49. Powledge, T. M., and Fletcher, J.: Guidelines for the ethical, social and legal issues in prenatal diagnosis. N. Engl. J. Med. *300:*168–172, 1979.
50. Reigel, D. H.: Tethered spinal cord. Concepts Pediatr. Neurosurg. *4:*142–164, 1983.
51. Reigel, D. H., and McLone, D. G.: Myelomeningocele: operative treatment and results—1987. Concepts Pediatr. Neurosurg. *8:*41–50, 1988.
52. Sharrard, W. J. W., Zachary, R. B., Lorber, J., et al.: A controlled trial of immediate and delayed

closure of spina bifida cystica. Arch. Dis. Child. *38:*18–22, 1963.
53. Sharrard, W. J. W.: The segmental innervation of the lower limb muscles in man. Ann. R. Coll. Surg. *35:*106–122, 1964.
54. Shurtleff, D. B., Hayden, P. W., Loeser, J. D., et al.: Myelodysplasia: a decision for death or disability. N. Engl. J. Med. *291:*1005–1011, 1974.
55. Soare, P. L., and Raimondi, A. J.: Intellectual and perceptual motor characteristics of treated myelomeningocele children. Am. J. Dis. Child. *131:*199–204, 1977.
56. Sutton, L. N., Charney, E. B., Bruce, D. A., and Schut, L.: Myelomeningocele—the question of selection. Clin. Neurosurg. *33:*371–382, 1986.
57. Wealthall, S. R., Whittaker, G. E., and Greenwood, N.: The relationship of apnoea and stridor in spina bifida to other unexplained infant deaths. Dev. Med. Child Neurol. *16:*107–116, 1974.
58. Williams, B., and Fahy, G.: A critical appraisal of "terminal ventriculostomy" for the treatment of syringomyelia. J. Neurosurg. *58:*188–197, 1983.
59. Yen, S., and MacMahon, B.: Genetics of anencephaly and spina bifida. Lancet *2:*623–626, 168.

OCCULT SPINAL DYSRAPHISM AND TETHERED CORD

Developmental defects involving the caudal portion of the neural tube constitute a major source of disability among children and adults. These spinal dysraphisms may be divided into two types: (1) *spina bifida cystica,* which includes the familiar myelomeningocele and meningocele, as described previously, and is clinically obvious at birth; and (2) *spina bifida occulta* in which the underlying neural anomaly is masked by a covering of full-thickness skin—the external signs are often subtle, and symptoms may not develop until later childhood or even adulthood as the result of spinal cord tethering. Included in this latter group are such diverse entities as lipomyelomeningocele, hypertrophied filum terminale, congenital dermal sinus, neurenteric cyst, diastematomyelia, and anterior sacral meningocele (Table 11–2). Early recognition of these lesions is important to the clinician, since they are progressive and prophylactic operative treatment is indicated in most cases.[5–7]

Table 11–2. INCIDENCE OF SPINAL DYSRAPHISM AT THE CHILDREN'S HOSPITAL OF PHILADELPHIA

Myelomeningocele		132
Occult spinal dysraphism		
Lipomyelomeningocele	34	
Diastematomyelia	7	
Congenital dermal sinus	14	
Hypertrophied filum	3	
Anterior meningocele	2	
Total	60	

Embryology

After closure of the neural tube, the fetal spine is covered by ectoderm and the low lumbar and sacrococcygeal segments have not developed.[11] At this point, the caudal end of the neural tube blends with a large aggregate of undifferentiated cells, the *caudal cell mass.* A series of vacuoles in this mass coalesce and achieve continuity with the central canal of the previously formed neural tube (at roughly 29 days' gestation), a process called *canalization.* The third phase involves *retrogressive differentiation,* during which the previously formed tail structures undergo a precise, ordered necrosis, leaving only the filum terminale, the coccygeal ligament, and the terminal ventricle of the conus as remnants by 11 weeks. Cell rests with potential for differentiation may be left within these structures, accounting for the development of lipomas, hamartomas, and the rare malignancy occasionally found in association with occult spinal dysraphism. Failure of the caudal cell mass to regress presumably gives rise to the hypertrophied filum terminal.

The bony vertebrae develop subsequently. The sacrococcygeal vertebrae also undergo regressive changes to decrease the number of segments originally present. Some vertebral malformations found in conjunction with neural defects arise during this period and may be part of a more generalized complex of anomalies involving other structures, such as the rectum and bladder.

Pathogenesis

Symptoms may be caused in several ways. Abnormal formation of the spinal cord and roots during embryogenesis may result in permanent deficits manifest at birth, as seen in myelomeningocele. Second, local masses growing within the rigid bony spinal canal may compress the conus medullaris or cauda equina and thus cause mechanical distortion or ischemia, with consequent dysfunction of these neural elements in a progressive fashion.[6, 7, 9]

This may account for the acceleration of symptoms seen in some patients with significant weight gain in whom a lipoma enlarges in proportion to other body fat stores.

Finally, symptoms may be produced by traction on the spinal cord. Early in embryonic development there is a progressive and rapid ascent of the conus within the bony spinal canal owing to faster growth of the vertebral bodies compared with the spinal cord.[2] This so-called "ascent of the conus" in children is, in fact, slight, being only one segment—from the third to the second lumbar body—in the period from the 26th week of intrauterine life until maturity.[15] Nonetheless, if the conus is tethered to the bony spinal canal, as often occurs in dysraphic states, there is loss of mobility of the conus during spinal flexion and extension. Experimentally, spinal cord tethering has been shown to interfere with spinal cord energy metabolism,[16] and is probably the major cause of progressive neural damage in older children and adults with dysraphic lesions.[3]

Clinical Manifestations

Bony spina bifida occulta at the L5–S1 level is a common radiologic finding in children and adults and is usually associated with no symptoms or signs. Unless other findings are present, no further evaluation or treatment is required. Signs of clinically significant spina bifida occulta may be in the form of cutaneous, neurologic, orthopedic, or urologic abnormalities (Table 11–3).

Table 11–3. PRESENTING SYMPTOMS AND SIGNS OF OCCULT SPINAL DYSRAPHISM

	%
Foot deformity	39
Scoliosis	14
Gait abnormality	16
Leg weakness	48
Sensory abnormality	32
Urinary incontinence	36
Recurrent UTI	20
Fecal incontinence	32
Cutaneous abnormality	48

Adapted from James, H. E., and Walsh, J. W.: Spinal dysraphism. Curr. Probl. Pediatr. *11*:1–25, 1981.

Cutaneous Syndrome

Cutaneous abnormalities indicative of an underlying spinal dysraphism are situated on or near the midline, usually in the lumbosacral region. A wide variety of abnormalities are seen (Table 11–4).

A striking finding is the hairy patch (hypertrichosis), also known as "faun's tail," which always occurs in the midline. It may be small but more commonly is a wide, diamond-shaped patch in the lumbar or lower thoracic area (Fig. 11–5). Frequently, the patient's mother has trimmed the hair for years before presentation to the physician. If the dysraphism is in the cervical or upper thoracic region, there is usually a smaller patch of silky hair.[13] The underlying abnormality may not be confined to the area of the hairy patch, and it is important to examine the entire spine. There is no association of hypertrichosis with any particular intraspinal anomaly.[6, 7]

Subcutaneous lipomas at or near the midline of the lumbosacral spine may indicate an underlying intradural lipoma. They are nontender, poorly circumscribed soft masses of fat that are continuous with the normal subcutaneous tissue and with the intraspinal portion of a lipomyelomeningocele. The overlying skin is either normal, hairy, or dimpled and there may be an associated angioma or skin tag (Fig. 11–6). Other conditions, however, may present as skin-covered masses overlying the caudal spine (Table 11–5). Often, an older patient will give a history of having had the superficial mass removed for cosmetic reasons.

Pigmented nevi may be red to brown in color with mottling. Cutaneous port-wine angiomas in the suboccipital area ("stork bites") are usually not significant. Hemangiomas in the lumbosacral area are frequently associated with an underlying dysraphic state.

Atretic meningoceles may also be seen, consisting of a central area of thin, pearly skin

Table 11–4. CUTANEOUS ABNORMALITIES IN OCCULT SPINAL DYSRAPHISM

	No. of Patients
Subcutaneous skin-covered mass (lipoma)	24
Hairy patch	7
Spinal aplasia cutis	4
Rudimentary tail (caudal appendage)	2
Dermal sinus/dimple	10
Nevus/angioma	1
Asymmetric gluteal fold	3

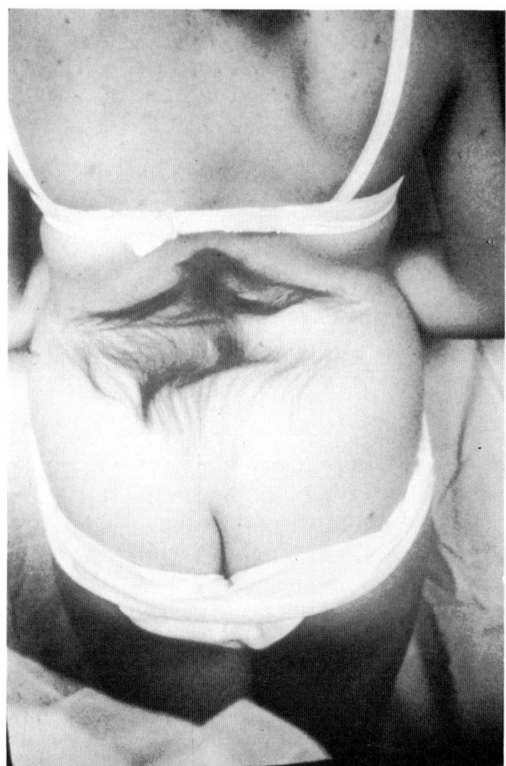

Figure 11–5. Hypertrichosis in a young woman, indicating a tethered cord.

surrounded by a halo of red, pink, or brown. These represent myelomeningoceles or meningoceles that have healed spontaneously. Dimples at the tip of the coccyx are a frequent finding in normal newborns and usually have no significance. Deep dimple-like depressions higher in the spine may be the external stigma of an epithelialized tract that connects with the filum terminale, spinal cord, or intraspinal dermoid cyst and require further investigation.

Neurologic Syndrome

Muscle weakness and gait disturbance is usually apparent at 2 years of age when a child begins to walk. On examination, there may be striking muscular atrophy and leg length asymmetry. The deep tendon reflexes may be normal, increased, or absent, giving the pattern of a mixed upper and lower motor neuron lesion. Patchy sensory loss is found, particularly in the distal leg and perineum. Pain in the back with a radicular component is frequent in the older child or adult.[12]

Table 11–5. DIFFERENTIAL DIAGNOSIS OF SKIN-COVERED LESIONS OVERLYING THE CAUDAL SPINE

Myelocystocele
Meningocele
Lipomyelomeningocele
Sacrococcygeal teratoma
Duplication of rectum
Abscess
Hemangioma
Bony malformation/tumor
Epidermoid/dermoid
Pilonidal cyst
Chondroma
Neuroblastoma
Glioma
Chordoma
Hamartoma

Orthopedic Syndrome

The most frequent orthopedic finding is unilateral or bilateral cavovarus deformity of the foot, with or without leg length discrepancy (Fig. 11–7). There may also be "claw toes." The abnormal gait is the result of orthopedic deformity and muscular weakness. It is pre-

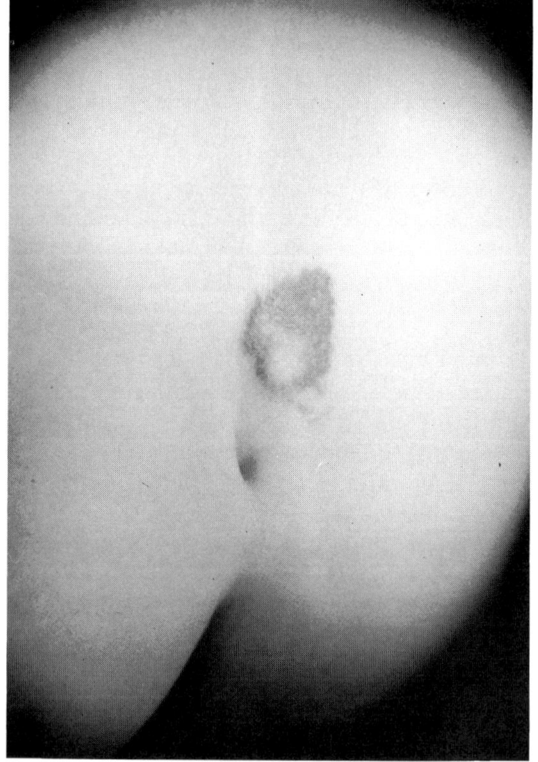

Figure 11–6. Lumbosacral hemangioma with a congenital dermal sinus tract below.

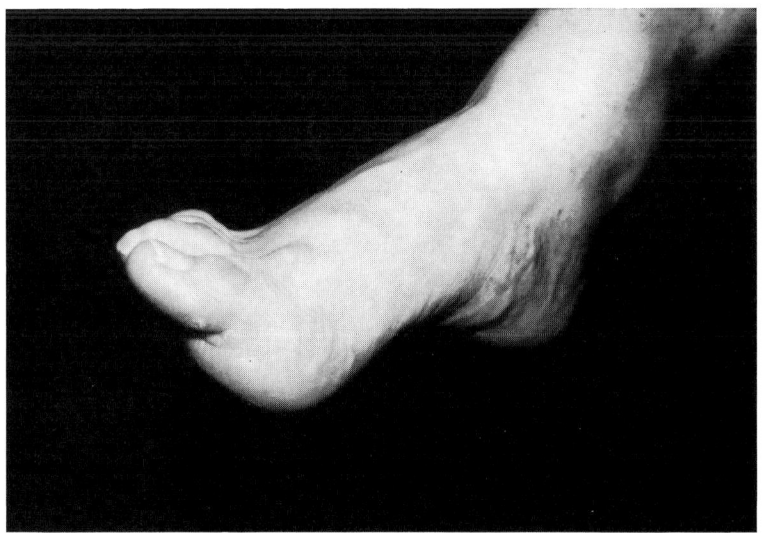

Figure 11–7. Foot deformity with tethered cord. The high arch is typical and may also be accompanied by hammer toes and leg length inequality.

sumed that the foot deformity is due to lack of, or weak innervation of, antagonistic muscles of the lower extremity.[14] Scoliosis, especially if rapidly progressive or accompanied by pain, may also suggest an underlying spinal cause.

Urologic Syndrome

Occult spinal dysraphism should always be considered when one encounters infants with an abnormal voiding pattern, new-onset urinary or fecal incontinence in a previously toilet-trained child, or urinary tract infection in a child of any age. Most infants with occult spinal dysraphism have normal results on urodynamic testing, as opposed to older children.[10] This underscores the importance of recognizing the syndrome as early as possible so that prophylactic surgery can be performed.

Radiologic Investigation

In the relatively recent past, plain x-ray,[9] myelography,[1] and CT[8] were the procedures of choice for evaluating spinal dysraphism. MRI has all but replaced these older studies, since it is easily performed, even in young children and infants, and provides detailed information regarding soft tissues. Bony anatomy is poorly seen but is of secondary importance in planning an operative approach for most lesions. In some cases of tethering due to a hypertrophied filum terminale, MRI may be equivocal or negative, and if a high clinical suspicion exists a supine myelogram and follow-up metrizamide CT study may still be warranted.[4] Postoperative studies may be difficult to interpret. A tethered cord may be suspected when the conus lies at the L2–L3 level or below in a child or adult or if the conus is dorsally displaced. The conus rarely ascends significantly after successful surgery, and even in asymptomatic patients the conus is shown to be dorsally displaced postoperatively. Thus, although MRI is currently the best screening test for spinal cord tethering, it may not be useful for ruling out postoperative retethering.

Ultrasonography has been used to screen both young infants suspected of having tethered cords and also postoperative patients. A lack of pulsation in the latter suggests retethering.

References

1. Anderson, F. M.: Occult spinal dysraphism. A series of 73 cases. Pediatrics *55*:826–834, 1975.
2. Barson, A. J.: The vertebral level of termination of the spinal cord during normal and abnormal development. J. Anat. *106*:489, 1970.
3. Bassett, R. C.: The neurologic deficit associated with lipomas of the cauda equina. Ann. Surg. *131*:109–116, 1950.
4. Brophy, J. D., Sutton, L. N., Zimmerman, R. A., et al.: Magnetic resonance imaging of lipomyelomeningocele and tethered cord. Neurosurgery *25*:336–340, 1989.
5. Ingraham, F. D., Swan, H., Hamlin, H., et al.: Spina

Bifida and Cranium Bifidum. Cambridge, MA, Harvard Press, 1944.
6. James, C. C. M., and Lassman, L. P.: Spinal dysraphism. Arch. Dis. Child. *35*:315, 1960.
7. James, C. C. M., and Lassman, L. P.: Spinal Dysraphism—Spina Bifida Occulta. New York, Appleton-Century-Crofts, 1972.
8. James, H. E., and Oliff, M.: Computed tomography in spinal dysraphism. J. Comput. Assist. Tomogr. *1*:391–397, 1977.
9. James, H. E., and Walsh, J. W.: Spinal dysraphism. Curr. Probl. Pediatr. *11*:1–25, 1981.
10. Keating, M. A., Rink, R. C., Bauer, S. B., et al.: Neurological implications of the changing approach in management of occult spinal lesions. J. Urol. *140*:1301, 1988.
11. Lemire, R. J., Loeder, J. D., Leech, R. W., et al.: Normal and Abnormal Development of the Human Nervous System. Hagerstown, MD, Harper & Row, 1975, pp. 71–83.
12. Pang, D., and Wilberger, J. E., Jr.: Tethered cord syndrome in adults. J. Neurosurg. *57*:32–47, 1982.
13. Schut, L., Pizzi, F., and Bruce, D. A.: Occult spinal dysraphism. *In* McLaurin, R. L. (ed.): Myelomeningocele. New York, Grune & Stratton, 1977, pp. 349–368.
14. Sharrard, W. J.: The mechanism of paralytic deformity in spina bifida. Cerebr. Palsy Bull. *4*:310, 1962.
15. Till, K.: Spinal dysraphism: a study of congenital malformations of the lower back. J. Bone Joint Surg. *51*:415–422, 1969.
16. Yamada, S., Zinke, D. E., and Sanders, D.: Pathophysiology of "tethered cord syndrome." J. Neurosurg. *54*:494–503, 1981.

Specific Entities

Lipomyelomeningocele

The term "lipomyelomeningocele" is misleading in that it suggests herniation of neural elements through the bony defect, which is not usually the case. Some authors have used the term "lipoma of the cauda equina," but in fact the fatty mass is invariably attached to the conus medullaris or filum terminale rather than to the cauda equina. "Leptomyelolipoma," perhaps the most accurate term anatomically, has not gained popularity.

Emery and Lendon divided the fatty tumors related to neurospinal dysraphism into three types:[5]

1. *Fibrolipoma of the filum terminale,* in which the lipoma is attached to the intrathecal or extrathecal elements of the filum.
2. *Dural fibrolipoma,* in which the fatty tissue infiltrates the dura but remains free from the spinal cord.
3. *Leptomyelolipomas,* which are large fatty masses that are continuous with the subcutaneous fat of the gluteal region and penetrate through a defect in the lumbosacral spine, fascia, and dura to insert into the conus medullaris. The fat frequently intermingles with the spinal cord and roots.

The second type is of no clinical importance. The other two may present a technical challenge for the surgeon. Chapman further classified lipomyelomeningoceles into those that insert caudally and those that insert dorsally.[4] If the lipoma inserts onto the dorsal surface of the conus, there is usually a substantial subcutaneous mass, which may be asymmetric. Along the lateral interface of the attachment of the lipoma to the spinal cord, the dura and pia are also fused (Fig. 11–8). Sensory roots emerge just anterior to this latter line of fusion. As a result, neither the sensory roots nor the motor roots are actually within the lipoma. Alternatively, the lipoma may join the conus at its caudal extremity. The remaining mass may then lie entirely within the spinal canal or extend dorsally through the spina bifida defect (Fig. 11–9). The fatty tumor may replace the filum terminale, or there may be a separate filum that lies anteriorly. The nerve roots usually lie ventral to the fatty mass but may lie within the fibrous ventral portion of the mass itself. Although transitional forms may occur, this scheme is helpful in planning an operative

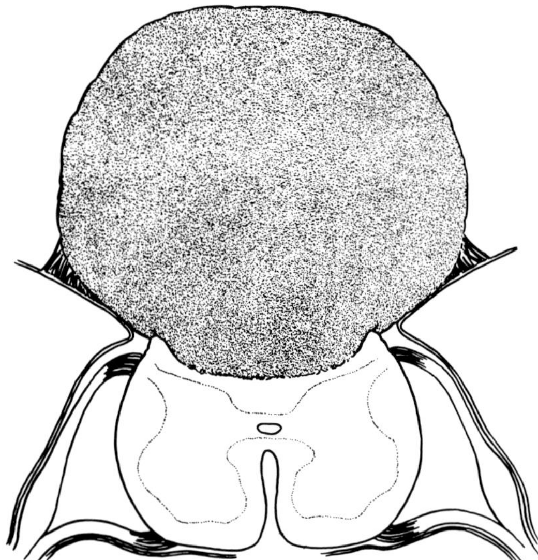

Figure 11–8. Cross-sectional anatomy of a dorsally inserting lipomyelomeningocele. There is a broad lateral attachment between the lipoma and the lateral dura. Nerve roots emerge anterior to the fatty mass.

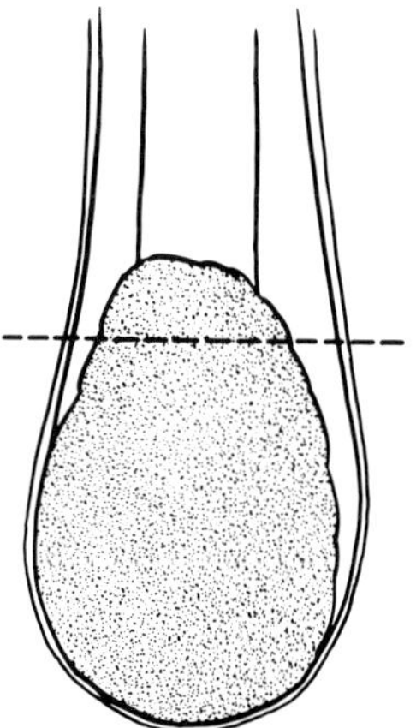

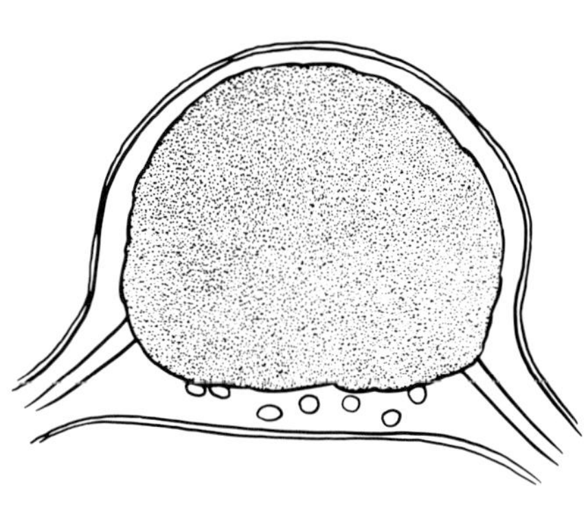

Figure 11–9. Caudally inserting lipomyelomeningocele. *Right,* The lipoma inserts on the low-lying conus. *Left,* Cross section through the lipoma, below the level of the cord. Nerve roots of the cauda equina usually pass ventrally.

approach, and MRI frequently provides information about which type a patient has.

The usual presentation of lipomyelomeningocele varies according to the age of the patient. Newborns (up to age 1 year) typically present with a skin-covered lumbosacral mass (Fig. 11–10). There may be associated hair, sinuses, tags, or nevi. Children 1 year of age or older present with progressive signs or symptoms of the tethered spinal cord, as previously described. Adults may present with back pain and sciatica or acute neurologic deterioration associated with lifting, exercise, or assuming positions of spinal flexion.

MRI should be performed in both sagittal and axial planes. Fatty tumors are readily visualized on T1-weighted images as areas of increased signal intensity because of their short relaxation times. The conus will be low, extending to the caudal portion of the thecal sac. The lipoma may insert dorsally (Fig. 11–11) or caudally (Fig. 11–12) and may or may not include the filum (Fig. 11–13). Not infrequently, an associated syrinx or hydromyelic cavity may be seen within the terminal spinal cord, corresponding to a dilated terminal ventricle (Fig. 11–14). A large neurogenic bladder may also be seen.

Urologic evaluation is recommended for all patients and should include ultrasonography of bladder and urodynamic studies.

All children with skin-covered lumbosacral masses, with or without associated neurologic, urologic, or orthopedic abnormalities, should be explored, preferably in infancy. The surgeon must be prepared to manage a lipomye-

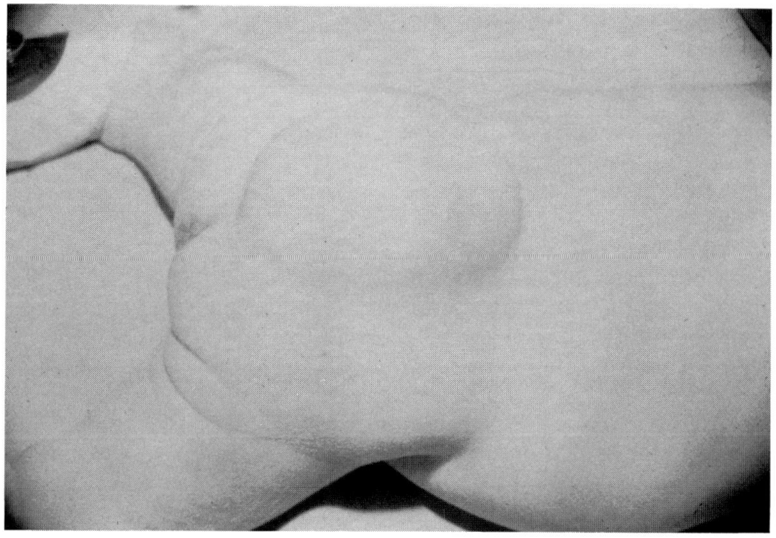

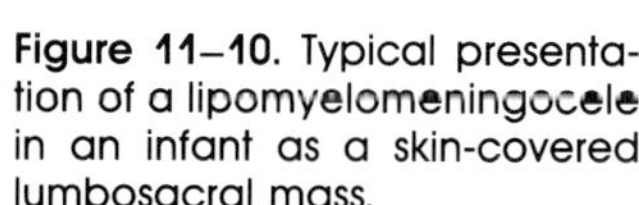

Figure 11–10. Typical presentation of a lipomyelomeningocele in an infant as a skin-covered lumbosacral mass.

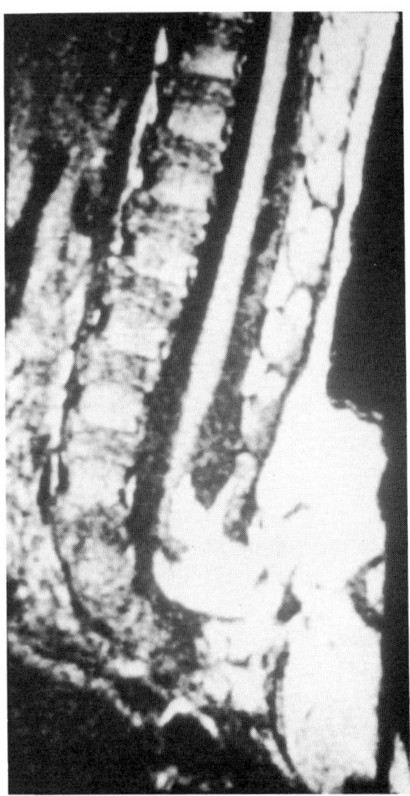

Figure 11–11. T1-weighted sagittal MRI scan of a dorsally inserting lipomyelomeningocele. The cord is low lying and the lipoma inserts broadly along its dorsal aspect. The lipoma exits the spinal canal and connects with a large subcutaneous lipoma.

lomeningocele properly before undertaking the exploration of any midline spinal mass, to avoid damaging neural structures. The first operative procedure stands the best chance of success, as scar formation and distorted anatomy found at reoperation only compound the difficulties inherent in the procedure. Children with the tethered cord syndrome should have prophylactic surgery at the time the lesion is discovered. Till in 1973 advised against prophylactic surgery, but most subsequent authors strongly favor it.[4, 6, 9] The adult patient with a lipomyelomeningocele and nonprogressive symptoms may be followed nonoperatively, although this situation is uncommon. The patient should be warned of the possibility that permanent worsening may occur.

The goals of surgery are (1) to untether the spinal cord from either the lipoma itself, the filum terminale, or both; (2) to remove the lipomatous mass insofar as this is possible to prevent retethering and to relieve direct compression—it is also desirable to decrease the size of the subcutaneous mass for cosmetic reasons; and (3) to reconstruct the dural canal to prevent CSF leakage and to allow sufficient room for the neural elements. This last goal often requires a dural patch graft. The surgeon must provide sufficent room to allow the conus to float freely within the dural sac and thereby prevent retethering due to surgical scarring.

General anesthesia is used. Muscle relaxants may be employed because nerve stimulation is not usually helpful. In difficult situations some authors have employed somatosensory evoked potential monitoring, bladder manometry, or rectal sphincter electromyelography (EMG) to avoid damage to roots,[4, 7, 8] but these adjuncts have not been proved useful.

The pediatric patient is placed in the prone position with towel rolls underneath the chest and iliac crest to allow the abdomen to hang freely. Adult patients are placed in the kneel-

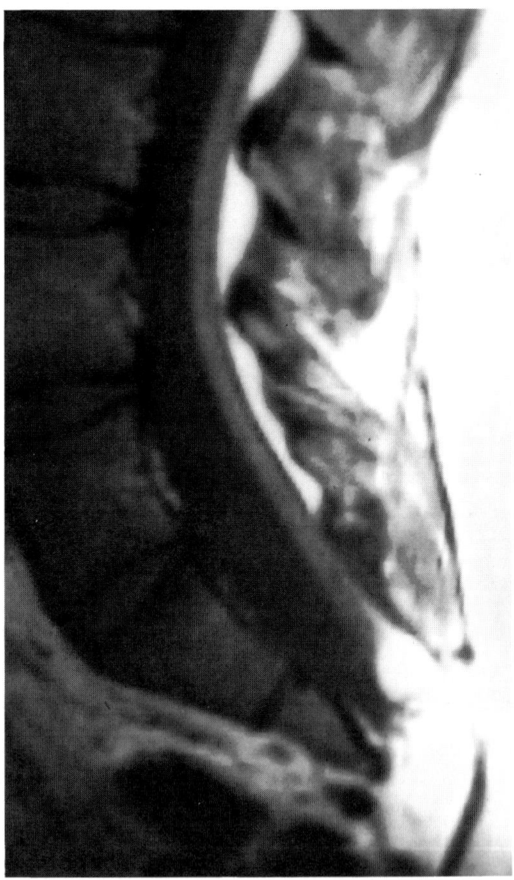

Figure 11–12. T1-weighted sagittal MRI scan of a caudally inserting lipomyelomeningocele. The lipoma tethers the conus to the caudal end of the thecal sac.

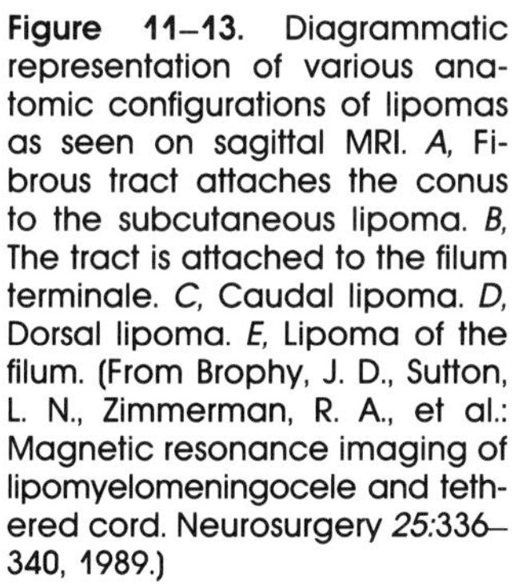

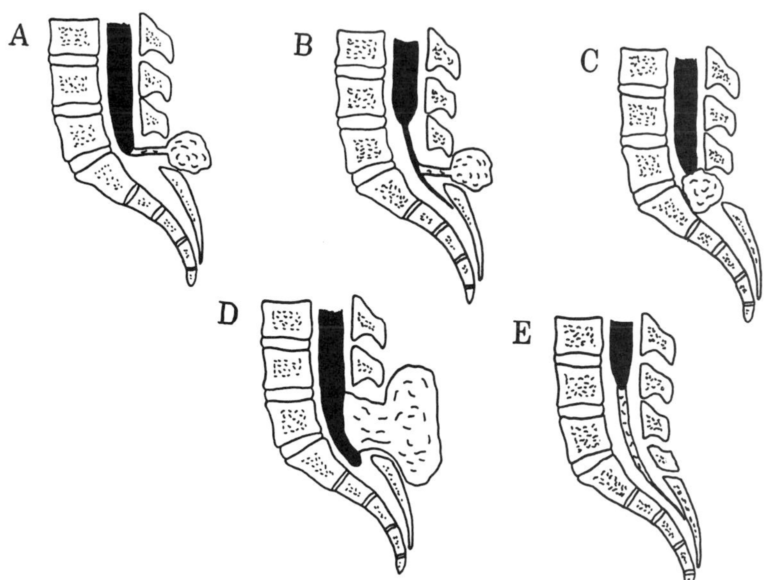

Figure 11–13. Diagrammatic representation of various anatomic configurations of lipomas as seen on sagittal MRI. *A*, Fibrous tract attaches the conus to the subcutaneous lipoma. *B*, The tract is attached to the filum terminale. *C*, Caudal lipoma. *D*, Dorsal lipoma. *E*, Lipoma of the filum. (From Brophy, J. D., Sutton, L. N., Zimmerman, R. A., et al.: Magnetic resonance imaging of lipomyelomeningocele and tethered cord. Neurosurgery *25*:336–340, 1989.)

ing position with a binder to support the buttocks. The operative site is scrubbed with an iodine solution, and after this is damp dried, a transparent adhesive plastic drape impregnated with iodine is applied over the skin. A separate plastic "apron" excludes the anus from the operative field. In our opinion, prophylactic antibiotics are not necessary and may actually result in a more serious infection from opportunistic microorganisms in the event of a CSF leak postoperatively.

Magnification with 3.5× loupes or the operative microscope is helpful. An elliptic skin incision surrounding the subcutaneous mass is made along a vertical axis, hemostasis being obtained by applying straight mosquito hemostats. The ellipse must be narrow enough to allow skin closure at the end of the procedure. The subcutaneous tissue is then incised in a circumferential fashion down to the lumbodorsal fascia (Fig. 11–15). When an anatomic cleavage plane becomes evident, the lipoma is mobilized medially by blunt dissection with the use of a sponge and periosteal elevator, so that the stalk can be visualized as it traverses the fascial defect. A self-retaining retractor is inserted, and the lowest intact laminar arch above the bony defect is palpated. The fascia over this spinous process is opened with the cutting cautery, and the laminae are exposed. A laminectomy of this segment is carried out, exposing the underlying normal dura (Fig. 11–16). It may be helpful at this point to amputate the large subcutaneous mass with the skin attached at the level of its stalk.

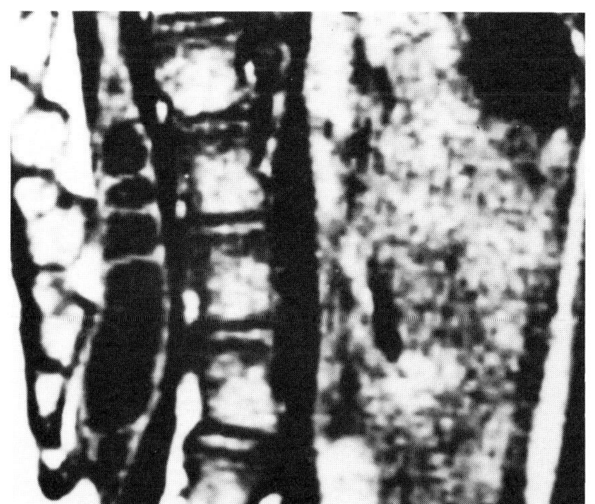

Figure 11–14. T1-weighted sagittal MRI of a caudal lipoma. There is also a large multiseptated hydromyelia within the lower spinal cord.

Starting at the level of normal dura cephalad to the mass, the epidural fat is melted with the bipolar cautery until the dural defect with fatty tissue extruding through it is encountered. A midline dural opening is made above the defect, exposing the spinal cord (Fig. 11–16). As the dural opening is carried inferiorly toward the defect, a transverse band of thick fibrous tissue is noted at the rostral end of the lipoma stalk, which acts to kink the spinal cord. This

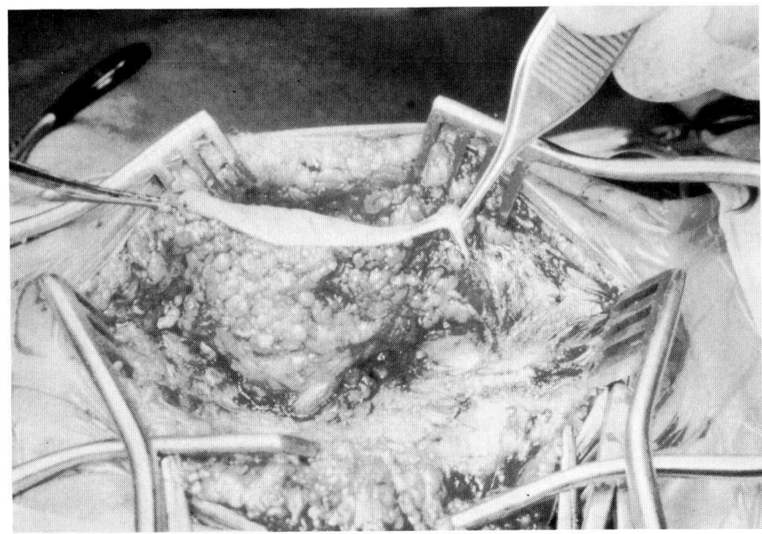

Figure 11–15. Initial operative exposure of a lipomyelomeningocele. A vertically oriented elliptic skin incision has been made, and the subcutaneous lipoma followed to the fascial defect where it enters the spinal canal.

is opened widely along with the dura. The dural opening is extended caudally on either side of the exiting lipoma circumferentially.

At this point, the lipoma will usually be found to correspond to one of the two types described by Chapman.[4] Lipomas that insert into the conus dorsally can be removed from the dorsal aspect of the cord in a plane superficial to the lateral lines of fusion of lipoma, conus, and meninges, with the nerve roots emerging anteriorly. Simultaneously, the lines of fusion are divided laterally, first on one side and then on the other, with bipolar cautery and microscissors or a knife blade over a dissector (Fig. 11–17). The operating microscope and laser have been helpful in shaving down the mass of the lipoma. The filum is identified and divided.

Lipomas that insert caudally into the conus must be sectioned distal to any functional roots (Fig. 11–18). It is not necessary to remove all the gross lipoma: to attempt this risks damage to the conus and nerve roots. Simple division of the lipoma releases the point of tethering and fulfills the goal of the operation. After the lipoma has been largely removed from the spinal cord, it is sometimes possible to reapproximate the pial edges of the cord to reconstitute the normal tubular configuration. This, of course, does not in any way improve neu-

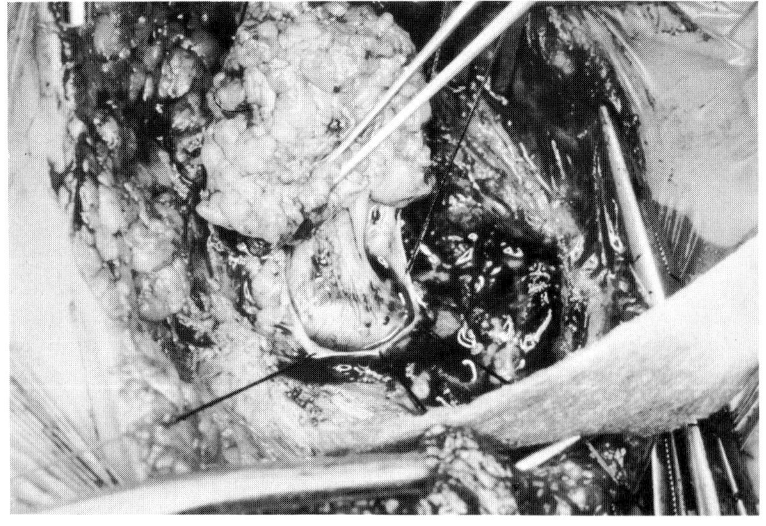

Figure 11–16. A one-level laminectomy has been performed superior to the spina bifida defect *(right)* and the dura opened. The lipoma can be seen inserting at the caudal end of the spinal cord and connecting with the subcutaneous fat.

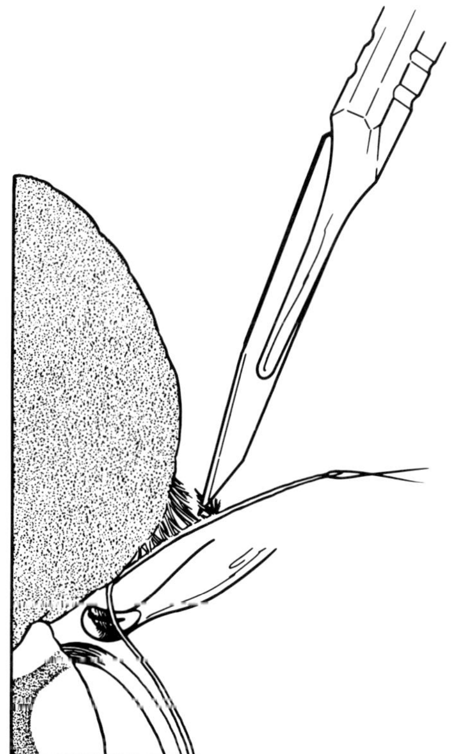

Figure 11–17. The lateral attachment between the lipoma and the dura is sharply divided, while a dissector protects the underlying nerve roots.

rologic function but may serve to prevent retethering. If a terminal syrinx is seen on the preoperative MRI, a midline myelotomy may be performed to provide communication with the subarachoid space.

When the cord is free of adhesions, the dura is closed. In some cases, the dura may be approximated and closed with a running locked suture of 4-0 nylon. In many situations, however, this results in stricture of the canal, with the likelihood of scar formation and retethering. If there is any doubt, an elliptic graft of lyophilized dura is reconstituted by soaking in sterile saline for 30 minutes and is sutured to the dural edges in a watertight fashion with a 5-0 or 6-0 nonabsorbable suture (Fig. 11–19). Often the superficial subcutaneous tissue layers in the closure are inadequate for a truly watertight closure, and the dural repair becomes of primary importance to avoid a CSF fistula. The patient is placed in steep reverse Trendelenburg position and a Valsalva maneuver is carried out to make sure the closure is adequate.

The fascia is closed in the usual fashion if possible. If a large fascial defect prevents approximation, lateral fascial flaps are elevated and reflected medially, as in the fascial closure in the standard myelomeningocele repair. In closing the skin it may be advisable to tack the subcutaneous layer to the underlying fascia to obliterate any dead space. The skin itself is closed with interrupted mattress sutures of 4-0 nylon, which are left in for two weeks.

Patients are kept prone for 72 hours with the head lower than the buttocks. Those who experience difficulty with voiding in the immediate postoperative period are treated with judicious urinary catheterization to prevent unnecessary straining that might threaten the dural closure. Infants are diapered below the dressing to avoid fecal soiling of the incision. Postoperative antibiotics are not necessary.

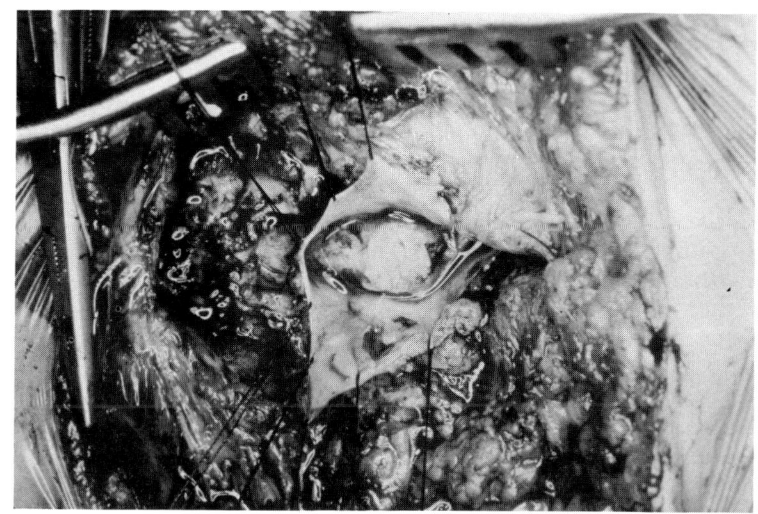

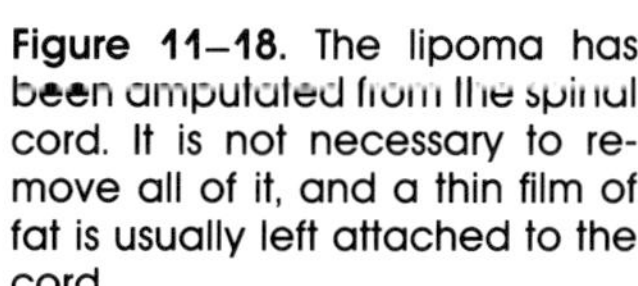

Figure 11–18. The lipoma has been amputated from the spinal cord. It is not necessary to remove all of it, and a thin film of fat is usually left attached to the cord.

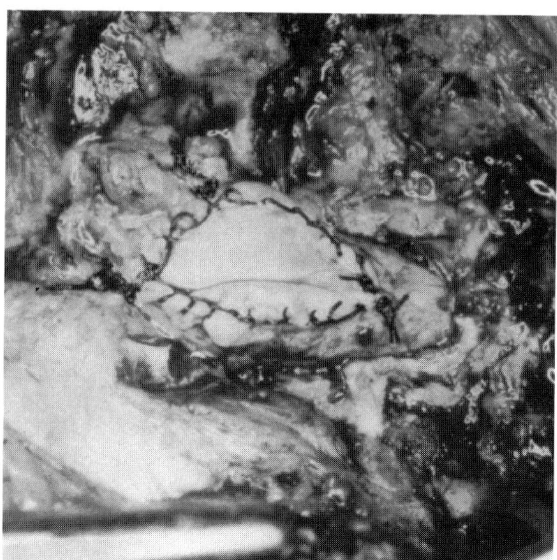

Figure 11–19. A watertight dural closure is essential, using a graft if necessary.

Patients, particularly those in whom a significant mass has been left, are cautioned to avoid excessive weight gain. They often require urologic or orthopedic referral as well as close neurosurgical follow-up.

Surgery is relatively safe, and in our series no deaths have resulted. The major postoperative complications have been CSF leaks, as it is difficult at times to obtain good tissue for surgical repair. A persistent subcutaneous collection or frank leak requires reexploration of the operative site and meticulous closure. We have found that a week with an external spinal drainage catheter carefully inserted above the lamina defect through a Tuohy needle is useful in protecting the closure after reexploration. Persistent fever with sterile CSF cultures and a cellular reaction postoperatively may reflect a mild allergic reaction to the lyophilized dural graft. This may persist for several months if untreated, but usually resolves with a short course of steroids.

Reexploration of previously operated lipomyelomeningoceles is tedious. Tissue planes are obliterated and nerve roots often pass within the substance of the lipoma and scar tissue. For this reason, definitive surgery is required at the primary procedure.

Surgical treatment for lipomyelomeningocele is basically prophylactic and is aimed at preventing progression of fixed deficits or development of new deficits in the infant and asymptomatic child or adult. Data documenting the progressive nature of untreated lipomyelomeningocele are compelling. Hoffman and colleagues reported 12 patients who initially were neurologically and functionally intact and were untreated or inappropriately treated.[6] Only one of these patients remained intact, whereas the others deteriorated over time. After appropriate repair there was a halt in further deterioration, but few patients actually improved in function. Patients who are discovered at a younger age (because of cutaneous abnormality) are far more likely to remain symptom free if they undergo appropriate surgery than are those in whom surgery is deferred.[2, 9]

In perhaps 20 per cent of patients an appropriate operation is followed by improvement in stance and gait, and in about 25 per cent there may be improved bowel or bladder function.[1] Deformities of the feet usually do not improve and may continue to worsen even after successful surgery, as abnormal muscular innervation and gait lead to progressive deformity. Continued orthopedic surveillance and physical therapy are indicated.

Surgery is relatively safe. In Anderson's series only two of 33 patients had worsening of foot weakness after surgery and four experienced worsening of urinary incontinence.[1] In Hoffman's later series there was no functional deterioration after surgery and the only complications were CSF leakage and superficial wound infections.[6]

There is now substantial evidence that occult dysraphic states occur in association with an increased incidence of classic neural tube defects among family members (myelomeningocele, anencephaly). In fact, the risk of a sibling having a neural tube defect if the index patient harbors an occult dysraphic state approaches the risk expected if the index patient also suffered from a major neural tube defect. Patients with lipomyelomeningoceles and their families should therefore be offered formal genetic counseling and screening procedures for neural tube defects.

References

1. Anderson, F. M.: Occult spinal dysraphism. A series of 73 cases. Pediatrics *55*:826–834, 1975.
2. Bruce, D. A., and Schut, L.: Spinal lipomas in infancy and childhood. Childs Brain *5*:192, 1979.

3. Carter, C. O., Evans, K. A., and Till, K.: Spinal dysraphism: genetic relations to neural tube malformations. J. Med. Genet. *13*:343–350, 1976.
4. Chapman, P. H.: Congenital intraspinal lipomas. Anatomic considerations and surgical treatment. Childs Brain *9*:37–47, 1982.
5. Emery, J. L., and Lendon, R. G.: Lipomas of the cauda equina and other fatty tumors related to neurospinal dysraphism. Dev. Med. Child Neurol. *20*:62–70, 1969.
6. Hoffman, H. J., Taecholarn, C., Hendrick, E. B., et al.: Lipomyelomeningoceles and their management. Concepts Pediatr. Neurosurg. *5*:107–117, 1985.
7. James, H. E., Mulcahy, J. J., Walsh, J. W., et al.: Use of anal sphincter electromyography during operations on the conus medullaris and sacral nerve roots. Neurosurgery *4*:521–523, 1979.
8. McLone, D. G., Mutluer, S., and Naidich T. P.: Lipomyelomeningoceles of the conus medullaris. Concepts Pediatr. Neurosurg. *3*:170–177, 1983.
9. Schut, L., Pizzi, F., and Bruce, D. A.: Occult spinal dysraphism. *In* McLaurin, R. L. (ed.): Myelomeningocele. New York, Grune & Stratton, 1977, pp. 349–368.

Anterior Sacral Meningocele

Anterior meningocele is a relatively rare condition in which there is a herniation of the dural sac through a defect in the anterior surface of the spine, usually in the sacrum. The sac is composed of an outer dural membrane and an inner arachnoid membrane. It contains CSF and occasionally neural elements. If the sac is large, it may present as a pelvic mass.

Since its original description in 1837 by "a distinguished surgeon" who preferred to remain anonymous,[3] approximately 200 cases have been reported. The varied presentations may bring patients to the attention of a wide range of specialists including urologists, proctologists, gynecologists, pediatric surgeons, orthopedic surgeons, and neurosurgeons. When the condition is properly diagnosed and treated, the cure rate is high; if it is improperly managed, meningitis may result in death.

Most anterior sacral meningoceles are congenital, as evidenced by their frequent appearance in infants and young children, the associated anomalies of pelvic organs, and the familial incidence. Unlike the typical posterior myelomeningocele, there is no accompanying hydrocephalus or association with Chiari malformations. The embryogenesis of the lesion is not clear. Possibilities include

1. Defective dural development, resulting in a defect through which the arachnoid herniates, leading to pulsations that erode the bone.[6]
2. Partial or complete agenesis of the anterior sacral elements, which would account for the association with other abnormalities of fusion such as bicoronate uterus and duplication of the vagina or abnormalities of the renal pelvis.[2]
3. Acquired weakness of the dura, as described with Marfan's syndrome[10] or von Recklinghausen's disease.[5]

The lesion is far more common in women than in men, but in children the sex incidence is approximately equal. Most likely, there is really no sex prediliction, and the lesion simply remains undetected in many adult males.[2]

Most of the clinical manifestations are caused by pressure of the sac on adjacent pelvic structures such as the rectum, bladder, uterus, and sacral nerve roots. Constipation is the most common symptom, particularly in infants and children. Many patients report use of laxatives and enemas. Urinary difficulties may be due to direct pressure of the mass or to pressure on sacral nerve roots. Midline lumbosacral back pain occurs in some patients and may radiate to the perineal area or inner thighs. Some patients report relief after a bowel movement. Headache may be due to either high or low intracranial pressure. Classically, the headache begins in childhood with sudden onset with Valsalva maneuver, as during straining or defecation. In later life it may accompany coitus.[5, 8] The headache is reproduced when the pelvic mass is compressed on digital examination. When the patient stands, the meningocele fills with fluid, which may cause a secondary low-pressure headache. Meningitis may be either septic or aseptic. Bacterial meningitis may be spontaneous owing to microperforations of the rectum allowing passage of bacteria into the sac, or may result from traumatic rupture of the sac during childbirth. Meningitis may also result from attempted needle aspiration of the sac. Aseptic meningitis has been described, presumably from irritation due to an associated dermoid.[7] In women of childbearing age, anterior meningocele may result in obstructed labor or rupture of the sac during delivery.[5]

The cardinal sign is a smooth, cystic mass palpable on rectal or pelvic examination. It is usually adherent to the sacrum. Only when the mass is enormous is it detectable on routine abdominal examination. The differential diagnosis of such masses includes dermoids, chordomas, and osseous or metastatic tumors.[12]

Radiologic evaluation of the sacrum usually demonstrates some abnormality, classically the "scimitar" sacrum. The anteroposterior roentgenogram shows a well-circumstribed lucent defect on one side of the sacrum corresponding to the sac, and there is no surrounding bony destruction.[5] Urologic contrast studies often show compression of the bladder and uterus and duplication of the ureters or renal pelvis. Myelography is a critical diagnostic test and should be done with water-soluble contrast media to show a small communication between the subarachnoid space and the meningocele sac. If there is doubt whether a communication exists, a postmyelogram CT scan of the pelvis is indicated.[4, 7] MRI is a useful screening test, and in patients in whom communication of the sac with the lumbar theca is clearly visible, no further studies may be required (Fig. 11–20).

Surgical treatment of symptomatic lesions is generally advised because there is no possibility of spontaneous regression, and in untreated patients there is a 30 per cent mortality rate owing to pelvic obstruction at the time of labor or to erosion into the rectum followed by meningitis.[2, 5] The asymptomatic lesion may be followed without the need for surgery if there is no possibility of pregnancy and if the lesion does not enlarge on repeated rectal examination.

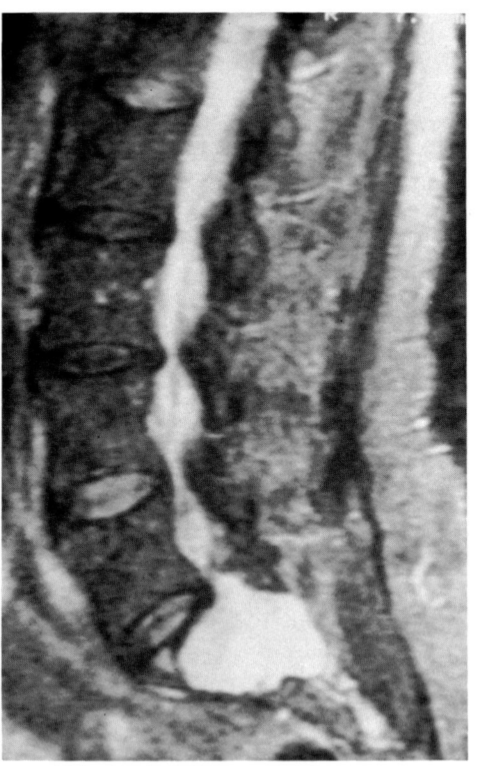

Figure 11–20. T2-weighted midsagittal MRI scan showing a small anterior sacral meningocele.

Aspiration through the rectum or vagina or percutaneously should not be performed. If a cyst is discovered at laparotomy for other reasons and CSF is obtained on aspiration, the operation should be terminated and radiologic studies performed to define the extent of the lesion and the nature of its communication with the subarachnoid space.

Surgical treatment via laparotomy has been described,[2] but most modern authors favor sacral laminectomy as the initial approach, as initially described by Adson.[1] This approach allows visualization of the intraspinal contents and resection of adhesions or division of an abnormal filum terminale. Nerve roots can be protected and there is usually good visualization of the opening into the meningocele to allow suturing. The goal of surgery is to untether the spinal cord, decompress the sac, and obliterate the CSF fistula. It is not necessary to remove the lining of the pelvic cyst, which may be densely adherent to the rectum. If the dura is fragile or cannot be mobilized sufficiently to allow suture even with a fascial graft, a posterior pelvic operation or laparotomy should be performed with the assistance of an experienced abdominal surgeon.

The technique of sacral laminectomy has been reviewed by several authors.[4, 9, 11] Antibiotic coverage and a bowel preparation are begun 48 hours before surgery in case the rectum is inadvertently entered during the procedure. Under general anesthesia, the patient is placed in the prone position with the chest and abdomen supported, and the anus draped out of the field with a plastic sheet. A lumbosacral laminectomy is performed from L5 to S4 and the posterior dura opened longitudinally (Fig. 11–21). Nerve roots within the dural canal are carefully retracted laterally, and the filum terminale is divided, exposing the anterior defect in the dura leading to the sac. If no roots enter the sac and the neck is narrow, CSF may be aspirated from the sac and the anterior dura oversewn with 4-0 nonabsorbable

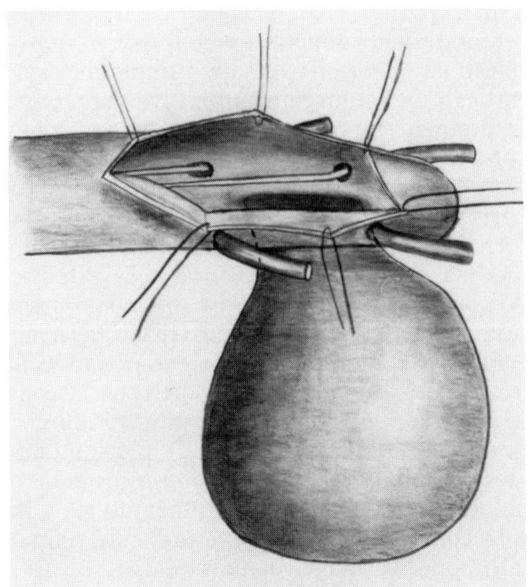

Figure 11–21. Diagrammatic representation of an anterior sacral meningocele (bones are not shown for clarity). The posterior dura has been opened, exposing the ventral defect, which communicates with the sacral mass.

suture (Fig. 11–22). If the sac inserts caudally and is merely a terminal extension of the dural canal without nerve roots within it, the terminal sac may be simply amputated and the caudal sac reconstructed. If the anterior defect is wide and cannot be mobilized into the field sufficiently for primary closure, digital collapse of the sac through the rectum as the sac is ligated may be helpful, or a fascial graft may be sewn to the edges of the defect. If roots exit through the osteum, the dura will have to be plicated around them to permit their exit. If it proves impossible to close a widened stalk, a second procedure with an abdominal approach is necessary. The posterior dura is closed in a watertight fashion. Postoperatively, special care must be taken to protect the wound from fecal contamination, and stool softeners may be given to prevent straining.

Should an abdominal procedure be required, the lithotomy position is used.[2] After a urethral catheter is placed, a midline incision is extended from the symphysis pubis to above the umbilicus. The procedure is then carried out like an abdominoperineal resection of the rectum. The wall of the meningocele is exposed by opening the peritoneum on the right side of the rectum, and then dissected between the wall of the cyst and the fibrous capsule, keeping the sac intact. When the base has been identified, the sac is opened and nerve roots are identified. The meningocele is then resected at its base, leaving enough membrane to effect a watertight closure. The incision is closed without drains.

Surgical results reported in the recent literature have been generally good. Complications include meningitis or neurologic deterioration in cases in which nerve roots have been found within the sac.

References

1. Adson, A. W.: Spina bifida cystica of the pelvis: diagnosis and surgical treatment. Minn. Med. *21*:468–475, 1938.
2. Amacher, A. L., Drake, C. G., and McLaughlin, A. D.: Anterior sacral meningocele. Surg. Gynecol. Obstet., *126*:986–994, 1968.
3. Bryant, T.: Case of deficiency of the anterior part of the sacrum with a thecal sac in the pelvis, similar to the tumour of spina bifida. Lancet *1*:358, 1837.
4. Mapstone, T. B., White, R. J., and Takaoka, Y.: Anterior sacral meningocele. Surg. Neurol. *16*:44–47, 1981.

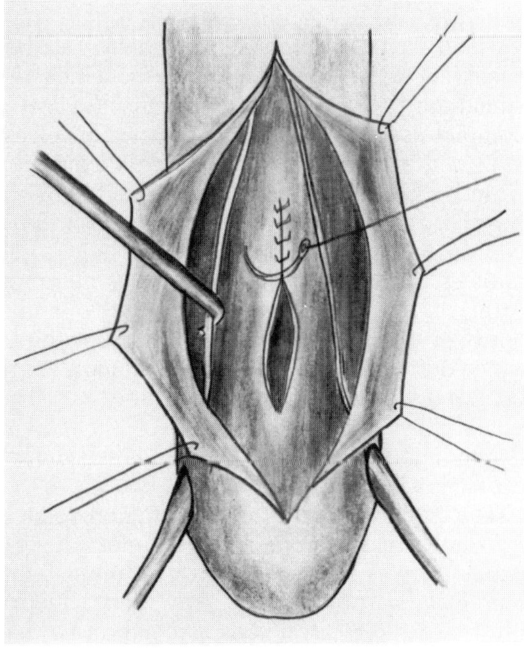

Figure 11–22. Anterior sacral meningocele. The ventral dural defect is closed with a running suture. Large defects require a graft.

5. Oren, M., Lorber, B., Lee S. H., et al.: Anterior sacral meningocele. Report of 5 cases and review of the literature. Dis. Colon Rectum *20*:492–505, 1977.
6. Palazzoli, A.: Rilievi climici e patogenetici su un caso di meningocele sacrale occulto simulante un ernia discale. Bol. Soc. Med. Chir. *17*:203–225, 1963.
7. Quigley, M. R., Schinco, F., and Brown, J. T.: Anterior sacral meningocele with an unusual presentation. J. Neurosurg. *61*:790–792, 1984.
8. Rowlands, B. C.: Anterior sacral meningocoele: report of 2 cases. Br. J. Surg. *43*:301, 1955.
9. Smith, H. P., and Davis, C. H.: Anterior sacral meningocele: two case reports and discussion of surgical approach. Neurosurgery *7*:61–67, 1980.
10. Strand, R. D., and Eisenberg, H. M.: Anterior sacral meningocele in association with Marfan's syndrome. Radiology *99*:653–654, 1971.
11. Villarejo, F., Scavone, C., Blazquez, M. G., et al.: Anterior sacral meningocele: review of the literature. Surg. Neurol. *19*:57–71, 1983.
12. Vogel, E.: Anterior sacral meninogocele as a gynecologic problem. Obstet. Gynecol. *36*:766–768, 1970.

Diastematomyelia

The term "diastematomyelia" refers to a congenital cleft or splitting of the spinal cord. The word derives from the Greek *diastema* (cleft) and *myelos* (medulla). Diastematomyelia thus refers to the split in the spinal cord and not, as frequently misapplied, to the intervening bony or cartilaginous spur that often separates the two hemicords. It is to be distinguished from diplomyelia, which, strictly speaking, refers to a condition in which the spinal cord is completely duplicated (i.e., two complete sets of anterior and posterior horns, with anterior and posterior roots emerging from both medial and lateral surfaces of both hemicords). If diplomyelia truly exists as a clinical entity it is extremely rare, and some authors maintain that diplomyelia is merely a form of diastematomyelia.[18] The two hemicords in diastematomyelia may exist within a single dural envelope, or, more commonly, are enclosed within separate dural tubes.[12, 14] The defect may be at any spinal level but is most common in the lower thoracic or upper lumbar areas.[12, 15, 17, 24]

The embryogenesis of diastematomyelia is not fully understood, but the most logical explanation is that suggested by Bremer[2] and amplified by others.[1, 3, 18] Any viable theory must explain the frequent association of diastematomyelia with vertebral anomalies, spina bifida, and gut malformations and the equal involvement of both the ventral and dorsal aspects of the neural tube.

In early embryonic development, the neurenteric canal connects the yolk sac (primitive intestinal cavity) with the amniotic cavity through the proliferating primitive knot, which is destined to become the brain and spinal cord. If this canal or an accessory canal persists, the entodermal lining of the yolk sac can herniate through the fistula and split the notochord, neural tube, and migrating mesenchymal elements that are to form the vertebrae. A temporary persistence of this communication results in hemivertebrae: if the herniated ectoderm continues to differentiate it results in a neurenteric cyst, and if the tract attaches to the gut, intestinal malrotation or duplications may result. The cuff of pluripotential mesenchymal cells that condense around the entodermal sinus determines the nature of the split cord. The mesenchyme may differentiate into bone, cartilage, or fibrous tissue to form the median septum, which may or may not induce its own investing meninges. A thin membranous septum may be mistaken for a true diplomyelia. Whether or not the hemicords possess medial rootlets depends on the location of the neural crest cells within the spinal cord. If they are far lateral and therefore unaffected by the split, only one set of dorsal roots will develop on the lateral aspect of the hemicord. If the cell mass is bisected by the split, each hemicord will have its own set of paramedian dorsal roots. If the neurenteric tract persists further dorsally to involve the cutaneous ectoderm, a true myelomeningocele will occur. This is also the explanation for the cutaneous signature that often accompanies the malformation.

Because normal ascent of the spinal cord continues through this sequence of events, the septum usually lies cranial to the vertebral defect, and the septum is found at the caudal end of the cleft at surgery.

Clinically, diastematomyelia occurs predominantly in females.[15, 24] The condition may be asymptomatic or may present with symptoms of spinal cord dysfunction or scoliosis. The clinical findings are thus no different from those found in other cases of spina bifida occulta. Most patients have a midline thoracic or lumbar cutaneous abnormality. The incidence ranges between 50 and 80 per cent.[5, 13–15, 24] The level of the skin lesion does not necessarily correspond to the level of the diastematomyelia. The most common finding is a hairy patch (40 per cent), but other abnormalities may include dimples, hemangiomas, lipomas, sinus tracts, or myelomeningocele/meningocele.[15]

Virtually all patients develop a significant congenital spinal deformity[12, 14, 24] averaging 60 degrees during the growth years. The incidence increases with age throughout childhood and is more likely to occur with higher lesions.[12] Scoliosis is widely attributed to the associated vertebral anomalies such as hemivertebrae, spina bifida, or spinal canal widening rather than to spinal cord dysfunction. The incidence of diastematomyelia among patients with congenital scoliosis is estimated to be 4.9 per cent.[24] The type of scoliosis is nonspecific, apart from the equal incidence of right- or left-sided curves, and thus some authors have recommended myelography before surgical treatment in all patients with congenital scoliosis.[15, 24]

Neurologic symptoms occur as a result of spinal cord tethering and may not arise until adulthood. Symptoms are those typical of the tethered cord syndrome, including back pain, gait disturbance, muscular atrophy or deformity of the calf or foot, and spasticity or sensory abnormalities below the level of the lesion, with trophic skin changes. Urologic abnormalities occur in about 50 per cent of cases.[6] These abnormalities are nonspecific, and other disease entities such as spinal cord tumor, Friedreich's ataxia, and syringomyelia must be considered.[13] The traction force exerted on the spinal cord may even result in brain stem or spinal cord symptoms as the result of an acquired Arnold-Chiari malformation.[4] Similarly, the spinal traction associated with corrective casts for scoliosis or operative intervention may lead to precipitous paraparesis.[23] Late deterioration in adults has been reported after a blow to the back,[11] after saddle block anesthesia,[6] or simply with associated spondylosis.[6] Adult patients may also demonstrate progressive myelopathy without a precipitating event, which may recover after surgery.[7, 22]

The classic roentgenographic appearance of diastematomyelia is a fusiform interpedicular widening of the spinal canal on the anteroposterior view with a midline oval bony mass projecting posteriorly from the vertebral body (Fig. 11–23). Usually the spur is not visible on lateral views.

Particularly in early infancy, the spur may not be visible and may not be in continuity with the vertebral body or laminae, supporting the view that the septum is calcified from a separate ossification center.[12] Even in childhood and adult cases, however, the septum may be cartilaginous and invisible on plain x-rays. In such cases, widening of the neural canal should alert the clinician to the possibility of the diagnosis, and in general the adjacent pedicles should not be widened, as would be seen with an expanding intraspinal tumor.[15] In addition to the widened canal, spina bifida is frequently associated, as are other vertebral anomalies. Scoliosis and kyphosis are common and their incidence increases with age.[12] This observation reinforces the importance of early detection, since the chance of scoliosis developing increases the longer that patients are left without treatment.

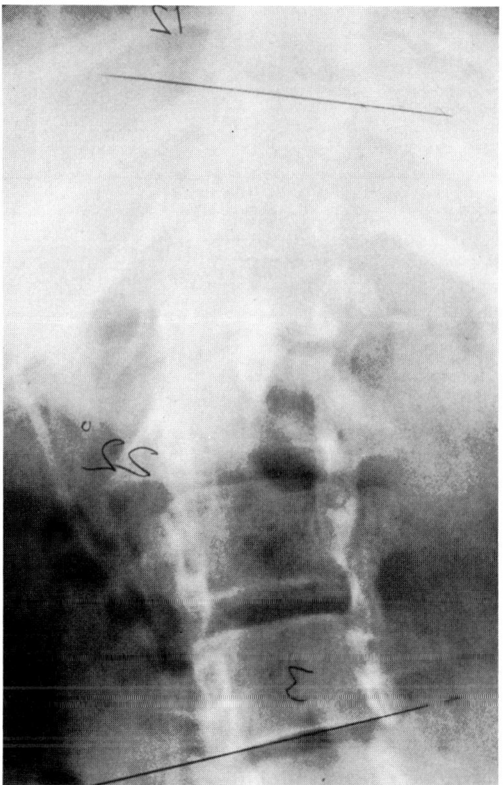

Figure 11–23. Anteroposterior plain spine x-ray film showing a bony diastematomyelia at L1.

Myelography will confirm the diagnosis, define the extent of the split in the cord, and detect associated problems, such as a low-lying conus, a prominent filum terminale, or lipoma. Further definition can be accomplished by postmetrizamide CT through the area of the abnormality (Fig. 11–24).

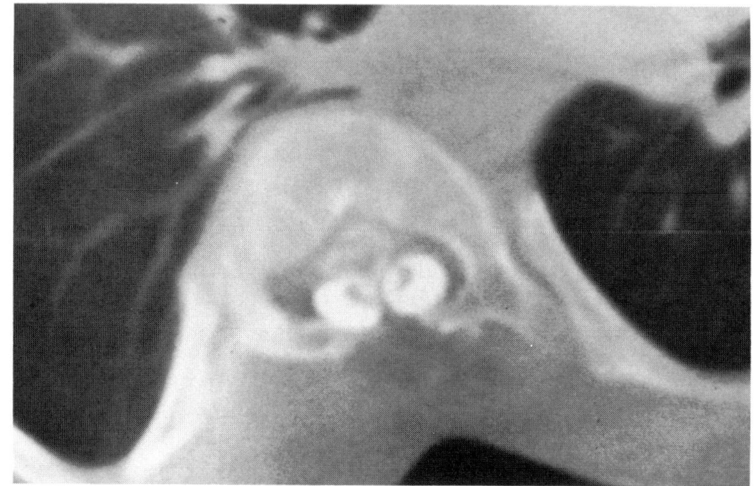

Figure 11–24. Axial metrizamide CT scan through diastematomyelia. Two separate dural sleeves are seen, with the two hemicords within them. The bony spur is anterior.

MRI is probably the current procedure of choice for evaluation of diastematomyelia (Fig. 11–25).[21] A coronal study will show the split nicely, but sagittal views may not show each hemicord separately and the study may mistakenly be considered normal. Severe scoliosis may make MRI difficult to interpret as the twisted cord weaves in and out of the imaging plane. In these cases, myelography with axial CT slices after the injection of contrast material is the procedure of choice. The entire spine should be evaluated for the possibility of secondary lesions, such as an associated tight filum terminale, lipoma, or dermoid cyst or a second spur.

Indications for surgery include progressive neurologic deficit and prophylactically before treatment of scoliosis. Application of a cast or halo pelvic traction for severe kyphoscoliosis may result in paraplegia if the point of tethering is not relieved.[23] Similarly, it is advisable to remove the bony spike as a separate procedure before operative correction of scoliosis.[15, 24] Although it would be technically feasible to perform both procedures at a single sitting, removal of the septum may result in early loss of evoked potentials owing to spinal cord manipulation, which would reduce the safety of the orthopedic procedure.[18] In addition, instrumentation of the spine is best avoided with intradural procedures when there is a possibility of a CSF leak.

Management of the asymptomatic patient with diastematomyelia remains controversial. Matson and colleagues[16] and others[9, 10, 17] urged that asymptomatic children and those who are neurologically stable should undergo prophylactic surgery within the first two years of life, and cited tethering as the cause of progressive symptoms. Other authors pointed out that surgery carries potential risk of neurologic worsening[24] and noted that a significant number of patients with diastematomyelia remain asymptomatic (or with fixed deficit) throughout growth, thus favoring a conservative approach.[3, 5, 14] A compromise would be to consider the relationship of the septum to the intermedullary cleft[8] in deciding the likelihood of progression due to tethering. The asymptomatic patient may thus be followed nonoperatively if the septum is separated from the inferior portion of the cleft, but if the septum is at the caudal end of the cleft, prophylactic surgery is advisable. The role of surgery in a patient with a cleft but no apparent septum is also unclear. In such patients there appears to be no reason for tethering, but Pang[18] found that at operation these patients may have an unrecognized midline fibrous partition, and recommended that this lesion be treated as though a septum were present. Finally, the indications for surgery in the patient with myelomeningocele and associated diastematomyelia are unclear, although it seems logical to explore such a patient and untether the cord in the face of progressive symptoms referable to the lesion.

The surgical technique described by Matson

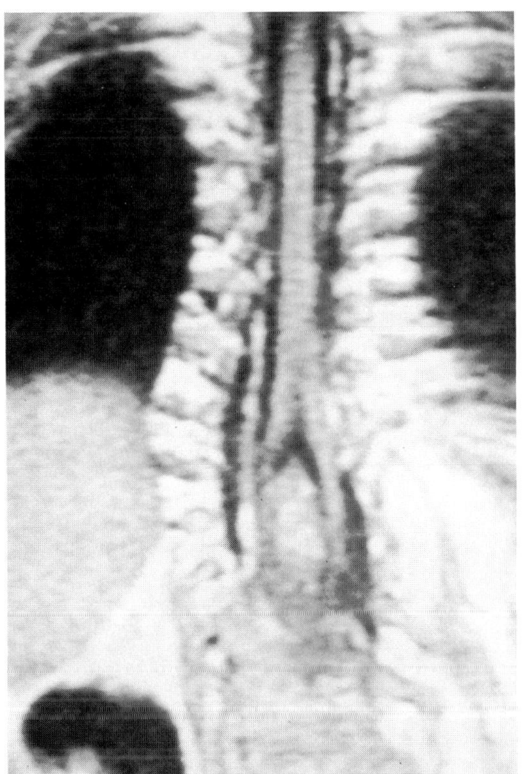

Figure 11–25. T1-weighted MRI scan in the coronal plane shows the hemicords separating around the diastematomyelia. Note that there is a CSF density cleft superior to the bony spur, but the spinal cord tightly hugs the inferior margin of the spur, suggesting tethering.

and colleagues[16] and Meacham[17] is employed. The use of intraoperative evoked potential recording[19] and rectal manometry[20] has been described but their value is unproved. In the thoracic spine, the level of the lesion is marked by x-ray film before the procedures. The patient is positioned as for a standard laminectomy. The paraspinal muscles on each side of the midline are freed and retracted laterally as in any standard laminectomy, but vigorous blunt dissection with a periosteal elevator is avoided, since a spina bifida may coexist with the bony septum. The laminectomy is initiated at least one segment above and below the septum and carried out around the bony spike itself, exposing the dural cleft. The cleft usually extends cephalad to the spur, but hugs it tightly caudaully. A septal elevator is used to free the septum from the surrounding dura, and the superficial portion of the septum is removed by a rongeur or the highspeed drill with a diamond burr within the investing dural sheath, which serves to protect the spinal cord. The inferior portion of the spur may extend anterior to the spinal cord at the inferior portion of the cleft, and in this case final removal is deferred until the dural compartment has been opened. The epidural venous plexus surrounding the bony spur and deep to the two hemicords may be substantial and should be controlled with bipolar cautery as the spur is removed. Once the cleft is decompressed and the cord moves cephalad, bleeding may be difficult to control.[21]

The dura is opened circumferentially around the cleft and all intradural adhesions at the cleft side are divided (Fig. 11–26). The island of dura and the remainder of the spike are then removed to the level of the anterior spinal canal (Fig. 11–27). A small midline myelotomy at the caudal portion of the cleft may be required to accomplish this.

It is neither necessary nor desirable to close the anterior dura. The posterior dura is closed

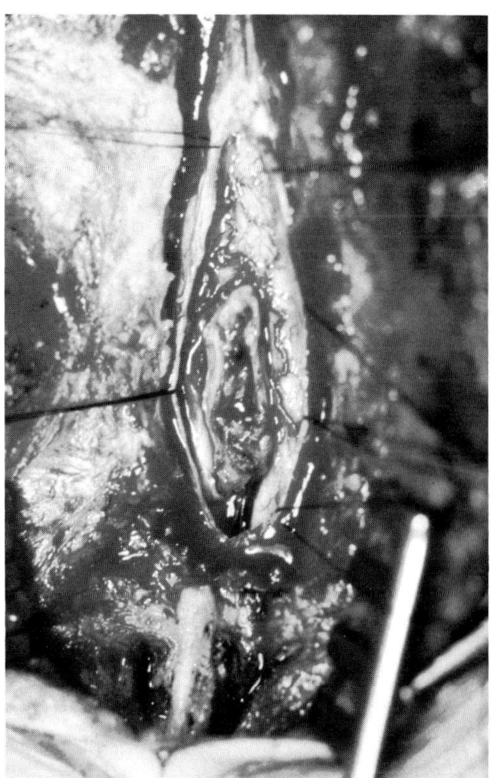

Figure 11–26. Operative exposure of diastematomyelia. The dura has been opened around the bony spur, which has been partially removed.

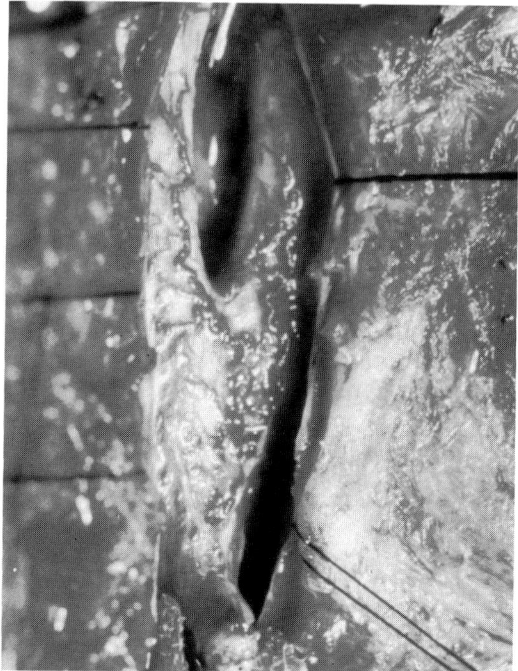

Figure 11–27. The bony spur and dural cuff have been excised. It is not necessary to close the anterior dura.

in a watertight closure, with a graft if necessary. If an associated tight filum is suspected, the laminectomy is carried inferiorly to expose it, or a separate laminectomy is performed.

The procedure should be considered largely prophylactic, although there may be improvement in some symptomatic patients.[7, 14, 16, 22] Complications include CSF leakage and worsening of neurologic status. Failure to improve or late deterioration after operation may be due to failure to entirely remove the tethered spur, failure to address a second lesion, or (rarely) regrowth of the septum.[20]

References

1. Bently, J. F. R., and Smith, J. R.: Developmental posterior enteric remnants and spinal malformations. The split notochord syndrome. Arch. Dis. Child. *35:*76–86, 1960.
2. Bremer, J. L.: Congenital Anomalies of the Viscera. Cambridge, MA, Harvard University Press, 1957.
3. Cohen, J., and Sledge, C. B.: Diastematomyelia. An embryological interpretation with report of a case. Am. J. Dis. Child. *100:*257–263, 1960.
4. Davis, E. D.: Diastematomyelia with early Arnold-Chiari syndrome and congenital dysplastic hip. Clin. Orthop. *52:*179–185, 1967.
5. Eid, K., Hochberg, J., and Saunders, D. E.: Skin abnormalities of the back in diastematomyelia. Plast. Reconstr. Surg. *63:*534–539, 1979.
6. English, W. J., and Maltby, G. L.: Diastematomyelia in adults. J. Neurosurg. *27:*260–264, 1967.
7. Freeman, L. W.: Late symptoms from diastematomyelia. J. Neurosurg. *18:*538–541, 1961.
8. French, B. N.: Midline fusion defects and defects of formation. *In* Youmans, J. R. (ed.): Neurological Surgery. 3rd ed. Philadelphia, W. B. Saunders Co., 1990, pp. 1081–1235.
9. Guthkelch, A. N., Jones, R. A. C., and Zierski, J.: Diastematomyelia. Dev. Med. Child. Neurol. *13:*137–138, 1971.
10. Guthkelch, A. N.: Diastematomyelia with median septum. Brain *97:*729–742, 1974.
11. Hamby, W. B.: Pilonidal cyst, spina bifida occulta and bifida spinal cord. Report of a case with review of the literature. Arch. Pathol. *21:*831–838, 1963.
12. Hilal, S. K., Marton, D., and Pollack, E.: Diastematomyelia in children. Radiographic study of 34 cases. Neuroradiology *112:*609–621, 1974.
13. James, C. C. M., and Lassman, L. P.: Diastematomyelia and the tight filum terminale. J. Neurol. Sci. *10:*193–196, 1970.
14. James, C. C. M., and Lassman, L. P.: Diastematomyelia. A critical survey of 24 cases submitted to laminectomy. Arch. Dis. Child. *39:*125–130, 1964.
15. Keim, H. A.: Diastematomyelia and scoliosis. J. Bone Joint Surg. *55A:*1425–1435, 1973.
16. Matson, D. D., Woods, R. P., Campbell, J. R., et al.: Diastematomyelia (congenital clefts of the spinal cord): diagnosis and surgical treatment. Pediatrics *6:*98–112, 1950.
17. Meacham, W. F.: Surgical treatment of diastematomyelia. J. Neurosurg. *27:*78–85, 1967.
18. Pang, D.: Tethered cord syndrome: newer concepts. *In* Neurosurgery Update II. Chicago, McGraw-Hill Book Co., 1991, pp. 336–344.
19. Pang, D., and Casey, K.: Use of an anal sphincter pressure monitor during operations on the sacral spinal cord and nerve roots. Neurosurgery *13:*562–568, 1983.
20. Pang, D., and Parrish R. G.: Regrowth of diastematomyelic bone spur after extradural resection. J. Neurosurg. *59:*887–890, 1983.
21. Reigel, D. H.: Sacral agenesis and diastematomyelia. *In* McLaurin, R. (ed.): Pediatric Neurosurgery. Surgery of the Developing Nervous System. New York, Grune & Stratton, 1982, pp. 79–94.
22. Seaman, W. B., and Schwartz, H. G.: Diastematomyelia in adults. Radiology *70:*692–695, 1957.
23. Shorey, W. D.: Diastematomyelia associated with dorsal kyphosis producing paraplegia. J. Neurosurg. *12:*300–305, 1955.
24. Winter, R. B., Haven, J. J., Moe, J. H., et al.: Diastematomyelia and congenital spinal deformities. J. Bone Joint Surg. *56A:*27–39, 1974.

Neurenteric Cyst

Although neurenteric cysts are quite rare, they are well-described entities consisting of cystic structures within the spinal canal or anterior to the vertebral bodies in the mediastinum, abdomen, or neck. Ventral cysts may have connections by means of a stalk to the meninges and spinal cord through a tunnel-like defect in the vertebral bodies.[2, 11] The cyst wall resembles foregut tissue histologically, and in the literature these lesions are also referred to as enterogenous cysts.[4, 8, 10, 12, 13]

Early in the development of the human embryo there is a communication between the yolk sac (destined to become the gut) and the dorsal surface of the embryo called the neurenteric canal. This fistulous tract transiently connects the future enteric cavity with the neural groove in the region of the coccyx. Bremer pointed out that abnormal accessory neurenteric canals may persist cephalad to the coccygeal tip and can give rise to cysts along the persistent tract.[1] The tract also gives rise to associated vertebral anomalies: a widened vertebral body resulting from bony proliferation in an attempt to fill the gap following disappearance of the tract, or a circular defect in the vertebral body produced by the persistent tract that forces bone to form around it. Because the accessory neurenteric tract can be enlongated and stretched during growth, the canal may become divided into noncommunicating diverticula that lie at some distance from each other; for example, in the thoracic cavity and spinal canal.[13] The tendency for the cysts to lie to the right of the vertebral column has been ascribed to the developmental process of gastric and gut rotation.[13]

Neurenteric cysts within the spinal canal or ventral masses are similar pathologically. They may have thick, well-defined capsules or delicate, clear walls that may cause confusion with spinal arachnoid cysts.[12] They are typically described as strawberry-colored[7, 9] and when in the spinal canal may be intradural-extramedullary[2, 8, 12] or intramedullary.[7, 13] The cyst fluid is usually described as clear or milky and quite gelatinous. There may or may not be a ventral dural defect.

Histologically, the cyst wall typically is formed of endodermal ciliated columnar epithelium resting on a basement membrane and may contain gastric parietal and chief cells or mucin-producing goblet cells.[9] The epithelial cells are positive for material compatible with mucin on periodic acid–Schiff stains.

Neurenteric cysts are usually detected in childhood,[5, 7, 8, 11, 13] although adult patients have been reported.[2, 4, 8, 12] In early childhood the lesion may present as a chest or abdominal mass or as a neck mass with tracheal compression, or may be detected because of vertebral anomalies seen on x-ray film.

Patients in whom the lesion is suspected typically have had plain x-rays that may show widening of the neural canal, cleft vertebrae, or fusion of vertebral segments.[11] An anterior soft tissue mass may be seen in the chest, neck, or abdomen, and the association of such a mass with vertebral anomalies should suggest the diagnosis. The presence of the classic circular defect through the vertebral body is not essential. Patients in whom the diagnosis is suspected should undergo MRI and myelography with water-soluble contrast and postmyelogram CT to define the bony anatomy and establish the presence or absence of a communication between the spinal canal and a ventral mass (Fig. 11–28).

Adults and older children tend to present with signs of spinal cord compression in the cervical or thoracic regions. In addition to motor weakness, burning dysesthesias may occur aggravated by coughing or sneezing or recumbency.[2, 8, 13] Rarely, the neurenteric fistula may lead to meningitis with bowel organisms.[6, 10] Associated malrotation of the gut[13] and diaphragmatic hernia[11] may be found.

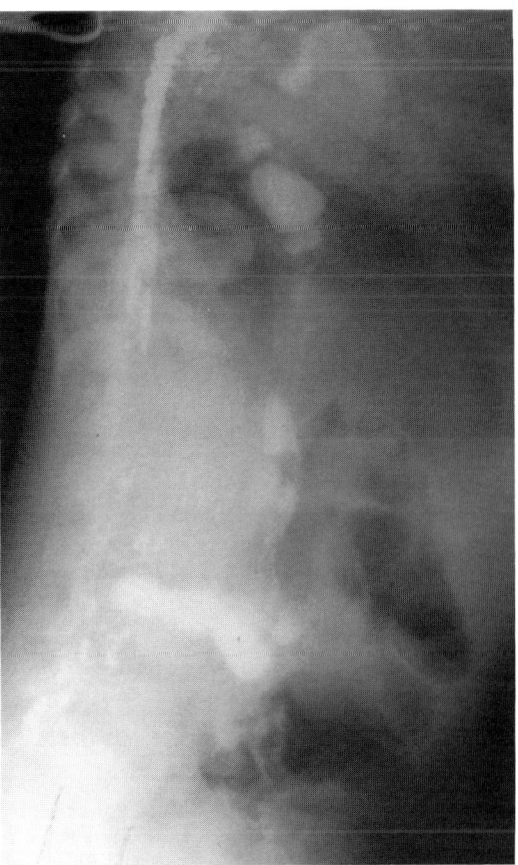

Figure 11–28. Lateral myelogram of a neurenteric cyst. The contrast material flows through a tract communicating anteriorly at L2–L3 and fills the bowel.

The treatment of neurenteric cysts varies with location and presentation. The intraspinal lesion can be corrected first, at a separate procedure, or as part of a combined procedure, such as thoracotomy, to excise the prevertebral lesion. Since the spinal mass is largely cystic, a wide laminectomy is usually adequate, because cyst drainage and conservative resection of cyst wall adherent to the spinal cord appear to eradicate the cyst. A cyst-subarachnoid shunt has been described,[13] but the thick nature of the fluid and its possible irritation of the meninges make this unlikely to be useful in most cases. If there is an anterior dural defect, this may be plugged with a muscle or fascial graft from a posterior approach, or ligated or sutured if a thoracotomy is performed.[3]

Patients generally show recovery of neurologic function if the deficit is not severe at the time of operation. Recurrence has been noted after incomplete resection,[2] but its incidence is unknown because follow-up of reported cases has been short.

References

1. Bremer, J. L.: Dorsal intestinal fistula, accessory neurenteric canal, diastematomyelia. Arch. Pathol. *54:*132–138, 1952.
2. Dorsey, J. F.: Intraspinal and mediastinal foregut cyst compressing the spinal cord. Report of a case. J. Neurosurg. *24:*562–567, 1966.
3. French, B. N.: Midline fusion defects and defects of formation. *In* Youmans, J. R. (ed.): Neurological Surgery. 3rd ed. Philadelphia, W. B. Saunders Co., 1990, pp. 1081–1235.
4. Harriman, D. G. F.: An intraspinal enterogenous cyst. J. Pathol. Bacteriol. *75:*413–419, 1958.
5. Holcomb, G. W., and Matson, D. P.: Thoracic neurenteric cyst. Surgery *35:*115–121, 1954.
6. Jackson, F. E.: Neurenteric cysts. Report of 2 cases of neurenteric cyst with associated meningitis and hydrocephalus. J. Neurosurg. *18:*678–682, 1961.
7. Knight, G., Griffiths, T., and Williams, I.: Gastrocystoma of the spinal cord. Br. J. Surg. *42:*635–638, 1954.
8. Laha, R. K., and Huestis, W. S.: Intraspinal enterogenous cyst: delayed appearance following mediastinal cyst resection. Surg. Neurol. *3:*67–70, 1975.
9. Levin, P., and Antin, S. P.: Intraspinal neurenteric cyst in the cervical area. Neurology *14:*727–730, 1964.
10. Millis, R. R., and Holmes, A. E.: Enterogenous cyst of the spinal cord with associated intestinal reduplication, vertebral anomalies, and a dorsal dermal sinus. Case report. J. Neurosurg. *38:*73–77, 1973.
11. Newhauser, E. B. D., Harris, G. B. C., and Berrett, A.: Roentgenographic features of neurenteric cysts. Am. J. Roentgenol. *79:*235–240, 1958.
12. Scoville, W. B., Manlapaz, J. S., Otis, R. D., et al.: Intraspinal enterogenous cyst. J. Neurosurg. *20:*704–706, 1963.
13. Silvernail, W. I., and Brown, R. B.: Intramedullary enterogenous cyst. Case report. J. Neurosurg. *36:*235–238, 1972.

Congenital Dermal Sinus and Dermoid Cysts

The term "dermal sinus" describes a group of congenital malformations in which a tubular tract lined with squamous epithelium extends from the skin overlying the spine inward to varying depths. Termination of the sinus may be in the subcutaneous tissue, bone, dura, subarachnoid space, or filum terminale; within an intradural dermoid expansion; or within a neuroglial mass inside the spinal cord. These cysts may occur in the occipital region of the head or at any level of the spine above the coccygeal area, but are most commonly in the lumbosacral area, where they may be confused with pilonidal sinuses or coccygeal dimples that have no connection with the spinal canal.

In early development the terminal portion of the neural tube and the coccygeal vertebrae are intimately related, and perhaps fused to the overlying epithelium. As the spine begins to elongate, the sacrococcygeal ligament applies traction on the overlying skin, producing a dimple in the skin overlying the sacrococcygeal region. There is no connection with the spinal canal, and these sacral dimples are reported to occur in about 4 per cent of children.[5] No treatment is necessary except local cleanliness.[4] The embryonic defect in true congenital dermal sinus is believed to occur early in fetal life at the time the ectoblast differentiates into cutaneous and neural ectoderm.[10] According to this theory, the cleavage between the two layers of ectoderm is incomplete at this point, giving rise to the sinus, and as the neural groove closes to create the neural tube, cutaneous ectodermal elements are invaginated within the neural tube, which may subsequently develop into an intraspinal dermoid growth. As the conus ascends, the sinus tract elongates. When there is an associated defect of mesodermal organization around the tract, spina bifida results. More superficial sinus tracts that do not penetrate to the spinal canal are explained as failure of fusion of the cutaneous ectoderm after it has separated from the neuroectoderm.[1] Pilonidal sinuses are acquired lesions in adults and are believed to result from repeated trauma or an inflammatory reaction secondary to penetration of broken strands of hair. It is possible that some pilonidal sinuses in adults represent chronic infection within a superficial congenital dermal sinus, and therefore the distinction between these entities may be blurred. In practice, the term "pilonidal sinus" should be reserved for acquired lesions in adults. The incidence of true congenital dermal sinus is about one in 2500 births.[7]

Congenital dermal sinuses may be detected during the course of routine examination of an infant or child or deliberately sought after recurrent bouts of meningitis.[3, 9] The sinus presents in the skin as a deep depression, usually in the lumbar region, which may be accompanied by nevi or hypertrichosis (see Fig. 11–6). Occasionally, multiple sinuses are encountered. There may be a history of an accompanying purulent or clear discharge. Local infection of the sinus tract with staphylococci or *Escherichia coli* is common. The opening of the sinus tract is invariably in the midline[1, 4] and may be extremely small. Such a sinus opening occurring above the sacrococcygeal region should be explored and excised. Probing and injection of dyes are inadvisable.

Patients may also present with signs of spinal cord or cauda equina compression, from either an expanding dermoid within the spinal canal[2] or an intraspinal abscess.[8] Whether the condition is of gradual or sudden onset, the patient may present with lower extremity weakness, sphincter incontinence, or root irritation and meningismus. Pain in the back and legs is usual with abscess formation or meningitis due to rupture of the irritating contents of the dermoid cyst. In chronic cases, motor weakness, foot deformity, and reflex changes occur. The young child may simply refuse to walk.

Prophylactic surgery is performed as early as possible to excise the entire tract.[1, 4, 6, 9] MRI is indicated in patients in whom there is clinical evidence of spinal cord compression, to determine the extent of abscesses or dermoids. In asymptomatic patients the lesions may simply be explored and the tract followed to its termination. The surgeon undertaking such an operation must be prepared to carry out an extensive intradural dissection, since the tract may extend for a considerable distance.

The operation is begun with an elliptic skin incision surrounding the sinus opening and any abnormal skin surrounding it. The tract is sharply dissected and followed through the fascia. A laminectomy is performed if the tract appears to continue to the dura. If the tract attaches to the dura, the dura is opened lateral to the entrance point and the intradural contents are inspected. Any intradural tract must be followed to its termination, even if this involves an extensive laminectomy to the conus, since remaining tissue has the capacity to grow into a large dermoid inclusion. Intradural cysts are completely removed without violating the capsule if possible. If the cyst has ruptured or is infected, a dense arachnoiditis with scarred nerve roots will prevent complete excision. In this event, judicious intracapsular removal of purulent material and dermoid elements is performed, but no attempt is made to remove the scarred capsule wall from the nerve roots. A watertight dural closure is made except in patients in whom closure would compress residual infected dermoid cyst material, in which case the dura may be left open and the muscle and fascia are closed.

References

1. Amador, L. V., Hankinson, J., and Bigler, J. A.: Congenital dermal sinuses. J. Pediatr. *47:*300, 1955.
2. Bailey, I. C.: Dermoid tumors of the spinal cord. J. Neurosurg. *33:*676–681, 1970.
3. Cardell, B. S., and Laurance, B.: Congenital dermal sinus associated with meningitis. Report of a fatal case. Br. Med. J. *2:*1558–1561, 1951.
4. Cheek, W. R., and Laurent, J. P.: Dermal sinus tracts. Concepts Pediatr. Neurosurg. *6:*63–75, 1985.
5. Howorth, J. C., and Zachary, R. B.: Congenital dermal sinuses in children—their relation to pilonidal sinuses. Lancet *2:*10–14, 1955.
6. Matson, D. D., and Jerva, M. J.: Recurrent meningitis associated with congenital lumbosacral dermal sinus tract. J. Neurosurg. *25:*288–297, 1966.
7. McIntosh, R., Merritt, K. E., Richards, M. R., et al.: The incidence of congenital malformations. A study of 5,964 pregnancies. Pediatrics *14:*505–521, 1954.
8. Mount, L. A.: Congenital dermal sinus as a cause of meningitis, intraspinal abscess and intracranial abscess. J. A. M. A. *139:*1263–1267, 1949.
9. Perloff, M. M.: Congenital dermal sinus complicated by meningitis. Report of a case. J. Pediatr. *44:*73–76, 1954.
10. Walker, A. E., and Bucy, P. C.: Congenital dermal sinuses: a source of spinal meningeal infection and subdural abscesses. Brain *57:*401–421, 1934.

Filum Terminale Syndrome

The hypertrophied filum terminale constitutes a relatively uncommon cause of the tethered cord syndrome. In its pure form, the conus is bound into a low position by a thickened filum terminale, but more complex variations include filum lipomas, traction bands, and so-called "meningocele manque," a term used to describe aborted or atrophic meningocele sacs that tether the conus.[5]

Patients present with a typical tethered cord syndrome. Cutaneous abnormalities are noted in approximately half of the patients[3] and may consist of a sinus tract, a hairy nevus, a hemangioma, an accessory appendage, or an area of atretic skin. Other symptoms include orthopedic deformity (scoliosis, leg or foot atrophy), progressive weakness, or urologic dysfunction (urinary incontinence, bladder distention, loss of perineal sensation). Back pain is often prominent in teenage and adult patients. The condition is rarely familial.[6]

Radiologic investigation usually shows a simple posterior lumbosacral spina bifida, but may reveal other vertebral anomalies. Further work-up consists of studies to evaluate the level of the conus, and may include MRI or supine myelography with CT. Barson measured the level of conus termination in normal infants and children and reported that on average the adult level (L1–L2) is reached by 2 months of age.[2] A conus tip below the L2–L3 interspace in a child over 5 years old is definitely abnormal. A filum thicker than 2 mm at myelography is also abnormal (Fig. 11–29). Although MRI may suggest the diagnosis with the finding of a low conus on sagittal and axial views, the filum itself may be poorly seen. If the clinical history is suggestive, a supine myelogram with a follow-up metrizamide CT scan is worthwhile even in the face of a normal MRI study.

Prophylactic surgery is recommended at the time the entity is discovered in order to prevent progression of symptoms and relieve chronic back pain.[7] A laminectomy is performed above or below the bifid segment, and the dura is opened. The filum is coagulated and sectioned as low as possible. In some reported cases, clips placed at the cut ends of the filum have separated by as much as 2.5 cm on postoperative x-ray films.[3] If it proves difficult to clearly identify the filum, it can be either electrically stimulated or followed to its termination by performing an extensive sacral laminectomy.

The results of surgery are favorable in relieving back pain and preventing the progression of existing deficits, and often some longstanding neurologic deficits may improve. In Anderson's series, urinary incontinence improved in 14 of 33 patients, and weakness and numbness of the legs lessened postoperatively in one third.[1] Back and leg pains were relieved in virtually all patients in several series.[1, 4, 7]

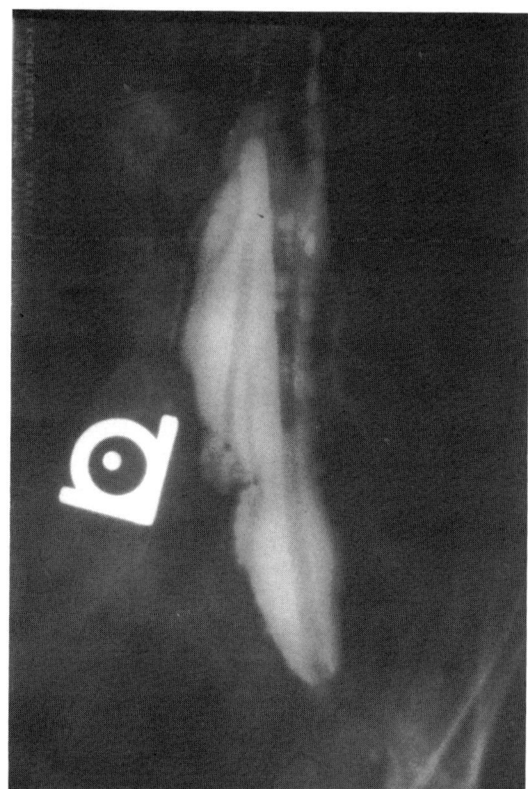

Figure 11–29. Lateral lumbar myelogram showing a thickened filum, extending to the end of the caudal sac. This might not have been seen on MRI.

References

1. Anderson, F. M.: Occult spinal dysraphism. A series of 73 cases. Pediatrics *55:*826–841, 1975.
2. Barson, A. J.: Vertebral level of termination of spinal cord during normal and abnormal development. J. Anat. *106:*489–497, 1969.
3. Fitz, C. R., and Harwood-Nash, D. C.: The tethered conus. Am. J. Roentgenol. *125:*515–523, 1975.
4. Hoffman, H. J., Hendrick, E. B., and Humphreys, R. P.: The tethered spinal cord. Its protean manifestations, diagnosis and surgical correction. Childs Brain *2:*145–153, 1976.
5. James, C. C. M., and Lassman, L. P.: Spinal Dysraphism—Spina Bifida Occulta. New York, Appleton-Century-Crofts, 1972.
6. Love, J. G., Daly, D. D., and Harris, L. E.: Tight filum terminale. Report of the condition in three siblings. J. A. M. A. *176:*115–117, 1961.
7. Pang, D., and Wilberger, J.: Tethered cord syndrome in adults. J. Neurosurg. *57:*32–47, 1982.

CHAPTER

12

SPINAL DISORDERS ASSOCIATED WITH SKELETAL DYSPLASIAS AND METABOLIC DISEASES

Vernon Tolo, M.D.

Some may call this subject orthopedic trivia. None of these conditions are found in a large segment of patients, and the numbers of syndromes and subclassifications at times seem almost endless. At a recent count there were over 120 different types of short stature syndromes described, and metabolic defects are being discovered regularly as techniques in molecular biology enable researchers to define defects in nucleic acid sequencing. It is a truism that one looks only for what one knows. Because of this, it is important for physicians and surgeons to know the features of these spinal disorders to allow early recognition of spinal problems, particularly in conditions in which spinal deformity generally progresses and may lead to spinal cord compression. Because the natural history of spinal disorders in each syndrome is often so different, it is important initially to establish as accurate a diagnosis as possible.

Skeletal dysplasia syndromes may often be identifiable at birth. To establish an appropriate diagnosis, it is necessary to correlate physical findings, family history, and selected radiographic studies. In short stature syndromes secondary to metabolic causes, further serum and urine laboratory studies, as well as biopsy material, also require consideration.

The physical findings most important in the identification phase relate to body length and body proportions. Infants under the fifth percentile with all other family members in the midsize range obviously require further workup. With regard to body proportions, skeletal dysplasias can roughly be divided into those with short limbs and a relatively normal trunk and those with a short trunk and relatively normal limbs. If an infant has short limbs, it is helpful to determine whether the shortening affects the proximal limb (rhizomelia), the forearm or lower leg (mesomelia), or the distal limb segment (acromelia) primarily. X-rays of the limbs may allow distinction between mainly epiphyseal or mainly metaphyseal involvement, even in infants. If a short trunk dominates the physical findings, one can assume spinal involvement of some type. This spinal involvement initially is usually platyspondyly, although later increasing trunk shortness may be related to spinal deformity. X-rays of the infant's spine, particularly the lateral view, may often provide specific clues to the correct diagnosis. Additional useful physical findings include facial features, hand and foot abnormalities, and angular deformity of the extremities. Combining the physical and radiographic findings with a geneticist's consultation should allow for earlier recognition of the correct syndrome, so that the appropriate spinal problems can be more closely observed and the family can benefit from early genetic counseling regarding having further children.

SKELETAL DYSPLASIAS

Achondroplasia

Recognizable at birth, achondroplasia is the most common skeletal dysplasia requiring treatment for spinal disorders. Short limbs of the rhizomelic variety are present and characteristic facial features of frontal bossing and nasal bridge depression enable this early diagnosis. Head size is often large compared with other body segments. Spinal x-rays at birth demonstrate narrowing of the interpediculate distances in the lumbar spine, which helps to confirm the diagnosis.

At birth, the achondroplastic infant has hypotonic musculature, and the parents should be advised to expect a delay in motor developmental milestones. In general, independent sitting occurs at about 9 months of age and independent walking at about 18 months in achondroplasia, whereas the normal child sits by about 6 months and walks by 1 year of age. Whether this generalized hypotonia is constitutional or the result of a neurologic deficit remains unclear. Adding to the speculation that some of the hypotonia may result from spinal cord compression is the relative frequency of sleep apnea in achondroplastic infants, at times leading to sudden unexpected death.[32] Sleep apnea monitors should be used for the first several months in many of these infants. If sleep apnea appears clinically, the achondroplastic infant needs to be evaluated thoroughly for the first of many potential spinal conditions: foramen magnum stenosis.[10, 34] This evaluation includes longitudinal clinical observation, computed tomography (CT) of the foramen magnum, somatosensory evoked potentials, and polysomnography (sleep laboratory studies for apnea and oxygen desaturation).[30] Possible causes of infant apnea include foramen magnum compression, upper airway obstruction, and small thoracic cage size. Although chest circumference is generally below the third percentile in these children, this measurement is the same in infants with or without apneic problems, so this is unlikely to be the cause. Midface hypoplasia, if severe, may cause snoring and upper airway respiratory compromise. However, the most commonly implicated cause of this infant apnea is cervical cord compression at the foramen magnum, where CT and magnetic resonance imaging (MRI) studies have repeatedly demonstrated a marked decrease in cross-sectional area of the foramen. While the sagittal dimension is relatively normal, the loss of area results from the severe side-to-side foraminal narrowing demonstrated.

Studies have divided this compression into two major types: the first involves cervical cord compression from direct impingement of the posterior rim of the foramen magnum, and the second is caused by the posterior foramen magnum rim invaginating into the ring of the atlas. These authors stressed that this compression is of the high cervical cord, not of the brain stem itself.[49] Autopsy studies noted histologic changes in the upper cervical spinal cord similar to those seen in the central cord syndrome, and some authors believe that if one avoids placing the head in hyperextension, the risk of spinal cord compression is lessened.[52] Another later result of foramen magnum compression may be cervical cord syringomyelia.[15]

On CT scans it has been demonstrated that there is uniformly some degree of foramen magnum compromise in virtually all achondroplastic children, 96 per cent of whom have a foramen magnum area even smaller than 3 standard deviations from the mean.[49] How and whom to treat, however, remains unsettled. One study of 32 achondroplastic children showed 28 per cent with a history of apnea and 22 per cent with abnormal sleep study results, both of which improved in the six children who had foramen magnum decompression.[30] More recently, foramen magnum decompression has been reported to be more safely and successfully performed when combined with external ventricular drainage to manage the abnormal cerebrospinal fluid (CSF) dynamics in this compressive condition.[8] Some authors are strong advocates of foramen magnum decompression in this setting, but others maintain that if appropriate sleep monitoring is continued until the child is 2 or 3 years of age, there will be a natural relative increase in the foramen magnum size with growth, thus relieving enough of the compression to avoid the need for surgical treatment.[50]

Reported mortality and morbidity rates from foramen magnum decompression are thought by these authors to be greater than if no treatment except monitoring is performed. It is rarely necessary to perform foramen magnum decompression in older children or in adults.

The principal spinal disorder in the rest of the achondroplastic cervical spine is spinal stenosis. A small spinal canal is present from birth, but signs or symptoms of spinal cord compression in the lower cervical spine are not noted until middle age or later.[18] Spinal cord or nerve root compression results from osteophytes that develop with degenerative disc changes. The cumulative effect of previous small cervical spine dimensions and osteophyte compression leads to a neurologic deficit that may require treatment. If pain or sensory changes are the only findings, conservative care with a cervical orthosis and anti-inflammatory agents can initially be used. However, if a motor deficit is present and pain is unrelieved by nonoperative treatment, laminectomy at multiple levels is needed.[30, 33] Preoperative myelography, CT, or MRI defines the levels of compression most clearly. Laminectomy is generally needed for three vertebral levels on each side of the most compressed segment(s), generally meaning that the entire cervical spine below the axis will require laminectomy. Posterior or anterior cervical fusion is rarely needed after laminectomy, but if it becomes necessary to perform these laminectomies in the skeletally immature, as in nonachondroplastic children, there is an increased risk of cervical kyphosis developing with growth. Atlantoaxial instability has been reported in achondroplasia but is rare.[11, 13]

Of all the spinal segments, the middle and upper thoracic spine is the least involved in spinal deformity or cord compression. The most common spinal deformity and neurologic problems occur in the thoracolumbar and lumbar spinal areas. It is in early childhood that a thoracolumbar kyphosis first develops (Fig 12–1*A*). When an achondroplastic infant sits, a total spinal kyphosis is generally noted, at least partly owing to the generalized hypotonia. Although some have advocated only reclined sitting to avoid the development of this thoracolumbar kyphosis,[12] the author does not believe this to be necessary. In over 90 per cent of children, the thoracolumbar kyphosis improves without treatment as the standing position is assumed and lumbar lordosis develops. The x-ray film may show relative anterior wedging of the thoracolumbar vertebrae, but this generally resolves as standing and walking proceed, with a filling in of the anterior aspects of the vertebral body or bodies at the thoracolumbar apex. Bracing has limited value for control of the kyphosis and is poorly tolerated by many children. Because of their short limbs, it is difficult if not impossible to reach the feet with a conventional thoracolumbar-sacral orthosis (TLSO) in place. An orthosis that utilizes a soft front while supporting the kyphosis has been reported to be successful,[21, 38, 39, 51] although proper patient selection for bracing remains problematic. Some have advocated stretching exercises for hip flexion contractures as a means to decrease lumbar lordosis and in turn control thoracolumbar kyphosis, but documentation of the effectiveness of this passive stretching program is difficult.[37]

In the few children in whom the thoracolumbar kyphosis does not resolve, either naturally or with orthotic assistance, the author advocates anterior and posterior spinal fusion of the kyphotic segment any time after age 4 or 5 years (Fig. 12–1*B*).[45] From an analysis of the early x-ray films of patients who later develop severe thoracolumbar kyphosis and neurologic deficits, it appears that persistent wedging has been present at this early age. Using this approach at this age, the kyphotic deformity can be generally corrected better, leading to prevention of localized increased kyphosis. Whether this early fusion will also decrease the later need for decompressive lumbar laminectomy cannot yet be determined. Fusion of the kyphosis in patients under the age of 2 years has been reported to lead to hypoplastic vertebral bodies in the fused area,[36] but this has not been noted in my patients who are only a few years older.

In these young children, the surgical technique favored by the author involves a combined anterior and posterior spinal fusion on the same operative day. The anterior discectomies are performed first. With the patient in the same lateral decubitus position, the posterior spine is exposed in the kyphotic region. Spinous process wires with Drummond buttons can generally be safely inserted and are wired to adjacent spinous process wires in an alternating fashion. Attempts to use a Luque rectangle or a similar configuration made from a Rush rod have led to loss of somatosensory

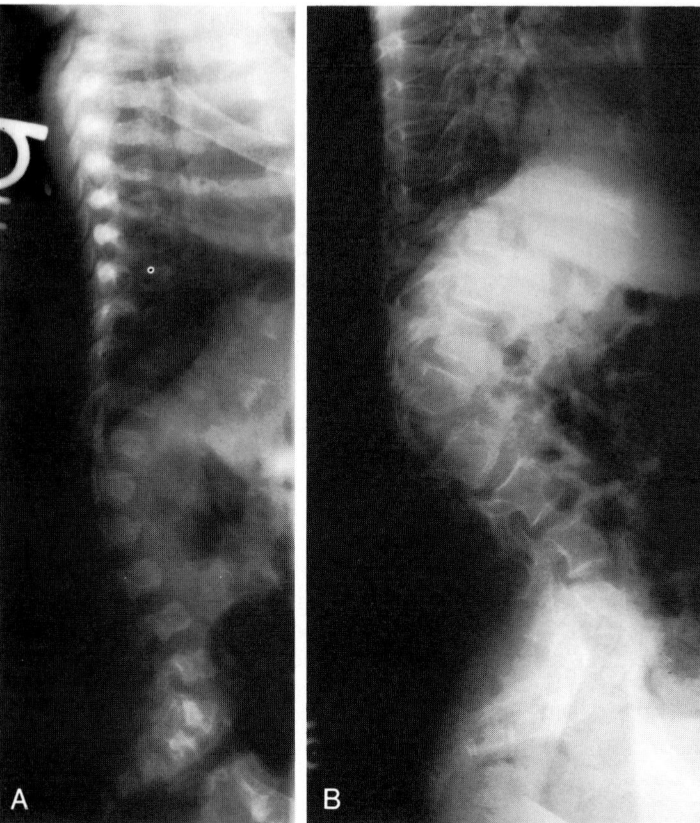

Figure 12–1. *A*, Lateral spinal radiograph at 6 months of age demonstrates early thoracolumbar kyphosis. Most of these deformities resolve by 2 or 3 years of age. If the apical vertebra remains wedged by age 5 or 6 years, surgery is recommended. *B*, Lateral radiograph (same child as *A*) of spine at age 10 years demonstrating persistent wedging of L1 at the thoracolumbar junction, which requires anterior and posterior spinal fusion.

evoked potentials in several patients and have been largely abandoned because of this risk of iatrogenic neurologic injury.[45] After posterior wiring and fusion have been completed to obtain some correction, the anterior rib strut graft is inserted under compression to further stabilize the correction. A body jacket cast is used six months postoperatively. Some have advocated bed rest until fusion, but the author allows walking in the cast as tolerated. Casts may require frequent changing to allow for accurate fitting to the dysplastic trunk and to accommodate extremity movement (Fig. 12–2).

Although clinically the principal thoracic and lumbar problem in preadolescent achondroplastic children is kyphosis, neurologic compromise is the most common spinal disorder in teenagers and adults. Lutter and Langer[26] divided these neurologic manifestations into four types:

I. Progressive, insidious onset.
II. Intermittent claudication.
III. Nerve root compression.
IV. Acute onset of paraplegia.

Types I and II are the most common. In Type I, there is a slow but progressive onset of back pain, associated with lower extremity paresthesias and sensory loss. Urologic function is often impaired, subclinically at first but later leading to incontinence.[47] In the Type II patient, there is also a rather slow and progressive onset of symptoms, with the patient first noting a decreased ability to walk distances. Pain and weakness in the legs results from the standing position and this is relieved by sitting, squatting, leaning forward, or lying down. The initial neurologic examination may be normal after the patient has been sitting in the waiting room for a time, but with this type of complaint, a repeat examination should be performed after having the patient walk or stand until symptoms recur. Often, such an examination elicits weakness not noted on the initial examination. The excessive lumbar lordosis of achondroplasia, combined with the stenotic lumbar canal, leads to less capacity of the spinal canal during standing than when the lumbar spine is flexed in sitting, squatting, or forward-bending positions.[37] Neurologic abnormalities may involve both lower extremities symmetrically or there may be uneven involvement. Type III patients have more obvious unilateral radicular signs and symptoms. A positive straight leg raising (SLR) test is found in Type III, whereas this test is negative in Type II patients. Confirmation of this type is by myelography or MRI. In Type IV, acute paraparesis or paraplegia occurs, at times associated with trauma. Generally, these patients have had some symptoms suggestive of Types I or II before the acute neurologic deficit.

If neurologic deficits are suspected from the history or demonstrated by examination, further imaging studies are indicated to localize the abnormal area(s). Most commonly, the interpediculate distance is significantly narrowed while the anteroposterior dimension is relatively normal, until osteophytes from disc degeneration protrude into the spinal canal.[27] Classically, myelography has been the most productive in delineating the levels of spinal cord and cauda equina compression. In achondroplasia, a myelogram is best performed through a cisternal, rather than a lumbar, puncture.[43] Because of the stenotic lumbar spine, it is difficult to insert the needle safely at this level. In addition, if any fluid is removed or leaks through the puncture site, it is possible to increase the neurologic deficit, particularly when kyphosis is present, by exacerbation of the anterior cord compression that may be present. If there is kyphosis, the patient should be placed supine for part of the examination to allow a better evaluation of dye flow over the kyphosis apex. Use of CT scans with myelograms allows for a better determination of the number of levels that require decompressive laminectomy. MRI has the obvious advantages of being free of radiation and being noninvasive, but in the author's experience the

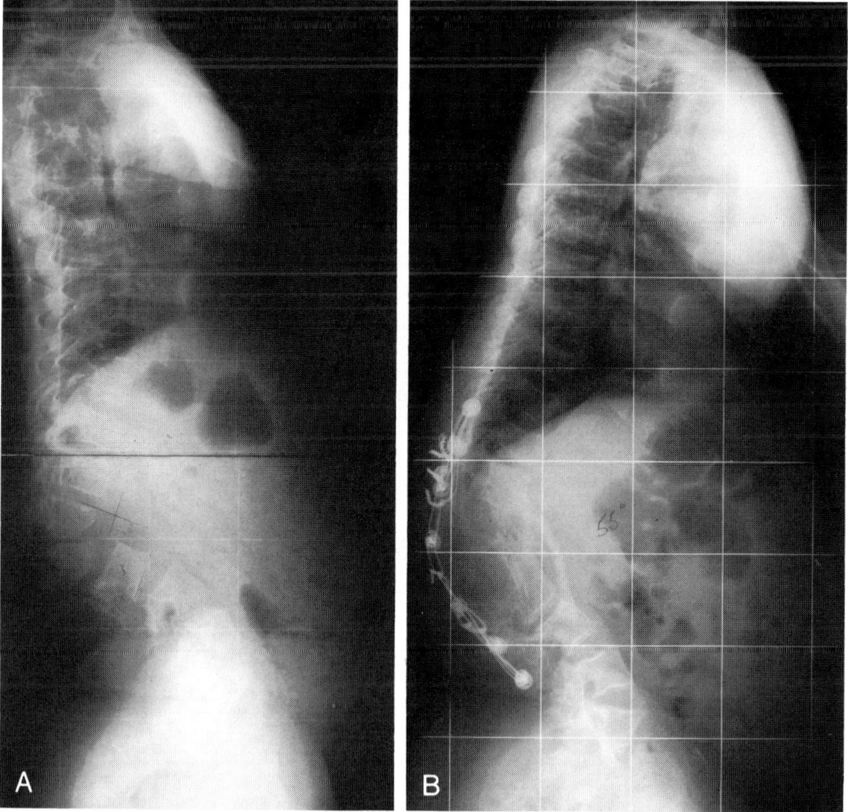

Figure 12–2. *A*, Lateral spinal radiograph demonstrating 90-degree thoracolumbar kyphosis in a 12-year-old boy with achondroplasia. *B*, Lateral spinal radiograph two years after anterior and posterior spinal fusion with posterior wiring demonstrating a residual but nonprogressive 55-degree kyphosis. It appears this tension-band wiring technique has both a simpler cast immobilization and less risk of causing iatrogenic neurologic injury in achondroplasia kyphosis than have other posterior instrumentation methods.

extent and degree of stenosis can usually be better demonstrated by myelography with CT.

The selection of the surgical procedure(s) best suited to the individual achondroplastic patient depends on the physical and imaging findings. In a Type III patient, a limited laminectomy and disc excision with foraminotomy generally suffice. More commonly, however, in the other types, multilevel decompressive laminectomy is the surgical treatment of choice.[42] Whether concurrent fusion is needed usually depends on the degree of kyphosis present at the time of laminectomy.

In the presence of thoracolumbar kyphosis and lumbar stenosis, it is often difficult to determine the exact level of neurologic compromise. As a general principle, if depressed reflexes and leg weakness are present, lumbar laminectomy appears to suffice. However, if hyperreflexia is present, together with leg weakness and sensory changes, anterior spinal cord decompression at the apex of the kyphosis is recommended in addition to the multilevel lumbar laminectomies.

In achondroplastic patients without kyphosis but with neurologic defects secondary to the stenosis, multilevel laminectomy is the treatment of choice (Fig. 12–3).[2, 42] Because of the severe stenosis present in these patients, with the concurrent loss of most of the subarachnoid space, special precautions are required to complete the laminectomy more safely.[47] It is important to avoid placing rongeurs inside the spinal canal at the time of laminectomy in view of the risk of increased neurologic deficit postoperatively. Uematsu and colleagues advocated a revised approach to decrease the complications of dural tears, increased neurologic deficit, and pseudomeningocele formation.[47] This approach uses a high-speed burr to transect the laminae just medial to the facet, after which the lamina segment is lifted dorsally. After unroofing the lumbar canal, further foraminotomies can more safely be performed. Closure using the paraspinous muscles to obliterate the dead space left by the extensive laminectomy appears to decrease the later development of pseudomeningoceles that may lead to later neurologic deterioration. These authors also stressed the need to perform multilevel decompressions, with a typical laminectomy extending from T9 to the sacrum.[47] Fusion is rarely needed if no thoracolumbar kyphosis is present. If there is kyphosis of

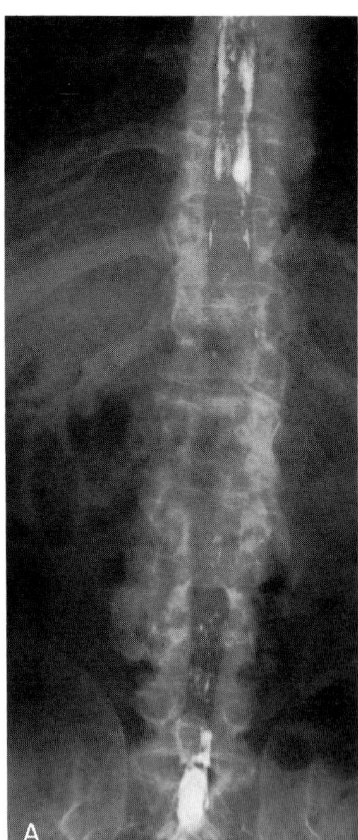

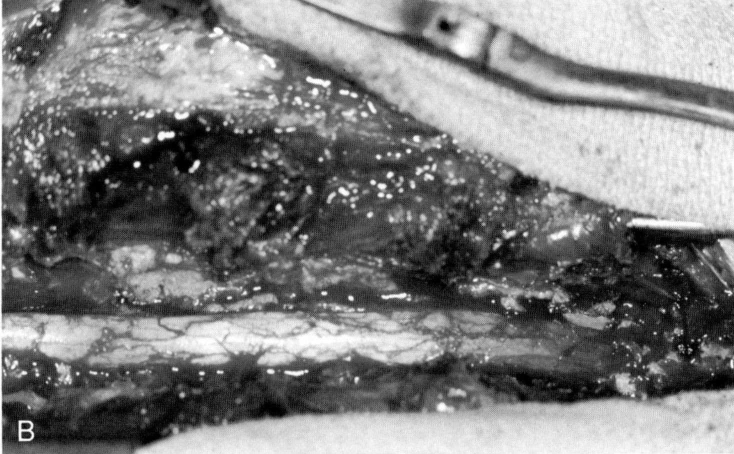

Figure 12–3. Radiograph *(A)* and photograph *(B)* of multilevel laminectomy generally needed for spinal stenosis in achondroplasia. If multiple levels are not included, recurrence of symptoms a few months after limited decompression is common.

more than 40 or 50 degrees, lateral fusion at the same time as laminectomy is indicated to prevent progressive kyphosis. Larger kyphotic deformities require both anterior and posterior fusion.[45]

In patients with kyphosis and lumbar spine stenosis, both disorders being a possible cause of the underlying neurologic deficit,[14] two-stage anterior decompression-fusion and posterior fusion is needed.[35, 45] It is in these patients, with long-standing progressive kyphosis, that minimal correction is feasible. Anterior disc removal and fusion, with or without spinal cord decompression, constitute the initial stage, followed one week later by posterior decompression and lateral fusion. It is possible to use 5- and 6-mm pedicle screws with Cotrel-Dubousset (C-D) instrumentation to allow for more secure correction in achondroplasia, but preoperative CT scans should be used to demonstrate sufficient pedicle size if use of this instrumentation is contemplated.

In older children, adolescents, and adults with progressive kyphosis but no neurologic deficit, anterior and posterior spinal fusion is generally carried out as a two-stage procedure. Anterior discectomy and fusion with a strut graft is followed one week later by posterior spinal fusion. In several attempts to instrument the spine posteriorly, the author has noted loss of somatosensory evoked potentials after instrumentation.[45] One should never insert hooks or wires into the stenotic lumbar canal. Even with interspinous wires attached to a Luque rectangle, with all instrumentation outside the spinal canal, iatrogenic neurologic injury rates are extremely high. As noted previously, interspinous wires applied as tension bands appear to be safer and allow for some internal stabilization. Spinal cord monitoring during any attempts at correction or decompression in achondroplasia is mandatory to decrease the risk of permanent impairment.[28, 45]

Diastrophic Dysplasia

Another syndrome that can be recognized at birth, diastrophic dysplasia, encompasses patients with classic diastrophic dwarfism and those with diastrophic variants. Inherited as an autosomal recessive disorder, this syndrome is rare. Characteristic diagnostic features include micromelia with marked short stature, "hitch-hiker thumb" due to proximal placement of the thumb, severe clubfeet, and, within a few weeks of birth, a "cauliflower deformity" of the ears secondary to calcification in the external ear cartilage.[48] Intelligence is normal. A cleft palate occurs in about 25 per cent of these children.

Several spinal findings may be noted. Cervical spine spina bifida is uniformly present, although symptoms directly related to this anatomic feature do not seem to occur.[5, 17] Atlantoaxial instability has not been reported and foramen magnum compression is not seen. The principal cervical spine abnormality in this syndrome is kyphosis,[16, 20] which typically occurs in the midcervical region. Many young children with diastrophic dysplasia have a mild degree of midcervical kyphosis and most resolve.[5] The reason for progression of this kyphosis in a few patients is unclear, but the presence of bifid spinous processes in this syndrome may play a role. In the few patients in whom the kyphosis does not resolve spontaneously, wedging of the apical vertebrae occurs. If this x-ray finding is present, surgical treatment is warranted. As the kyphosis becomes severe, spinal cord compression may occur, and death has been reported to have resulted from this.[19] At autopsy, neuropathologic examination has demonstrated neurolytic changes in the anterior columns from progressive spinal cord compression.

The goal of treatment is obviously to detect the progressive kyphosis early. Both anterior and posterior cervical fusion are indicated for optimal stabilization. A halo-brace can be effectively used to help obtain some initial correction as well as to immobilize the cervical spine postoperatively until fusion is solid. Whether or not there is a neurologic defect, laminectomy has no place in the treatment of this cervical kyphosis.

In the thoracic spine, kyphoscoliosis is the primary spinal disorder. Approximately 40 per cent of these children develop scoliosis of a mild to moderate degree that requires little or no orthotic treatment and no surgery. About 30 per cent develop severe, progressive thoracic scoliosis that is associated with a sharply angular thoracic kyphosis at the same level. In a review of 43 patients with diastrophic dysplasia,[46] it was noted that if significant kyphoscoliosis was to be present, the spinal deformity could be noted before the age of 4 years.

Treatment is difficult. The goal is basically

partial control of the kyphoscoliosis until the child is mature enough to undergo spinal fusion. Orthotic treatment is useful if there is any flexibility of the spinal deformity on bending films. In the more rigid and progressive curves, tomography of the apex of these kyphoscolioses often demonstrates a wedging or failure of formation or segmentation of a portion of the apical vertebral body, resembling tomographic findings in congenital kyphosis or scoliosis.[46] In young children with progressive spinal deformity, submuscular posterior spinal instrumentation has been used to help control the scoliosis while the limited growth proceeds (Fig. 12–4). Observation in children with diastrophic dysplasia appears to indicate that spinal growth is complete by age 10, so that spinal fusion can be recommended earlier than in other children. If it is necessary to fuse a younger child's spine surgically, combined anterior and posterior fusion is indicated to avoid the "crankshaft" phenomenon that leads to increased spinal deformity, despite posterior fusion, by continued growth in the anterior column of the spine.

Another spinal feature of diastrophic dysplasia is a marked lumbosacral lordosis. The sacrum itself may become increasingly lordotic with growth, and the lordosis is exaggerated by posterior vertebral body wedging that occurs at L5; it is further amplified by the flexion contractures always present at the hips. In some diastrophic patients the anteroposterior radiograph demonstrates interpediculate narrowing at the lumbosacral area. Even though myelograms may confirm narrowing at this level, the stenosis does not occur higher in the lumbar spine and rarely requires decompressive laminectomy, even in conjunction with the severe lumbosacral lordosis.[46]

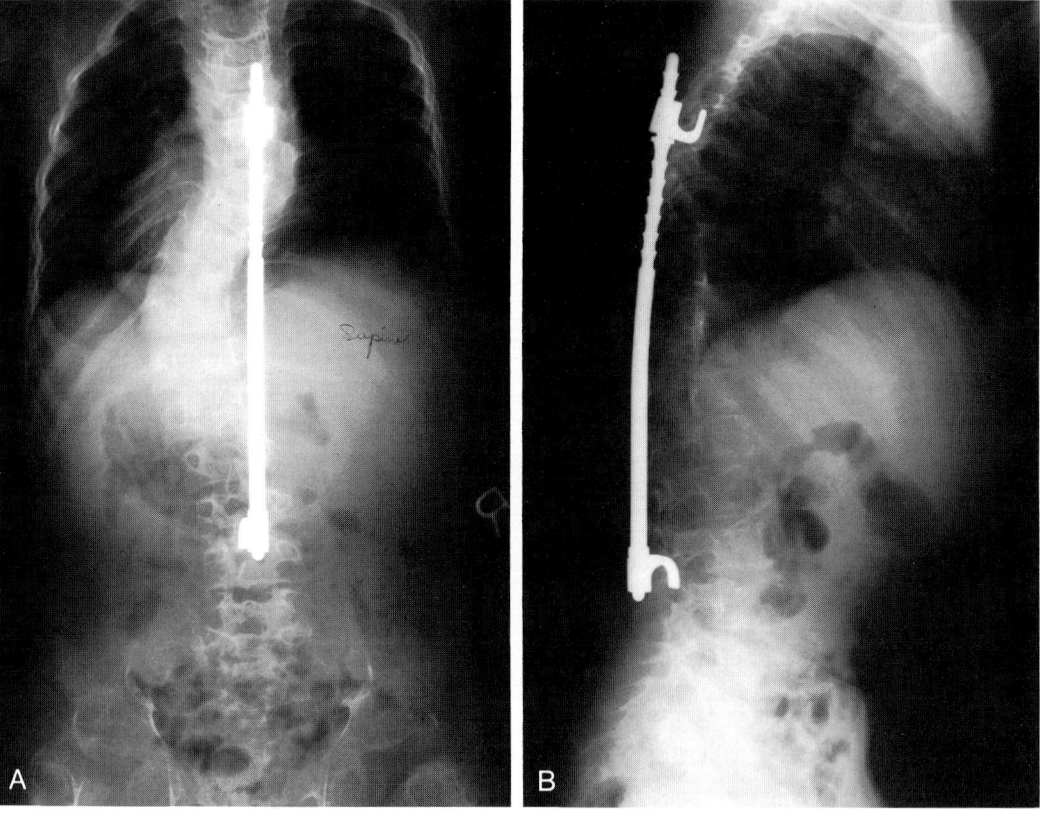

Figure 12–4. *A*, Anteroposterior spinal radiograph of a 5-year-old boy with diastrophic dysplasia. Scoliosis was corrected from 70 to 40 degrees by this submuscular rod without fusion. Although braces must still be worn after these rods, they are useful in this condition in which young children frequently have severe progressive scoliosis. Definitive instrumentation and fusion can usually be accomplished at age 9 or 10 years. *B*, This radiograph demonstrates the progressive kyphosis that often occurs above the distraction instrumentation without fusion, if multiple lengthenings are necessary.

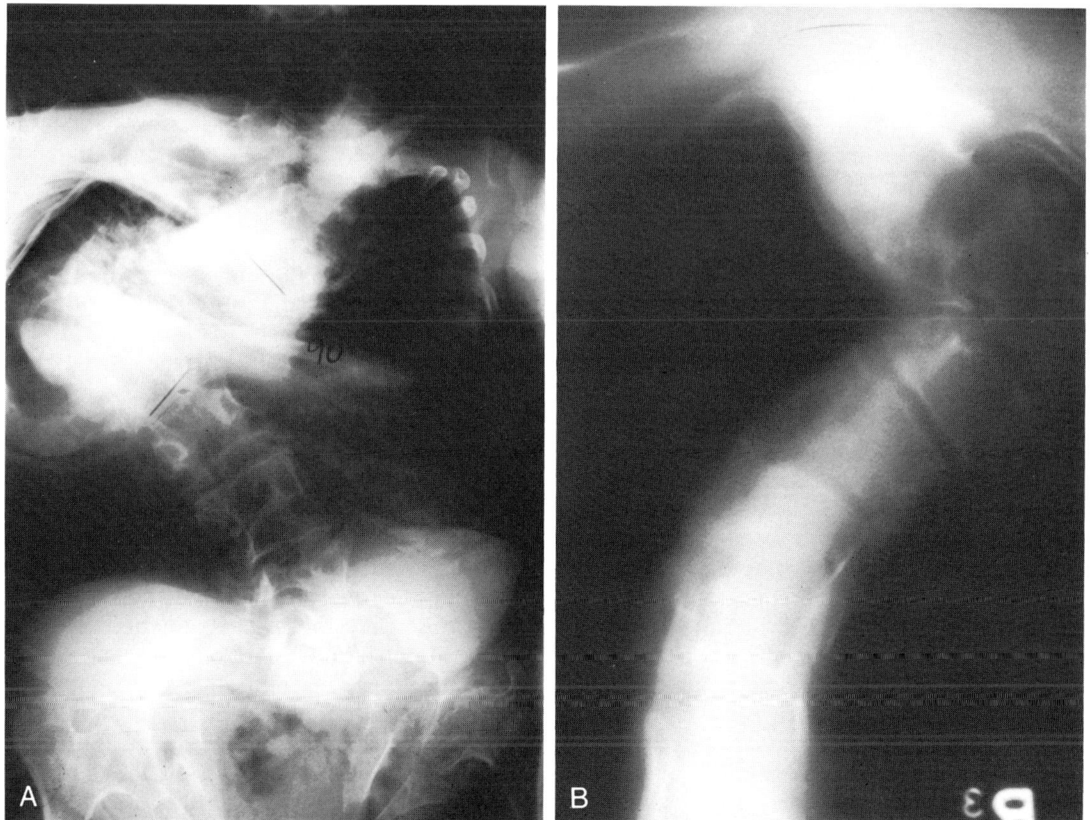

Figure 12–5. *A*, Anteroposterior spinal radiograph of a female with diastrophic dysplasia, a condition in which some of the most severe scoliosis and kyphosis seen with skeletal dysplasias are present. *B*, Tomogram of the thoracic spine in a child with diastrophic dysplasia. This demonstrates a finding common in this condition when severe scoliosis is present at a young age. The resemblance to a congenital kyphoscoliosis may help explain why progression may be so rapid and eventual curve magnitude so severe.

Some of the most severe cases of kyphoscoliosis the author has seen have been in patients with diastrophic dysplasia (Fig. 12–5). Even though some of these severe spinal deformities have caused swallowing difficulties from the aberrant path of the esophagus, neurologic signs and symptoms related to spinal cord compression are exceedingly rare. In other severe, sharply angular kyphotic conditions, in patients with normal or short stature, spinal cord compression is generally anticipated. In the diastrophic group, however, the primary neurologic problem that occurs is iatrogenic, secondary to surgical attempts to straighten the spinal deformity. These severe curves are minimally flexible and any attempts at instrumentation must use spinal cord monitoring to help avoid overdistraction with instrumentation. If marked kyphosis is present, combined anterior and posterior spinal fusion is needed. It is, of course, preferable to detect the spinal deformity early, follow the progress of the deformity carefully, and then fuse the curve at an appropriate time, rather than allow the deformity to progress unchecked. The spinal canal is of sufficient size to accept the appropriately sized implants of the standard posterior spinal instrumentation systems (e.g., Harrington, Wisconsin).

Spondyloepiphyseal Dysplasia (SED)

The two forms of this condition, spondyloepiphyseal dysplasia congenita and spondyloepiphyseal dysplasia tarda, are distinct from each other.

SED tarda is inherited as an X-linked recessive condition affecting males only. Children with this form appear to have normal body proportions at birth. The diagnosis generally is not made until late childhood or early adolescence, by which time there has been a virtual halt to spinal growth. Radiographs demonstrate platyspondyly with a characteristic vertebral body shape consisting of a hump-shaped build-up of bone in the central and posterior aspects of the vertebral body, with delayed ossification of the vertebral ring apophysis. A common feature of this syndrome is premature osteoarthritis, particularly of the hips, that may require total joint arthroplasty in early adult life. Low back pain may result from the combination of disc degenerative changes and the lumbar lordosis present, at least in part due to the hip disease. Scoliosis and kyphosis appear to be rare.

Of more concern from the spinal point of view is SED congenita. Recognizable at birth, this condition is inherited in an autosomal dominant manner.[41] The primary diagnostic features include a short-trunk type of dwarfism, delayed ossification of the vertebral bodies, and coxa vara. The hands and feet are of relatively normal size. Extremity x-ray films show delayed ossification of the proximal femora and irregularities of both the epiphyseal and metaphyseal regions in the long bones. A commonly associated finding is retinal detachment, so periodic ophthalmologic examination is important during childhood.

In the cervical spine of children with SED congenita, atlantoaxial instability is the most commonly encountered problem, found in 30 to 40 per cent.[20] Although these infants may have low muscle tone, this hypotonia should resolve. Failure to attain motor milestones progressively should direct the orthopedist's attention to the cervical spine, because atlantoaxial instability in this condition may be found in infancy or early childhood. One should remember when interpreting x-ray studies, however, that normally there is increased flexibility in a young child's spine. Flexion-extension lateral cervical spine x-rays should be obtained to evaluate the atlantoaxial area if there is delayed motor development and if neurologic symptoms and signs are present, and before anesthesia is given for other surgical procedures. If instability is present on plain x-ray films, an MRI scan in the flexed and extended positions allows excellent evaluation of neural compression at the high cervical area, in this way better determining the urgency of surgical treatment.

If atlantoaxial instability is present, posterior fusion is needed to protect the cervical spinal cord. Fusion is accomplished more safely with a halo-brace or halo-cast to immobilize the upper cervical spine (Fig. 12–6*A*). The halo is applied preoperatively (Fig. 12–6*B*). The author has successfully utilized the halo in children with SED as young as 15 months. The younger the child, the more skull fixation pins are needed, six to eight being most commonly employed. Torque screwdrivers are used to tighten to only 3 to 4 psi in the very young. Once the halo is applied, the atlantoaxial area is reduced, with radiographic confirmation. The child is anesthetized in the halo-brace, and fiberoptic bronchoscopes are very useful to allow safe endotracheal tube placement without undue patient discomfort. In fusing the upper cervical spine, care should be taken to expose only those levels needed to accomplish stabilization, since simple exposure of multiple levels in children may lead to spontaneous unintended fusion of these exposed levels. If possible, atlantoaxial fusion is preferable to including the occiput in the fusion, but in children under the age of 5 years the posterior arch of the atlas is often unossified, making wire stabilization of this single segment more difficult. Even though wiring of the axis to either the atlas or the occiput does provide some internal stability, the author prefers maintaining the halo-brace as external support for three months after surgery. Laminectomy is rarely necessary at the time of fusion and should never be the only treatment for the upper cervical cord compression caused by atlantoaxial instability.

In the thoracic and lumbar spine, stenosis is not a problem. Spinal deformity may occur. Thoracolumbar kyphosis, although not common, may appear in conjunction with the platyspondyly that is uniformly present and is the cause of the short trunk in this syndrome. Progressive scoliosis can sometimes be successfully managed with the usual spinal deformity orthoses, but fitting and tolerance are difficult with the short trunk in this syndrome. If the scoliosis is progressive, posterior spinal instrumentation and fusion can safely be used without the need for customized implant construction. As with nondwarf spinal deformity, spinal cord monitoring should be used intraoperatively.

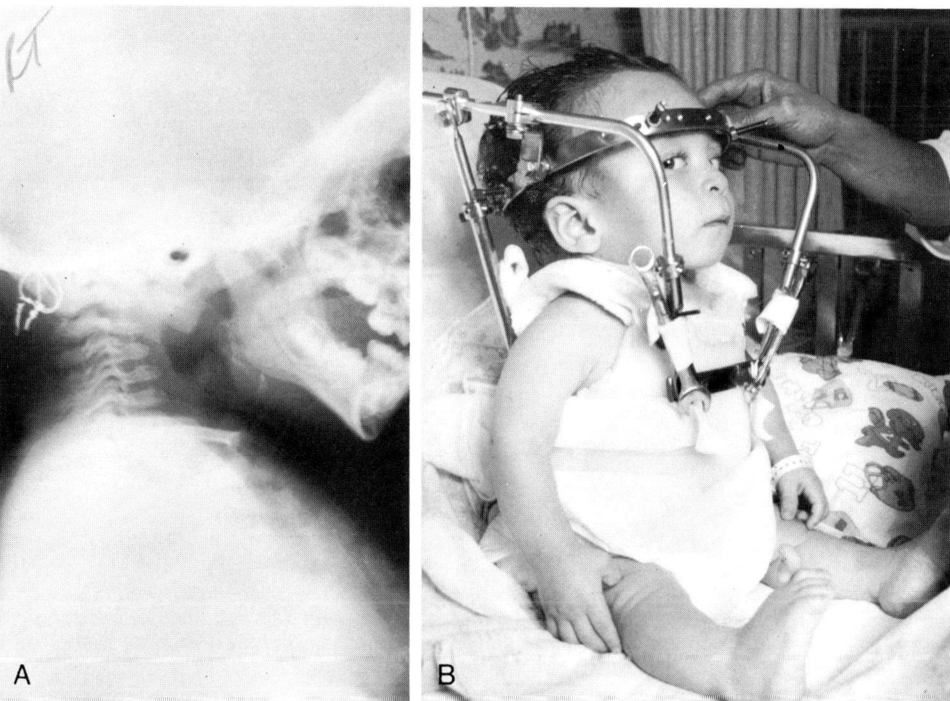

Figure 12–6. *A*, Lateral cervical spine radiograph demonstrates occipitoaxial wiring and fusion in an 18-month-old boy with spondyloepiphyseal dysplasia. Atlantoaxial instability was present on flexion-extension lateral neck radiographs. A flexion magnetic resonance imaging study demonstrated spinal cord compression. After fusion, motor development of both upper and lower extremities improved dramatically. *B*, An 18-month-old boy with spondyloepiphyseal dysplasia had occipitoaxial fusion for atlantoaxial instability. Reduction was obtained preoperatively by this halo-brace, which was left on intraoperatively and for three months postoperatively. In children of this age, six or eight halo-pins are generally necessary for fixation.

Pseudoachondroplastic Dysplasia

Inherited generally in an autosomal dominant manner, this short-limbed form of dwarfism usually is not diagnosed until the child is 1 or 2 years old. Although the body proportions are similar to those found in achondroplasia, there should be no confusion between these syndromes. In pseudoachondroplasia, there is a normal face, long bone x-rays demonstrate both epiphyseal and metaphyseal abnormalities, and spinal x-rays show flattened vertebral bodies with a central, anterior tongue–like projection, as well as no interpediculate narrowing in the lumbar spine.[9] Premature osteoarthritis and angular deformity of the lower extremity are the primary orthopedic problems needing attention.

In the spine, some vertebral body flattening is present, despite the relatively normal trunk height. Lumbar lordosis may be marked, at least in part due to the flexion deformity of the hips. In the initial stages, this lordosis can be improved by appropriate proximal femoral extension osteotomies, but it becomes fixed with increasing age. Kyphosis of the thoracic and thoracolumbar regions may develop in preadolescence and adolescence. Initially this kyphosis is relatively flexible and appears to form as a compensatory sagittal curve to balance the lumbar lordosis, but later structural deformity may require surgical treatment if anterior vertebral wedging at several levels occurs. The kyphosis seen here is not usually associated with apical vertebral wedging of only one or two vertebrae at the thoracolumbar area, as is common in achondroplasia. Scoliosis has also been reported in this syndrome, but there are no particular distinguishing features of this deformity. If spinal instrumentation is needed, the spine and spinal canal are of relatively normal size and any type of

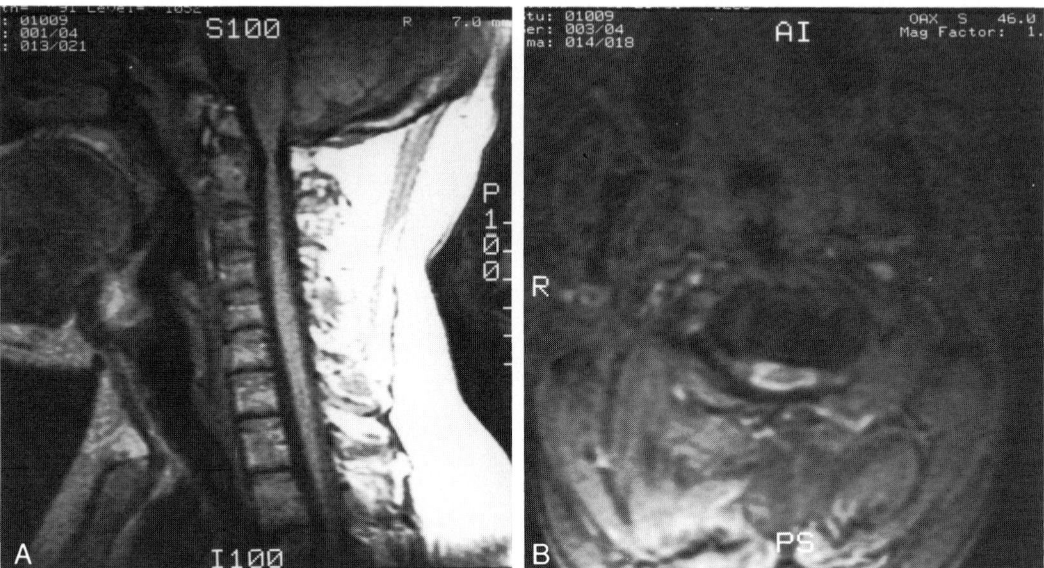

Figure 12–7. *A* and *B*, Magnetic resonance imaging study of the cervical spine in a male with pseudoachondroplasia demonstrates marked narrowing of the spinal cord at the atlantoaxial level, with flattening of the spinal cord seen on transverse cuts. Flexion-extension lateral cervical spine radiographs demonstrated 9 mm of atlantoaxial motion. Posterior atlantoaxial fusion is needed in these cases.

spinal instrumentation implants used in normal-sized patients can be safely used in this disorder. Just as the peripheral joints demonstrate significant laxity that often interferes with function, atlantoaxial instability has been noted in some of these children and requires radiographic evaluation (Fig. 12–7).

MUCOPOLYSACCHARIDOSES

Seven different syndromes have been described with abnormal metabolism of mucopolysaccharides. Spinal manifestations of importance are rare or absent in Type III (Sanfilippo's syndrome), Type VII, and Type I-S (MPS V or Scheie's syndrome), although concentric dural thickening leading to neurologic deficits has been noted in the cervical spine in Type I-S disease.[40] In the remaining types, short-trunk dwarfism is generally seen, and the most common spinal abnormalities are kyphosis of the thoracic and thoracolumbar spine and atlantoaxial instability. Specific diagnosis is established by appropriate serum and urine studies, and by culture of either fibroblasts or leukocytes to elucidate the specific mucopolysaccharide abnormality. It is important to establish the exact diagnosis, because the prognosis and natural history of each condition is different, varying from death in childhood to survival into late adult life. Similarly, the severity of the spinal abnormality varies from one syndrome to another. Research continues on the feasibility of gene therapy to correct the underlying enzymatic defects.

Mucopolysaccharidosis I (Hurler's Syndrome)

Although they appear normal at birth, short stature becomes apparent in these patients in the first two or three years of life. Thoracolumbar kyphosis is generally seen early, and lateral spinal x-rays demonstrate anterior beaking of other vertebral bodies. By 2 years of age, corneal clouding, coarse facial features with large tongue and lips, stiff joints, and herniae are present and both motor and mental deterioration are seen after this time. Laboratory studies demonstrate excessive dermatan sulfate and heparan sulfate secretion. Although the kyphosis tends to persist, surgical treatment is not indicated, because most of these children die by age 10 years. Atlantoaxial instability may be present.[7, 44]

Mucopolysaccharidosis II (Hunter's Syndrome)

Athough the urinary laboratory findings in this syndrome are the same as in Hurler's syndrome, the clinical findings are much milder and the mode of inheritance is X-linked recessive, affecting only males. These children appear normal at birth and grow normally for about two years. As with other physical manifestations, vertebral changes are milder and generally do not require treatment, but the lumbar kyphosis may be marked.[3] Survival in Hunter's syndrome may reach well into adult life, although many die by age 20 of cardiopulmonary problems.

Mucopolysaccharidosis IV (Morquio's Syndrome)

For the first year or two of life, growth and development in Morquio's syndrome is normal. An early finding that should attract the orthopedist's attention is thoracolumbar kyphosis, with wedging of the apical thoracolumbar vertebrae. This should not be confused with congenital kyphosis, because radiographs of the spine also demonstrate anterior vertebral beaking at other spinal levels. As the child becomes older, short stature becomes detectable, together with genu valgum, pectus carinatum, and corneal clouding. Laboratory findings include increased keratan sulfate in the urine and a defect in *N*-acetyl-hexosamine 6-sulfate sulfatase in fibroblasts. Decreased exercise tolerance with lower extremity weakness may be attributed to the genu valgum deformity, but generally results from spinal cord compression due to atlantoaxial instability that results from odontoid aplasia or hypoplasia.[6, 20, 25, 30] This instability generally occurs in early childhood, but tends to be clinically noted somewhat later than the atlantoaxial instability in spondyloepiphyseal dysplasia congenita.

Upper cervical posterior fusion is needed to regain stability and protect the spinal cord. Before any lower extremity realignment surgery is performed, flexion-extension lateral cervical x-ray films should be obtained. Treatment of the thoracolumbar kyphosis consists primarily of serial observation and x-rays; a spinal orthosis is useful to prevent progression in children with evident worsening. Surgical fusion of the thoracolumbar kyphosis is not usually needed. Patients with Morquio's syndrome can survive to adulthood, but many die by age 20 owing to cardiopulmonary disease or sequelae from neurologic deficits. Earlier awareness and diagnosis of the atlantoaxial instability should prevent the neurologic deficits (Fig. 12–8).

Mucopolysaccharidosis VI (Maroteaux-Lamy Syndrome)

Also normal at birth, these children have short-trunk dwarfism noted by age 2 or 3 years. There is normal intelligence, although many of the physical features may resemble Hurler's syndrome. Laboratory findings demonstrate increased urinary excretion of dermatan sulfate and arylsulfatase B deficiency in fibroblasts and white blood cells. Vertebral flattening is seen and there is kyphosis in the thoracolumbar or lumbar spine. If persistent apical vertebral wedging in the kyphotic area is progressive with growth, combined anterior and posterior spinal fusion is feasible, although implants within the spinal canal may lead to iatrogenic neurologic deficits.

MISCELLANEOUS SYNDROMES

Kniest's Syndrome. Abnormal-appearing limbs and characteristic x-ray findings allow this syndrome to be diagnosed in infancy, although the long bone x-ray results have been confused with metatropic dwarfism in the past.[4, 24] Life expectancy is normal, as is intelligence. Extremity deformities make walking difficult and often require realignment osteotomies to improve motor function. Excessive lumbar lordosis appears to result from a combination of hip flexion contractures and inherent lumbar spine position, and may be partially improved by extension osteotomy at the hip. Kyphoscoliosis is frequently progressive at an early age. If marked, the scoliosis requires instrumentation and fusion to prevent increased pulmonary compromise. Atlantoaxial instability has been noted in this syndrome, and if documented by flexion/extension lateral cervical spine x-rays, is adequately treated by upper cervical fusion.

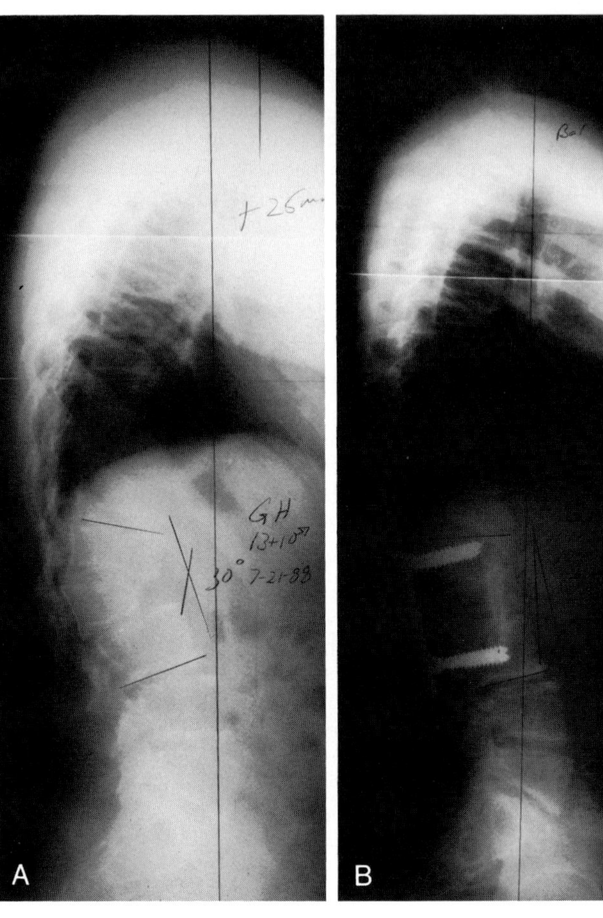

Figure 12–8. *A* and *B*, Lateral spinal radiographs before and seven months after laminectomy and spinal fusion in a teenager with thoracolumbar kyphosis associated with Morquio's syndrome. Although most of the kyphotic deformities in this syndrome are minimally progressive or nonprogressive, careful follow-up with growth is needed. Surgical treatment is indicated with progressive kyphosis despite bracing and when abnormal neurologic signs and symptoms are present. If a neurologic deficit is present, the atlantoaxial region should be evaluated carefully. Instability here is common in Morquio's syndrome. (Courtesy of Marc A. Asher, M.D., Kansas City, KS.)

Metatropic Dysplasia. In this rare syndrome, there is an apparent change in body proportions with increasing age, at least partly due to progressive scoliosis. At birth, these infants have short limbs and a slender, long trunk. As growth progresses, the trunk becomes increasingly short, owing to the vertebral body flattening and the increasing spinal deformity. Life expectancy usually extends to early adulthood. The progressively severe scoliosis is difficult to manage. Early orthotic treatment is warranted, but if this is unsuccessful, instrumentation without fusion should be considered in early childhood. Definitive posterior instrumentation and fusion are needed when other methods are unable to control the scoliosis progression.

Mucolipidoses. Thoracolumbar kyphosis has been noted in mucolipidosis Types II and III. In Type II, the physical features are similar to those in Hurler's syndrome. Spinal abnormalities include thoracolumbar kyphosis, anterior vertebral body beaking, and scoliosis. Although spinal orthotic care may be indicated in some patients, surgery is not recommended, because these children usually die by age 5 years. In Type III, the biochemical abnormality is similar to that found in Type II, but the clinical manifestations are milder and life expectancy is well into adult life. Progressive thoracolumbar kyphosis may be present, and surgical treatment of anterior and posterior fusion with spinal instrumentation is indicated in these patients. Carpal tunnel syndromes requiring median nerve release are common in adolescence.

Chondrodysplasia Punctata. Also known as Conradi-Hünermann syndrome, this condition is characterized by short limbs, flat facial features, and radiographic findings of punctate calcification at the ends of the long bones. Atlantoaxial instability may occur at an early age and has been reported to have led to early death from cervical cord compression.[1] Scoliosis is common, appearing in early childhood and often progressing. If orthotic control is not feasible, spinal instrumentation is necessary, since life expectancy and intelligence are normal if the patient survives the newborn period.

Camptomelic Dysplasia. In this rare disorder, bowing of the long bones is present at birth, as is scoliosis or kyphoscoliosis. No orthopedic treatment is needed, because almost all die in infancy.

Parastremmatic Dysplasia. This short-trunk form of dwarfism is very rare. There is angular deformity of the lower extremities and radiographic findings of both epiphyseal and metaphyseal changes. Spinal x-ray films show flattened vertebral bodies with irregular end-plate ossification. Kyphoscoliosis is present in virtually all and, if of sufficient magnitude, requires orthotic and/or surgical treatment, as patients survive to adulthood.

Spondyloepimetaphyseal Dysplasia With Joint Laxity. The development of severe progressive kyphoscoliosis during infancy is noted in this disorder. If it is left untreated, death in early childhood due either to spinal cord compression sequelae or to cardiorespiratory failure has been noted in most patients.[23]

Spondylometaphyseal Dysplasia, Kozlowski Type. The diagnosis of this condition, a short-trunk form of dwarfism, is not usually established until preschool age. Platyspondyly is present and kyphosis is common. Life expectancy is normal and kyphosis treatment is indicated if progression can be proved.[22]

SUMMARY

In the future, genetic engineering will probably reverse the defects present in many of the syndromes discussed, as information from ongoing molecular research is rapidly accumulating that makes it possible to pinpoint the exact abnormalities that cause these conditions. However, that day is several years away. In the meantime, it is necessary that when we see a patient with short stature, an accurate diagnosis is first obtained, to allow us to watch for expected spinal problems in each of these syndromes. Early diagnosis of these spinal conditions will lead to less functional loss for these patients, and appropriate spinal care will avoid unnecessary disability. These syndromes are not common, but each patient is a unique individual who will benefit from this approach and will be helped to become a well-integrated, contributing member of society.

References

1. Afshani, E., and Girdany, B. R.: Atlanto-axial dislocation in chondrodysplasia punctata: report of the findings in two brothers. Radiology *102*:399–401, 1972.
2. Alexander, E., Jr.: Significance of the small lumbar spinal canal: cauda equina compression syndromes due to spondylosis. Part 5: Achondroplasia. J. Neurosurg. *31*:513–519, 1969.
3. Benson, P. F., Button, L. R., Fensom, A. H., and Dean, M. F.: Lumbar kyphosis in Hunter's disease (MPS II). Clin. Genet. *16*:317–322, 1979.
4. Bethem, D., Winter, R. B., Lutter, L., et al.: Spinal disorders of dwarfism. Review of the literature and report of eighty cases. J. Bone Joint Surg. *63A*:1412–1425, 1981.
5. Bethem, D., Winter, R. B., and Lutter, L.: Disorders of the spine in diastrophic dwarfism. A discussion of nine patients and review of the literature. J. Bone Joint Surg. *62A*:529–536, 1980.
6. Blaw, M. F., and Langer, L. O.: Spinal cord compression in Morquio-Brailsford disease. J. Pediatr. *74*:593–600, 1969.
7. Brill, C. B., Rose, J. S., Godmilow, L., et al.: Spastic quadriparesis due to C1–C2 subluxation in Hurler syndrome. J. Pediatr. *92*:441–443, 1978.
8. Carson, B., Winfield, J., Wang, H., et al.: Surgical management of cervicomedullary compression in achondroplastic patients. *In* Nicoletto, B., Kopits, S. E., Ascani, E., and McKusick, V. A. (eds.): Human Achondroplasia: A Multidisciplinary Approach. New York, Plenum Press, 1988, pp. 207–214.
9. Ford, M., Silverman, F. N., and Kozlowski, K.: Spondyloepiphyseal dysplasia (pseudoachondroplastic type). J. Roentgenol. Radium Ther. Nucl. Med. *86*:462–472, 1961.
10. Fremion, A. S., Garg, B. P., and Kalsbeck, J.: Apnea as the sole manifestation of cord compression in achondroplasia. J. Pediatr. *104*:398–401, 1984.
11. Gulati, D. R., and Rout, D.: Atlantoaxial dislocation with quadriparesis in achondroplasia: case report. J. Neurosurg. *40*:394–396, 1974.
12. Hall, J. G.: Kyphosis in achondroplasia: probably preventable. J. Pediatr. *112*:166–167, 1988.
13. Hammerschlag, W., Ziv, I., Wald, U., et al.: Cervical instability in an achondroplastic infant: case report. J. Pediatr. Orthop. *8*:481–484, 1988.
14. Hancock, D. O., and Phillips, D. G.: Spinal compression in achondroplasia. Paraplegia *3*:23–33, 1965.
15. Hecht, J. T., Butler, I. J., and Scott, C. I., Jr.: Long-term neurological sequelae in achondroplasia. Eur. J. Pediatr. *143*:58–60, 1984.
16. Hensinger, R. N.: Kyphosis secondary to skeletal dysplasias and metabolic disease. Clin. Orthop. *128*:113–128, 1977.
17. Herring, J. A.: The spinal disorder in diastrophic dwarfism. J. Bone Joint Surg. *60A*:177–182, 1978.

18. Kahonovitz, N., Rimoin, D. L., and Sillence, D. O.: The clinical spectrum of lumbar spine disease in achondroplasia. Spine 7:137–140, 1982.
19. Kash, I. J., Sane, S. M., Samaha, F. J., and Briner, J.: Cervical cord compression in diastrophic dwarfism. J. Pediatr. *78*:862–865, 1974.
20. Kopits, S. E.: Orthopaedic complications of dwarfism. Clin. Orthop. *114*:153–179, 1976.
21. Kopits, S. E.: Thoracolumbar kyphosis and lumbosacral hyperlordosis in achondroplastic children. *In* Nicoletti, B., Kopits, S. E., Ascani, E., and McKusick, V. A. (eds.): Human Achondroplasia: A Multidisciplinary Approach. New York, Plenum Press, 1988, pp. 241–255.
22. Kozlowski, K. S.: Chondrodysplasia spondylometaphysealis. Birth Defects *11*:183–185, 1975.
23. Kozlowski, K., and Beighton, P.: Radiographic features of spondylo-epimetaphyseal dysplasia with joint laxity and progressive kyphoscoliosis. Review of 19 cases. Fortschr. Roentgenstr. *141*:337–341, 1984.
24. Lachman, R. S., Rimoin, D. L., Hollister, D. W., et al.: The Kniest syndrome. Am. J. Roentgenol. Radium Ther. Nucl. Med. *123*:805–814, 1975.
25. Lipson, S. J.: Dysplasia of the odontoid process in Morquio's syndrome causing quadriparesis. J. Bone Joint Surg. *59A*:340–344, 1977.
26. Lutter, L. D., and Langer, L. O.: Neurologic symptoms in achondroplastic dwarfs—surgical treatment. J. Bone Joint Surg. *59A*:87–92, 1977.
27. Lutter, L. D., Lonstein, J. E., Winter, R. E., and Langer, L. O.: Anatomy of the achondroplastic lumbar canal. Clin. Orthop. *126*:139–142, 1977.
28. McPherson, R. W., North, R. B., Udvarhelyi, G. B., and Rosenbaum, A. E.: Migrating disc complicating spinal decompression in an achondroplastic dwarf: intraoperative demonstration of spinal cord compression by somatosensory evoked potentials. Anesthesiology *61*:764–767, 1984.
29. Morgan, D. F., and Young, R. F.: Spinal neurological complications of achondroplasia. Results of surgical treatment. J. Neurosurg. *52*:463–472, 1980.
30. Nelson, J., and Thomas, P. S.: Clinical findings in 12 patients with MPS IV A (Morquio's disease): further evidence for heterogeneity. Part III: Odontoid dysplasia. Clin. Genet. *33*:126–130, 1988.
31. Nelson, F. W., Hecht, J. T., Horton, W. A., et al.: Neurological basis of respiratory complications in achondroplasia. Ann. Neurol. *24*:89–93, 1988.
32. Pauli, R. M., Scott, C. I., Jr., Wassman, E. R., Jr., et al.: Apnea and sudden unexpected death in infants with achondroplasia. J. Pediatr. *104*:342–348, 1984.
33. Pyeritz, R. E., Sack, G. H., and Udvarhelyi, G. B.: Cervical and lumbar laminectomy for spinal stenosis in achondroplasia. Johns Hopkins Med. J. *146*:203–206, 1980.
34. Reid, C. S., Pyeritz, R. E., Kopits, S. E., et al.: Cervicomedullary compression in young patients with achondroplasia: value of comprehensive neurologic and respiratory evaluation. J. Pediatr. *110*:522–530, 1987.
35. Sculco, T. P., and Levine, D. B.: Thoracolumbar kyphosis in achondroplasia (with spinal cord compression). N. Y. State J. Med. *76*:426–429, 1976.
36. Sensenbrenner, J. A.: Achondroplasia with hypoplastic vertebral bodies secondary to surgical fusion. Birth Defects *10*:356–357, 1974.
37. Siebens, A. A., Hungerford, D. S., and Kirby, N. A.: Curves of the achondroplastic spine: a new hypothesis. Johns Hopkins Med. J. *142*:205–210, 1978.
38. Siebens, A. A., Hungerford, D. S., and Kirby, N. A.: Achondroplasia: effectiveness of an orthosis in reducing deformity of the spine. Arch. Phys. Med. Rehabil. *68*:384–388, 1987.
39. Siebens, A. A., Kirby, N., and Hungerford, D. S.: Orthotic correction of sitting abnormality in achondroplastic children. *In* Nicoletti, B., Kopits, S. E., Ascani, E., and McKusick, V. A. (eds.): Human Achondroplasia: A Multidisciplinary Approach. New York, Plenum Press, 1988, pp. 313–320.
40. Sostrin, R. D., Hasso, A. N., Peterson, D. I., and Thompson, J. R.: Myelographic features of mucopolysaccharidoses: a new sign. Radiology *125*:421–424, 1977.
41. Spranger, J., and Wiedemann, H. R.: Dysplasia spondyloepiphysaria congenita. Helv. Paediatr. Acta *21*:598–611, 1966.
42. Streeten, E., Uematsu, S., Hurko, O., et al.: Extended laminectomy for spinal stenosis in achondroplasia. *In* Nicoletti, B., Kopits, S. E., Ascani, E., and McKusick, V. A. (eds.): Human Achondroplasia: A Multidisciplinary Approach. New York, Plenum Press, 1988, pp. 261–273.
43. Suss, R. A., Udvarhelyi, G. B., Wang, H., et al.: Myelography in achondroplasia: value of a lateral C1–2 puncture and non-ionic, water-soluble contrast medium. Radiology *149*:159–163, 1983.
44. Thomas, S. L., Childress, M. H., and Quinton, B.: Hypoplasia of the odontoid with atlanto-axial subluxation in Hurler's syndrome. Pediatr. Radiol. *15*:353–354, 1985.
45. Tolo, V. T.: Surgical treatment of kyphosis in achondroplasia. *In* Nicoletti, B., Kopits, S. E., Ascani, E., and McKusick, V. A. (eds.): Human Achondroplasia: A Multidisciplinary Approach. New York, Plenum Press, 1988, pp. 257–259.
46. Tolo, V. T., and Kopits, S. E.: Spinal deformity in diastrophic dysplasia. Orthop. Trans. 7:31–32, 1983.
47. Uematsu, S., Wang, H., Hurko, O., and Kopits, S. E.: The subarachnoid fluid space in achondroplastic spinal stenosis: the surgical implications. *In* Nicoletti, B., Kopits, S. E., Ascani, E., and McKusick, V. A. (eds.): Human Achondroplasia: A Multidisciplinary Approach. New York, Plenum Press, 1988, pp. 275–281.
48. Walker, B. A., Scott, C. I., Hall, J. G., et al.: Diastrophic dwarfism. Medicine (Baltimore) *51*:41–59, 1972.
49. Wang, H., Rosenbaum, A. E., Reid, C. S., et al.: Pediatric patients with achondroplasia: CT evaluation of the craniocervical junction. Radiology *164*:515–519, 1987.
50. Wassman, E. R., Jr., and Rimoin, D. L.: Cervicomedullary compression with achondroplasia (letter). J. Pediatr. *113*:411, 1988.
51. Winter, R. B., and Herring, J. A.: Kyphosis in an achondroplastic dwarf. J. Pediatr. Orthop. *3*:250–252, 1983.
52. Yang, S. S., Corbett, D. P., Brough, A. J., et al.: Upper cervical myelopathy in achondroplasia. Am. J. Clin. Pathol. *68*:68–72, 1977.

CHAPTER

13

DISCITIS

Jeffery L. Stambough, M.D.
Eugene L. Saenger, M.D.

Although a myriad of terms have been applied to the syndrome of radiographic single-level disc space narrowing, fever, and elevated erythrocyte sedimentation rate, the term discitis is the most widely used[3, 12, 17, 18, 21, 24, 25, 28, 31] and is credited to Eric Price of Melbourne, Australia.[23, 26] Perhaps Smith and Taylor[34] were among the first to describe this clinical entity, but it was Saenger[31] who first described the syndrome in detail, emphasizing its now classic radiographic criteria. While the exact etiology and management remain open to some controversy, the prognosis is that of a self-limiting benign disorder with no serious late sequelae. The syndrome of discitis has been reviewed in several large series, and the term most accurately applies to patients in the first or second decades of life.[33, 35, 37]

Spinal sepsis may be divided into three major categories: vertebral osteomyelitis (pyogenic and nonpyogenic), epidural abscess, and discitis. Discitis is more self-limiting and is most probably an inflammatory process involving the pediatric intervertebral disc and adjacent vertebral end plates. Discitis must be differentiated from adult osteomyelitis and disc space infection as well as vertebral osteomyelitis in the pediatric population.[7, 14, 15, 22, 30]

PATHOPHYSIOLOGY

The exact cause of discitis is not known but an infectious etiology is assumed in most cases. Trauma may play an ancillary role in predisposing the vertebral end plates to the infectious or inflammatory process.[5] Various authors reviewed the vascular anatomy of the intervertebral disc and cartilaginous end plates.[5, 30, 34, 38, 39] In the pediatric disc, abundant anastomoses of interosseous arterioles, which are lacking in the adult disc, are identified. In adults these anastomoses are diminished, but the vascular supply of the vertebral end plates shows a prominence of interosseous end arteries. Wiley and Trueta documented a rich arterial blood supply to the vertebral body in both pediatric and adult populations.[39] Coventry and colleagues and Whalen and associates defined the vascular anatomy related to the cartilaginous end plates and immature intervertebral disc.[5, 38] These authors demonstrated cartilage canals that are direct vascular canals crossing the cartilaginous end plates supplying blood and nutrients to the annulus fibrosus and intervertebral disc. The disc remains avascular throughout life. Furthermore, Whalen and associates showed a glomerular configuration of the cartilage canals consisting of an arteriole, tufts of sinusoidal capillaries, and recurrent venules (Fig. 13–1). The cartilage canals begin to disappear in late adolescence, assuming their final adult form (Figs. 13–1, 13–2). The process of inflammatory discitis appears to start centrally in the intervertebral disc region and spreads radically toward the periphery (Fig. 13–2).

Bacteria can be demonstrated in some pa-

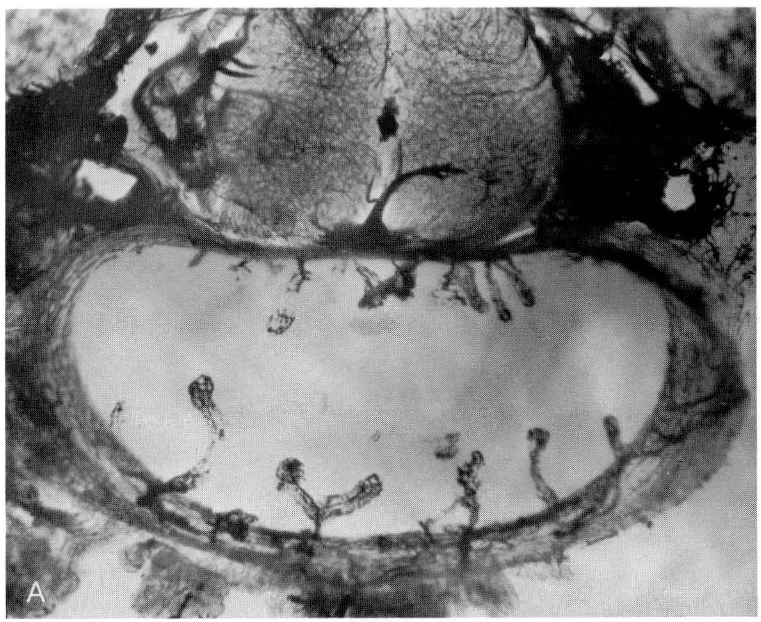

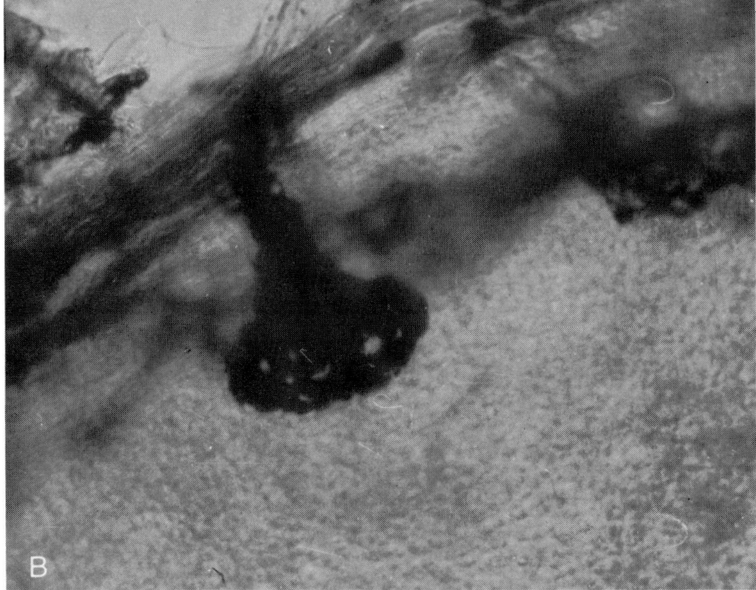

Figure 13–1. Cartilage canals in the intervertebral end plates of a 3-day-old perinatal rabbit. The rabbit was injected with a mixture of latex and India ink and cleared in a solution of tributyl-tricresyl phosphate for transillumination. *A,* The coronal section of the blood supply to the chondroepiphysis and *B,* a magnified view of a singular cartilage canal with its accompanying vessels. (Courtesy of Wesley Parke, Ph.D., Department of Anatomy, University of South Dakota, Vermillion, SD.)

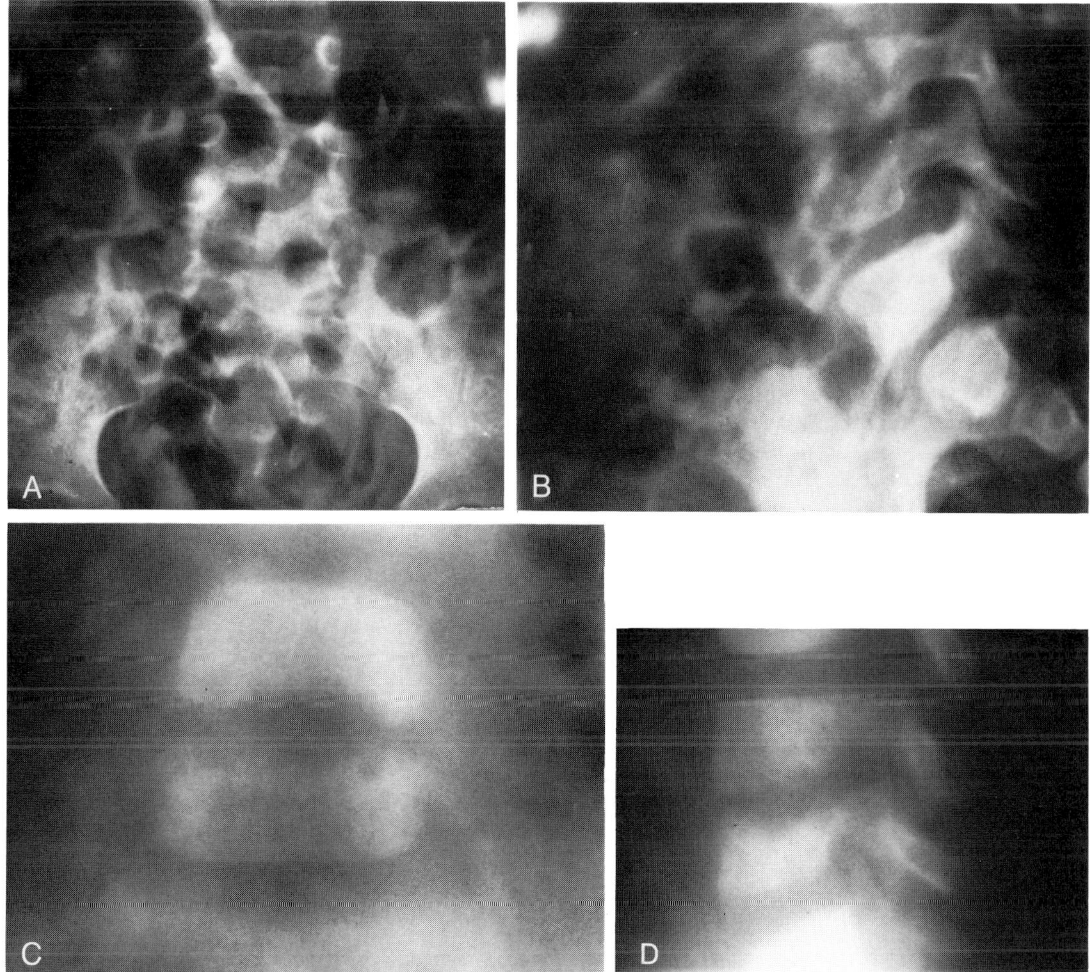

Figure 13–2. A 3-year-old black female presented with a low-grade fever and refused to stand or walk. Anteroposterior *(A)* and lateral *(B)* radiographs show disc space narrowing and vertebral end plate erosions at the L4–L5 level. Anteroposterior *(C)* and lateral *(D)* tomograms further delineate these changes. The erosions are more prominent centrally, equally involving both sides of the L4–L5 intervertebral disc.

tients by either blood culture or biopsy (open or closed). The most common organism cultured continues to be *Staphylococcus aureus*; other organisms are rarely reported. When cultures or biopsies have been performed, approximately 30 to 50 per cent of patients show positive bacteriology at some time during their clinical course.[33, 35, 37]

CLINICAL PRESENTATION

Discitis has a peak incidence at about 6 years of age. There are no sex or race predilections. The lumbar spine is involved much more commonly than the thoracic or cervical regions. Most children are in good health before the onset of the clinical symptoms without a prodromal syndrome or bacterial source being identified. They usually present with a very-low-grade fever (99° to 100°F). Although they demonstrate no systemic symptoms, very young children may be quite irritable. There is a spectrum of clinical features directly dependent on age and duration of symptoms, but not necessarily on the level of spine involved.[19] Common chief complaints are back pain, abdominal pain, hip and thigh pain, nocturnal discomfort, and refusal to stand or walk. In a retrospective review of 41 patients, Wenger and associates found that back pain was most common in children over the age of 9 years.[37]

Difficulty in standing or walking was seen most commonly in children under 3 years of age. Abdominal complaints were more common in the 3- to 9-year-old age group.

Physical findings also depend on age.[36] The most common early findings are localized spinal tenderness, loss of lordosis, and limitation of spinal motion. Abdominal tenderness or loss of hip motion, with or without pain, also commonly occurs. A positive Gowers sign has also been described.[13] Refusal to stand or walk is noted most commonly in very young patients. Puig Guri provided three observations to differentiate the so-called hip joint syndrome from inflammatory changes in the spine.[29] The first shows that there is usually no posterior hip pain on palpation in spinal diseases. On the other hand, tenderness is usually located over the greater trochanter in hip disorders. Patients who suffer from hip joint problems tend to have pain on extension but not on flexion. The differential diagnosis of discitis includes mechanical derangements of the spine, lumbar disc herniations, painful spondylolysis or spondylolisthesis, acute disc space calcification, juvenile rheumatoid arthritis, pelvic or sacroiliac joint infections, neoplasms of the vertebral bodies or spinal canal, vertebral osteomyelitis, urinary tract infections or pyelonephritis, neurologic syndromes including Guillain-Barré syndrome, appendicitis, pancreatitis, and vertebral changes simulating Scheuermann's disease.[2, 4, 9, 16] The chief differential diagnoses of inflammatory changes of the intervertebral disc are developmental anomalies and vertebral osteomyelitis.[27]

The only consistently positive laboratory finding is an elevation in the erythrocyte sedimentation rate (ESR), which is usually two to three times normal. The white blood cell (WBC) count may be increased in recalcitrant or late cases. Cerebrospinal fluid analysis and culture, as well as other laboratory tests, have consistently been normal. Tuberculin skin test results are also normal, but should be performed in all patients in whom discitis is suspected. In patients in whom biopsy has been performed, histologic changes are consistent with inflammatory or infectious processes of the intervertebral disc and surrounding tissues.[33–35, 37]

RADIOLOGY

Radiographic changes remain the sine qua non of the diagnosis of discitis,[31] lagging behind clinical symptoms by two to three weeks.[20] Grunebaum and colleagues divided the radiographic findings into four phases: latent (onset of symptoms), acute (two to four weeks), healing (two to three months), and late (months to years).[10] Most series report radiographic changes by the time the patient presents to the hospital or physician.[35, 37] The sequence of radiographic changes begins with irregularities in the vertebral end plates involving both sides of the disc progressing to variable degrees of disc space narrowing or ankylosis. A variable degree of restoration of intervertebral disc height is observed, depending in part on the patient's age, as the inflammatory process begins to resolve.[31] Some disc space narrowing occurs in all cases, but ankylosis, anterior wedging, mild scoliosis, and vertebra magna are less consistently encountered (Fig. 13–3*A–C*).[2, 33]

Technetium Tc-99m diphosphonate bone scanning remains the procedure of choice and the gold standard for screening of suspicious or early cases of discitis.[1] Bone scans are positive within days of the inflammatory changes and predate all radiographic changes. Although very sensitive, the bone scan is not specific for discitis alone (Fig. 13–3*D*). Gallium 67 citrate scanning is less helpful and takes longer to become positive.[8, 33] Magnetic resonance imaging (MRI) may replace bone scanning as a screening test as the availability and cost of the test approach that of bone scans (Fig. 13–3*E*, *F*). Typical T1- and T2-weighted image changes are noted on MRI. The adjacent vertebral end plates and marrow are darker on the T1-weighted images. These changes enhance and become whiter (brighter) on T2-weighted images. MR scans also have the advantage of ruling out intraspinal tumors and disc disease, which are processes in the differential diagnosis of patients presenting with back pain. Computed tomography (CT) scans are best reserved for recalcitrant cases or patients in whom paraspinal or epidural abscesses are suspected.[32]

MANAGEMENT

The management of discitis begins with early and prompt diagnosis based on a high index of suspicion in young patients presenting with back pain, abdominal pain, or hip and lower extremity symptoms. Blood cultures and tuberculin skin tests are indicated in all patients

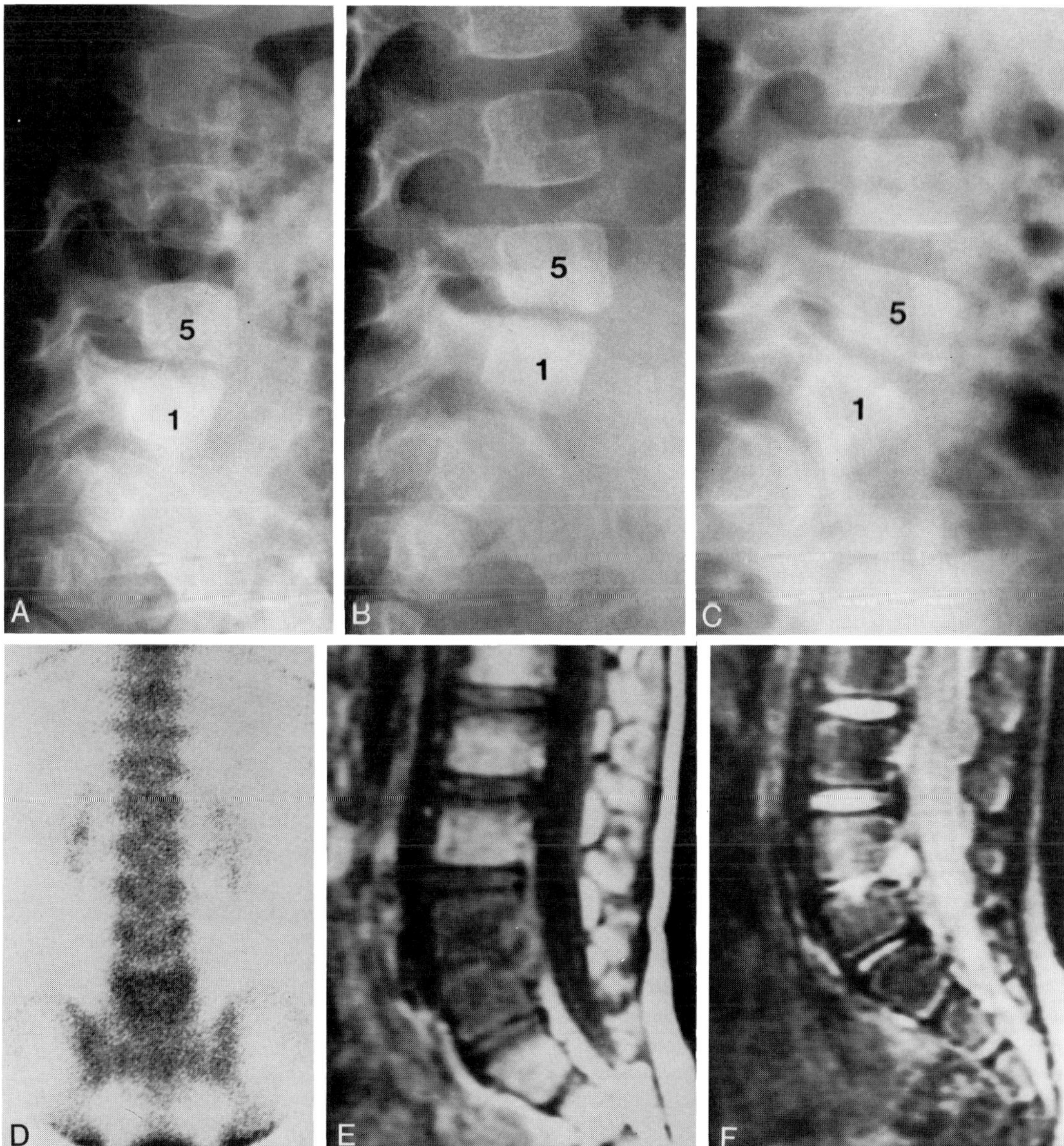

Figure 13–3. A 4-year-old white female is evaluated for vague abdominal complaints and back pain. The erythrocyte sedimentation rate is 42 mm per hour. White blood cell count is normal. Lateral radiographs show disc space narrowing and end plate irregularity at the L5–S1 intervertebral disc level over a 12-month period; on presentation *(A)*, at two months *(B)*, and at 18 months *(C)*. A technetium Tc-99m diphosphonate bone scan at the time of presentation showed diffuse increased uptake at the L5–S1 level *(D)*. *E*, T1- and *F*, T2-weighted magnetic resonance imaging (MRI) shows changes in the vertebral body bone marrow and adjacent vertebral end plates at the L5–S1 level. The signal changes present on T1-weighted images enhance on T2-weighted images. Note the extensive epidural reactive tissue, which is thought to be common in these cases and does not require surgical decompression. (Courtesy of Donald Kirk, M.D., Department of Radiology, Children's Hospital and Medical Center, University of Cincinnati, Cincinnati, OH.)

suspected of having discitis.[33, 35, 37] The blood culture is more likely to be positive early in the clinical course and in older age groups.[37] Monitoring of oral temperatures and ESR is also mandatory. Closed biopsy is indicated if the clinical course suggests a poor response to conservative care, recurrence of symptoms despite adequate care, or continued systemic toxicity and high fever despite treatment.[27] Closed biopsy is also recommended in geographic areas where tuberculosis or fungal infections are common.[37] Open biopsy should be reserved for surgical drainage and debridement. Despite some debate over the management of discitis, spinal rest with or without immobilization is the cornerstone of management. Menelaus observed that rest is the most important factor that alters the natural history and speeds the resolution regardless of the stage of the disease.[23] Braces, casts, or other immobilization techniques are best reserved for older patients or patients not responding to the initial two to three weeks of bed rest. Younger patients usually respond to bed rest alone.[27, 33, 35, 37]

The use of antibiotics is recommended (1) in cases with positive bacteriologic results from blood cultures or biopsy, (2) empirically in patients with poor clinical response to rest or immobilization alone, (3) in patients with elevated WBC counts, (4) in patients with constitutional symptoms and high fever, and (5) in patients with neurologic sequelae (very rare). Some authors advocate the empiric use of antibiotics in all cases, but most reserve these for the above indications.[2, 3, 12, 15, 16, 18, 22–24, 26, 27, 31, 33–35, 37] The duration of antibiotic therapy should be four to six weeks, starting with intravenous administration until clinical symptoms abate, then converting to oral antibiotics to complete the regimen. A methicillin-resistant antibiotic is the best choice if bacteriology and sensitivity results are not available.[37]

PROGNOSIS

In most cases, the prognosis for discitis is for complete resolution of the symptoms in nine to 22 weeks without recurrence in long-term follow-up.[3, 12] Although radiographic changes may persist, no late sequelae have been identified in relation to these. Surgery is rarely required but should be offered in recalcitrant or recurrent cases, if there are symptoms or signs of sepsis despite adequate antibiotic treatment, or to patients in whom paraspinal abscesses are identified.[23]

References

1. Atkinson, R. N., Paterson, D. C., Morris, L. L., and Savage, J. P.: Bone scintigraphy in discitis and related disorders in children. Aust. N.Z. J. Surg. *48*:374–377, 1978.
2. Boston, J., Jr., Bianco, A., Jr., and Rhodes, K. H.: Disc space infections in children. Orthop. Clin. North Am. *6*:953–964, 1975.
3. Bremner, A. E., and Neligan, G. A.: Benign form of acute osteitis of the spine in young children. Br. Med. J. *1*:856–860, 1953.
4. Bunnell, W. P.: Back pain in children. Orthop. Clin. North Am. *13*:587–604, 1982.
5. Coventry, M. B., Ghormley, R. K., and Kernohany, J. W.: Intervertebral disc: its microscopic anatomy and pathology. J. Bone Joint Surg. *27*:105–115, 1945.
6. Doyle, J. R.: Narrowing of the intervertebral-disc space in children. J. Bone Joint Surg. *42A*:1191–1200, 1960.
7. Edelman, R. R., Shoukimas, G. N., Stark, D. D., et al.: High-resolution surface-coil imaging of lumbar disk disease. A.J.R. *144*:1123–1129, 1985.
8. Eismont, F. J., Bohlman, H. H., Soni, P. L., et al.: Vertebral osteomyelitis in infants. J. Bone Joint Surg. *64B*:32–35, 1982.
9. Fischer, G. W., Popich, G. A., Sullivan, D. E., et al.: Diskitis: a prospective diagnostic analysis. Pediatrics *62*:543–548, 1978.
10. Greene, T. L., Hensinger, R. N., and Hunter, L. Y.: Back pain and vertebral changes simulating Scheuermann's disease. J Pediatr. Orthop. *5*:1–7, 1985.
11. Grunebaum, M., Horodniceanu, C., Mukamel, M., et al.: The imaging diagnosis of nonpyogenic discitis in children. Pediatr. Radiol. *12*:133–137, 1982.
12. Jamison, R. C., Heimlich, E. M., Miethke, J. C., and O'Laughlin, B. J.: Nonspecific spondylitis of infants and children. Radiology *77*:355–367, 1961.
13. Kelfer, H., and Haller, J. S.: Gowers' sign in diskitis. Am J. Dis. Child. *136*:555, 1982.
14. Kemp, H. B. S., Jackson, J. W., Jeremiah, J. D., and Hall, A. J.: Pyogenic infections occurring primarily in intervertebral discs. J. Bone Joint Surg. *55A*: 698–714, 1973.
15. Kulowki, J.: Pyogenic osteomyelitis of the spine. J. Bone Joint Surg. *18*:343–364, 1936.
16. La Rocca, H: Intervertebral disc space inflammation in children. In Rothman, R. H. and Simeone, F. A. (eds): The Spine. 2nd ed. 1982, pp. 766–767.
17. Lascari, A. D., Graham, M. H., and MacQueen, J. C.: Intervertebral disc infection in children. J. Pediatr. *70*:751–757, 1967.
18. Littleton, H. R., and Rhoades, H. R.: Septic discitis: report of a case and review of the literature. J. Am. Osteopath. Assoc. *79*:544–546, 1980.
19. Leahy, A. L., Fogarty, E. E., Fitzgerald, R. J., and Regan, B. F.: Discitis as a cause of abdominal pain in children. Surgery *95*:413–414, 1984.

20. Matthews, S. S., Wiltse, L. L., and Karbeling, M. J.: A destructive lesion involving the intervertebral disk in children. Clin. Orthop. *9*:162–168, 1957.
21. Mayer, L.: An unusual case of infection of the spine. J. Bone Joint Surg. *7*:957–968, 1925.
22. McCain, G. A., Harth, M. H., Bell, D. A., et al.: Septic discitis. J. Rheumatol. *8*:100–109, 1981.
23. Menelaus, M. B.: Discitis, an inflammation affecting the intervertebral discs in children. J. Bone Joint Surg. *46B*:16–23, 1964.
24. Milone, F. P., Bianco, A. J., Jr., and Divins, J. C.: Infections of the intervertebral disc in children. J.A.M.A. *181*:1029–1033, 1962.
25. Moes, C. A. F.: Spondylarthritis in childhood. Am. J. Roentgenol. *91*:578–587, 1964.
26. O'Brien, T. M., and McManus, F.: Discitis—the irritable back of childhood. Ir. J. Med. Sci. *152*:404–408, 1983.
27. Peterson, H.: Disc-space infection in children. Instructional Course Lectures *32*:50–60, 1983.
28. Pritchard, A. E., and Thompson, A. L.: Acute pyogenic infections of the spine in children. J. Bone Joint Surg. *42B*:86–89, 1960.
29. Puig Guri, J.: Pyogenic osteomyelitis of the spine: differential diagnosis through clinical and radiographic observations. J. Bone Joint Surg. *28*:29–35, 1946.
30. Ratcliffe, J. F.: Anatomic basis for the pathogenesis and radiologic features of vertebral osteomyelitis and its differentiation from childhood discitis: a microanteriographic investigation. Acta Radiolog. [Diagn.] (Stockh.) *26*:137–143, 1985.
31. Saenger, E. L.: Spondylarthritis in children. Am. J. Roentgenol. *64*:20–31, 1950.
32. Sartoris, D. J., Moskowitz, P. S., Kaufman, R. A., et al.: Childhood discitis: computed tomographic findings. Radiology *149*:701–707, 1983.
33. Scoles, P. V., and Quinn, T. P.: Intervertebral discitis in children, and adolescents. Clin. Orthop. *162*:31–36, 1982.
34. Smith, R. F., and Taylor, T. K. F.: Inflammatory lesions of intervertebral discs in children. J. Bone Joint Surg. *49A*:1508–1520, 1967.
35. Spiegel, P. G., Kengla, K. W., Isaacson, A. S., and Wilson, J. C.: Intervertebral disc-space inflammation in children. J. Bone Joint Surg. *54A*:284–296, 1972.
36. Sullivan, C. R., and Symmonds, R. E.: Disk infections and abdominal pain. J.A.M.A. *188*:655–658, 1964.
37. Wenger, D., Bobechko, W., and Gilday, D.: The spectrum of intervertebral disc-space infection in children. J. Bone Joint Surg. *60A*:100–108, 1978.
38. Whalen, J., Parke, W. W., Mazur, J. M., and Stauffer, E. S.: The intrinsic vasculature of developing vertebral end plates and its nutritive significance to the intervertebral discs. J. Orthop. *5*:403–410, 1985.
39. Wiley, A. M., and Trueta, J.: The vascular anatomy of the spine and its relationship to pyogenic vertebral osteomyelitis. J. Bone Joint Surg. *41B*:796–809, 1959.

CHAPTER

14

JUVENILE AND ADOLESCENT SCOLIOSIS

Robert B. Winter, M.D.
John E. Lonstein, M.D.

CONGENITAL SCOLIOSIS

Definitions

Congenital scoliosis is scoliosis caused by specific congenitally anomalous vertebrae, which must be identified on x-ray films or magnetic resonance imaging (MRI) or at the time of surgery. Scoliosis in an infant who does not have these congenital anomalies should not be called "congenital scoliosis." Care should be taken to call lateral curvatures of the spine "scoliosis," whereas posterior curvatures are kyphosis and anterior curvatures are lordosis. Many congenital scolioses contain a component of kyphosis or lordosis, and should be labeled kyphoscoliosis or lordoscoliosis when these definitions fit. A rib hump due to rotation is not a kyphosis, and the term kyphoscoliosis should be reserved specifically for patients having an abnormal posterior curvature of the spine in addition to scoliosis.

Classification and Natural History

Congenital scoliosis is classified according to the types of anomalies. This is the most useful and functional classification. The main subdivisions relate to defects of formation and defects of segmentation. Defects of formation are failures of the hemimetameric developmental process to form all or part of vertebral segments. The extreme cases are of total absence of vertebrae such as in sacral agenesis and caudal regression syndromes. At the other end of the spectrum are wedged vertebrae, when there is a deficient but not totally absent half of one vertebra. The most classic form of formation defect is the hemivertebra, in which the one hemimetamere has failed to form and the other is present. It should always be remembered that the pathology consists of the absence on one side, not the presence of the hemimetamere on the opposite side.

The second major subclassification is defects of segmentation: failures of the normal segmentation process. If unilateral, these result in a unilateral unsegmented bar; if just posterior, in posterior laminar synostosis with lordosis; if anterior, in an anterior unsegmented bar with kyphosis. If there is a total defect of segmentation, front, back, right, and left, this is called a "bloc" vertebra and there is no deformity other than the lack of vertical growth in that area (Fig. 14–1).

The natural history of the spine deformity depends to a great extent on the anomalies

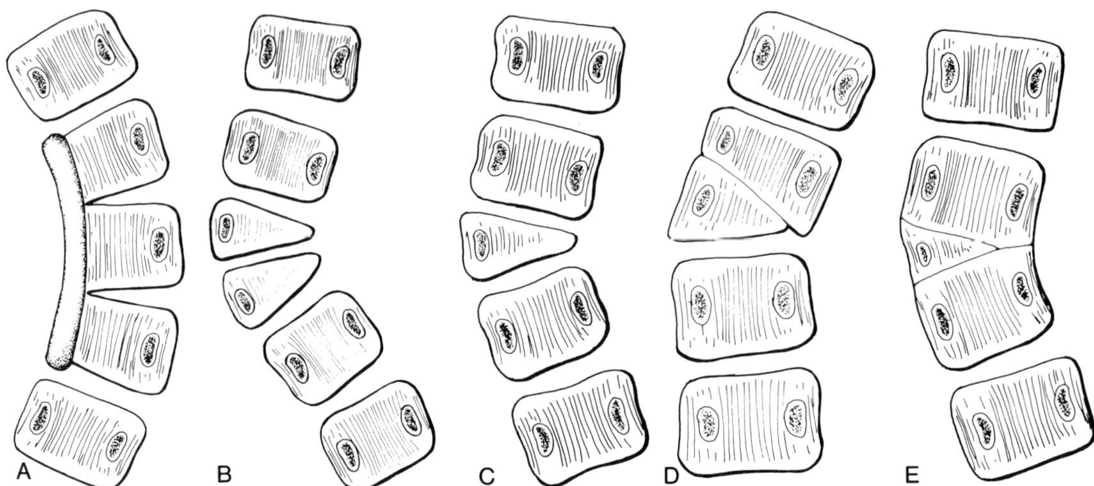

Figure 14–1. *A*, The classic unilateral unsegmented bar. The concave side cannot grow, but the convex side has very healthy growth. Thus, the prognosis for severe progression is very high. *B*, Double convex "free" hemivertebrae demonstrating marked hypoplasia of growth tissue in the concavity and virtually normal growth on the convexity. The prognosis is very poor. *C*, A single "free" (full-segmented) hemivertebra. The prognosis is poor but not as poor as that of either *A* or *B*. *D*, A semisegmented hemivertebra. The prognosis is guarded because there may or may not be growth discrepancy. *E*, A nonsegmented hemivertebra. There is no growth discrepancy and, therefore, little change of curve progression.

present. This is the single most important factor in whether or not a curve is going to be progressive. Certain defects are known to be always progressive, the most classic of these being an unsegmented bar in which there is a failure of segmentation on the one side of the spine, but on the opposite side healthy development of tissue with good discs, good pedicles, and good vertebral formation. This situation is so universally progressive, and usually severely so, that its recognition demands immediate treatment. To allow progressive deformity to occur in the face of a unilateral unsegmented bar is to allow an unnecessary deformity. At the other end of the spectrum are the total bloc vertebrae that do not produce any curvature of the spine but only shortening; these, of course, do not need any immediate treatment. In between are many variations of the natural history from extremely progressive to minimally progressive or nonprogressive. Often these are extremely difficult to predict. Rather than memorizing a list of progressive versus nonprogressive problems, it is always better to look at high-quality radiographs and then decide on which side the growth factors are balanced. If there is an obvious discrepancy of growth factors, progressive curvature is highly likely, whereas if the growth factors are balanced, progressive curvature is relatively unlikely. Almost nothing can be taken for certain, and it is only by very careful periodic follow-up that the true natural history of a given patient can be delineated. There are several articles on the natural history of congenital scoliosis, but the reader is referred to the classic article by McMaster and Ohtsuka.[6]

Hemivertebrae cause a considerable problem in estimation of their prognosis. Some can produce extremely severe curves, whereas others produce no progression at all. Over many years of experience, it has become obvious that the "free" hemivertebra (a hemivertebra with healthy discs above and below and with a healthy pedicle) is at the greatest risk for progression.[8] A hemivertebra that is fused to one or more of its adjacent vertebrae has much less likelihood of progression. A hemivertebra fused to both its adjacent vertebrae has no chance of progression.

A few words about the monitoring of patients are in order. Particularly in young children, standing or sitting x-rays are very unreliable owing to the movements of the child and poor postural mechanisms. Furthermore, bone detail is not as good as in a supine film. Therefore, in young children (up to about age 4), we routinely take supine x-rays. This allows a better comparison between repeat views, better views of the details of bone development, and better measurements, while making possible better judgments about the natural history potential.

Measurement of congenital scoliosis is often difficult because of the distortion of the traditional anatomic landmarks. It is best to select a pair of pedicles at the top and the bottom of the curve, to use the two points on the upper contour of the pedicle superiorly and the lower contour of the pedicle inferiorly, and to create the lines from these four points. When reviewing subsequent x-rays, these same pairs of pedicles should be used, and extremely careful measurements made. If the child is progressing at the rate of 5 degrees per year and is being seen twice a year, one is expected to appreciate a progression of only 2.5 degrees per visit, which is almost impossible owing to measurement variations. It is therefore important to review all the x-ray films taken from the first visit until the current one, in order to determine whether progression is taking place or not.

Caution is necessary with a scoliosis patient whose measurements are not changing but who is developing increasing lordosis or kyphosis. This necessitates periodic taking of lateral views as well as posteroanterior views (Figs. 14–2 to 14–4).

Genetics, Associated Disorders, and Other Anomalies

Patients with congenital scoliosis are very different from those with idiopathic scoliosis because of the different genetics and different pattern of associated problems. In idiopathic scoliosis there is a very strong genetic tendency, whereas in congenital scoliosis there is a very low hereditary tendency. There has been very little work on the inheritance of congenital scoliosis, but the classic article by Wynne Davies should be reviewed.[16] She

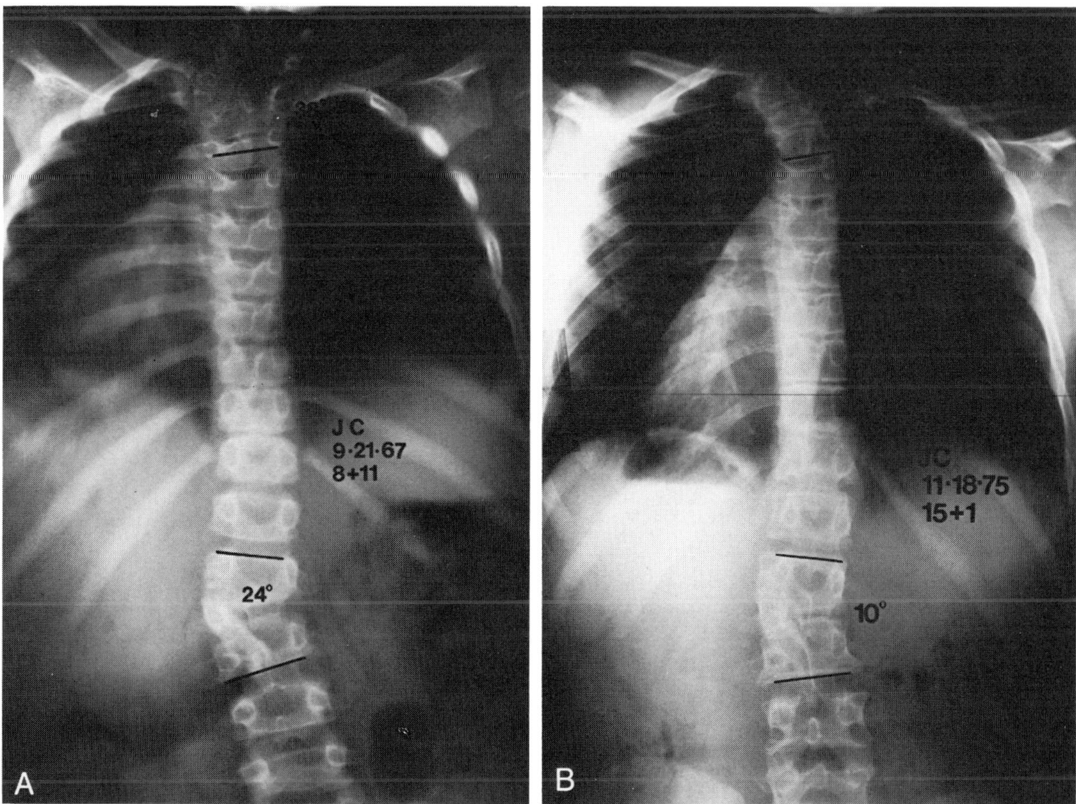

Figure 14–2. *A*, A midlumbar semisegmented hemivertebra with a 24-degree curve at age 8 years, 11 months. *B*, The same patient at age 15 years. No treatment had been given. The curve spontaneously improved to 10 degrees. It is now apparent that the convex side was nonsegmented, but the concave side had growth potential.

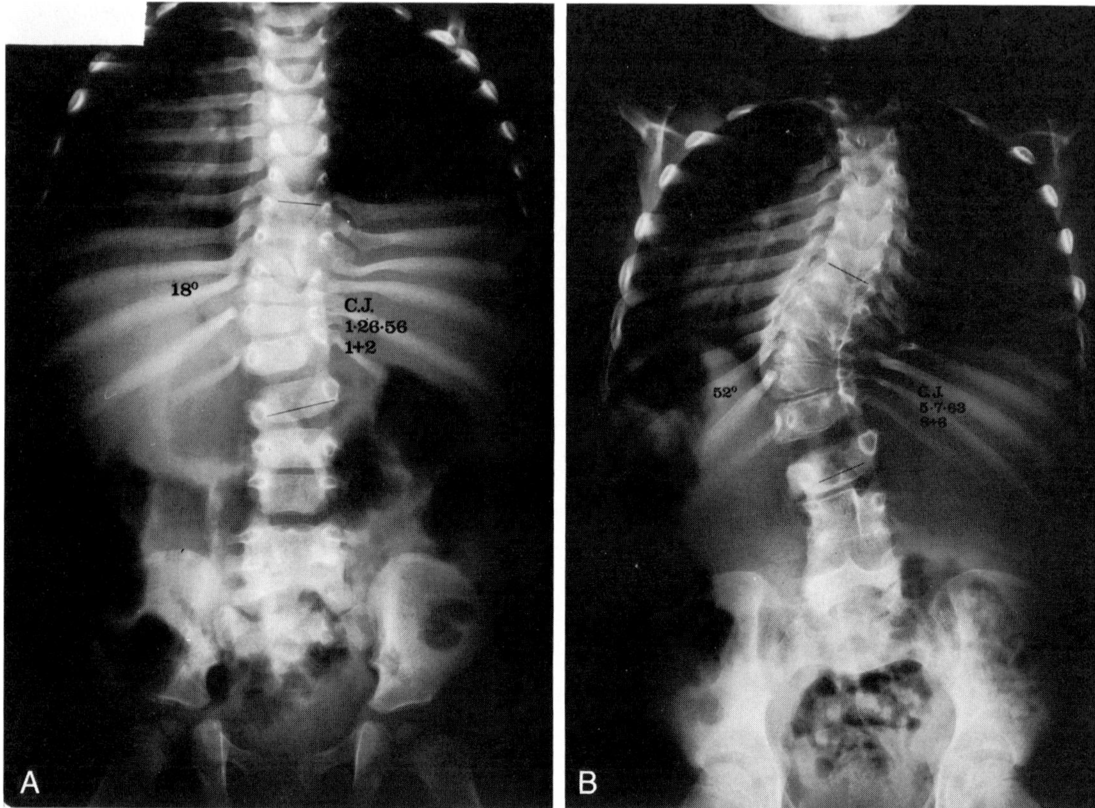

Figure 14–3. *A*, This 1-year-old boy had 18-degree scoliosis and multiple areas of segmentation defects but no hemivertebrae. Although there is a unilateral bar at T9–T12 on the right, the growth potential on the left is not normal. *B*, By age 8 years, the curve was 52 degrees. This is an increase of 44 degrees over a 7-year period or a change of 6 degrees per year or 3 degrees every six months. (See Fig. 14–12 for a case of much more rapid progression due to a bar.)

noted close correlation between congenital scoliosis and neural tube defects, particularly in the child with multiple anomalies rather than a single anomaly. At our center we have not found that relationship to be so strong. Of 1250 patients with congenital spine deformity reviewed in 1981, only 12 had a positive family history of congenital scoliosis, an incidence of only 1 per cent. Only seven of these patients had relatives with neural tube defects.

Many other anomalies can occur in the patient with congenital scoliosis. Highest on the list are anomalies of the genitourinary tract. In several series in which routine intravenous pyelograms were obtained in all patients with congenital scoliosis, an incidence of about 25 per cent of these anomalies was found. Many of these were single kidneys, duplicated ureters, crossed renal ectopia, and so forth, conditions of interest but not of potential danger to the child. However, in about 5 per cent of the patients there was obstructive uropathy, ureterovesicular obstruction being the most common of these. In many children, kidney function was salvaged by early recognition of these potentially lethal problems. Today intravenous pyelograms are not always used, since renal ultrasonography and MR scans can provide almost equivalent information with less difficulty and risk.

Many other anomalies can occur in addition to the renal problems. Congenital heart defects are common, as are Sprengel's deformity, Klippel-Feil deformity, Goldenhar syndrome, full or hemisacral agenesis, anal atresia, and others. There is very little correlation between the area of the spine involved by the congenital anomalies and the other anomalies involved. For example, Klippel-Feil syndrome in which there are segmentation defects in the cervical spine has the highest incidence of renal abnormalities.

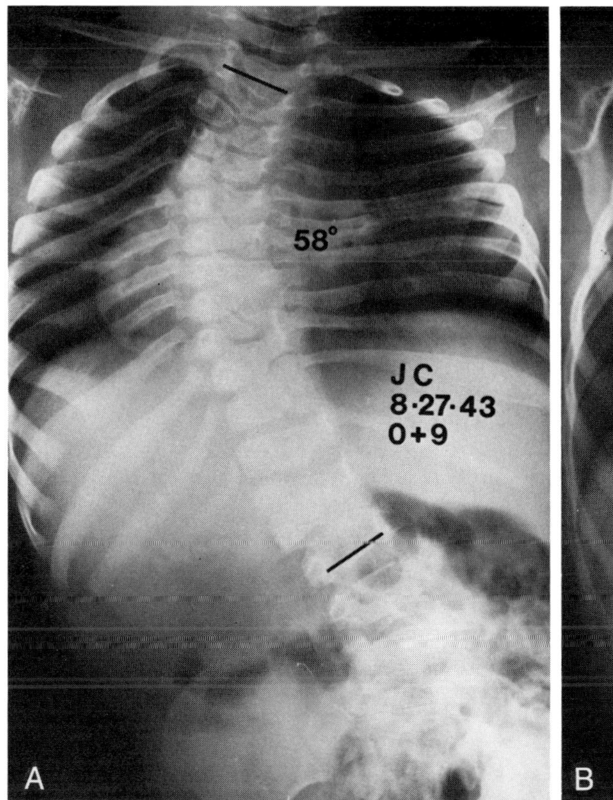

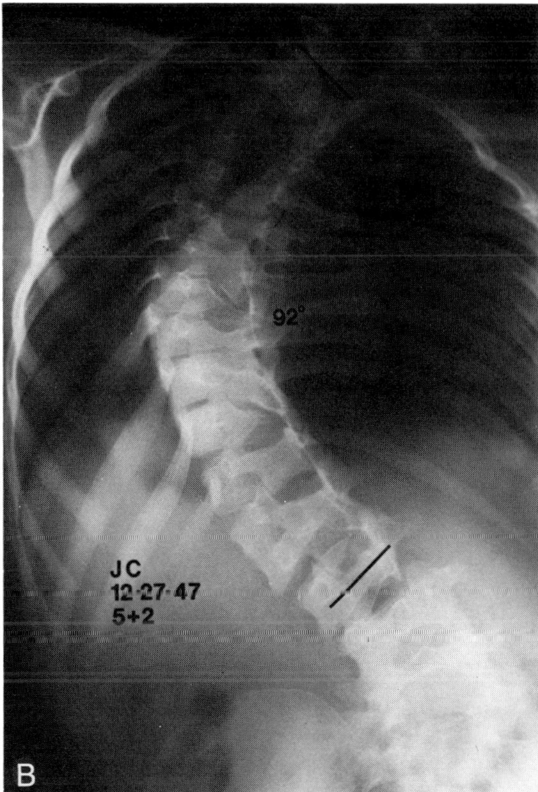

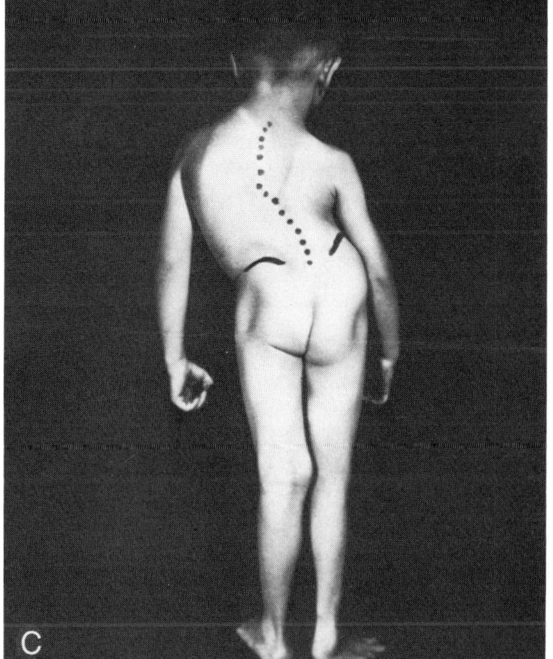

Figure 14–4. *A*, This 9-month-old boy already had a 58-degree, long scoliosis at T1–L2. There are 13 left ribs and 11 right ribs. *B*, By age 5 years, the curve had increased to 92 degrees. Congenital scoliosis often increases severely during the first few years of life. *C*, The clinical appearance at age 5 years.

Finally, one must remember the very close association between the spinal cord and the vertebrae. Very many patients have abnormalities of the spinal cord in association with anomalies of the vertebrae. Diastematomyelia and filum terminale are the two most common of these. Formerly, myelography was required to detect these problems, but MRI has made most of the myelograms unnecessary. In very severe deformities, MRI is less than optimal, since the slicing technique can miss the obvious pathology, whereas the myelogram can show the lesion clearly. Often more than one anomaly is present. For example, we noted eight examples of both diastematomyelia and tight filum terminale in the same patient. Syringomyelia can occur in association with these congenital cord anomalies, and is best seen on MRI (Figs. 14–5 and 14–6).

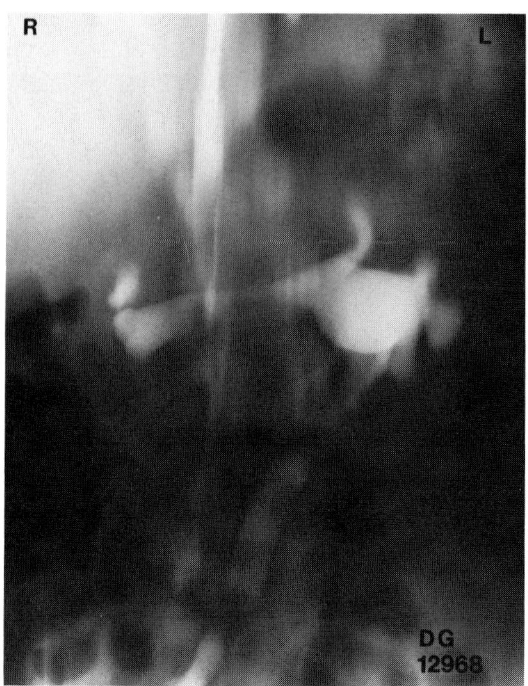

Figure 14–5. A tomogram of an intravenous pyelogram shows a horseshoe kidney, a single ureter, hydroureter, and hydronephrosis due to ureteral-vesical stenosis. These findings were detected on a routine study because of congenital scoliosis.

Nonoperative Treatment

Unlike idiopathic scoliosis, for which bracing can be very effective, very few cases of congenital scoliosis lend themselves well to brace treatment. Congenital kyphosis and congenital lordosis are totally refractory to brace treatment. The only congenital scolioses that do well in braces are long curves that have good flexibility. These are curves where there is usually an area of mild anomalies, then a couple of healthy, mobile discs, then another anomaly, then another two or three mobile discs, and then another anomaly. The other area where bracing is effective is in the secondary curves above or below a primary congenital curve.

The brace of choice is the Milwaukee brace, since it avoids constriction of the thorax. Children below the age of adolescence have very soft ribs, and the traditional underarm braces that may be effective for idiopathic scoliosis are very damaging to the chest cage of these young children. A significant shoulder elevation is best treated with a shoulder ring attached to the Milwaukee brace, and head support pads can be added if there is a head tilt, to create a neutral head position. Only the Milwaukee brace and its modifications can do this.

The best guide, therefore, to whether or not a brace will be effective is the flexibility of the curve as determined by bending or traction x-rays. Usually the brace is worn to delay a fusion until a more suitable time, rather than to avoid surgery entirely.[9]

No other known form of nonoperative treatment has any effect on congenital spine deformity. Exercises, manipulation, calisthenics, and electrical stimulators have all been total failures.

Operative Treatment

There are many different forms of operative treatment for congenital scoliosis, and all have their place. Because of this, there can be confusion on the part of the treating surgeon over which is best for a given patient at a given time. The complete and versatile surgeon will be fully capable in all the different methods and will therefore try to select the best one for the individual patient. The challenge is to know which is the best.

Posterior Spine Fusion Without Instrumentation

This is the basic "gold standard" of congenital scoliosis surgery. It should be thought of first, and if it is the best procedure, it should

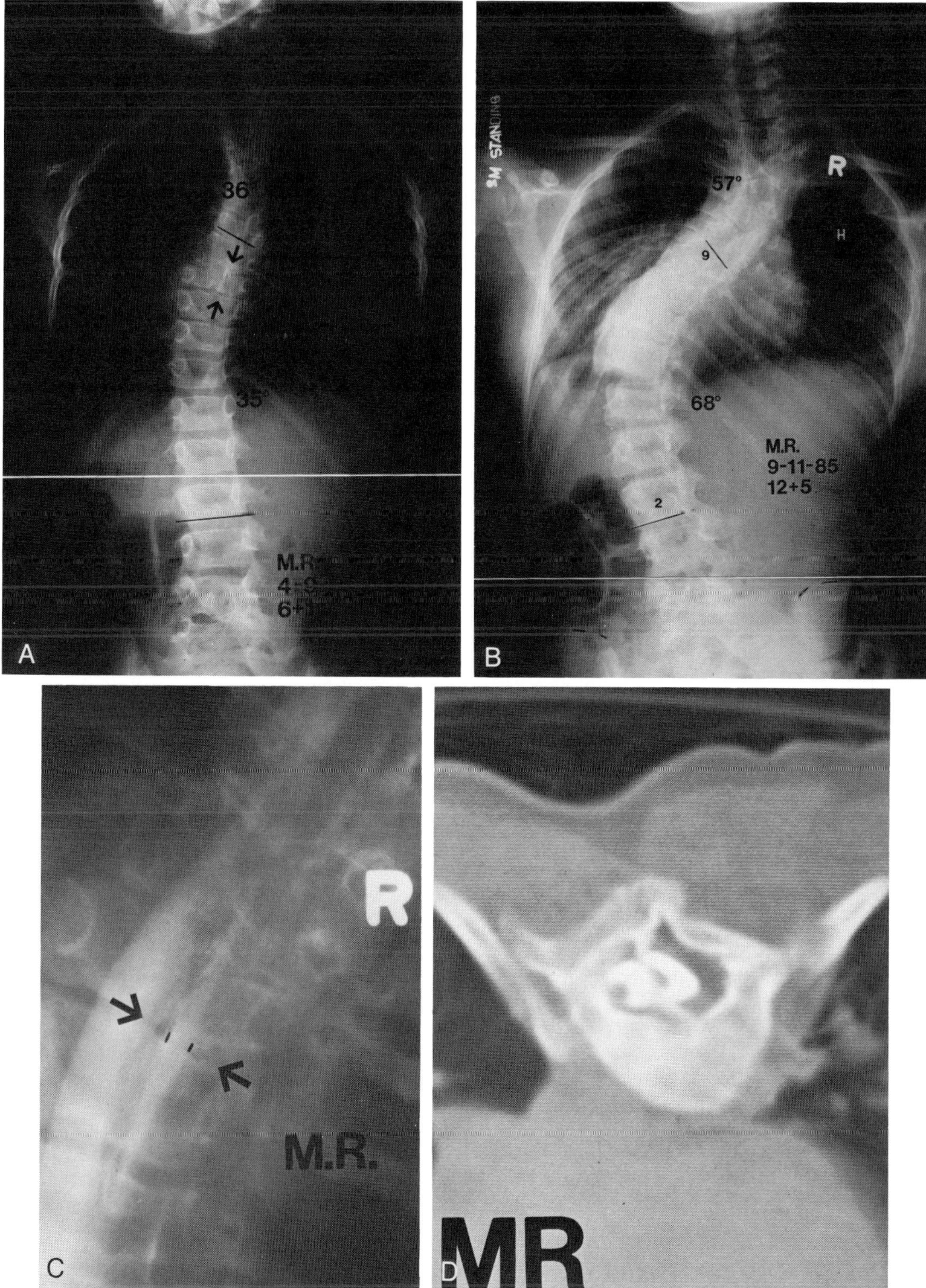

Figure 14–6. *A*, This girl was observed at another institution at age 6 years. She had 36- and 35-degree curves. A midline spur at T8–T9 is indicated by the arrows. No treatment was given. *B*, Six years later, the upper curve was 57 degrees and the lower, 68 degrees. Because of vertebral rotation, the spur is no longer visible. *C*, A water-soluble myelogram shows well the split cord. *D*, A computed tomographic scan of the myelogram shows well the two hemicords and a narrow bony septum. This was removed before corrective surgery for the scoliosis.

be performed. All others should be weighed against it. The technique is simple. The spine posteriorly is exposed with a very wide exposure to the tips of the transverse processes. The ribs should not be exposed. The facet joints are then removed thoroughly, the laminae and transverse processes are vigorously decorticated, an abundant bone graft is applied, and the wound is closed. Correction of the deformity is achieved externally by casting or bracing. This should not be thought of as a "fusion in situ" but rather as correction and fusion, since in almost every patient some correction can be achieved. A good posterior spine fusion creates a wide thick fusion mass that will be resistant to bending and torsion over the years. It is difficult to obtain a large thick fusion mass in a young child because there is very little local bone and a very meager supply of autogenous donor bone. In such circumstances one should use bank bone of some type and place the maximal amount of bone graft in the wound that still enables the fascia to be closed. If the fascia is easily closed, not enough bone has been added.

The patient should be immobilized completely by the appropriate cast or brace until the fusion is absolutely solid. Although a soft fusion may occur in four to six months, a strongly trabeculated fusion will not occur for about one year, particularly if bank bone has been used, since it takes longer to incorporate into the body.

The common mistakes made in this operation are failure (1) to select the proper area for the fusion, (2) to create a large and thick enough fusion mass, (3) to apply the most appropriate type of corrective cast or brace (especially the use of underarm casts when a full Risser cast including the neck should be used), and (4) to realize that there is a pseudarthrosis, thus allowing deterioration to take effect.

Posterior spine fusion is the best technique for the cervical spine, where other techniques are very difficult or impossible. In the major cervical curves, the halo cast is the best for obtaining correction and immobilization (Fig. 14–7).

Posterior Spine Fusion With Instrumentation

In this, the same basic procedure described above is supplemented by the use of some type of instrumentation. Originally this consisted of Harrington rods and for many years there was no other supplemental device. Finally came the Luque and more recently the Cotrel-Dubousset instrumentation. The chief advantage of the instrumentation was that a slightly better correction was achieved than by casting or bracing alone, and that the internal fixation of the bones secured a better union, along with the advantage of having a less restrictive cast or brace after the surgery. At no time did the presence of the instrumentation detract from the need for a very thorough fusion technique and abundant bone grafting.

The main negative aspect of the instrumentation was the higher paraplegia rate associated with their use. In several reviews by the Scoliosis Research Society of the mortality and morbidity rates of scoliosis, congenital spine deformity always was perceived as the most likely to cause trouble with the use of rods. This is presumably due to the more frequent tethering of the spinal cord, the anomalies of the neural arches, and the presence of areas of stenosis. Certainly, instruments should never be used unless first it has been proved by MRI or myelography that there is no diastematomyelia or tethered cord, and second that a wake-up test is used during surgery to monitor the leg function immediately after the rods are inserted. The author (RW) recently operated on a girl about 8 years of age and decided to use a small distraction rod, using the 3/16-inch threaded Harrington rod with two small pediatric hooks. There had been a negative myelogram preoperatively. The spine was very gently distracted. A wake-up test was performed and the patient was unable to move her feet despite accurate hand commands. The rod was immediately relaxed so that there was no distractive tension on it, and she still could not move her feet. The author therefore immediately cut the rod and removed the lower hook, but she still could not move her feet. Finally, the upper hook located at T6 was maneuvered out, and she immediately was able to move her feet. Thus, the presence of the hook in the spinal canal at the T6 level was the cause of the paralysis, and not a distraction effect.

The author does not consider that electronic spinal cord monitors are accurate enough of themselves, and therefore a wake-up test is always performed. In this particular case we went ahead with the fusion and used an old-

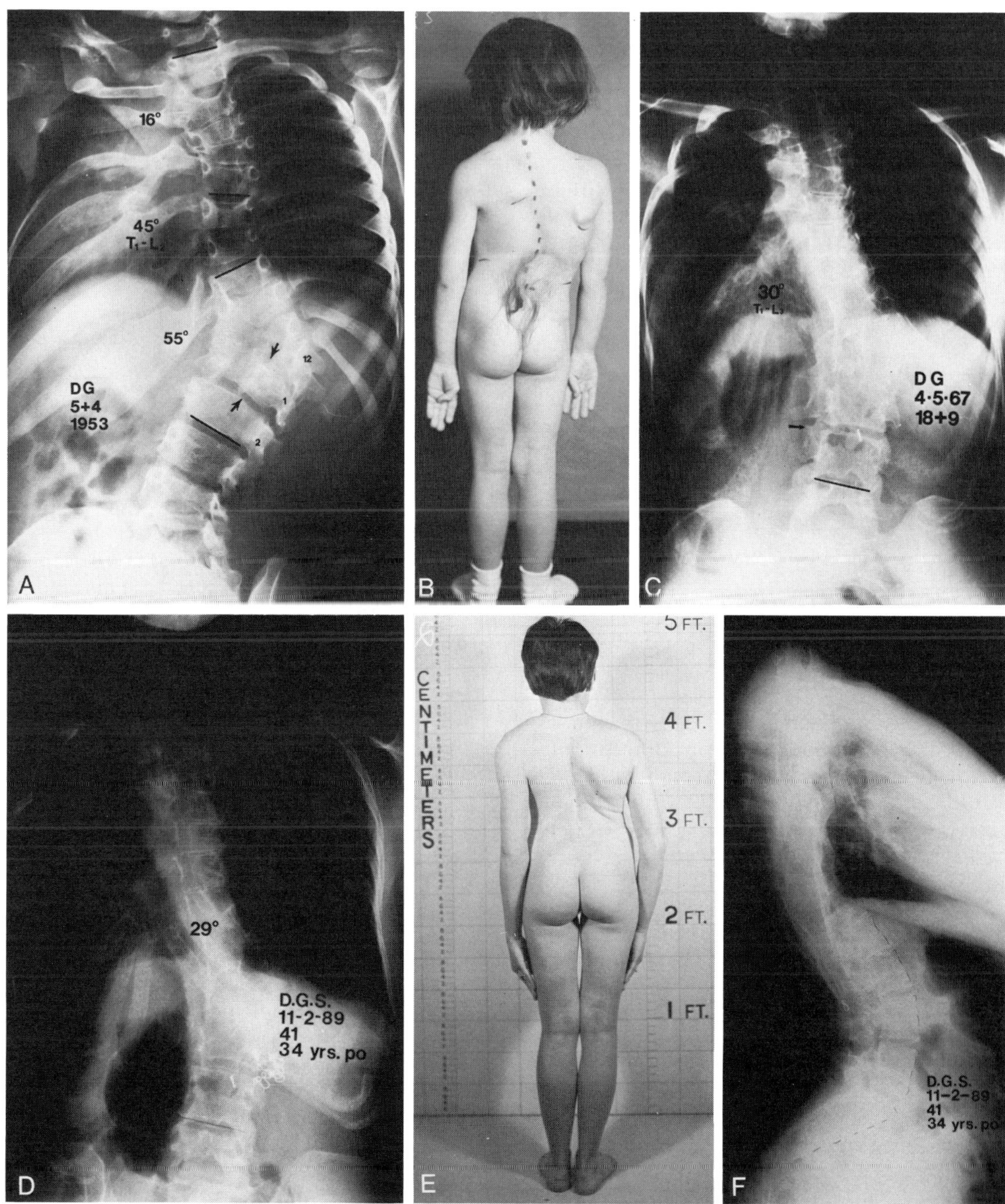

Figure 14–7. *A*, This girl was first seen at Gillette Children's Hospital, St. Paul, in 1953 at age 5 years. She had a very complex scoliosis plus a midline spur (*arrows*) but was neurologically normal. *B*, Clinical photography shows the classic hair patch of a dysraphic spine. *C*, She underwent cast correction and posterior fusion at age 6 years while in the care of Dr. John H. Moe. The patient is seen here at age 18 years with a 30-degree curve. *D*, Despite the long fusion (T2–L3) at age 6 years, the clinical appearance is excellent. *E*, At age 41 years, 34 years after surgery, correction has been maintained. She has no low back or neck pain. *F*, At age 41 years, the view is normal. Early fusion did not create lordosis.

fashioned Risser cast for correction and maintenance. The end result was quite good.

Many errors have been made through the use of rods, the most common being the attempt to use rods in small children with soft bone when, in fact, an equivalent or even a better result could have been obtained with a cast or brace. Because of the very common use of instrumentation in spine surgery these days, there is a tendency to think that all corrective surgery must be done with some type of metallic device. This is not the case, and congenital scoliosis is the most glaring example of this (Fig. 14–8).

Combined Anterior and Posterior Spine Fusion

One of the negative aspects of posterior spine fusion alone, whether done with or without rods, is the fact that the growth plates anteriorly, the powerful growth forces that cause the deformity, are not surgically touched. This can sometimes result in late bending and torsional deformity (the "crankshaft" phenomenon). This can be prevented by eliminating the growth plates anteriorly by combined anterior and posterior surgery.

This is usually done under the same anesthetic. It is preferable to do the front first, by removing an appropriate rib to expose the area of the curvature, by ligation of the segmental vessels in that area, by subperiosteal stripping of the spine, and then by removal of the disc and growth plates via curettement. The rib removed for the thoracotomy is placed in a trough rongeured out of the vertebral bodies, and the periosteum is resutured. This has benefits in addition to the removal of the growth plates, since it gives a greater assurance of solid fusion without pseudarthrosis; because the discs are removed, there can be greater mobility in the curvature, allowing a better correction. A chest tube is inserted, the chest is closed, the patient is turned prone, and the standard posterior spine fusion is performed with or without instrumentation, depending on the circumstances. If a cast is to be used, it can often be put on during the same anesthetic procedure even though there is a chest tube in place.

Combined anterior and posterior fusion is used much more now than in the past. Familiarity and comfort with anterior spine surgery has made this possible. In most children there is very little morbidity from the anterior approach, and only in those with extremely severe deformities and markedly reduced pulmonary function is there much danger.

The one circumstance in which anterior fusions are contraindicated is in the very young child with a kyphotic deformity, when we want the anterior growth plates to continue to function in the face of a solidly fused spine posteriorly, and therefore progressive correction of kyphosis can take place by this posterior growth arrest (Fig. 14–9).

Convex Growth Arrest Procedures

Although these procedures (convex epiphysiodesis) have been available for a very long time, they have only recently achieved popularity. This is largely due to the ability to perform routine anterior surgery without significant morbidity to the child. The concept is exciting in that we want to arrest the pathologic growth of the convexity, and allow whatever growth is possible on the concavity to continue to take place. If significant growth is available, the curve can spontaneously correct itself over time.

The technique is much the same as for combined anterior and posterior fusion, differing only in that only the convex half of the spine is fused both front and back. Care must be taken to fuse the entire curve plus one healthy segment above and below the pathologic area. Postoperatively, maximal correction should be obtained with a cast or brace and the spine held until the fusion is solid, which takes at least six to eight months. After that, no further treatment is necessary and the patient must be carefully observed. Because the fusion mass is narrower, pseudarthrosis may occur and refusion is a possibility. Instrumentation customarily is not used, although a subcutaneous rod can be used posteriorly and then removed a year later. This is done only when the rod would provide a significant amount of correction compared with the casting technique.

The results of this procedure have been reported from England by Andrew and Piggott[1] and from the United States by Winter and colleagues.[14] Not all cases have had a good result, since it is very difficult to predict in

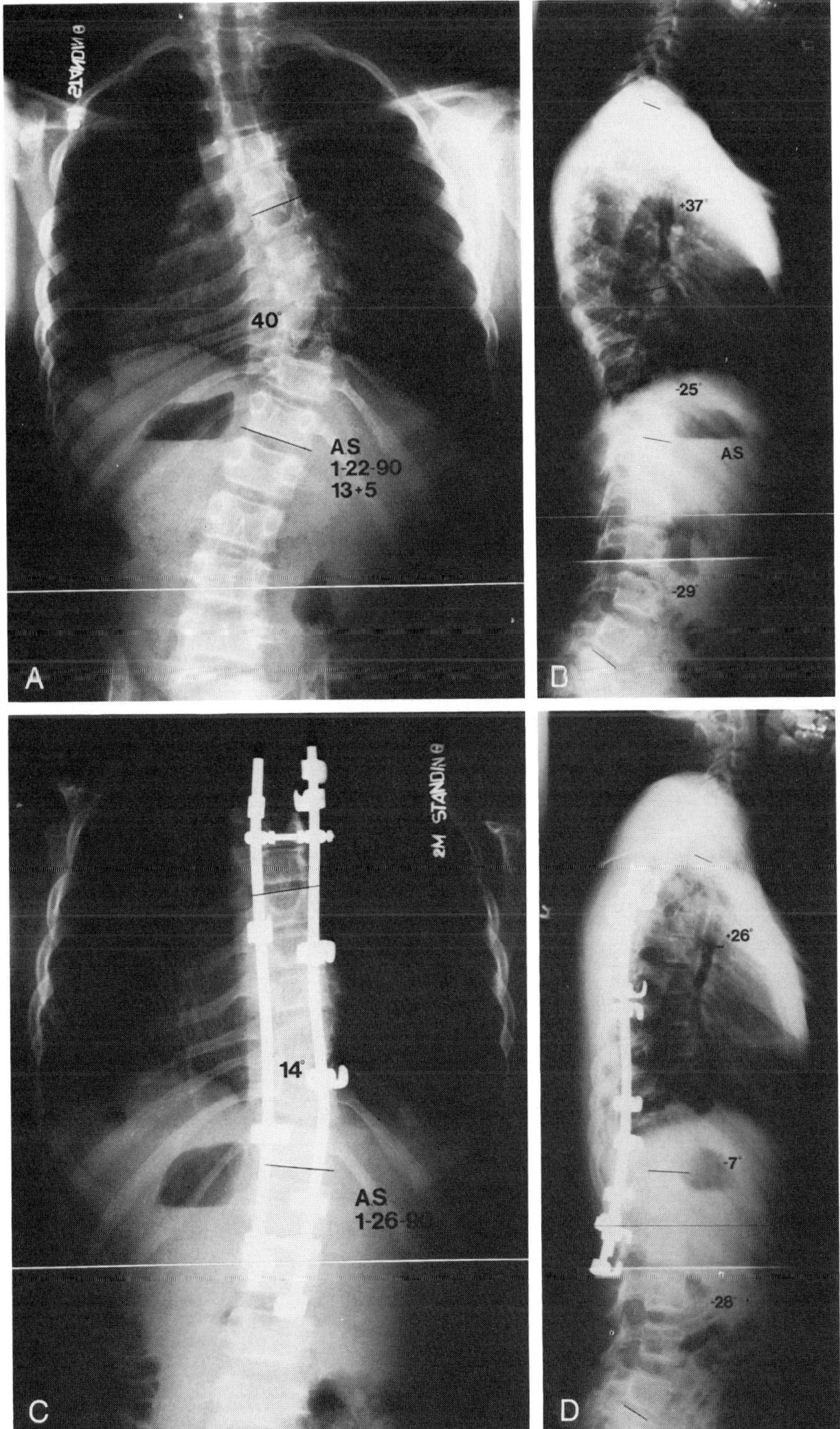

Figure 14–8. *A*, This 13-year-old boy had progressive congenital scoliosis of 40 degrees. The lateral film shows a compound thoracic spine, kyphotic in the upper half and lordotic in the lower half. *C*, The treatment was a posterior spine fusion with Cotrel-Dubousset rods (5 mm). The scoliosis was corrected to 14 degrees. *D*, The sagittal contour was also corrected, improving both the upper thoracic kyphosis and the lower thoracic lordosis. (No anterior procedure was done because the patient was a follower of Jehovah's Witnesses, prohibiting blood transfusion.)

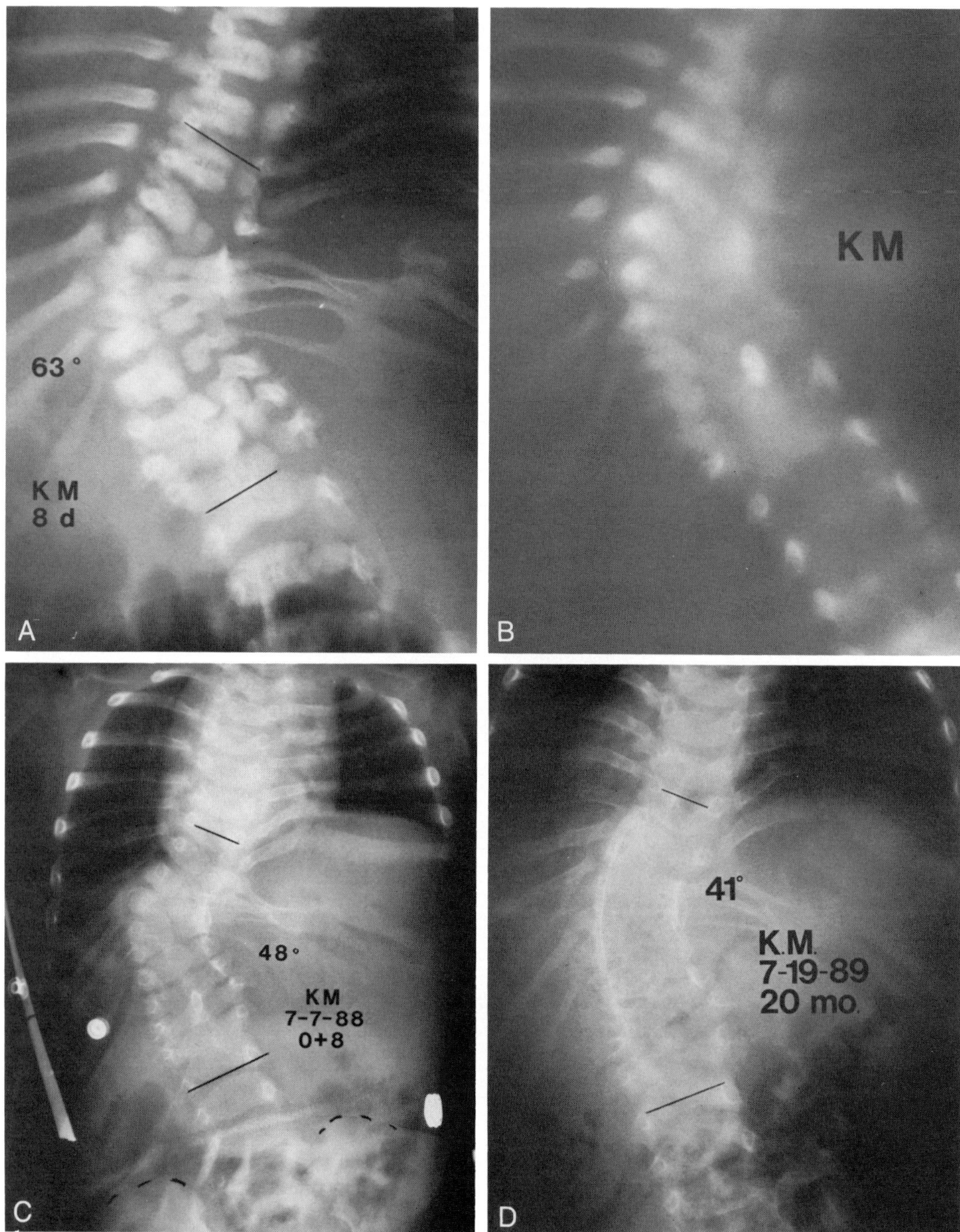

Figure 14–9. *A*, At birth, this girl had a 63-degree curve. An obvious unilateral unsegmented bar as well as interpediculate widening is seen. *B*, A tomogram and magnetic resonance imaging confirmed the diastematomyelia spur. *C*, She was treated during her first year of life with a Kallabis brace. In the brace, the curve was 48 degrees at age 8 months. *D*, At age 12 months, she underwent removal of the spur followed a week later by combined anterior and posterior spine fusion. The patient is seen here eight months after surgery with a solid fusion and 41-degree curve. Correction was achieved with a Milwaukee brace.

advance which patients are going to have decent growth on the concavity of the curve. Even if this concave growth does not take place, a good anterior and posterior fusion has been achieved and the curvature fully stabilized. This procedure should not be used in patients who have significant kyphosis, since the anterior portion of the fusion may aggravate the kyphosis. The great advantage of this technique is its simplicity, the very low blood loss, and the very low risk (Fig. 14–10).

Hemivertebra Excision

Hemivertebra excision has been available for a long time, having first been performed in Australia in 1921. Despite this long experience, there are very few reports of significant follow-up. This tends to indicate that although the procedure appears exciting at first, the results have not been as good as expected. The only exception is the excellent paper by Leatherman and Dickson.[5]

Hemivertebra excision is a direct attack on the pathology of the curvature and must be thought of as a wedge osteotomy at the apex of the curve. It should be remembered that the entire curve must always be fused, and if one is making the effort to go anteriorly to remove the hemivertebra, one should also take out any other discs and growth plates anteriorly that might exist in the curve area. This enhances the correction and certainly the arthrodesis.

Technically the hemivertebra is removed anteriorly and must be removed right back to the dural sac. The anterior half of the pedicle is removed via the anterior approach. Either under a second anesthetic or under the same anesthesia, the patient is turned prone and the posterior portion of the hemivertebra is excised, including the posterior half of the pedicle and transverse process. The wedge is then closed. This can be done by instrumentation if the bones are large enough, or by casting if the bones are too small and soft. Once again, it is emphasized that the entire curve must be fused. A cast or brace is used until the fusion is solid.

There is a neurologic risk rate with hemivertebra excision, and the blood loss is significantly higher than with anterior and posterior fusion or growth arrest surgery.

When the operation is done in the area of

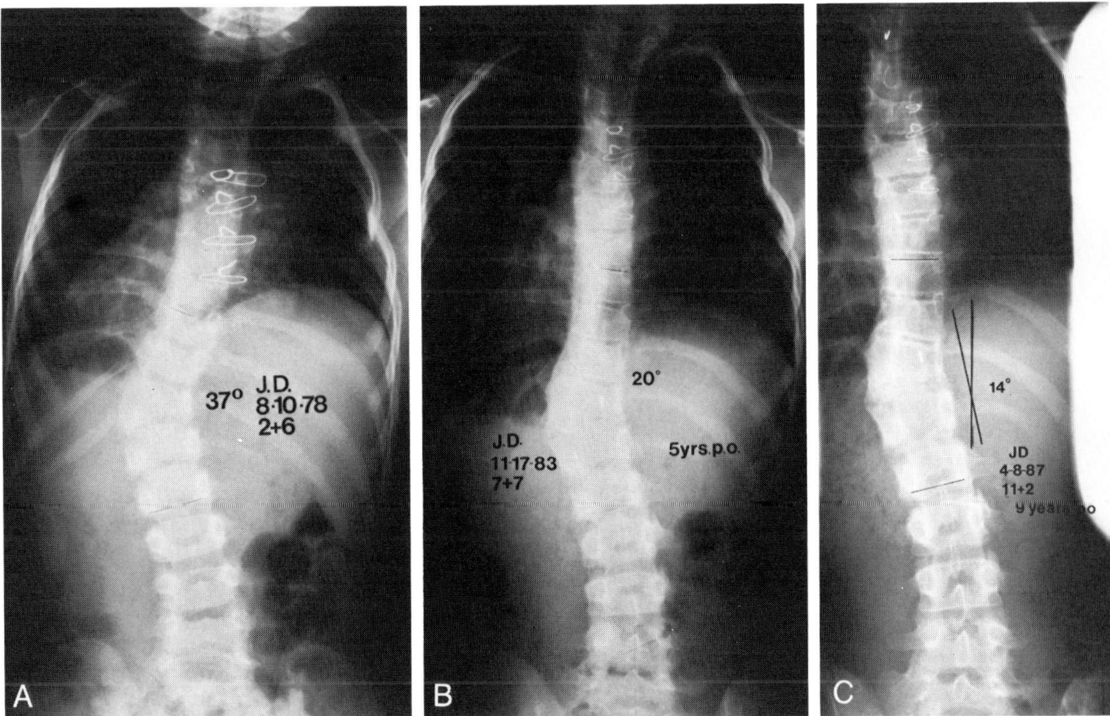

Figure 14–10. *A*, This 2½-year-old girl had progressive scoliosis related to a left T12 hemivertebra. *B*, Five years after surgery, the curve was 20 degrees. *C*, Nine years after surgery, the curve was 14 degrees.

the cauda equina, a common experience, one has to be careful that the pedicle coming down from above as the wedge is closed does not press unduly on the exiting nerve root. This nerve root must be watched at all times, and if there is excessive pressure the pedicle should be totally or partly removed. The author (RW) has noted this complication in two of 43 hemivertebra excisions done by our group (Fig. 14–11).

Vertebrectomy

Vertebrectomy is the most radical of all procedures for congenital scoliosis. It is the deliberate removal of two or more vertebrae in their entirety, including pedicles from both sides, laminae, and bodies. This is done deliberately in order to create mobility but at the price of instability. Customarily the anterior procedure is done first, and then the patient is turned over and the posterior part done either a week later or the same day. It is suggested that there be a waiting period between the front and back procedure to allow the blood supply of the spinal cord to accommodate itself. At the time of the posterior procedure, when the remaining stabilizing structures are excised, extremely firm internal fixation must be achieved on the table before the patient is awakened. This is a neurologically risky procedure that must be accompanied by appropriate spinal cord monitoring and wake-up tests. It should be reserved for the most severe deformities.

Combined Procedures

In general, many congenital scoliosis patients have a variety of congenital anomalies and need a variety of procedures. For example, we can combine an apical hemivertebra excision with epiphysiodesis above and below it, or we can combine bilateral posterior fusion in one area with combined anterior and posterior growth arrest surgery in a different area of the spine.

Sometimes, one is confronted with a difficult congenital spine disorder that does not lend itself well to any kind of instrumentation owing to the size of the bones, the shape of the curve, or some other complication. These can often be very major curves and very challenging. For these, the author (RW) performs a very radical anterior approach to the curvature, excising all of the discs in the curve area and all of the growth plates, along with some bone above and below each disc. This is then coupled with a similar procedure posteriorly, with a very radical facetectomy, bilateral fusion, and the addition of large amounts of bone graft. The patient may then be slowly corrected by traction; this is one of the very few times when halofemoral traction is still used. This is the ultimate monitor of the spinal cord, since the patient is awake at all times, correction taking place gradually, with any alteration of neurologic function being detected immediately. When a maximal correction has been achieved, the patient is placed in a cast to hold the alignment until solid. This may require several months of bed rest (Fig. 14–12).

Spinal Dysraphism

A special discussion of this condition is necessary. Earlier it was mentioned that a high percentage of patients with congenital scoliosis have tethered and anomalous spinal cords. How should these be addressed when treating the curvatures? If a child has a tethered spinal cord but a totally normal neurologic status, and if no corrective surgery is planned for the spine, we do not believe that the tether or spur should be removed. We know of many patients who lived their whole childhood with a well-established diastematomyelia and yet had no trouble at all. This requires an extremely careful observational approach, with periodical monitoring of the scoliosis at least twice a year, careful neurologic examinations at each visit, careful urologic evaluation to make sure that there is no evidence of neurogenic bladder, and activities such as sports and other exercises to make sure the child is fully functional.[4, 7]

There can be a dysraphic spinal cord without progressive scoliosis. In such a case, removal of the tether or spur is dependent on the patient's functional status and neurologic examinations. Finally, many patients present with significant curvatures who also have a dysraphic spinal cord. Usually, some kind of corrective maneuver for the curvature is desirable, and in such cases the tethering structure should be removed first by the neurosurgeon. This may mean the excision of a diastematomyelia spur, the release of a filum terminale, or both. Treatment of the curvature should

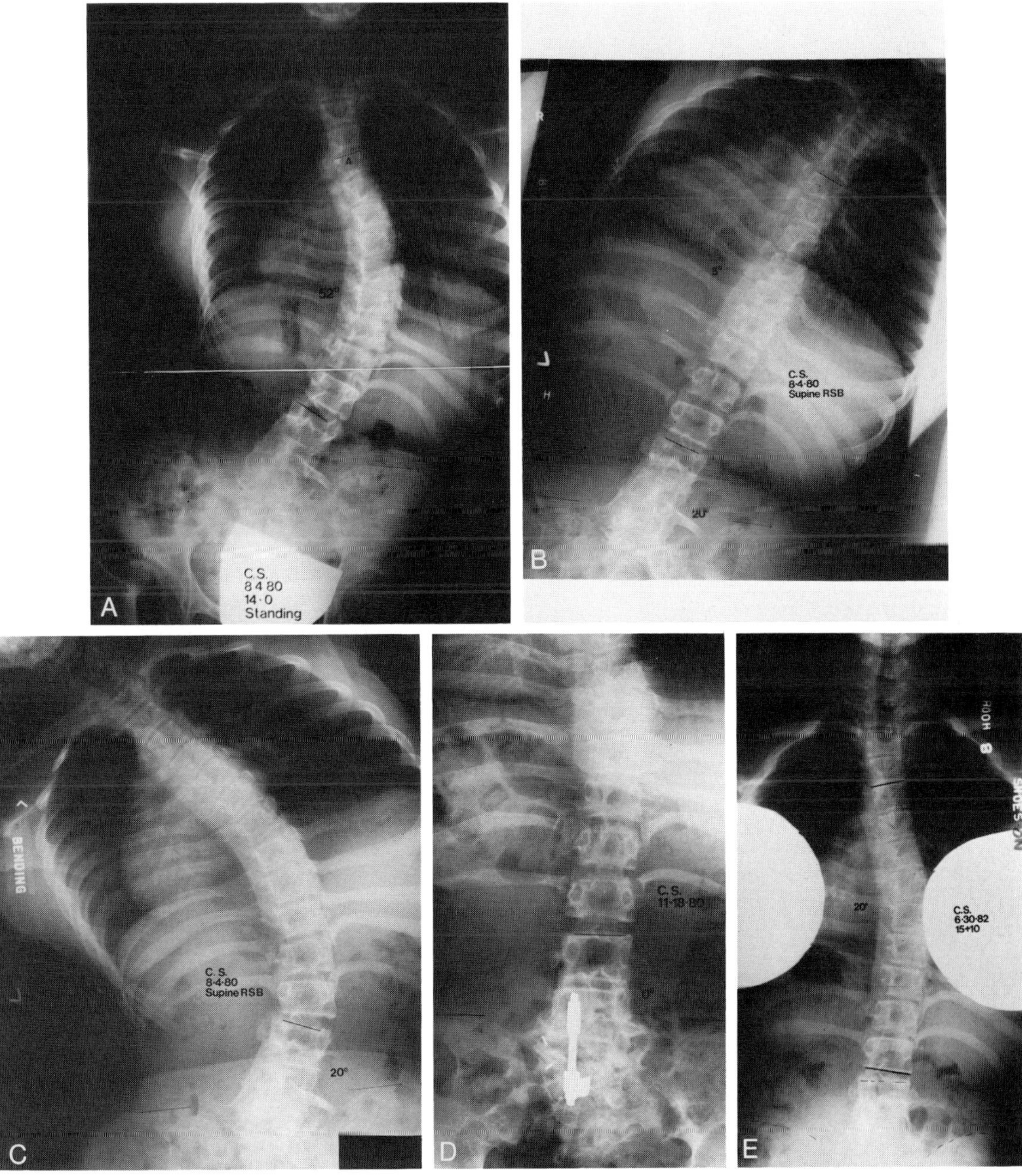

Figure 14–11. *A*, This 14-year-old girl had marked and increasing lateral torso deviation and 52-degree scoliosis. *B*, On the supine right-side bending film, the 52-degree scoliosis is fully corrected. *C*, On the spine left-side bending film, the rigid 20-degree lumbosacral curve is evident. *D*, After an L5 hemivertebra excision and fusion, the 20-degree lumbosacral curve was fully corrected (supine film). *E*, A two-year follow-up (standing) shows the excellent overall result.

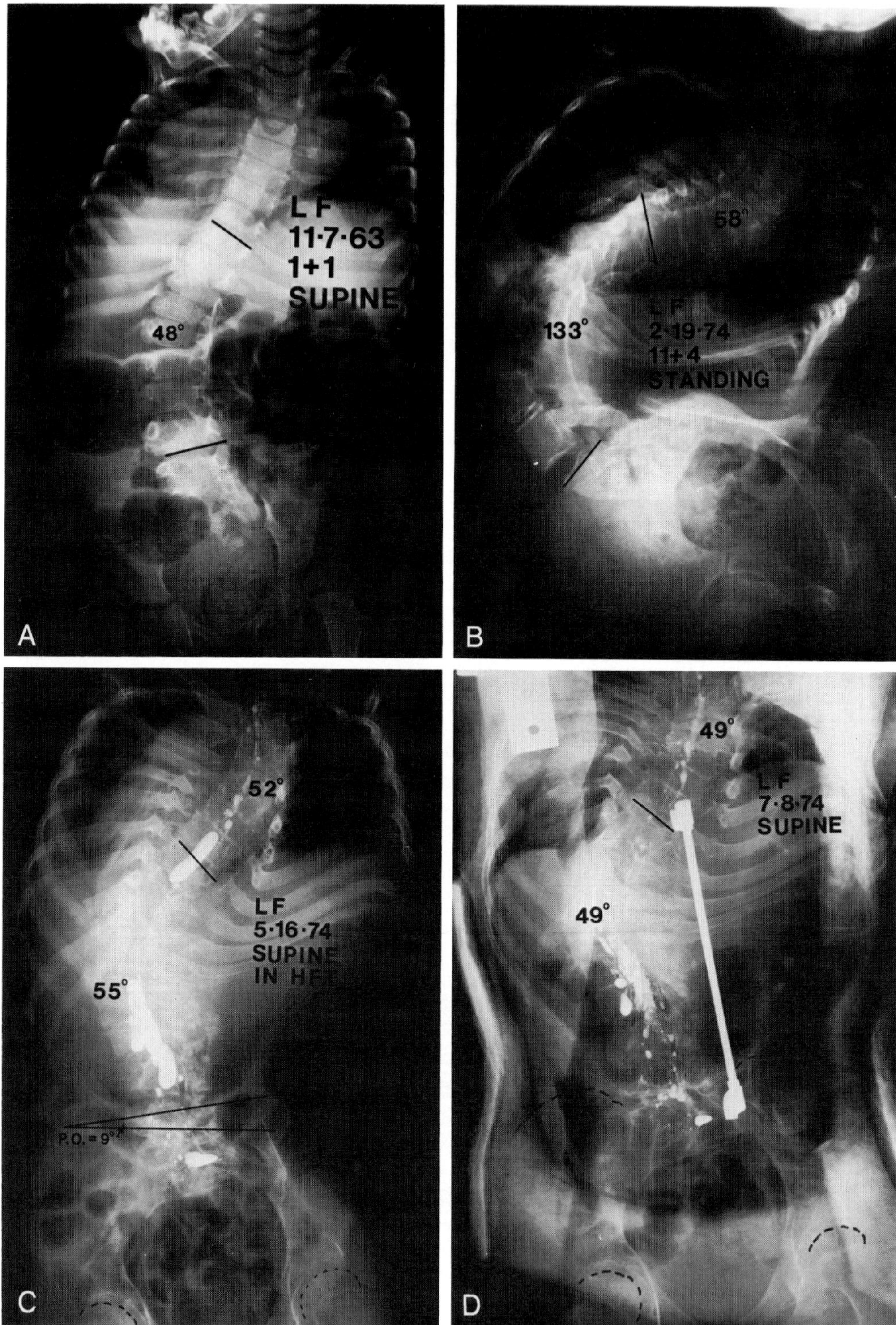

Figure 14–12. *A,* This 1-year-old girl with a 48-degree curve due to a unilateral unsegmented bar T11–S1 was observed at another institution. *B,* After ten years of "observation," the curve measured 133 degrees with severe pelvic obliquity. *C,* Treatment consisted of radical anterior discectomy, fusion from T10 to S1, complete resection of the unsegmented bar, and right leg femoral halo traction with correction gradually to 55 degrees. *D,* After maximal traction improvement, the patient underwent reoperation with Harrington rod insertion, posterior fusion, femoral traction pin removal, and halo-casting.

not be instituted until after the neurosurgical release has been done and the neurologic status of the patient reassessed. Simultaneous treatment is not recommended.

References

Congenital Scoliosis

1. Andrew, T., and Piggott, H.: Growth arrest for progressive scoliosis, combined anterior and posterior fusion of the convexity. J. Bone Joint Surg. *67B:*193–197, 1985.
4. Hood, R. W., Riseborough, E., Nehme, A., et al.: Diastematomyelia and structural spinal deformities. J. Bone Joint Surg. *62A:*520–528, 1980.
5. Leatherman, K. D., and Dickson, R. A.: Two-stage corrective surgery for congenital deformities of the spine. J. Bone Joint Surg. *61B:*324–328, 1979.
6. McMaster, J. F., and Ohtsuka, K.: The natural history of congenital scoliosis; a study of 251 patients. J. Bone Joint Surg. *64A:*1128–1147, 1982.
7. McMaster, M. J.: Occult intraspinal anomalies and congenital scoliosis. J. Bone Joint Surg. *66A:*588–601, 1984.
8. McMaster, M. J., and David, C. V.: Hemivertebra as a cause of scoliosis; a study of 104 patients. J. Bone Joint Surg. *68B:*588–595, 1986.
9. Winter, R. B., Moe, J. H., MacEwen, G. D., and Peon-Vidales, H.: The Milwaukee brace in the nonoperative treatment of congenital scoliosis. Spine *1:*85–96, 1976.
11. Winter, R. B.: Congenital Deformities of the Spine. New York, Thieme Stratton, 1983.
12. Winter, R. B., Moe, J. H., and Lonstein, J. E.: Posterior spinal arthrodesis for congenital scoliosis: an analysis of the cases of 290 patients 5–19 years old. J. Bone Joint Surg. *66A:*1188–1197, 1984.
14. Winter, R. B., Lonstein, J. E., Denis, F., and Sta.-Ana de la Rosa, H.: Convex growth arrest for progressive congenital scoliosis due to hemivertebrae. J. Pediatr. Orthop. *8:*633–638, 1988.
15. Winter, R. B.: Congenital spine deformity: what's the latest and what's the best? Spine *14:*1401–1409, 1989.
16. Wynne-Davies, R.: Congenital vertebral anomalies: aetiology and relationship to spina bifida cystica. J. Med. Genet. *12:*280–288, 1975.

IDIOPATHIC SCOLIOSIS

Idiopathic scoliosis is the most common form of spinal deformity seen. By definition it is a lateral curvature of the spine, occurring in an otherwise healthy child, for which no recognizable etiology exists. In these children there is no evidence of an underlying neurologic or muscular disorder, and radiographically there are no developmental vertebral abnormalities. It is divided into three categories, depending on the age at which it is first detected: infantile, juvenile, and adolescent. Infantile idiopathic scoliosis has its onset before age 3 years. Juvenile idiopathic scoliosis first appears between age 3 years and puberty, and adolescent idiopathic scoliosis, the most common type, is first detected after puberty.

Prevalence

Two terms are often confused in discussing the number of cases of a disease in the population: incidence and prevalence. Incidence refers to the rate of occurrence of new cases of a disease or disorder in a population, and is expressed as new cases per 1000 population per year. Conversely, prevalence refers to the number of a population with the disease or disorder, and is expressed as number of cases per 1000 population. All studies of scoliosis refer to the prevalence of scoliosis.

Early prevalence studies were either radiographic reviews or reviews of children referred for scoliosis treatment, and thus biased toward larger curves. Subsequent studies have been on school screening programs, which have shown a wide range of prevalence, 0.3 to 15.3 per cent.[10, 24, 54, 124, 130, 139, 198, 243] These vast differences reflect detection methods, different populations of children examined radiographically, and differing definitions of scoliosis. When only curves over 10 degrees are considered, the prevalence rates average 1.5 to 3 per cent.[10, 130, 137, 243] The rates vary as to the degree of curvature, as shown in Table 14–1.[27, 181, 214] This can be summarized as follows: curves over 10 degrees have a prevalence of 20 to 30 per 1000, those over 20 degrees 3 to 5 per 1000, and those over 30 degrees 2 to 3 per 1000.

There is a variation in the different types of idiopathic scoliosis regarding prevalence. Infantile idiopathic scoliosis has been relatively common in Great Britain but is rare in North America. The relative frequencies of the different types of idiopathic scoliosis have been changing in Great Britain. In a study of 157 consecutive patients with idiopathic scoliosis seen in Edinburgh between 1968 and 1971, 41 per cent had infantile curves, 7 per cent juvenile curves, and 52 per cent adolescent curves. Since that time there has been a change in these frequencies. Of the 153 patients with idiopathic scoliosis seen at the same clinic in

Table 14–1. PREVALENCE OF SCOLIOSIS BY DEGREE

Authors	No. of Patients	Patients with Curvatures (%)			
		>5°	>10°	>20°	>30°
Bruszewski and Kamza[27]	15,000	3.8	3.0	0.46	0.15
Rogala et al.[199]	14,999	4.3	—	0.3	0.3
Kane and Moe[109]	75,290	—	—	—	0.13
Patynski et al.[181]	5000	—	2.6	—	0.12
Shands and Eisberg[206]	50,000	1.9	1.4	0.3	0.29
Strayer[214]	928*	—	5.0	2.0	0.75

*All female.
From Bunnell, W. P.: The natural history of idiopathic scoliosis. Clin. Orthop. *229*:21, 1988.

the years 1980 to 1983, 4 per cent had infantile curves, 7 per cent juvenile curves, and 89 per cent adolescent curves.[150] These relative frequencies approach the frequencies in North America. In a survey of 208 patients in Boston, 0.5 per cent had infantile curves, 10.5 per cent juvenile curves, and 89 per cent adolescent curves.[195] A similar change was reported in Germany.[145, 146]

Etiology

By definition the etiology of idiopathic scoliosis is as yet unknown. Many theories exist as to the cause, and these are divided into those for the infantile and those for the adolescent types.

Infantile Idiopathic Scoliosis

Infantile idiopathic scoliosis, as stated, is more common in Europe. It occurs more frequently in boys, with a left thoracic curve predominating. In a family study conducted in Edinburgh by Wynne-Davies,[244, 245] she found a genetic tendency but thought the etiology to be multifactorial. Plagiocephaly is common in infantile idiopathic scoliosis. This is a change in shape of the skull, with the side of flattening and posterior occipital prominence corresponding to the convex side of the spinal curvature. The plagiocephaly, like the scoliosis, was not present at birth and developed within the first six months of life. This suggests a postural causation of both the plagiocephaly and the spinal curvature.

Wynne-Davies also found associated factors in her family review.[244] These included congenital dislocation of the hip, congenital heart disease, and mental deficiency. In addition, the mothers were older, with a higher incidence of hernias among relatives. Some of these findings are also reported in other series.[35, 42, 73, 100, 129]

Adolescent Idiopathic Scoliosis

Idiopathic scoliosis has been attributed to a wide variety of conditions from subclinical poliomyelitis to nutrition. Many other lines of research have focused attention on the genetic aspect, growth aspects, structural and biomechanical changes in discs and muscle, and central nervous system changes.

Family studies by Wynne-Davies[243, 244] and numerous population studies[47, 48, 74, 142, 197] pointed to a hereditary factor to account for the well-known familial pattern. The mode of inheritance is uncertain, being regarded as autosomal dominant or as sex-linked with incomplete penetrance and variable expressivity. This may explain the equal sex distribution in large school screening studies. However, for large curves needing treatment, girls predominate.[24, 199] It has been calculated that if both parents have idiopathic scoliosis, the chance of their offspring requiring treatment is 50 times that of the normal population.[142, 243]

Growth has a definite role in scoliosis. Curves progress rapidly during the adolescent growth spurt, which occurs around age 12 in girls and a year or two later in boys.[62] The crucial year is the year before menarche, the onset of menstruation.[21, 237] A Swedish study found that girls with adolescent idiopathic scoliosis were significantly taller than their normal peers. This was *not* seen in boys with scoliosis, nor in girls at younger ages.[236, 237] These girls started their growth spurt earlier, grew for a longer period, and had a skeletal age more advanced than that of normal girls.[176]

Increased levels of growth hormone in girls with scoliosis compared with normals has been found by Skogland and Miller[212] and others,[234] but Misol and colleagues could not confirm these findings.[158] The increased growth hormone and somatomedin levels would explain the early prolonged growth spurt in adolescent girls with idiopathic scoliosis.

Some authors have found structural changes in the spine. Many have reported decreased glucosaminoglycan (GAG) levels in the nucleus pulposus of the apical discs of patients with idiopathic scoliosis, with a concomitant rise in collagen levels.[74, 112, 183, 186] They concluded that these changes were secondary to the abnormal stresses placed on the disc by the curvature. This "effect rather than cause" theory was confirmed by studies on other types of scoliosis.[179, 218]

Nordwall and Wilner tested collagen in ligaments and tendons in patients with idiopathic scoliosis, comparing them with normal individuals.[177] They were unable to find any difference with respect to elastic stiffness, tensile strength, or elongation to failure. Similar findings were reported by Waters and Morris,[228] making a mechanical disorder of collagen unlikely as the cause of idiopathic scoliosis.

The muscles have been implicated in the etiology of idiopathic scoliosis. Electromyographic studies have been inconclusive. Most investigators found increased activity on the convexity,[33, 194, 255] but others found no difference.[95, 127] In addition, investigators found more Type I or slow-twitch (red, anaerobic) muscle fibers on the convexity of the apical level in idiopathic scoliosis.[70, 71, 101, 213, 224] Abnormalities were also found in muscle spindles;[13, 250] muscle histochemistry;[212, 249] sarcolemma;[116] calcium, phosphorus, and zinc concentrations in paravertebral muscles;[249] and platelets as they relate to skeletal muscle.[75] Whether all these abnormalities found are secondary to the curve or whether they exist before the development of scoliosis is unknown, but most authors think the former is the case.

Because of the association of scoliosis with neurologic disorders, an abnormality of the central nervous system (CNS) is an attractive etiologic theory. Research has concentrated on equilibrium and postural mechanisms. Investigating righting reflexes, drift reaction, and optokinetic nystagmus, Yamada and colleagues[246–248] found equilibrium dysfunction in patients, but it was not specific for idiopathic scoliosis. They also showed spontaneous nystagmus in a group of highly progressive idiopathic curves.[247] This has been confirmed by other authors.[49, 56, 208] Postural and equilibrium abnormalities and vestibular dysfunction have been shown in other studies.[74, 94, 97, 200, 201, 226, 250] It thus appears that there may be a postural equilibrium abnormality in idiopathic scoliosis, and some authors have suggested that it lies in the brain stem.

In summary, it appears that the etiology of idiopathic scoliosis is multifactorial; no single causative factor has been found. There may be two separate mechanisms: one that causes idiopathic scoliosis and the second related to curve progression. Genetic, growth, chemical, and neuromuscular factors all seem to be involved. Theories of pathomechanics have been postulated[5] where the mild CNS abnormality is genetically determined. With increased growth and altered viscoelasticity of discs, the spine is biomechanically less stable, making it susceptible to changes in postural equilibrium. The interrelation of these factors will determine whether the curve is nonprogressive and how much progression will occur, or perhaps will result in straightening of the curve.

Natural History

In the natural history of idiopathic scoliosis, there are three important questions. What are the effects of untreated scoliosis? What percentage of cases progress? Is it possible to predict which curves will progress?

Studies show the deleterious effects of the untreated severe curve in adults[19, 41, 169, 175, 229, 230] in terms of progression of the curve in adulthood, pain associated with the curve, reduced respiratory function with cor pulmonale, and socioeconomic effects.

Progression of the Curve. Curve progression has been shown to occur after skeletal maturity.[18, 41, 61, 229, 230] The two best long-term studies are those of Weinstein and Ponseti[229] and Ascani and colleagues,[8] the results of which were very similar, as seen in Table 14–2. In general, curves under 30 degrees at skeletal maturity tend not to progress in adult life regardless of curve pattern. Many curves do progress in adulthood, particularly the thoracic curves of 50 to 80 degrees at maturity, the lumbar component of double thoracic and lumbar curves and thoracolumbar curves.

Table 14–2. AVERAGE CURVE PROGRESSION AFTER MATURITY

Pattern	Progression	
	*Iowa City Group**	*Italian Group†*
Thoracic	17°	17°
Lumbar	10°	16°
Thoracolumbar	18°	14°
Double thoracic–lumbar	14°	13°
	14°	16°
All patterns	13°	15°

*A total of 102 patients, average curve 50 degrees, average follow-up 40 years.

†Multicenter, 187 patients, average follow-up 34 years.

From Weinstein, S. L.: The natural history of scoliosis in the skeletally mature patient. *In* Dickson, J. H. (ed.): Spinal Deformities. Vol. 1. Philadelphia, Hanley & Belfus, 1987, pp. 195–212.

Back Pain. The overall incidence of back pain in adult scoliosis patients has been shown to be the same as that found in the general population.[229, 230] Swedish long-term studies also showed no greater number of disability pension recipients with scoliosis than without this disorder.[102, 119, 169, 175] This contrasts with the fact that the most common indication for surgery in adult scoliosis is back pain.

Some differences have been found among scoliosis patients. The incidence of frequent or daily backache was slightly higher in the scoliosis patients in the Iowa study compared with controls.[229] Patients with lumbar or thoracolumbar curves, especially with rotatory translation at the lower end of the curve, had a slightly higher incidence of backache compared with patients with other curve patterns.[229] Thus, it appears that although there is no higher incidence of back pain in scoliosis patients, the pain intensity and frequency are greater with certain curve patterns at risk.

Pulmonary Function. Pulmonary function is reduced in thoracic curves with a direct correlation between decreasing vital capacity and increasing curve severity.[15, 85, 87, 107, 128, 143, 207, 230, 231, 254] The two long-term Swedish studies reported a higher mortality rate, especially from cor pulmonale and in patients over the age of 40 in thoracic scoliosis.[169, 175] These studies described patients diagnosed in their twenties and thirties who probably had severe curves. This is emphasized by the long-term study of Kolind-Sørensen,[119] who reported that the mortality rate in idiopathic scoliosis for curves of 40 to 100 degrees was comparable with that in the general population, but that in curves of over 100 degrees, the mortality rate doubled.

Socioeconomic Effects. The data on the socioeconomic effects are controversial. Some series suggest profound problems including poor self-image, a greater percentage unemployed or on disability pensions, and a lower marriage rate.[76, 169, 175] The Iowa group in contrast reported few of these problems.[41, 185, 229, 230] A high percentage of patients in one series, however, were self-conscious of their appearance and some were even embarrassed by it.[76] These differences can be explained by different cultural backgrounds and societal expectations, geographic differences in disability compensation, and the great variations in each person's self-perception and self-confidence.

Infantile Idiopathic Scoliosis

As stated, most curves are left-sided and develop in the thoracic spine before the age of 2 years. In series from the classic article of James,[106] it was shown that 55 to 60 per cent occur in boys and almost 90 per cent are left thoracic curves.[105, 129, 205] The most interesting finding in these latter studies was that 30 to 90 per cent resolved spontaneously. These are referral series and most authors concluded that overall the rate of spontaneous resolution is 90 per cent. This divides infantile idiopathic scoliosis into resolving and progressive types. The progressive type had all progressed to curves of 70 degrees or more by the age of 10 years.[105, 106, 205]

Efforts were made to differentiate between the progressive and the resolving types,[42, 245] but these were unsuccessful until the work of Mehta in 1972.[153] She noticed a relationship between the apical vertebrae of the thoracic curve and the ribs, called the rib-vertebra angle. This angle is formed by a line perpendicular to the end plate of the apical vertebrae and a line drawn along the center of the rib. The difference between the angle on the convex and on the concave sides is the rib-vertebra angle difference (RVAD) (Fig. 14–13). Mehta also noted the relationship between the head of the rib and vertebral body. There may be no overlap, called Phase 1 by Mehta, or the rib head may overlap the vertebral body, Phase 2 (Fig. 14–14).

In Mehta's study of 138 cases of infantile idiopathic scoliosis,[153] 86 curves were in Phase

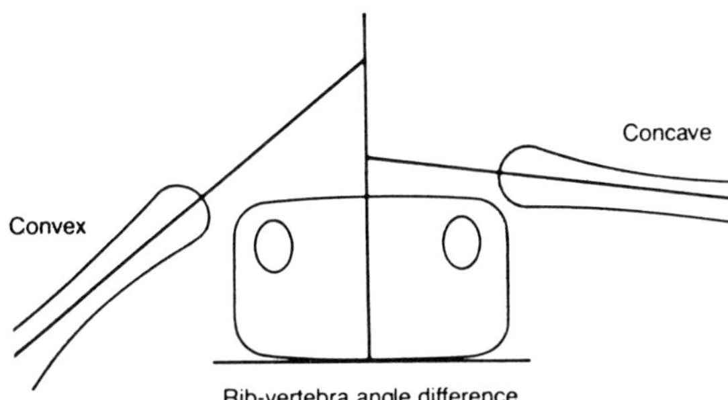

Figure 14–13. The rib-vertebra angle difference (RVAD) of Mehta, calculated by subtracting the convex value from the concave value at the apical vertebra of a thoracic curve. (From Koop, S. E.: Infantile and juvenile idiopathic scoliosis. Orthop. Clin. North Am. *19*:332, 1988.)

1. Of these, 46 resolved and 40 progressed. The average RVAD of the resolving group was 11.7 degrees (as high as 27 degrees), and 83 per cent of these curves had an RVAD of less than 20 degrees. In the remainder of the resolving curves the RVAD decreased in time, despite the Cobb measurement. The average RVAD of the progressive group was 25.5 degrees (range 18 to 38 degrees), and 84 per cent had an RVAD of greater than 20 degrees. In all cases in Mehta's study, if the apical rib head was in Phase 2, progression was certain and the RVAD was not necessary. These findings were confirmed by Ceballos and associates.[36] In addition, Mehta subdivided progressive infantile idiopathic scoliosis into benign and malignant forms. Both demonstrated rapid worsening in the first five years of life, gradual progression in the juvenile years, and marked deterioration in the adolescent years. The malignant form has more rapid progression in the first five years of life and is more difficult to manage. The difficulty in treating this latter type was confirmed by McMaster and MacNicol.[149]

Juvenile Idiopathic Scoliosis

The proportion of children with idiopathic scoliosis detected between the ages of 3 years and puberty is 12 to 21 per cent.[106, 114, 165, 185] There is a gradual change in this group from the infantile type with more boys under the age of 6, after which girls predominate. The thoracic curves are left-sided in boys and right-sided in girls. Juvenile idiopathic scoliosis is divided into nonprogressive and progressive curves. In general, when over 30 degrees, most

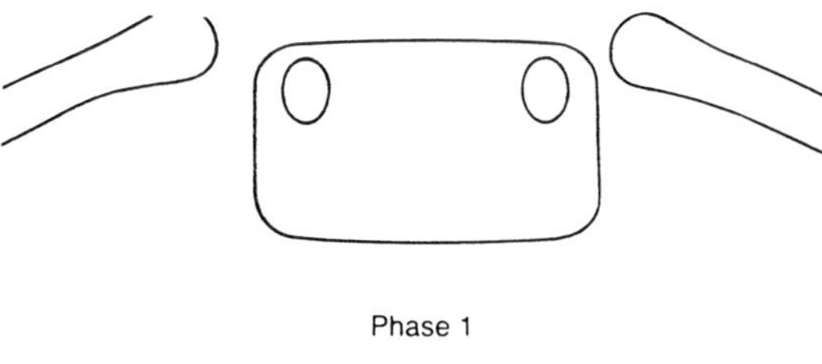

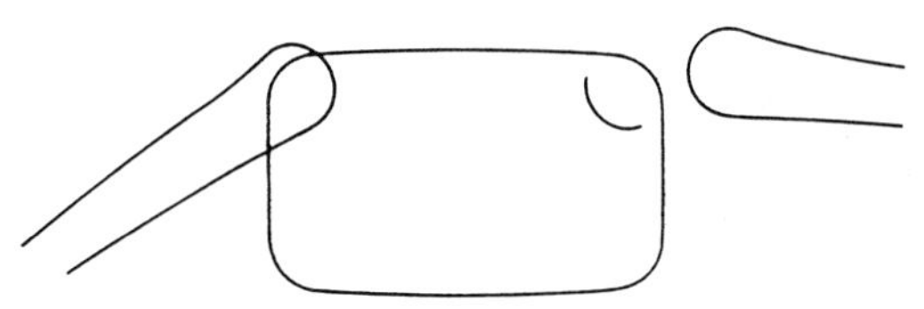

Figure 14–14. Apical vertebra phases of Mehta. Phase 2 implies that progression is under way and will continue. (From Koop, S. E.: Infantile and juvenile idiopathic scoliosis. Orthop. Clin. North Am. *19*:333, 1988.)

curves are progressive. In the curves first detected under age 6, most curves are progressive, and after this progression falls to two thirds in the late juvenile years. The RVAD of Mehta was not useful in predicting progression in the juvenile.[221]

Adolescent Idiopathic Scoliosis

The information in this age group is much greater owing to school screening studies. The sex ratio of children with curves detected on school screening is nearly 1:1,[130, 137] while most of those with large curves requiring treatment are girls (Table 14–3).[9, 24, 25, 32, 109, 130, 131, 199, 206, 222, 235, 244, 251] In this screened population, most

Table 14–3. PREVALENCE OF ADOLESCENT IDIOPATHIC SCOLIOSIS (AGES 10–16 YEARS)

	Prevalence	
Cobb Angle	*At-Risk Population (%)*	*Female-to-Male Ratio*
>10°	2.0–3.0	1.4:2.1
>20°	0.3–0.5	5.4:1
>30°	0.1–0.3	10:1
>40°	<0.1	

Reproduced with permission from Weinstein, S. L.: Adolescent idiopathic scoliosis: prevalence and natural history. Instr. Course Lect. *38*:115–126, 1988. Park Ridge, IL, American Academy of Orthopaedic Surgeons.

curves are small and only a small percentage require active treatment.[8, 24, 25, 131, 136, 199, 235]

The overall incidence of progression in this series is different from that in the younger age groups. In infantile and juvenile years, when a curve progresses, progression continues. In the adolescent, this is not necessarily the case. If a curve increases from 22 to 28 degrees, it is unknown whether this progression will continue and what the final curve will be. Will the curve continue progressing at a slower rate and stop at 35 degrees, or will progression be linear? The other problem is the definition of progression. Is it a 5- or 10-degree increase? Is the time in which the progression occurs noted? In addition, some series are of untreated cases and in others treatment is instituted after a 5- or 10-degree change.

The overall incidence of progression varies widely, as seen in Table 14–4. These series are all on smaller curves or on curves detected on school screening. Certain factors were found to be related to the incidence of progression:

1. Sex. As noted above, progression is more common in girls.[30, 31, 38, 198]

2. Age. As originally described by Duval-Beaupère, there is a relationship between curve progression and age, with a rapid rise in progression at the onset of the adolescent growth spurt.[62] This has been shown in idiopathic scoliosis, with an increased incidence of progression in younger adolescents.[30, 31, 38, 131]

3. Menarche. Progression has been found to be less common after menarche. In Lonstein and Carlson's series, 32 per cent of patients with progressive curves and 68 per cent of those with nonprogressive curves had reached menarche by the first visit.[131]

4. Risser sign. The Risser iliac apophysis ossification sign[196] has been found to be related to progression. This radiographic sign is a sign of skeletal maturity. The cartilage apophysis ossifies from anterior to posterior, and Risser divided this ossification into four quarters, 1 to 4, 0 being no ossification visible and 5 being fusion of the ossified cap to the ilium. The incidence of progression has been shown to decrease as the Risser sign increases.[30, 38, 131]

5. Curve pattern. The incidence of progression is related to curve pattern.[30, 38, 77, 131] In general, double curves progress more frequently than single curves. The curves that have the highest incidence of progression usually are the double thoracic pattern, the double thoracic and lumbar pattern, and the single right thoracic curve. The curve with the lowest incidence of progression is the single lumbar curve.

6. Curve magnitude. The incidence of progression increases with increasing curve magnitude.[30, 38, 77, 78, 131, 184, 229]

Numerous other factors and radiographic measurements have been found not to correlate with progression, including Mehta's RVAD.[30, 38, 131, 153, 203]

These factors have been combined to give useful tables for reference. Nachemson and associates calculated probabilities of progression based on curve magnitude and age (Table 14–5),[167] and Lonstein and Carlson used curve magnitude and the Risser sign (Table 14–6).[131] In general, the younger the child as evidenced by age, Risser sign of 0 or 1, and premenarchal status, the greater is the incidence of progression, and the larger the curve, the greater is the incidence of progression.

Attempts to predict progression in adolescents (as in infantile idiopathic scoliosis) have been unsuccessful. With electromyography of paraspinal muscles,[189] rotational prominence,[187] vertebral rotation,[7] and multiple

Table 14–4. TOTAL INCIDENCE OF PROGRESSION

	No. of Patients	Progression (%)	Curve
Brooks[25]	134	5.2	—
Rogala et al.[199]	603	6.8	—
Clarisse[38]	110	35	10°–29°
Fustier[77]	70	56	<30°
Bunnell[30]	326	20	<30°
		40	>30°
Lonstein and Carlson[131]	727	23	5°–29°

From Lonstein, J. E.: Risk of progression of idiopathic scoliosis in skeletally immature patients. Spine: State of Art Reviews, Vol. 1, No. 2, 1987.

Table 14–5. PROBABILITIES OF PROGRESSION BASED ON CURVE MAGNITUDE AND AGE

Curve Magnitude at Detection	Age (yrs)		
	10–12 (%)	*13–15 (%)*	*16 (%)*
<19°	25	10	0
20°–29°	60	40	10
30°–39°	90	70	30
>60°	100	90	70

Reproduced with permission from Weinstein, S. L.: Adolescent idiopathic scoliosis: prevalence and natural history. Instr. Course Lect. *38*:115–126, 1988. Park Ridge, IL, American Academy of Orthopaedic Surgeons.

Table 14–6. PROBABILITIES OF PROGRESSION BASED ON RISSER GRADE AND CURVE MAGNITUDE AT DETECTION

	Curve Magnitude	
Risser Grade	*5°–19°*	*20°–29°*
0–1	22%	68%
2–4	1.6%	23%

From Lonstein, J. E., and Carlson, J. M.: The prediction of curve progression in untreated idiopathic scoliosis during growth. J. Bone Joint Surg. *66A*:1061–1071, 1984.

radiographic measurements,[30, 38, 131, 153, 203] no prediction could be made. Using Tables 14–5 and 14–6 or the predictive factor of Lonstein and Carlson,[131] a general idea of the incidence of progression can be obtained. This is important for counseling the family and arranging follow-up.

Clinical Presentation

With the advent of school screening for spinal deformities, this became the usual method of referral of these children. In addition, the spine is checked by the family physician (family practitioner or pediatrician) on the yearly preschool physical examination or the physical required before participation in school athletics. Sometimes parents notice a back asymmetry, or it is detected by the first physical education staff or coaches at school.

In the school the screening is easily and quickly performed by a trained school nurse or physical education teacher. Children are examined in the Adams position (Fig. 14–15)[1] and are checked from ages 10 to 16. Girls wear a halter top and boys are checked with shirt removed. The child stands with feet together and knees straight, and bends forward at the waist with arms hanging and palms opposed. The examiner, at the head of the child, compares the two sides of the thoracic and lumbar areas for symmetry. Very minor differences between the two sides can thus be appreciated. If a definite difference is detected, the child is referred to the family physician. After rechecking the child, when a definite asymmetry is confirmed, a standing spine radiograph is taken. With the diagnosis of scoliosis, the child is referred to a general orthopedic surgeon, an orthopedic surgeon specializing in spine problems, or a Crippled Children's Clinic. Further assessment, including clinical and roentgenographic evaluation, follows.

Orthopedic Examination

The orthopedic examination (Fig. 14–16) of a patient with scoliosis should be detailed. A careful history must be taken and should include inquiries as to pain, neurologic symptoms, family history, growth spurt, and menarche. All diseases known to be associated with a high incidence of scoliosis (connective tissue diseases, neurologic disorders) should be ruled out. Once the history is completed, an examination of the patient is undertaken. The patient should be undressed except for a pair of underpants and a loose gown open in the back. The examiner should view the entire body from the front, side, and rear, noting (1) scapular asymmetry and unilateral prominence, (2) waist asymmetry or fullness, (3)

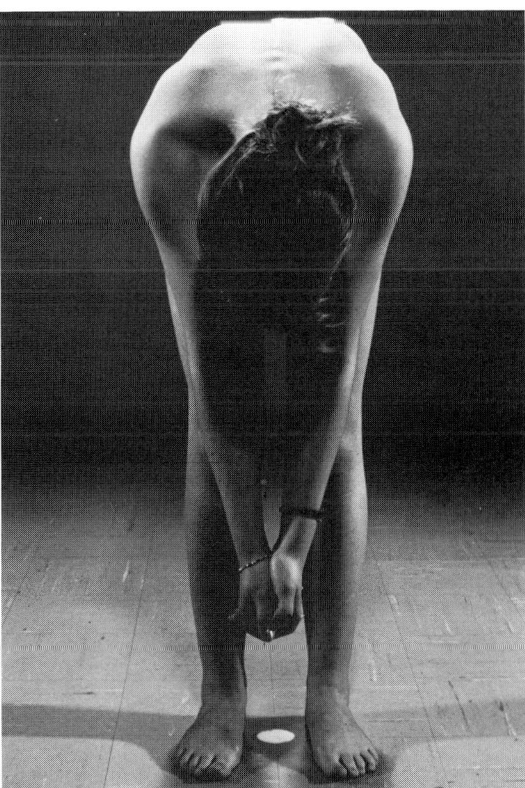

Figure 14–15. Adams forward bending test. The girl is standing with feet together, knees straight, and hands together. The examiner looks down the back comparing the two sides. Asymmetry in the thoracolumbar area with a left prominence is shown.

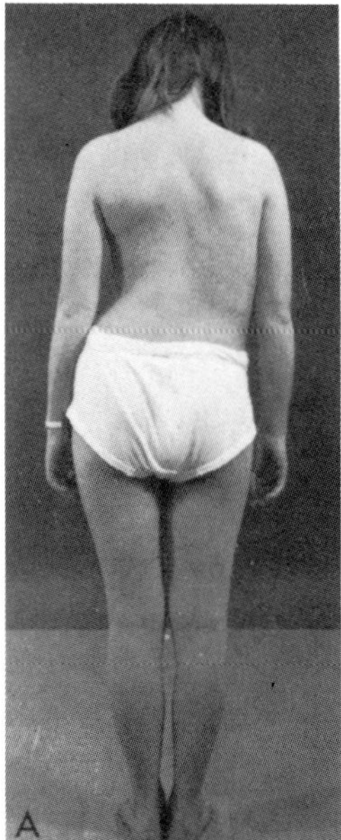

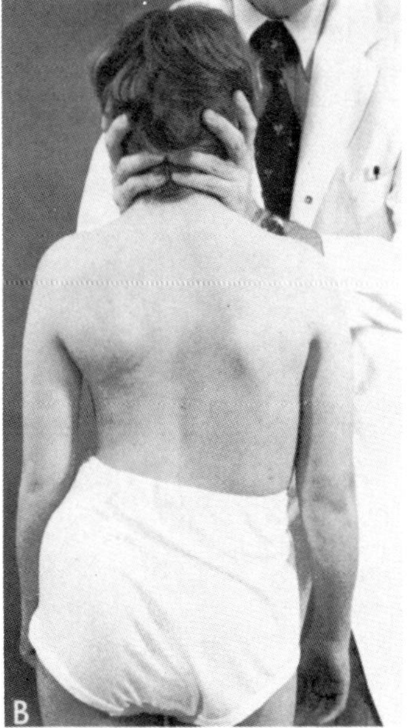

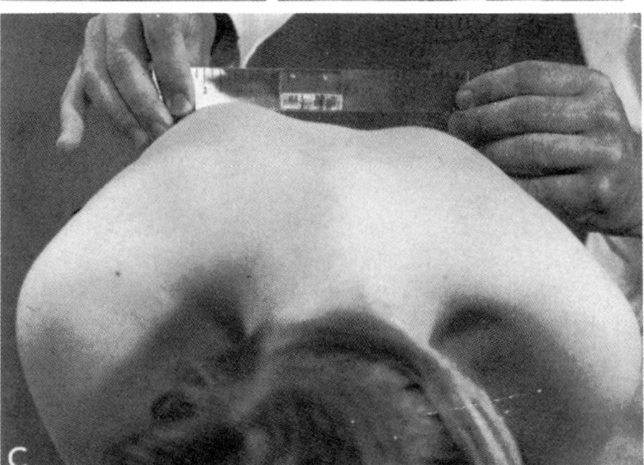

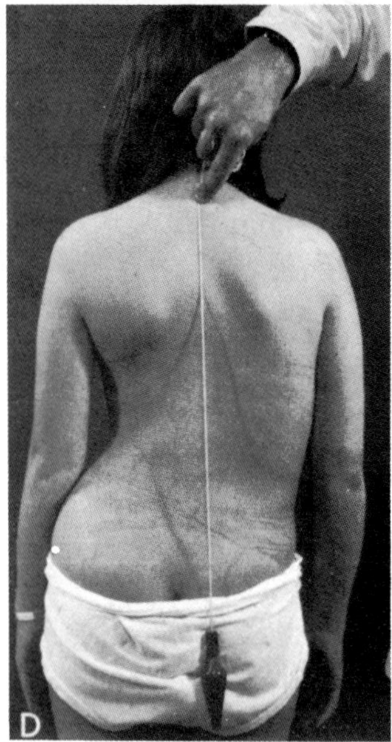

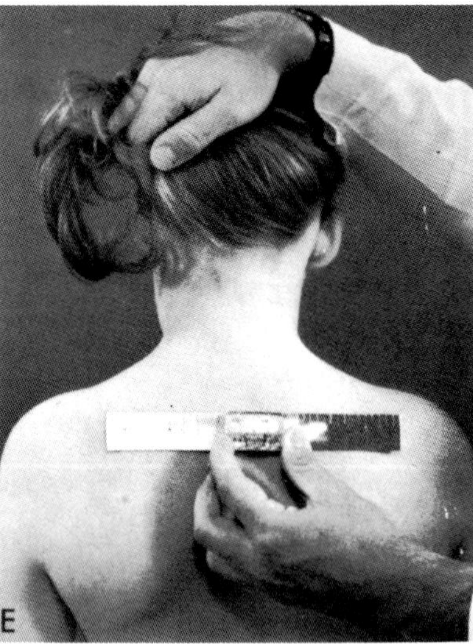

Figure 14–16. *A,* The patient must be viewed from a short distance to fully evaluate the deformity. From the rear view *all* clothing should be removed when permissible. Here is shown a typical right thoracic idiopathic curve. Note the lowering of the right shoulder, the fullness and scapular prominence over the right thorax, the decreased distance between the arm and the right thorax, and the increased distance between the left arm and thorax. The left pelvis seems higher than the right, but this is due to flank fullness on the right and flank depression on the left. The pelvis is level, and the "high hip" commonly referred to by parents is apparent, not real. The thorax is depressed on the left. *B,* Mobility of the spine can be quickly checked by hand suspension. *C,* The difference in the height of the thoracic cage should be recorded with a spirit level at the same distance from the spine. This is best determined in the thorax with the patient bent toward the examiner. The lumbar prominence is best checked from behind. One must be certain that the arms are dropped vertically and that the fingertips are together. *D,* A plumb line dropped from the midocciput or from the seventh (prominence) cervical vertebra demonstrates a list of the body toward the right. The distance from the gluteal crease to the line of deviation should be recorded. *E,* Shoulder level and low neck asymmetry should be checked and recorded.

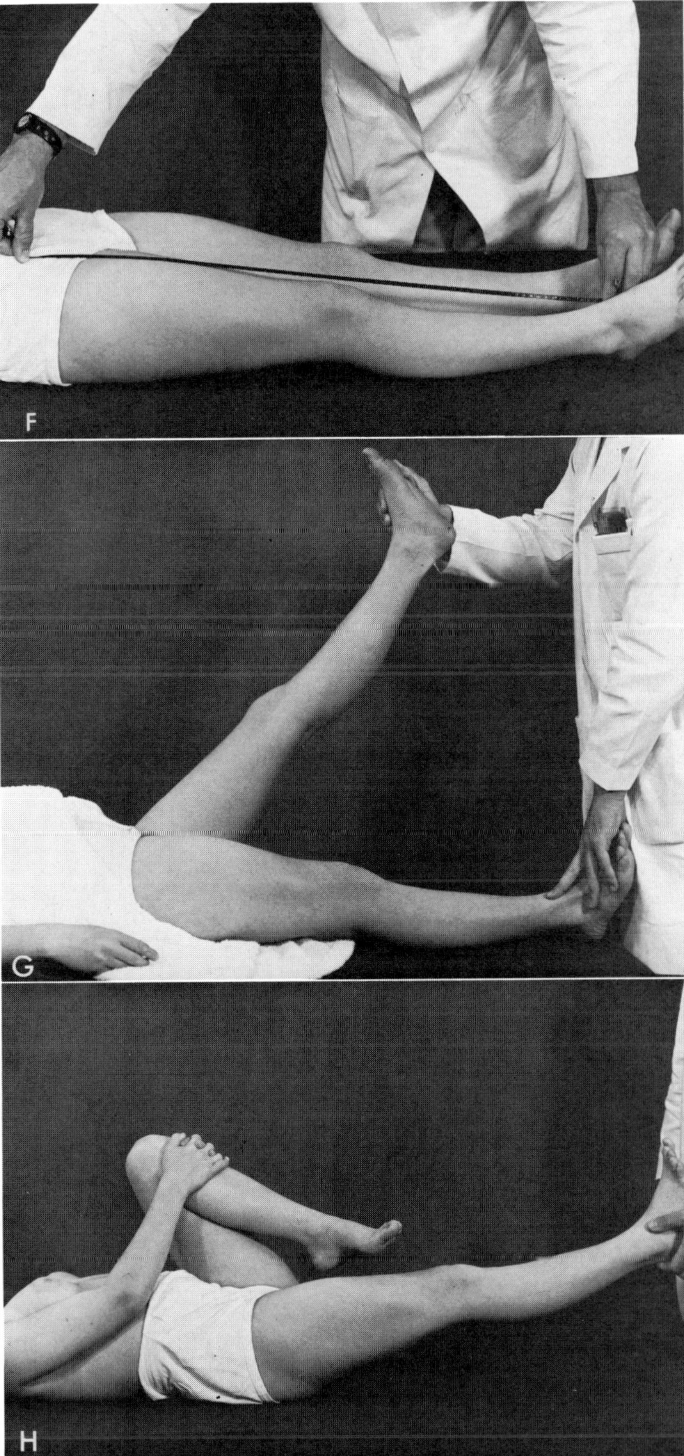

Figure 14–16 *Continued F,* The length of the lower extremities should be measured as accurately as possible. *G,* Tightness of the hamstrings, pectoral muscles, and heel cords should be recorded. *H,* Always check for hip flexion contractures.

Illustration continued on following page

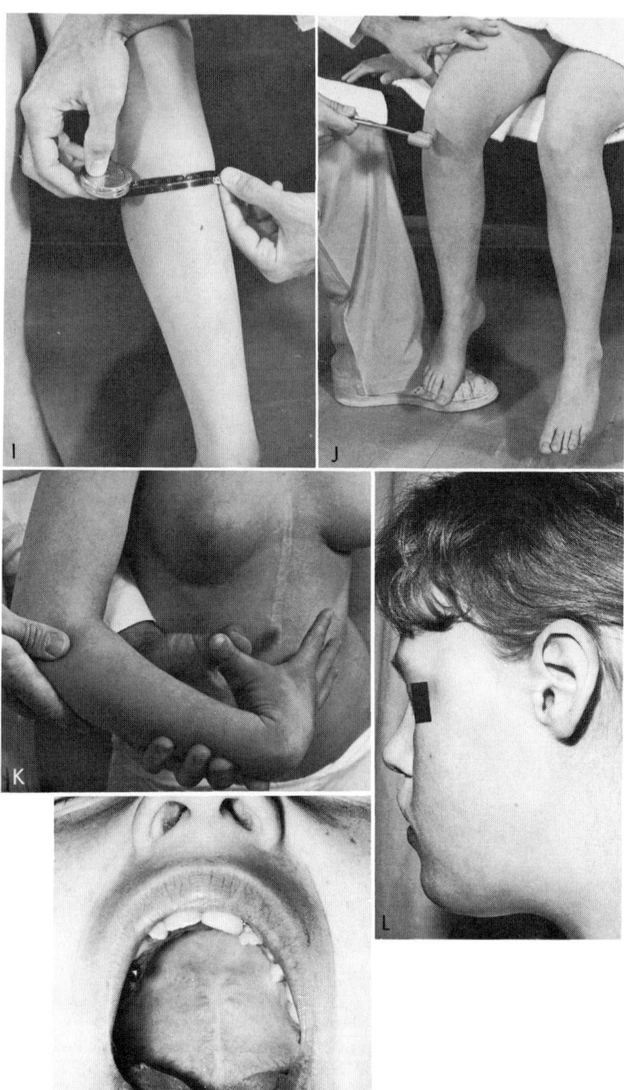

Figure 14–16 *Continued I,* Evidence of atrophy or hypertrophy should be determined by measurement. *J,* A complete neurologic evaluation should be made of every patient. *K,* All skin discolorations (café-au-lait) and scars (cardiac or other surgery) should be noted and recorded. Hypermobility of fingers and thumb should be tested. *L,* Abnormalities of the ears, nose, eyes, and extremities should be carefully noted. *M,* Abnormalities of bite, teeth, and palate should be recorded. The wearing of corrective orthodontic appliances should be recorded.

shoulder level, and (4) asymmetry in the distance between the arms and the torso. The patient is then asked to bend forward toward the examiner, dropping both arms vertically and holding the fingertips together, and the examiner notes any asymmetry of the rib case or lumbar area. A high rib cage on one side is invariably indicative of a thoracic curvature (Fig. 14–17). Asymmetry in the height of the lumbar area likewise denotes a rotational prominence of the lumbar spine, and hence spinal deformity. The height of the rib or lumbar prominence should be recorded. The way the patient bends forward is important: the child should bend straight forward without any deviation. Any persistent deviation to one side indicates an intraspinal irritative lesion (osteoid osteoma, bone or cord tumor) and warrants further tests (bone scan, computed tomography [CT], MRI). A plumbline should be dropped from the lower cervical spinous process at C7, and the distance from the vertical string to the gluteal cleft is a measurement of spinal imbalance. The patient is then requested to bend to each side. Extreme spinal spasm with inability to bend normally from side to side may be indicative of an intraspinal irritative lesion, such as a spinal cord tumor,

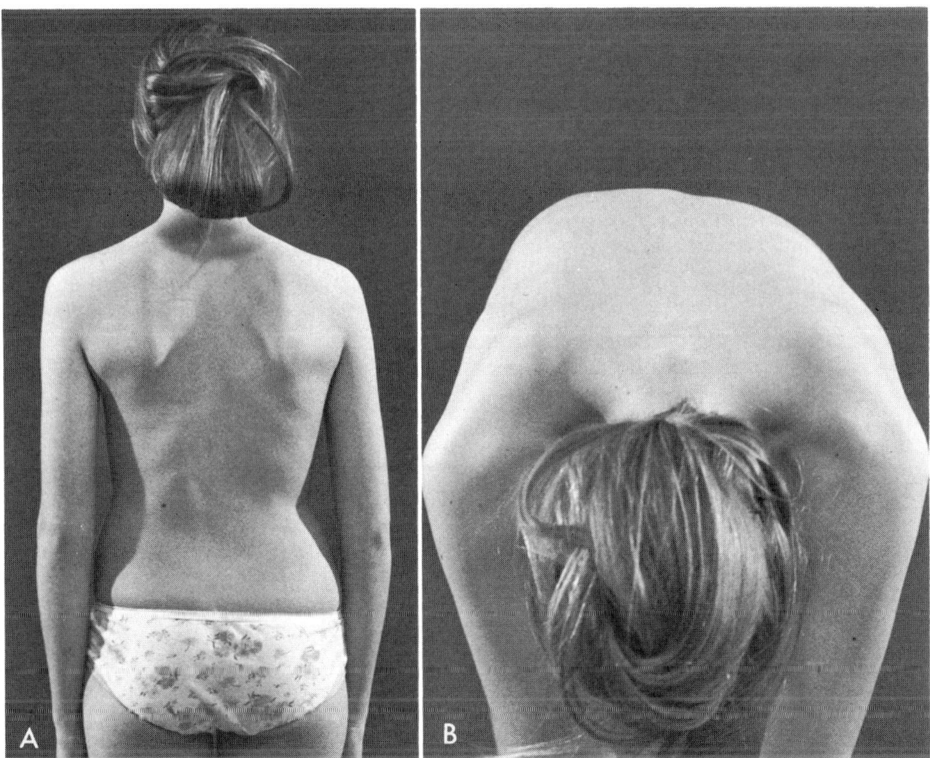

Figure 14–17. Careful examination by a school nurse resulted in early diagnosis of this curvature (10 degrees). Note the spine asymmetry in the flexed position *(B)*.

osteoid osteoma, or a herniated disc. The skin is examined for pigmented lesions, subcutaneous tumors, hairy patches, angiomas, and scars. Café au lait spots may be a manifestation of generalized neurofibromatosis. A hairy patch over the sacrum or lower lumbar spine is indicative of diastematomyelia until proved otherwise, and abnormal scarring with extreme elasticity may be a manifestation of Ehler-Danlos syndrome. Abnormalities of the extremities, appendages, mouth, and palate should be noted, and joint motions and contractures, especially in the hips, recorded. Measurements of leg lengths and circumferences and straight leg raising (SLR) tests should be carried out. Tight hamstrings with low back pain and spasms may be a manifestation of spondylolisthesis. Finally, a complete and careful neurologic examination, especially of the lower extremities, should be carried out and recorded. The patient's intelligence and mental status should be noted, and sitting and standing heights taken and recorded along with the arm span.

An assessment of physical maturity is important. This consists of Tanner grading of secondary sex characteristics in both sexes,[210] as well as noting the presence of axillary hair in boys, in whom this appearance coincides with the decreased slope of the growth curve.

Roentgenographic Evaluation

Roentgenographic evaluation of a child with spinal deformity is essential. In a young child, the entire spine and pelvis may be visualized on a 14 × 17 inch (36 × 43 cm) film. In older children and adolescents, longer films are necessary: 14 × 36 inches (36 × 91 cm). The whole spine is seen on the roentgenograph, and the relationship between the head, shoulders, upper trunk, and pelvis may be appreciated. Unnecessary exposure to x-rays should be avoided, and the technique used should reduce organ dosage as much as possible.[5, 51, 52, 82, 188] Only essential radiographs should be taken, with each examination tailored to the patient's problem. The x-ray beam should be collimated to reduce scatter. Beam filters give uniform radiographic density and filter unnecessary radiation. The use of faster radiographic films and intensifying screens (quanta rare earth screen) both aid in reducing exposure. The gonads are shielded and breast dosage is reduced by use of the posteroanterior (PA) position[5, 52, 171] or lead shields in the anteroposterior (AP) position.[82]

For patients being evaluated, only a standing PA view is necessary, additional views being taken as indicated. Supine side bending views are taken to evaluate curve flexibility and are indicated only when treatment (bracing or surgery) is prescribed. Traction roentgenograms may prove helpful if the patient has a severe curvature (greater than 70 degrees). In these patients, side bending views may not give a true indication of the flexibility of the deformity. A lateral standing view is taken before treatment so that the spine can be visualized in three dimensions, and also to evaluate hyper- or hypokyphosis. Any abnormalities noted in the lumbosacral area might be better delineated with a Ferguson view, which gives a true AP view of the lumbosacral joint. Any evidence of spondylolysis or spondylolisthesis necessitates oblique views in the lumbosacral area.

Radiographically, any abnormality suggests a diagnosis other than idiopathic scoliosis. Any apparent bony abnormality warrants further views (supine cone down view or tomography). Interpediculate widening raises the suspicion of an intraspinal lesion, and myelography or MRI is indicated. Since most thoracic curves are right-sided (see below), any left thoracic curve is evaluated for another etiology with a careful neurologic examination and MRI scan. The most frequent causes of this curve are an Arnold-Chiari malformation or syringomyelia.

Curve Evaluation

In the standing view, the curve pattern is identified (see below). Each curve is measured by the Cobb method (Fig. 14–18).[39] The end vertebrae are determined; these are the last ones that are tilted into the concavity of the curvature being measured. When they are parallel, the one farthest from the apex of the curve is the end vertebra. Once the caudal and cranial end vertebrae of each curve are identified, the curvature is measured by drawing a line along the end plate of the upper vertebra and another along the end plate of the lower vertebra. If these end plates are indistinct, the pedicle may be used instead. The angle formed by these two lines is measured and consists of the curve measurement. All curvatures should be measured. In double curves, the lower end vertebra of the upper curve is the upper end vertebra of the lower curve. Vertebral rotation may be determined by the method of Nash and Moe and may be graded I to IV, depending on the severity of rotation,[172] or may be measured by the Pedriolle technique.[182]

Skeletal Maturity

Skeletal maturity is measured not only by the patient's physiologic appearance but also radiographically by the bone age, iliac epiphysis, and vertebral ring apophysis. The bone age is determined by comparison of the wrist and hand roentgenogram with the standards found in the Greulich and Pyle atlas.[86] The ossification of the iliac apophysis is evaluated, and graded according to Risser. The vertebral ring epiphysis may be noted on the lateral roentgenogram of the vertebra; this consists of a separate ossification area that fuses to the vertebral body once vertebral maturation is complete. This appears to coincide well with complete cessation of vertebral growth.

Curve Patterns

The curves in idiopathic scoliosis fall into specific curve patterns that are classified as defined by the Terminology Committee of the Scoliosis Research Society. They are classified as to the site of the apical vertebra, and the curve patterns are as follows:

- Single high thoracic
- Single thoracic
- Single thoracolumbar
- Single lumbar
- Double major thoracic and lumbar
- Double major thoracic
- Double major thoracic and thoracolumbar
- Multiple patterns

A major curve is the structural and deforming curve, the curve that requires treatment, whereas a minor curve is less structural and

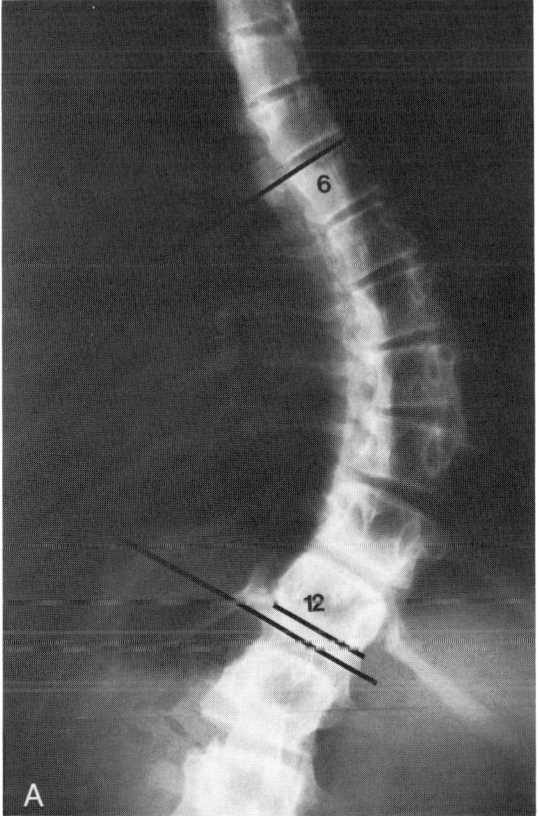

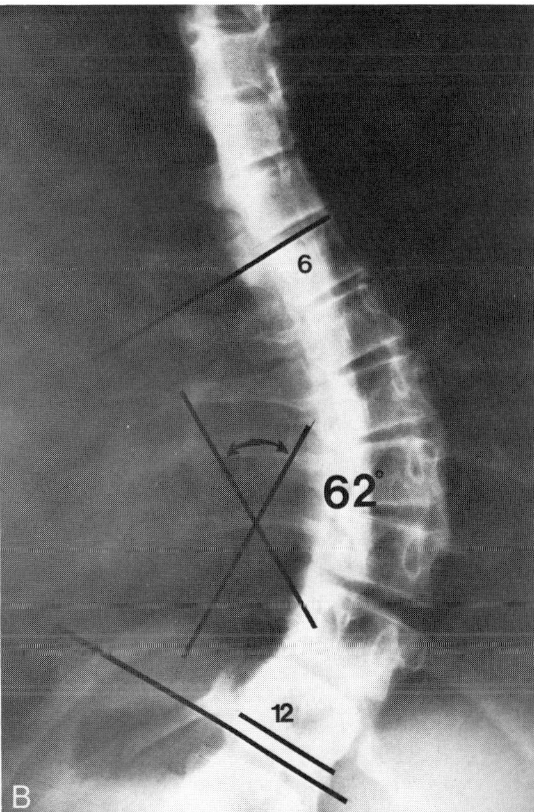

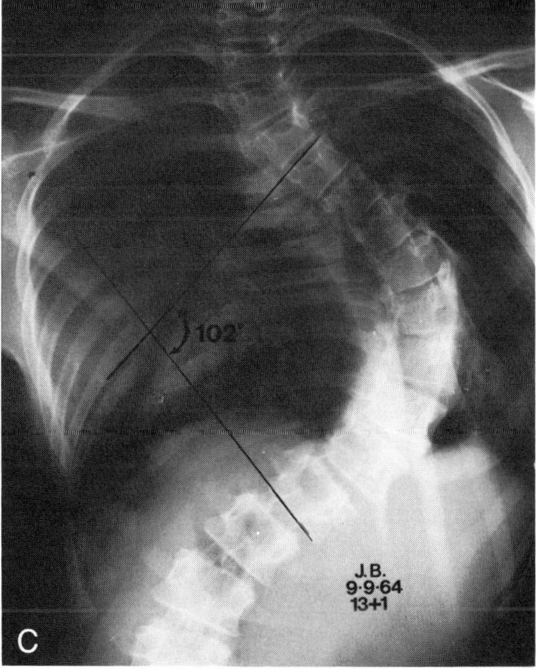

Figure 14–18. Cobb measurement of scoliosis. The end vertebrae (i.e., the vertebrae maximally tilted into the concavity of the curve) are chosen (T6 and T12). Lines are drawn at the end plates of these vertebrae *(A).* Note that at T12 an alternate line at the lower margin of the pedicles is shown. Using a protractor, lines at right angles to the end vertebral lines are drawn, and the angle formed by these lines is measured *(B).* In a larger curve the angle formed by the end vertebral lines can be directly measured *(C).* (From Bradford, D. S., Lonstein, J. E., Moe, J. H., et al.: Moe's Textbook of Scoliosis and Other Spinal Deformities, 2nd ed. Philadelphia, W. B. Saunders Co., 1987, p. 73.)

deforming and is often called a compensatory curve. To balance the torso, most of the major curves above are accompanied by compensatory curves.

Single High Thoracic Curve. The apex is in the high thoracic spine and the curve is usually a left thoracic curve. The upper vertebra is usually T1 or T2, but occasionally may be C7. There may be a lower thoracic compensatory curve, or an upper curve can be present alone. This pattern has been erroneously referred to as a cervicothoracic curve. This curve is associated with a high left thoracic prominence, as well as prominence of the trapezius neck line and occasionally elevation of the left shoulder.

Single Thoracic Curve. This is one of the most common and one of the most deforming patterns. The apex lies within the thoracic spine and is most commonly T8 or T9. The upper end vertebra can be from T4 to T6 and the lower end vertebra from T11 to L2, the most common being T5 to T12. The great majority (95 per cent) are right thoracic, so that any left thoracic curve is viewed with suspicion and warrants further evaluation. The spine in the area of this curve is often more lordotic, showing hypokyphosis or true lordosis on the lateral radiograph.

There is often a compensatory curve below, which may be as large as the thoracic curve and may cause confusion with the double major right thoracic left lumbar pattern. There are different types of right thoracic curves, as described by King and colleagues[117] and discussed below. The right shoulder is elevated, there is decompensation to the right, and there is a thoracic prominence whose magnitude varies. The amount of the prominence is not related to the magnitude of the thoracic curve or to the vertebral rotation.[26]

Single Thoracolumbar Curve. The apex of this curve is at T12 or L1, or the intervening disc, with the upper apex from T8 to T10 and the lower end vertebra usually L3. Most are right-sided with compensatory thoracic and lumbar curves. There is decompensation with loss of the waist fold on the convexity and accentuation on the concavity, plus an associated rotational prominence on forward bending.

Single Lumbar Curve. The apex is usually L2, with the upper end vertebra from T11 to L1 and the lower end vertebra L4 or L5. Most of the lumbar curves are convex left, and there is a compensatory curve above and below. There is decompensation, with marked distortion of the waistline similar to a thoracolumbar curve, and in addition there is a lumbar prominence on forward bending.

Double Major Thoracic and Lumbar Curves. This pattern consists of a thoracic and lumbar curve, both nearly the same magnitude with similar rigidity on supine side bending evaluation. The thoracic curve is usually convex right, with an apex at T7 or T8, upper end vertebra T4 to T6, and lower end vertebra T10 to T12. The left lumbar curve below has an apex at L2 and extends to L4, occasionally to L5. Because the curves are fairly equal in magnitude, the cosmetic appearance is good, with minimal decompensation and level shoulders. On forward bending there is both a right thoracic and a left lumbar prominence. This pattern is confused with the right thoracic curve with a compensatory lumbar curve, but differences exist both clinically (decompensation, shoulder level, and prominences) and radiographically (flexibility).

Double Major Thoracic Curve. This is typically a high left thoracic and a lower right thoracic curve and was first described by Moe.[163] The upper curve is short, with an apex at T3 or T4, and extends from T1 or T2 to T5 or T6. The lower curve extends to T11 to L2. The upper curve elevates the neck line and often the shoulder, and on forward bending there is both a high left and a lower right thoracic prominence. The upper curve is very structural on side bending view. This pattern is often not appreciated owing to use of a smaller cassette for radiographs that do not show the whole spine, and failure to obtain bending views of the high left curve.

Double Major Thoracic and Thoracolumbar Curves. This pattern usually consists of a right thoracic and a left thoracolumbar curve. The thoracic curve has an apex at T6 or T7 and extends from T4 to T9 or T10. The lower curve usually extends to L3 and has an apex at the disc between T12 and L1. Clinically the balance is good but the waistline is uneven. The thoracic prominence is usually less than the thoracolumbar prominence.

Multiple Curves. Multiple curves in a pattern do occur but are infrequent. The benign nature of these curves has been shown by Travaglini;[223] progression is rare and thus treatment is usually unnecessary.

Treatment

Infantile Idiopathic Scoliosis

The greater proportion of these children have nonprogressive curves, and thus this distinction is important. With vertebral rib relationship in Phase 1 and an RVAD of less than 20 degrees, the prognosis is good. The child is observed with follow-up radiographs at three- to four-month intervals. If resolution occurs, follow-up should continue until maturity at one-year intervals, because relapse can occur. With larger initial curves up to 30 or 35 degrees, a second evaluation is performed three months later. If the RVAD decreases, observation continues; if it increases, with or without curve increase, active treatment is instituted.

Active treatment is thus indicated for progressive curves (Mehta Phase 2 or RVAD of over 20 degrees) or curves that have an increased RVAD or curve magnitude under observation. The initial treatment is always nonoperative. Treatment is started immediately and further deterioration prevented. Under anesthesia, a well-fitting cast is applied and regularly reapplied until maximal curve correction has been obtained. At this stage a Milwaukee brace is fitted with full-time bracing (23 hours out of 24). The Milwaukee brace is preferable to a thoraco-lumbar-sacral-orthosis (TLSO). The circumferential TLSO causes rib pressure and results in a tubular thorax with reduction in pulmonary function; the Milwaukee brace prevents this. Occasionally a child presents with a very flexible curve. A Kallabis splint can be applied to a small child, with a change to a Milwaukee brace as soon as the child is large enough. This can be as early as 8 to 12 months of age and depends on the expertise of the orthotist. In most patients bracing continues full time until the adolescent growth spurt, when control is lost and spinal fusion is necessary.

Mehta reported that some curves falling into the progressive category may not require surgery because of excellent and lasting correction obtained by repeated casting.[151, 152] The casting is continued until the RVAD is zero and for six months thereafter, and then the brace is fitted. If correction is maintained in the brace, it is possible to wean the child out of and even discontinue the brace. The child is observed until maturity for relapse, which can occur. Mehta and Morel[151] observed that if the curve is totally corrected before the pubertal growth spurt, there is no relapse during adolescence. If full correction is not obtained, relapse can occur.

In some patients curve control cannot be maintained with bracing, and then the option of surgical stabilization needs consideration. In the older juvenile this may be an option, but it must be remembered that a fused portion of spine does not grow, and thus stunting of trunk growth results. An alternative is instrumentation without fusion. End fusions, as described by Marchetti and Faldini,[144] are performed with insertion of a Harrington or Moe rod without concomitant fusion. The spine is exposed only in the area of the end fusions, special small-blade pediatric hooks are used, and the rod is inserted under the muscle fascia or subcutaneously. The spine is still protected with a Milwaukee brace, with rod lengthenings every six months and replacements every 12 to 18 months. With this technique, additional spinal growth is obtained and fusion is delayed.[160]

In some patients, because of a larger or more rigid curve, instrumentation without fusion is difficult. In these cases the rigid apical area of the curve, as seen on a traction film, can be treated by hemiepiphysiodesis and posterior hemiarthrodesis. This is performed at the same time as the end fusion and rod insertion, and allows control of the curve apex with continued growth at the curve limits.

When fusion becomes necessary because of a loss of control with curve increase, in the late juvenile years or adolescence, the choices are between posterior fusion alone and a combined anterior and posterior fusion. McMaster and colleagues showed that curve progression[149] and, more important, increased rotation occur[93] with a posterior fusion alone. If the fusion is not substantial, the anterior growth causes curve increase. With a strong substantial fusion the posterior growth ceases. The vertebral bodies continue to increase in height, but lordosis is prevented by the bulk of the posterior fusion. The bodies increase in height, and disc spaces narrow. At this stage the continued anterior growth causes the bodies to rotate on the posterior fusion mass (the "crankshaft" effect). This causes curve increase on measurements and, more important, increase in rib prominence. This is prevented by the use of a combined anterior and posterior spinal fusion in the juvenile or early adolescent years.

Juvenile Idiopathic Scoliosis

In general, curves under 25 degrees are observed in juveniles. With curve increase, active treatment is indicated. Curves presenting under age 6 are treated very similarly to those of the infantile type as discussed above, i.e., serial casting, bracing, use of subcutaneous rod with end fusion, and also hemiarthrodesis and hemiepiphysiodesis and combined anterior and posterior fusions.

Curves first detected in the latter part of the juvenile years that are over 25 degrees or have shown documented progression should be treated. Nonoperative treatment with the Milwaukee brace is the treatment of choice, as discussed above. The brace is worn full time for 18 months to two years and then the control achieved is assessed. If there is good control of the curvature with reduction to under 20 degrees, part-time bracing is instituted. A radiograph is taken after the child has been out of the brace for four hours. If the control is maintained, brace-wearing time is reduced to 20 hours per day. Three months later a radiograph is taken six hours after the brace is removed: with continued control, more time, i.e., six hours, is allowed out of the brace. This is repeated, with increasing time out of the brace until the child wears the brace only while sleeping. With continued stability, an attempt is made to leave the child out of the brace. If no curve increase occurs, brace use may be discontinued, even though the child has not yet reached the growth spurt. Continued observation for relapse is necessary until maturity, so that treatment can be promptly reinstituted.

When weaning is unsuccessful or the curve in the brace is over 30 degrees, full-time bracing continues until the pubertal growth spurt. At this time curve control can be maintained, and bracing continues until maturity. If curve increase occurs at this time, a spinal fusion is indicated. In some patients, in spite of an excellent bracing program, the curve may increase before the growth spurt. In these cases the instrumentation without fusion program,[120] with or without apical hemiepiphysiodesis and hemiarthrodesis, may be indicated.

The success of nonoperative treatment varies. Figueiredo and James[72] reported a 56 per cent surgical rate, while Tolo and Gillespie[221] described only a 16 per cent rate and Lonstein and Winter[135] a 50 per cent rate. In the last-named series it was seen that children weaned before adolescence had slightly smaller curves and were younger when treatment was started. On the other hand, those who required bracing until maturity had larger curves and were older at the start of bracing.

The surgical decisions regarding selection of fusion area are the same as in the adolescent. The role of anterior fusion in the younger adolescent to prevent curve increase and the "crankshaft" effect is important.[93] For maximal benefit of curve stabilization and cosmetic improvement, greater use is probably indicated.

Adolescent Idiopathic Scoliosis

When an adolescent presents with idiopathic scoliosis, after a full physical evaluation has been made to exclude other causes of scoliosis and a standing radiograph taken, the important facts for decision making have been collected. These are the child's growth potential (age, Tanner grading, menarche in girls, axillary hair appearance in boys, and Risser sign) and curve characteristics (curve pattern and magnitude).

The choices for treatment are observation, nonoperative or operative. In general, all curves over 45 to 50 degrees in the adolescent are treated operatively. For curves under 45 degrees the first question is: "Is the child still growing?" In a child near or at the end of growth, the curve is followed for progression. Larger curves that progress require surgical stabilization. Some progression can be accepted in smaller curves as the child matures, as long as the curve remains under 40 degrees and the progression does not continue. In these cases a repeat standing PA roentgenogram is obtained every six to 12 months until maturity and cessation of growth.

When the child is still growing, treatment depends on the curve magnitude. First, it needs to be emphasized that there is *no* role for exercise alone in these cases. Although exercises have been used for many years in many centers, there is no report documenting the beneficial effect of exercise with improvement in progressive curves.

With a curve under 25 degrees in the growing child, and no history, the curve is followed for progression. A repeat roentgenogram is taken after six to eight months if the initial curve is under 20 degrees, and after three to four months for larger curves. A 5-degree change is called progression, and for some smaller curves a 10-degree change is necessary. If the curve progresses, nonoperative treatment is indicated. With no progression, observation continues to maturity. Not all progressive curves require treatment, as not all progression is equal, the rate of progression being important. A 12-year-old girl with Risser 0 grading who has progression from 20 to 28 degrees over six months needs treatment. On the other hand, a 12-year-old graded Risser 0 who has progression from 22 to 34 degrees over three years while she matures, and is one year post menarche and Risser 4, does not need treatment.

An actively growing child with a curve of 25 to 40 degrees, or curves with documented progression, requires nonoperative treatment. The choices of nonoperative treatment are electrical stimulation or orthotic therapy.

Electrical Stimulation. Electrical stimulation of the muscles on the convexity of the curve has been advocated for adolescent idiopathic scoliosis. This has been by means of implanted[21, 96] or surface[11, 12, 26, 108, 147, 148] electrodes. Initial studies of transcutaneous stimulation showed good results, but these included patients still under treatment, very few being mature and off treatment.[11, 12, 26, 147, 178] Many smaller studies have questioned these good results.[2, 23, 215] A review[132] of over 200 patients who had completed treatment showed that the results obtained, with failures defined as surgery or a 5-degree or more curve increase from pretreatment to follow-up, were not different from what could be expected from natural history predictions. This study took into account that the protocol for the stimulator required progression before treatment was initiated. The stimulator thus is not a choice for nonoperative treatment, since it does not affect the natural history.

Orthotic Treatment[113, 239]

Milwaukee Brace.[133] The first successful orthosis for the treatment of adolescent idiopathic scoliosis was the Milwaukee brace (cervico-thoraco-lumbo-sacral orthosis, or CTLSO). It was first developed in 1945 by Drs. Walter Blount and Al Schmidt for the postoperative treatment of postpoliomyelitis scoliosis. It was specifically designed for the treatment of thoracic deformity by the use of a lateral force at the apex of the curve, coupled with a longitudinal force. It is this lack of constrictive forces on the thorax that makes this orthosis the ideal for treating thoracic curves. It is often forgotten, in our enthusiasm to provide low-profile orthoses, that the prime reason for the treatment of thoracic scoliosis is preservation of pulmonary function.

The principles of manufacture are well covered in the monograph of Blount and Moe.[20] The primary indication is for a single right thoracic curve or a double curve pattern with a right thoracic component. This, as stated above, is seen in an actively growing child (Risser 0, 1, or 2) with a documented progressive curve or an initial curve of between 25 or 30 and 40 degrees. Occasionally a young child with a Risser grading of 0 and a curve of 40 to 50 degrees can be successfully treated in a Milwaukee brace.

The Milwaukee brace consists of a molded pelvic section (custom molded or manufactured—"Boston brace system"[68]) with two posterior uprights and one anterior upright, connected to a neck ring that has a thorax mold and two occipital pads (Fig. 14–19). Pads are added to the brace, depending on the curve pattern: a trapezius pad for a high thoracic curve, a thoracic pad for a thoracic curve, combination of an oval pad and a lumbar pad for a thoracolumbar curve, and a lumbar pad for a lumbar curve. Attention must be paid to the sagittal view, with the thoracic pad positioned under the posterior upright for hyperkyphosis, and lateral to the upright with no outrigger anteriorly for hypokyphosis.

The brace is worn full time with time out for bathing, swimming, physical education, and sports. This totals a maximum of two to four hours a day, and thus brace wearing is 20 to 22 hours daily. Part-time bracing has been suggested by Green[83] and others, but their series are small with no long-term results. Follow-up is every four months with radiographs in the brace at each visit and appropriate brace adjustments for growth. At the end of growth, as evidenced by no height increase, a Risser 4 grading, and the patient being 12 to 18 months post menarche, weaning is started. A radiograph is taken four hours after the brace is removed. If the curve control is maintained, this amount of time is allowed out of the brace. This is repeated every visit with an additional four hours out until the child wears the brace only while sleeping (usually during

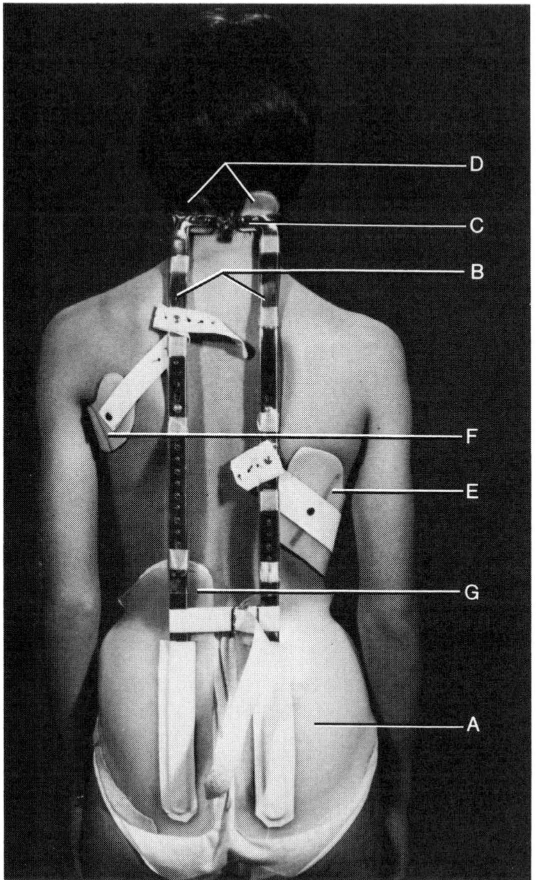

Figure 14–19. Milwaukee brace for a right thoracic left lumbar double curve. The pelvic section (A) has two posterior uprights (B) and one anterior upright attached superiorly to a neckring (C) with two occipital pads posteriorly (D) and a throat mold anteriorly. Attached to the uprights are a right thoracic pad (E) and a left axillary sling (F). The left lumbar pad is under the plastic of the lumbar extension of the pelvic section (G).

the last six to 12 months of treatment). This regimen has given the best results (see below) (Figs. 14–20, 14–21).

Thoracolumbar Sacral Orthoses (TLSO). This group of orthoses can be divided into the higher underarm type that comes up to one or both axillae, used for thoracic curves, and the lower type that extends to the lower thoracic area, used for thoracolumbar or lumbar curves. In many centers the high TLSO is used extensively,[13, 14, 29, 89, 155, 193] but most results are short term or preliminary. Many still believe, because of the open design and minimal thoracic compression in the Milwaukee brace, that this is the best choice for thoracic curves, the low TLSO being reserved for thoracolumbar or lumbar curves.

The low TLSO (Fig. 14–22) has a lumbar pad for lumbar curves. The indications for treatment, wearing schedule, and weaning are the same as for the Milwaukee brace for thoracic curves (Fig. 14–23). It must be remembered that these curves are less common and progress less frequently.

Results. Before the results of orthotic treatment are discussed, it must be realized that there are problems with reported studies. There is no matched untreated control group, and studies do not compare results of bracing with studies of natural history. Many studies evaluate results of curve responses to the brace rather than response of the curve patterns, e.g., the thoracic curve in double curve patterns is analyzed together with the single right thoracic curve.

Most studies discuss averages, which disposes of the variation in groups. All age groups, juvenile and adolescent, are combined and all curve magnitudes, 20- and 40-degree curves, assessed together. In averaging results the true picture is not seen. For example, if ten curves start out at 30 degrees before treatment, and at the end five curves are of 20 degrees and five of 40 degrees, this would be

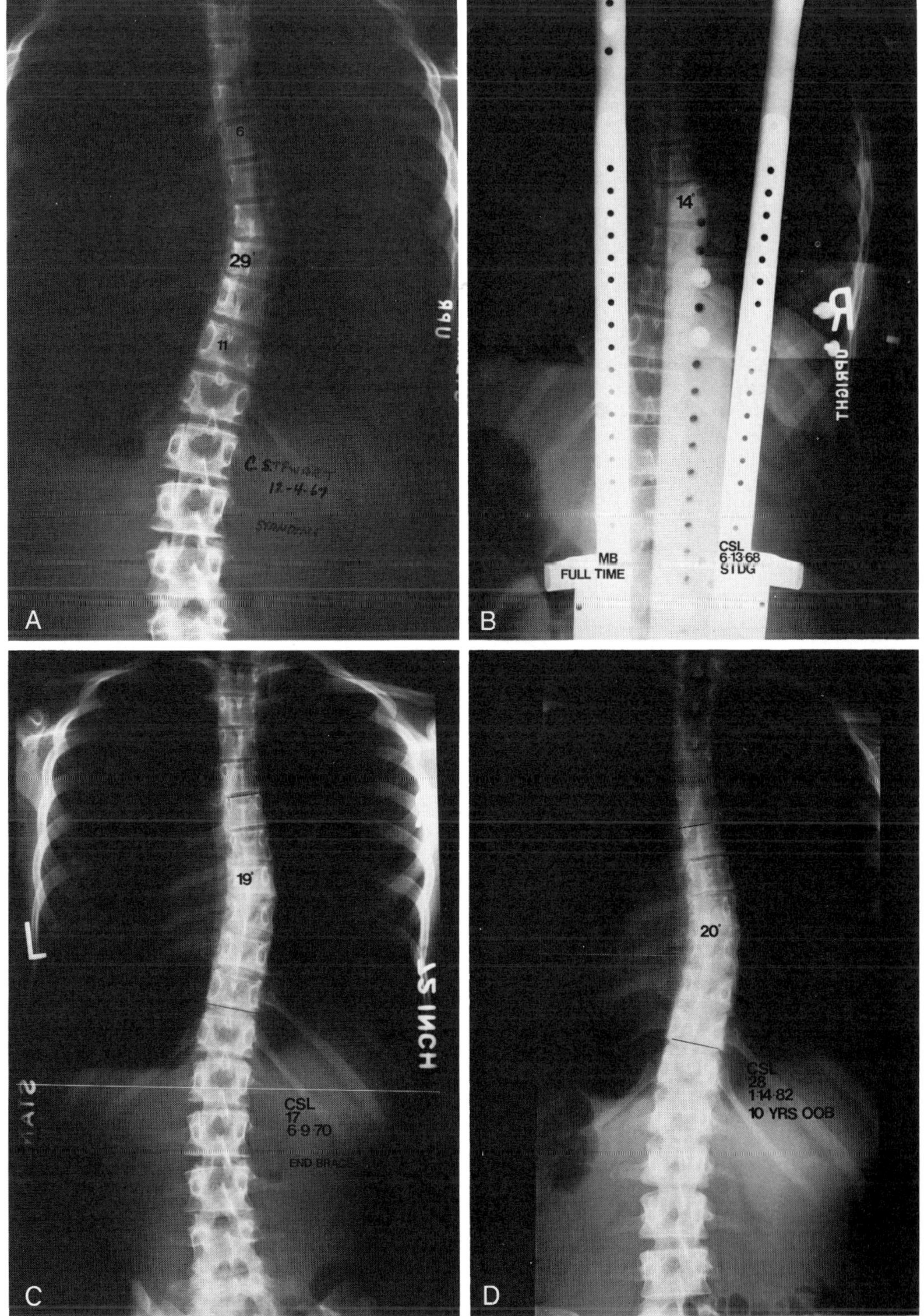

Figure 14–20. C. S. presented at age 14 years with a right thoracic curve of 29 degrees *(A)*. A Milwaukee brace was fitted with excellent correction in the brace to 14 degrees *(B)*. At the end of brace wearing 3½ years later, the curve correction was maintained at 19 degrees *(C)*. Ten years later there was no loss, the curve measuring 20 degrees *(D)*.

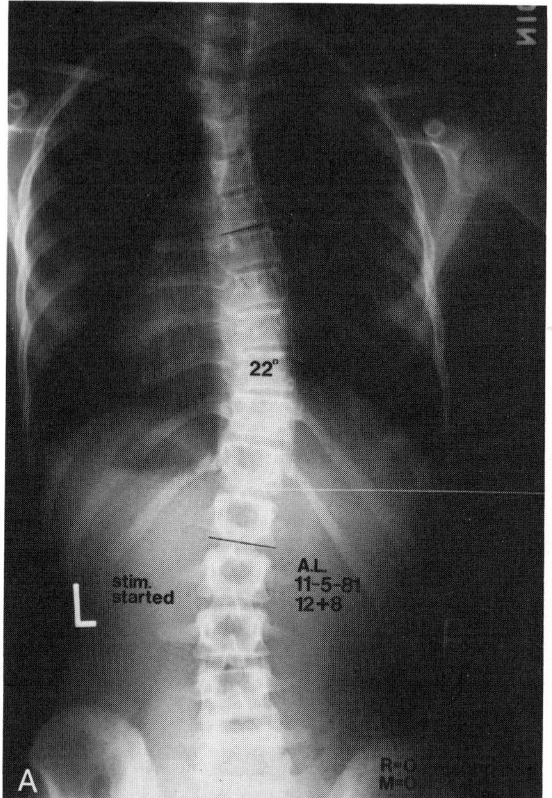

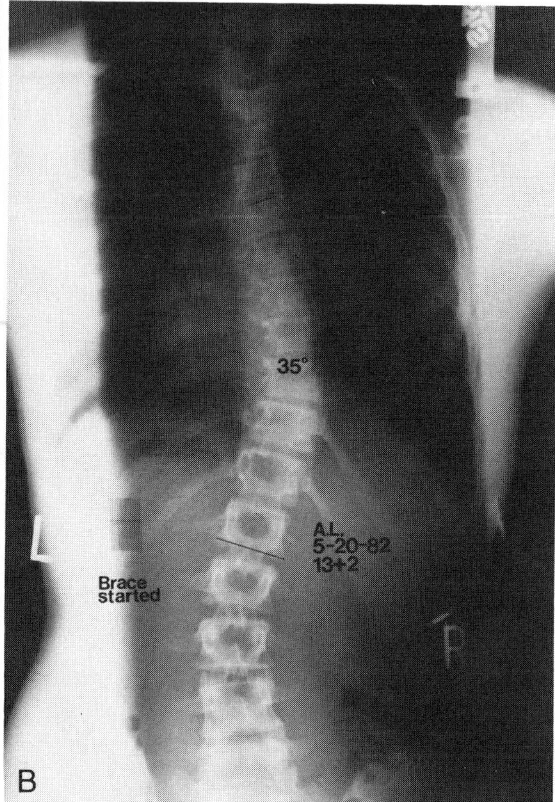

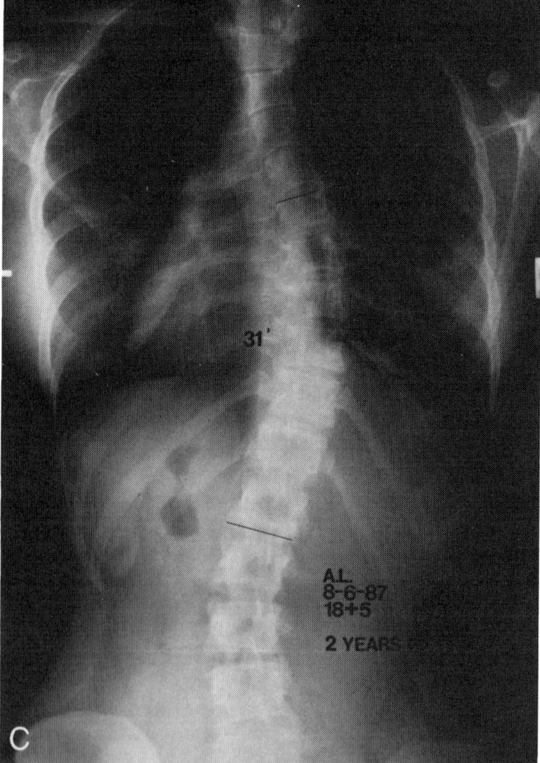

Figure 14–21. A. L. presented at age 12 years, 8 months with a curve of 22 degrees that had shown documented progression. She was immature, being premenarchal with a Risser sign of 0 *(A)*. The transcutaneous stimulator was prescribed. After six months' use it was seen that progression continued, the curve now measuring 35 degrees *(B)*. A Milwaukee brace was prescribed and worn full time. After three years of brace wearing, the brace was discontinued. Two years later the curve was still controlled, and measured 31 degrees *(C)*. This case represents failure of the stimulator, with subsequent brace success in preventing continued progression.

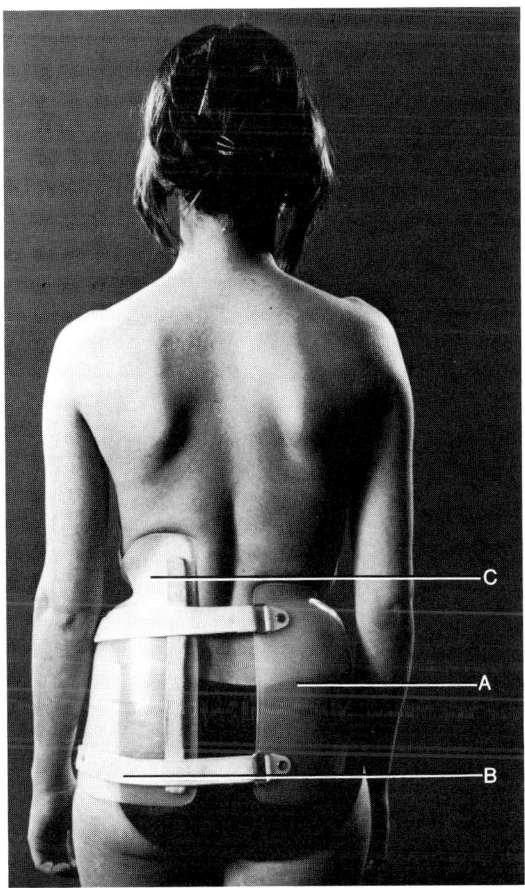

Figure 14–22. Thoracolumbosacral orthosis (TLSO) for a single left lumbar curve. The pelvic section *(A)* has a left trochanteric extension *(B)* with the lumbar pad under the left lumbar extension of the orthosis *(C)*.

reported as "average initial curve, 30 degrees and average final curve, 30 degrees"—no change, which obviously is not the true picture. Large standard deviations exist, and the results must reflect this.

The definition of "good" or "bad" results is difficult. Surgery is described as a failure of treatment, but the indications vary with time and also from center to center, making comparisons difficult. An increase of 5 degrees or more is regarded as a bad result, but not all increases are the same. If a curve increases from 38 to 44 degrees and surgery is needed, this is a bad result. But what about an increase from 30 to 36 degrees with no change thereafter, and a stable curve?

With the above limitations in mind, the Milwaukee brace results will be reviewed. The best are from the long-term studies of Mellencamp and colleagues,[154] Carr and associates,[34] Moe and Kettleson,[159] Edmonson and colleagues,[66, 67] Keiser and Shufflebarger,[114] Shufflebarger and associates,[210] Salanova,[202] Emans and colleagues,[68] and Lonstein and Winter.[134] All these studies show similar results. There is initial improvement with the Milwaukee brace, which can be as much as 50 per cent in the first six to nine months of treatment. After this there is gradual loss of improvement, so that at the end of bracing the average curve is about 15 per cent better than the pre-brace curve. After five or more years out of the brace, the average curve is about the same as the initial pre-brace curve. As noted above, the averages can be misleading.

Only one study has compared the results with the natural history and has concentrated on curve patterns rather than on curves. Lonstein and Winter[134] reviewed 1020 adolescents treated with the Milwaukee brace, with 54 per cent of patients having more than two years' follow-up after stopping use of the brace (average 6.2 years). Two thirds of the prebrace curves were between 20 and 39 degrees. The overall surgical rate was 22 per cent, the most frequent indications for surgery being initial response in the brace and then curve increase, or no improvement in the brace. The surgical rate was similar for the main curve patterns, being slightly higher with the double thoracic pattern. The rate increased with increasing curve magnitude, especially for curves over 30 degrees.

The results were compared with natural history studies. Curve increase was defined as those cases needing surgery plus those cases that at follow-up were 5 or more degrees larger than the prebrace curve. The single right thoracic curves of 20 to 39 were analyzed. For curves of 20 to 29 degrees the Milwaukee brace results showed an increase in 30 per cent with Risser grading 0 or 1 and 11 per cent with Risser 2 or more, compared with natural history figures of 68 and 23 per cent, respectively. For curves of 30 to 39 degrees the Milwaukee brace results were 39 per cent (Risser 0 to 1) and 18 per cent (R2+), showing curve increase compared with natural history predictions of 57 and 43 per cent, respectively. All these figures are half of the natural history predictions, indicating that the Milwaukee brace alters the natural history of idiopathic scoliosis.

There are few studies of TLSO results for lumbar and thoracolumbar curves.[57, 68, 240]

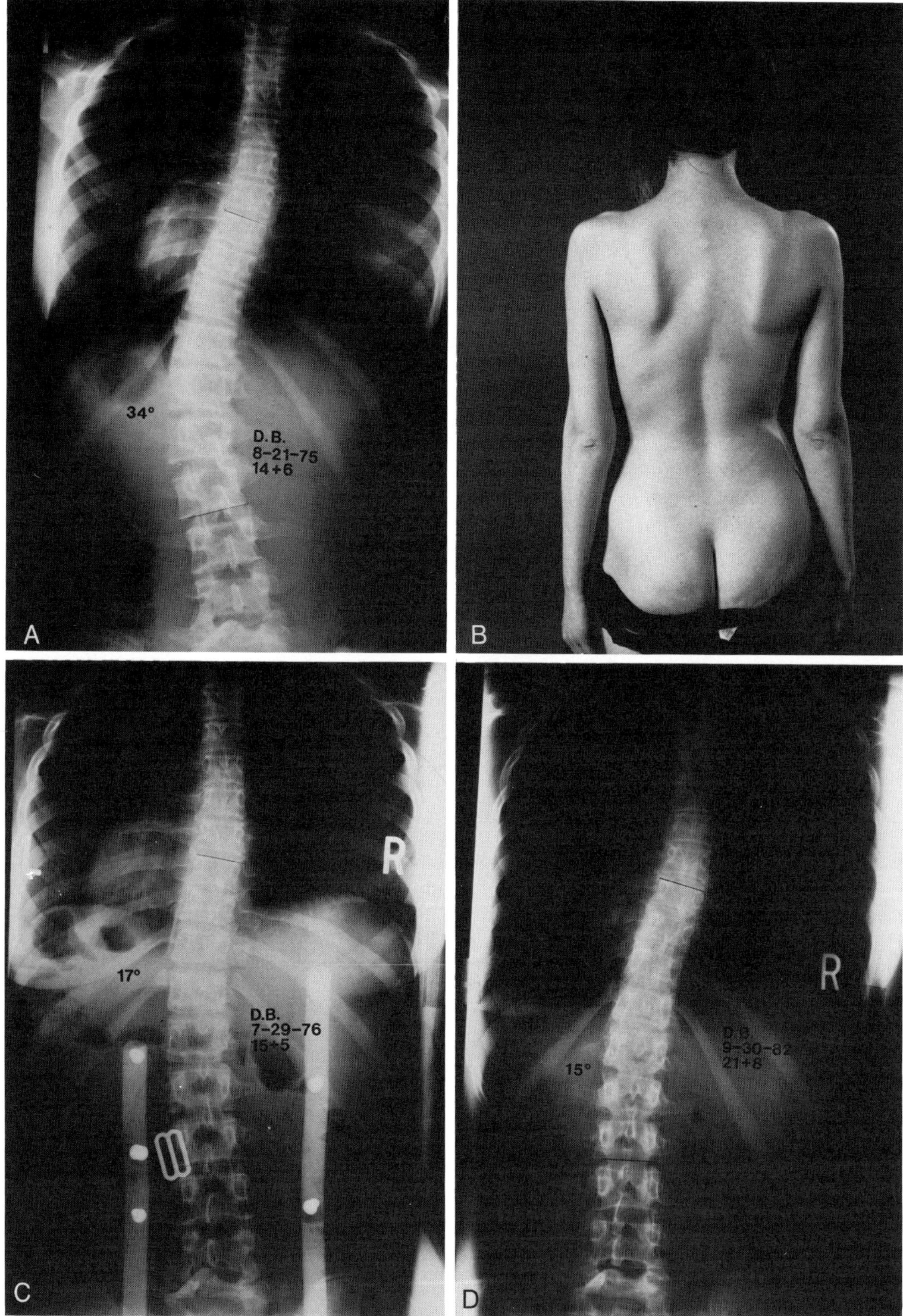

Figure 14–23. D. B. presented at age 14 years, 6 months with a 34-degree left thoracolumbar curve *(A)*. She was fitted with a TLSO as she was still growing and had a curve that was deforming her waistline *(B)*. In the TLSO the curve was corrected to 17 degrees *(C)*. The brace was worn for 3½ years. After the patient had been out of the brace for two years, the curve at age 21 years, 8 months was stable at 15 degrees *(D)*.

These show good control of these curves, with an extremely low fusion rate. In these curves, efforts are made to avoid surgery, because fusion of the lumbar spine reduces spinal motion.

Operative Treatment

The indications for operative treatment in adolescents are: (1) a child still actively growing presenting with a 40- to 45-degree curve, (2) progression in a child undergoing nonoperative therapy, or (3) curves over 50 to 60 degrees in a mature adolescent. The decision for surgery cannot be based on the Cobb measurement alone: other factors must be taken into account. The age of the child, and thus the growth potential and possibility of progression in adolescence and adulthood, are important. A 45-degree curve in an 11-year-old premenarchal female has a high likelihood of progressing, whereas the same curve in a 17-year-old is unlikely to progress in the late adolescent years and in adulthood. The clinical appearance is important. The rotational prominence and presence of thoracic hypokyphosis or true lordosis have a bearing on the chances of successful brace therapy, and in a curve of 35 degrees or more may tip the scale to surgery rather than bracing. The clinical appearance when there is a markedly unbalanced decompensated torso must also be considered.

Preoperative Evaluation

Preoperative evaluation includes a full examination and neurologic evaluation. Once surgery is recommended, radiographs in addition to the standing PA view are necessary. A lateral view is obtained so that the spine can be appreciated in three dimensions. Supine side bending views are obtained of each curve to assess its flexibility. In curves of over 60 degrees, a traction view is more accurate in determining flexibility. In the presence of increased thoracic kyphosis, a hyperextension view shows the flexibility of the kyphosis.

Pulmonary function testing is performed on larger thoracic curves of over 60 degrees. It is also necessary in cases of marked thoracic lordosis, owing to the demonstrated adverse effect of these curves on breathing ability.[242] Preoperative casting, with surgery performed in the cast, was the standard operative technique until the early 1970s;[90, 92, 165] this allowed safe correction, and with Cotrel traction was thought to increase the amount of correction. However, studies showed that Cotrel traction did not increase the amount of curve correction possible or decrease the complications.[18, 53, 65, 79, 125, 168] Second, the advent of spinal cord monitoring[69, 225] supplied a way to monitor spinal cord function during correction, thus preventing overdistraction and possible neurologic loss. In general, the spine has a certain amount of flexibility, which is well seen on a supine film with maximal active side bending. This is the amount of "give" the spine has and a good indication of the amount of correction to be expected at surgery. Traction, usually halo gravity, does play a role in patients with severe curves and pulmonary compromise. Here the traction allows partial correction of the deformity, allowing the abdominal contents to fall out of the chest cage and thus permitting more efficient diaphragmatic action. This allows for active pulmonary toilet, with improvement in pulmonary status, allowing surgery to be performed. This is unusual in idiopathic scoliosis and occurs much more frequently in neuromuscular conditions.

Decision Making

In the process of spinal fusion, certain decisions have to be made: the curves to be fused, the levels to be fused, the instrumentation needed, and the surgical approach. It must be remembered that the aim of surgical treatment is correction and stabilization of the curvature, with prevention of future progression. This should be performed as safely as possible, maximizing the clinical and radiographic results.

Selection of Fusion Area

The selection of fusion area involves the questions: Which curve to fuse? Which levels to fuse? The decision is made after analyzing the clinical appearance and the standing and bending views. Using these, the curve pattern is identified. All major curves need to be fused. The most common errors seen are (1) failure to recognize the thoracic curve with a flexible compensatory curve below, mistakenly calling this a double major curve pattern; and (2) failure to recognize the double thoracic pattern. Articles by King and colleagues[117, 118] described the curve patterns in thoracic idiopathic scoliosis (Table 14–7) and are an important addition to the literature.

The choice of levels to be fused is based on careful analysis of curve patterns by Moe[164, 165] and Goldstein,[80, 81] using vertebral rotation to select the fusion area.[22, 80, 81, 164, 165] These authors suggested that the levels of fusion extend from the neutrally rotated vertebra above to the neutrally rotated vertebra below, vertebral rotation being determined by the Nash and Moe method.[170] In addition, the lower vertebra has to be balanced over the sacrum, falling into the stable zone of Harrington.[91, 92] Thus, the surgical decision is generally made after analysis of the standing and side bending views and the clinical appearance, especially rotational prominences, which all determine the curve pattern. Then, on the standing view, all vertebrae of the major curve need to be fused from neutral vertebra to neutral vertebra, and the lower fusion vertebra must lie on the midsacral line, i.e., be the stable vertebra. There are two exceptions to these rules. First, in fusion of a thoracolumbar or lumbar curve anteriorly, the fusion is less than the measured curve. Second, in long thoracic curves extending to L5 (King Type IV) or in some double curves with L5 still rotated into the curve, the fusion can be stopped at L4, short of the neutral vertebra.

The reliability of these rules was shown by King and colleagues in a review of 405 cases of thoracic and thoracic and lumbar scoliosis treated by Moe and the other surgeons in the Twin Cities.[117] The most important finding supported Moe's concept of selective fusion of the thoracic curve only with a flexible lumbar curve (King Type II) (Fig. 14–24). In these cases the lumbar curve spontaneously balances the fused thoracic curve. The saving of mobile lumbar segments is important since Cochran and associates[40] showed an increase of low back pain with fusion into the low lumbar spine. The importance of fusion to neutral vertebrae and with the lower vertebra falling on the midsacral line was also confirmed. The article also emphasized the appreciation of the double thoracic pattern. These rules have been found to apply irrespective of the posterior instrumentation system used.

The spine must be appreciated in three dimensions when selecting the fusion area. When there is thoracic hyperkyphosis, this deformity needs to be addressed in the fusion. Thus, the fusion area must encompass all the vertebrae to be fused considering the scoliosis and all the vertebrae to be fused considering the sagittal view.

Table 14–7. CURVE PATTERNS

Type I
- S-shaped curve in which both thoracic and lumbar curves cross midline
- Lumbar curve is larger than thoracic curve
- Lumbar curve is less flexible than thoracic when thoracic curve is larger than lumbar curve

Type II
- S-shaped curve; both thoracic and lumbar curves cross midline
- Thoracic curve equal to or greater than lumbar curve
- Lumbar curve more flexible than thoracic curve

Type III
- Thoracic curve where lumbar curve does not cross midline

Type IV
- Long thoracic curve in which L4 tilts into thoracic curve

Type V
- Double thoracic curve with T1 tilted into convexity of upper thoracic curve
- Upper thoracic curve structural on side bending

From King, H. A.: Selection of fusion levels for posterior instrumentation and fusion in idiopathic scoliosis. Orthop. Clin. North Am. *19*:247–255, 1988.

Instrumentation and Approach

Since the development of the Harrington rod and its introduction in 1960,[92] instrumentation has been standard in spinal fusions. The rod gives additional correction and internal stability, allowing ambulation, while the fusion incorporates with a lower pseudarthrosis rate. The original instrumentation introduced by Harrington consisted of a distraction rod on the concavity of the curve and a compression rod on the convexity.[92] Many surgeons, including Moe,[162, 166, 190] used only the distraction rod (Fig. 14–25). Modifications of the system developed with the addition of a device for transverse traction (DTT) by Cotrel and associates[43] and Armstrong and Connock,[6] sublaminar wires,[98, 211, 219, 220, 238, 241] and spinous process wires[58, 59, 84, 90, 191, 238] attached to a Harrington distraction rod with the addition of a convex Luque C rod (Wisconsin system).[28, 40, 92] Luque instrumentation was used in some centers for the treatment of idiopathic scoliosis.[4, 16, 17, 28, 40, 44, 92] The newest instrumenta-

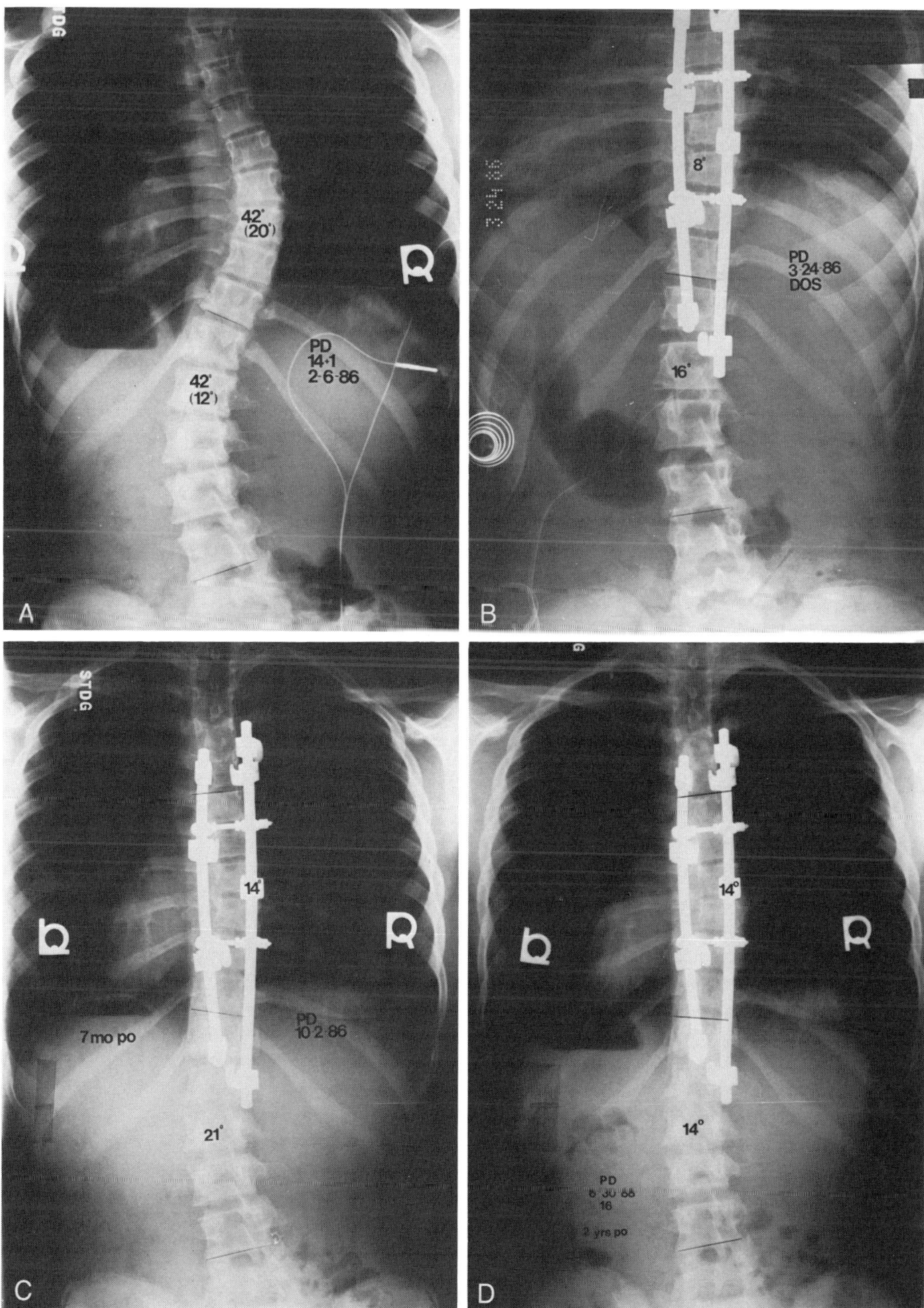

Figure 14–24. P. D. at age 14 years, 1 month had failed stimulator treatment and progressed to a 42-degree right thoracic and 42-degree left lumbar curve. The lumbar curve was more flexible, correcting to 12 degrees, and thus she had a right thoracic curve with a compensatory left lumbar curve—a false double major curve *(A)*. She underwent a posterior fusion and CD instrumentation of the right thoracic curve alone with correction to 8 degrees on the day of surgery *(B)*. She was not braced postoperatively. A seven-month postoperative lumbar curve measured 21 degrees, a worrisome increase *(C)*. With no treatment, at two years postoperatively the curves were balanced at 14 degrees *(D)*. With progression of the lumbar curve a TLSO may be used to control it.

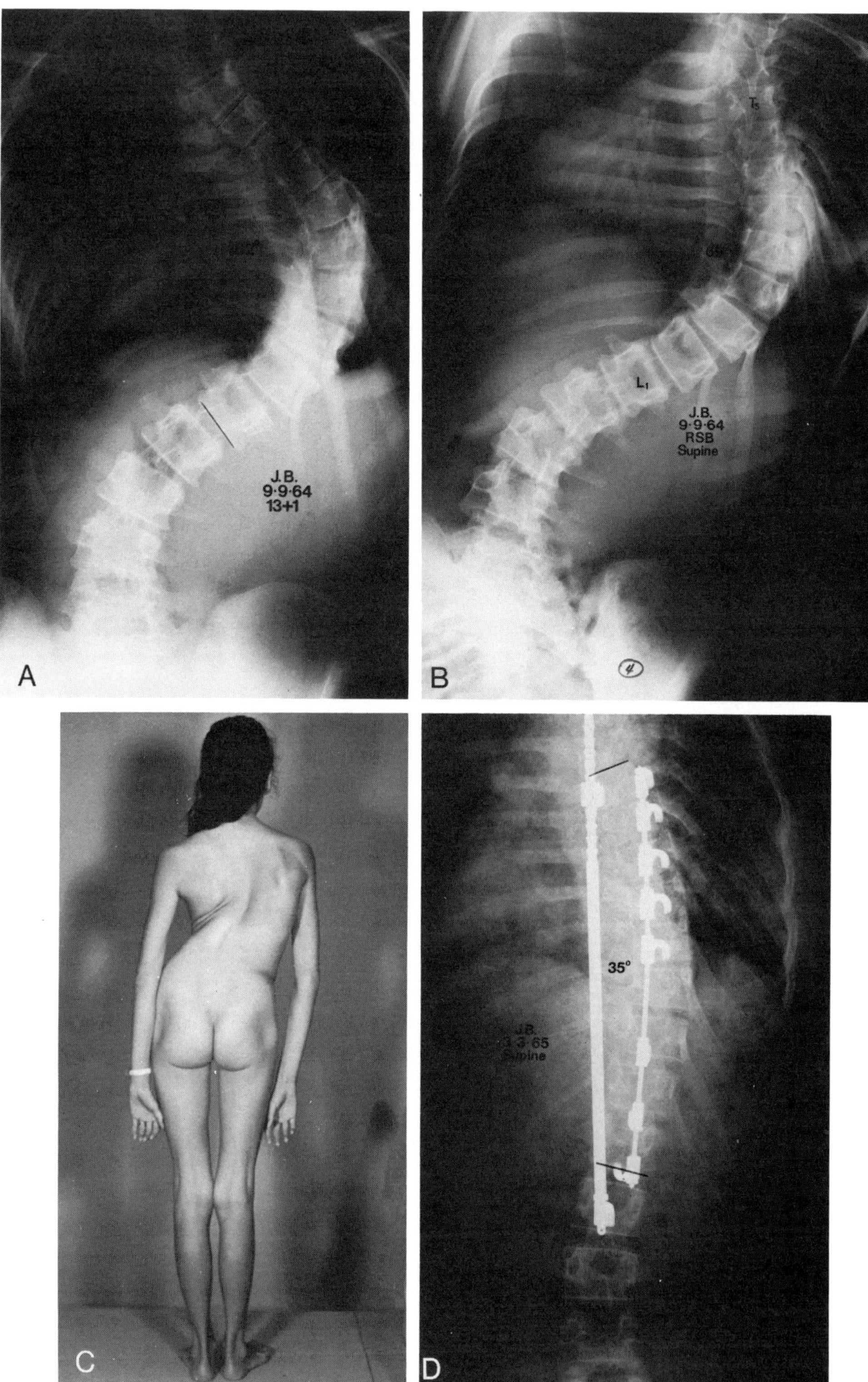

Figure 14–25. J. B. presented at age 13 years, 1 month with a 102-degree right thoracic curve *(A)*, which corrected to 69 degrees on a right side bending film *(B)*. Clinically the deforming nature of the curve is seen *(C)*. She was treated with a series of preoperative casts and operated on in a cast. She underwent a spinal fusion from T4 to L2, and the correction on the day of surgery was 35 degrees *(D)*.

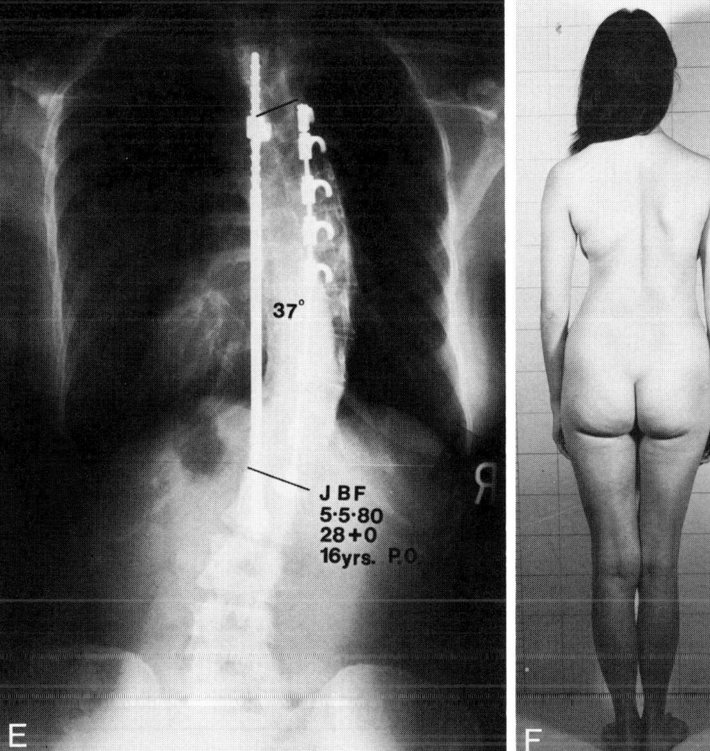

Figure 14–25 *Continued* She was treated ambulatorily in a postoperative cast for nine months. Sixteen years postoperatively the fusion is solid and correction maintained at 37 degrees *(E)*. The improved clinical appearance is seen in this back view four years after surgery *(F)*.

tion that has gained popularity is that of Cotrel and Dubousset (the C-D system).[45, 46, 50, 60, 192, 209] It is noted that these instrumentation systems are all for the posterior approach, the Dwyer[63, 64, 104, 156] and the Zielke system[103, 110, 111, 161, 252, 253] being used with an anterior approach.

A wide variety of options thus exist for the scoliosis surgeon, which makes decision making difficult. In evaluating these options, each system must be viewed from different aspects, as discussed by Akbarnia.[3] Among these are the capability of three-dimensional correction, rigidity of fixation, safety, preservation of spinal mobility, technical complexity, cost, and ease of postoperative care. In addition, there are factors related to the patient that affect the choice. These include the curve magnitude and location, sagittal alignment, cosmetic appearance, and patient size.

Three-dimensional Correction

It must be remembered that scoliosis is a three-dimensional deformity, and thus the effect of the instrumentation on the spine in three dimensions must be considered. The effect of instrumentation on the correction of the scoliosis is the usual manner of assessment used, i.e., using the Cobb measurement. In general, corrections of 40 to 70 per cent are reported.[28, 37, 138, 157] It has also been seen that distraction reduces the sagittal contour, i.e., thoracic kyphosis and lumbar lordosis.[28, 40]

The addition of a compression rod increases stability and can reduce thoracic kyphosis.[157] The addition of sublaminar wiring has been shown, with a square-ended Harrington rod, to improve thoracic hypokyphosis or lordosis, with an average improvement of 19 degrees in one study.[157, 241] With the use of spinous process wiring, Drummond and colleagues[59, 174] and other authors[40, 92] demonstrated maintenance of thoracic kyphosis, with an improvement of 4 to 10 degrees.

There are very few studies comparing different instrumentation systems.[37, 115, 157] That of Mielke and colleagues compared the treatment of thoracic idiopathic scoliosis with four systems: (1) the Harrington distraction rod alone, (2) with the addition of a compression rod, (3) with subsequent addition of a DTT, and (4) the distraction rod with sublaminar wires.[157] The average preoperative curve was comparable, and there was no difference in the postoperative correction obtained or maintained at follow-up. The only difference was in the sagittal correction with reduced thoracic hyperkyphosis with the Harrington distraction and compression rods, and improvement in thoracic lordosis with the use of a Harrington distraction rod and sublaminar wires.

The C-D system, because of rotation of the rod on the concavity, with rotation of the curve apex, has the capability of three-dimensional correction (Fig. 14–26). A comparison of all these systems and their effect on the spine in three dimensions is important. Adequate follow-up is essential before this assessment is possible.

It must be remembered that distraction is more effective with curves over 56 degrees, while a transverse force is more effective for smaller curves.[232] This effect, plus the desired effect on the sagittal profile, needs to be considered in the choice of instrumentation.

Rigidity of Fixation

The quality of fixation determines the correction obtained at surgery and the subsequent loss at follow-up. In general, the more fixation points, the more stable is the fixation with reduced hook dislodgment, and reduced loss of correction at follow-up. In general, the loss of correction at follow-up varies greatly, from 2 to 11 per cent. The better the quality of fixation, the less rigid is the immobilization required postoperatively, and with some systems no postoperative immobilization is needed.[44–46, 59, 60] Added fixation shortens immobilization time and leads to faster incorporation of the fusion.

Safety

The safety of the instrumentation to be used is important, especially with regard to neurologic complications. With use of distraction in the Harrington system, it has been shown that overdistraction is the danger. MacEwen and associates[141] reported a 0.5 per cent incidence of neurologic deficits in idiopathic scoliosis. With the use of sublaminar wires a higher rate was reported by Wilber and colleagues (17 per cent),[220, 233] but Winter and associates[241] reported no neurologic deficits in their series.

A comparison of cord injuries was made in the 1987 Morbidity Reports to the Scoliosis Research Society.[204] The overall incidence of cord problems in idiopathic scoliosis was 0.26 per cent. With sublaminar wires the rate was 0.86 per cent, with C-D instrumentation 0.60 per cent, and with the Harrington distraction rod 0.23 per cent. These newer systems thus carry a potentially higher neurologic rate than the Harrington distraction rod group. This may be because this represents early experience with these newer systems, but this higher neurologic rate must be taken into account in the choice of instrumentation.

Preservation of Spinal Mobility

In general the thoracic spine is not made for motion, and thus a fusion does not reduce spinal motion. The lumbar spine is the mobile portion of the spine, and any fusion into the lumbar spine will reduce lumbar motion. This decreases the number of motion segments between the fusion and the pelvis, and has been shown to increase the possibility of back pain and degenerative changes in the long term.[40, 227]

When lumbar or thoracolumbar curves are fused, fusion posteriorly usually has to extend to L4. An alternative is the anterior approach with the use of instrumentation: Dwyer initially[63, 64, 156, 191] and later the Zielke instrumentation.[110, 111, 161, 204, 252] The ideal curve for this is a thoracolumbar and occasionally a lumbar curve. If there is a thoracic curve above, this needs to be flexible. Since only the structural central area of the curve needs fusion, using the Zielke instrumentation, one or two motion segments can be saved (Fig. 14–27).

Technical Complexity

With the introduction of new instrumentation systems, the technical complexity tends to increase. With each system, experience is needed to be able to use the system effectively and also to assess its role in spinal fusions. These play a role in the spinal surgeon's decision making.

Cost

The cost of the newer systems is high. In some cases this needs to be considered in the choice of instrumentation. This increased cost is offset by a possibly reduced period of post-

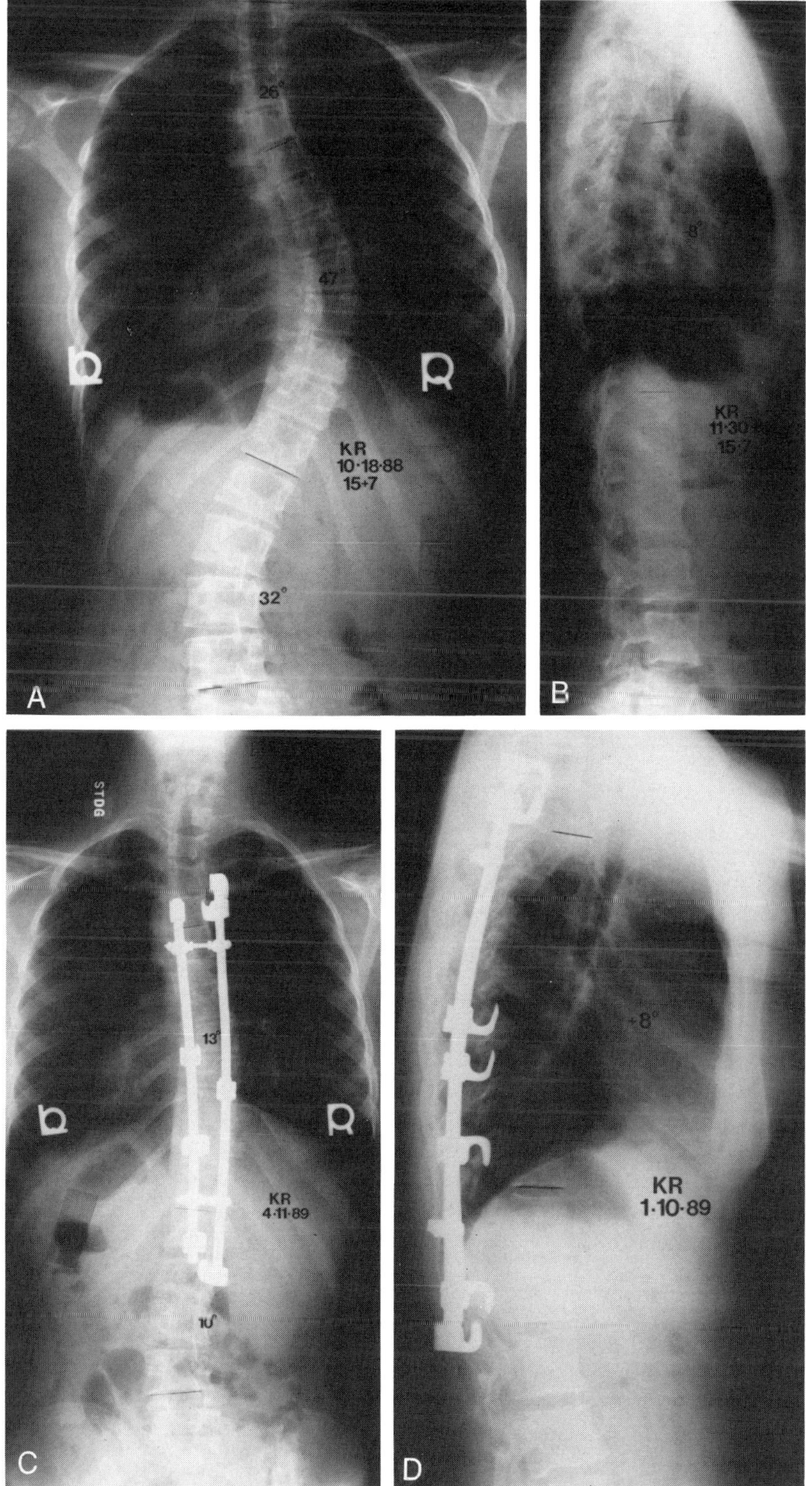

Figure 14–26. K. R. presented at age 14 years, 7 months with a single right thoracic curve of 47 degrees *(A)*. A lateral view showed thoracic lordosis of −8 degrees *(B)*. She underwent a posterior fusion from T4 to L1 with C-D instrumentation, with correction to 13 degrees *(C)*. There is improvement in the sagittal plane of 16 degrees, the kyphosis measuring +8 degrees *(D)*.

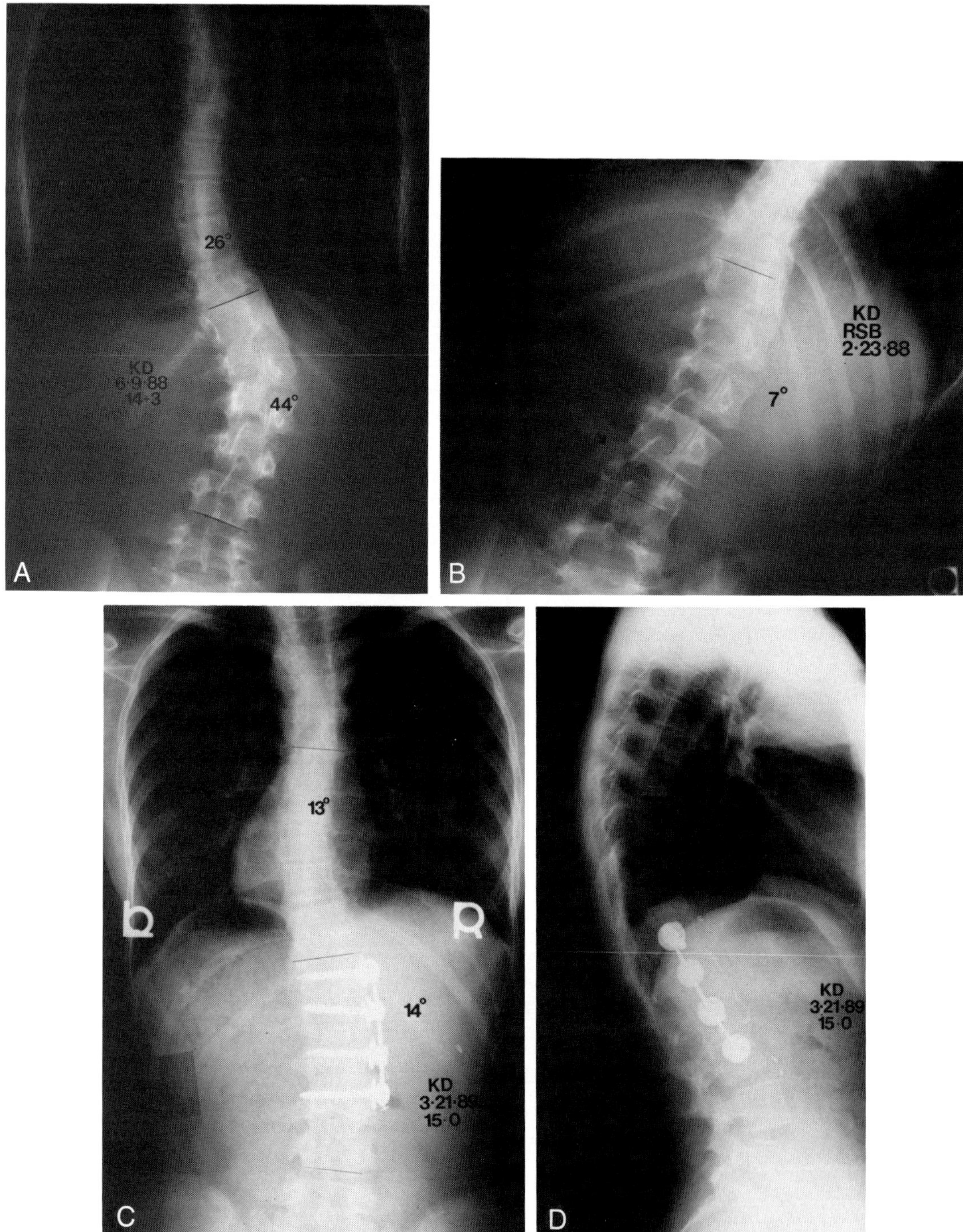

Figure 14–27. K. D. failed stimulator treatment with progression of her lumbar curve to 44 degrees *(A)*. The left thoracic curve corrected to 3 degrees and the lumbar curve to 7 degrees on side bending *(B)*. She underwent an anterior fusion and Zielke instrumentation from T12 to L3 and was treated postoperatively in a TLSO. Nine months after surgery the fusion is solid with balanced curves of 13 and 14 degrees *(C)* and maintenance of the lumbar lordosis without kyphosis in the instrumented area *(D)*.

operative immobilization and the savings if such immobilization is not required.

Patient Factors

The choice of instrumentation depends on the type of patient and the curve characteristics. An obese or large patient needs additional fixation and a system that does not require postoperative immobilization. Larger curves are more effectively treated by a distraction type of instrumentation rather than one using a transverse force, the latter being better for smaller (and longer) curves. The location and the sagittal contour, i.e., the amount of kyphosis or lordosis, are also important in the choice of instrumentation, as is the ability of each system to reduce the rotational prominence.

Choice of Instrumentation

The choice of instrumentation, taking all the above into consideration, is also affected by the curve location and the sagittal contour.

A single thoracic curve with normal thoracic lordosis can be instrumented with a contoured Harrington distraction rod, with or without sublaminar wires, the Wisconsin system or the C-D system (Fig. 14–27). If the sagittal contour is more kyphotic, the best systems are combination of a Harrington distraction and compression rods, the C-D system or the Wisconsin system. When there is thoracic hypokyphosis or true lordosis, the C-D system or a Harrington distraction rod with a square end and sublaminar wires is best to restore the sagittal contour to normal (Fig. 14–26).

A single thoracolumbar curve is best treated with an anterior fusion using Zielke instrumentation, so that lumbar motion segments are saved with a shorter fusion (Fig. 14–27).[180] In single lumbar curves, it is usually not possible to save motion segments, but whenever possible an anterior approach with Zielke instrumentation to save a level should be the procedure of choice. In this pattern it is important when a posterior approach is performed to use the system that does *not* distract the lumbar spine and reduce lumbar lordosis, i.e., the C-D system.

The double thoracic pattern is best treated with the C-D system, the Wisconsin system, or a Harrington distraction rod with sublaminar wires (Fig. 14–28). The sagittal contour affects the choice of system and its application. The other double curves (double thoracic and lumbar or double thoracic and thoracolumbar patterns) offer the same choices as above for the double thoracic curve. In these, maintenance of thoracic kyphosis and lumbar lordosis is essential (Fig. 14–29). In some cases of double thoracic and thoracolumbar curves, it is possible to save motion segments with a combined anterior fusion and Zielke and posterior fusion with instrumentation.

It must be emphasized that all these instrumentations are adjunctive and *not* the procedure. The procedure being performed is a spinal fusion, and meticulous fusion technique is essential. This includes careful exposure to the tips of the transverse processes in the thoracic and lumbar areas, excision of facets, and packing with autologous iliac bone graft. Some authors have reported use of bank bone or fusion without decortication.[55] The effectiveness of these variations is unproved in studies on a significant number of patients with adequate follow-up.

An essential part of any instrumentation system use is careful monitoring of neurologic function intraoperatively, with the Stagnara wake-up test or electronic spinal cord monitoring using somatosensory evoked potentials (SSEP).[88, 170, 173] Any change in neurologic function needs to be promptly diagnosed and treated, with reduction of distraction and/or removal of the hardware. Work on motor evoked potentials is being undertaken and may in the future play a role in spinal cord monitoring.[126] The efficacy of these monitoring techniques needs to be determined by large studies comparing all three methods.

Approach

There are three approaches for fusion and instrumentation. The most common is the posterior approach. An anterior approach is used with single thoracolumbar (or lumbar) curves when a Zielke is used and motion segments are saved from being included in the fusion area. In these cases the fusion area is only the structural central part of the curve and is shorter than the measured curve on the standing PA radiograph.

A combined approach (anterior plus posterior) is used for the large thoracic curve that is a rapidly progressive adolescent variety, or for the neglected juvenile case. The anterior

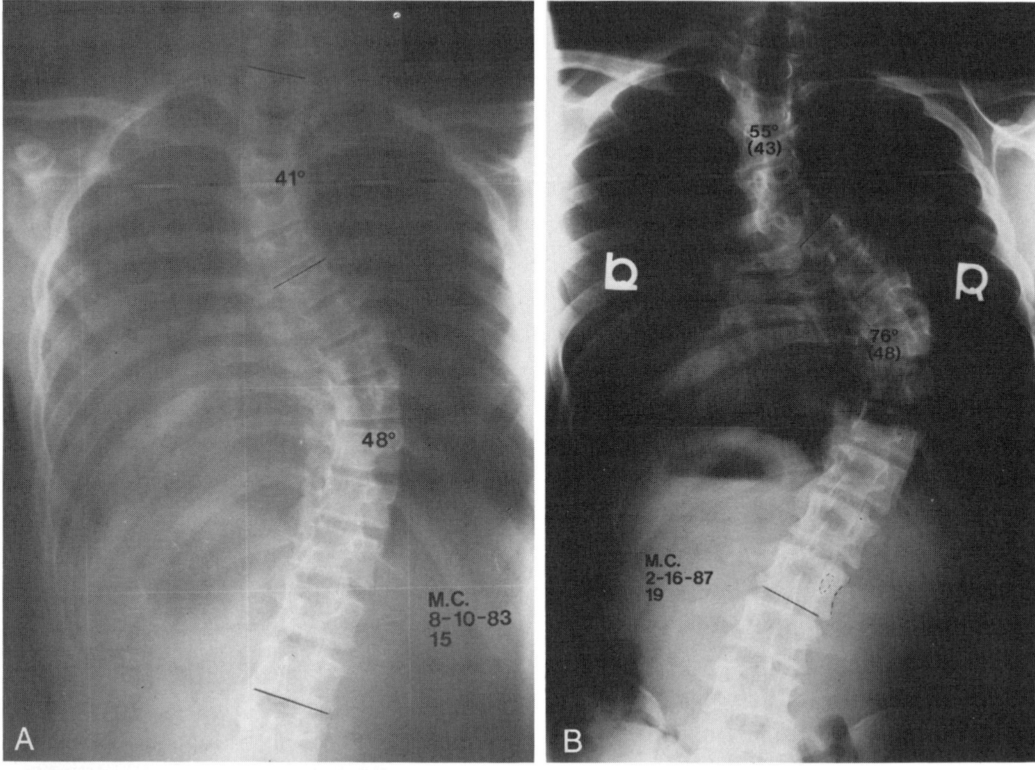

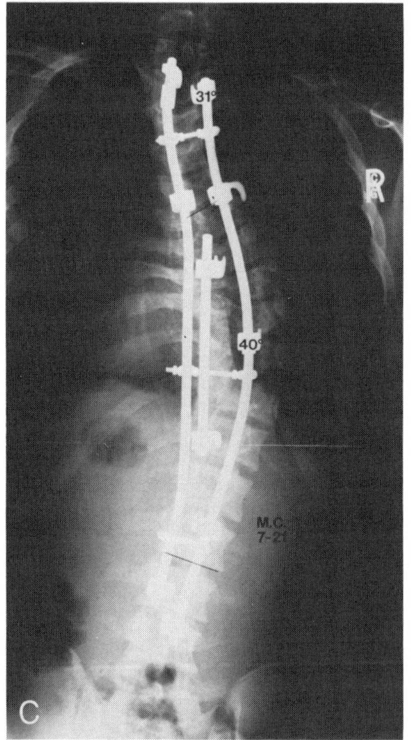

Figure 14–28. M. C. presented at age 15 years with a double thoracic curve of 41 and 48 degrees *(A)*. He was not treated and it progressed to 55 and 76 degrees *(B)*. He underwent a posterior fusion with C-D instrumentation of both curves. Note the use of an additional distraction rod for the rigid right thoracic curve *(C)*.

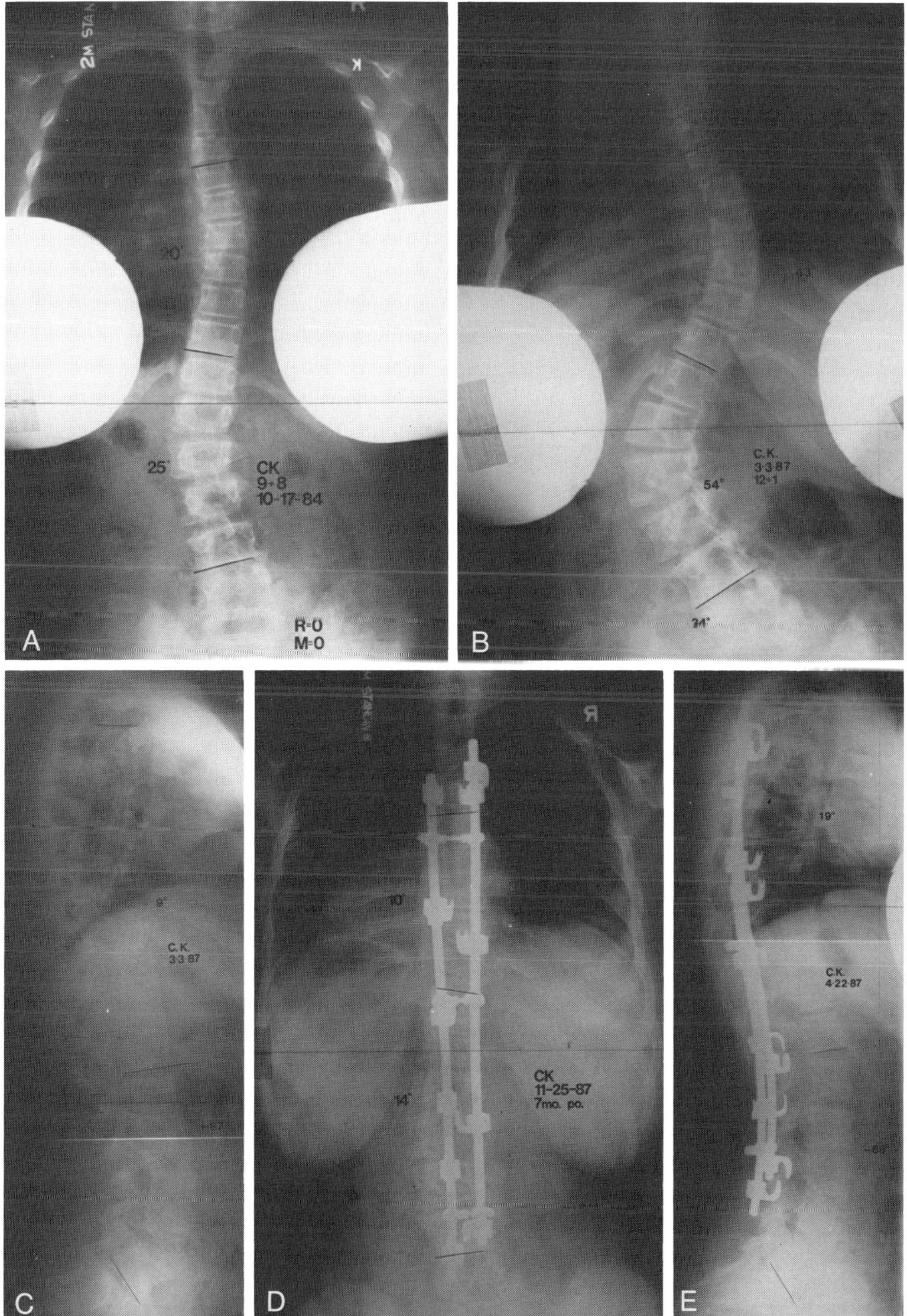

Figure 14–29. C. K. originally presented with a 20-degree right thoracic and 25-degree left lumbar curve at age 9 years, 8 months *(A)*. She was lost to follow-up and presented at age 12 years, 1 month with curves of 43 and 54 degrees *(B)*. The curves were flexible on side bending, correcting to 15 and 20 degrees. A lateral x-ray showed thoracic hypokyphosis of 9 degrees *(C)*. She underwent a posterior fusion with C-D instrumentation of both curves and at seven months postoperatively the fusion was solid with curves of 10 and 14 degrees *(D)*. A lateral x-ray shows improvement in the thoracic hypokyphosis and maintenance of the lumbar lordosis *(E)*.

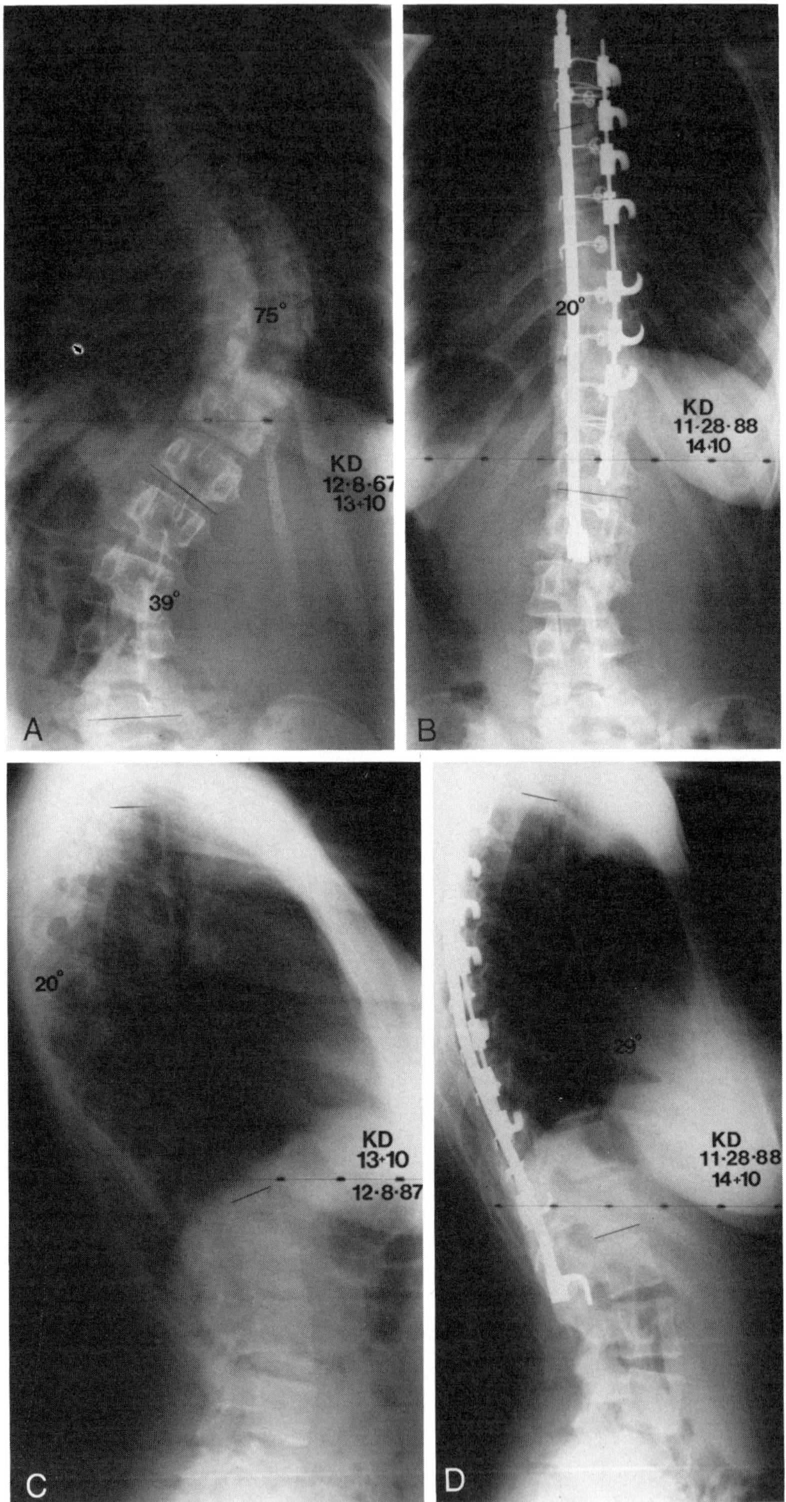

Figure 14–30. K. D. presented at age 13 years, 10 months with a 75-degree right thoracic curve *(A)*. She underwent a posterior fusion with a Harrington distraction rod with Drummond spinous process wires plus a Harrington compression rod, with correction to 20 degrees *(B)*. The lateral radiograph showed a preoperative thoracic kyphosis of 20 degrees *(C)*, which was maintained with surgery *(D)*. (Reprinted with kind permission of Dr. A. Crawford.)

approach is via the convexity of the curve and consists of disc excisions with perhaps a wedge of vertebral end plate, and packing of bone in the disc spaces for an anterior fusion. In very rare cases with extremely large curves (usually a neglected infantile or early juvenile curve), an apical vertebrectomy is necessary to aid curve correction. The second stage, performed one week later or under the same anesthesia, consists of posterior fusion with instrumentation, usually with osteotomy of spontaneously fused facet joints. Additional distraction is necessary on the concavity with multiple distraction rods (Harrington or C-D systems) (Fig. 14–30).

Other indications for the combined approach are uncommon in adolescent idiopathic scoliosis. These include the presence of rigid thoracic hyperkyphosis, which requires an anterior release and fusion. Another indication is the double thoracic and thoracolumbar curve, which can be treated via an anterior approach and Zielke instrumentation and posterior fusion and instrumentation to save lumbar motion segments.[122]

Postoperative Immobilization

With the addition of alternative fixation techniques to the surgeon's armamentarium, it was initially thought that postoperative immobilization was unnecessary. With the Luque system[123] or the Harrington distraction rod with sublaminar wires,[157] this assumption proved to be false. In these systems there was a greater loss of correction and a higher pseudarthrosis rate. Initial reports on the Wisconsin and C-D systems without the use of postoperative immobilization described excellent maintenance of correction and no increase in the pseudarthrosis rate.

After the fusion procedure, a decision needs to be made regarding postoperative immobilization. When postoperative immobilization is necessary, a cast or brace is used. With the advent of newer plastics, an under-arm TLSO is usually the device of choice. The model is taken three to five days after surgery. Depending on the stability of the instrumentation fixation and the preference of the surgeon, the model is taken with the patient either supine (on a Risser table) or standing. The orthosis is worn day and night, with time out for showering.

Postoperative immobilization is continued until the fusion is solid. This is seen on supine oblique radiographs where the fusion mass is visualized in profile. A solid fusion is present when there is a continuous mass of bone alongside the spine, and the facet joints are obliterated, demonstrating a solid facet fusion. This takes approximately four months in most adolescents but may take up to six or even eight months with larger curves, or for unknown reasons. Thus, the immobilization is discontinued when the fusion is solid and not after a fixed number of calendar weeks.

The postoperative activity level varies greatly, depending on the surgeon performing the procedure and the treatment protocols. It also depends on whether immobilization is used postoperatively.

References

Idiopathic Scoliosis

1. Adams, W.: Lectures on Pathology and Treatment of Lateral and Other Forms of Curvature of the Spine. London, Churchill Livingstone, 1865.
2. Akbarnia, B. A., and Keppler, L.: Lateral electrical surface stimulation for the treatment of adolescent idiopathic scoliosis. An analysis based on progression risk. J. Pediatr. Orthop. *6:*369, 1986.
3. Akbarnia, B. A.: Selection of methodology in surgical treatment of adolescent idiopathic scoliosis. Orthop. Clin. North Am. *19:*319–329, 1988.
4. Allen, B. L., Jr., and Ferguson, R. L.: The Galveston experience with L-rod instrumentation of adolescent idiopathic scoliosis. Clin. Orthop. *229:*59–69, 1988.
5. Andersen, P. E., Jr., Andersen, P. E., and van der Kooy, P.: Dose reduction in radiography of the spine in scoliosis. Acta Radiol. [Diagn.] (Stockh.) *23:*251–253, 1982.
6. Armstrong, G. W. D., and Connock, S. H. G.: A transverse loading system applied to a modified Harrington instrumentation. Clin. Orthop. *108:*70–75, 1985.
7. Armstrong, G. W. D., Livermore, N. B., III, Suzuki, N., and Armstrong, J. G.: Nonstandard vertebral rotation in scoliosis screening patients. Its prevalence and relation to the clinical deformity. Spine *7:*50–54, 1982.
8. Ascani, E., Bartolozzi, P., Logroscino, C. A., et al.: Natural history of untreated idiopathic scoliosis after skeletal maturity. Spine *11:*784–789, 1986.
9. Ascani, E., Giglio, G. C., and Salsano, V.: Scoliosis screening in Rome. *In* Zorab, P. A., and Siegler, D. (eds.): Scoliosis. London, Academic Press, 1980, pp. 39–44.

10. Asher, M., Green, P., and Orrick, J.: A six year report: spinal deformity screening in Kansas school children. J. Kans. Med. Soc. *81:*968–571, 1980.
11. Axelgaard, J., and Brown, J. C.: Lateral electrical stimulation for the treatment of progressive idiopathic scoliosis. Spine *8:*242–260, 1983.
12. Axelgaard, J., Nordwall, A., and Brown, J. C.: Correction of spinal curvatures by transcutaneous electrical muscle stimulation. Spine *8:*463–481, 1983.
13. Bassett, G. S., Bunnell, W. P., and MacEwen, G. D.: Treatment of idiopathic scoliosis with the Wilmington brace. Results in patients with a twenty to thirty-nine degree curve. J. Bone Joint Surg. *68A:*602–605, 1986.
14. Bassett, G. S., and Bunnell, W. P.: Influence of the Wilmington brace on spinal decompensation in adolescent idiopathic scoliosis. Clin. Orthop. *223:*164–169, 1987.
15. Bergofsky, E. H., Turino, G. M., and Fishman, A. P.: Cardiorespiratory failure in kyphoscoliosis. Medicine *38:*263–317, 1959.
16. Bersoin, M., Bollini, G., Hornuns, H., et al.: Is the Cotrel-Dubousset really universal in the surgical treatment of idiopathic scoliosis? J. Pediatr. Orthop. *8:*45–48, 1988.
17. Birch, J. G., Herrins, J. A., Roach, J. W., and Johnston, C. E.: Cotrel-Dubousset instrumentation in idiopathic scoliosis. A preliminary report. Clin. Orthop. *227:*24–29, 1988.
18. Bjerkreim, I., Carlsen, B., and Korsell, E.: Preoperative Cotrel traction in idiopathic scoliosis. Acta Orthop. Scand. *53:*901–905, 1982.
19. Bjure, J., and Nachemson, A.: Non-treated scoliosis. Clin. Orthop. *93:*44–52, 1973.
20. Blount, W. P., and Moe, J. H.: The Milwaukee Brace. 2nd ed. Baltimore, Williams & Wilkins Co., 1980.
21. Bobechko, W. P., Herbert, M. N., and Friedman, H. G.: Electrospinal instrumentation for scoliosis: current status. Orthop. Clin. North Am. *10:*927–941, 1979.
22. Bradford, D. S., Lonstein, J. E., Moe, J. H., et al.: Moe's Textbook of Scoliosis and Other Spinal Deformities. 2nd ed. Philadelphia, W. B. Saunders Co., 1987.
23. Bradford, D. S., Tanguy, A., and Vanselow, J.: Surface electrical stimulation in the treatment of idiopathic scoliosis: preliminary results in 30 patients. Spine *8:*757, 1983.
24. Brooks, H. L., Azen, S. P., Gerberg, E., et al.: Scoliosis: a prospective epidemiological study. J. Bone Joint Surg. *57A:*968–972, 1975.
25. Brooks, H. L.: Current incidence of scoliosis in California. *In* Zorab, P. A., and Siegler, D. (eds.): Scoliosis. London, Academic Press, 1980, pp. 7–12.
26. Brown, J. C., Axelgaard, J., and Howson, D. C.: Multicenter trial of a noninvasive stimulation method for idiopathic scoliosis. Orthop. Tran. *7:*10, 1983.
27. Bruszewski, J., and Kamza, Z.: The incidence of scoliosis on the basis of serial radiography. Chir. Narzadow. Ruchu. Ortop. Pol. *22:*1156, 1957.
28. Bunch, W. H.: Posterior fusion for idiopathic scoliosis. Instruc. Course Lect. *34:*140–152, 1985.
29. Bunnell, W., MacEwen, J., and Jayakumar, S.: The use of plastic jackets in the non-operative treatment of idiopathic scoliosis. J. Bone Joint Surg. *62A:*31, 1980.
30. Bunnell, W. P.: The natural history of idiopathic scoliosis before skeletal maturity. Spine *11:*773–776, 1986.
31. Bunnell, W. P.: The natural history of idiopathic scoliosis. Clin. Orthop. *229:*20–25, 1988.
32. Burwell, R. G., James, N. J., Johnson, F., et al.: The rib hump score: a guide to referral and prognosis? J. Bone Joint Surg. *64B:*248, 1982.
33. Butterworth, T. R., and James, C.: Electromyographic studies in idiopathic scoliosis. South. Med. J. *62:*1008–1010, 1969.
34. Carr, W. A., Moe, J. H., Winter, R. B., et al.: Treatment of idiopathic scoliosis in the Milwaukee brace: long term results. J. Bone Joint Surg. *62A:*599–612, 1980.
35. Ceballos, R., Ferrer-Torrelles, M., Castillo, F., and Fernandez-Paredes, E.: Prognosis in infantile idiopathic scoliosis. J. Bone Joint Surg. *54B:*648–655, 1972.
36. Ceballos, T., Ferrer-Torrelles, M., Castillo, F., et al.: Prognosis in infantile idiopathic scoliosis. J. Bone Joint Surg. *62A:*863–875, 1980.
37. Christodoulou, A. G., Prince, H. G., Webb, J. G., and Burwell, R. G.: Adolescent idiopathic thoracic scoliosis. A prospective trial with and without bracing during postoperative care. J. Bone Joint Surg. *69B:*13–16, 1987.
38. Clarisse, P. H.: Pronostic evolutif des scolioses idiopathiques mineures de 10 degrees à 29 degrees, au periode de croissance. Thesis, Lyon, France, 1974.
39. Cobb, J.: Instructional Course Lecture—Outline for Study of Scoliosis. Vol. V. Am. Acad. Orthop. Surg., 1948.
40. Cochran, T., Irstam, L., and Nachemson, A.: Long-term anatomic and functional changes in patients with adolescent idiopathic scoliosis treated by Harrington rod fusion. Spine *8:*576–583, 1983.
41. Collis, D. K., and Ponseti, I. V.: Long-term follow-up of patients with idiopathic scoliosis not treated surgically. J. Bone Joint Surg. *51A:*425–445, 1969.
42. Connor, A. N.: Developmental anomalies and prognosis in infantile idiopathic scoliosis. J. Bone Joint Surg. *51B:*711–712, 1969.
43. Cotrel, Y., Denis, F., Galante, H., et al.: Bilan actuel des 250 premieres arthrodeses vertebrales pour scoliose par greffon tibial, Harrington et Dispostif de traction transversale (DTT). Communication au Congres du GES, St. Etienne, 1976.
44. Cotrel, Y., Dubousset, J., and Guillaumat, M.: New universal instrumentation in spinal surgery. Clin. Orthop. *227:*10–23, 1988.
45. Cotrel, Y., and Dubousset, J.: New segmental posterior instrumentation of the spine. Orthop. Trans. *9:*118, 1985.
46. Cotrel, Y., and Dubousset, J.: Nouvelle technique d'ostéosynthèse rachidienne segmentaire par voie postérieure. Rev. Chir. Orthop. *70:*489–495, 1984.
47. Cowell, H. R., Hall, J. N., and MacEwen, G. D.: Familial patterns of idiopathic scoliosis. J. Bone Joint Surg. *51A:*1236, 1969.
48. Cowell, H. R., Hall, J. N., and MacEwen, G. D.: Genetic aspects of idiopathic scoliosis. Clin. Orthop. *86:*121–131, 1972.

49. Crisfield, R. J.: Scoliosis with progressive external ophthalmoplegia in four siblings. J. Bone Joint Surg. *56B:*484–489, 1974.
50. Denis, F.: Cotrel-Dubousset instrumentation in the treatment of idiopathic scoliosis. Orthop. Clin. North Am. *19:*291–311, 1988.
51. DeSmet, A., Fritz, S. L., and Asher, M. A.: A method for minimizing the radiation exposure from scoliosis radiographs. J. Bone Joint Surg. *63A:*156, 1981.
52. DeSmet, A. A., Goin, J. E., Asher, M. A., and Scheuch, H. G.: A clinical study of the differences between the scoliotic angles measured on PA vs AP radiographs. J. Bone Joint Surg. *64A:*489–493, 1982.
53. Dickson, R. A., and Leatherman, K. D.: Cotrel traction, exercises, casting in the treatment of idiopathic scoliosis. A pilot study and prospective randomized controlled clinical trial. Acta Orthop. Scand. *49:*46–48, 1978.
54. Dickson, R. A., Stamper, P., Sharp, A. M., and Harken, P.: School screening for scoliosis: cohort study of clinical course. Br. Med. J. *73:*265–268, 1980.
55. Dubousset, J., Graf, H., Miladi, L., et al.: Spinal and thoracic derotation with CD instrumentation. Orthop. Trans. *10:*36, 1986.
56. Dodd, C. A., Fergusson, C. M., Freedman, L., et al.: Allograft versus autograft bone in scoliosis surgery. J. Bone Joint Surg. *70B:*431–434, 1988.
57. Dretakis, E. K., and Kondoyannis, P. N.: Congenital scoliosis associated with encephalopathy in five children of two families. J. Bone Joint Surg. *56A:*1747–1750, 1974.
58. Drogt, J., Winter, R. B., and Lonstein, J. E.: Results of TLSO treatment of adolescent idiopathic lumbar and thoracolumbar scoliosis. A.A.O.S., San Francisco, CA, 1987.
59. Drummond, D. S., Guadagni, J., Keene, J. S., et al.: Interspinous process segmental spinal instrumentation. J. Pediatr. Orthop. *4:*397–404, 1984.
60. Drummond, D. S.: Harrington instrumentation with spinous process wiring for idiopathic scoliosis. Orthop. Clin. North Am. *19:*281–289, 1988.
61. Duriez, J.: Évolution de las scoliose idiopathique chez l'adulte. Acta Orthop. Belg. *33:*547–550, 1967.
62. Duval-Beaupère, G.: Pathogenic relationship between scoliosis and growth. *In* Zorab, P. A. (ed.): Scoliosis and Growth. Proceedings of a Third Symposium, London, November 1970. Edinburgh, Churchill Livingstone, 1971, pp. 58–64.
63. Dwyer, A. F., Newton, N. C., and Sherwood, A. A.: An anterior approach to scoliosis. Clin. Orthop. *62:*192, 1969.
64. Dwyer, A. F.: Experience in anterior correction of scoliosis. Clin. Orthop. *93:*191, 1977.
65. Edgar, M. A., Chapman, R. H., and Glasgow, M. M.: Preoperative correction in adolescent idiopathic scoliosis. J. Bone Joint Surg. *64B:*530–535, 1982.
66. Edmonson, A., and Morris, J. T.: Followup study of Milwaukee brace treatment in patients with idiopathic scoliosis. Clin. Orthop. *126:*58–61, 1983.
67. Edmonson, A., and Smith, G. R.: Long-term followup study of Milwaukee brace treatment in patients with idiopathic scoliosis. Orthop. Trans. *7:*10–11, 1983.
68. Emans, J. B., Kaelin, A., Bancel, P., et al.: The Boston brace system for idiopathic scoliosis; follow-up results in 295 patients. Spine *11:*792–801, 1986.
69. Engler, G. L., Spielholz, N. J., Bernhard, W. N., et al.: Somatosensory evoked potentials during Harrington instrumentation for scoliosis. J. Bone Joint Surg. *60A:*528–532, 1978.
70. Fidler, M. W., Jowett, R. L., and Troup, J. D. G.: Histochemical study of the function of multifidus in scoliosis. *In* Zorab, P. A. (ed.): Scoliosis and Muscle. Proceedings of a Fourth Symposium, London, November 1973. London, W. Heinemann Medical Books, 1974, pp. 184–192.
71. Fidler, M. W., and Jowett, R. L.: Muscle imbalance in the aetiology of scoliosis. J. Bone Joint Surg. *58B:*200–201, 1976.
72. Figueiredo, U. M., and James, J. I. P.: Juvenile idiopathic scoliosis. J. Bone Joint Surg. *63B:*61–66, 1981.
73. Fillio, N. A., and Thompson, M. W.: Genetic studies in scoliosis. Proceedings of the Scoliosis Research Society. J. Bone Joint Surg. *53A:*199, 1971.
74. Fisher, R. L., and DeGeorge, F. V.: Idiopathic scoliosis: an investigation of genetic and environmental factors. J. Bone Joint Surg. *49A:*1006, 1967.
75. Floman, Y., Liebergall, M., Robin, G. C., and Eldor, A.: Abnormalities of aggregation, thromboxane A2 synthesis, and ^{14}C serotonin release in platelets of patients with idiopathic scoliosis. Spine *8:*236, 1983.
76. Fowles, J. V., Drummond, D. S., L'Ecuyer, S., et al.: Untreated scoliosis in the adult. Clin. Orthop. *134:*212–217, 1978.
77. Fustier, T.: Evolution radiologique spontanée des scolioses idiopathiques de moins de 45 degrees en periode de croissance. Étude graphique retrospective de cente dossiers du Centre d'adaptation fonctionnelle des Massues. Thesis, Université Claude-Bernard, Lyon, France, 1980.
78. Gardner, A.: Evolution and progression in nonoperated idiopathic scoliosis. Spine (in press).
79. Goldberg, C., Dowling, F., Blake, N. S., and Regan, B. F.: A retrospective study of Cotrel dynamic spinal traction in the conservative management of scoliosis. Ir. Med. J. *74:*363–365, 1981.
80. Goldstein, L. H.: Surgical management of scoliosis. J. Bone Joint Surg. *48A:*167–196, 1966.
81. Goldstein, L. H.: The surgical management of scoliosis. Clin. Orthop. *35:*95–115, 1964.
82. Gray, J. E., Hoffman, A. D., and Peterson, H. A.: Reduction of radiation exposure during radiography for scoliosis. J. Bone Joint Surg. *65A:*5–12, 1983.
83. Green, N.: Part time bracing of adolescent idiopathic scoliosis. J. Bone Joint Surg. *68A:*738–742, 1986.
84. Guadagni, J., Drummond, D., and Breed, A.: Improved postoperative course following modified segmental instrumentation and posterior fusion for scoliosis. J. Pediatr. Orthop. *4:*405–408, 1984.
85. Gucker, T.: Changes in vital capacity in scoliosis: preliminary report of effects of treatment. J. Bone Joint Surg. *44A:*469–481, 1962.
86. Greulich, W. W., and Pyle, S. I.: Radiographic Atlas of Skeletal Development of the Hand and Wrist. 2nd ed. Stanford, CA, Stanford University Press, 1959.

87. Gzioglu, K., Goldstein, L. A., Femi-Pearse, D., et al.: Pulmonary function in idiopathic scoliosis: comparative evaluation before and after orthopaedic correction. J. Bone Joint Surg. *50A:*1391–1399, 1968.
88. Hall, J. E., Levin, C. R., and Sudhir, K. G.: Intraoperative awakening to monitor spinal cord function during Harrington instrumentation and spine fusion: description of procedure and report of three cases. J. Bone Joint Surg. *60A:*528–536, 1978.
89. Hanks, G. A., Zimmer, B., and Nogl, J.: TLSO treatment of idiopathic scoliosis. An analysis of Wilmington jacket. Spine *13:*626–629, 1988.
90. Harrington, P. R.: Surgical instrumentation for management of scoliosis. J. Bone Joint Surg. *42A:*1448, 1960.
91. Harrington, P. R.: Technical details in relation to the successful use of instrumentation in scoliosis. Orthop. Clin. North Am. *3:*49–67, 1972.
92. Harrington, P. R.: Treatment of scoliosis, correction and internal fixation by spine instrumentation. J. Bone Joint Surg. *44A:*591–610, 1962.
93. Hefti, F. L., and McMaster, M. J.: The effect of the adolescent growth spurt on early posterior spinal fusion in infantile and juvenile idiopathic scoliosis. J. Bone Joint Surg. *65B:*247–254, 1983.
94. Henriksson, N. G.: En översikt i vestibulär otoneurologi. Lund, Sweden, Studentlitteratur, 1966.
95. Henssge, J.: Electromyographischer Beitrag zum Skoliosen-problem. Fortschr. Med. *82:*665–668, 1964.
96. Herbert, M. H., and Bobechko, W. P.: Paraspinal muscle stimulation for the treatment of idiopathic scoliosis in children. Orthopedics *10:*1125–1132, 1987.
97. Herman, R., Maulucci, R., Stuych, J., et al.: Vestibular functioning in idiopathic scoliosis. Orthop. Trans. *3:*218, 1979.
98. Herring, J. A., Fitch, R. D., Wenger, D. R., et al.: Segmental instrumentation: a review of early results and complications. Orthop. Trans. *8:*172, 1984.
99. Herring, J. A., and Wenger, D. R.: Segmental spinal instrumentation: a preliminary report of 40 consecutive cases. Spine *7:*285–298, 1982.
100. Hooper, G.: Congenital dislocation of the hip in infantile idiopathic scoliosis. J. Bone Joint Surg. *62B:*447–449, 1980.
101. Hoppenfeld, S.: Histochemical findings in paraspinal muscles of patients with idiopathic scoliosis. *In* Zorab, P. A. (ed.): Scoliosis and Muscle. Proceedings of a Fourth Symposium, Brompton Hospital, London, Nov. 1973. S.I.M.P. Research Monograph No. 4, Spastics International Medical Publications, London, Wm. Heinemann Medical Books, 1974, pp 113–114.
102. Horal, J.: The clinical appearance of low back disorders in the city of Gothenburg, Sweden: comparisons of incapacitated probands with matched controls. Acta Orthop. Scand. *118*(Suppl.):1–109, 1969.
103. Horton, W. C., Holt, R. T., Johnson, J. R., and Leatherman, K. D.: Zielke instrumentation in idiopathic scoliosis: late effects and minimizing complications. Spine *13:*1145–1149, 1988.
104. Hsu, L. C., Zucherman, J., Tang, S. C., et al.: Dwyer instrumentation in the treatment of adolescent idiopathic scoliosis. J. Bone Joint Surg. *64B:*536–541, 1982.
105. James, J. I. P., Lloyd-Roberts, G. C., and Pilcher, M. F.: Infantile structural scoliosis. J. Bone Joint Surg. *41B:*719–735, 1959.
106. James, J. I. P.: Idiopathic scoliosis: the prognosis, diagnosis, and operative indications related to curve patterns and the age at onset. J. Bone Joint Surg. *36B:*36–49, 1954.
107. Kafer, E. R.: Respiratory and cardiovascular functions in scoliosis. Bull. Eur. Physiopathol. Respir. *13:*299–321, 1977.
108. Kahanovitz, N., and Weiser, S.: Lateral electrical surface stimulation (LESS) compliance in adolescent female scoliosis patients. Spine *11:*753–755, 1986.
109. Kane, W. J., and Moe, J. H.: A scoliosis prevalence study in Minnesota. Clin. Orthop. *69:*216–218, 1970.
110. Kaneda, K., Fujiya, N., and Satch, S.: Results with Zielke instrumentation for idiopathic thoracolumbar and lumbar scoliosis. Clin. Orthop. *205:*195–203, 1986.
111. Kaneda, K., Satoh, S., and Fujiya, N.: Analysis of results with Zielke instrumentation for thoracolumbar and lumbar curvature. Nippon Seikeigeka Gakkai Zasshi *59:*841–851, 1985.
112. Kazmin, A. I., and Merkureva, R. V.: Role of disturbances of glucosaminoglycan metabolism in the pathogenesis of scoliosis. Ortop. Travmotol. Protez. *32:*87–91, 1971.
113. Kehl, D. K., and Morrissy, R. T.: Brace treatment in adolescent idiopathic scoliosis. An update on concepts and technique. Clin. Orthop. *229:*34–43, 1988.
114. Keiser, R. P., and Shufflebarger, H. S.: The Milwaukee brace in idiopathic scoliosis: evaluation of 124 completed cases. Clin. Orthop. *118:*19, 1976.
115. Khan, A., Shank, M., and Snyder, M.: A comparison of Luque versus Harrington instrumentation techniques in adolescent idiopathic scoliosis. Orthop. Trans. *7:*431, 1983.
116. Khosla, S., Tredwell, S. J., Day, B., et al.: An ultrastructural study of multifidus muscle in progressive idiopathic scoliosis: changes resulting from a sarcolemmal defect at the myotendinous junction. J. Neurol. Sci. *46:*13, 1980.
117. King, H. A., Moe, J. H., Bradford, D. S., et al.: The selection of fusion levels in thoracic idiopathic scoliosis. J. Bone Joint Surg. *56A:*1302–1313, 1983.
118. King, H. A.: Selection of fusion levels for posterior instrumentation and fusion in idiopathic scoliosis. Orthop. Clin. North Am. *19:*247–255, 1988.
119. Kolind-Sørensen, V.: A follow-up study of patients with idiopathic scoliosis. Acta Orthop. Scand. *44:*98, 1973.
120. Koop, S. E., Winter, R. B., Lonstein, J. E., et al.: Spinal instrumentation without fusion in progressive spinal deformity of childhood. Presented at the Annual Meeting of the American Academy of Orthopaedic Surgeons, Las Vegas, Nevada, February 1989.
121. Koop, S. E.: Infantile and juvenile idiopathic scoliosis. Orthop. Clin. North Am. *19:*331–337, 1988.
122. Korovessis, P.: Combined VDS and Harrington in-

strumentation for treatment of idiopathic double major curves. Spine *12:*244–250, 1987.

123. Leatherman, K. D., Johnson, J., Holt, R., et al.: A clinical assessment of 357 cases of segmental spinal instrumentation. *In* Luque, E. R. (ed.): Segmental Spinal Instrumentation. Thorofare, NJ, Slack, 1984.
124. Leaver, J. M., Alvik, A., and Warren, M. D.: Prescriptive screening for adolescent idiopathic scoliosis: a review of the incidence. Int. J. Epidemiol. *11:*101–111, 1982.
125. Letts, R. M., Palakar, G., and Bobecko, W. P.: Preoperative skeletal traction in scoliosis. J. Bone Joint Surg. *57:*616–619, 1975.
126. Levy, W. J., York, D. H., McCaffrey, M., et al.: Motor-evoked potentials from transcranial stimulation of the motor cortex in man. Neurosurgery *16:*287–302, 1984.
127. Lihvar, G. T., Putilova, A. A., Tabin, V. I., and Uleschenko, V. A.: Statistical and correlation analysis of electrical muscle activity in congenital scoliosis. Ortop. Travmotol. Protez. *36:*9–14, 1975.
128. Lindh, M., and Bjure, J.: Lung volumes in scoliosis before and after correction by the Harrington instrumentation method. Acta Orthop. Scand. *46:*934–948, 1975.
129. Lloyd-Roberts, G. C., and Pilcher, M. F.: Infantile structural scoliosis in infancy; a study of the natural history of 100 patients. J. Bone Joint Surg. *47B:*520–523, 1965.
130. Lonstein, J. E., Bjorklund, S., Wanninger, M. H., et al.: Voluntary school screening for scoliosis in Minnesota. J. Bone Joint Surg. *64A:*481–488, 1982.
131. Lonstein, J. E., and Carlson, J. M.: The prediction of curve progression in untreated idiopathic scoliosis during growth. J. Bone Joint Surg. *66A:*1061–1071, 1984.
132. Lonstein, J. E., Willson, S., Beattie, C., et al.: Result of stimulator treatment of 219 cases of adolescent idiopathic scoliosis. Presented at the Annual Meeting of the Scoliosis Research Society, Baltimore, MD, October 1988.
133. Lonstein, J. E., and Winter, R. B.: Adolescent idiopathic scoliosis. Nonoperative treatment. Orthop. Clin. North Am. *19:*239–246, 1988.
134. Lonstein, J. E., and Winter, R. B.: Milwaukee brace treatment of adolescent idiopathic scoliosis—review of 939 patients. Presented at the Annual Meeting of the Scoliosis Research Society, Baltimore, MD, October 1988.
135. Lonstein, J. E., and Winter, R. B.: Milwaukee brace treatment of juvenile idiopathic scoliosis. Presented at the Annual Meeting of the Scoliosis Research Society, Baltimore, MD, October 1988.
136. Lonstein, J. E.: Natural history and school screening for scoliosis. Orthop. Clin. North Am. *19:*227–237, 1988.
137. Lonstein, J. E.: Screening for spinal deformities in Minnesota schools. Clin. Orthop. *126:*33–42, 1972.
138. Lovallo, J. L., Banta, J. V., and Renshaw, R. S.: Adolescent idiopathic scoliosis treated by Harrington rod distraction and fusion. J. Bone Joint Surg. *68:*1326–1330, 1986.
139. Low, S. D., Chew, E. C., Kung, L. S., et al.: Ultrastructures of nerve fibers and muscle spindles in adolescent idiopathic scoliosis. Clin. Orthop. *174:*217, 1983.
140. Luque, E. R.: Segmental spinal instrumentation for correction of scoliosis. Clin. Orthop. *163:*192–198, 1982.
141. MacEwen, G. D., Bunnell, W. P., and Sriram, K.: Acute neurological complications in the treatment of scoliosis. J. Bone Joint Surg. *57A:*404–408, 1975.
142. MacEwen, G. D., and Cowell, H. R.: Familial incidence of idiopathic scoliosis. J. Bone Joint Surg. *52A:*405, 1970.
143. Makley, J. T., Herndon, C. H., Inkley, S., et al.: Pulmonary function in paralytic and non-paralytic scoliosis before and after treatment: a study of sixty-three cases. J. Bone Joint Surg. *50A:*1379–1390, 1968.
144. Marchetti, P. G., and Faldini, A.: End fusions in the treatment of severe progressing or severe scoliosis in childhood or early adolescence. Orthop. Trans. *2:*271, 1978.
145. Mau, H.: Etiology of idiopathic scoliosis. Reconstr. Surg. Traumatol. *13:*184–190, 1972.
146. Mau, H.: The changing concept of infantile scoliosis. Int. Orthop. *5:*131–137, 1981.
147. McCollough, N. C., Friedman, H., and Bracale, R.: Surface electrical stimulation of the paraspinal muscles in the treatment of idiopathic scoliosis. Orthop. Trans. *4:*29, 1980.
148. McCollough, N. C.: Nonoperative treatment of idiopathic scoliosis using surface electrical stimulation. Spine *11:*802–804, 1986.
149. McMaster, M. J., and MacNicol, M. F.: The management of progressive infantile idiopathic scoliosis. J. Bone Joint Surg. *61B:*36–42, 1979.
150. McMaster, M. J.: Infantile idiopathic scoliosis: can it be prevented? J. Bone Joint Surg. *65B:*612–617, 1983.
151. Mehta, M. H., and Morel, G.: The non-operative treatment of infantile idiopathic scoliosis. *In* Zorab, P. A., and Siegler, D. (eds.): Scoliosis. London, Academic Press, 1979, pp. 71–84.
152. Mehta, M. H.: Infantile idiopathic scoliosis. *In* Dickson, R., and Bradford, D. S. (eds.): Management of Spinal Deformities. Boston, Butterworths, 1984, p. 114.
153. Mehta, M. H.: The rib-vertebra angle in the early diagnosis between resolving and progressive infantile scoliosis. J. Bone Joint Surg. *54B:*230–243, 1972.
154. Mellenkamp, D. D., Blount, W. P., and Anderson, A. J.: Milwaukee brace treatment of idiopathic scoliosis: late results. Clin. Orthop. *126:*47–57, 1977.
155. Michel, C. R., Caton, J., Allegre, G., et al.: The place of a four piece spinal support in the conservative treatment of 700 cases over 10 years. Orthop. Trans. *7:*131, 1983.
156. Michel, C. R., Onimus, M., and Kohler, R.: The Dwyer operation in the surgical treatment of scoliosis. Rev. Chir. Orthop. *63:*237–255, 1977.
157. Mielke, C. H., Lonstein, J. E., Denis, F., et al.: Comparative analysis of methods for surgical treatment of adolescent idiopathic scoliosis. Orthop. Trans. *12:*237, 1988.
158. Misol, S., Ponseti, I. V., Samaan, N., and Bradbury, J. T.: Growth hormone blood levels in patients

with idiopathic scoliosis. Clin. Orthop. *81:*122–125, 1970.
159. Moe, J. H., and Kettleson, D. N.: Idiopathic scoliosis: analysis of curve patterns and the preliminary results of Milwaukee brace treatment in 169 patients. J. Bone Joint Surg. *52A:*1509–1533, 1970.
160. Moe, J. H., Kharrat, K., Winter, R. B., et al.: Harrington instrumentation without fusion plus external orthotic support for the treatment of difficult problems in young children. Clin. Orthop. *185:*35–45, 1984.
161. Moe, J. H., Purcell, G. A., and Bradford, D. S.: Zielke instrumentation (VDS) for the correction of spinal curvature. Analysis of results in 66 patients. Clin. Orthop. *180:*133–153, 1983.
162. Moe, J. H., Sundberg, B., and Gustilo, R.: A clinical study of spine fusion in the growing child. J. Bone Joint Surg. *46B:*784–785, 1964.
163. Moe, J. H.: Methods and technique of evaluating idiopathic scoliosis. *In* American Academy of Orthopaedic Surgeons Symposium on the Spine. St. Louis, C. V. Mosby Co., 1969, pp. 196–240.
164. Moe, J. H.: Methods and techniques of evaluating idiopathic scoliosis. *In* American Academy of Orthopaedic Surgeons Symposium on the Spine. St. Louis, C. V. Mosby Co., 1969, pp. 196–240.
165. Moe, J. H.: Methods of correction and surgical techniques in scoliosis. Orthop. Clin. North Am. *3:*17–48, 1972.
166. Moe, J. H.: Modern concepts of treatment of spinal deformities in children and adults. Clin. Orthop. *110:*137–153, 1969.
167. Nachemson, A., Lonstein, J. E., and Weinstein, S. L.: Report on Prevalence. Natural History Committee of Scoliosis Research Society, Denver, 1982.
168. Nachemson, A., and Nordwall, A.: Effectiveness of preoperative Cotrel traction for correction of idiopathic scoliosis. J. Bone Joint Surg. *59A:*504–508, 1977.
169. Nachemson, A.: A long-term follow-up study of nontreated scoliosis. Acta Orthop. Scand. *39:*466–476, 1968.
170. Nash, C. L., and Brown, R. H.: The intraoperative monitoring of the spinal cord function: its growth and current status. Orthop. Clin. North Am. *10:*919–926, 1979.
171. Nash, C. L., Gregg, E. D., Brown, H. R., and Pillia, M. S.: Risk of exposure to x-rays in patients undergoing long term treatment for scoliosis. J. Bone Joint Surg. *61A:*371–380, 1979.
172. Nash, C. L., and Moe, J. H.: A study of vertebral rotation. J. Bone Joint Surg. *51A:*223–229, 1969.
173. Nash, C. L., and Brown, R. H.: Current concepts review: spinal cord monitoring. J. Bone Joint Surg. *71A:*627–630, 1989.
174. Neuwirth, M. G., and Drummond, D. S.: The results of interspinous segmental instrumentation in the sagittal plane. Orthop. Trans. *12:*258, 1988.
175. Nilsonne, U., and Lundgren, K. D.: Long-term prognosis in idiopathic scoliosis. Acta Orthop. Scand. *39:*456–465, 1968.
176. Nordwall, A., and Wilner, S.: A study of skeletal age and height in girls with idiopathic scoliosis. Clin. Orthop. *110:*6–10, 1975.
177. Nordwall, A.: Studies in idiopathic scoliosis relevant to etiology, conservative and operative treatment. Acta Orthop. Scand. (Suppl.)*150:*1–178, 1973.
178. O'Donnell, C. S., Bunnell, W. P., Betz, R. R., et al.: Electrical stimulation in the treatment of idiopathic scoliosis. Clin. Orthop. *229:*107–113, 1988.
179. Oegema, T. R., Bradford, D. S., Cooper, K. M., and Hunter, R. E.: Comparison of the biochemistry of proteoglycans isolated from normal idiopathic scoliotic and cerebral palsy spines. Spine *8:*378, 1983.
180. Ogilivie, J. W.: Anterior spine fusion with Zielke instrumentation for idiopathic scoliosis in adolescents. Orthop. Clin. North Am. *19:*313–317, 1988.
181. Patynski, J., Szcezekot, J., and Szwaluk, F.: The incidence of scoliosis. Chir. Narzadow. Ruchu. Ortop. Pol. *22:*111, 1957.
182. Pedriolle, R.: La Scoliose. Paris, Maloine SA Editeur, 1979.
183. Pedrini, V. A., Ponseti, I. V., and Dohrman, S. C.: Glycosaminoglycans of intervertebral disc in idiopathic scoliosis. J. Lab. Clin. Med. *82:*938–950, 1973.
184. Picault, C., deMauroy, J. C., Mouilleseaux, B., and Diana, G.: Natural history of idiopathic scoliosis in girls and boys. Spine *11:*777–778, 1986.
185. Ponseti, I. V., and Friedman, B.: Prognosis in idiopathic scoliosis. J. Bone Joint Surg. *32A:*381–395, 1950.
186. Ponseti, I. V., Pedrini, V., and Dohrman, S.: Biochemical analysis of intervertebral discs in idiopathic scoliosis. J. Bone Joint Surg. *54A:*1793, 1972.
187. Ponte, A.: Prognostic evaluation of vertebral rotation in small idiopathic curves. Orthop. Trans. *6:*6–7, 1982.
188. Raia, R. J., and Kilfoyle, R. M.: Minimizing radiation exposure in scoliosis screening. Appl. Radiol. *11:*45–55, 1982.
189. Redford, R. B., Butterworth, T. R., and Clements, E. L., Jr.: Use of electromyography as a prognostic aid in the management of idiopathic scoliosis. Arch. Phys. Med. Rehabil. *50:*433–438, 1969.
190. Renshaw, T. S.: The role of Harrington instrumentation and posterior spine fusion in the management of adolescent idiopathic scoliosis. Orthop. Clin. North Am. *19:*257–267, 1988.
191. Resina, J., and Ferreira-Alvez, A.: A technique for correction and internal fixation for scoliosis. J. Bone Joint Surg. *5B:*159–165, 1977.
192. Richards, B. S., and Johnston, C. E., 2nd: Cotrel-Dubousset instrumentation for adolescent idiopathic scoliosis. Orthopedics *10:*649–654, 1987.
193. Riddick, M., and Price, C.: Time modified brace wear—an effective alternative treatment regimen. Presented at the 19th Annual Meeting of the Scoliosis Research Society, Orlando, FL, September 1984.
194. Riddle, H. V. F. V., and Roaf, R.: Muscle imbalance in the causation of scoliosis. Lancet *1:*1245–1247, 1975.
195. Riseborough, E. J., and Wynne-Davies, R.: A genetic survey of idiopathic scoliosis in Boston, Massachusetts. J. Bone Joint Surg. *55A:*974–982, 1973.
196. Risser, J. C.: The iliac apophysis: an invaluable sign in the management of scoliosis. Clin. Orthop. *11:*111–119, 1958.
197. Robin, G. C., and Cohen, T.: Familial scoliosis. J. Bone Joint Surg. *57B:*146–147, 1975.

198. Rogala, E. J., Drummond, D. S., and Gurr, J.: Scoliosis: incidence and natural history. A prospective epidemiological study. J. Bone Joint Surg. *60A:*173–176, 1978.
199. Rogala, E. J., Drummond, D. S., and Gurr, J. F.: Scoliosis: incidence and natural history. A prospective epidemiological study of 22,584 school children. Presented at the Annual Meeting of the Scoliosis Research Society, Ottawa, Ontario, September 1976.
200. Sahlstrand, T., Petruson, B., and Nachemson, A.: an electronystagmographic study of the vestibular function in patients with idiopathic scoliosis. Presented at the Annual Meeting of the Scoliosis Research Society, Ottawa, Ontario, September 1976.
201. Sahlstrand, T., and Petruson, B.: A study of labyrinthine function in patients with adolescent idiopathic scoliosis. Acta Orthop. Scand. *50:*759, 1979.
202. Salanova, C.: Late results of Milwaukee brace treatment of idiopathic scoliosis. Orthop. Trans. *10:*2, 1986.
203. Schultz, A. B., Ciszewski, D. J., DeWald, R. L., et al.: Spine morphology as a determinant of progression tendency in idiopathic scoliosis. Orthop. Trans. *3:*52, 1979.
204. Scoliosis Research Society: Morbidity and Mortality Committee Report, 1987.
205. Scott, J. C., and Morgan, T. H.: The natural history of infantile idiopathic scoliosis. J. Bone Joint Surg. *37B:*400–413, 1955.
206. Shands, A. R., Jr., and Eisberg, H. B.: The incidence of scoliosis in the state of Delaware: a study of 50,000 minifilms of the chest made during a survey for tuberculosis. J. Bone Joint Surg. *37A:*1243–1249, 1955.
207. Shannon, D. C., Riseborough, E. J., Valenca, L. M., et al.: The distribution of abnormal lung function in kyphoscoliosis. J. Bone Joint Surg. *52A:*131–144, 1970.
208. Sharpe, J. A., Silversides, J. L., and Blair, R. D. G.: Familial paralysis of horizontal gaze. Neurology *25:*1035–1040, 1975.
209. Shufflebarger, H. L., and Clark, C.: Cotrel-Dubousset instrumentation in adolescent idiopathic scoliosis. Orthop. Trans. *11:*49, 1987.
210. Shufflebarger, H. S., Keiser, R. P., and King, W.: Non-operative treatment of idiopathic scoliosis: a 10-year study. Orthop. Trans. *7:*11, 1983.
211. Silverman, B. J., and Greenbarg, P. E.: Internal fixation of the spine for idiopathic scoliosis using square-ended distraction rods and lamina wiring (Harrington-Luque technique). Bull. Hosp. Joint Dis. Orthop. Inst. *44:*41–55, 1984.
212. Skogland, L. B., and Miller, J. A. A.: Growth related hormones in idiopathic scoliosis. Acta Orthop. Scand. *51:*779, 1980.
213. Spencer, G. S. G.: Muscle and enzyme staining in scoliosis. *In* Zorab, P. A. (ed.): Scoliosis and Muscle. Proceedings of a Fourth Symposium, London, November 1973. London, W. Heinemann Medical Books, 1974, pp. 103–112.
214. Strayer, L. M., III: The incidence of scoliosis in the post-partum female on Cape Cod. J. Bone Joint Surg. *55A:*436, 1973.
215. Sullivan, J. A., Davidson, R., Renshaw, T. S., et al.: Further evaluation of the Scolitron treatment of idiopathic adolescent scoliosis. Spine *11:*903–906, 1986.
216. Tanner, J. M.: Growth and endocrinology of the adolescent. *In* Gardner, L. I. (ed.): Endocrine and Genetic Diseases of Childhood. 2nd ed. Philadelphia, W. B. Saunders Co., 1975, pp. 14–64.
217. Tanner, J. M.: Some main features of normal growth in children. *In* Zorab, P. A. (ed.): Proceedings of a Third Symposium, London, November 1970. Edinburgh, Churchill Livingstone, 1971, pp. 14–25.
218. Taylor, T. K. F., Ghosh, P., and Bushell, G. R.: The contribution of the intervertebral disc to the scoliotic deformity. Clin. Orthop. *156:*79, 1981.
219. Thometz, J. G., and Emans, J. B.: A comparison between spinous process and sublaminar wiring combined with Harrington distraction instrumentation in the management of adolescent idiopathic scoliosis. J. Pediatr. Orthop. *8:*129–132, 1988.
220. Thompson, G. H., Wilber, P. G., Shaffer, J. W., et al.: Segmental spinal instrumentation in idiopathic scoliosis. Spine *10:*623–630, 1985.
221. Tolo, V. T., and Gillespie, R.: The characteristics of juvenile idiopathic scoliosis and results of its treatment. J. Bone Joint Surg. *60B:*181–188, 1978.
222. Torell, G., Nordwall, A., and Nachemson, A.: The changing pattern of scoliosis treatment due to effective screening. J. Bone Joint Surg. *63A:*337–341, 1981.
223. Travaglini, F.: Multiple primary idiopathic scoliosis. Ital. J. Orthop. Traumat. *1:*67–80, 1975.
224. Tsairis, P.: A histochemical study of paraspinal muscles in idiopathic scoliosis. *In* Zorab, P. A. (ed.): Scoliosis and Muscle. Proceedings of a Fourth Symposium, London, November 1973. London, W. Heinemann Medical Books, 1974, pp. 115–120.
225. Vauzelle, C., Stagnara, P., and Jouvinroux, P.: Functional monitoring of spinal cord activity during spinal surgery. Clin. Orthop. *93:*173–178, 1973.
226. Von Duensing, F., and Schaefer, K. P.: Die Aktivität einzelner neurone im Bereich der Vestibulariskerne bei Horizontalbeschleunigungen unter besonderer Berücksichtigung des vestibulären Nystagmus. Arch. Psychiat. Z. Neurol. *198:*225–252, 1958.
227. Wasylenko, M., Skinner, S. R., Perry, J., et al.: An analysis of posture and gait following spinal fusion with Harrington instrumentation. Spine *8:*840–845, 1983.
228. Waters, R. L., and Morris, J. M.: An in vitro study of normal and scoliotic interspinous ligaments. J. Biomech. *6:*343–348, 1973.
229. Weinstein, S. L., and Ponseti, I. V.: Curve progression in idiopathic scoliosis. J. Bone Joint Surg. *65A:*447–455, 1983.
230. Weinstein, S. L., Zavala, D. C., and Ponseti, I. V.: Idiopathic scoliosis: long-term followup and prognosis in untreated patients. J. Bone Joint Surg. *63A:*702–712, 1981.
231. Westgate, H. D., and Moe, J. H.: Pulmonary function in kyphoscoliosis before and after correction by the Harrington instrumentation method. J. Bone Joint Surg. *51A:*935–946, 1969.
232. White, A. A., and Panjabi, M. M.: Clinical biomechanics of the spine. Philadelphia, J. B. Lippincott Co., 1978, p. 105.

233. Wilber, R. G., Thompson, G. H., Shaffer, J. W., et al.: Postoperative neurological deficits in segmental spinal instrumentation. J. Bone Joint Surg. *66A:*1178–1198, 1984.
234. Willner, S., Nilssone, K. O., Kastrup, K., and Bergstrand, C. G.: Growth hormone and somatomedin A in girls with adolescent idiopathic scoliosis. Acta Paediatr. Scand. *65:*547–552, 1976.
235. Willner, S., and Udén, A.: A prospective prevalence study of scoliosis in southern Sweden. Acta Orthop. Scand. *53:*233–237, 1982.
236. Willner, S.: Factors contributing to structural scoliosis. University of Lund. Thesis, Lund, Sweden, Studentlitteratur, 1972.
237. Winner, S.: A study of height, weight and menarche in girls with idiopathic structural scoliosis. Acta Orthop. Scand. *46:*71–83, 1975.
238. Winter, R. B., and Anderson, M. N.: Spinal arthrodesis for spinal deformity using posterior instrumentation and sublaminar wiring: 100 consecutive personal cases. Int. Orthop. *9:*239–245, 1985.
239. Winter, R. B., and Carlson, M. J.: Modern orthotics for spinal deformities. Clin. Orthop. *126:*74, 1977.
240. Winter, R. B., Lonstein, J. E., Drogt, J., and Noren, C. A.: The effectiveness of bracing in the nonoperative treatment of idiopathic scoliosis. Spine *11:*790–791, 1986.
241. Winter, R. B., Lonstein, J. E., VandenBrink, K., et al.: The surgical treatment of thoracic adolescent idiopathic scoliosis with a Harrington rod and sublaminar wires. Orthop. Trans. *11:*89, 1987.
242. Winter, R. B., Lovell, W., and Moe, J. H.: Excessive thoracic lordosis and loss of pulmonary function in patients with idiopathic scoliosis. J. Bone Joint Surg. *57A:*972, 1975.
243. Wynne-Davies, R.: Genetic and other factors in etiology of scoliosis. Doctoral Thesis, University of Edinburgh, 1973.
244. Wynne-Davies, R.: Familial (idiopathic) scoliosis. A family survey. J. Bone Joint Surg. *50B:*24–30, 1968.
245. Wynne-Davies, R.: Infantile idiopathic scoliosis. Causative factors, particularly in the first six months of life. J. Bone Joint Surg. *57B:*138–141, 1975.
246. Yamada, K., Ikata, T., Yamamoto, H., et al.: Equilibrium function in scoliosis and active corrective plaster jacket for the treatment. Tokushima J. Exp. Med. *16:*1–7, 1969.
247. Yamada, K., Yamamoto, H., Tamura, T., and Tezuka, A.: Development of scoliosis under neurological basis, particularly in relation with brainstem abnormalities. J. Bone Joint Surg. *56A:*1764, 1974.
248. Yamada, K., and Yamaoto, H.: Equilibrium function in scoliosis and active corrective plaster jacket for treatment. Am. Digest Foreign Orthop. Lit., Third Quarter, *VI*182–185, 1972.
249. Yarom, R., Robin, G. C., and Gorodetsky, R.: X-ray fluorescence analysis of muscles in scoliosis. Spine *3:*142, 1978.
250. Yekutiel, M., Robin, G. C., and Yarom, R.: Proprioceptive function in children with adolescent idiopathic scoliosis. Spine *6:*560, 1981.
251. Zaoussis, A. L., and James, J. I. P.: The iliac apophysis and the evolution of curves in scoliosis. J. Bone Joint Surg. *40B:*442–453, 1981.
252. Zielke, K., Stunkat, R., and Beaujean, F.: Ventrale derotations—spondylodesis. Author's translation. Arch. Orthop. Unfallchir. *85:*257–277, 1976.
253. Zielke, K.: Ventral derotation spondylolisthesis. Results of treatment of cases of idiopathic lumbar scoliosis. Author's translation. Z. Orthop. *120:*320–329, 1982.
254. Zorab, P. A., Prime, F. J., and Harrison, A.: Lung function in young persons after spinal fusion for scoliosis. Spine *4:*22–28, 1979.
255. Zuk, T.: Role of spinal and abdominal muscles in the pathogenesis of scoliosis. J. Bone Joint Surg. *44B:*102–105, 1962.

CHAPTER

15

NEUROMUSCULAR SCOLIOSIS

Jonathan F. Camp, M.D.
Dennis Wenger, M.D.
Scott Mubarak, M.D.

GENERAL PRINCIPLES

Compared with idiopathic scoliosis, neuromuscular scoliosis is unique in several important ways:

1. *Large Progressive Curves Early in Life.* Neuromuscular scoliosis begins to progress from the time of disease onset or neurologic insult. As many of these conditions originate in the prenatal period, associated spinal deformity may progress to a magnitude requiring treatment in infancy or early childhood.

2. *Early Onset of Curve Stiffness.* Early loss of spinal flexibility may result from muscle or soft tissue contracture formation as in arthrogryposis, or persistent asymmetric muscle tone as in cerebral palsy.

3. *Curve Progression During Adulthood.* During adolescence, progression of neuromuscular spinal deformity is partly linked to rapid spine growth. Neuromuscular curves, however, can progress independent of growth before adolescence, as well as after adolescence into adulthood. Late curve progression in cerebral palsy (CP) may be secondary, in part, to markedly delayed bone age, with bone growth continuing into the late teens and early twenties. In neurologically static conditions (CP, myelodysplasia, poliomyelitis, and spinal cord injury), progression in adulthood may also be secondary to asymmetric muscle tone or increasing body weight and trunk height, which may overwhelm the poorly supported spine. In conditions that are progressive neurologically (e.g., Duchenne muscular dystrophy) an even more dramatic progression of spinal deformity is anticipated.

4. *Long Curves with Pelvic Obliquity.* Neurologic curves frequently involve two to four more spinal segments than idiopathic curves, and because of their thoracolumbar pattern, pelvic obliquity is common.

5. *Increased Complications.* From a surgical standpoint, patients with neuromuscular disorders have several unique features that increase operative risk. They have a higher risk of infection.[8] The bone is softer, which increases the risk of instrumentation failure and postoperative pseudarthrosis. Surgical blood loss is often greater because of adherent paraspinous muscles that do not strip from the bone well and do not contract down on bleeding arterioles. Blood loss is also increased because of the increased length of fusion and increased operative time, with the frequent necessity of sacropelvic instrumentation and fusion. Pulmonary complications are certainly greater in this group of patients. Because of diaphragmatic and intercostal muscular weakness, postoperative ventilatory support is often necessary. In patients with severe respiratory

compromise, e.g., as in spinal muscular atrophy, diaphragmatic surgery at the time of anterior spinal fusion is discouraged. Pre- and postoperative bracing and casting is poorly tolerated in most patients with neuromuscular disorders because of decreased intelligence, poor cooperation, skin insensitivity and weakness, spasticity, or athetosis that may lead to skin pressure problems.

These factors combine to make scoliosis in neuromuscular patients the most difficult and complicated of all spinal deformities to manage.

Classification

Our classification of neuromuscular scoliosis is based on two factors: the progressive nature of a disorder and the origin of the condition from upper motor neuron areas, lower motor neuron areas, or muscle. As prototypes of the various categories we will discuss examples of:

- I. Upper motor neuropathy
  - A. Nonprogressive
    - 1. Cerebral palsy
    - 2. Acquired paralysis
  - B. Progressive
    - 1. Friedreich's ataxia
    - 2. Charcot-Marie-Tooth disease
- II. Lower motor neuropathy
  - A. Nonprogressive
    - 1. Poliomyelitis
    - 2. Myelomeningocele
  - B. Progressive
    - 1. Spinal muscular atrophy
- III. Myopathic
  - A. Nonprogressive
    - 1. Arthrogryposis
  - B. Progressive
    - 1. Duchenne muscular dystrophy

General Treatment Principles

There are three major treatment options for patients with scoliosis: observation, bracing, and fusion.

Observation and Bracing

Only minor neuromuscular curves under 20 degrees can be safely observed. Once the curve has reached 20 degrees and progression is documented, treatment should be considered. Even though most neuromuscular scoliosis continues to progress despite brace use, bracing can be a temporizing measure to allow spinal growth and preserve upper extremity function with maintenance of trunk balance while eventual spinal arthrodesis is awaited. Muscular dystrophy is an exception to this bracing philosophy because bracing allows further deterioration of pulmonary function, making the eventual surgery more dangerous.

Since most progressive neuromuscular curves are thoracolumbar, an under-arm brace can often be used. In very young children, soft thoracolumbar Plastazote body jackets with a rigid shell can provide needed support (Fig. 15–1). Older patients require more rigid materials such as Kydex or Orthoplast. In older children with poor voluntary trunk control, an element of spine control can be achieved with "passive" total contact orthoses. These braces are fitted to the body contours without corrective molds. A more effective "dynamic" molded thoracolumbar orthosis (TLSO) can be used in children who possess enough motor control to pull away from the brace and its corrective contours. Reclined custom sitting spine orthoses can be effective in severely affected patients with no head control or sitting balance (Fig. 15–2).

Fusion

Traditionally, fusion is considered in patients who experience functional compromise as a result of progressive spinal deformity. The authors do not feel completely comfortable with the traditional definition of function, which is often restricted in context to sitting, ambulation, or purposeful upper extremity activity. We consider it inappropriate that patients who do not fit into this functional definition should be allowed to progress without treatment when involved caretakers and parents struggle with their care or believe them to be in pain. Surgery of the spine and hips is indicated in patients in whom comfortable seating and even lying in bed is compromised by distorted body contours or chronic skin breakdown. Obviously, when a spinal deformity has progressed to a point where surgical risks outweigh realistic benefits, the surgeon

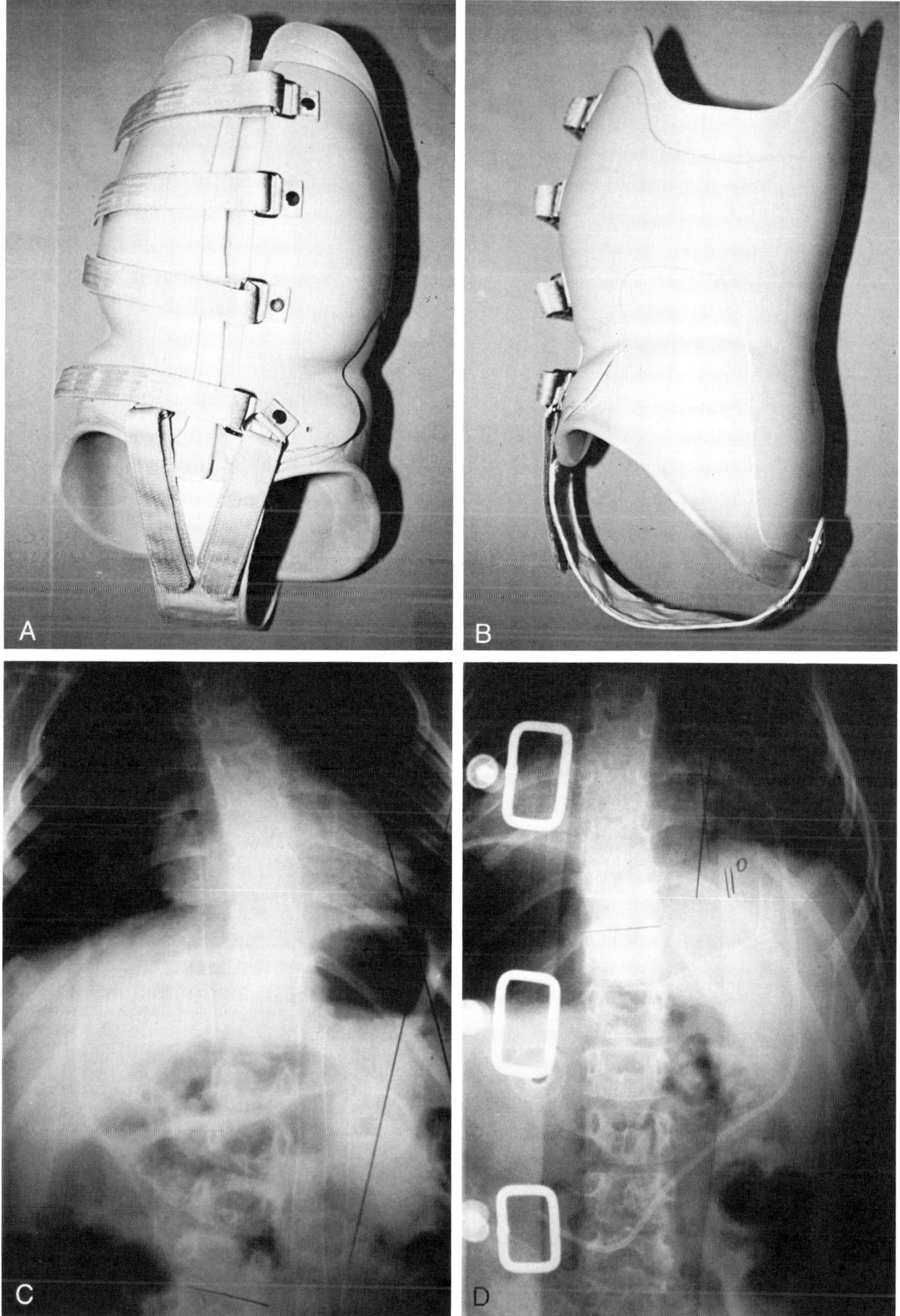

Figure 15–1. *A, B,* Plastazote body jacket with Kydex shell. *C, D,* In and out of brace films demonstrating correction despite the soft nature of the material.

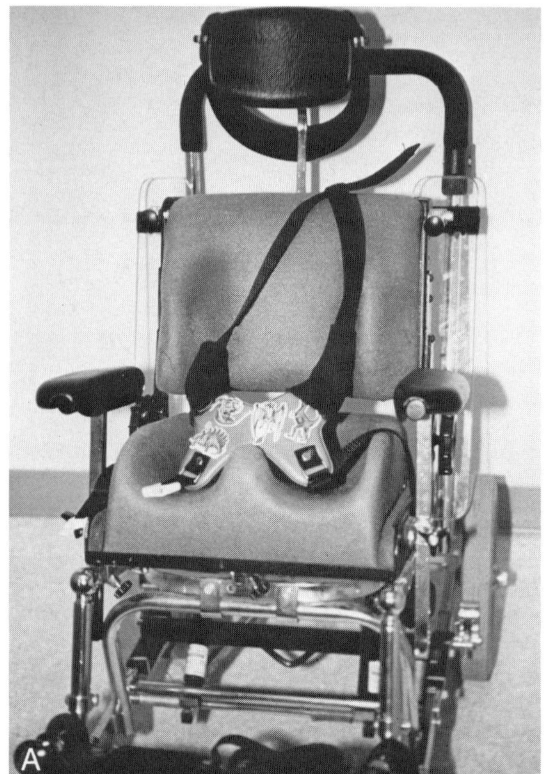

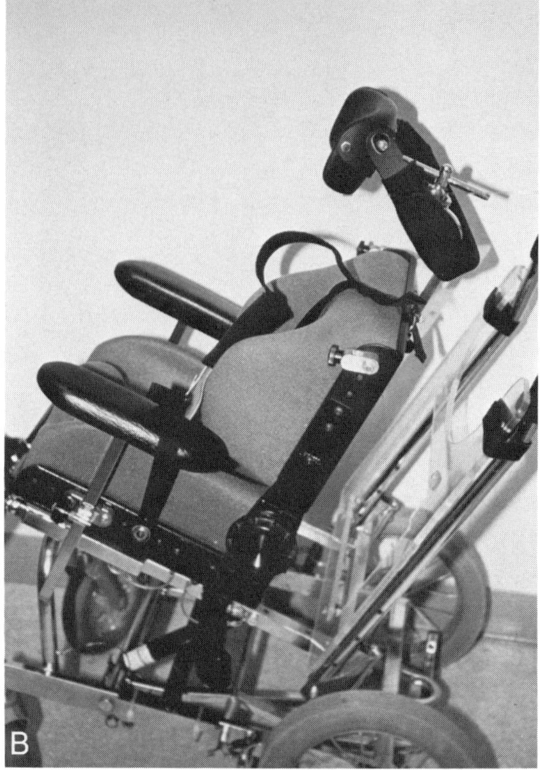

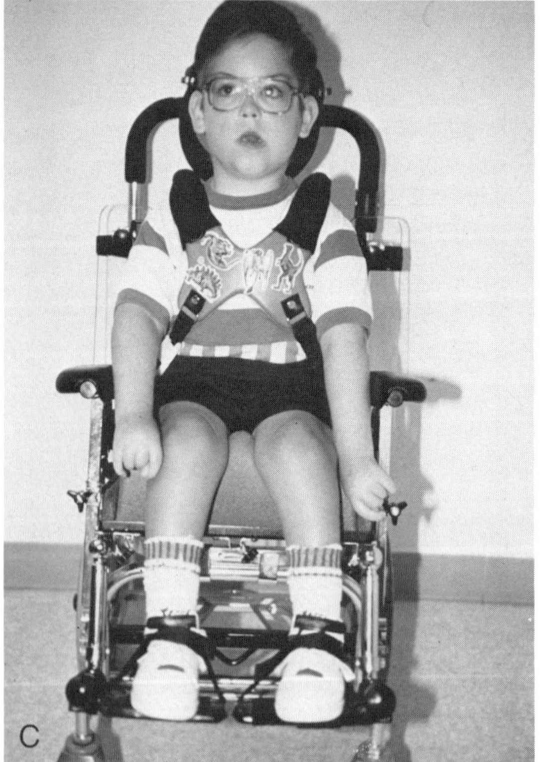

Figure 15–2. *A* to *C*, Reclined sitting spinal orthosis molded for spinal correction; reclined for gravity head control.

and the parents should both agree that surgery be withheld.

When indicated, posterior segmental instrumentation and fusion is generally the technique of choice, augmented by anterior fusion for large rigid curves or those with significant pelvic obliquity.

Preoperative Considerations

Every patient with a neuromuscular disorder should receive the benefits of a team approach in preparation for surgery.

Neurologic. A neurologist can assist in the confirmation of the neurologic diagnosis and ensure that proper medications are appropriately monitored and adjusted both before and after surgery. Patients taking phenytoin (Dilantin) may have softer bones. In our experience, valproic acid use can be associated with increased intraoperative and postoperative bleeding.

Cardiopulmonary. A cardiopulmonary evaluation should be considered in patients with progressive disorders (Duchenne muscular dystrophy, spinal muscular atrophy, Friedreich's ataxia) or any neuromuscular patients' disorder in which there is a curve greater than 90 degrees and cardiopulmonary compromise is suspected. This evaluation should include pulmonary function testing, arterial blood gas analysis, chest radiographs where indicated, as well as cardiac echo to assess cardiac function. Nickel and colleagues[11, 12] stated that patients with vital capacities of less than 30 per cent are likely to require postoperative respiratory support, and recommended that surgery take place before such a severe degree of pulmonary compromise. Anticipating prolonged respiratory dependence after surgery, Brown and associates[4] recommended preoperative tracheostomy in patients without voluntary cough reflex and a vital capacity of less than 30 per cent. Bradford[3] preferred indwelling endotracheal tubes for as long as necessary. Although no particular test can determine with 100 per cent reliability the need for prolonged postoperative respiratory support, we feel that the inability to generate a cough reflex is a significant predictor of the need for such prolonged support.

Gastrointestinal and Nutritional. Hiatal hernia and esophageal reflux are common in CP patients and should be surgically corrected preoperatively to minimize aspiration risks.

Nutrition should be maximized orally or via gastric tube if necessary. The patients' nutritional status bears directly on their ability to resist infection and heal a surgical incision. A patient with little or no subcutaneous tissue is also more at risk for skin pressure problems resulting from prominent bones and surgical implants.

Hematologic. As part of the preoperative preparation, baseline complete blood count (CBC), bleeding studies (PT, PTT, platelet count, bleeding time) and use of autologous or designated donor blood are recommended to minimize concerns regarding potential transmission of disease from blood bank blood.

Radiologic. Complete preoperative evaluation of a patient with a spinal deformity includes lateral and anteroposterior (AP) spine films. The static radiographs should be obtained in the functional upright sitting or standing position if feasible. For sitting patients we recommend a seat known as the muscular dystrophy throne developed at the Hospital for Sick Children in Toronto (Fig. 15–3).[9] If the patient can stand, a posteroanterior (PA) view is taken.

A Stagnara view may help document the true curve magnitude in a very rotated spine. Complete analysis of the curvature requires assessment of spine rotation and may have an influence on the extent of fusion. Because convex right curves are rotated in a direction opposite to curves with a convexity to the left, a true kyphosis may exist at the point of rotational transition between two major lordotic curves. Fusion should extend beyond this functional kyphosis.

Physician-assisted bending or traction films taken in the supine position are very important in assessing curve flexibility. In ambulatory patients with curves extending into the lumbar spine, standing, physician-monitored bending films should be obtained to assess the spontaneous flexibility of compensatory curves and noninvolved lumbar segments. As fusion to the sacrum should usually be avoided in walking patients, these latter films help determine the appropriate inferior level of fusion. The surgeon should evaluate pelvic obliquity, if present, as well as the flexibility of a lumbosacral curve if present. If the L5–S1 disc does not level to within 15 degrees of horizontal, sacropelvic fusion should be considered.

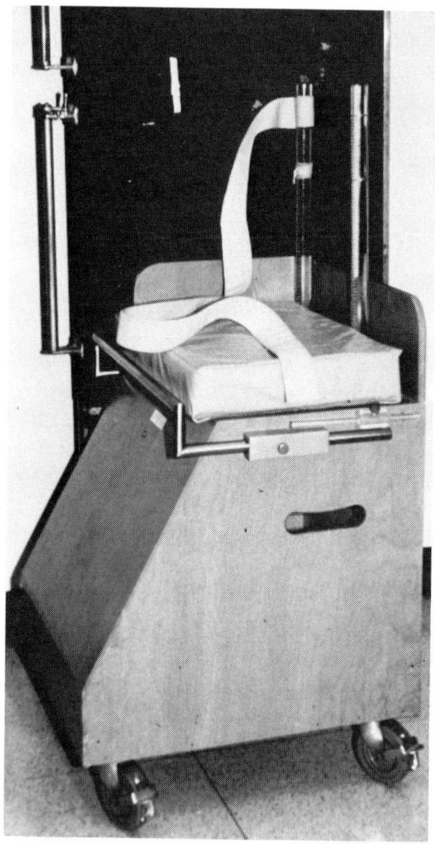

Figure 15–3. Muscular dystrophy throne developed at the Hospital for Sick Children in Toronto to obtain standardized upright sitting x-ray films. (From Koreska, J., Schwentker, E. P., and Albisser, A. M.: A simple method for obtaining accurate and reproducible bi-plane spinal radiographs. Presented at the 28th Annual Conference on Engineering in Medicine and Biology, New Orleans, September 20–24, 1975. © 1975 IEEE.)

Intraoperative Considerations

Blood Conservation. The use of a cell saver is recommended to decrease the need for postoperative blood products. In our experience there is some risk of underestimating total blood loss with the use of the cell saver, because blood loss cannot be measured by standard operating room techniques. Constant communication between surgeon and anesthesiologist is therefore necessary to determine when to transfuse non–cell saver blood. Devices are now available for recovery of transfusable blood to continue into the postoperative period through wound drains (Davol Autotransfuser Stryker, ConstaVac).

Somatosensory Evoked Potentials. With the advent of brain stem somatosensory evoked potentials (BSEP), reliable monitoring of the severely involved patient can be performed. We strongly recommend its use in these patients to prevent further compromise of their neurologic condition (Fig. 15–4).[1, 10]

Instrumentation Principles. Fusion inferiorly to the pelvis is generally considered in any nonwalking or spastic patient with rigid pelvic obliquity greater than 15 degrees (iliac crest relative to lumbar spine). The contribution of hip contractures to pelvic obliquity should be assessed and surgically addressed. Whether the hips or spine are approached as a first stage depends on the contribution of the hip contractures to the pelvic obliquity, and from a practical standpoint the ability to position the patient adequately for spine surgery.

Segmental posterior instrumentation and fusion is preferred for most neuromuscular disorders. Luque instrumentation is the standard of segmental fixation. Cotrel-Dubousset (C-D) or Texas Scottish Rite (TSRH) instrumentation may be appropriate in some instances, because it can be effectively extended to the pelvis by means of the Galveston technique (Fig. 15–5), sacral screws (Fig. 15–6), and iliosacral screws (Fig. 15–7).[2, 5, 7, 13] We prefer the Galveston technique, which is biomechanically superior and associated with less postoperative failure.[5] Derotation can be accomplished while still using the Galveston technique for pelvic fixation with two sets of rods, one set for the spine and one for the pelvis. After the derotation maneuver has been performed with the spinal set, the two sets are connected using C-D dominoes or TSRH cross-locking plates (Fig. 15–5*B*). Additional indications for combined anterior and posterior spinal fusion have been clarified recently by Dubousset and colleagues.[6] They have demonstrated the need for anterior spinal fusion in young Risser 0 patients to control the continued progression caused by the anterior growth plates growing around a solid posterior fusion (crankshaft phenomenon). In addition, many patients with neuromuscular disorders require anterior fusion regardless of the status of skeletal maturity because of the inability to correct the curve adequately with posterior fusion alone and in order to decrease the potential for pseudarthrosis.

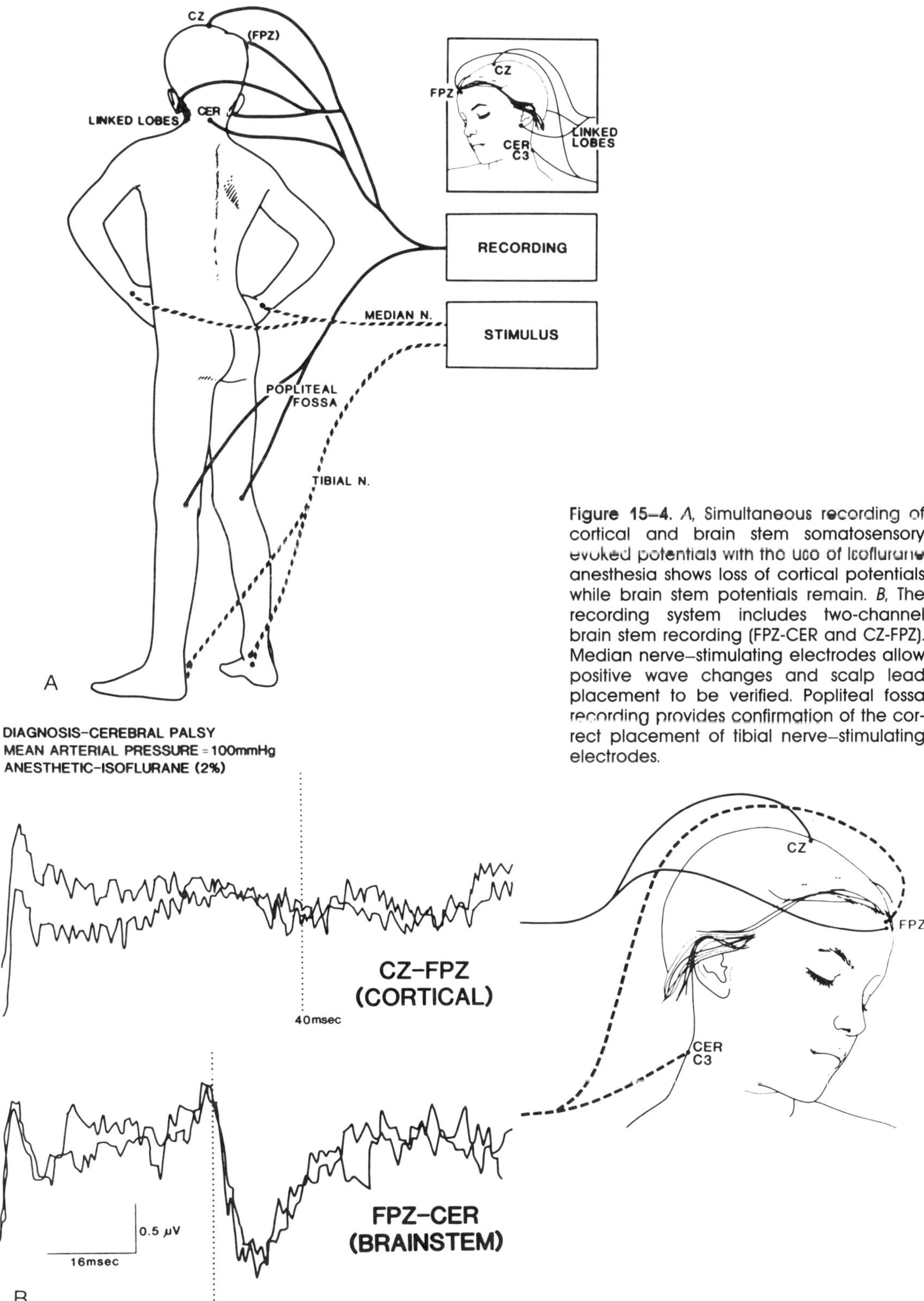

Figure 15–4. *A*, Simultaneous recording of cortical and brain stem somatosensory evoked potentials with the use of isoflurane anesthesia shows loss of cortical potentials while brain stem potentials remain. *B*, The recording system includes two-channel brain stem recording (FPZ-CER and CZ-FPZ). Median nerve–stimulating electrodes allow positive wave changes and scalp lead placement to be verified. Popliteal fossa recording provides confirmation of the correct placement of tibial nerve–stimulating electrodes.

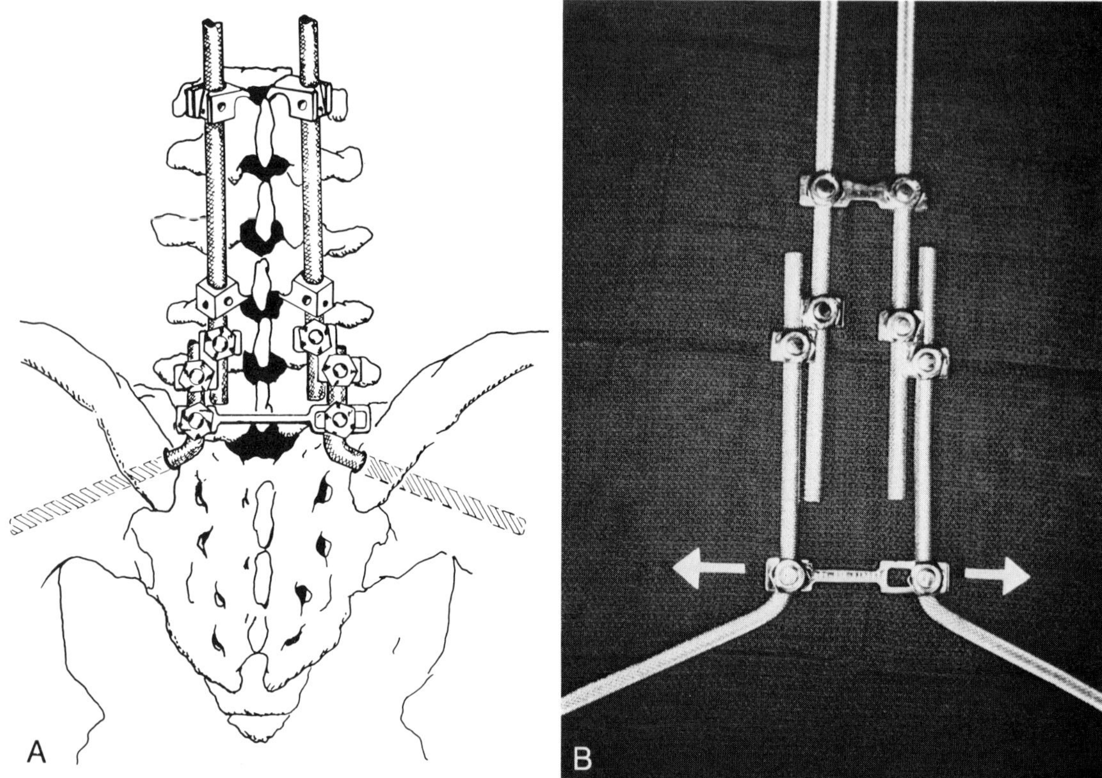

Figure 15–5. *A, B,* Cotrel-Dubousset (C-D) Galveston pelvic instrumentation technique using two sets of C-D rods, one set in the pelvis and one in the spine connected by TSRH cross-locking plates, the most inferior of which is set in distraction to hold the instrumentation in the pelvis.

CEREBRAL PALSY

Cerebral palsy (CP) is a term applied to conditions in which interference with control of the developing motor system results from static lesions within the brain,[23] sustained frequently around the time of birth from anoxic insult. It has become the most common neuromuscular condition in the Western world and has replaced poliomyelitis as the prototype of neuromuscular spine deformity.[3, 16, 22, 24]

Scoliosis Risk Factors in CP

Spasticity predisposes a CP patient to develop scoliosis. Dickson[23] found the incidence of scoliosis to be highest in spastic patients over primarily athetoid patients (50 per cent versus 25 per cent) and a rate ten times higher in spastic patients compared with primarily ataxic patients.

The extent of neural involvement is also

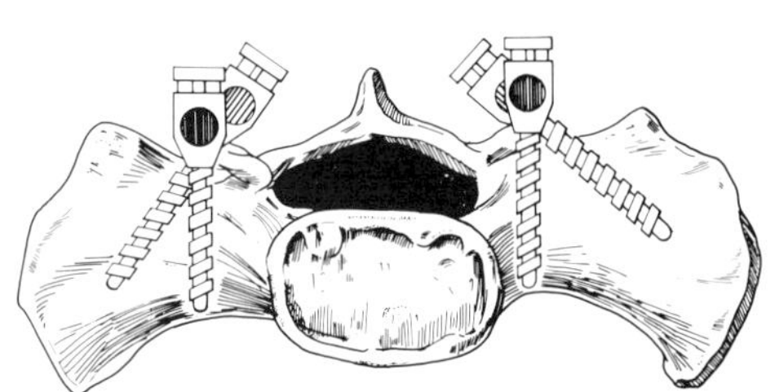

Figure 15–6. C-D sacral screw technique with divergent sacral screws at S1.

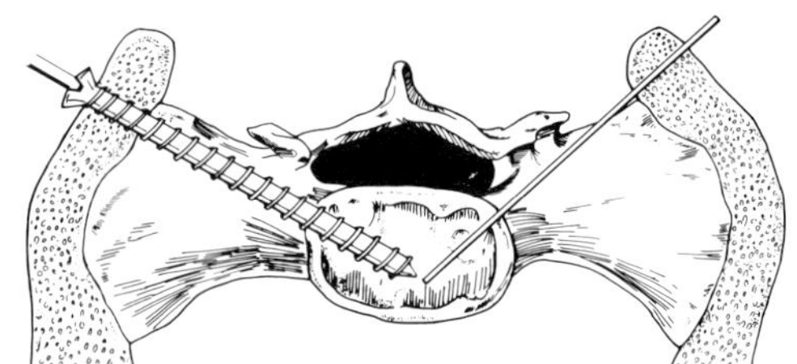

Figure 15–7. C-D iliosacral screws using cannulated C-D bone screws through two cortices of ilium and into the sacrum.

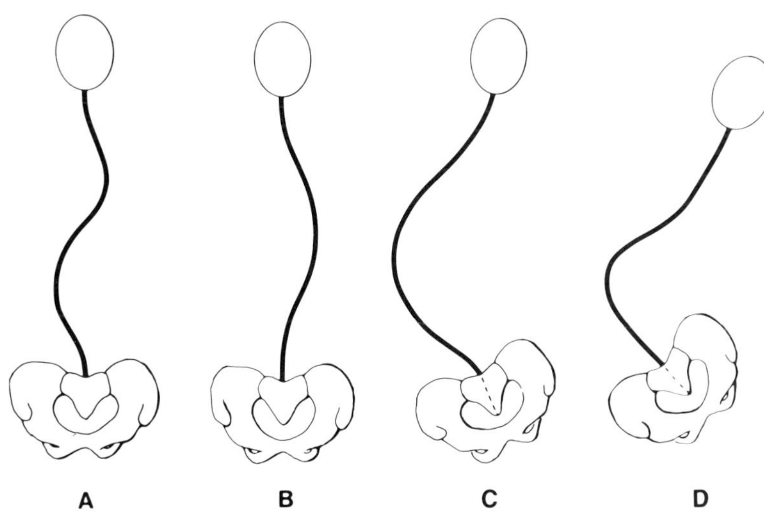

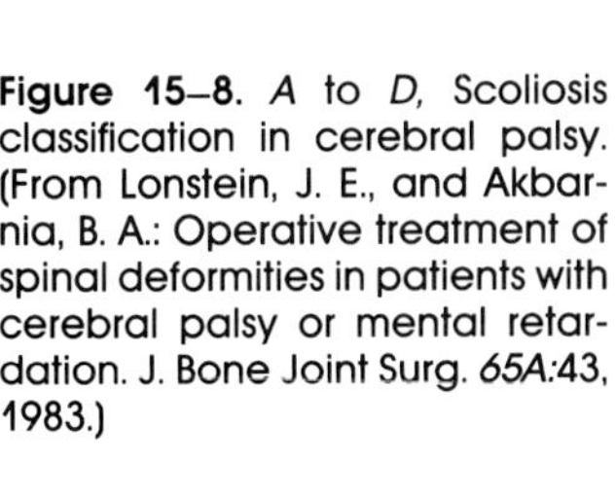
Figure 15–8. *A* to *D,* Scoliosis classification in cerebral palsy. (From Lonstein, J. E., and Akbarnia, B. A.: Operative treatment of spinal deformities in patients with cerebral palsy or mental retardation. J. Bone Joint Surg. *65A:*43, 1983.)

correlated to scoliosis incidence. In the most severely affected institutionalized quadriplegics, there is an almost universal incidence of spinal deformity. Madigan and Wallace[37] found a 75 per cent incidence and Samilson and Bechard[41] noted 94 per cent in 206 patients. Severely involved institutionalized diplegic patients have a 68 per cent incidence of scoliosis,[37] whereas scoliosis incidence in the less involved ambulatory diplegics and hemiplegics varies from 6 to 10 per cent. It should be noted, however, that even this seemingly low incidence is still three to five times that of idiopathic scoliosis[29, 42] in the general population.

Classification

Lonstein and Akbarnia[32] classified scoliosis in CP into four categories based on the presence or absence of pelvic obliquity and the presence of associated single or double curves (Fig. 15–8). They noted that long "C" curves with pelvic obliquity generally occurred in a more severely involved nonambulatory patient with spasticity. The "S" curves occurred more frequently in sitting or walking patients with little spasticity. These "S" curves likewise appeared more idiopathic in nature, often without associated pelvic obliquity.

Allen and Ferguson[14] believed that more functional patients have an S-shaped curve because their balance when sitting requires compensatory curve formation to keep the pelvis and head vertically balanced. In support of Allen and Ferguson's assumption of a milder neurologic involvement in CP patients with double curves, Horstmann and Boyer,[29] in a study of 2000 CP patients at the Dupont Institute, found that the double or triple curves carry a prognosis more similar to that of idiopathic scoliosis, and progress less predictably into adulthood than the single, long thoracolumbar curves characteristic of more severe involvement. Severely involved patients with a developmental level less than six months seldom attain independent sitting balance. They therefore do not sense that their head is out of proper alignment and do not develop compensatory curves to bring the shoulders and head over the pelvis.

Pathophysiology

The development of scoliosis in CP is thought to result in part from persistent primitive reflex patterns (Fig. 15–9) as well as asymmetric tone in the paraspinous and intercostal muscles. Pelvic obliquity from contractures about the hip plays a role in scoliosis development; however, it is often difficult to isolate this as a contributing factor because the pelvic obliquity and the scoliosis often develop simultaneously.

Placing weak-trunked quadriplegics into artificial upright sitting positions without appropriate spinal support may encourage gravity-related kyphosis and scoliosis. This suspicion was raised by Madigan and Wallace[37] as they compared the 75 per cent incidence of scoliosis

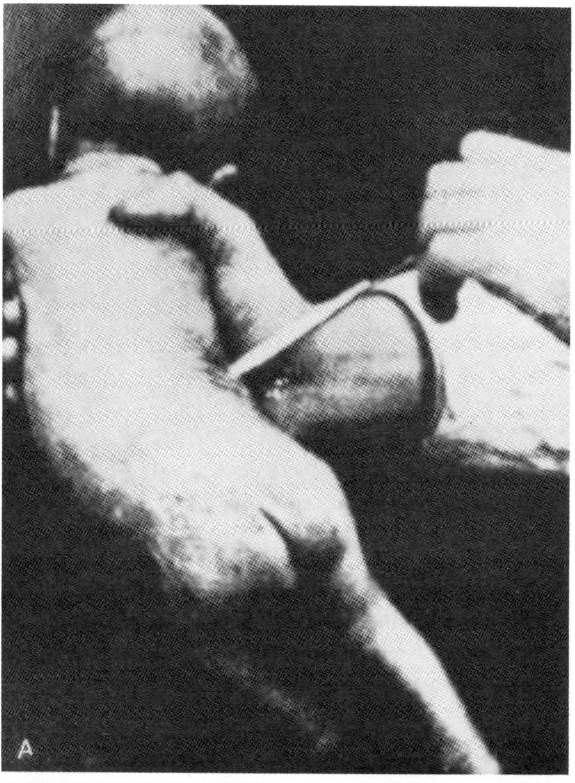

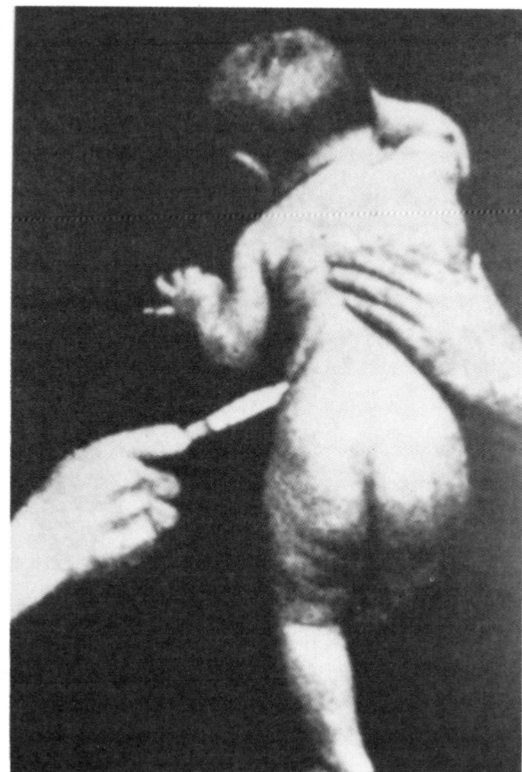

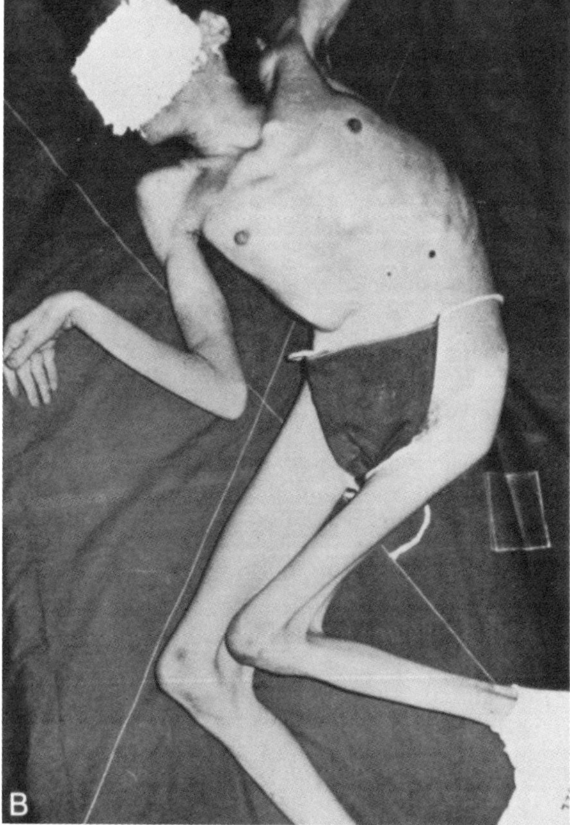

Figure 15–9. *A*, Galante reflex as possible etiology of scoliosis in CP. *B*, Persistent Galante reflex posture in an adolescent CP patient. (From Samilson, R. L., and Bechard, R.: Scoliosis in cerebral palsy: incidence, distribution of curve patterns, natural history and thoughts on etiology. Current Practice in Orthopedic Surgery. St. Louis, C. V. Mosby Co., 1973, pp. 186, 200.)

in a predominantly institutionalized population of spastic quadriplegics made up of "prop sitters" with a population of spastic quadriplegics with a 25 per cent incidence of scoliosis where a similar practice of prop sitting was not pursued.

Natural History

Curve progression is related to the risk factors listed above and, like idiopathic scoliosis, is also related to the amount of growth remaining in the spine and the magnitude of the existing curve. Because progression of spinal deformity begins at onset of the neuromuscular condition, CP patients have a much longer time to progress, with a potential for larger curves than patients of similar age with idiopathic scoliosis. This period of potential curve progression is further prolonged because these patients often maintain open growth plates into their late teens or early twenties. In adults, Thometz and Simon[47] found that larger curves progress faster than smaller curves; they noted a curve progression of 0.8 degrees per year in curves less than 50 degrees and 1.4 degrees per year in curves greater than 50 degrees.

Treatment

Bracing

Historically, CP patients have been excluded from nonoperative treatment because of their poor tolerance of manipulative casting and their inability to perform exercises that were thought to be important to ensure success with casting therapy.[3] Dynamic bracing as a treatment modality has not been as successful in neuromuscular deformity as in idiopathic scoliosis. Dynamic bracing in idiopathic scoliosis attempts to gain a three-point fixation on the curve with molded pads, and operates in part on the premise that the patient voluntarily pulls away from the prominent points of brace contact. CP patients often do not have this degree of voluntary control. Skin breakdown and pain may result. Bleck[16] and Bradford[3] recommended passive bracing with total torso contact, since it matches the native configuration of the torso, supporting it without prominent padding or brace molding. Even this type of passive bracing approach can be problematic for CP patients with spasticity or a motion disorder, as they press against the brace, often causing skin breakdown or overpowering the soft materials used to avoid skin breakdown. Both Bleck[16] and MacEwen[36] found the Milwaukee brace to be poorly tolerated in these patients because of the neck ring. In an ambulatory population, Bleck found that the ring was poorly tolerated because it altered equilibrium enough to unbalance the patient. This can make the ambulatory patient a sitter and require the sitting patient to use upper extremities for balance. MacEwen had to discontinue the use of a rigid under-arm Wilmington brace in 38 of 41 patients because of skin problems and breakdown.

In 68 patients, Zimbler and associates[49] found that children under 10 years old with curves under 40 degrees tolerated the brace well enough to justify its limited use. They recommended the use of softer materials to limit potential skin problems. We prefer a Plastazote jacket for our young, generally hypotonic quadriplegic patients. This orthosis is well tolerated, soft, and comfortable and in most cases is adjustable and will fit the patient for several years (see Fig. 15–1). For more rigid curves a Kydex or a hard plastic TLSO is necessary and seems to be well tolerated (Fig. 15–10). In more severely involved patients without sitting balance or head control, Bradford[3] recommended sitting spinal orthosis systems (SSO), which incorporate corrective pad placement in a semireclined position (see Fig. 15–2). Systems of this nature work most effectively on curves with more weakness than spasticity that are gravity affected in the more upright supported sitting position. However, young patients quickly outgrow these units and we recommend their use in older patients growing less rapidly.

Considering all approaches to bracing, most authors found that bracing provides only temporary control of the deformity, delaying fusion until adequate spinal growth has been attained.

Indications for Surgery

Lonstein and Renshaw[33] recommended observation of curves under 30 degrees in immature CP patients and observation of curves under 50 degrees in mature CP patients. They suggested that curves be treated with bracing or surgery, depending on the patient's mental

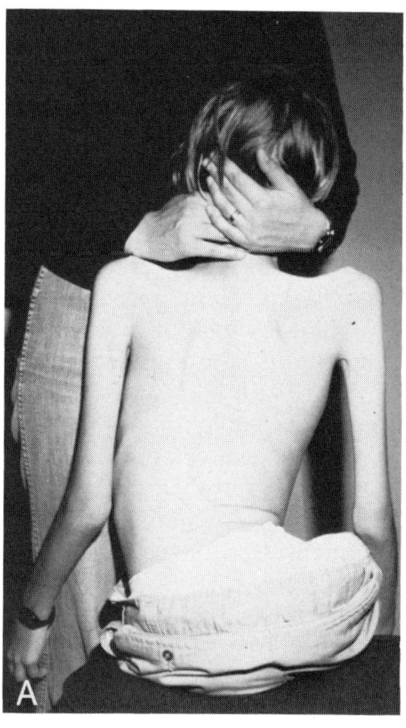

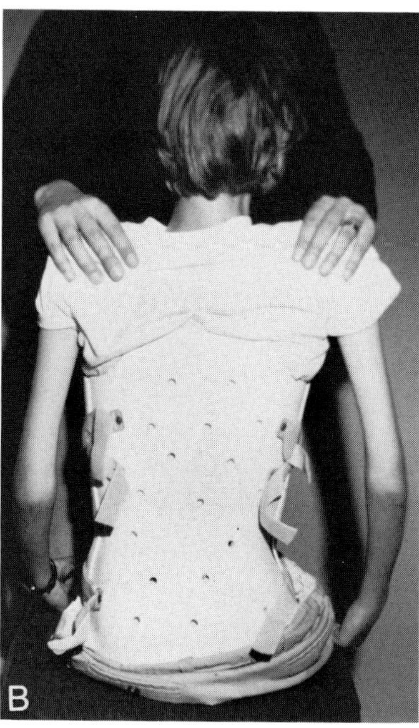

Figure 15–10. *A, B,* Kydex underarm orthosis in an older child.

status. In a child with normal intelligence, a curve of 40 to 50 degrees would be fused, as opposed to a child with marked mental retardation whose curve would be allowed to progress to 80 degrees before fusion was recommended. Loss of function secondary to trunk deformity, pelvic obliquity, and loss of spinal balance are the accepted, traditional indications for treatment of a spinal deformity in neuromuscular disorders.

It is a simple task to define the loss of function that occurs in a walking patient who stops walking, or a sitting patient who now needs upper extremities support for balance. Loss of function, however, is less clear in the mentally retarded, noncommunicating spastic quadriplegic patient with scoliosis who may at best be a dependent sitter. Some authors assume that these patients have no function and recommend that their deformity be allowed to progress untreated because it does not compromise classic function in terms of ambulation or sitting. This suggests that these authors feel that curves in mentally retarded patients do not alter their function. Function in this most severely affected group of patients consists of a comfortable existence in a seated position. We feel that a patient confined to bed because of severe scoliosis and pelvic obliquity loses function and quality of life if decubitus ulcers result in pain and osteomyelitis, or if restricted pulmonary mechanics result in pneumonia with predictable morbidity and mortality. The expense and convenience of care is likewise optimized if spinal deformity is controlled in these patients. We propose that the numerical Cobb angle indicators for surgery should be equally stringent in all CP patients, regardless of mental status. We agree with Bradford[3] in recommending a more aggressive surgical approach to the severely involved quadriplegic patient, especially where interested caretakers and parents are involved.

Contraindications to Surgery

Contraindications to fusion are few. Bonnett and colleagues[18] suggested that patients with severe athetosis have an unacceptably high pseudarthrosis rate and should be carefully assessed. These patients are very difficult to brace postoperatively because they tend to "wear themselves out" on the brace. Rather than denying surgery to the athetoid individual, anterior and posterior instrumentation and fusion with optional postoperative external immobilization may be indicated for this particular group.

Techniques

In 1942 Haas[27] published one of the first references to surgical intervention in neuromuscular scoliosis: a case report describing muscle and fascial transfers to obtain spinal correction (Fig. 15–11). He reported complete and permanent correction in one patient. With the introduction of the Harrington rod in 1962, use of this instrumentation with fusion of the CP spine became the standard. Series using only Harrington rods and posterior spinal fusion have been associated with high incidences of pseudarthrosis (19 to 40 per cent),[15, 45] moderate initial correction (20 to 57 per cent),[15, 44, 45, 49] and loss of correction ranging from 14 to

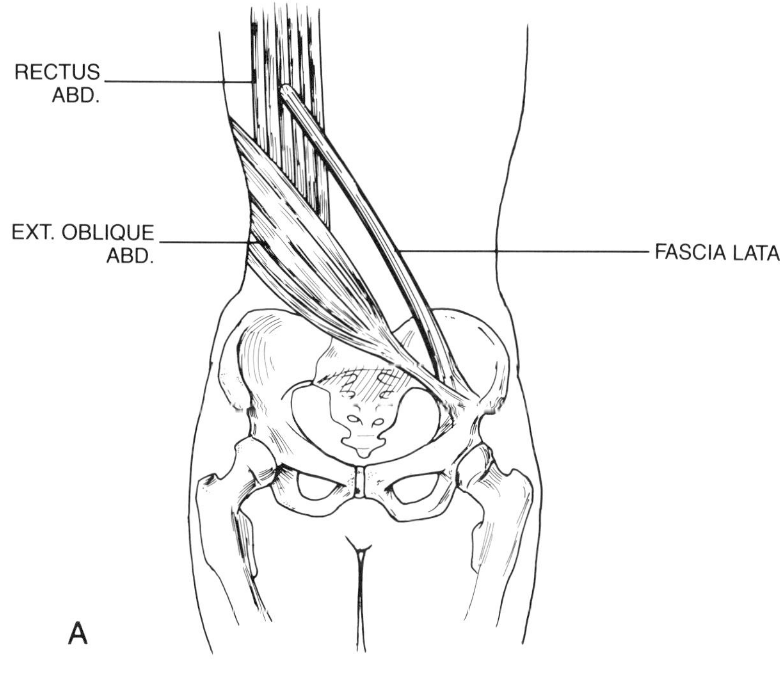

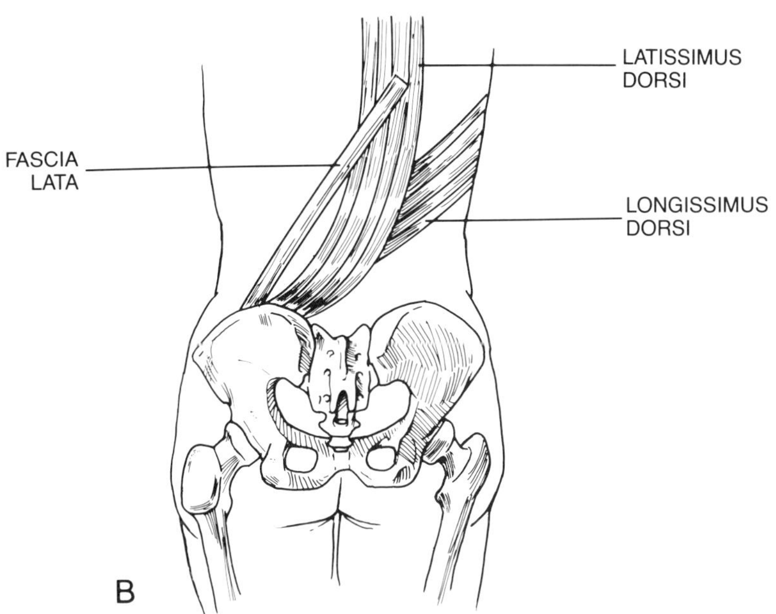

Figure 15–11. Anterior *(A)* and posterior *(B)* muscle transfers to balance and correct scoliosis. (From Haas, S. L.: Spastic scoliosis and obliquity of the pelvis. J. Bone Joint Surg. *24*:775, 1942.)

28 per cent.[44, 45] After Harrington rod instrumentation, most patients require bed rest and bracing or casting for up to one year. With the introduction of segmental spinal instrumentation in the form of Luque[34] and Wisconsin[25] instrumentation, major advances were made in the biomechanical stability and correction of these very deformed spines. Contouring Luque spinal rods after the technique introduced by Allen and Ferguson[14, 26] allowed the rods to be fixed to the pelvis, providing the surgeon with a more effective method of controlling pelvic obliquity. These segmental instrumentation systems have been shown to be stable enough that no brace or cast is felt to be necessary postoperatively.[26] With the exception of athetoid patients, patients surgically fused and instrumented into the sacrum or pelvis, or patients with poor bone stock, this concept generally can be applied to the CP patient. This is a tremendous advantage because postoperative casting carries the potential for skin and pulmonary complications.

In a small series in 1982 Allen and Ferguson[14] demonstrated that anterior fusion did not decrease pseudarthrosis rates in patients fused posteriorly with Luque segmental instrumentation. They studied ten patients, five who were treated with Luque only and five who were treated with Luque plus Dwyer, and found no pseudarthrosis in either group. They did note an increased correction in the anterior and posterior fusion group of 2.2 degrees per segment. In 1983 Ferguson[26] confirmed the increased correction with anterior release (64 per cent) and fusion, followed by posterior segmental instrumentation and fusion, and demonstrated that no brace was routinely required postoperatively despite the potentially destabilizing anterior surgery.

Sponseller and associates,[43] using a neurologically safer Wisconsin system, found that segmental spinous process bony fixation was adequate to achieve correction and fusion in CP. They fused 21 of their 38 patients anteriorly in addition to using the posterior Wisconsin instrumentation. Some of these anterior fusions were done without Dwyer instrumentation. They found only one nonunion in the entire series. This suggests, as do the 1982 and 1983 Allen and Ferguson studies, that with the increased mechanical stability of the segmental posterior instrumentation, anterior instrumentation may not increase the fusion potential over anterior fusion without instrumentation followed by posterior segmental instrumentation and fusion.

We feel anterior instrumentation and fusion, however, is more important if less stable nonsegmental Harrington rod fixation is used posteriorly. Comparing Harrington rod and anterior instrumentation combinations used in CP, Bonnett and colleagues[18] found a 40 per cent pseudarthrosis rate in 10 patients with posterior fusion using Harrington rod instrumentation, a 72 per cent rate when only anterior fusion with Dwyer instrumentation was used, and no pseudarthrosis with circumferential spinal fusion in five cases with Dwyer instrumentation being used anteriorly and Harrington rod instrumentation used posteriorly. Bonnett and colleagues also noted an increased correction of 62 per cent in the anteroposterior fusion group, compared with a 48 per cent correction in the Dwyer only group and a 30 per cent correction in the Harrington rods only group.

Using Dwyer and Harrington, these excellent results with anteroposterior instrumentation and fusion were repeated by Stanitski and associates[44] in 13 patients with a 71 per cent correction rate and no pseudarthrosis, and by Brown and associates[20] in 17 patients who showed a 60 per cent correction with a pseudarthrosis rate of 18 per cent. Brown and associates again suggested that although Dwyer instrumentation and anterior fusion alone may be adequate in idiopathic scoliosis, it is not adequate alone for neuromuscular spinal deformity. This was reconfirmed by Hall and colleagues, who demonstrated a 25 per cent pseudarthrosis rate with use of only Dwyer instrumentation and anterior fusion.[28] As shown, the use of either Harrington rods posteriorly or Dwyer anteriorly alone is inadequate. Combined, they approach the results of circumferential fusion and Luque rod instrumentation, but require more extensive bracing and casts postoperatively.

Looking only at fusion rates and spinal stability, studies have suggested that the Zielke anterior instrumentation system,[21] with posterior Luque rods and cross links, may further increase stability and fusion rate.[35] Work by Johnston and associates in a goat model suggested that this increased instrumentation stability is associated with early increased fusion mass strength.[30]

Brown and associates[20, 46] showed that if an anterior system of instrumentation is chosen,

Zielke used with Harrington posteriorly corrects more (77 per cent vs. 60 per cent) with a lower pseudarthrosis rate (5 per cent vs. 18 per cent) than the Dwyer and Harrington instrumentation combination. Bleck,[16] Broom and colleagues,[19] and Lonstein and Renshaw[33] discouraged the use of anterior instrumentation in the form of either Dwyer or Zielke before posterior fusion, because this particular technique may limit the correction obtained through the posterior instrumentation, as well as potentially causing kyphosis in the lumbar spine if used in that area. Lumbar kyphosis is particularly detrimental, according to Bleck,[16] because it transfers all the weight on the forward-flexed pelvis to the ischial tuberosities, as opposed to the thighs.

It is too early to know if using stronger segmental Luque, C-D, or TSRH instrumentation will necessitate instrumented anterior fusions to achieve and maintain correction and minimize pseudarthrosis rates. It is our feeling that anterior instrumentation in this circumstance is superfluous.

Extent of Fusion. Broom and associates showed that the extent of fusion superiorly in the CP patient should be at least to T4, to prevent the possibility of kyphosis above the instrumented curve (Fig. 15–12).[19]

Preoperative Traction. Longitudinal traction is an efficient means of correcting spinal deformities of greater than 53 degrees.[19] For lesser curves, transverse forces at the apex of the curve are biomechanically more efficient. For severe curves, Bradford[3] found halo gravity traction a useful technique for short periods if the cranial bone stock is good, if the spine is supple, and if there is no cervical or cervicothoracic instability. He also recommended its use to assess pulmonary function improvement with curve correction, and to obtain increased correction between anterior and posterior fusion stages. Bradford, on the other hand, advised against its use, believing that it weakens the patient and delays surgery.[3] In the occasional robust patient we have found that it is possible with prolonged traction to demonstrate dramatic improvement in spinal alignment if this is combined with appropriate anterior release and fusion (Fig. 15–13).

Pelvic Obliquity

Pelvic obliquity is a three-dimensional malalignment of the pelvis in relation to the lumbar spine. The resulting excessive skin pressure secondary to uneven ischial weight bearing can be a source of discomfort and can cause pressure sores and osteomyelitis. Appropriate hip releases and spinal fusion to the sacrum or pelvis should be considered for a significant pelvic obliquity, in order to maintain a balanced spine with a level pelvis. There is little agreement on the etiology or treatment of pelvic obliquity. Muscle releases and/or osteotomy may be required to alleviate the infrapelvic component, in addition to correction and fusion of the suprapelvic scoliosis. If the pelvis is not level, anterior and posterior lumbosacral fusion is generally recommended in order to mobilize the pelvis enough to correct the obliquity. Lonstein and Akbarnia[32] reviewed 68 patients with CP, classifying the curves into two types, with Type 2 curves involving an oblique pelvis. They recommended fusion to the pelvis in the spastic, quadriplegic, nonambulatory patient even if the pelvis is not oblique. We have found it necessary on occasion to extend instrumentation to the pelvis of patients with progressive pelvic obliquity who were previously fused only to the lower lumbar spine, because their obliquity initially corrected on bend films (Fig. 15–14). In contrast, O'Brien and Yau[38] felt that if L4 levels with L5, fusion to L4 is sufficient; if the L4–L5 disc can be leveled, L5 will subsequently pull the pelvis around because of the large, strong iliolumbar ligaments. Saer and associates[40] found 49 per cent correction of pelvic obliquity and no pseudarthrosis in adults fused anteriorly and posteriorly to the pelvis.

Fusion to the pelvis in ambulatory patients has been condemned because it is thought to compromise ambulation. However, Boachie-Adgei and colleagues[39] used Luque instrumentation in 46 patients with CP. The spine of six ambulatory patients is fused inferiorly to the pelvis; none lost the ability to ambulate postoperatively. In this series, the anterior plus posterior spinal fusion patients had 55 per cent correction of pelvic obliquity and did not require a postoperative cast or brace.

Kyphosis and Lordosis

Sagittal plane deformity, in the form of kyphosis in CP, can be secondary to two factors: first, gravity acting on a hypotonic weak trunk, and second, pelvic tilt or extension

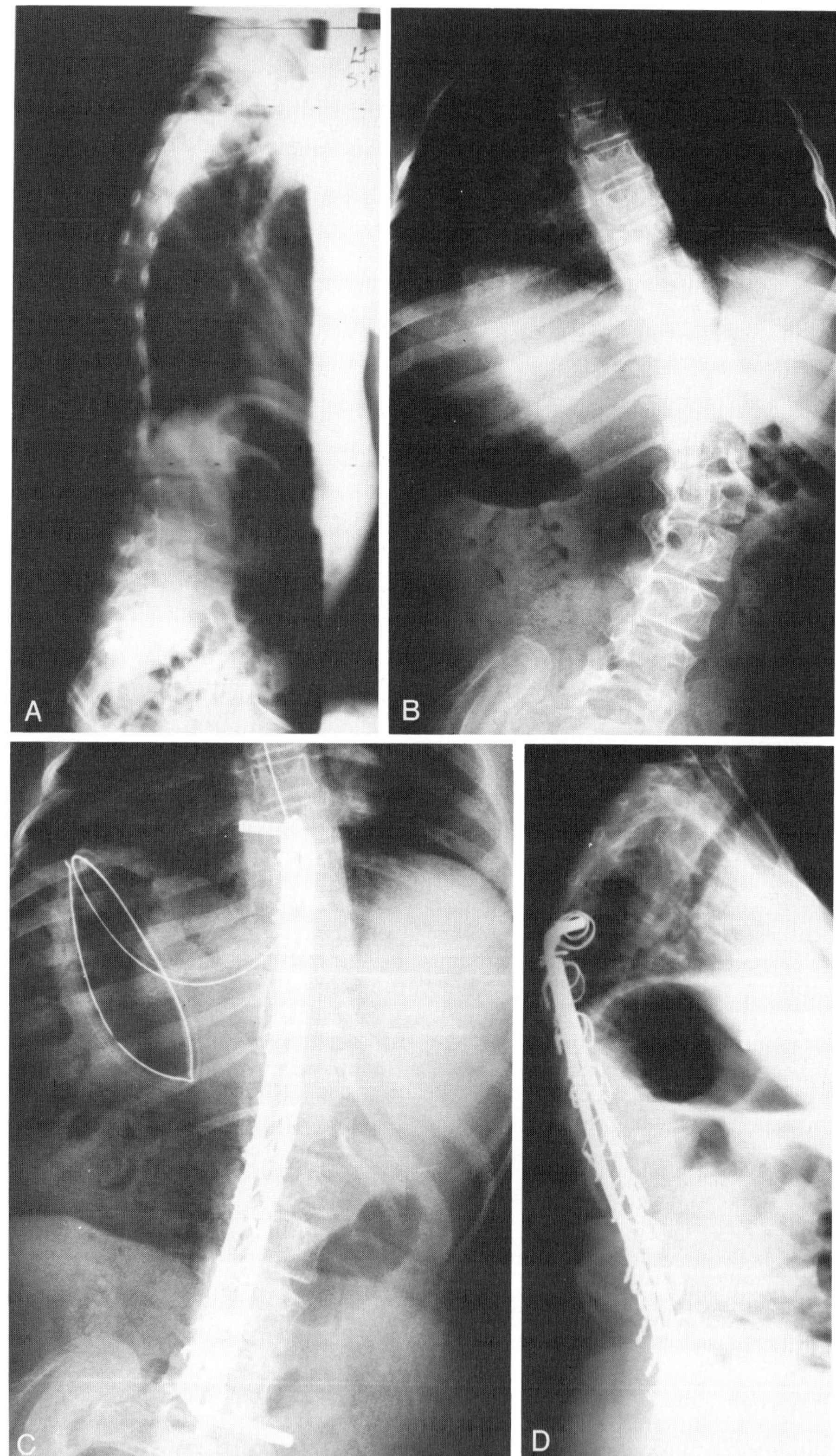

Figure 15–12. Sequence of x-rays in a female with spinal muscular atrophy fused to only T6 superiorly demonstrating increasing thoracic kyphosis after instrumentation. *A, B,* Preoperative posteroanterior and lateral views. *C, D,* Immediately postoperative posteroanterior and lateral views.

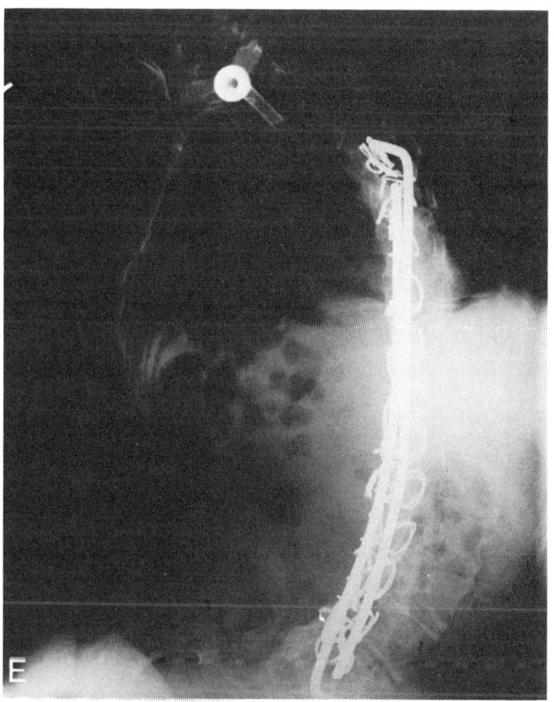

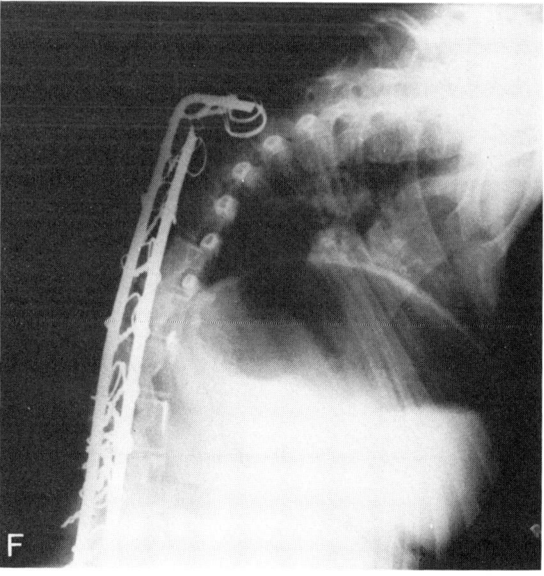

Figure 15–12 *Continued E, F,* Posteroanterior and lateral views five years after surgery.

secondary to tight hamstrings.[17] Bleck[16] believed that tight hamstrings, causing the patient to slip forward in the wheelchair, cause kyphosis because the individual then has a tendency to lean forward to allow the head to be centered over the pelvis in the sagittal plane. Bleck did not consider that kyphosis is necessarily a disabling condition, and felt that bracing adds another handicap; consequently, he did not recommend treating kyphosis with a brace. More than 60 degrees of thoracic kyphosis is abnormal; Bleck recommended fusion for kyphosis greater than 80 degrees.

Thoracic lordosis is infrequently seen as an isolated component of spinal deformity. It is more often seen as a component of significant idiopathic scoliosis. The advantage of segmental C-D or TSRH spinal instrumentation in treatment of this deformity is the sagittal correction made possible by increasing the kyphosis. Distraction C-D or TSRH is very effective in treating thoracic lordosis in conjunction with segmental posterior ligament sectioning and facet capsulotomies. Maximal correction is possible only with a staged anterior discectomy if the deformity is rigid (Fig. 15–15).

Authors' Recommendations

For gravity-dependent mild scoliosis or hypotonic kyphosis in children under 10 years of age, we recommend a Plastazote body jacket. This supports the spine, assists head control, and is very well tolerated by the patient. It usually last more than two years before the patient outgrows it. For more rigid curves between 30 and 50 degrees or in less rapidly growing patients over the age of 12, a rigid total-contact orthosis should be tried. Although less well tolerated, it provides better correction and may delay surgery.

Anterior fusion should be considered in rigid curves greater than 60 degrees, in Risser 0 patients, or in cases of rigid pelvic obliquity. In severe curves that require anterior spinal fusion, we feel that the stability and corrective potential of C-D, TSRH, or Luque segmental instrumentation is such that anterior instrumentation may not be routinely required. In this circumstance, anterior instrumentation, especially Zielke, may inhibit further correction by the segmental posterior instrumentation.

It has also been our experience that the quality of the bone in the vertebral bodies of patients with cerebral palsy is so poor that often the vertebral screws fail by pulling out of the bone at the point of anterior correction. Several intraoperative treatment techniques have proved useful in maximizing the stability of fixation as well as the potential for solid

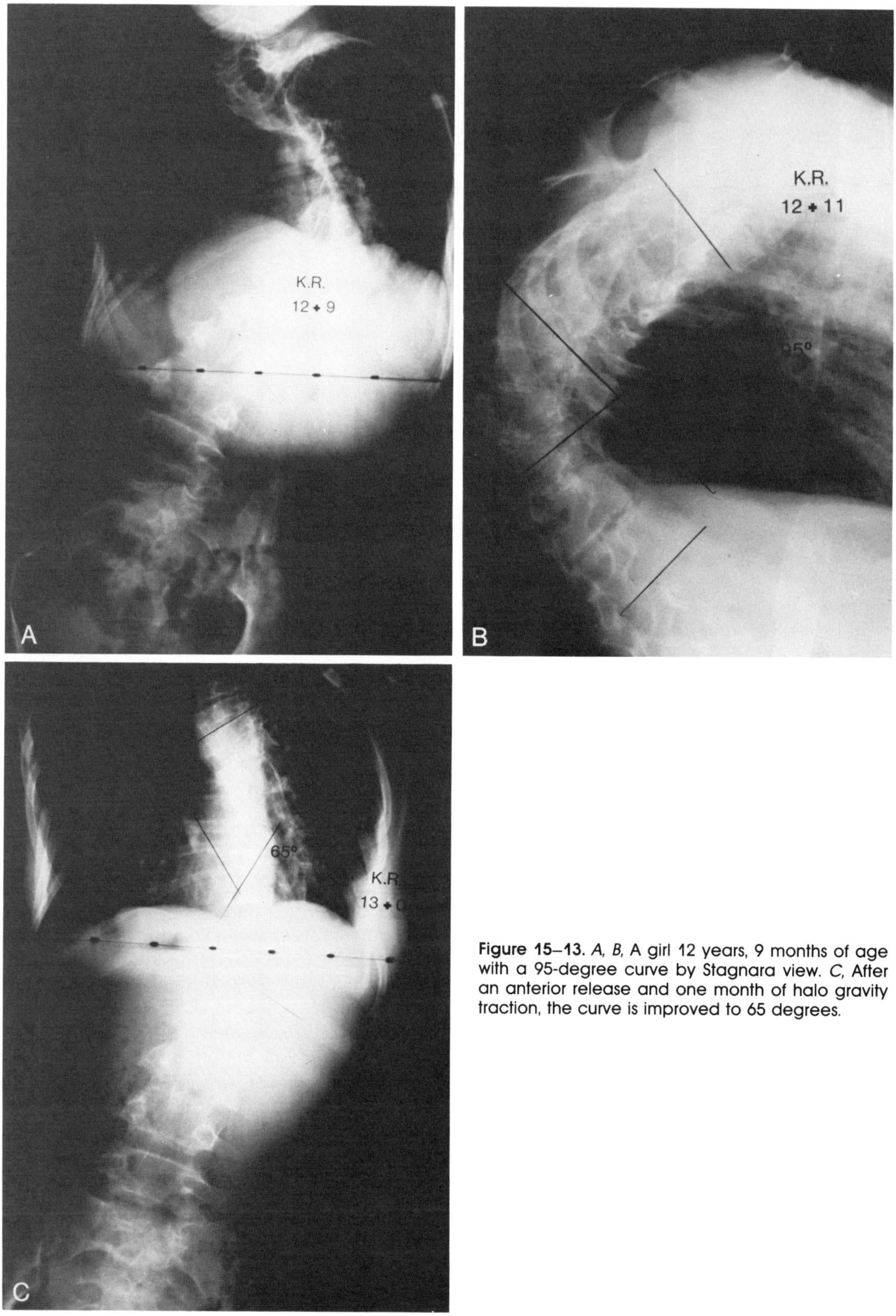

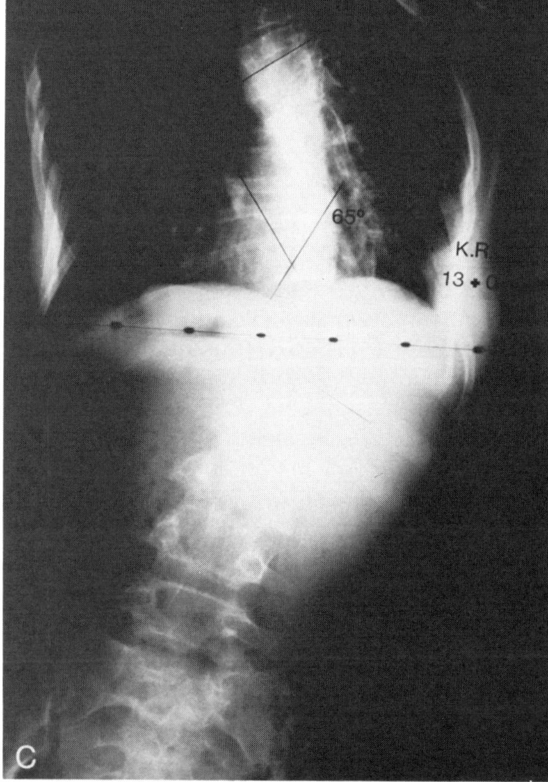

Figure 15–13. *A, B,* A girl 12 years, 9 months of age with a 95-degree curve by Stagnara view. *C,* After an anterior release and one month of halo gravity traction, the curve is improved to 65 degrees.

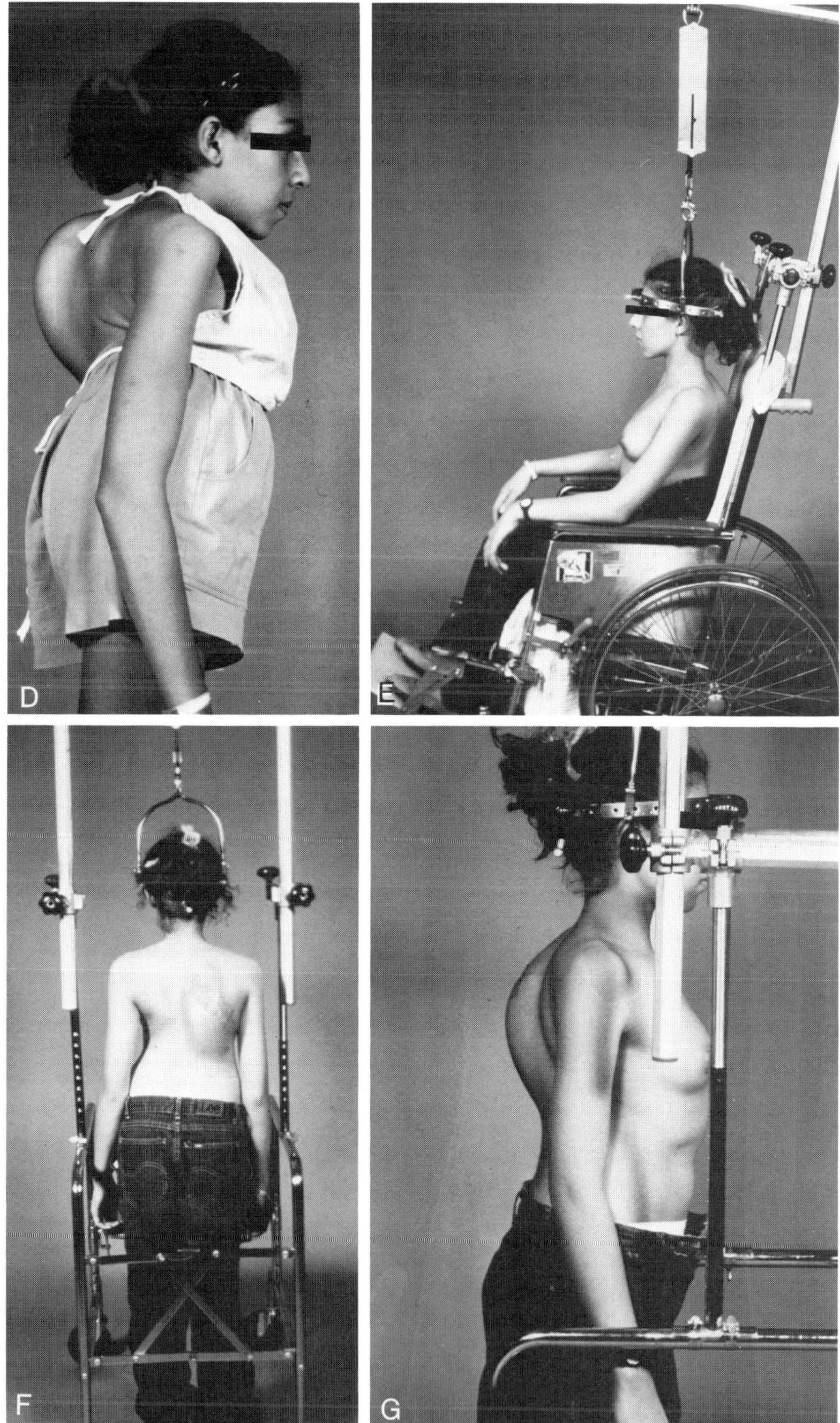

Figure 15–13 *Continued D*, Preoperative clinical appearance. *E*, Sitting in halo traction apparatus in traction. Note the use of a spring scale that can be overcome by pushing up with the arms if the patient notices any neurologic changes. *F*, *G*, Standing in halo traction device just before posterior fusion. Note the clinical improvement at the conclusion of three months of traction.

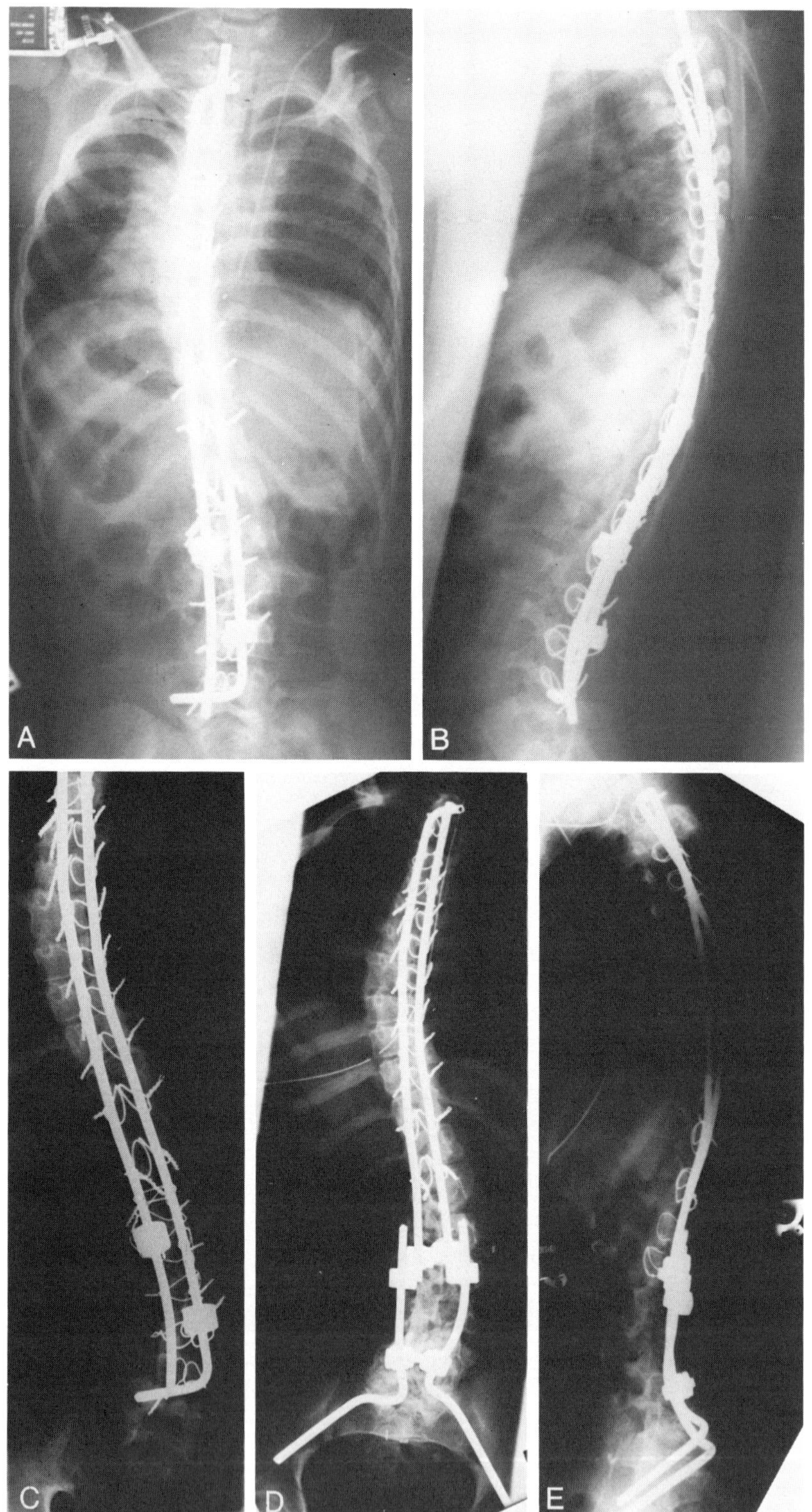

Figure 15–14. *A* to *E*, Progression of pelvic obliquity after posterior fusion, not including the pelvis. Note that the initial instrumentation leveled the pelvis. Progression of pelvic obliquity required revision, with extension to the pelvis using the Galveston technique.

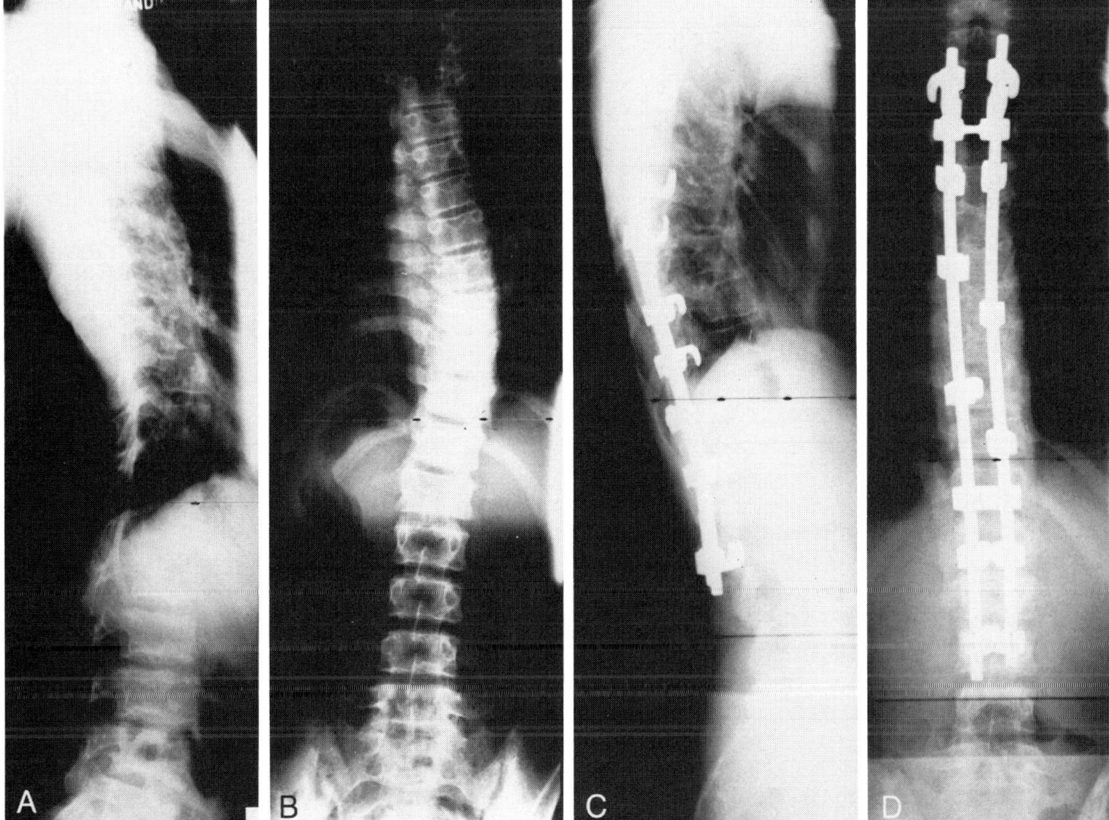

Figure 15–15. *A* to *D*, Patient with thoracic lordosis treated with C-D instrumentation in distraction, showing excellent correction.

fusion. It is our recommendation that, if Luque instrumentation is used, the ¼-inch Luque rod be used in larger patients to maximize the biomechanical stability, especially if the residual curve is large enough to diminish the biomechanical stability of the instrumentation.

A technique we have found useful in preventing kyphosis above the most superiorly instrumented level when Luque instrumentation is used is fusion one level higher than extent of instrumentation because the laminotomy at the superiormost instrumented level causes a loss of tension band effect of the supraspinous and interspinous ligaments at that level with potential kyphosis.

C-D or TSRH instrumentation may now be used in selected cases of neuromuscular scoliosis with extension of the instrumentation to the pelvis using sacral, iliosacral, or Galveston techniques (Fig. 15–16).[2]

The advantage of C-D or TSRH instrumentation in this particular population is that the segmental fixation can be obtained with hooks and sublaminar wires. Strategic hook placement allows distraction to take place, a much more biomechanically effective correction technique than the Luque system, which pulls the spine into a corrected position through its sublaminar fixation without direct distraction.[48]

The authors feel that all sitting CP patients should be fused inferiorly to include the pelvis even if their obliquity is correctable because of continued muscle imbalance and persistent Galante reflex. After fusion to the sacrum, it is important to obtain maximal postoperative control over the sacropelvic unit to improve the chances of fusion. It is therefore our recommendation that any patient with poor bone stock or a motion disorder with fusion to the pelvis be braced or casted with one thigh included for three to six months.

ACQUIRED PARALYSIS: TRAUMA, TUMOR

Paralysis is a devastating condition in children. Every year in the United States there

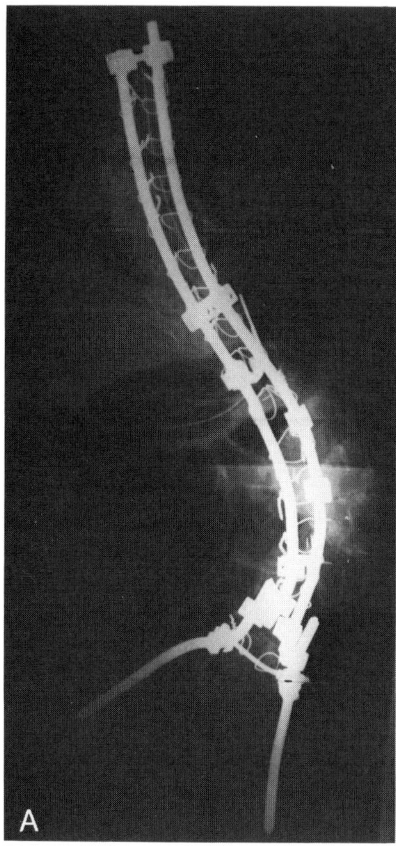

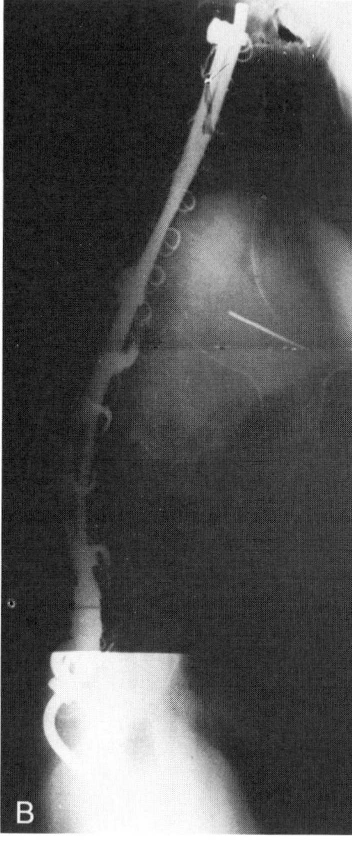

Figure 15–16. *A, B,* A 16-year-old patient with CP and a 110-degree curve who underwent a two-stage procedure with anterior release and fusion, followed by posterior fusion to the sacrum using C-D instrumentation, segmental wires, and Galveston technique for pelvic fixation.

are an estimated 11,200 new spinal cord injuries,[55] 1065 of which are reported to occur in persons under the age of 15.[53] An estimated 80 per cent of these children survive. These data indicate that the annual U.S. incidence of paralysis from acute spinal cord injury is greater than the incidence of paralytic poliomyelitis from 1964 to 1973 (448 cases). Children with paralysis from spinal cord injury have a very high risk of developing spinal deformity with growth. Studies have shown that scoliosis develops in 92 to 100 per cent of this patient population.[51, 52, 54, 56, 57, 59]

Acquired paralysis in children is most often secondary to trauma, but in younger children it can be secondary to spinal infection or tumor. Banniza von Bazan and Paeslock[50] demonstrated in 116 patients that there is a higher incidence of spinal deformity resulting from infection and tumor in children under the age of 8 years; those over 8 were more likely to have acquired paralysis from spinal trauma.

The etiology of scoliosis in the paralytic postinjury patient is multifactorial, the greatest contributor being the effects of gravity on a weakened spinal column. Malcolm[58] suggested that the deformity in part may result from a malunion of underlying bony fractures or chronic instability after fracture. A malunion with deformity may be progressive despite solid bony healing, secondary to compressive growth plate suppression on the concavity of the curve. Renshaw[61] suggested that additional factors contributing to spinal deformity are asymmetric trunk muscle tone, muscular paralysis, and hip contractures. The vertebral osteoporosis prevalent in adults generally does not play a major role in this type of progressive pediatric spinal deformity.

The strongest determinant of spinal deformity incidence is the age of the child at the time of paralysis. The younger the patient, the more likely is it that deformity will result. Mayfield and associates[59] showed a 100 per cent incidence of spinal deformity in children who became paralytic in preadolescence, as opposed to a 40 per cent incidence after the adolescent growth spurt. Lancourt and colleagues[56] noted the onset of scoliosis in 16 of 20 spinal cord injury patients under the age of 10.

The more cephalad the level of paralysis, the higher is the incidence of scoliosis. Liedholt and associates[57] found a 100 per cent incidence of scoliosis in 25 patients with injuries above T10. Only 16 of 26 developed scoliosis when paralysis levels were from T11 to L1, and four of seven when below L2. McSweeney[60] noted that the lesions below the conus medullaris were not associated with spinal deformity. He also found that patients with incomplete lesions had more severe deformity because of asymmetric trunk muscle weakness. Lancourt and colleagues[56] reviewed the influence of laminectomy on spinal deformity after onset of paraplegia. They found that a laminectomized patient did not show a higher incidence of deformity, but in comparison to nonlaminectomized patients experienced a more rapid progression after the onset of spinal deformity.

Treatment

Renshaw[61] stated: "It is important to assume that all children with spinal cord injury are developing a paralytic spinal deformity until proven otherwise" and affirmed that the trunk of the paraplegic patient should be controlled as soon as deformity is detected. The initial approach to deformity prevention logically should be perfect reduction of the initial injury, with the goal of maximal structural integrity of the vertebral column. Prevention of major joint contractures about the hip and knees, as well as efforts to reduce spasticity, can be instrumental in preventing pelvic obliquity. Six of the 40 patients of Mayfield and associates were placed in braces to control their spinal deformity.[59] Five of the six needed posterior spinal fusion, but reached the ages of 10 to 12 years before surgery. Mayfield and associates recommended that bracing be instituted for 20 degrees of spinal deformity, with the goal of allowing the patient to reach age 10 before surgery. Bradford was more aggressive, recommending that all patients should be braced while upright even before deformity develops, in the hope of preventing it.[3]

Renshaw recommended posterior fusion when the scoliosis curve reaches 40 degrees and the kyphosis 60 degrees.[61] Anterior release should be performed on a kyphotic or scoliotic curve that is rigid, or greater than 60 degrees. Bedbrook[51] found anterior and posterior fusion to be the most reliable approach to arrest progression and obtain a fusion in paralyzed patients.

Authors' Recommendations

In acquired paraplegia, we recommend early bracing as soon as a progressive curve is noted, certainly at 20 degrees. With quadriplegia, bracing is usually necessary to allow the child to be upright after the injury.

Traditionally, segmental Luque wiring has been the instrumentation of choice for posterior spinal fusion in paralytic patients. C-D or TSRH instrumentation, however, may be able to secure greater correction of pelvic obliquity, particularly if supplemented with sublaminar wires as needed, depending on bone quality. If C-D or TSRH instrumentation is chosen, sacropelvic fixation can be achieved using the techniques described in the section on "Cerebral Palsy."

FRIEDREICH'S ATAXIA

Friedreich's ataxia was described by Friedreich in 1863.[64] It is characterized histologically by progressive degeneration of the spinocerebellar tracts and it is usually inherited as an autosomal recessive trait.

Geoffroy and colleagues[65] in 1976 proposed criteria for diagnosis of Friedreich's ataxia based on primary and secondary symptoms. The primary symptoms include onset of progressive ataxia before age 20, dysarthria, decreased vibratory and position sense, muscle weakness, and deep tendon areflexia. Secondary symptoms include pes cavus, scoliosis, a positive Babinski sign, and the presence of cardiomyopathy.

Affected children are usually diagnosed at about age 9 years, but the range is 3 to 16 years. They generally become wheelchair-bound by age 15[62, 63] and die from complications of cardiomyopathy by their midthirties.[67]

Scoliosis occurs in a relatively high percentage of patients with Freidreich's ataxia (75 to 100 per cent).[68, 70, 71] The cause is thought to be related to the ataxia and disturbance of equilibrium, a condition that also may be operative in idiopathic scoliosis.[69, 70, 72]

Although scoliosis in Friedreich's ataxia is

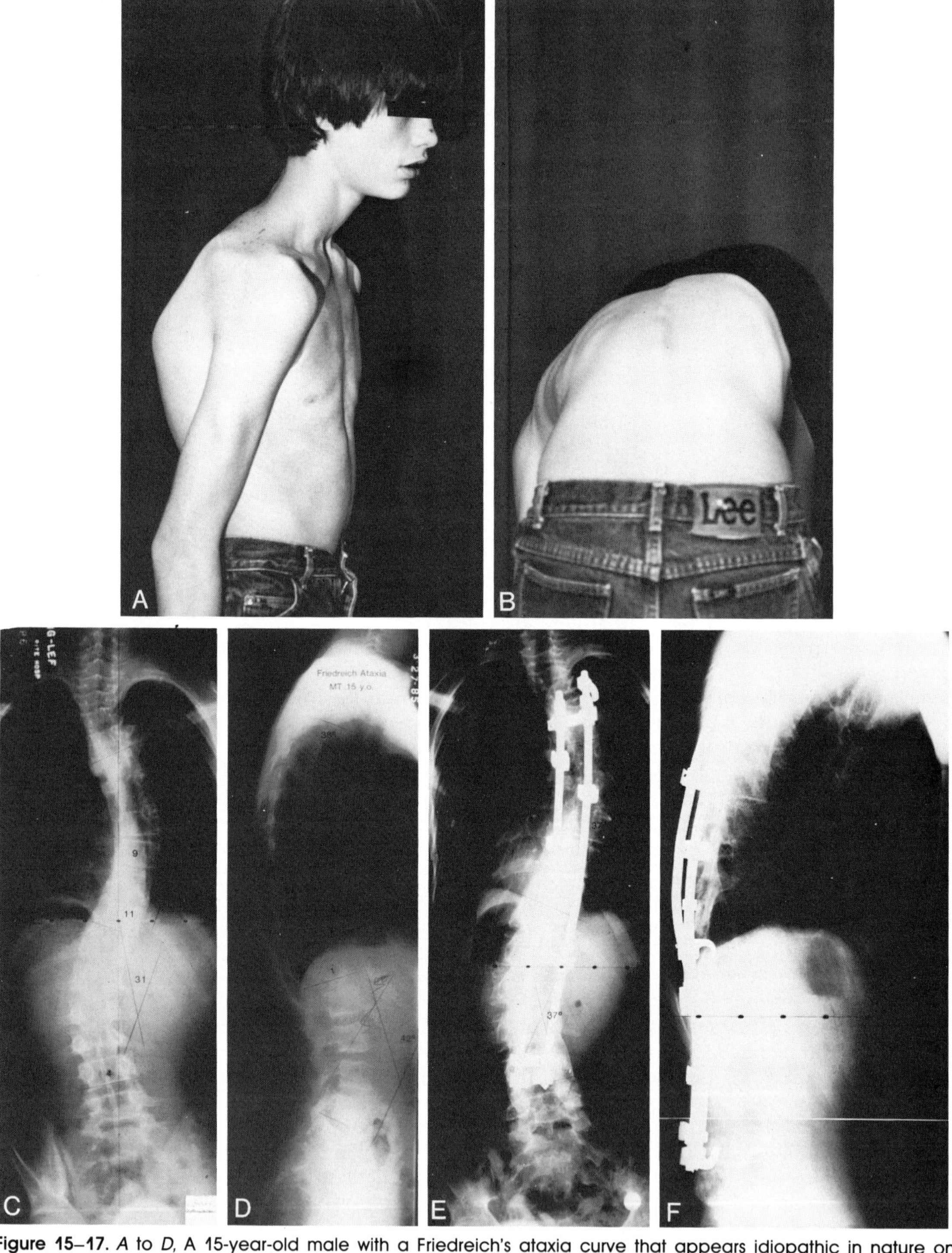

Figure 15–17. *A* to *D*, A 15-year-old male with a Friedreich's ataxia curve that appears idiopathic in nature on x-ray and clinical examination. *E, F,* C-D instrumentation and fusion demonstrating excellent correction fused as an idiopathic curve.

classified as neuromuscular, it appears to have idiopathic characteristics and to behave like idiopathic scoliosis in many respects (Fig. 15–17*A* to *D*). In 78 patients, LaBelle and associates[68] found only a 14 per cent incidence of the classic neuromuscular-type thoracolumbar curve with associated pelvic obliquity. Contrary to previous observations suggesting that scoliosis in Friedreich's ataxia always progresses into adulthood,[24, 62, 66] these curves are now thought to be nonprogressive in patients with onset of scoliosis after puberty, another characteristic similar to idiopathic scoliosis.[68] LaBelle and associates found no relationship between severity of ataxia and severity of scoliosis or curve progression.

Treatment

Bracing is tolerated poorly by ambulatory patients with Friedreich's ataxia because it compromises torso balance. We do not recommend bracing, because it has not been shown to affect the natural history in patients with progressive curves.[62, 63, 68] Both LaBelle and associates[68] and Cady and Bobechko[62] documented progression in all braced patients. This lack of response to bracing therapy is thought to result from an inability to pull away from the brace secondary to truncal ataxia.

When surgery is indicated, the procedure of choice is posterior instrumentation and fusion. LaBelle and associates[68] recommended fusion for all curves over 60 degrees, observation for curves under 40 degrees, and fusion for curves of 40 to 60 degrees, depending on the age of the patient and evidence of progression of the curve.

Authors' Recommendations

Because scoliosis with Friedreich's ataxia is so similar to idiopathic scoliosis, we recommend surgical treatment similar to that for idiopathic scoliosis. Fusion is indicated for curves over 40 degrees in immature patients (Risser 0 to 3) and between 50 and 60 degrees in adults. Fusion to the sacrum should be discouraged in patients with Friedreich's ataxia as in those with idiopathic scoliosis, because the mobility of the pelvis is an important determinant of balance in ambulatory patients.

Harrington instrumentation has been successful in achieving fusion. However, it has a tendency to compromise the sagittal contours of the spine and therefore may compromise ambulation in ataxic patients. We recommend the use of C-D or TSRH instrumentation for rigid segmental spinal fixation with maintenance of natural contours (Fig. 15–17*E, F*); it alleviates the necessity of postoperative bracing, allowing easier ambulation.

CHARCOT-MARIE-TOOTH DISEASE

Charcot-Marie-Tooth disease is a hereditary, demyelinating motor and sensory neuropathy symmetrically affecting peripheral nerves, motor nerve roots, and spinal cerebellar tracts.[75] Charcot and Marie in France[73] and Tooth in England[77] are credited with the original description of this condition in 1886. Dyck[75] in 1968 classified it into seven major clinical forms. The clinical description of Charcot-Marie-Tooth disease in this chapter will deal only with the most common classic presentation (Type I), although the risk of scoliosis is thought to be equal in all groups.

I. Classic Charcot-Marie-Tooth (CMT), hypertrophic form
   A. Roussy-Lévy syndrome, areflexic dystaxia (classic CMT with tremor)
II. Neuronal form of CMT
III. Hypertrophic neuropathy of infancy (Déjérine-Sottas disease)
IV. Refsum's disease
V. Progressive paraplegia
VI. Similar to Type I with optic atrophy
VII. Similar to Type II with retinitis pigmentosa

Charcot-Marie-Tooth disease affects males more frequently than females, although affected females are often more severely involved. Inheritance patterns are most commonly described as autosomal dominant.[74]

The condition usually becomes clinically apparent in the second decade, generally in the form of mild loss of coordination and progressive development of cavus feet and claw toes. This is thought to be secondary to weak peroneal muscles, foot intrinsics, and ankle dorsiflexors.[76] Patients never lose bowel or bladder control and rarely lose ambulation. Intelligence remains normal, as does life expectancy.

Treatment

Hensinger and MacEwen[66] reported 69 patients with Charcot-Marie-Tooth disease of whom seven had scoliosis (10 per cent). Two patients were observed, two were successfully treated in Milwaukee braces, and two failed Milwaukee brace treatment. Three patients underwent posterior spinal fusion with no complications. Daher and colleagues,[74] in a series of 12 patients with scoliosis, found five who were appropriate for observation. Two of three patients were controlled well in a Milwaukee brace, and five, including the patient with brace failure, were fused posteriorly. Two pseudarthroses were reported, only one of which required refusion.

Authors' Recommendations

Both Daher and colleagues[74] and Hensinger and MacEwen[66] recommended that scoliosis associated with Charcot-Marie-Tooth disease be managed with the same techniques used for idiopathic scoliosis, including the effective use of bracing, the same indications for fusion level, and the same postoperative management. When surgery is indicated, Bradford prefers segmental instrumentation without postoperative brace or cast.[3] We agree and have found C-D and TSRH instrumentation to work well in the few selected patients with Charcot-Marie-Tooth disease who require spinal fusion for progressive scoliosis.

POLIOMYELITIS

Poliomyelitis is an acute viral illness that affects the anterior horn cells of the spinal cord and brain stem nuclei. The offending neurotropic viruses include poliovirus Types 1, 2, and 3, coxsackievirus, and echovirus. Exposure is through the oral-fecal route. The virus spreads through the respiratory and gastrointestinal tracts, and then is blood-borne to the central nervous system. Paralysis occurs in only 1 to 2 per cent of those with clinically evident illness, resolving in a large percentage within the first six to 12 months. In the prevaccine era those most frequently affected were children aged 5 to 14 years. Today unimmunized infants are those most at risk to contract poliomyelitis.

Colonna and VanSaal in 1941[78] determined that the risk of a poliomyelitis patient developing scoliosis was approximately 30 per cent. Spinal deformity in poliomyelitis results from trunk involvement with asymmetric intercostal, abdominal, and paraspinous muscle paralysis. Pelvic obliquity secondary to asymmetric muscle paralysis of the pelvic girdle muscles is also a causative factor. Irwin[79] described a mechanism whereby a contracted iliotibial band (an abductor) can cause pelvic obliquity and subsequent scoliosis. The prognosis for worsening of the spinal deformity has been correlated to the degree of weakness and age at curve onset.[80]

Spinal deformities in poliomyelitis are generally long, "C"-shaped curves with associated pelvic obliquity. However, other curve patterns are seen involving the lumbar or thoracic spine[3] in an isolated manner.

Treatment

As with most neuromuscular scoliosis, bracing has not been shown to alter the natural history significantly. Bracing may, however, be beneficial in allowing continued spinal growth in very young patients with flexible curves. Leong and associates[81] recommended that bracing be instituted in this particular situation at 20 degrees. Risser[84] described the use of serial casting to obtain correction, followed by posterior in situ fusion through a cast window and subsequent long-term casting.

Delay of fusion until the end of growth is not recommended in young patients with progressive curves, because this would put the patient at risk for dramatic progression during rapid growth as an adolescent. Brown and colleagues[4] recommended that bracing cease and surgical intervention be considered for Cobb angles of 40 to 50 degrees with documented progression in the brace, even if the patient is not yet prepubertal (boys, age 12; girls, age 10).

There is controversy over the use of preoperative traction in this condition. Leong and associates[81] recommended halofemoral and halo traction for curves greater than 100 degrees. Bradford[3] stated that preoperative traction has a very limited role in his practice. In very large spinal curves, he said that it is neither helpful nor indicated except in curves associated with cardiopulmonary compromise, where traction may demonstrate a possible reversibility of pulmonary dysfunction and improve the patient's general status before surgery.

Swank and colleagues[85] reported a series of 20 patients with cor pulmonale and curvatures of 90 to 200 degrees. The best results of halo traction were in the poliomyelitis population. Average vital capacity increase was from 595 to 1000 ml, arterial oxygenation increased from an average of 55 to 64 mm Hg, and PCO_2 decreased from an average of 52 to 43 mm Hg.

Our experience has been that very large curves may benefit significantly from halo traction, applied between the anterior and posterior stages. To be effective, traction may need to be used over a prolonged period, six to 12 weeks (Fig. 15–18). Patients can be maintained in the walker halo traction or wheelchair halo traction during the day, with a standard "fish scale" to adjust traction magnitude (see Fig. 15–13). This allows the patient to push away with the upper extremities from the traction weight if pain or neurologic symptoms develop. Traction at night can be effected through the use of free weights on the halo apparatus, using a Trendelenburg bed position or split mattress–type horizontal traction.

Reports of anterior or posterior arthrodeses alone for neuromuscular scoliosis in poliomyelitis have demonstrated inferior results with regard to curve correction and pseudarthrosis.[81, 82] Circumferential spinal arthrodesis using anterior and posterior fusion is indicated in most curves except those very few flexible curves without pelvic obliquity, for which almost full correction can be obtained with posterior fusion alone. Posterior instrumentation and fusion using Luque rods with sublaminar wires have become the standard. Anterior release and fusion have been shown to improve curve and pelvic obliquity correction, as well as decrease the incidence of pseudarthrosis. O'Brien and associates[82] in an early series of three patients found 88 per cent curve correction with no pseudarthrosis using anterior Dwyer and posterior Harrington rod instrumentation. Using anterior Zielke instrumentation and posterior Harrington rods in 19 patients, Swank and colleagues[85] found a 77 per cent spinal curve correction with only one pseudarthrosis. Pelvic obliquity corrected from an average of 23 degrees preoperatively to 6 degrees postoperatively. Leong and associates[81] demonstrated dramatic decreases in the pseudarthrosis rate: 25 to 7 per cent in patients with thoracic curves and 50 to 12 per cent in patients with thoracolumbar curves with the use of anterior Dwyer and posterior Harrington rod instrumentation and fusion.

Ferguson and Allen obtained 64 per cent spinal correction and 67 per cent pelvic obliquity correction using segmental spinal instrumentation posteriorly and anterior release and fusion without instrumentation.[26] The obvious advantage of this technique is that routine postoperative bracing is not required and by using strong segmental posterior instrumentation, instrumentation anteriorly may not be needed.

Authors' Recommendations

We recommend posterior segmental fusion in patients with curves greater than 40 degrees. Anterior fusion should be performed in Risser 0 children who otherwise satisfy surgical medications to prevent the "crankshaft" phenomenon and in patients with rigid curves greater than 60 degrees. If anterior instrumentation is felt to be necessary, the Zielke system is preferable because it has less potential to cause kyphosis than the Dwyer and because the semirigid rod may be more structurally stable. When anterior instrumentation is placed, it is more likely to maintain its correction as the bone is generally much stronger and holds vertebral screws better than in CP. The only potential disadvantage of its use may be a decreased capacity to further correct the curvature and rotation using posterior segmental spinal instrumentation as a staged procedure (Fig. 15–19). As in CP, the present alternatives for posterior segmental spinal instrumentation (Luque, TSRH, and C-D) with their dramatic corrective powers have such structural stability that anterior instrumentation may be superfluous.

Fusion level selection in the poliomyelitis spine should include all rotated vertebral bodies in the cephalad and caudad deformity. The top and bottom of the fusion areas should lie within Harrington's stable zone, which on occasion may require fusion into the cervical spine.[83] Fusion to the pelvis should be considered in all patients who have significant rigid pelvic obliquity, but caution should be used, especially in ambulatory patients, because in-

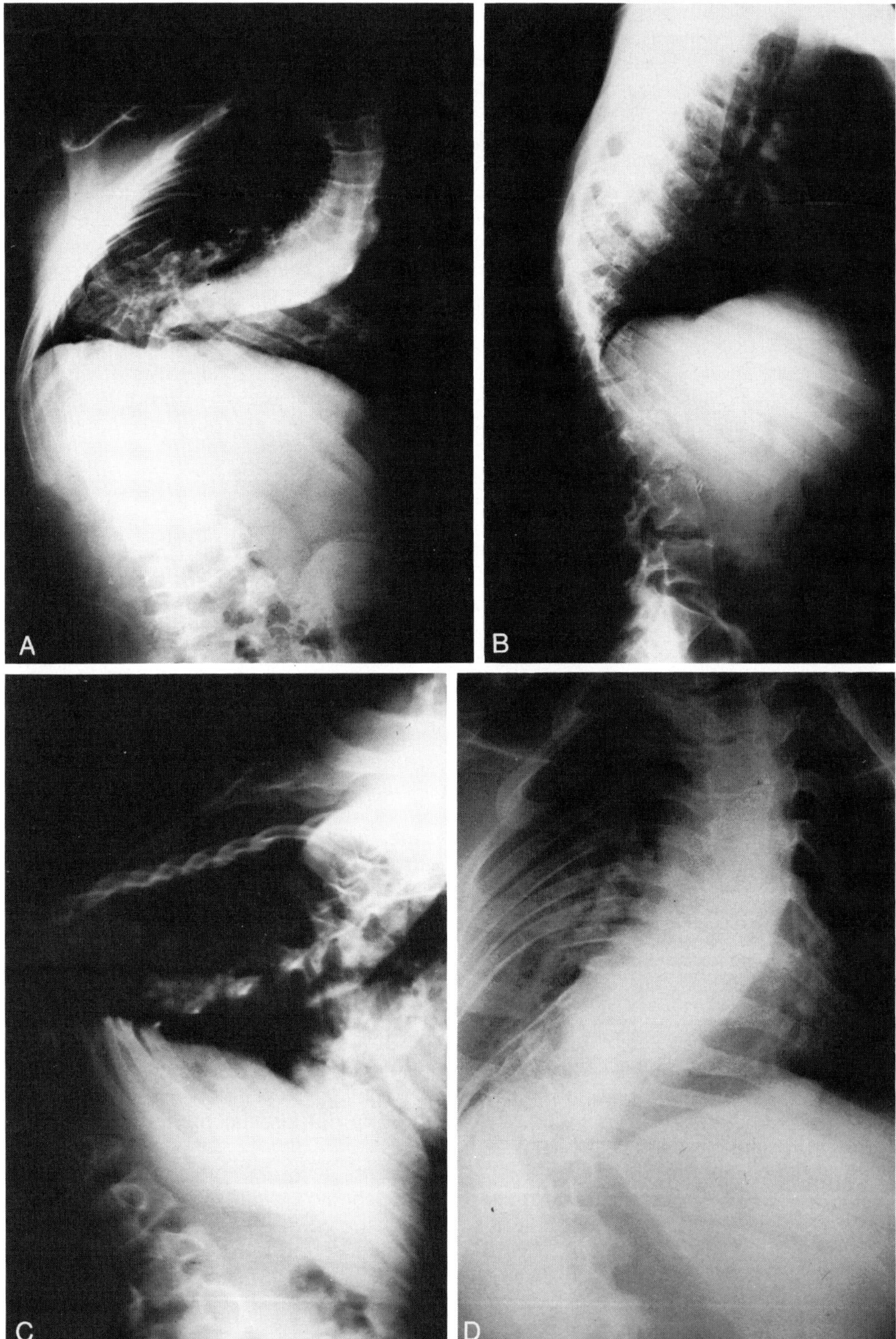

Figure 15–18. *A, B,* A 17-year-old ambulatory male with severe scoliosis and pelvic obliquity. The upper curve measures 84 degrees; the lower curve, 90 degrees. *C,* Stagnara view measuring 140 degrees. *D,* Two weeks after anterior release and fusion T3–L3 in 20 pounds of halo traction. The curve measures 70 degrees.

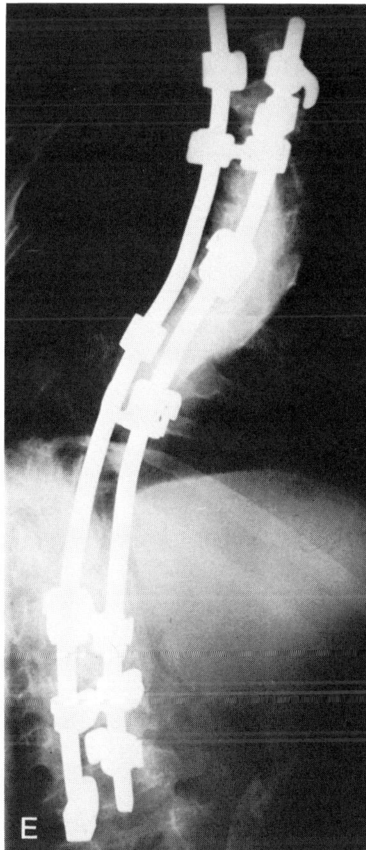

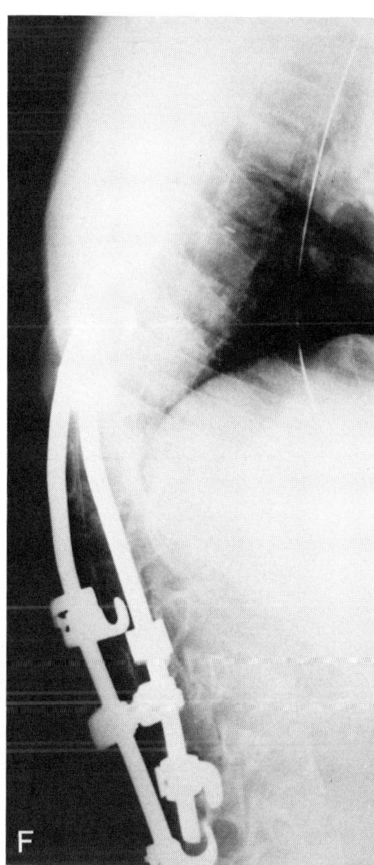

Figure 15–18 *Continued E, F,* C-D instrumentation T3–L4 with curve correction to 60 and 80 degrees, respectively.

dependent ambulation and mobility is facilitated by a flexible lumbosacral junction (see Fig. 15–18).

When in a case of severe pelvic obliquity it is necessary to achieve pelvic correction and fusion, we recommend anterior release and fusion across the L5 disc space. This is in contrast to the recommendations of Leong and associates,[81] who suggested anterior fusion only to L5 followed by posterior fusion and instrumentation to the pelvis. Anterior fusion to the sacrum can be achieved by retracting the bifurcated iliac vessels to each side and directly approaching the L5–S1 interspace between the bifurcation. As in CP, once pelvic fixation is achieved, postoperative casting or bracing should be considered by means of a spica with a single leg-thigh extension for three to six months.

If a major component of pelvic obliquity originates from hip contractures, their release may correct the pelvic obliquity enough to eliminate the necessity of fusion to the sacrum, and makes bracing easier. Irwin[79] suggested confirming the contribution of tensor fascia lata tightness to the pelvic obliquity by flexing, abducting, and externally rotating the extremity. If the pelvis levels, there is significant infrapelvic contribution to the pelvic obliquity and releases are beneficial.

In general, our recommended treatment of scoliosis in poliomyelitis is similar to that for CP, keeping in mind the importance of leaving mobile lumbar segments in an ambulatory patient without significant pelvic obliquity.

SPINAL DEFORMITY IN MYELOMENINGOCELE

Scoliosis and kyphosis in myelomeningocele (MM) are among the most difficult to treat of all spinal deformities in children (Fig. 15–20). Many more children now present with progressive deformity because vigorous early med-

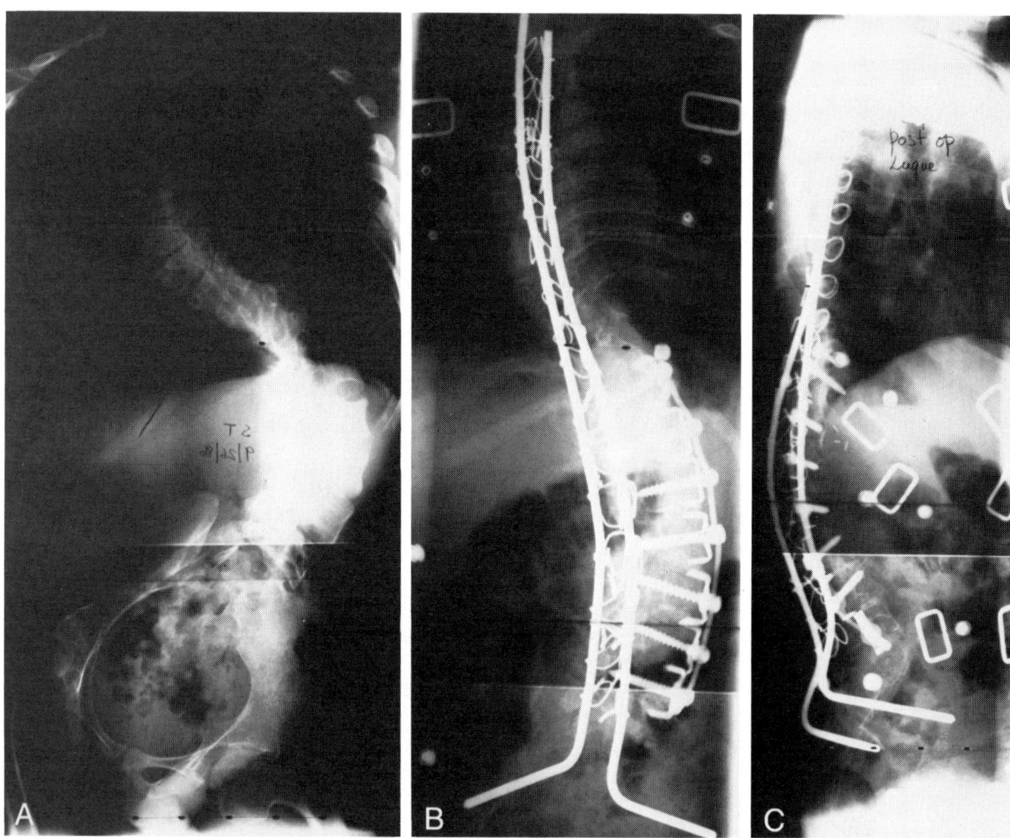

Figure 15–19. *A, B,* A 16-year-old nonambulatory male with polio-related scoliosis. The lower curve measures 90 degrees; the upper curve, 70 degrees. *C,* Curves measure 40 and 30 degrees, respectively, after anterior Dwyer and posterior Luque instrumentation to the pelvis.

ical and neurosurgical intervention has improved survival rates, allowing the children to mature, thus allowing time for the spine to deform. Drennan and colleagues noted scoliosis in 52 per cent of MM patients by age 15 years, with a 100 per cent incidence in patients with a level at T12 or higher.[87]

The MM spine is more complex than that in typical neuromuscular scoliosis (CP, muscular dystrophy). In addition to spastic or weak "guidewires" (muscles), there may also be missing posterior elements as a cause of trunk collapse and congenital scoliosis, which in itself can lead to curve progression. The congenital component of the spinal deformity may require separate early treatment.

Children with MM and progressive congenital scoliosis should have early in situ fusion, just as for congenital scoliosis in an otherwise normal child. The pure neuromuscular component may not require treatment until later.

MM patients may have a tethered spinal cord that can cause rapid curve progression. Unfortunately, most MM patients have some variation of cord tethering as a residual of the MM and its neurosurgical closure and repair. In patients with unexpected rapid curve progression, the possibility of a tethered cord, hydromyelia, or increased trunk spasticity (hypertonicity) should be considered as a cause. Studies such as magnetic resonance imaging (MRI) or myelography may help to define anatomy, but determining the causal relationship between the abnormal neural anatomy and curve progression may be difficult. Thoughtful teamwork with a neuroradiologist, neurologist, and neurosurgeon will help to clarify these issues. Surgical release of a tethered cord is only occasionally effective in reversing rapid progression of scoliosis in MM.[87]

Other factors contributing to the complexity of MM scoliosis include hip flexion, adduction,

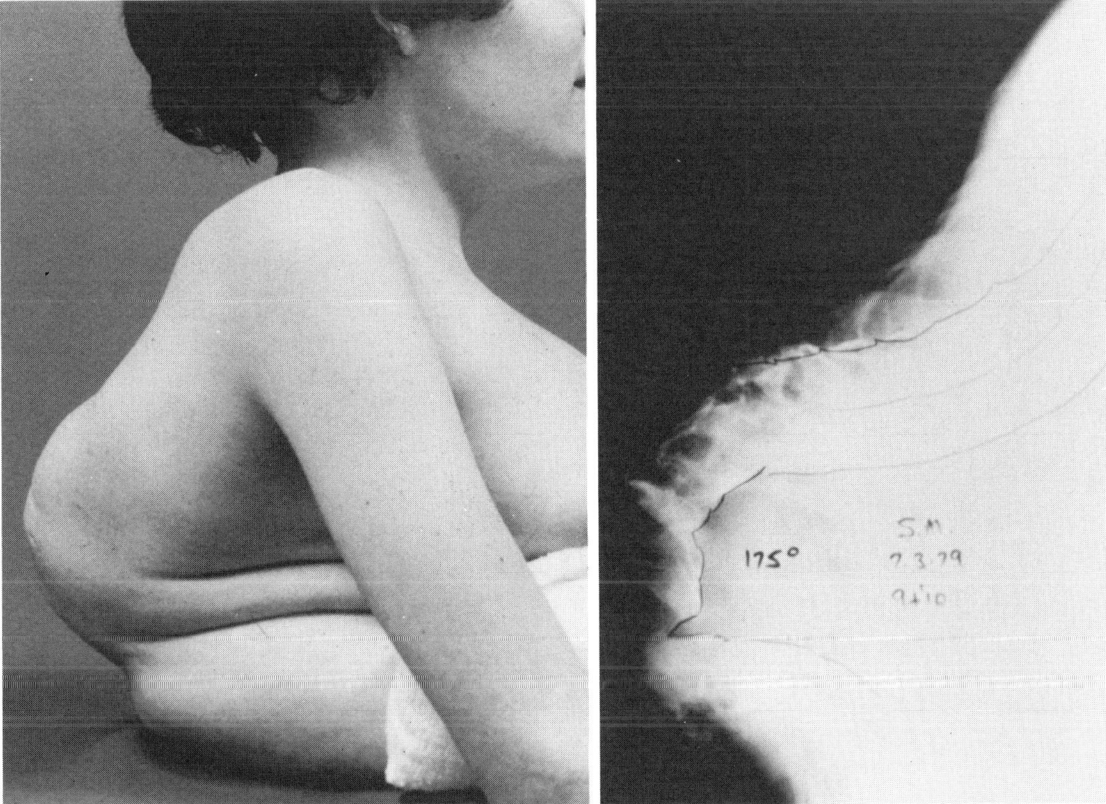

Figure 15–20. Lateral clinical and radiographic view of a child with severe kyphosis secondary to a midthoracic level myelomeningocele (MM). The marked bony deformity and absence of normal trunk muscle strength characterizes the magnitude of the problem facing the surgeon who plans surgical correction.

or abduction contractures, especially if they are asymmetric. A significant amount of lumbar scoliosis can be produced by a severe hip abduction contracture.

Patient Evaluation

Patients with MM should undergo an orthopedic evaluation every six to 12 months that includes spinal examination in both the upright and supine positions. Many other factors must be considered in these evaluations.

Flexion and Abduction Contractures. If the child has a significant hip flexion-abduction contracture producing lumbar lordosis and scoliosis (typically convex toward the side of the abduction contracture), the hip contracture should be surgically released before attempts at either brace control or surgical correction of the spine (Fig. 15–21).

Trunk Spasticity. Residual trunk and lower extremity spasticity due to isolated distal cord reflex function can cause rapid scoliosis progression. Patients with this condition can sometimes be helped by rhizotomy of nerve roots on the affected side.[88] Failure to consider this procedure in severe cases may doom attempts at brace or surgical stabilization.

Radiography. The first examination includes sitting spine radiographs to document curve severity and to determine the congenital components. Sitting radiographs are performed annually in routine cases, and more frequently in patients with high-risk congenital components or rapidly progressive curves.

Treatment of Scoliosis

After dealing with or ruling out associated problems (tethered cord, spasticity, congenital curve), one is often left with a progressive curve that must eventually be treated. In gen-

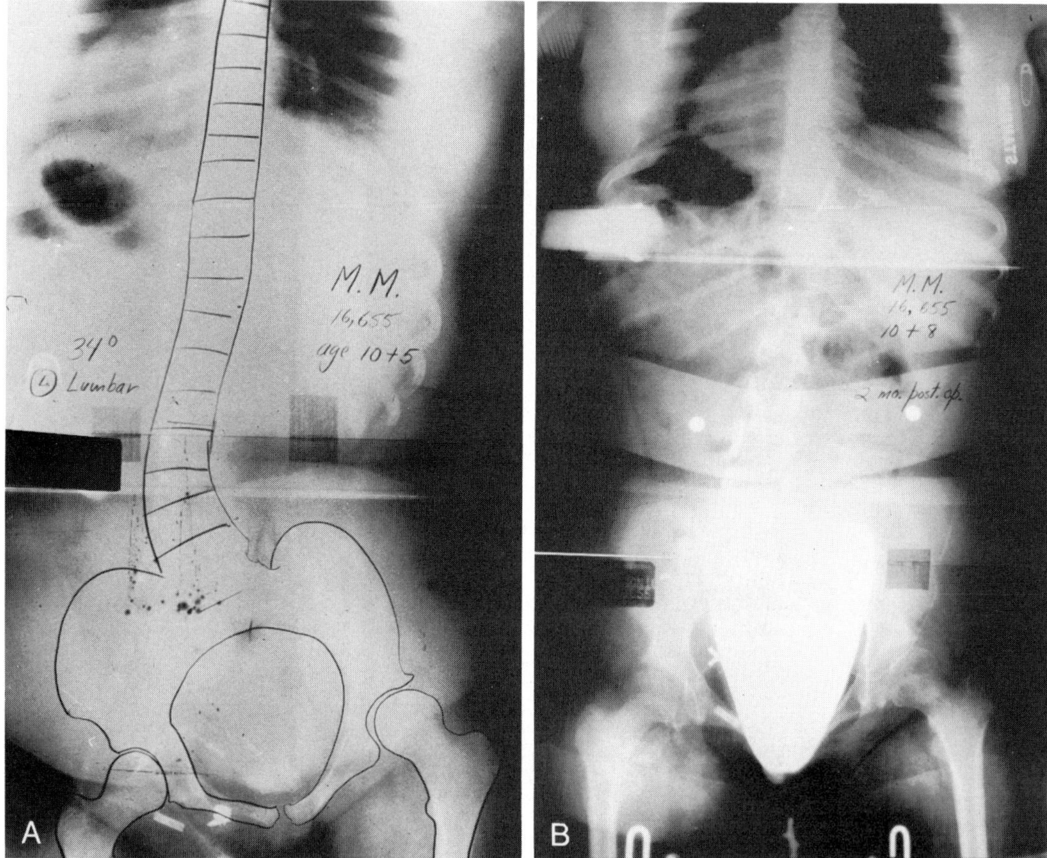

Figure 15–21. *A*, Left lumbar curvature in a 10-year-old with lumbar level MM and a left hip flexion-abduction contracture. *B*, Two months after surgical release of the flexion and abduction contracture. The curvature caused by the now released contracture has disappeared.

eral, if the curve progresses to 25 to 30 degrees or more, it should be braced. Although nonoperative treatment is usually a temporizing measure, patients do benefit from bracing. The goal is not to correct the curve but instead to slow curve progression until the child has achieved adequate trunk height to allow a reasonable adult truncal self-image. Thus, whenever possible, bracing is used to postpone surgery until age 10 to 12 years. A few patients escape surgery entirely, and some have to undergo fusion earlier because of severe progressive deformity.

Bracing is difficult because the children are often obese and difficult to fit. Previously, urinary diversion via ileostomy, with stomal bags attached to the trunk, made bracing even more difficult. Decreased trunk sensation can also be a problem. Despite these factors, most children can achieve reasonable trunk control by wearing a well-molded plastic under-arm jacket. A brace with a single opening (anterior or posterior) seems to give the best control, although a bivalved brace may be easier to place in a handicapped child. More complex devices, such as the Newington suspension jacket, can be tried in problematic cases, but specialized devices are more difficult to fit and maintain.

The brace should provide modest correction, as confirmed by sitting radiographs taken with the brace on. Subsequent films are taken every six months, alternating in-brace and out-of-brace films to provide data as to the brace's effectiveness and the curve's progression.

As noted, the goal is to delay spinal fusion until adequate spinal growth has been achieved. With meticulous bracing, surgery may be delayed until age 12 years. If, however, scoliosis progresses to greater than 40 to 50 degrees on the in-brace film, earlier fusion must be considered to avoid truncal deformity so great as to prevent adequate subsequent surgical correction.

With kyphosis, bracing is also difficult because of the risk of skin breakdown over the prominent kyphosis. A well-designed and padded brace can be tried but often fails, in which case surgical correction may be considered after age 5 to 6 years.

The indications for surgical correction of MM scoliosis are curve progression to more than 40 to 50 degrees with failure of brace control. Progressive congenital curves are treated by either in situ fusion or, in selected cases, anterior and posterior hemiepiphysiodesis as described by Winter and colleagues.[91]

Instrumentation and fusion for lordosis and scoliosis is more difficult than in other types of neuromuscular scoliosis because of the absence of posterior elements and poor skin quality. Also, wound infections are more common. In a review of 38 patients,[90] Ward and colleagues confirmed the previous recommendations of Osebold and associates[89] that both anterior and posterior fusion are required to achieve predictable long-term correction.

Anterior Fusion

The anterior fusion is very important in MM because the anterior spine provides a large surface for bony fusion (vertebral end plates) in the lumbar levels. By contrast, the deficient posterior elements at these levels provide minimal contact surface for bone grafting. The anterior disc excision and fusion is performed first, approaching from the convex side. A thoracoabdominal retroperitoneal approach, taking down the diaphragm, is usually required. In most cases the preoperative plan is to extend the fusion to the pelvis; thus, an attempt should be made to fuse the L5–S1 disc space anteriorly. As previously mentioned, this is most easily done by retracting the common iliac artery and vein laterally (toward the surgeon) with the disc exposed midline below the Y bifurcation of the great vessels. The great vessels are retracted medially (away from the surgeon) for all other disc levels.

A complete disc excision plus removal of vertebral end plate is performed at all levels, sparing only the posterior annulus fibrosus. The excised rib is cut into small pieces and used as bone graft. This can be supplemented with freeze-dried bank bone when the rib graft is inadequate. The iliac crest can be used as a bone graft source but is often inadequate in MM.

The only real question regarding the anterior approach is whether or not instrumentation is required (Dwyer, Zielke). With the advent of segmental posterior instrumentation (Luque, TSRH, C-D, pedicle screw systems), anterior instrumentation has become less essential. In a small series of MM patients we found little difference in the fusion rate or curve correction with combined surgery (anterior plus posterior fusion) whether or not anterior instrumentation was used.[90] In patients with a lumbar curve and fixed pelvic obliquity as a part of the curve, instrumentation does provide somewhat better correction of the obliquity (Fig. 15–22). The anterior procedure is usually performed one to two weeks before the posterior fusion. In certain patients, it may be possible to perform both the anterior and the posterior fusion on the same day (particularly for anterior and posterior hemiepiphysiodesis).

Posterior Fusion

Successful spinal fusion in MM requires posterior instrumentation and fusion, in addition to anterior fusion. The posterior fusion is difficult because of poor skin quality, the open spinal column, and lack of normal posterior elements for instrument attachment. With any type of posterior instrumentation, maintenance of a physiologic magnitude of lumbar lordosis is encouraged to shift weight bearing anteriorly on to the midthigh level, away from the ischial tuberosities.

Most authors have advised fusion to the pelvis in MM. Lindseth[88] contended that this is necessary only if there is a component of kyphosis in the lumbar spine or if the L5–S1 interspace is part of the lumbar curve. He noted an increased incidence of ischial ulcers in patients left with residual pelvic obliquity and fusion to the pelvis, probably because the rigid, long, curved segment prevents easy shifting of weight between ischial tuberosities. We have noted similar problems and no longer believe that fusion to the pelvis eliminates the possibility of ischial ulcers, especially if pelvic obliquity persists. We have spared the lowest lumbar disc levels in several athletic MM teenagers (participants in wheelchair tennis or basketball) with generally satisfactory results (Fig. 15–23). Problems with this approach include difficulty in finding a distal instrument attach-

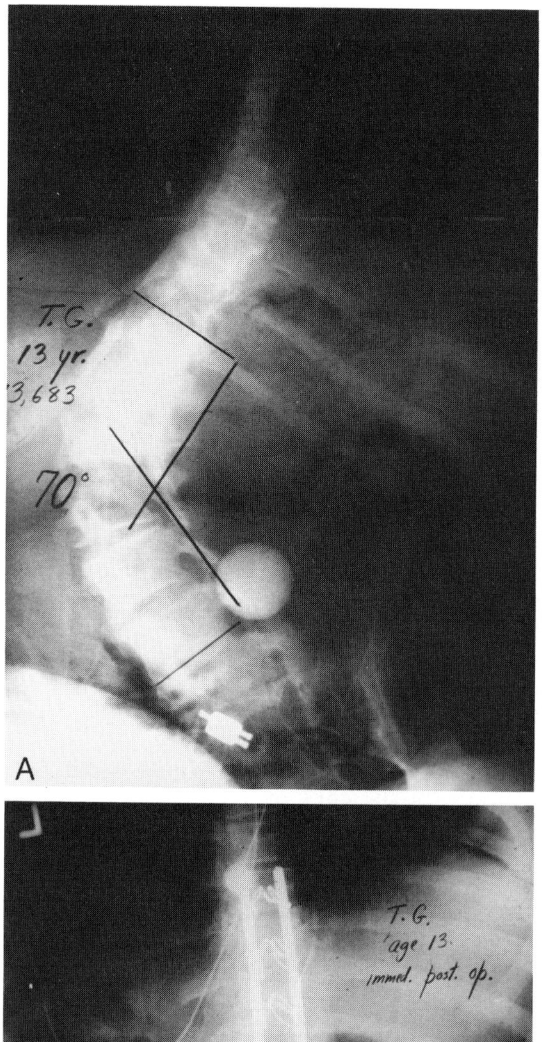

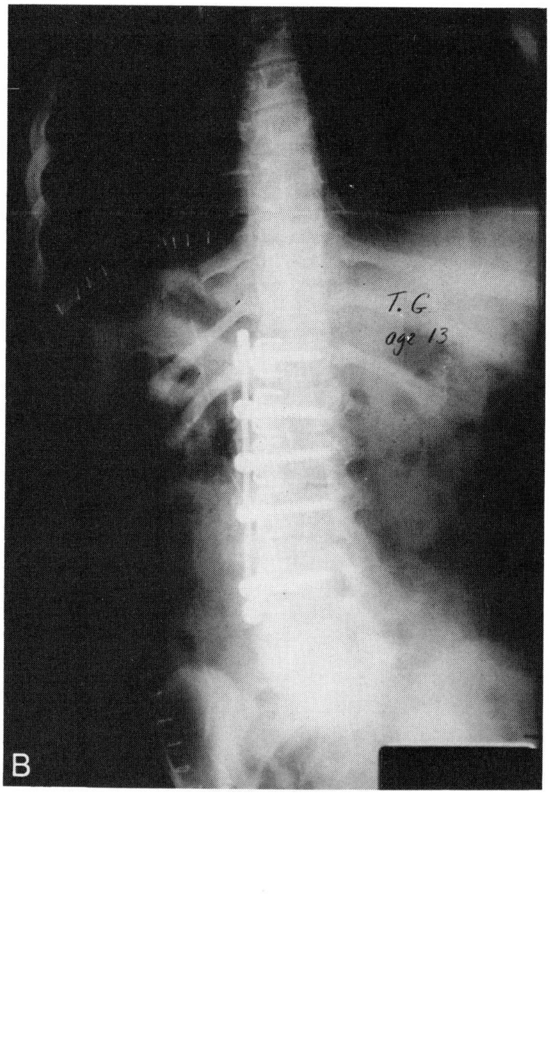

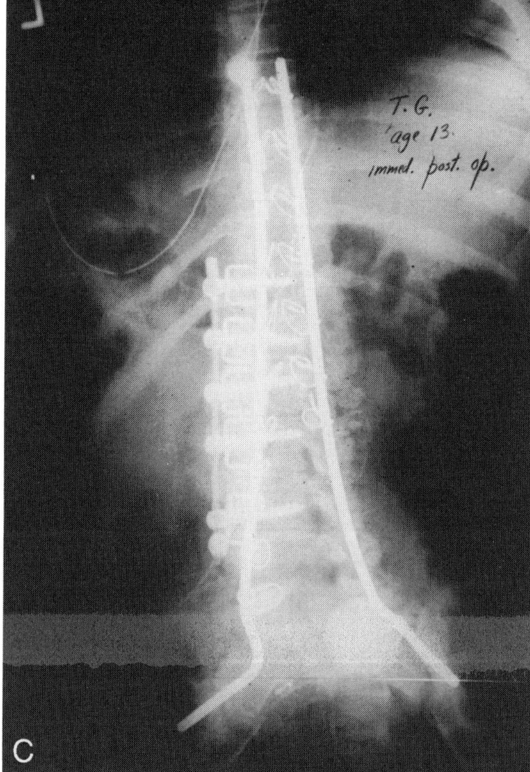

Figure 15–22. *A*, Preoperative radiograph of a 13-year-old with high lumbar level MM and marked scoliosis plus pelvic obliquity. *B*, Note the correction of pelvic obliquity gained by the first stage of surgery (anterior fusion), in which Dwyer instrumentation was used. *C*, Correction after completion of the second stage (posterior fusion with the Galveston-Luque method).

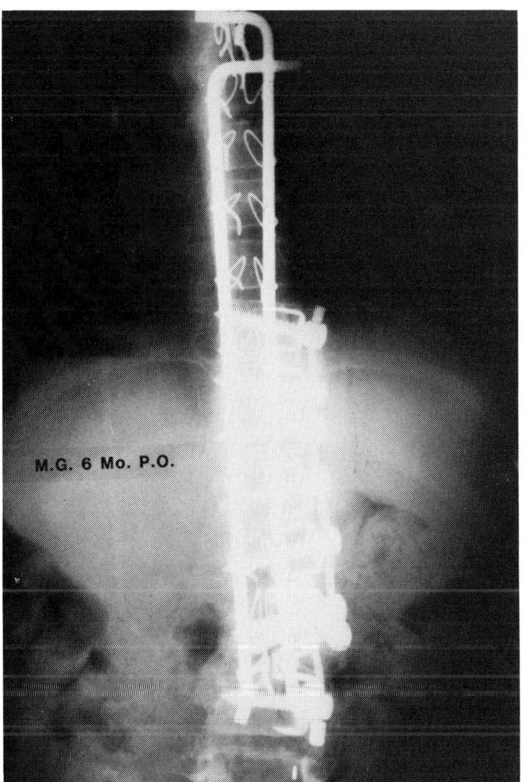

Figure 15–23. Postoperative radiographs in an athletic 13-year-old male with high lumbar level MM who had relentless curve progression. He was fused only to the lumbar level, anterior Dwyer plus posterior Luque instrumentation being used to maintain trunk mobility.

ment site (pedicle screws may help) and risk of curve progression. Clearly, the most predictable approach is fusion to the pelvis.

Luque segmental instrumentation has radically improved the results of posterior scoliosis fusion in all types of neuromuscular scoliosis, but to a lesser degree in MM because of the poor posterior attachment sites. The Galveston modification of the original Luque method of pelvic attachment, plus development of methods for attaching segmental wires to pedicles, residual laminae, and residual osteochondral processes in the open lumbar spine, has made Luque's segmental wiring method more applicable to MM scoliosis.

The fusion should be long, usually above T4 proximally and to the pelvis distally. We use an inverted Y incision that is midline proximally, bifurcating at the level where the spine opens and continuing distally to the ilium on either side. To avoid necrosis, the midline distally based flap must not be undermined. The entire spine is exposed and laminar wires are passed under each normal lamina proximally. Distally, wires are passed around the osteochondral processes or pedicles as described by Allen and Ferguson (Fig. 15–24).[86]

The posterior crest of the ilium is exposed on both sides and prepared for Galveston-type attachment to the pelvis by drilling a hole between the inner and outer table of the ilium (Fig. 15–25). The Luque rods are carefully contoured to fit the corrected spine, providing significant lumbar lordosis as well as scoliosis correction. The rods are inserted with the spine and pelvis manually corrected as the wires are tensioned with the jet wire tightener. The TSRH cross lockers can be added to the rods, both to stabilize the two rods into a single unit and to provide lateral forces at the distal end to help maintain the rods in the wing of the ilium.

All facets are excised, the spine is decorticated, and bone graft is added. This is usually freeze-dried bank bone, since the ilium can provide only moderate bone if the Galveston pelvic fixation is to be left undisturbed. Most patients fused with Galveston-Luque instrumentation develop the so-called "windshield wiper" effect around the portion of the rod implanted in the ilium, confirming that the sacroiliac joint remains mobile (Fig. 15–26). The horizontal distraction on the rods as they enter the pelvis with the use of the TSRH cross lockers may decrease this rod motion. True fusion to the pelvis (to the wing of the ilium rather than just to the sacrum) can be achieved by suturing the detached iliac crest apophysis to the transverse process area of the spine at L4 or L5 and filling the created triangle with bone graft (Fig. 15–27).

Postoperative Immobilization

Pseudarthrosis is common in fusions to the pelvis, and we still advise the conservative immobilization protocol that we developed for patients treated by anterior disc excision and posterior Harrington instrumentation. This includes 12 weeks of sitting in a semireclining wheelchair (Fig. 15–28) and use of a plastic orthosis extending down the thigh on one side 23 hours a day. After 12 weeks the thigh extension is removed and the patient is allowed to sit fully upright (and walk if a walker). The spine is protected for a total of six to 12 months

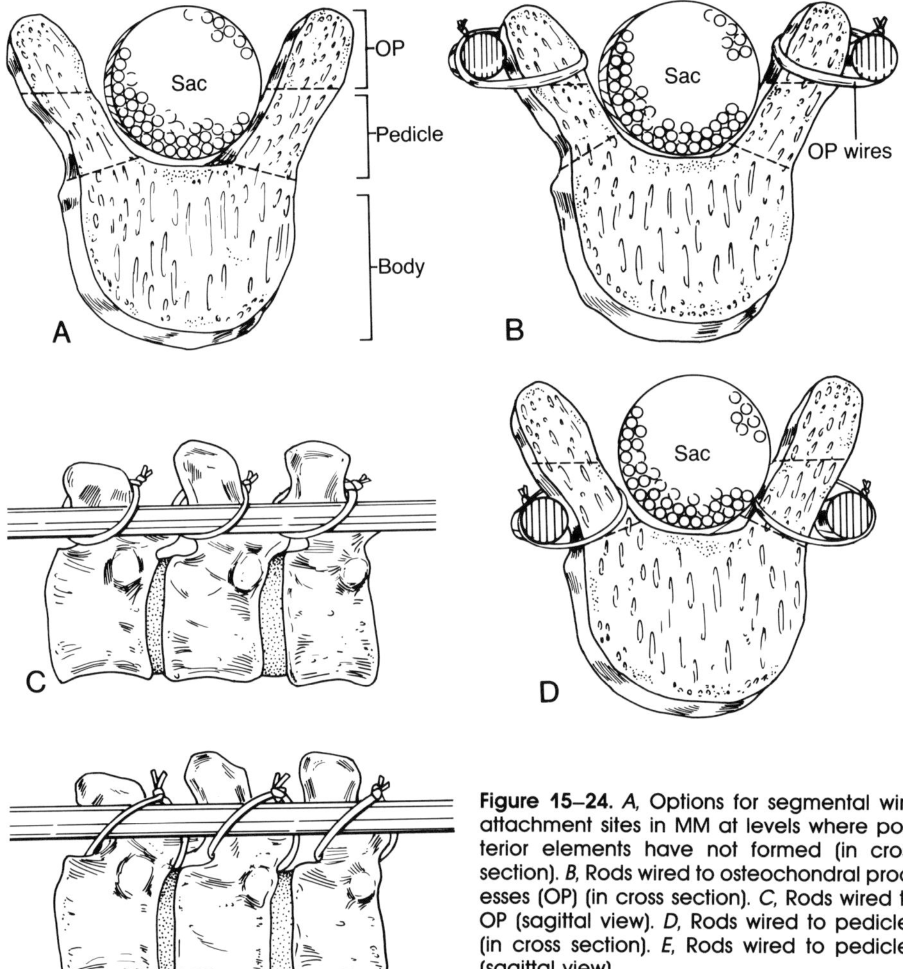

Figure 15–24. *A,* Options for segmental wire attachment sites in MM at levels where posterior elements have not formed (in cross section). *B,* Rods wired to osteochondral processes (OP) (in cross section). *C,* Rods wired to OP (sagittal view). *D,* Rods wired to pedicles (in cross section). *E,* Rods wired to pedicles (sagittal view).

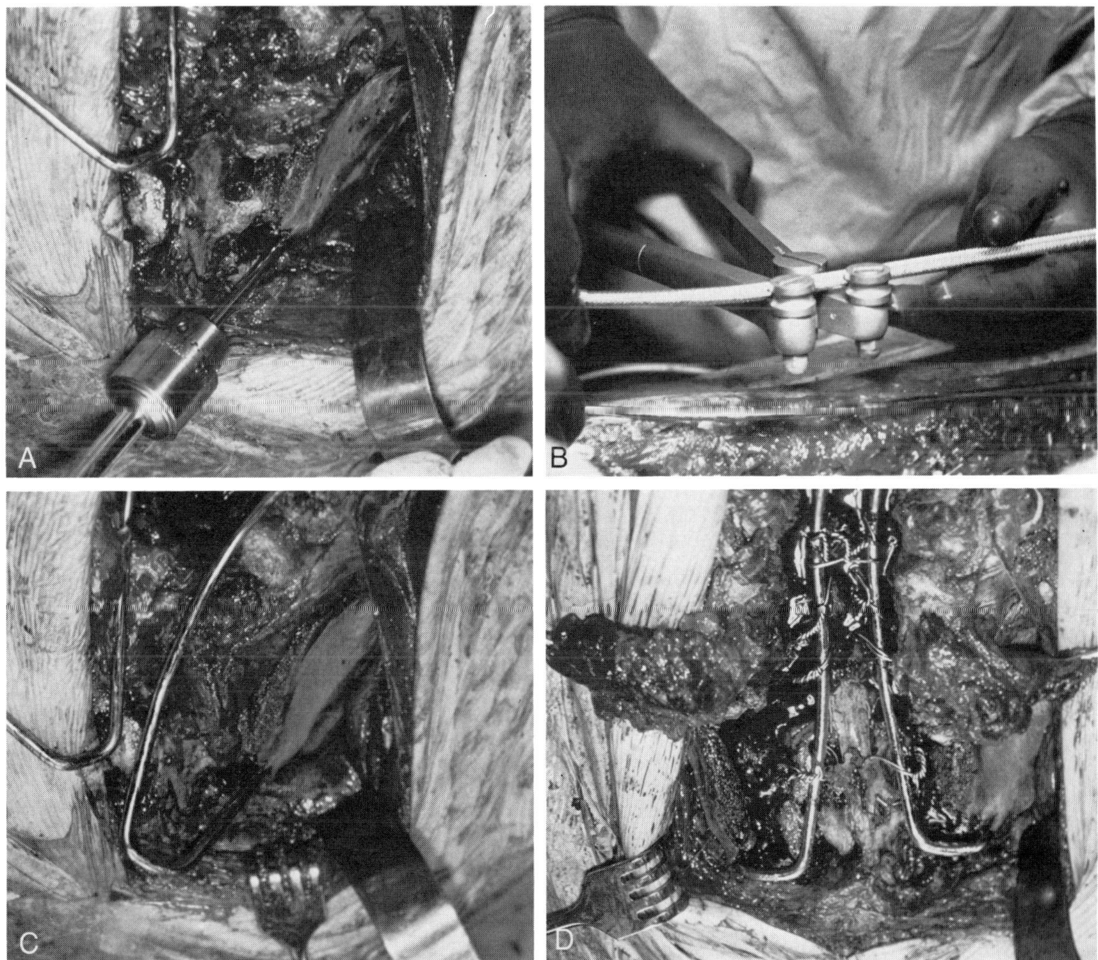

Figure 15–25. *A,* Drilling between the inner and outer table at the ilium in preparation for Luque-Galveston instrumentation to the pelvis. *B,* The French rod bender is invaluable for producing lordosis in the rods that are to be implanted. *C,* Introduction of contoured rods into the previously drilled holes. *D,* Both rods now inserted with segmental wires in place (for Luque-Galveston fusion to the pelvis).

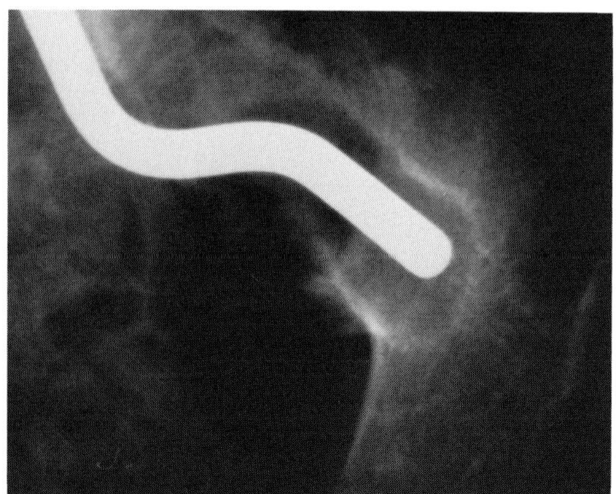

Figure 15–26. Radiolucent area (windshield wiper effect) around a rod within the wiring of the ilium two years after Luque-Galveston instrumentation to the pelvis.

postoperatively, the orthosis being worn while the child is upright.

Complications

Many patients have minor complications such as urinary tract infections or minor wound dehiscence. Major complications, including massive wound infection, instrumentation failure, and pseudarthrosis, are more common in MM scoliosis than in idiopathic scoliosis or other neuromuscular conditions. By attending to detail and applying all that is currently known about MM scoliosis surgery (careful anterior and posterior fusion, segmental attachment, cautious remobilization), the major complication rate can be reduced to 15 per cent or less.[90] Achievement of this goal requires the services of the most experienced scoliosis surgeons.

Kyphosis

As already noted, bracing is extremely difficult in the severe kyphosis associated with MM. Progressive kyphosis is the rule. Because surgical correction is complex and difficult, many children are left untreated and seem to function reasonably well, although skin breakdown over the kyphosis and poor trunk height remain as problems. Indications for surgery include progressive kyphosis, skin breakdown over the kyphosis, and concern regarding the cosmetic effect of severe trunk shortening.

Kyphosis in MM can be corrected, but the procedure is among the most challenging of all spinal deformity corrective operations. Intra- or perioperative death is frequent enough to give pause to all who treat this disorder. Death can occur from uncontrolled bleeding or problems with cerebrospinal fluid (CSF) dynamics.

The advent of segmental spinal instrumentation has made kyphectomy plus fusion at least moderately predictable. The ideal age for surgery has not been clarified, and we usually wait until the patient is 6 to 10 years old. The segmental attachment must extend well into the thoracic spine to control the large sagittal plane bending moments. Therefore, some spinal growth before fusion is desirable.

Basic principles include a long midline posterior approach with exposure of five or six levels of normal closed laminae proximally and distal exposure down to the midsacral level. The sac and cord are resected, care being taken to repair the dura slightly distal to and separate from the cord transaction to avoid tying off

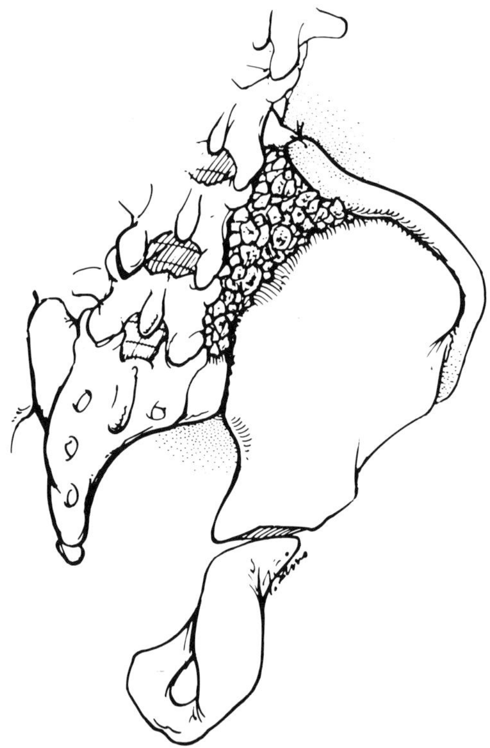

Figure 15–27. Elevating the medial 3 to 4 cm of iliac crest apophysis and suturing it to the spine at the L4 level provides a triangle where bone graft can be packed. This technique increases the chance of a stable fusion because it includes not only the sacrum but also the wiring at the ilium.

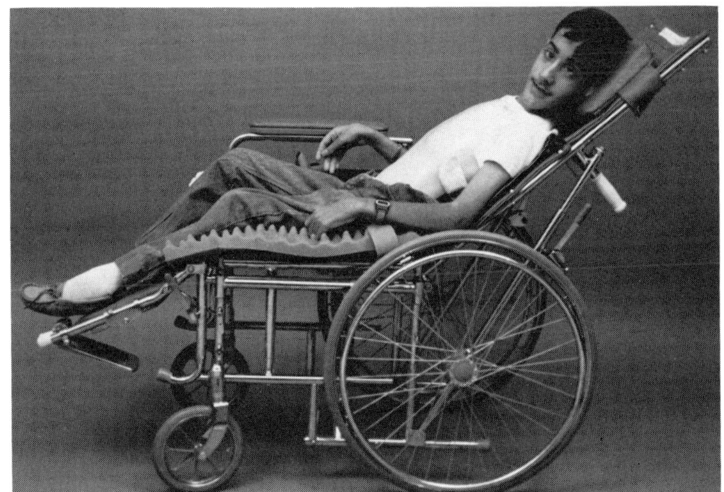

Figure 15–28. Semireclining wheelchair position used for the first three months after spinal fusion that extends to the pelvis.

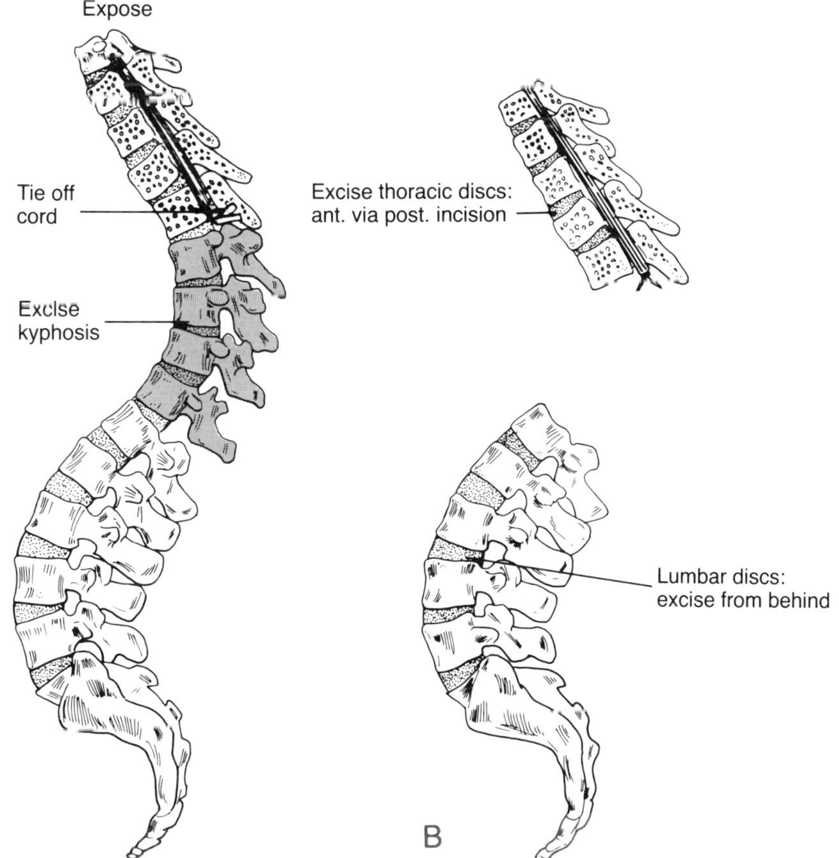

Figure 15–29. *A*, Sagittal plane diagram describing the sequence for lengthening. The spine is exposed, the dural sac tied off, and a segment of bone excised. *B*, To improve the mobility of the remaining segments, discs can be excised and the lower two or three pairs of ribs can be sectioned at their origins.

Illustration continued on following page

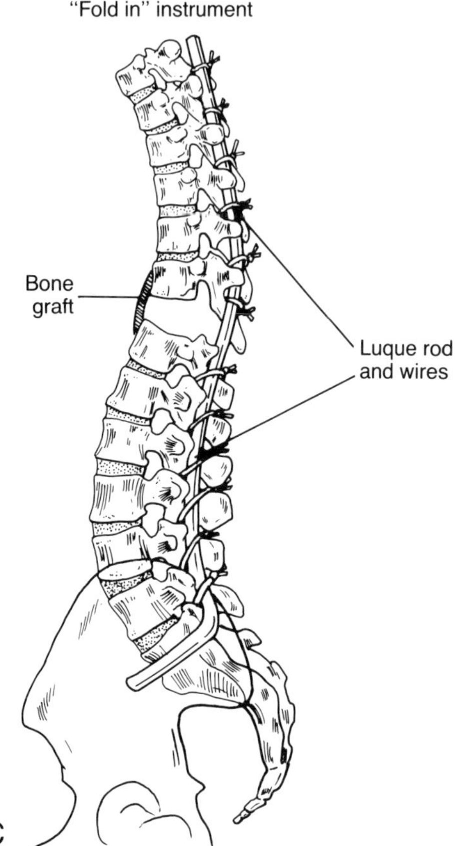

Figure 15–29 *Continued C,* The two segments are then "folded inward" and wired to the previously contoured rods.

the central canal and disturbing CSF dynamics (Fig. 15–29).

The spine is then prepared for segmental attachment by passing laminar wires under all normal laminae proximally (often T6 to T12) and around the osteochondral processes in the distal lumbar area. The iliac wings are drilled to accept Galveston-style Luque rods. The rods are then contoured. All of this is done before the spinal osteotomy, because the bleeding encountered with osteotomy may force a rapid finish. Being fully prepared (wires passed, iliac wings drilled, rods contoured) may make the difference between closing with the spine corrected and agonizing defeat (closing without correction and instrumentation).

The vertebral bodies making up the cranial two thirds of the kyphosis are excised, allowing one to "fold in" the remaining proximal and distal spinal segments. Often ribs 10 to 12 must be transected bilaterally to free the proximal segment enough so that the spine will fold inward. The rods are then positioned posterior to the infolded segments and wired in place. The excised vertebrae provide adequate bone graft, applied both anteriorly and posteriorly.

Variations on this theme include use of pediatric size C-D hooks on 3/16-inch Luque rods and possible use of pedicle screws. Other variations include complex rod contouring to engage the superior and anterior sacral alar surfaces, rather than placing the rods between the tables of the iliac wing.

Postoperative immobilization is even more restrictive than for MM scoliosis surgery, with both thighs incorporated into a body jacket for the first 12 weeks, followed by gradually increased mobilization.

By following meticulous guidelines and applying recently developed segmental techniques, experienced MM scoliosis surgeons can venture into MM kyphosis correction with reasonable success (Fig. 15–30).

SPINAL MUSCULAR ATROPHY

The term spinal muscular atrophy (SMA) describes a spectrum of conditions caused by degeneration of the anterior horn cells of the spinal cord and brain stem in childhood, resulting in symmetric muscle paralysis of the trunk and proximal musculature.[104] It is usually autosomal recessive, with males usually more severely involved than females. Werdnig in 1891[108] and Hoffmann in 1893[101] described what is now recognized as Werdnig-Hoffmann infantile spinal muscular atrophy, a condition that is often fatal by age 3 years. Kugelberg and Welander in 1956[102] described a milder juvenile form, with onset up to age 15.

The spectrum of disease in SMA can be classified by age and maximal functional attainment into four categories.[95, 96, 105] Type I (Werdnig-Hoffmann) has an onset within the first six months. This group is characterized by lack of achievement of head control or sitting balance. Intermediate Types II and III have an onset at six to 24 months. Type II is defined by the achievement of sitting balance only. A Type III patient achieves walking capability with aids but cannot run or climb stairs normally. The function of all children deteriorates from their point of maximal function, with the exception of some patients with Type IV (Ku-

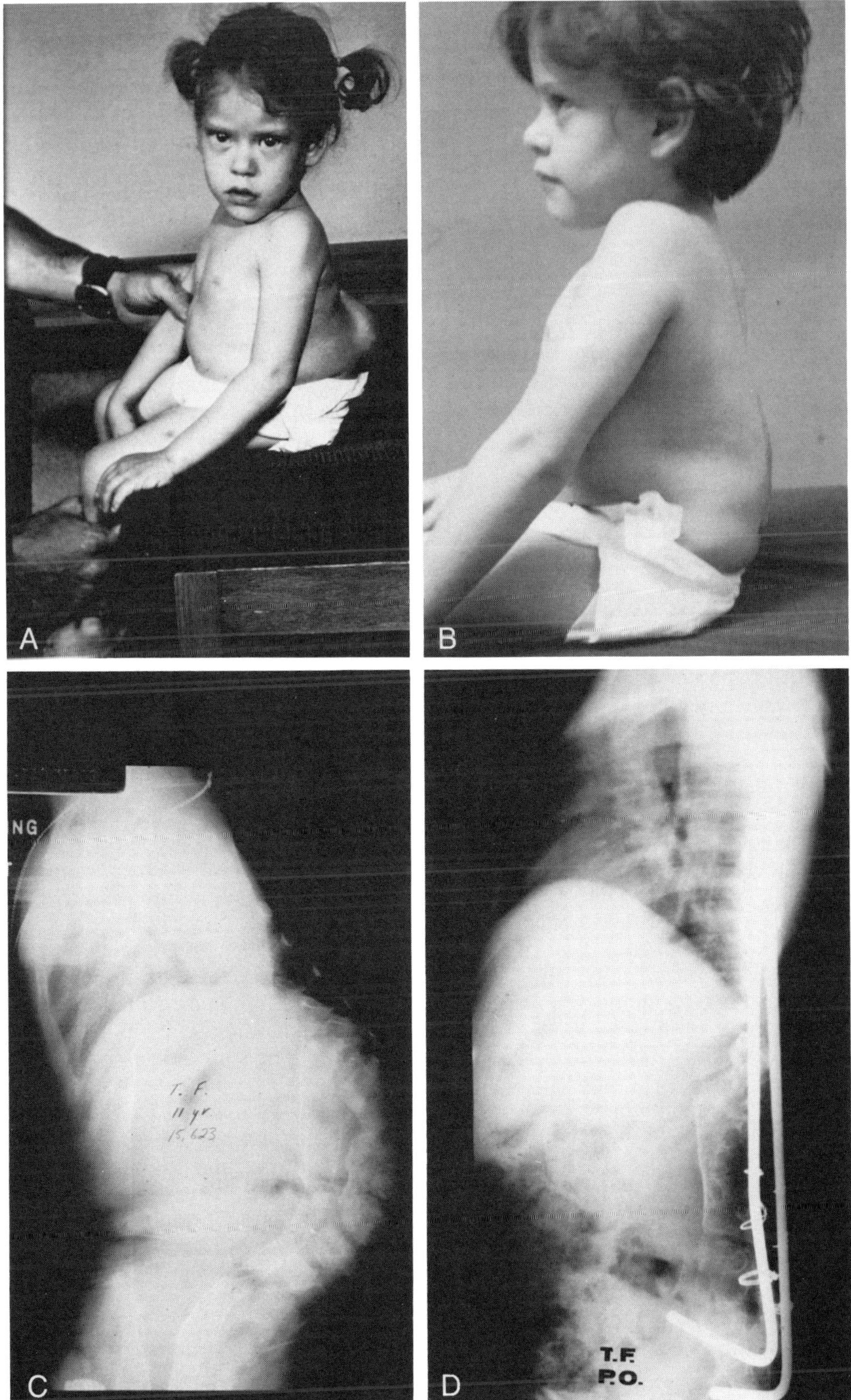

Figure 15–30. *A, B,* Pre- and postoperative views of a 6-year-old girl whose MM kyphosis was corrected surgically. *C, D,* Pre- and postoperative two-year follow-up radiographs of an adolescent with MM kyphosis, connected by single-stage kyphectomy, fusion, and segmental instrumentation.

gelberg-Welander), who attain relatively normal ambulatory function. On occasion, patients have been described as remaining static for extended periods.[96]

As reflected by the combined classification schema of Evans,[98] the best predictor of prognosis is age and the extent of clinical disease at onset. Patients affected with Werdnig-Hoffmann are in the minority, as 80 per cent of all SMA patients survive into adulthood and achieve sitting ability.[97]

The clinical disease is characterized by severe weakness (proximal greater than distal), flaccidity, and areflexia. Normal sensation is preserved, as is intelligence. Normal serum enzyme and aldolase levels differentiate this process from primary myopathies. Nerve conduction velocities are normal, EMG studies show denervation of muscle, and biopsy shows nerve and muscle atrophy.[106]

Schwentker and Gibson[106] reported scoliosis as the most severe problem in patients who survive. Once scoliosis appears, it is invariably progressive,[96] with an earlier onset, higher frequency, and more rapid progression in the nonwalker.[106] All patients with Types I, II, and III have a curve of 15 degrees or greater. Only those most minimally involved patients with juvenile onset (Type IV) may be spared spinal deformity.[93, 105] Since Werdnig-Hoffmann is usually fatal at an early age, scoliosis, though present, is not generally treated. These patients may benefit from part-time use of a lightweight (e.g., Plastazote) body jacket to support sitting balance. Average onset of scoliosis can be as early as 2 to 4 years in the intermediate forms,[66, 92] for which aggressive bracing and surgical treatment is indicated, with an average age of fusion of 12 to 13 years.[66, 106]

Most curves are the classical neuromuscular long "C" with a thoracolumbar apex, often associated with pelvic obliquity.[106]

Treatment

Bracing is not well tolerated by patients with spinal muscular atrophy because of the collapsing nature of the curve and their inability to pull away from the brace because of weakness. Discomfort is generated by the normal sensate skin being pressed against the hard surface of the brace. Children with SMA can also experience respiratory compromise with bracing. They are diaphragmatic breathers, and the brace limits abdominal expansion and diaphragmatic excursion. Braces that are back opening without abdominal pressure may be tolerated better. Despite this relative intolerance, bracing is employed by most authors.[100, 102] Shapiro and Bresman[107] considered that bracing delays eventual fusion, which serves to gain trunk height, and the patient likewise has larger bones to instrument. They feel that bracing provides truncal stability and balance necessary to free the upper extremities of the sitting patient for activities of daily living. A brace should accommodate the patient's excessive lordosis, as opposed to the lumbosacral kyphosis that is generally built into a brace for an idiopathic scoliosis patient. If the lordotic lumbosacral spine of an SMA patient is "tucked" into kyphosis, he will fall forward. In the walking patient, a brace in too much lumbosacral kyphosis may curtail ambulation.

Despite the advantages of truncal stability and increased function in a brace, scoliosis in SMA tends to progress.[100, 106] In 52 cases of Type II SMA, Granata and associates found an 8 degree per year increase in curve magnitude despite brace use. They likewise demonstrated a significant increase in curve progression when a mildly involved patient stops walking. In 13 nonwalking SMA patients they found a 3 degree per year curve progression. Mildly involved walking patients showed only a 0.6 degrees per year progression.

As in poliomyelitis, preoperative traction in severe curves is somewhat controversial.[92, 96] Daher and colleagues[96] suggested that it is unnecessary and may cause muscle weakness; they found pulmonary function improvement of 9 per cent in only one patient. Using halo traction, Aprin and associates[92] had excellent results in two patients, with a functional vital capacity increase of 30 to 40 per cent. They felt that this was secondary to decompressing the thorax from the abdominal contents. They recommended that proper corrective traction be used for no longer than two weeks, because most correction is obtained within this period, and prolonged traction further weakens the patient (Fig. 15–31).

As the experience with scoliosis in SMA increases, the Cobb angle indications for surgical intervention seem to progressively decrease. Zeller and colleagues found a 16 per cent less complication rate and greater correction if fusion was performed at about 37 de-

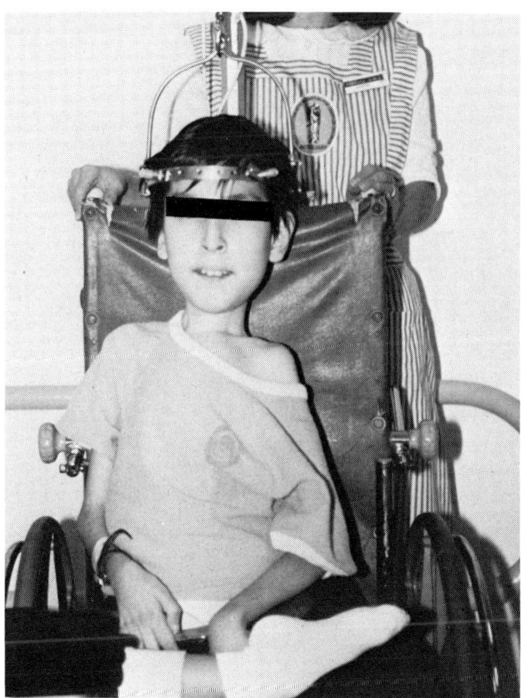

Figure 15–31. A 15-year-old male with spinal muscular atrophy (SMA) in halo gravity—"spring" traction—used preoperatively. There was only moderate return of pulmonary function yet he experienced dramatic subjective improvement while in traction.

grees, as opposed to an average 57 degrees.[109] Shapiro and Bresman[107] and Daher and colleagues[96] suggested that the patient be fused for curves over 40 degrees. Bonnett and associates[94] proposed the most aggressive approach, suggesting that fusion should be performed as soon as the curve loses flexibility and does not completely correct on side bending films. Fusion should be performed along the entire extent of the curve and should include the pelvis in all nonwalking patients.[96] Segmental instrumentation is the instrumentation of choice, so that postoperative bracing may be minimized. Anterior fusion should be avoided if possible because of potential pulmonary compromise.[98] Aprin and associates, however, suggested that anterior surgery can be well tolerated if the approach is limited to a single cavity (chest or abdomen) without cutting the diaphragm.[92]

Much like Duchenne muscular dystrophy, pulmonary function in many SMA patients continues to decrease independent of spinal deformity. As in Duchenne, worsening spinal curvature accelerates pulmonary deterioration.[103] Occupational and physical therapy evaluations by Furumasu and colleagues and Zeller and colleagues[99, 109] demonstrated that functional upper extremity improvement is unpredictable after spine fusion. These authors determined that gross motor lower extremity activities declined for two to five years postoperatively and stabilized. Upper extremity function improved slightly at five years, owing to increased use of upper extremity equipment. In contrast, Hensinger and MacEwen[66] found in 13 patients that none lost function if vigorous postoperative physical and respiratory therapy were pursued.

Authors' Recommendations

We use bracing in early flexible curves as soon as progression is documented. The goal in bracing is to temporize, allowing the child to achieve as much sitting height as possible. This may delay spinal fusion until approximately 10 to 12 years of age, unless the curve is uncontrollable by bracing and is more than 40 degrees. Surgical intervention with Luque segmental spinal instrumentation and fusion to the pelvis is the method of choice. In patients graded Risser 0, anterior fusion without diaphragmatic takedown should be considered in order to prevent the "crankshaft" phenomenon.[6]

ARTHROGRYPOSIS

Arthrogryposis was first described by Adolf W. Otto in 1847.[116] In 1905 Rosenkranz (quoted in reference 113) coined the term "arthrogryposis," which means curved or hooked joint. Stern in 1923[119] is credited with originating the term in most common use today: "arthrogryposis multiplex congenita."

Swinyard and Mayer[120] defined arthrogryposis multiplex congenita as an "expected and predictable response to a variety of agents and processes that creates generalized or local muscle weakness, making the limb vulnerable to mechanical limitation of movement."

Despite earlier literature suggesting relative trunk sparing,[115, 122] trunk involvement with scoliosis does occur. The incidence of spinal deformity in arthrogryposis has been reported to be as high as 42 per cent.[3, 110, 111, 114, 118, 121] Most of these curves are noted at birth or within the first year of life.[114] Curves are rigid

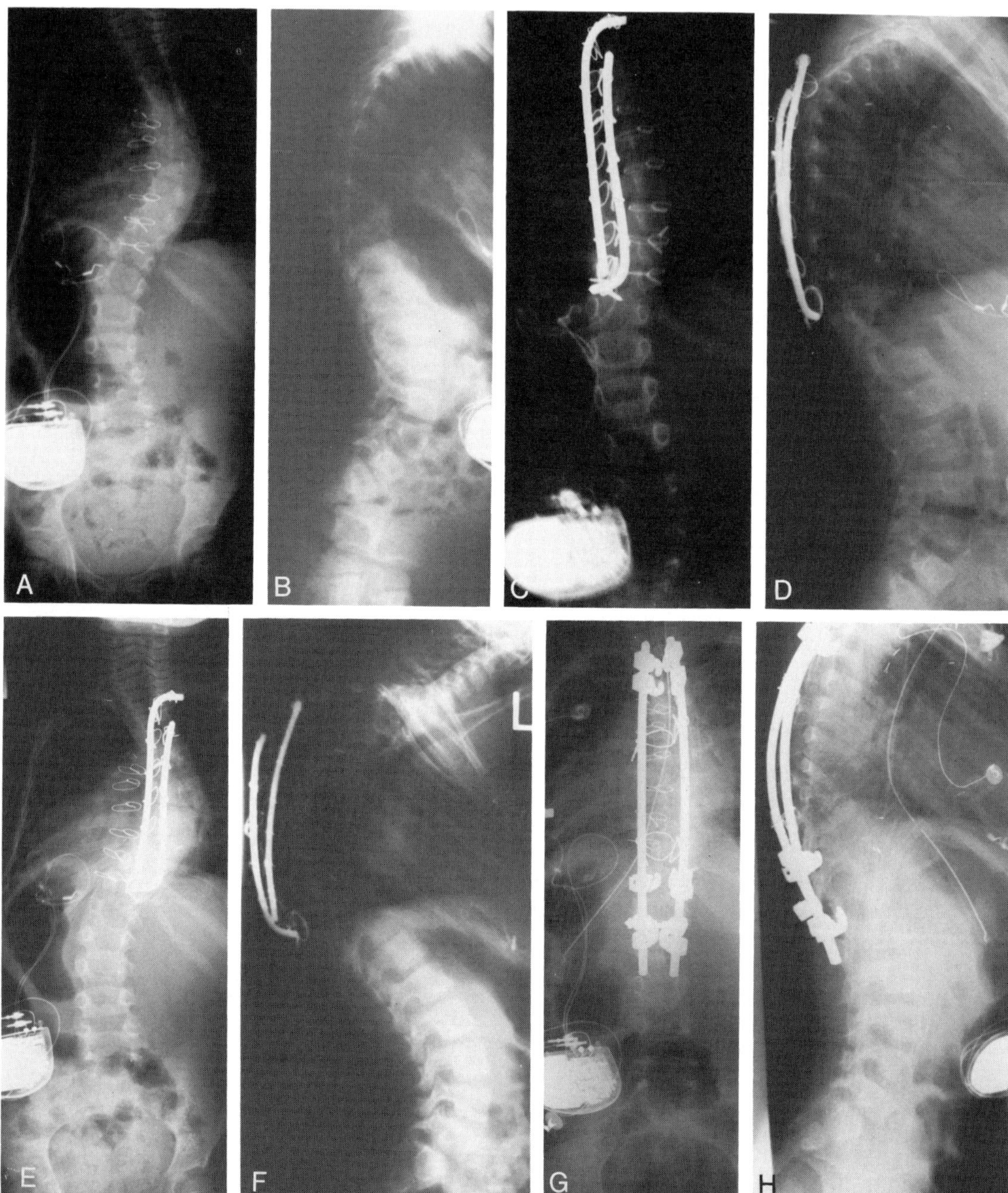

Figure 15–32. *A, B,* A 4-year-old boy with arthrogryposis and kyphoscoliosis. The right thoracic curve measures 45 degrees; the left lumbar curve measures 28 degrees with a 57-degree kyphosis. The deformity is progressive despite bracing. *C, D,* Anterior discectomy without fusion plus Luque instrumentation and wiring without fusion. Scoliosis was corrected to 20 degrees; the kyphosis was unchanged after surgery. *E, F,* View 1½ years after surgery with failure of Luque instrumentation, and progression of scoliosis to 47 degrees and kyphosis to 105 degrees. *G, H,* At 5 years, 9 months the patient underwent anterior discectomy and fusion followed by posterior osteotomies and C-D instrumentation with correction to 80 degrees kyphosis, 20 degrees scoliosis.

very early in their development and may require treatment in infancy. Most curves have paralytic characteristics, with associated congenital vertebral anomalies in 11 to 50 per cent of cases.[110, 111, 114, 117, 118] Those curves without congenital elements are often thoracolumbar in pattern, with pelvic obliquity.[114]

Children with arthrogryposis generally live long into adulthood, providing ample time for demonstration of the natural history of the spinal deformity. Significant potential for early progression has been documented.[111, 114]

Treatment

Bradford thought that bracing may help in early small curves, especially in younger children.[3] Siebold and associates,[117] in two of their six patients, were able to keep the curve magnitude less than 40 degrees. In the review by Herron and colleagues[114] of 88 patients with arthrogryposis, bracing was found to be ineffective. They demonstrated a 5 degree per year progression in brace patients, compared with 6.5 degrees per year in untreated patients. All brace-treated patients in this series eventually required fusion. Drummond and McKenzie[111] recommended fusion of patients with arthrogryposis at approximately 40 degrees. Instrumentation is an important part of the fusion process, as demonstrated by Herron and colleagues[114] who found that most of their patients fused through a cast without instrumentation had pseudarthrosis with loss of correction.

Attempts at posterior instrumentation without fusion have been made to allow for growth of the spine while maintaining correction. This internal bracing approach has been fraught with problems. In 16 patients, Eberle[112] found six with fractured Luque rods and four in whom the short limb of one or both of the L-shaped rods had rotated out of the pelvis, perforating the skin and resulting in infection and rod removal. At the time of review, the deformity of patients in his series was essentially unchanged in 15 of the 16 patients. Some success has been achieved using Harrington rods with rod lengthenings and/or exchange every six months, concurrent with Milwaukee bracing. Luque instrumentation without fusion has been very unsuccessful (Fig. 15–32).

The connective tissue of the arthrogrypotic patient is tough and tight and the bones are soft and osteoporotic. This limits correction of the curvature as well as the loss of correction after surgery. According to Siebold and associates,[117] the average correction lost with Harrington rod instrumentation was only 5 degrees, which may reflect the rigidity of soft tissues, inhibiting correction loss, rather than stability of fixation.

Treatment decisions regarding the congenital component of the scoliosis should be made according to recognized criteria for in situ fusion of congenital curves.

Authors' Recommendations

In patients with arthrogryposis there is a significant incidence of scoliosis that appears early and is often rigid, requiring early treatment. Bracing has achieved some success in flexible curves in young patients, but progression is unaffected in the larger, more rigid curves. We recommend bracing of noncongenital curves of up to 40 degrees of deformity, beginning at 20 degrees or when progression is documented, and segmental posterior instrumentation and fusion in patients who have demonstrated progression and have curve magnitudes over 40 degrees. Anterior fusion may be required for severe rigid curvature and pelvic obliquity, as well as curves in Risser 0 patients at risk for the "crankshaft" phenomenon. Fixation to the pelvis is mandatory to maintain torso alignment in patients with significant rigid pelvic obliquity.

DUCHENNE MUSCULAR DYSTROPHY

Duchenne muscular dystrophy is a sex-linked recessive disease characterized by progressive muscular weakness. Usually diagnosed between the ages of three and five years, labored ambulation subsequently develops and long leg bracing is required. Patients become wheelchair bound around 10 to 12 years of age (Fig. 15–33). Once this happens, a relentless progression of spinal deformity and associated decline in pulmonary function directly contribute to early death in the late teens or early twenties.

Wilkins and Gibson theorized two pathways of spinal deformity in Duchenne muscular dystrophy: a "stable" pathway characterized by a position of extension and an "unstable" path-

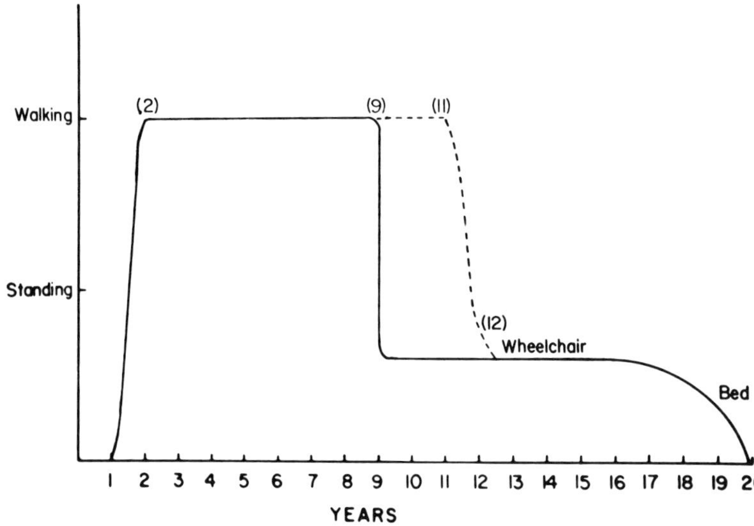

Figure 15–33. The natural history of Duchenne muscular dystrophy. The boys begin walking at around 1½ years of age. They usually require lower extremity surgery and bracing between 9 and 11 years of age to continue walking. They become wheelchair bound at around 12 years and subsequently develop scoliosis. (From Kurz, L. T., Mubarak, S. J., Schultz, P., et al.: Correlation of scoliosis and pulmonary function in Duchenne muscular dystrophy. J. Pediatr. Orthop. *3*:347, 1983.

way exhibiting progressive thoracolumbar kyphosis and scoliosis (Fig. 15–34).[144] A prophylactic electric wheelchair "spinal support system" was proposed to guide the early straight spine into a stable extended posture, thereby averting the need for operative intervention (Fig. 15–35).[126] Later authors, however, found that the attitude of the spine did not preclude progression of deformity[128] and that wheelchair spine support systems and braces only delay the onset of scoliosis.[125, 128, 139, 142]

It is clear from the literature that the incidence of progressive scoliosis is about 95 per cent in patients with Duchenne muscular dystrophy.[125, 135] Furthermore, the natural history of these curves is progression to more than

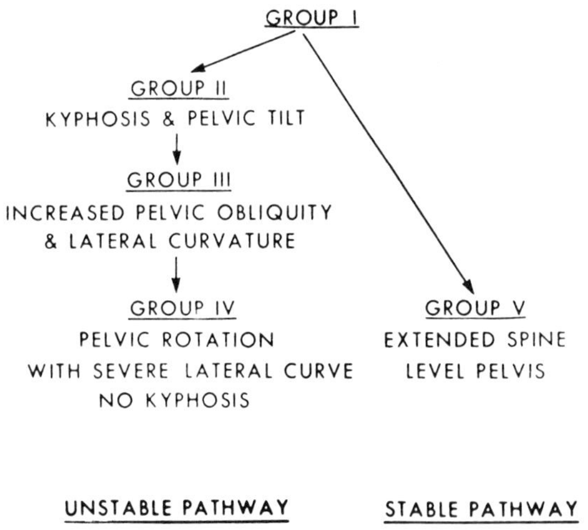

GROUP I

GROUP II
KYPHOSIS & PELVIC TILT

GROUP III
INCREASED PELVIC OBLIQUITY
& LATERAL CURVATURE

GROUP IV
PELVIC ROTATION
WITH SEVERE LATERAL CURVE
NO KYPHOSIS

GROUP V
EXTENDED SPINE
LEVEL PELVIS

UNSTABLE PATHWAY

STABLE PATHWAY

Figure 15–34. Stable and unstable pathways of spinal deformity in Duchenne muscular dystrophy (From Wilkins, K. E., and Gibson, D. A.: The patterns of spinal deformity in Duchenne muscular dystrophy. J. Bone Joint Surg. *58A*:24, 1976.)

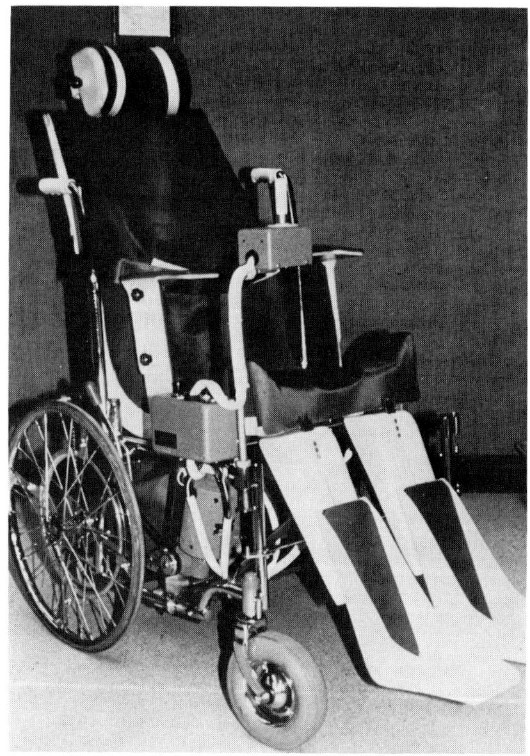

Figure 15–35. Toronto electric wheelchair spinal support system.

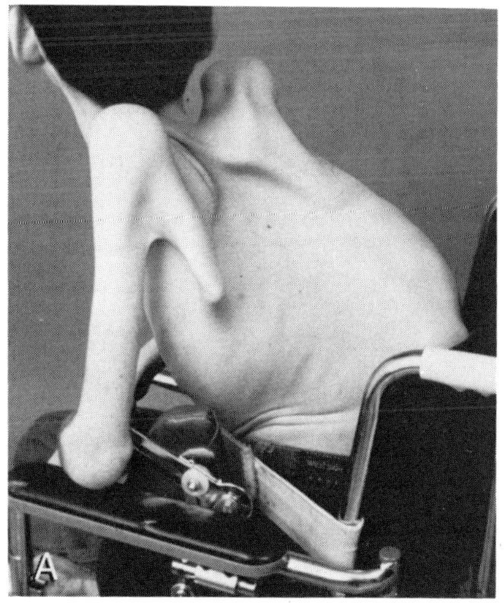

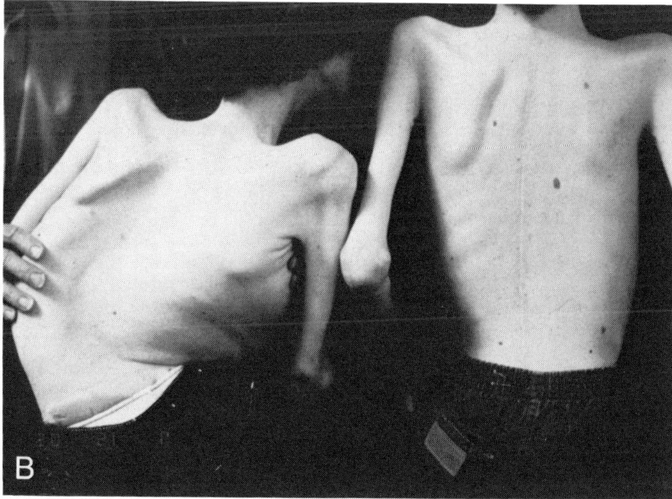

Figure 15–36. *A,* Example of severe neuromuscular scoliosis, not treated surgically, in the pre-Luque era. In this adolescent with muscular dystrophy, even wheelchair sitting is becoming difficult. *B,* Rear view of two brothers with severe neuromuscular scoliosis secondary to muscular dystrophy. The boy on the right underwent a successful Luque posterior spinal instrumentation and fusion and has good sitting balance. His older brother *(left)* already had lost so much pulmonary function that surgery could not be considered. He is unable to sit well, even with support.

100 degrees. This usually occurs within five years of the patient being wheelchair bound and greatly interferes with sitting and proper positioning in the wheelchair, caloric ingestion, cosmesis, and respiratory function (Fig. 15–36).

In idiopathic scoliosis, the degree of scoliosis shows a strong linear correlation, with a decline in percentage of predicted forced vital capacity (%FVC) and total lung capacity.[132, 140, 142, 143] Many authors concluded that in idiopathic scoliosis the degree of thoracic scoliosis is the most important factor causing a decline in these clinical parameters of pulmonary function. In contrast, a study of pulmonary function in patients with paralytic scoliosis showed much weaker correlations than those parameters of pulmonary function shown to be important in patients with idiopathic scoliosis.[132] This probably reflects a multifactorial influence on declining pulmonary function in patients with paralytic scoliosis, increasing scoliotic deformity being only one of these factors.

Although numerous studies have described the pulmonary function abnormality seen in patients with Duchenne muscular dystrophy,[124, 127, 129, 130, 131, 137, 138, 140] none has shown such a correlation with scoliosis until 1983, when we studied 25 patients with this condition.[133] We found that FVC peaked at approximately the age when standing ceased, then declined rapidly (Fig. 15–37). Percentage FVC was found to be the parameter of pulmonary function most strongly correlated with age and thoracic scoliosis measurements. Age and thoracic scoliosis together were better predictors of %FVC than either one alone. Each 1 year of age had approximately the same negative influence on %FVC as each 10 degrees of

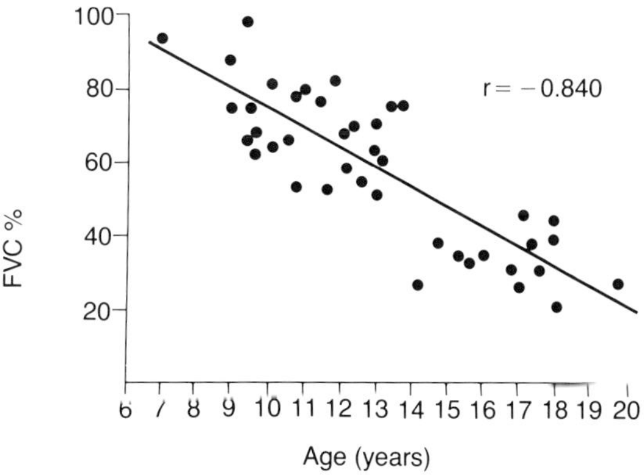

Figure 15–37. Percentage of forced vital capacity depicted on the axis and age in years; a patient with Duchenne muscular dystrophy on the X axis. Percentage FVC was found to be the parameter of pulmonary function that was most strongly correlated with age and thoracic scoliosis measurement. (From Kurz, L. T., Mubarak, S. J., Schultz, P., et al.: Correlation of scoliosis and pulmonary function in Duchenne muscular dystrophy. J. Pediatr. Orthop. *3*:347, 1983.)

thoracic scoliosis; both decreased %FVC by approximately 4 per cent. A regression equation for %FVC theorized that the patient whose scoliosis progression was halted by spinal instrumentation and fusion would, subsequent to the surgery, show a slower rate of decline of %FVC and that this rate is quantifiable and predictable and depends solely on the patient's advancing age.

Miller and colleagues[135] refuted these observations. These authors noted that the group with early spinal instrumentation had declining respiratory function that was the same as that in the group not treated. However, most of their patients were not instrumented until the scoliosis curve was greater than an average of 40 degrees. They also did not look exclusively at thoracic deformity in their statistical correlations. We have advocated early fusion when the curves approach 20 degrees and feel this may prevent further decline in pulmonary function secondary to the scoliosis.

Treatment

In 1982 Luque revolutionized the surgical treatment of paralytic scoliosis when he introduced segmental spinal instrumentation.[34, 134] This eliminated the need for prolonged postoperative immobilization, characteristic of Harrington instrumentation. The Galveston technique of pelvic instrumentation allowed stable spinal instrumentation of the pelvis.[123]

Because of these studies, it was generally recommended that instrumentation and fusion be carried out to the sacrum to prevent or correct pelvic obliquity. However, as Allen and Ferguson pointed out, pelvic fixation is technically a demanding procedure that requires increased operative time and increased risk of sacral nerve injury.[123] In 1984 Sussman suggested that fusion and fixation to the fifth lumbar level may be sufficient in Duchenne muscular dystrophy, but follow-up was limited.[139]

To define this issue, we prospectively studied two groups of patients, 12 undergoing instrumentation and fusion to the sacrum, and 10 having instrumentation to L5 only. In all patients, cephalad instrumentation and fusion was carried out to the high thoracic level (generally T2–T3). Average follow-up was 3½ years with minimal follow-up of two years in all living patients. There were no significant

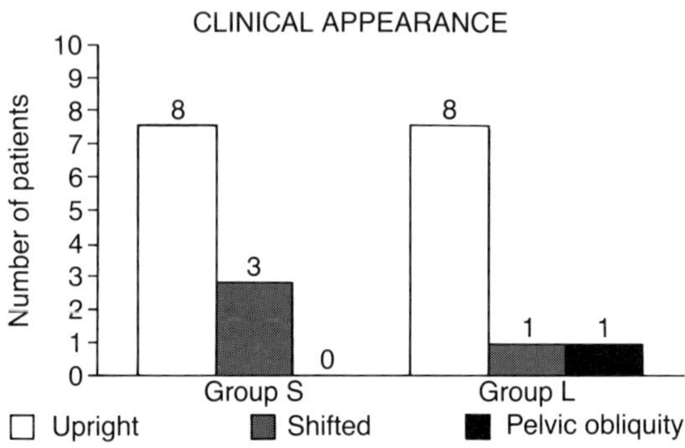

Figure 15–38. Fusion to the pelvis required in Duchenne muscular dystrophy. The clinical appearance between the Group S fusion to the sacrum (pelvis) and Group L fusion to L5 was essentially the same at four-year follow-up. (From Mubarak S., Morin, W., and Leach, J.: Spinal fusion in Duchenne muscular dystrophy—fixation and fusion to the sacrum? Orthop. Trans. *13:*169, 1989.)

differences in estimated blood loss or length of stay in the intensive care unit and hospital between the two groups. The operative time was approximately 30 minutes longer in patients fused inferiorly to include the pelvis or sacrum. Review of the patients' sitting balance and pelvic obliquity revealed only minor differences, with only one patient (whose preoperative curve was 50 degrees) developing a significant pelvic obliquity (Fig. 15–38). All other patients had no significant pelvic obliquity and remained in an upright or only slightly shifted position. We concluded that instrumentation to L5 is sufficient if treatment is initiated early (Fig. 15–39).

Authors' Recommendations

We have found the following treatment plan to be successful for patients with Duchenne muscular dystrophy. Spinal fusion is performed when curves reach 20 degrees and FVC is greater than 40 per cent. Preoperative FVC of less than 30 per cent is correlated with a high incidence of major respiratory complications.[130]

If progressive scoliosis collapse is halted with posterior spinal fusion, decline in %FVC would theoretically be slowed and be ultimately dependent on progressive weakness alone. Wheelchair spinal support systems and thoracolumbar bracing do not control these curves and only delay surgery until the pulmonary function is so low (less than 40 per cent FVC) that safe spinal instrumentation is not feasible.

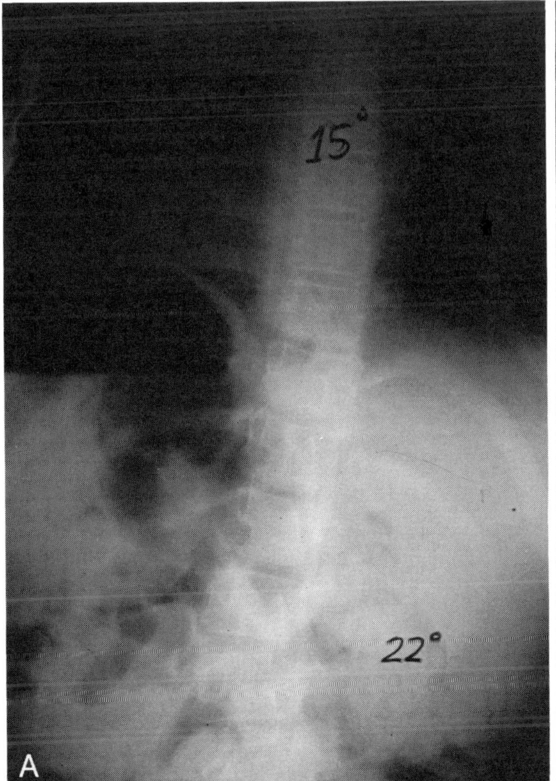

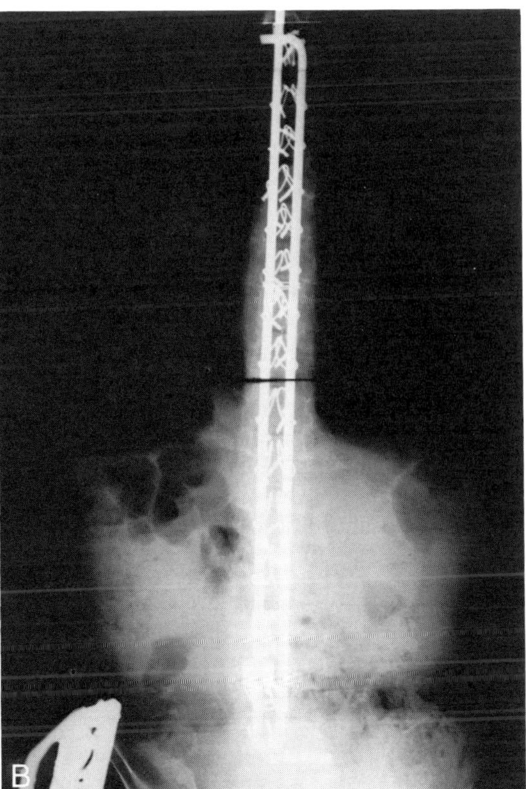

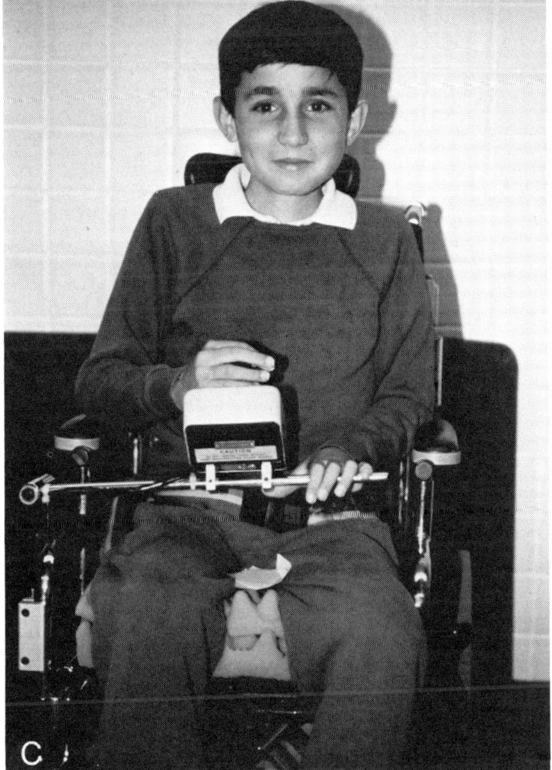

Figure 15–39. *A,* A 13-year-old male with Duchenne muscular dystrophy developed a 15-degree right thoracic, 22-degree left lumbar scoliosis. *B,* Five years after Luque segmental instrumentation to L5, he demonstrates a straight spine with no significant residual lumbar curve or pelvic obliquity. *C,* Clinical appearance five years postoperatively.

The surgical technique we recommend is Luque segmental instrumentation and posterior fusion from the high thoracic level (T2 or T3) down to L5. Usually, the intensive care unit stay is around two days and the average hospital stay about nine days. We recommend use of a lightweight Orthoplast body jacket for six months when the patient is upright.

If the pelvic obliquity is greater than 10 degrees and/or the scoliosis curve greater than 40 degrees, one should consider instrumentation to the pelvis to correct this obliquity and ensure a level pelvis.

The ultimate goal in the treatment of spinal deformity in Duchenne muscular dystrophy is the maintenance of upright sitting balance and maximal pain-free function. Many of our patients are now over 20 years of age with an upright posture, minimal wheelchair difficulties, and improved quality of life.

References

General Principles

1. Abel, M. F., Mubarak, S. J., Wenger, D. R., et al.: Brainstem evoked potentials for scoliosis surgery: a reliable method allowing use of halogenated anesthetic agents. J. Pediatr. Orthop. *10:*208, 1990.
2. Beurier, J., Dubousset, J., and Soudrie, B.: Evaluation of the pelvic fixation for spinal deformities in children at Saint Vincent de Paul Hospital in Paris during the last 20 years. Experiences about 155 cases. Paper 114. Scoliosis Research Society, Amsterdam, 1989.
3. Bradford, D. S.: Neuromuscular spinal deformity. *In* Bradford, D. S., Lonstein, J. E., Moe, J. H., et al. (eds.): Moe's Textbook of Scoliosis and Other Spinal Deformities. Philadelphia, W. B. Saunders Co., 1987, pp. 271–305.
4. Brown, J. C., Swank, F. C., Bradford, D. S., and Hensinger, R.: The Pediatric Spine. New York, Thieme & Stratton, 1985, pp. 251–272.
5. Camp, J. F.: Immediate complications of CD instrumentation to the sacropelvis: a clinical and biomechanical study. Paper 17. Scoliosis Research Society, Amsterdam, 1989.
6. Dubousset, J., Herring, J. A., and Shufflebarger, H.: Inevitable progression of scoliosis following posterior fusion alone in the immature spine: the crankshaft phenomenon. Paper 93. Scoliosis Research Society, Baltimore, 1987.
7. Dubousset, J., Guillaumat, M., and Cotret, Y.: Correction and fusion to the sacrum of pelvic obliquity with CD instrumentation in children and adults. Paper 28. Scoliosis Research Society, Hamilton, Bermuda, 1986.
8. Gershoff, W. F., and Renshaw, T. S.: The treatment of scoliosis in cerebral palsy by posterior spinal fusion with Luque rod segmental instrumentation. J. Bone Joint Surg. *70A:*41, 1988.
9. Koreska, J., Schwentker, E. P., and Albisser, A. M.: A simple method for obtaining accurate and reproducible bi-plane spinal radiographs. Presented at the 28th Annual Conference on Engineering in Medicine and Biology, New Orleans, September, 1975.
10. Mubarak, S. J., and Hicks, G. E.: Monitoring spinal cord function with brainstem somatosensory evoked potentials. Orthop. Trans. *9:*117, 1985.
11. Nickel, V., Perry, J., Afeldt, J., and Dale, C.: Elective surgery on patients with respiratory paralysis. J. Bone Joint Surg. *39A:*989, 1957.
12. Nickel, V., and Perry, J.: Respiratory evaluation of patients for major surgery. AAOS Instructional Course Lectures XVIII. St. Louis, MO, C. V. Mosby Co., 1961.
13. Passuti, N., Cistac, C., and Bainvel, J. V.: Fixation of severe neurologic scoliosis with pelvic obliquity with C.D. instrumentation. Technical problems and results (20 cases). Paper 113. Scoliosis Research Society, Amsterdam, 1989.

Cerebral Palsy

14. Allen, B. L., Jr., and Ferguson, R. L.: L-rod instrumentation for scoliosis in cerebral palsy. J. Pediatr. Orthop. *2:*87, 1982.
15. Balmer, G. A., and MacEwen, G. D.: The incidence and treatment of scoliosis in cerebral palsy. Dev. Med. Child. Neurol. *10:*447, 1968.
16. Bleck, E. E.: Orthopaedic Management in Cerebral Palsy. Philadelphia, J. B. Lippincott Co., 1987.
17. Bobath, K.: Neuropathology of cerebral infantile paralysis. Wien. Med. Wochens. *116:*736, 1966.
18. Bonnett, C., Brown, J. C., and Grow, T.: Thoracolumbar scoliosis in cerebral palsy. J. Bone Joint Surg. *58A:*328, 1976.
19. Broom, M. J., Banta, J. V., and Renshaw, T. S.: Spinal fusion augmented by Luque rod segmental instrumentation for neuromuscular scoliosis. J. Bone Joint Surg. *71A:*32, 1989.
20. Brown, J. C., Swank, S., and Specht, L.: Combined anterior and posterior spine fusion in cerebral palsy. Spine *7:*570, 1982.
21. Cohen, D. S., Swank, S. M., and Branon, J. C.: Spine fusion in cerebral palsy with L-rod segmental spinal instrumentation and analysis of single and two stage combined approach. Paper 77. Scoliosis Research Society, Baltimore, 1988.
22. Dept. of Health, Education and Welfare, National Institute of Neurologic Diseases and Blindness: Estimated number and cost of neurologic disabilities in the United States, 1968.
23. Leatherman, K. D., and Dickson, R.: The Management of Spinal Deformities. Boston, Wright Publications, 1988.
24. Drennan, J. C.: Orthopaedic Management of Neuromuscular Disorders. Philadelphia, J. B. Lippincott Co., 1983.
25. Drummond, D. S.: Harrington instrumentation with spinous process wiring for idiopathic scoliosis. Orthop. Clin. North Am. *19:*281, 1988.
26. Ferguson, R. L., and Allen, B. L., Jr.: Staged correction of neuromuscular scoliosis. J. Pediatr. Orthop. *3:*555, 1983.
27. Haas, S. L.: Spastic scoliosis and obliquity of the pelvis. J. Bone Joint Surg. *24:*775, 1942.

CHAPTER

16

JUVENILE KYPHOSIS

Howard S. An, M.D.
Richard A. Balderston, M.D.

Scheuermann's disease or juvenile kyphosis is caused by a wedge-shaped deformity of usually three to five vertebrae with characteristic roentgenographic changes. In 1920, Scheuermann first outlined these radiographic manifestations of the deformity, which included wedged vertebrae, Schmorl's nodules, and irregularity of the vertebral end plates.[59] In 1964, Sorenson further defined juvenile kyphosis as at least three adjacent vertebrae with wedging of 5 degrees or more in each vertebra.[60] These radiographic changes occur most commonly at the thoracic spine but the thoracolumbar or lumbar spine may also be involved.[3, 25, 29] Treatment depends on the extent of kyphotic deformity and the patient's symptoms.

Normal thoracic kyphosis ranges widely, but most people have kyphosis of between 21 to 33 degrees using the Cobb method.[52] Stagnara and associates studied 100 healthy subjects and noted normal kyphosis ranging to 45 degrees.[62] A growing child with a thoracic kyphotic deformity greater than 45 to 50 degrees should be investigated to rule out Scheuermann's disease or other causes of thoracic kyphosis. Any kyphosis at the thoracolumbar junction or in the lumbar spine is abnormal. The purpose of this chapter is to give a review of Scheuermann's disease—its pathoetiology, clinical findings, and nonoperative and operative treatments. Before discussing Scheuermann's disease, a classification of kyphosis, important in terms of the differential diagnoses of juvenile kyphosis, is presented.

CLASSIFICATION AND DIFFERENTIAL DIAGNOSES OF KYPHOSIS

Winter and Hall have classified kyphosis into 15 major groups (Table 16–1).[68] The most common type of kyphosis is round-back or postural kyphosis. During their adolescent growth spurt, children may assume poor postures that may aggravate postural kyphosis. Structural abnormalities are rare, but the curve may become structural if untreated for a prolonged period. This condition should easily be distinguished from Scheuermann's disease by the flexibility of the curve and the lack of roentgenographic abnormalities. Postural kyphosis is particularly common in adolescent girls, in that they assume a round-shouldered slouch to hide developing breasts. Education in proper sitting and standing posture is important. An exercise program or sometimes bracing is necessary to treat this condition.[6] The use of a brace may be indicated in patients with persistent symptoms and round-back postures despite education and exercise. Milwaukee brace treatment has been shown to be effective in these patients.[14]

Table 16–1. CLASSIFICTION OF KYPHOSIS (WINTER AND HALL)

I. Postural disorders
II. Scheuermann's kyphosis
III. Congenital disorders
  A. Failure of segmentation
  B. Failure of formation
IV. Paralytic
  A. Polio
  B. Anterior horn cell disease
  C. Upper motor neuron disease (e.g., cerebral palsy)
V. Myelomeningocele
VI. Posttraumatic
  A. Acute
  B. Chronic
  C. With or without cord damage
VII. Inflammatory
  A. Tuberculosis
  B. Other infections
VIII. Postsurgical
  A. Postlaminectomy
  B. Postexcision (e.g., tumor)
IX. Inadequate fusion
  A. Too short
  B. Pseudarthrosis
X. Postirradiation
  A. Neuroblastoma
  B. Wilms' tumor
XI. Metabolic
  A. Osteoporosis (juvenile or senile)
  B. Osteogenesis imperfecta
XII. Developmental
  A. Achondroplasia
  B. Mucopolysaccharidosis
  C. Other
XIII. Collagen disease (e.g., Marie-Strumpell)
XIV. Tumor (e.g., histiocytosis "X")
  A. Benign
  B. Malignant
XV. Neurofibromatosis

A rarer type of kyphosis is congenital kyphosis. Congenital kyphosis is further subdivided into three groups: Type I, in which failure of formation is evident anteriorly; Type II, in which failure of segmentation is present with resultant unsegmented bar; and mixed types, in which Types I and II are combined. Early diagnosis and prompt treatment are important when dealing with congenital kyphosis because of a high risk for severe curve progression. Tomography, myelography, computed tomography (CT), and magnetic resonance imaging (MRI) are helpful diagnostic aids. Type II lesions may go undetected until late childhood and may be confused with juvenile kyphosis. Type I lesions uniformly produce a severe kyphotic deformity if untreated. Winter and associates studied the natural histories of 20 patients with congenital kyphosis who had had no treatment during their growing years.[72] The average progression was 41 degrees during six years of observation, starting from the average of 48 degrees and ending at 89 degrees. Seven of 20 patients had curves over 110 degrees at the end of the observation period. Of 130 patients with congenital kyphosis, the authors reported 12 patients who had paralysis as a result of the natural history of the curve. All of these patients with paraplegia had Type I lesions. Myelography is required in congenital cases or in any deformity with neurologic involvement. MRI may replace myelography. The detection of a tethered cord or cord compression is critical for the successful management of these cases. Preoperative skeletal traction is contraindicated in congenital kyphotic patients because paraplegia may result.

Because of this devastating potential for grotesque deformity and paraplegia, most authors recommend early posterior fusion if the patients are younger than 5 years old and if the deformity is less than 55 degrees.[36, 45, 69] The surgical treatment of severe congenital kyphosis in patients older than 5 years usually consists of anterior and posterior fusion.[45, 67] Winter and associates studied 130 patients with congenital kyphosis and found out that without treatment, progression of the kyphosis averaging 7 degrees per year occurred.[72] Brace treatment was ineffective. Pseudarthrosis occurred in 15 of 28 patients who had posterior fusions, but only two of 16 patients who had anterior and posterior spine fusions developed pseudarthrosis. Another series was reported by Montgomery and Hall, who reviewed 34 consecutive patients treated surgically.[45] Eighteen patients had combined anterior and posterior fusion, 11 had an anterior fusion only, and five had a posterior fusion only. Neurologic deficit improved in six of eight cases postoperatively. They concluded that early surgical treatment is necessary in Type I lesions, anterior decompression is essential with neurologic deficit, and anterior and posterior fusion is the treatment of choice for kyphosis greater than 60 degrees.

Anterior cord decompression and strut fusion are difficult procedures and should be performed only by surgeons specifically trained in this work. The standard transthoracic approach is used, and the rib to be resected should correspond to the upper level of the deformity. Decompression of the cord includes removal of bone, disc material, and the posterior longitudinal ligament, allowing the spinal cord to move anteriorly.[17] Kyphosis reduction and strut bone grafting should be done in a meticulous manner to avoid graft dislodgement, graft fracture, and loss of correction.[12, 63] Bradford and associates reported a series of patients who received a vascularized pedicle rib graft for their kyphotic deformities, and the results are encouraging.[8, 11] Anterior fusions with strut grafts should always include interbody fusions at all levels within the strut, because continued growth at the disc may cause pseudarthrosis. Posterior fusion should not include distraction rods, because distraction of the spine may tether the spinal cord and cause paraplegia. In situ stabilization or compression instrumentation and fusion is recommended.

Paralytic kyphosis is usually due to neuromuscular diseases such as cerebral palsy, muscular dystrophy, and poliomyelitis. The deformity tends to be long and frequently associated with scoliosis.[16, 54] The primary problem is related to the lack of the extensor muscles. This lack of muscle control contributes to curve progression beyond skeletal maturity in these patients. Initial management should include spinal bracing to limit progression until the patient enters the early teenage years. Delaying fusion until the patient is in his or her early teenage years will allow proper trunk height. Most patients with paralytic kyphosis will eventually require a fusion. The entire curve should be included in the fusion, which should extend from the high thoracic area to the lumbar or sacral area. Luque rods with sublaminar wires and Galveston pelvic fixation techniques are the best methods of stabilization in these long neuromuscular curves. Anterior fusion is also necessary in patients with more severe fixed deformities, and in those in whom traction roentgenograms fail to balance the spine and the pelvis.

Myelomeningocele patients may have either congenital or paralytic kyphosis. Paralytic kyphosis is developmental and increases during growth. Management includes bracing and surgery, as in any other paralytic kyphosis. Spinal fusion in myelomeningocele patients is difficult because of the lack of posterior bony elements, osteopenia, and poor bone stock at the donor site. Many myelomeningocele patients therefore require both anterior and posterior fusions. Congenital kyphosis is present at birth and can produce an extreme kyphotic deformity. Excision of two to three vertebral bodies proximal to the apex of the deformity is carried out in patients over 3 years of age.[18, 26, 30, 32, 34, 38, 42] This is a formidable procedure that has a significant risk of extensive blood loss.

Kyphosis may develop secondary to trauma, inflammatory or infectious diseases, laminectomy, irradiation, tumors, metabolic diseases, collagen diseases, skeletal dysplasias, neurofibromatosis, neuropathy, and Klippel-Feil syndrome.[27, 31, 35, 41, 43, 44, 48, 49, 51, 55, 56, 66, 70, 71, 73] Careful history taking and thorough physical examination point to the obvious cause of kyphosis in most cases. Plain roentgenograms and special imaging studies further define the pathoetiologic process of the deformity. It is important to define the cause of the kyphotic deformity since treatment will vary accordingly. Evaluation should also include assessment of curve progression, curve magnitude, flexibility, and neurologic involvement. The end vertebrae of kyphosis should be accurately determined because a short fusion may lead the deformity to progress beyond the fusion site. A combined anterior and posterior fusion is usually required in severely affected patients in most cases.[24]

SCHEUERMANN'S DISEASE

Cause and Pathogenesis

Although the cause of Scheuermann's disease is still unknown, its pathogenesis has been outlined over the last several decades. In 1920, Scheuermann postulated that avascular necrosis of the cartilage ring apophysis of the vertebral body caused the disease process, but this theory has not been substantiated.[59] Bick and Copel noted in 1951 that the ring apophysis did not contribute to the longitudinal growth of the vertebrae.[2] Other investigators have failed to demonstrate evidence of avascular necrosis in histologic material. In 1930, Schmorl noted that kyphosis is produced by herniation of intervertebral material through the growth plates, but these "Schmorl's nodes" are nonspecific findings and are found in those with asymptomatic, normal spines.[33, 59a] Interestingly, the Schmorl node formation is usually in the anterior aspect of the vertebrae in Scheuermann's kyphosis, whereas in normal spines this node formation is more central, and in scoliotic spines it is posterior.[33] Herniation of the intervertebral discs through the weakened end plates may play a part in the pathogenesis of kyphotic deformity although it is probably not the inciting event.

There is no clear evidence that Scheuermann's kyphosis is associated with endocrine or metabolic abnormalities. Bradford and associates suggested that many patients with Scheuermann's kyphosis have a mild form of juvenile osteoporosis.[10] Lopez and associates compared ten untreated patients with thoracic Scheuermann's kyphosis with seven controls and found that the mean bone mineral density measured by single- and dual-photon absorptiometry was significantly lower in the Scheuermann's group.[37] Further research is needed to determine the pathoetiologic relationship between osteoporosis and Scheuermann's disease.

Mechanical or traumatic factors have been implicated in the pathogenesis of Scheuermann's disease. Scheuermann's changes in the thoracolumbar or lumbar areas appear to be related to strenuous physical activity.[3, 25] Thoracolumbar or lumbar types produce more pain and occur more commonly in men. Scheuermann's kyphosis in the thoracic spine with the apex at T8 is less clearly associated with mechanical factors or repeated traumas. Nonetheless, biomechanical factors definitely play a significant role in the progression of the kyphosis. The growing cartilage of the end plates is subject to compression forces that further suppress growth anteriorly, whereas tensile forces on the posterior aspect of the end plates enhance cartilaginous growth. As the kyphosis increases, the kyphotic moment arm increases even more. These biomechanical factors are important in the progression of the kyphotic deformity as well as in the treatment of kyphosis.

Gross and histologic findings of vertebral-body material removed through anterior surgery are of interest. The anterior longitudinal ligament is thickened and contracted, which contributes to the rigidity of deformity.[13] The vertebral body is wedged anteriorly, and the weakened end plate with disc protrusion is frequently observed. Histologic studies have demonstrated abnormalities in the end plate growth cartilage with stunted ossification. Electron micrographs have demonstrated deficient collagen fibers.[1] A disturbance of collagen or other matrix substance biosynthesis may be important in the pathoetiology of juvenile kyphosis. Although the cause remains obscure, matrix or collagen abnormalities in the end plate growth cartilage with resultant stunted endochondral ossification seem most plausible at this time. Mechanical factors are probably secondary but are important in aggravating the existing condition.

Clinical Findings

The prevalence of Scheuermann's disease varies from 0.4 to 8.3 per cent of the general population, depending on whether the diagnosis is based on clinical or radiographic criteria.[6] It seems to affect men and women equally, although different series report slight male or female predominance. The age of onset is difficult to determine, because roentgenographic changes are not evident until age 11. Most patients present in their early teenage years and complain of poor posture, fatigue, and pain near the kyphos.

As stated before, thoracic kyphosis or Type I deformities occur as a result of deformity, but thoracolumbar or lumbar kyphosis or Type II deformities occur around maturity with pain rather than deformity.[3, 25, 29] The typical patient with thoracic kyphosis has a relatively rigid thoracic deformity that becomes more apparent on forward flexion and partially corrects with hyperextension. Lumbar and cervical lordosis is typically increased as a compensatory mechanism, and the abdomen is prominent. As a consequence, normal pelvic tilt is exaggerated and straight leg raising is limited by hamstring tightness. Pain is an unusual presenting complaint in patients with thoracic Scheuermann's disease, but Sorenson has noted that the incidence of pain increases with the duration of the deformity.[60] Sorenson found that pain was present in over 50 per cent of 103 patients. The pain is usually aching and intermittent and rarely disabling. The site of pain is generally at the apex of the deformity and is nonradiating. If the pain is unusually constant and incapacitating, tumors such as osteoid osteoma and osteoblastoma or infection should be ruled out. Thoracic disc herniation or intraspinal tumors such as neurilemoma may be the cause of pain, particularly if neurologic deficit is present.

Most patients with Scheuermann's disease

are neurologically normal, but spinal cord compression secondary to thoracic disc herniation or severe kyphosis has been reported in patients with Scheuermann's disease.[4, 57, 74] Many patients with Scheuermann's disease have associated scoliosis. Deacon and associates analyzed 50 cases of thoracic Scheuermann's disease and demonstrated that a lateral curvature of the spine was present in 85 per cent.[22] The most common area of scoliosis was in the region of compensatory lordotic lumbar spine with vertebral rotation similar to the idiopathic scoliotic deformity. The average size was 14 degrees and progression was rare. Spondylolysis or spondylolisthesis may also be associated with Scheuermann's disease. Ogilvie and Sherman reported a 50 per cent incidence of asymptomatic spondylolysis in 18 patients who had Scheuermann's kyphosis.[50] Increased lumbar lordosis places increased stress on the pars interarticularis. Conversely, spondylolisthesis at L5–S1 can produce a severe lumbar lordosis and compensatory thoracic kyphosis. This round-back deformity may be confused with Scheuermann's kyphosis. The lumbosacral region should be carefully examined and radiographed if spondylolysis or spondylolithesis is suspected in patients with Scheuermann's disease.

In Type II (thoracolumbar or lumbar) kyphosis, pain is the presenting complaint in most patients. The incidence of pain has been reported to be 78 per cent.[33] On occasion, this disease may be confused with disc space infection.[19] In lumbar Scheuermann's disease, however, the pain is related to physical activity, and often a definite history of injury coincident with the onset can be elicited. Also, there is an increased prevalence rate of spondylolysis and spondylolisthesis in patients with Type II Scheuermann's kyphosis.

Roentgenographic Findings

The early roentgenographic findings of Scheuermann's disease include irregular end plates, Schmorl's nodes, and vertebral wedging. Vertebral wedging is the most specific radiologic finding of thoracic Scheuermann's disease (Fig. 16–1).[59] Sorenson's criterion of a minimum of three apical vertebrae wedged by at least 5 degrees has not been strictly followed for the diagnosis of Scheuermann's disease.[60]

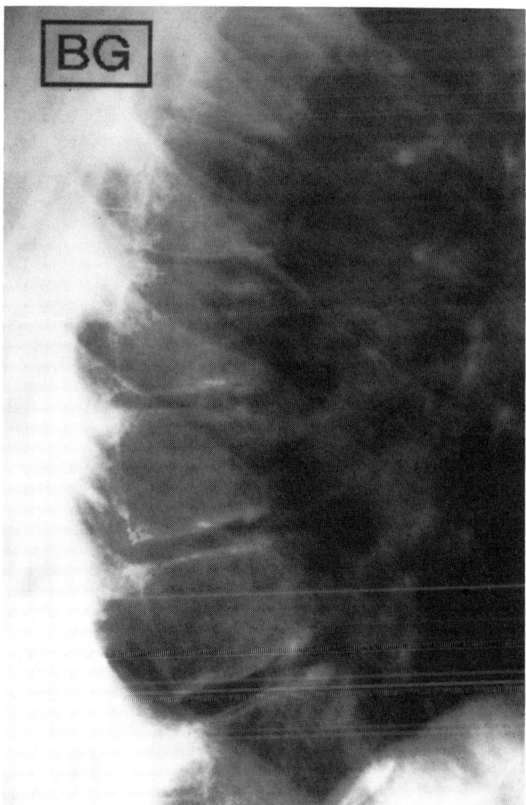

Figure 16–1. This lateral roentgenograph demonstrates the typical changes of Scheuermann's disease. The vertebrae show anterior body wedging, end plate irregularity, disc space narrowing, and small Schmorl's nodes. This patient is an adolescent.

Bradford's criterion is one or more vertebrae wedged 5 or more degrees, and Drummond's criterion is two or more wedged vertebrae.[6, 23] An increase in normal thoracic kyphosis above 45 degrees is another radiographic criterion for Scheuermann's disease. This angle is measured from the lines drawn from the superior border of the upper end vertebra and the inferior border of the lower end vertebra, as in the Cobb technique for measuring scoliosis.

Late radiographic changes in patients with Scheuermann's kyphosis may include syndesmophytes anteriorly and facet joint osteophytes posteriorly. These are arthritic changes in adults and may coincide with increasing back pain. To assess flexibility of the deformity, a hyperextension view should be obtained in patients who may require bracing or surgery. Radiographic findings in thoracolumbar or lumbar Scheuermann's disease include end plate irregularities that may be misinterpreted as infection. There is no significant deformity or vertebral wedging in the lumbar spine. Associated spondylolysis is best detected on oblique projections of the lumbar spine.

Treatment

The treatment of juvenile kyphosis is somewhat controversial. The natural history of untreated Scheuermann's disease is not clear. Sorenson has suggested that thoracic Scheuermann's disease has a favorable outcome and treatment is largely unnecessary.[60] Bradford favors active treatment to relieve present symptoms, to correct the cosmetic deformity, and to prevent potential progression and future development of back pain.[5, 6] We believe that treatment should be individualized according to the patient's primary concern, expectations, and compliance. Other important factors are the patient's age, the gender, and the magnitude and flexibility of the deformity. For example, a young female patient with significant cosmetic concerns should be treated. If the deformity is relatively supple and vertebral growth remains, bracing is preferred. If the deformity is rigid and greater than 75 degrees, operative treatment is offered. A male patient who has minimal cosmetic concerns and whose pain can be managed with nonsteroidal anti-inflammatory medications or exercises should not need bracing or surgery. Since the vertebral growth plates fuse at approximately 25 years of age, follow-up should be carried out until this age.

Nonoperative Treatment

Many patients with Scheuermann's kyphosis respond well to casting or bracing, and surgery is rarely necessary in these patients. Bracing should aim to restore the anterior vertebral body height, thereby reducing the kyphosis. The brace should also reduce the lumbar lordosis, which also helps to reduce thoracic kyphosis. A hyperextension cast may initially be applied in one or two stages if the deformity is relatively severe or rigid.

Although many types of braces are available, the Milwaukee brace has been the mainstay of treatment for juvenile kyphosis. In their review of 75 patients with Scheuermann's kyphosis who had completed Milwaukee brace treatment, Bradford and associates showed that vertebral wedging and kyphosis improved by 49 per cent and lumbar lordosis improved by 36 per cent.[14] The factors associated with worse results were kyphosis greater than 75 degrees, skeletal maturity, and increased vertebral wedging greater than 10 degrees. Sachs and associates reviewed the same patients with a longer follow-up time.[58] The long-term results at least five years after completion of the Milwaukee brace revealed improvement in 69 per cent of patients. Again, an initial kyphosis of 75 degrees or more was associated with worse results. These authors noted that the initial correction obtained during the active phase of brace treatment was partially lost over time. Montgomery and Erwin also studied 21 patients with Scheuermann's disease who wore the Milwaukee brace for 18 months.[46] They noted that the initial curve improved from an average of 62 to 41 degrees, but loss of correction averaging 15 degrees was noted over time. Leatherman and Dickson believe that the loss of correction is less if the orthosis is worn for a longer period.[33] They also stated that an orthosis with superstructure is unnecessary. They favor Boston-type braces, because they decrease and control the lumbar lordosis better. Boston-type braces are preferred over the Milwaukee brace for the thoracolumbar or lumbar types of Scheuermann's disease.

Exercises alone are rarely of benefit in the treatment of Scheuermann's kyphosis, but may be beneficial in conjunction with brace treatment. These exercises should consist of thoracic hyperextension to reduce kyphosis, and hamstring stretching and pelvic tilt to decrease lumbar lordosis. Exercises may be more beneficial if back pain is part of the patient's symptoms. Electric surface stimulation has been attempted as an alternative treatment for Scheuermann's kyphosis, but long-term results are unknown at this time. Electric stimulation has been disappointing in the treatment of idiopathic adolescent scoliosis and would probably have the same results for kyphosis. Therefore, electric treatment is not a viable alternative to bracing at this time.

Operative Treatment

The indications for surgery in thoracic Scheuermann's disease are rare. These may include significant rigid kyphosis above 75 degrees and unrelenting pain despite conservative treatment. These patients should be poor candidates for bracing. As stated previously, poor candidates for brace treatment are those with a rigid deformity greater than 75 degrees and those who are skeletally mature.

When indicated, surgical correction of kyphosis may be completed through an isolated posterior procedure if the deformity is relatively mild and flexible. This is a rare circumstance, since most patients with a relatively mild and flexible deformity respond well to bracing. If these patients refuse bracing, posterior compression instrumentation and fusion may be done. Drummond stated that if a kyphosis is less than 65 degrees or bending correction is less than 50 degrees, the posterior approach alone may be adequate.[23] Bradford and associates reported on 22 patients with Scheuermann's kyphosis in 1975 and concluded that posterior fusion with Harrington instrumentation relieved pain and improved deformity, but more than 5 degrees of correction was lost in 16 patients.[13] There were two pseudarthrosis and five instrumentation problems. Bradford and associates later reported on 24 patients with Scheuermann's kyphosis who underwent a combined anterior and posterior spine fusion.[9] All had a solid arthrodesis with good pain relief. Significant loss of correction was not observed in these patients. The authors concluded that a kyphosis of more than 70 degrees should have a combined anterior and posterior spine fusion. Herndon and associates also recommended a combined anterior and posterior fusion for patients with Scheuermann's kyphosis.[28] Speck and Chopin reported on 59 patients with Scheuermann's disease and concluded that posterior fusion alone is adequate in skeletally immature patients, but combined anterior and posterior surgery is recommended in skeletally mature patients.[61] Taylor and associates studied 27 adolescent patients with Scheuermann's kyphosis or round-back deformity who underwent posterior fusion and Harrington compression instrumentation.[64] As in Bradford's early series, good correction of deformity with pain relief was observed, but a mean loss of 5.7 degrees was noted at follow-up study. We believe that for the majority of patients who require surgery, a combined anterior and posterior fusion is necessary.[28, 47] Posterior fusion alone will result in loss of correction and pseudarthrosis in a significant number of cases.[9, 13]

Before operative techniques are discussed, the biomechanics of kyphosis correction should be mentioned (Figs. 16–2 to 16–5). With an increased kyphosis there are greater compression forces anteriorly and tensile forces posteriorly. Because under tension bone graft will be absorbed according to Wolff's law, anterior fusion is an essential part of kyphosis surgery. Instrumentation to correct kyphosis includes Harrington compression rods. In Scheuermann's kyphosis, the thickened and contracted anterior longitudinal ligament resists the correctional forces by compression instrumentation. By using the middle column as a hinge, posterior compression instrumentation distracts the anterior column and provides correction of the deformity. Use of multiple hooks and instrumentation of the entire kyphosis reduces the tendency of hook dislodgment. Use of Cotrel-Dubousset (C-D) instrumentation may be used to apply compression forces posteriorly, similar to Harrington compression rods. The C-D system also allows one to apply distraction and compression forces along the same rod. If desired, apical distraction can be applied to reduce associated scoliosis, and compression forces can be applied above and below the apex to reduce the tensile forces of the posterior column.

Operative Techniques. Meticulous technique and great care are important in the prevention of complications such as neural injury, pseudarthrosis, instrument failure, and loss of correction. Anterior transthoracic exposure and fusion for kyphosis are techniques that only skillful and experienced spinal surgeons should attempt in well-equipped medical centers with maximal support. Posterior instrumentation and fusion is most commonly achieved with use of compression Harrington rods or the C-D system. Use of Luque rods and sublaminar wires is associated with increased risk of neural injury, and has been reported with greater failures.[20] The entire kyphosis should be fused posteriorly, since inadequate fusion length may result in a deformity adjacent to the fusion area. Typically, fusion should extend from T2 or T3 to L1 or L2. During the anterior procedure, only five to six apical segments need to be fused. The purpose of the anterior discectomy and interbody fusion is to enhance correction and improve the fusion rate.

A transthoracic approach is used for anterior exposure, removing the rib corresponding to

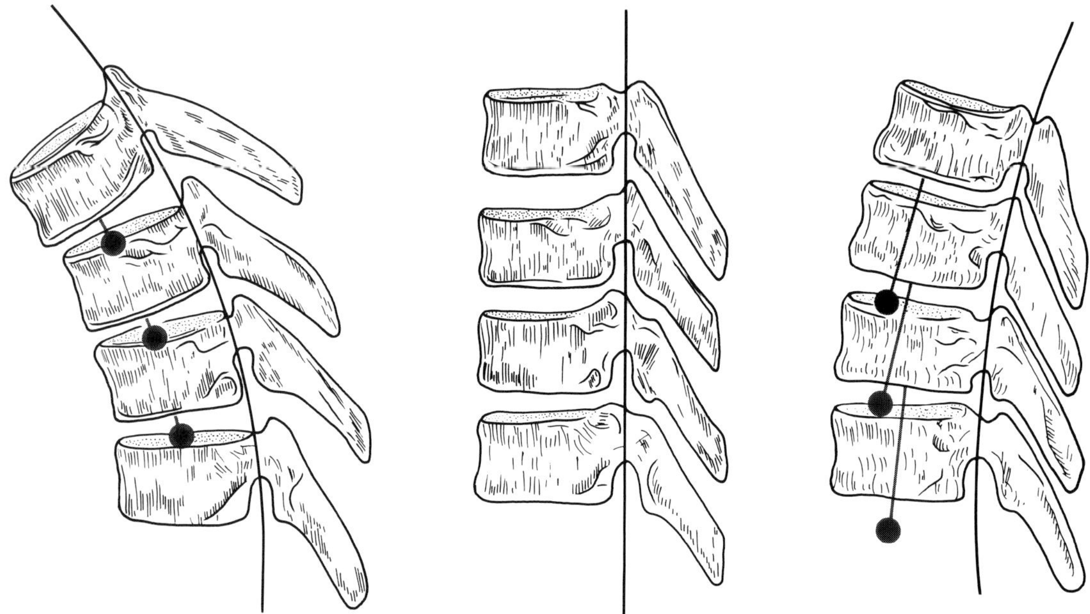

Figure 16–2. With flexion and extension of the spine, sagittal rotation normally occurs at about a point at the junction of the anterior and middle columns. Shortening of the posterior column must occur for the spine to extend.

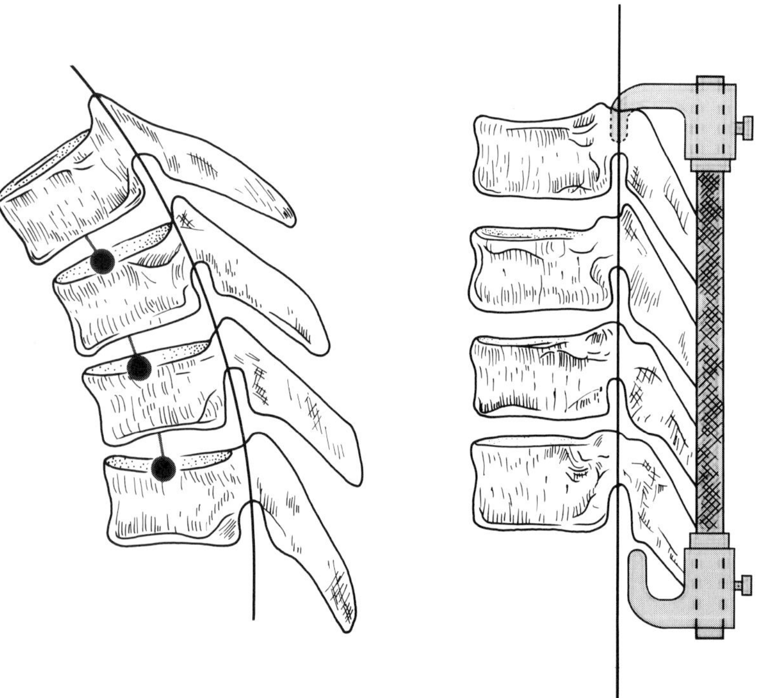

Figure 16–3. With increased kyphosis of the spine, compression instrumentation is effective in reducing angular deformity. With the center of sagittal rotation near the midpoint of the vertebral body, the best lever arm for control of spinal extension is the posterior column.

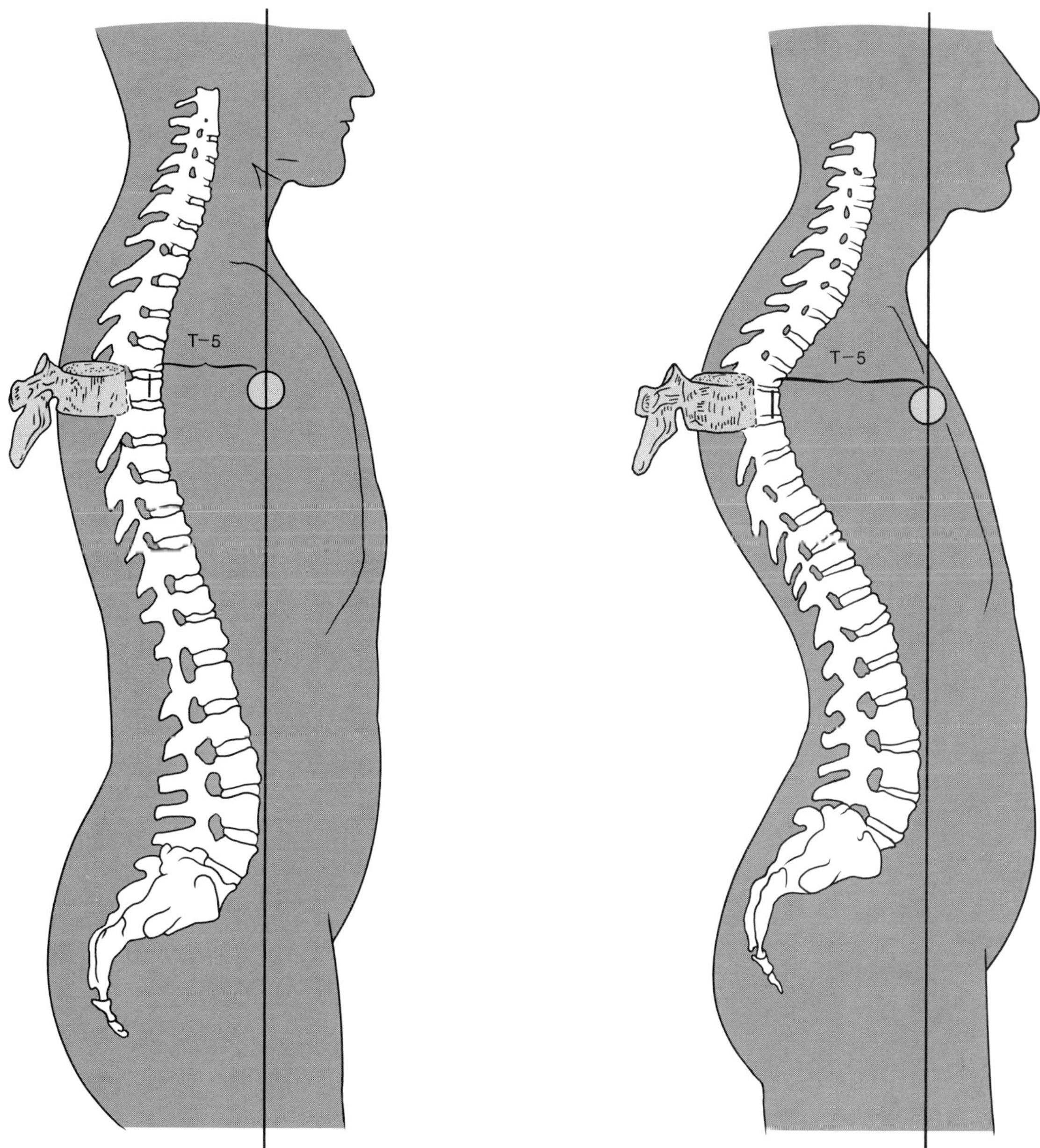

Figure 16–4. The line projected in the illustration is parallel to a plumb line through the center of mass of the body. With increased kyphosis, the moment arm between the thoracic vertebral bodies and the center of mass of the body increases. As the moment arm increases, there is a greater tendency for progressive deformity. Notice that the angular forces in the lumbar spine are much less than those in the thoracic spine.

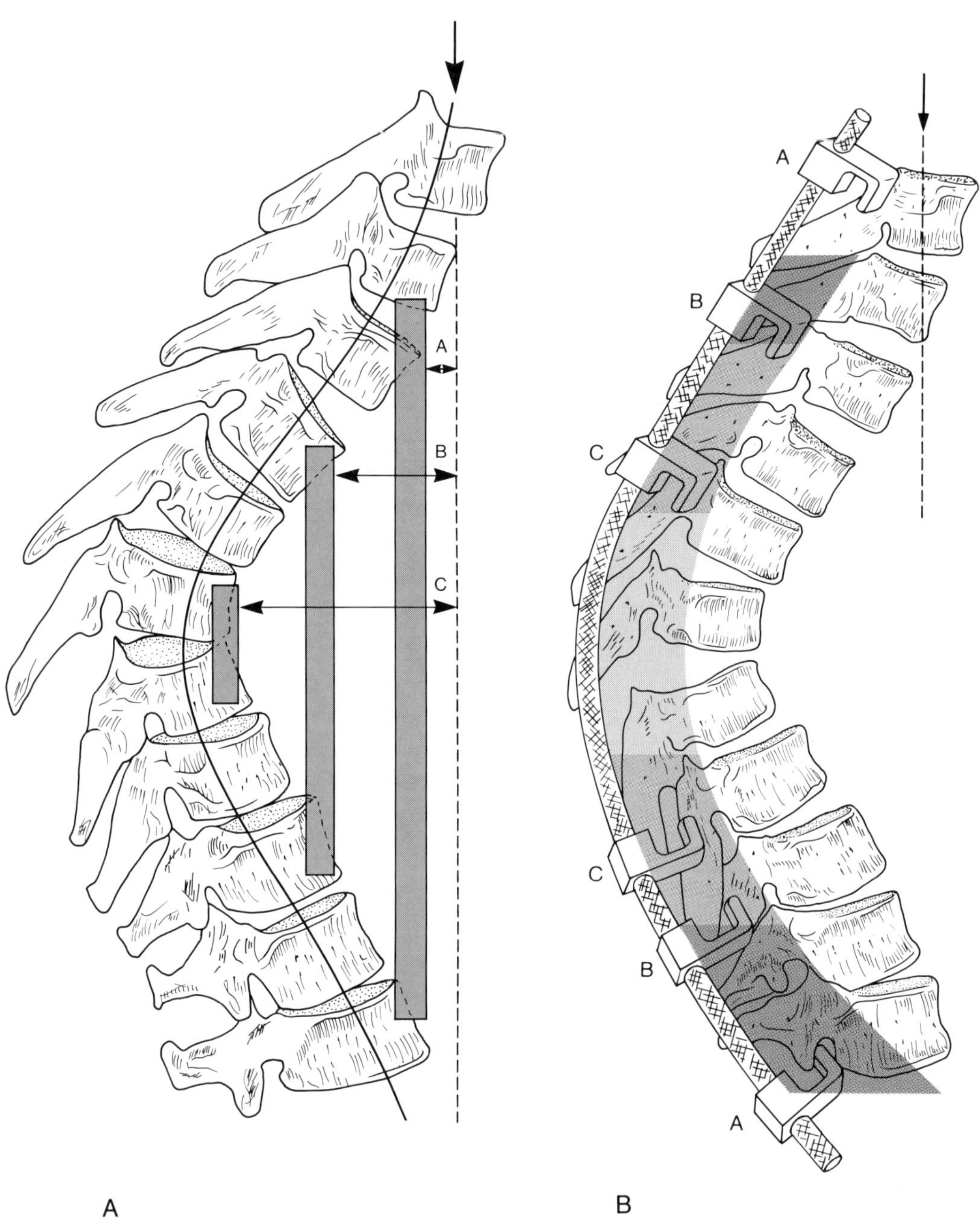

Figure 16–5. *A*, With anterior strut graft fusion, bone grafts are placed in compression, promoting bone healing. Strut graft C is closer to a plumbline through the center of mass and will have less tendency for angulation *above* the fusion than struts A or B. Strut A with no posterior supplementation will have the greatest tendency for progressive deformity above the fusion. *B*, The same principles apply for posterior fusions with compression instrumentation. Progressive lengthening of the posterior construct decreases the bending moment both above and below the fusion.

the upper portion of the kyphosis to be fused.[15] A right- or left-sided approach is feasible, but the spine should be approached from the convexity of the curvature if scoliosis is also present. For the thoracotomy approach, place the patient in the lateral decubitus position and move the upper arm forward. Insertion of a double-branched endotracheal tube into the right and left main stem bronchi is helpful to allow selective collapse of the lung. An axillary roll under the down arm is important to prevent compression of axillary neurovascular structures. The skin and subcutaneous tissues are opened from the lateral border of the paraspinous musculature to the sternocostal junction over the rib to be resected. After the pleura is incised, exposure of the vertebral column is performed by deflating the lung with a surgical laparotomy sponge. A rib spreader is used to widen the exposure. The lap sponge should be removed periodically to prevent atelectasis.

The segmental artery can be preserved in most cases if discectomy and interbody fusion only are performed. These vessels should be carefully identified and ligated if a strut graft is to be placed, however. The segmental artery must be ligated at the midportion of the vertebral body to preserve collateral circulation to the spinal cord.

After the spine is adequately exposed, removal of disc material is completed. All disc tissue must be removed to the posterior annulus and to the annulus on the opposite side. The vertebral end plates are removed to subchondral bleeding bone using a fine osteotome or angled curet. Minced rib can be used for the interbody fusion. If further correction is desired, each interspace may be spread with a laminar spreader, and a solid interbody graft may be inserted under compression. The rib or iliac crest may be used for bone graft sources.

Closure should begin by approximating the pleura over the spine. The chest tube should be placed in the posterior chest cavity to enhance drainage. The pleura and the ribs are approximated next. Multiple drill holes may be used in the caudad rib to place heavy sutures. This should prevent possible intercostal neuralgia caused by the closing sutures.

Posterior instrumentation and fusion is performed subsequently. Depending on the patient and surgeon's preference, this procedure may be performed at the same time or one week later. Our usual spinal deformity frame is the four-poster or Relton-Hall frame. By adjusting all posters with regard to the patient's width and height, pressure points are evenly distributed on the chest and iliac crests. One must avoid pressure on the brachial plexus and ulnar nerves. The arms should not abduct beyond 90 degrees. It is important that the abdomen be free of pressure to allow venous drainage of the lower extremities and to decrease blood loss during surgery.

Patients should donate two to three units of their blood the weeks before surgery. The intraoperative blood-cell saver system is also used whenever possible. Hypotensive anesthesia by the skilled anesthesiologist is also useful in decreasing operative blood loss.

Meticulous operative technique is most important to achieve successful fusion and prevent both operative and late complications. Initial subperiosteal dissection is done with the Cobb elevator, exposing the spinous processes, lamina, facets, and the tips of the transverse processes. Harrington compression rods are commonly used for Scheuermann's kyphosis. The heavy 3/16-inch threaded rods and multiple hooks should be used to increase overall stability. Five upper hooks and four lower hooks typically are necessary. Upper hooks may be applied to the transverse processes or the laminae. Application of upper hooks over the laminae is slightly more risky, but offers better protection against hook dislodgment. The lower hooks are usually applied under the lamina. The threaded contoured rods are then applied, and the hooks are seated with nuts. Crimping of the threads of the compression rods or the nuts is recommended to prevent hex-nut loosening (Fig. 16–6).[53] If associated scoliosis is present, a distraction rod should be inserted on the concave side and a compression rod on the convex side. Segmental instrumentation with sublaminar wires has also been used to correct kyphosis.[39, 40] The passage of sublaminar wires may be associated with increased neurologic risk, however. Under no circumstances should a compression system be used with a sublaminar wire. Tightening of a sublaminar wire produces anterior migration of the compression hook attached to the compression rod and may produce neurologic deficit. Boxed Luque rods are most commonly used with sublaminar wires. Although segmental instrumentation with sublaminar wires enhances the overall stability of the surgical

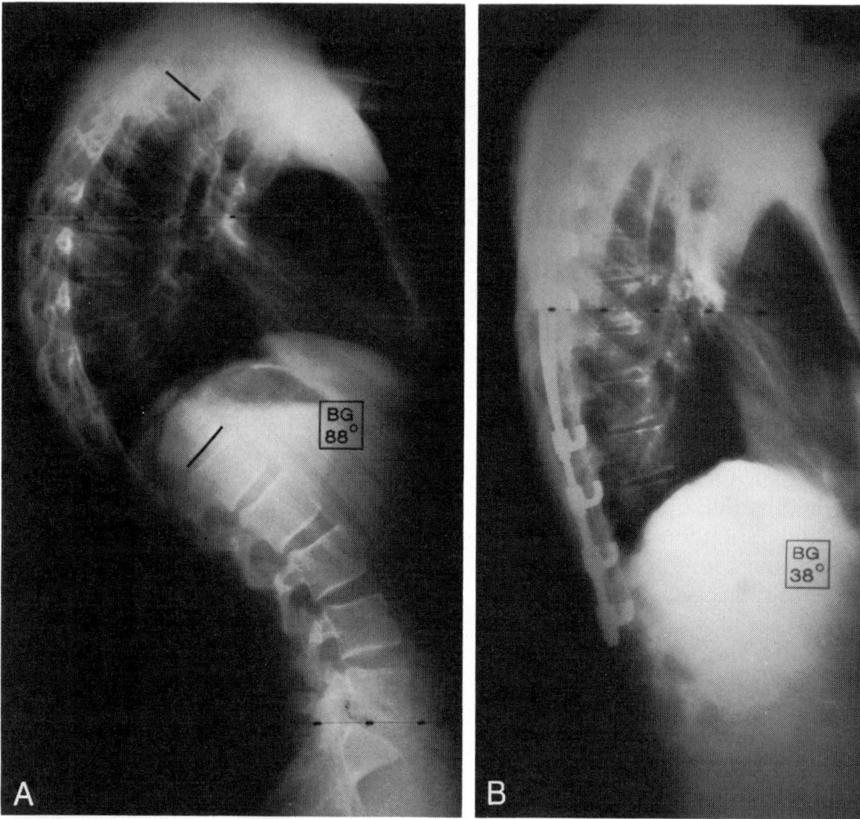

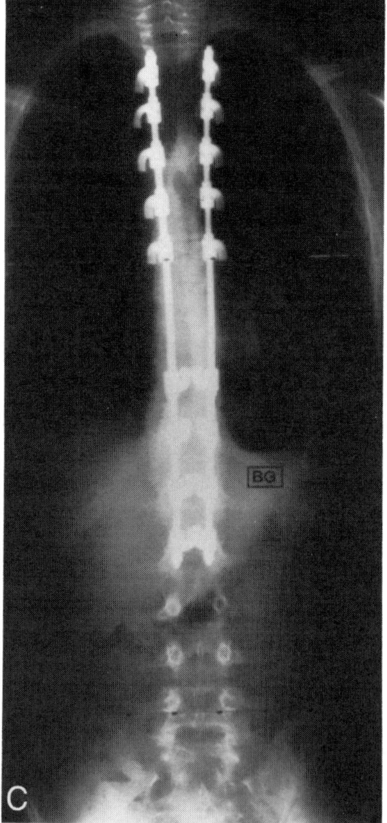

Figure 16–6. *A*, This 20-year-old male demonstrated progressive deformity and shows typical roentgenographic changes of Scheuermann's disease. The kyphosis is 88 degrees. *B*, After multilevel anterior discectomy and fusion, posterior instrumentation was accomplished with Harrington 3/16-inch heavy compression rods. A two-year follow-up film demonstrates 38 degree kyphosis. *C*, The upper hooks are anchored to the transverse processes, while the lower hooks are secured to the lamina.

construct, we believe that the use of postoperative orthosis is important in avoiding problems with fixation or loss of correction.

The C-D system has been applied for kyphosis surgery (Fig. 16–7). The surgical instrumentation and technique are complex and sufficient training is required for proper use of this system. This system may be used in a similar manner to the Harrington compression rods. Because of heavier rods and interconnecting bars, stability of this construct is enhanced. This system may also be applied to give apical distraction force and compression of the end vertebrae above and below the same rod if associated scoliosis is present. Undue force will fracture the lamina. One should obtain hands-on experience and training with other surgeons well versed in the techniques used.

Complications. Spinal cord injury is the most feared surgical complication, particularly during cord decompression through an anterior approach. Mechanical damage or vascular insult to the cord may result in paraplegia. Dural or spinal cord injuries from overaggressive disc excision or instrument penetration are technical errors that should be avoided. Vascular damage may be best prevented by avoiding ligation of the segmental vessels close to the intervertebral foramen. An anterior procedure between the fifth and ninth thoracic vertebrae must not be taken lightly, since circulatory compromise to the cord is possible when severe hypotension due to blood loss occurs. Neurologic compromise has also been associated with use of skeletal traction, particularly in congenital kyphosis. Skeletal traction is rarely necessary in patients with Scheuermann's disease.

Development of a pseudarthrosis may lead to progression of the kyphosis, loss of correction, or failure of surgical construct. Multiple factors should be considered in the development of pseudarthrosis after kyphosis surgery. First, fusion techniques must be meticulous. Meticulous decortication and massive bone graft cannot be overemphasized. Rigid stabilization with heavy Harrington compression rods or the C-D system is important. Postop-

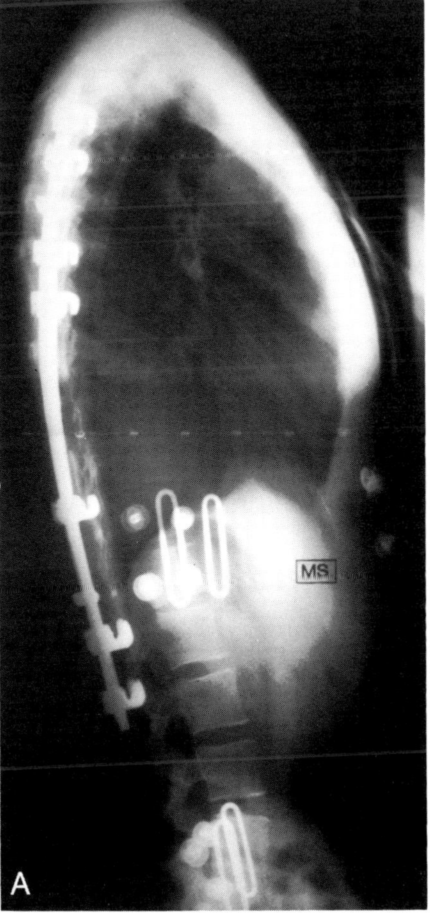

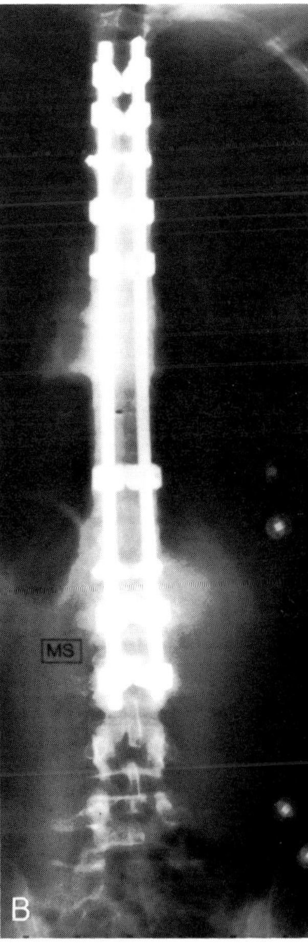

Figure 16–7. *A*, Correction of kyphosis may also be achieved with the Cotrel-Dubousset (C-D) device. Shortening of the posterior column must be accomplished by compression at multiple sites. *B*, One great advantage of the C-D device is the transverse fixator connecting the two rods to form a rectangular construct. The rotational stability of each rod is greatly enhanced

erative immobilization with a brace is also important. Most patients with significant kyphosis should have anterior fusion as well. Combined anterior and posterior fusions improve both overall corrections and fusion rates. Anterior grafting techniques are even more demanding. Inadequate disc and end plate removal lead to pseudarthrosis. A pseudarthrosis should be repaired if it is associated with loss of correction and instrument failure. More rigid constructs such as C-D rods may enhance fusion rates.

Inadequate fusion length may lead to deformity adjacent to the fusion mass. The entire kyphosis should be instrumented and fused. Instrument failures such as hook dislodgment and rod breakage are usually related to pseudarthrosis, but poor rod contouring, poor placement of hooks, and inadequate fusion length may be responsible. Meticulous surgical techniques are necessary to prevent these complications.

References

1. Aufdermauer, M., and Spycher, M.: Pathogenesis of osteochondrosis juvenilis Scheuermann. J. Orthop. Res. *4:*452–457, 1986.
2. Bick, E. M., and Copel, J. W.: Longitudinal growth of the human vertebra; contribution to human osteogeny. J. Bone Joint Surg. *33A:*783, 1951.
3. Blumenthal, S. L., Roach, J., and Herring, J. A.: Lumbar Scheuermann's: a clinical series and classification. Spine *12:*929–932, 1987.
4. Bradford, D. S.: Neurological complications in Scheuermann's disease. J. Bone Joint Surg. *51A:*657, 1969.
5. Bradford, D. S.: Juvenile kyphosis. Clin. Orthop. *128:*45–55, 1977.
6. Bradford, D. S.: Juvenile kyphosis. *In* Bradford, D. S., Lanstein, J. E., Moe, J. H., et al. (eds.): Scoliosis and Other Spinal Deformities. Philadelphia, W. B. Saunders Co., 1988, pp. 347–368.
7. Bradford, D. S., and Moe, J. H.: Scheuermann's juvenile kyphosis: a histologic study. Clin. Orthop. *110:*45–53, 1975.
8. Bradford, D. S.: Anterior vascular pedicle bone grafting for the treatment of kyphosis. Spine *5:*318–323, 1980.
9. Bradford, D. S., Ahmed, K. B., Moe, J. H., et al.: The surgical management of patients with Scheuermann's disease. J. Bone Joint Surg. *62A:*705–712, 1980.
10. Bradford, D. S., Brown, D. M., Moe, J. H., et al.: Scheuermann's kyphosis, a form of juvenile osteoporosis. Clin. Orthop. *118:*10, 1976.
11. Bradford, D. S., and Daher, Y. H.: The vascularised rib grafts for stabilisation of kyphosis. J. Bone Joint Surg. *68B:*357–361, 1986.
12. Bradford, D. S., Ganjavian, S., Antonious, D., et al.: Anterior strut-grafting for the treatment of kyphosis: review of experience with forty-eight patients. J. Bone Joint Surg. *64A:*680–690, 1982.
13. Bradford, D. S., Moe, J. H., Montalvo, F. J., and Winter, R. B.: Scheuermann's kyphosis: results of surgical treatment by posterior spine arthrodesis in twenty-two patients. J. Bone Joint Surg. *57A:*439–448, 1975.
14. Bradford, D. S., Moe, J. H., Montalvo, F. J., and Winter, R. B.: Scheuermann's kyphosis and roundback deformity: results of Milwaukee brace treatment. J. Bone Joint Surg. *56A:*740–758, 1974.
15. Bradford, D. S., Winter, R. B., Lonstein, J. E., and Moe, J. H.: Techniques of anterior spinal surgery for the management of kyphosis. Clin. Orthop. *128:*129–139, 1977.
16. Bunch, W. H., Smith, D., and Hakala, M.: Kyphosis in the paralytic spine. Clin. Orthop. *128:*107–112, 1977.
17. Chou, S. N.: The treatment of paralysis associated with kyphosis. Clin. Orthop. *128:*149–154, 1977.
18. Christofersen, M. R., and Brooks, A. L.: Excision and wire fixation of rigid myelomeningocele kyphosis. J. Ped. Orthop. *5:*691–696, 1985.
19. Cohn, S. L., Akbarnia, B. A., Luisiri, A., and Sundaram, M.: Disk space infection versus lumbar Scheuermann's disease. Orthopaedics *11:*330–335, 1988.
20. Coscia, M. F., Bradford, D. S., and Ogilvie, J. W.: Scheuermann's kyphosis—results in 19 cases treated by spinal arthrodesis and L-rod instrumentation. Presented at the Scoliosis Research Society, 1987.
21. Daher, Y. H., Lonstein, J. E., Winter, R. B., and Bradford, D. S.: Spinal deformities in patients with Friedreich's ataxia: a review of 19 patients. J. Ped. Orthop. *5:*553, 1985.
22. Deacon, P., Berkin, C. R., and Dickson, R. A.: Combined idiopathic kyphosis and scoliosis. J. Bone Joint Surg. *67B:*189–192, 1985.
23. Drummond, D. S.: Kyphosis in the growing child. Spine: State of the Art Review *1:*339–356, 1987.
24. Floman, Y., Micheli, L. J., Penny, N., et al.: Combined anterior and posterior fusion in seventy-three spinally deformed patients. Clin. Orthop. *164:*110–122, 1984.
25. Greene, T. L., Hensinger, R. N., and Hunter, L. Y.: Back pain and vertebral changes simulating Scheuermann's disease. J. Ped. Orthop. *5:*1–7, 1985.
26. Hall, J. E., and Poitras, B.: The management of kyphosis in patients with myelomeningocele. Clin. Orthop. *128:*33–40, 1977.
27. Hensinger, R. N.: Kyphosis secondary to skeletal dysplasia and metabolic disease. Clin. Orthop. *128:*115–128, 1977.
28. Herndon, W. A., Emans, J. B., Micheli, L. J., and Hall, J. E.: Combined anterior and posterior fusion for Scheuermann's kyphosis. Spine *6:*125–130, 1981.
29. Herring, J. A., and Hall, J. E.: A lucent lesion of the lumbar spine. J. Ped. Orthop. *3:*113–115, 1983.
30. Heydemann, J. S., and Gillespie, R.: Management of myelomeningocele kyphosis in the older child by kyphectomy and segmental spinal instrumentation. Spine *12:*37–41, 1987.
31. Hsu, L. C., Lee, P. C., and Leong, J. C. Y.: Dystrophic spinal deformities in neurofibromatosis. J. Bone Joint Surg. *66B:*495–499, 1984.
32. Leatherman, K. D., and Dickson, R. A.: Congenital

kyphosis in myelomeningocele, vertebral resection and posterior spine fusion. Spine *3:*22, 1978.
33. Leatherman, K. D., and Dickson, R. A.: The Management of Spinal Deformities: Scheuermann's Kyphosis. London, Butterworth & Co., 1988, pp. 123–136.
34. Linseth, R. E., and Stelzer, L.: Vertebral excision for kyphosis in children with myelomeningocele. J. Bone Joint Surg. *61A:*699–704, 1979.
35. Lonstein, J. E.: Postlaminectomy kyphosis. Clin. Orthop. *128:*93–100, 1977.
36. Lonstein, J. E.: Neurologic deficits secondary to spinal deformity: a review of the literature and report of 43 cases. Spine *5:*331–355, 1980.
37. Lopez, R. A., Burke, S. W., Levine, D. B., and Schneider, R.: Osteoporosis in Scheuermann's disease. Spine *13:*1099–1103, 1988.
38. Lowe, G. P., and Menelaus, M. B.: The surgical management of kyphosis in older children with myelomeningocele. J. Bone Joint Surg. *60B:*40–45, 1978.
39. Lowe, T. G.: Double L-rod instrumentation in the treatment of severe kyphosis secondary to Scheuermann's disease. Spine *12:*336–340, 1987.
40. Luque, E. R.: The correction of postural curves of the spine. Spine *7:*270–275, 1982.
41. Malcolm, B. W., Bradford, D. S., Winter R. B., and Chou, S. N.: Post-traumatic kyphosis. J. Bone Joint Surg. *53A:*891–899, 1981.
42. Mayfield, J. K.: Severe spine deformity in myelodysplasia and sacral agenesis. Spine *6:*498–509, 1981.
43. McBride, G. G., and Bradford, D. S.: Vertebral body replacement with femoral neck allograft and vascularized rib strut graft: a technique for treating post-traumatic kyphosis with neurologic deficit. Spine *8:*406–415, 1983.
44. Moe, J. H., and Van Dam, B. E.: Neurofibromatosis. *In* Bradford, D. S., et al. (eds.): Scoliosis and Other Spinal Deformities. Philadelphia, W. B. Saunders Co., 1988, pp. 329–346.
45. Montgomery, S. P., and Hall, J. E.: Congenital kyphosis. Spine *7:*360–364, 1982.
46. Montgomery, S. P., and Erwin, W. E.: Scheuermann's kyphosis—long-term results of Milwaukee brace treatment. Spine *6:*5–8, 1981.
47. Nerubay, J., and Katznelson, A.: Dual approach in the surgical treatment of juvenile kyphosis. Spine *11:*101–102, 1986.
48. O'Brien, J. P.: Kyphosis secondary to infectious disease. Clin. Orthop. *128:*56–64, 1977.
49. Ogilvie, J. W.: Spine deformity following radiation. *In* Bradford, D. S., Lonstein, J. E., Moe, J. H., et al. (eds.): Scoliosis and Other Spinal Deformities. Philadelphia, W. B. Saunders Co., 1988, pp. 547–554.
50. Ogilvie, J. W., and Sherman, J.: Spondylolysis in Scheuermann's disease. Spine *12:*251–253, 1987.
51. Piazza, M. R., Bassett, G. S., and Bunnell, W. P.: Neuropathic spinal arthropathy in congenital insensitivity to pain. Clin. Orthop. *236:*175–179, 1988.
52. Propst-Proctor, S. L., and Bleck, E. E.: Radiographic determination of lordosis and kyphosis in normal and scoliotic children. J. Ped. Orthop. *3:*344–346, 1983.
53. Purnell, M., Drummond, D. S., Keene, J. S., and Narechania, R.: Hex-nut loosening following compression instrumentation of the spine. Clin. Orthop. *203:*172–178, 1986.
54. Riddick, M. F., Winter, R. B., and Lutter, L. D.: Spinal deformities in patients with spinal muscle atrophy: a review of 36 patients. Spine *7:*476–483, 1982.
55. Riseborough, E. J.: Irradiation induced kyphosis. Clin. Orthop. *128:*101–106, 1977.
56. Roberson, J. R., and Whitesides, T. E., Jr.: Surgical reconstruction of late post-traumatic thoracolumbar kyphosis. Spine *10:*307–312, 1985.
57. Ryan, M. D., and Taylor, T. K. F.: Acute spinal cord compression in Scheuermann's disease. J. Bone Joint Surg. *64B:*409, 1982.
58. Sachs, B., Bradford, R., Winter, R., et al.: Scheuermann's kyphosis: Follow-up of Milwaukee-brace treatment. J. Bone Joint Surg. *69A:*50–57, 1987.
59. Scheuermann, H. W.: Kyfosis dorsalis juvenilis. Ugeskr. Laeger *82:*385, 1920.
59a. Schmorl, G.: Die Pathogenese der juvenilen Kyphose. Fortschr. Geb. Roentgenst. Nuklearmed. *41:*359, 1930.
60. Sorenson, K. H.: Scheuermann's Juvenile Kyphosis. Copenhagen, Munksgaard, 1964.
61. Speck, G. R., and Chopin, D. C.: The surgical treatment of Scheuermann's kyphosis. J. Bone Joint Surg. *68B:*189–193, 1986.
62. Stagnara, P., De Mauroy, J. C., Dran, G., et al.: Reciprocal angulation of vertebral bodies in a sagittal plane: approach to references for the evaluation of kyphosis and lordosis. Spine *7:*335–342, 1982.
63. Streitz, W., Brown, J. C., and Bonnett, C.: Anterior fibular strut grafting in the treatment of kyphosis. Clin. Orthop. *128:*140–148, 1977.
64. Taylor, T. C., Wenger, D. R., Stephen, J., et al.: Surgical management of thoracic kyphosis in adolescents. J. Bone Joint Surg. *61A:*496–503, 1979.
65. White, A. A., III, Panjabi, M. M., and Thomas, C. L.: The clinical biomechanics of kyphotic deformities. Clin. Orthop. *128:*8–17, 1977.
66. Whitesides, T. E., Jr.: Traumatic kyphosis of the thoracolumbar spine. Clin. Orthop. *128:*78–92, 1977.
67. Winter, R. B., Moe, J. H., and Lonstein, J. E.: The surgical treatment of congenital kyphosis: a review of 94 patients age 5 years or older, with 2 years or more follow-up in 77 patients. Spine *10:*224–231, 1985.
68. Winter, R. B., and Hall, J. E.: Kyphosis in childhood and adolescence. Spine *3:*285–308, 1978.
69. Winter, R. B., and Moe, J. H.: The results of spinal arthrodesis for congenital spinal deformity in patients younger than five years old. J. Bone Joint Surg. *64A:*419–432, 1982.
70. Winter, R. G. B., Moe, J. H., Bradford, D. S., et al.: Spine deformity in neurofibromatosis. J. Bone Joint Surg. *61A:*677–694, 1979.
71. Winter, R. B.: Dwarfs. *In* Bradford, Lonstein, J. E., Moe, J. H., et al. (eds.): Scoliosis and Other Spinal Deformities. Philadelphia, W. B. Saunders Co., 1988, pp. 522–547.
72. Winter, R. B., Moe, J. H., and Wang, J. F.: Congenital kyphosis: its natural history and treatment as observed in a study of one hundred and thirty patients. J. Bone Joint Surg. *55A:*223–256, 1973.
73. Winter, R. B., Moe, J. H., and Lonstein, J. E.: The incidence of Klippel-Feil syndrome in patients with congenital scoliosis and kyphosis. Spine *9:*363–366, 1984.
74. Yablon, J. S., Kasdon, D. L., and Levine, H.: Thoracic cord compression in Scheuermann's disease. Spine *13:*896–898, 1988.

CHAPTER

17

THORACIC AND LUMBAR SPINAL TRAUMA OF THE IMMATURE SPINE

Ronney L. Ferguson, M.D.

Trauma to the thoracic and lumbar spinal column and the neural elements is rare in childhood. Spinal cord injury in children represents 2 to 4 per cent of all admissions to large spinal trauma rehabilitation centers.[22, 23] Published reports dealing specifically with thoracic and lumbar spinal injury in this age group are scarce. Melzak reported that 29 of 4470 patients admitted to the National Spinal Injuries Centre, Stoke Mandeville Hospital with traumatic paraplegia between the years of 1948 and 1969 were under the age of 14 years, an incidence of 0.6 per cent.[38] Scher found a 0.9 per cent incidence of paraplegia in children between the ages of 2 and 12 years at the Conradie Hospital Spinal Injury Unit.[47]

Distinct patterns of injury occur that are characteristic of the immature spine. The purpose of this section is to delineate the differences between the traumatized mature and immature thoracic and lumbar spinal column. The anatomy, spectrum of injury, outcome after injury, treatment, and complications peculiar to the child will be emphasized.

ANATOMY

Vertebral Disc

The intervertebral disc consists of the nucleus pulposus, the annulus fibrosus, and the cartilaginous end plates. The differences between the immature and the mature intervertebral disc may account for variations in the injury patterns seen among different age groups.

The immature nucleus pulposus is characteristically more hydrophilic in nature than in the mature spine.[51] The larger water content causes it to act more efficiently as a hydraulic shock absorber between the vertebral bodies. Energy is more effectively absorbed when the spine is loaded. This may play a role in the lower incidence of vertebral body fractures seen in the immature spine. When vertebral body fractures do occur they are often centrally located, creating end plate fractures and Schmorl's nodes in the vertebral bodies.[3] Such fractures occur when the hydrophilic nucleus pulposus is loaded excessively and ruptures through the end plate of the vertebral body.[42, 44] The character of the nucleus pulposus begins to change as early as 7 to 8 years of age, when collagen begins to replace the water in the nucleus pulposus.[49] As the disc collagenizes, it becomes less elastic. Load concentration then occurs more readily at the periphery of the vertebral end plates, rather than being dissipated throughout the nucleus pulposus.[51] This may play a role in the greater number of osseous injuries seen in adolescents and adults. The higher incidence of Schmorl's nodes in children and adolescents versus adults may also be explained by this phenomenon.

The vertebral end plate of the immature spine is composed of two cartilaginous types: a hyaline cartilage adjacent to the nucleus pulposus and a physeal cartilage (a physis) adjacent to the bony vertebral body.[3] The physeal cartilage can be further categorized into a ring apophysis and an end plate physis. The ring apophysis traverses the circumference of the vertebral body, begins to ossify at age 7 to 8 years with complete ring formation by age 12, and begins to fuse with the vertebral body by age 14 to 15. Final closure occurs by age 21 to 25.[49] The ring apophysis accounts for growth of vertebral body breadth. The physeal portion of the end plate is responsible for vertical growth of the vertebral body. This physeal plate contains the architecture typical of a physis: a resting zone, proliferative zone, hypertrophic zone, and zone of primary and secondary spongiosa. Anatomic studies demonstrate that fractures occurring through the disc space in the immature spine traverse ". . . almost exclusively the two growth layers of the growth zone" of the physis, just as they do in long-bone physeal fractures.[3] The annulus fibrosus has not been found to fail in the immature spine.[3] After the seventh to eighth year of age, the end plate physis develops areas of degeneration typified by loss of nuclei in the cellular substance. Growth of vertebral body height ceases after skeletal maturity with closure of the physis. After physeal closure a weak "growth zone" no longer exists in the mature spine. Failure now occurs through the bony vertebral body or through the annulus fibrosus in the substance of the disc space.[42, 44] The changing injury patterns seen among child, adolescent, and adult patients can be explained in part by changing anatomy brought about by growth and maturation of the end plate.

The hyaline cartilage end plate functions as an interface with the nucleus pulposus and transmits load from it to the trabeculae and cortical rim of the vertebral body. As the child matures, the ratio of end plate volume to bony vertebral body volume decreases. The lumbar intervertebral disc changes shape from biconvex to biconcave between the ages of 2 to 7 years.[49] The concavity of the end plate may predispose to the development of end plate fractures or Schmorl's nodes when the immature spine is excessively loaded. Aufdermaur demonstrated in his necropsy study that end plate fractures were a frequent finding and often were not demonstrable on plain roentgenograms.[3] No sexual differences in either disc space development or in the sex ratio of spinal injuries without osseous disruption have been found.[53]

Vertebral Body

The height of lumbar and thoracic vertebral bodies in the child grow at a constant rate during childhood; however, the lumbar vertebrae tend to grow to a greater degree in breadth after age 2 years. Thus, the thoracic spine bears a greater load per unit area than the lumbar spine during a constant load. The notion that the breaking stress of vertebral body bone is constant implies that the ultimate strength of the vertebral bodies is largely a function of size, and may be one of the reasons spinal injuries are more common in the thoracic than lumbar spine in the child.[45]

The neural elements ascend to their normal levels in the spinal canal by the age of 1 year. The neurologic injury level in the immature thoracic and lumbar spinal column should be consistent with adult levels after 1 year of age. The spinal canal attains adult volume by age 6 years. Thus, encroachment on the spinal cord by spinal column deformity or fragmentation should be similar to the adult by this age. This may play a role in the higher incidence of complete spinal cord injuries occurring in children less than 8 years of age.

Mechanics of the Immature Spinal Column

Crothers has demonstrated in immature cadaveric spine studies that the childhood bony and ligamentous spinal column can be easily lengthened by as much as 5 cm before disrupting whereas the spinal cord and meninges lengthen approximately 1 cm before rupturing. Most of the meningeal ruptures occurred at the cervicothoracic junction.[14, 15] The spinal cord is well fixed in both the cervical and lumbar regions by roots and the dentate ligaments; however, the cervicothoracic junction has less support. Thus, the immature spinal column may not protect the spinal cord from injury if subjected to extreme distraction loads. Cervicothoracic junction spinal cord injury is relatively common in the child, especially in birth injuries and in injuries without radiographic evidence of spinal column disruption.

SPINAL COLUMN AND NEUROLOGIC INJURY IN THE THORACIC AND LUMBAR SPINE

Clinically evident thoracic and lumbar spinal trauma in children is rare. Although the true incidence is not known, large referral centers for spinal trauma report an incidence of 0.6 to 0.9 per cent of all spine trauma cases. Thoracic and lumbar spinal trauma constitutes 40 to 74 per cent of all immature spine injuries.[1, 10, 11, 26, 30, 38, 47, 53] Spine trauma in some children who do not have radiographically recognizable lesions and no neurologic lesion may go unrecognized. A greater awareness of this injury pattern may allow it to be recognized more frequently.

Spinal injury in children, as in adults, occurs secondary to significant trauma. The most common causes of traumatic spinal lesions in children are automobile and automobile–pedestrian accidents. Other high-impact events such as falls, sports-related activities, birth trauma, child abuse, and other major trauma cause spinal injury in the child. Associated injuries in children occur in approximately 50 per cent of cases.[1, 30] Males and females have an equal incidence of nonosseous injury but males predominate when osseous injury occurs.[53] Approximately 20 per cent of spinal trauma cases involving an osseous lesion in the thoracic and lumbar spine have an associated neurologic injury.[1] The incidence of concomitant spinal trauma and neurologic injury increases logarithmically with age.[1]

Thoracic and Lumbar Spinal Cord Injury without Osseous Injury

Spinal cord injury without obvious radiographic signs of spinal column disruption occurs commonly in the immature spine. The incidence of thoracic- and lumbar-level spinal cord injuries without obvious spinal column injury ranges from a reported 1 per cent to 55 per cent with a median of 42.5 per cent.[1, 3, 11, 30, 53] In adults this phenomenon is much rarer, occurring in 2 per 1000 spinal injuries.[47]

Pathophysiology

Proposed causes of spinal cord injury without detectable bony damage are numerous, but can rarely be proven.

Physeal End Plate Fracture. Aufdermaur reported on the cellular pathology, necropsy, and radiographic results in 12 of 100 spinal injuries coming to necropsy over an eight-year period.[3] The 12 reported cases ranged in age from birth to 18 years whereas the other 88 cases were adults. In only one of these cases was a fracture suspected before autopsy. The fractures were all found to traverse the "growth zone" of the cartilaginous end plates, with three fractures having minimal involvement of the primary spongiosa. In three cases the posterior ligamentous structures of the facet joints were disrupted, leading the authors to classify these as unstable fractures. In all three of these cases it was believed that the spinal injury was directly responsible for the death of the patient; all were cervical lesions. Five of the twelve injuries were in the thoracic or lumbar spine. In none of these cases was the annulus fibrosus disrupted. The author was able to reproduce a similar injury in the laboratory using immature spines with an axial distraction flexion force applied to the spine.[3] It would appear that one possible mechanism of spinal cord injury without obvious osseous injury could be when spinal column disruption occurs through the hypertrophic zone of the physis in the end plate with subsequent reduction. Minimal or no radiographic findings would be noted in this instance. Physeal injuries in long bones may have similar findings. Aufdermaur also noted that the end plates were invariably fractured, although this was not visible on plain radiographs.[3]

Stretch of the Spinal Cord. Crothers has described overstretching of the spinal column with subsequent injury to the spinal cord as a cause of paraplegia in children.[14, 15] Both necropsy and laminectomy data support the concept of cord injury without obvious spinal column disruption.[11, 24, 32, 34]

Other Mechanisms. In-folding of the ligamentum flavum can occur with a hyperextension injury, a mechanism demonstrated in the cervical spine that presumably can occur in the thoracolumbar spine as well.[2, 9, 48] Infarction of the spinal cord from disrupted blood supply, especially at the T4 to L1 levels of the anterior spinal cord where the collateral blood supply to the spinal cord is limited, could lead to spinal cord injury.[13, 32, 47] Acute prolapse of a thoracic disc or the protrusion of a cartilaginous end plate into the spinal canal have also been reported to cause spinal cord injury with normal plain radiographic findings.[47, 53]

Clinical Findings

Neurologic injury to the thoracic and lumbar spinal cord in the absence of obvious spinal column disruption may occur at birth secondary to the trauma of the birthing process or secondary to exogenous trauma.[3, 11, 26, 34, 53] Children with such injuries present at a mean age of 6 years, which is significantly younger than children with obvious spinal column damage.[53] A higher percentage of these younger patients also have complete injuries compared with those with concomitant osseous injury.[11, 13, 38, 53] Injuries without obvious spinal column disruption tend to occur at the cervicothoracic junction but may occur at any level in the spine.[53] Onset of neurologic symptoms can be delayed as long as four days after injury and such a delay may not be unusual.[41] Poorer neurologic recovery occurs in children under 8 years of age who have this lesion.[41] The cervicothoracic junction is also the most common level of spinal cord injury in children as the result of birth trauma. Such cord injury occurs three times more frequently during difficult breech deliveries. Reflex movement of the baby's extremities makes early diagnosis difficult, but the infant will eventually prove to have no volitional movement below the spinal cord injury in complete lesions. These children are often not diagnosed to have paraplegia or paraparesis until several months after birth. Birth injury paraplegia involving the upper thoracic spine often presents with frequent episodes of pneumonia secondary to poor respiratory effort caused by paralyzed intercostal and abdominal muscles.[34] All the sequelae of paraplegia and paraparesis are present in these children. Since by definition there are no radiographic findings on plain roentgenograms, the level of the injury must be discerned by physical examination. A complete history and physical examination of the child, including a complete neurologic examination with evaluation of bowel and bladder function and distal reflexes, must be performed initially and at frequent intervals to document possible progressive neurologic deterioration in the acute lesion.

Radiographic Evaluation

Multiple reports have demonstrated that complete neurologic injury can occur in the child without any abnormality on plain roentgenogram, tomogram, myelogram, computed tomographic (CT) scan, or in one case, magnetic resonance imaging (MRI) scan. Follow-up plain radiographs in these patients have not demonstrated subsequent fractures or other abnormalities.[47] Myelography has on occasion demonstrated a block at the level of the injury. MRI scan can demonstrate acute hemorrhage or edema in the spinal cord.[12] No report has confirmed MRI's diagnostic efficacy for this injury in the immature spine. Most authors with experience in childhood spine injuries do not recommend invasive radiographic studies of the spine. Ygnve and associates reported one case and the author has seen an additional case of paraparesis in a child in which the cartilaginous end plate fractured and extruded into the spinal canal. This lesion was not diagnosed on plain roentgenogram but was easily noted and analyzed by MRI scan. MRI scanning of children with neurologic injury and no obvious bony abnormalities in the spine should be considered in the evaluation of these injuries. Myelography with extravasation of the dye has prognostic value in that all patients with this finding demonstrated no recovery of function.[53]

Treatment

Conservative treatment is recommended in this group of spinal cord injury patients.[11, 34, 38, 41, 47, 53] Exploratory laminectomy has had no benefit in the few cases where it has been attempted other than to document spinal cord attenuation and injury once the dura was opened.[24, 32] Conservative care of the spine with immobilization for one to three weeks appears to be the treatment of choice. Surgical decompression of the spine should be considered when progressive neurologic deterioration occurs and a distinct lesion can be demonstrated radiographically.[53] Long-term spinal deformities have occurred secondary to spinal paralysis with resultant scoliosis, kyphosis, or lordosis. No short segment instability secondary to unrecognized motion segment disruption by trauma has been reported.[1, 11, 30, 38, 53] Laminectomy data have documented these lesions to occur both with posterior ligamentous disruption and without ligamentous disruption.[3, 11, 24, 32] Laminectomy has been documented to cause instability in some immature patients.[35]

Spinal injuries with Osseous or Ligamentous Disruption

Spinal fractures of the thoracic and lumbar spine presenting with obvious osseous or ligamentous disruption of the spinal column are reported to occur between 45 and 99 per cent of the time, with a median of 57.5 per cent of the cases reported.[1, 3, 11, 30, 53] The average age of patients with osseous injury is 16 years, significantly greater than those without osseous injury.[53]

Pathophysiology

Because these patients as a group are older, it is not surprising that their bony fracture patterns are similar to those reported in adult series. These osseous lesions usually fit well into present adult thoracic and lumbar spinal injury classifications. The criteria of Holdsworth, Denis, Ferguson and Allen, or McAfee and associates can be applied to both stable and unstable adolescent spine injuries.[19, 21, 28, 36]

Osseous injuries in the child may vary from those in the older adolescent spine because of the previously described anatomic differences. Childhood spinal injuries have a potential for physeal separations as a component of their injury, compared with predominantly bony and ligamentous injuries in the mature spine. This trend appears to be more prevalent in the younger child. Aufdermaur found that disc spaces were not disrupted in the immature spines.[3] The cartilaginous end plate separations represented physeal injuries of the end plate physis with potential extensions through the posterior ligaments when the traumatic forces were large.[3] Flexion–distraction dislocation of the spine that is considered unstable with poor healing potential in the adult may stabilize in the immature child.[19, 21, 28, 40] The child's physis may heal and continue to grow, establishing an anterior load path that is stable even in the face of posterior ligamentous disruption and elongation (Fig. 17–1). A comparison can be made to a Salter Harris Type I fracture of a long bone. This is unlike the adult injury where the dislocation of the spine will occur through the disc space by disrupting the annulus fibrosus and the posterior ligamentous complex.

The younger child with spinal column injury often presents with multiple levels of fracture within the end plate; the superior end plates are fractured twice as often as the inferior end plates (Figs. 17–2, 17–3). Compression fractures or Schmorl's nodes (Fig. 17–4) are usually minimal in nature. Restoration of vertebral body height will occur in children who have growth remaining in their vertebral physes or whose physes have not been damaged by the trauma of the spine injury.[29, 30]

Clinical Findings

The clinical symptoms are similar to those seen in adult spinal injury. Approximately 20 to 30 per cent of patients will have neurologic injury.[1, 30] Half of these patients have associated injuries.[1, 53] Males are more commonly involved than females.[1, 53] A thorough history and physical examination must be performed and all body systems included to detect associated injuries. The neurologic examination is mandatory at admission to the hospital and at frequent intervals after the injury to document both the neurologic status of the patient and any deterioration. Even patients with normal baseline neurologic examinations warrant frequent rechecking, since delayed neurologic deterioration may occur.[41] The initial examination should always include a rectal examination. In the neurologically involved pediatric patient, distal reflexes, such as the bulbocavernosus reflex, should be documented and all patients with significant spinal trauma should have bladder function evaluated. Either a check of the postvoid urine residual with an immediate postvoid straight catheterization, or urologic examination using a cystometrogram may be used. Bladder function evaluation is important not only to determine the neurologic

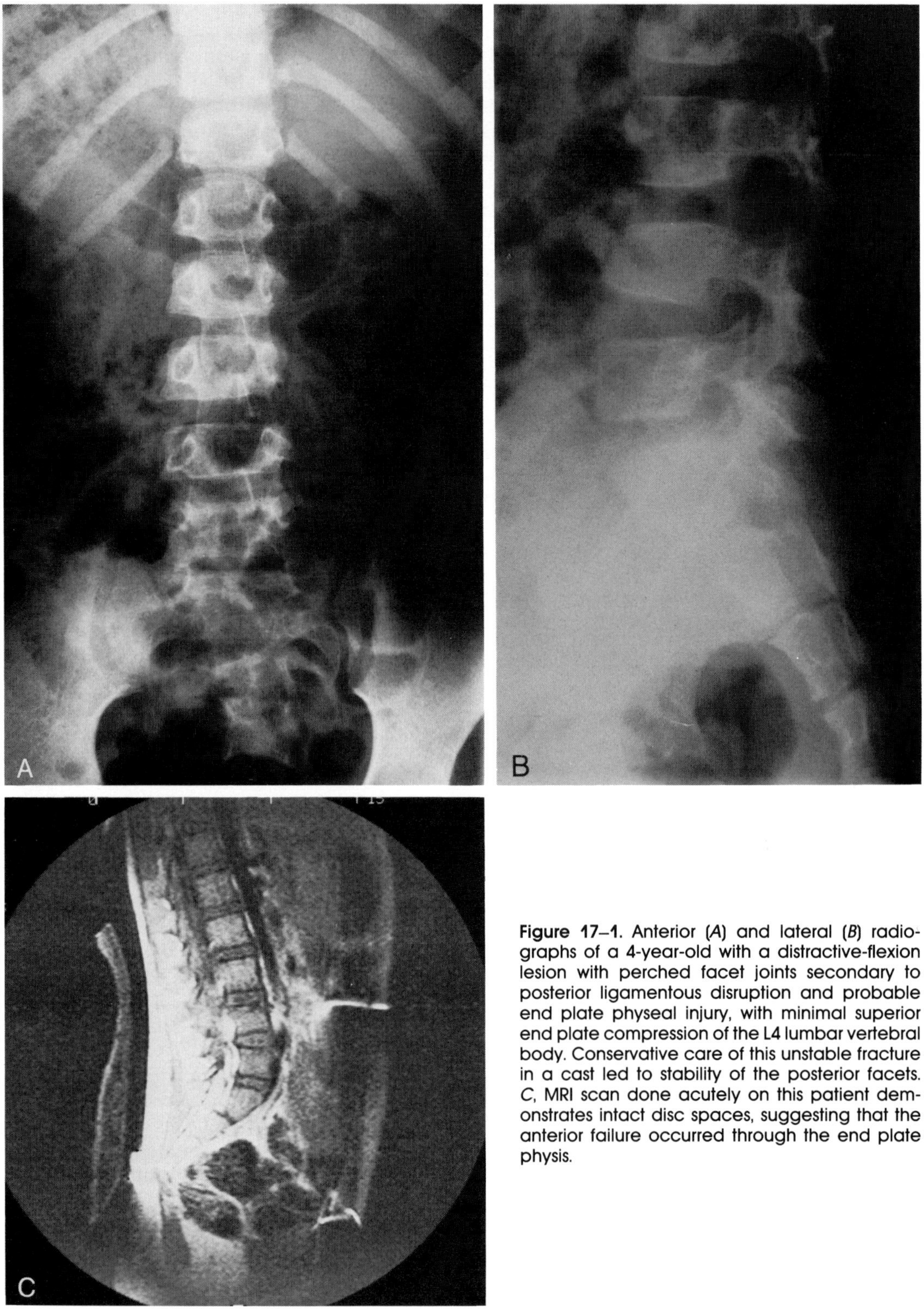

A

B

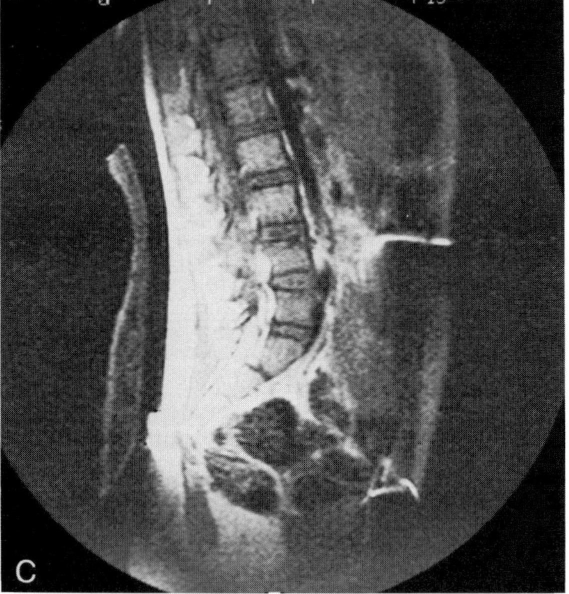

Figure 17–1. Anterior (*A*) and lateral (*B*) radiographs of a 4-year-old with a distractive-flexion lesion with perched facet joints secondary to posterior ligamentous disruption and probable end plate physeal injury, with minimal superior end plate compression of the L4 lumbar vertebral body. Conservative care of this unstable fracture in a cast led to stability of the posterior facets. *C*, MRI scan done acutely on this patient demonstrates intact disc spaces, suggesting that the anterior failure occurred through the end plate physis.

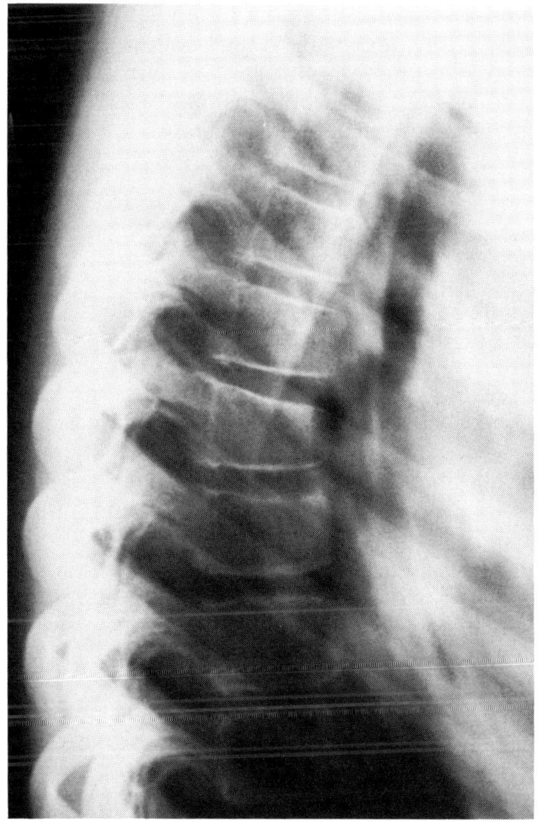

Figure 17–2. A compression fracture of a superior end plate in an immature thoracic vertebra.

status of the patient, but also to begin the patient on appropriate therapy for bowel and bladder management. Recovery from neurologic injury is poorer in children under 8 years of age than in older children.[10, 11, 13, 38, 41, 53]

Radiographic Evaluation

By definition this group of injuries will have positive plain radiographic findings. Since a larger proportion of the spinal column in the young child may be cartilaginous, it is advisable to study the spine with MRI scans to delineate the extent of the injury. The MRI scan can demarcate ligamentous disruption, cartilaginous displacements, disc space disruptions, spinal cord location, edema, and hemorrhage.[12] Such data can be helpful in judging stability of the thoracolumbar spinal fracture. MRI scans do not delineate bony detail well. Tomography may give some enhancement of the bony detail compared with plain radiographs and is not invasive. CT scans may also be used to enhance bony detail, especially in the transverse plane. Myelography, even with CT enhancement, is probably rarely warranted in childhood injuries.

Treatment

Judging stability of the thoracolumbar spine in these patients may be difficult, especially in the younger adolescent or child where the spine is still immature. Whether stability criteria for the adult spine are applicable to the child and young adolescent is uncertain. It is reasonable to assume that the adolescent lesion is similar to that in adults since the anatomy and mechanical properties of the spine are similar at these ages. The same criteria for stability should be used. Conservative versus operative treatment will depend on the philosophy and expertise of the institution where the adolescent is treated. Both conservative treatment and operative treatment with instrumentation have been used in this age group with satisfactory results. When surgical treatment is

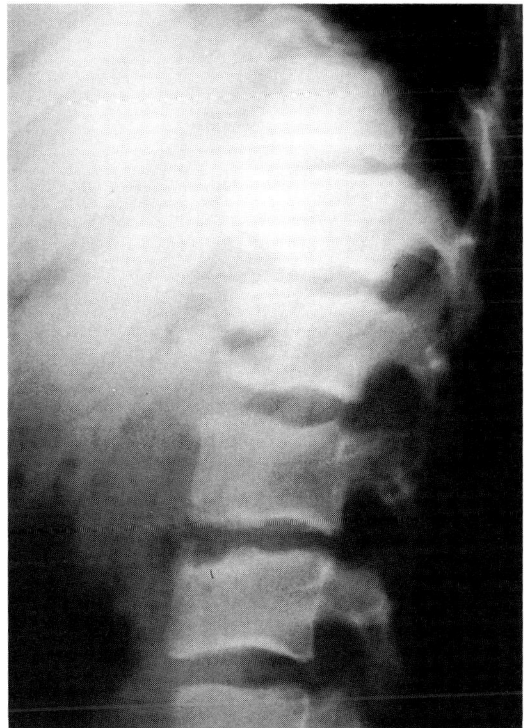

Figure 17–3. Compression fractures of both the superior and inferior end plates of immature thoracic vertebrae with Schmorl's nodes occurring at multiple levels.

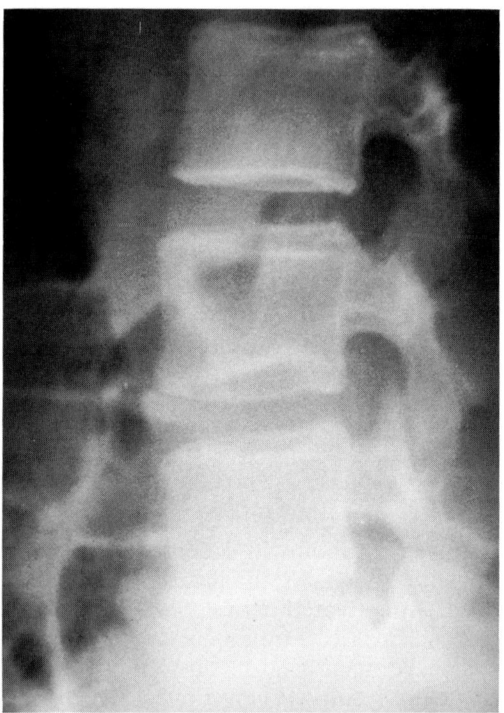

Figure 17–4. Schmorl's nodes in adjacent inferior and superior lumbar end plates in the lumbar spine.

deemed necessary in the unstable injury, care must be taken to ensure that the instrumentation will be of the appropriate size for the spine being instrumented.

In the younger child (eight years or less), conservative therapy should be the treatment of choice in stable spinal injuries and strongly considered in spinal injuries considered unstable, since many will have a physeal injury. On plain radiographs these injuries may appear to be unstable but they may have the potential to heal and become stable. Surgical intervention is indicated when instability persists after conservative care has been tried and shown to fail (Fig. 17–5). Flexion and extension x-rays of the injured spinal motion segment may be useful in judging the stability of the spine after treatment.

Operative decompression of the spine should be considered in any injury where it appears that the neurologic deficit is progressive and spinal deformity or bony encroachment on the neural elements may be the cause of deterioration. Chronic spinal instability after childhood spinal fractures characterized by continued pain has been shown to have no greater incidence than back pain in the general population after an average follow-up of 16 years, although significant local pain did occur in 4 per cent.[29] Chronic instability developing into progressive spinal deformity may require surgery to control spinal deformity.[18, 35, 43]

Complications

The complications of paraplegia and paraparesis, such as bowel and bladder dysfunction, skin insensitivity, thromboembolic disease, gastrointestinal dysfunction, and psychosocial problems are well known and documented. Between one third and one half of all immature patients sustaining a spine injury develop a major complication either acutely or at follow-up.[1, 11, 30, 53] Several complications secondary to spinal column fracture or spinal cord injury are specific to the immature spine. Differences in complication rates between the child and the adult spine injury patient also occur.

Musculoskeletal Deformities

Deformities in the child with spinal cord injury, as in the adult, occur secondary to muscle paralysis, spasticity, and contracture. But unlike the adult, the child also has growth as a potentially deforming force. This occurs secondary to a relative decrease in length of a spastic or contracted muscle faced with increasing length of the bone. If bony malalignment occurs, joint surfaces may also deform with growth, making correction of the deformity difficult or impossible. Prevention of deformities in children requires vigorous physical rehabilitation and occasionally surgery to correct deformities before joint malalignments become severe.[1, 10, 11]

Spinal Deformities

Ninety-seven to 100 per cent of children with a spinal cord injury incurred before the adolescent growth spurt develop a spinal column deformity.[18, 35, 43] Ninety-six per cent of the curves are progressive, with scoliosis occurring in 92 per cent, kyphosis in 64 per cent, and lordosis in 20 per cent. Sixty-eight per cent require surgery.[35] Those injured after the beginning of the adolescent growth spurt have a 52 per cent incidence of developing spinal

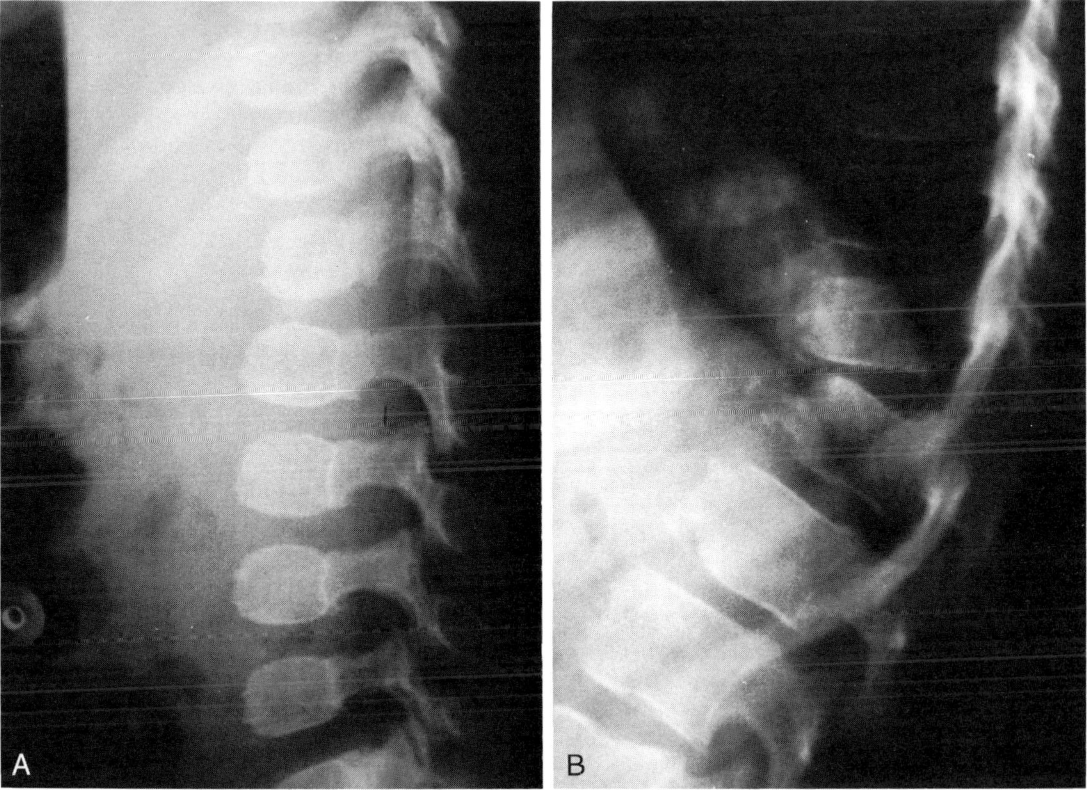

Figure 17–5. *A*, Distractive-flexion lesion of the lumbar spine in a 1-year-old child. This represents tension failure through both the ligaments posteriorly and the end plate physis anteriorly. This unstable injury would be expected to stabilize with conservative care. *B*, Distractive-flexion lesion at the thoracolumbar junction in an 8-year-old. Note the translation of the superior vertebral body on the inferior one. This represents an unstable injury that may or may not stabilize with conservative care. If conservative care was used, flexion-extension views would be necessary at the end of immobilization to prove the stability of the posterior ligaments.

deformities.[18] The apex of the curve always occurs below the level of the injury.[35] Spinal deformity can occur secondary to the paralysis of the spinal musculature, secondary to angular growth caused by asymmetric physeal closure, residual angulation of the injured motion segment, or a combination of these mechanisms.[18, 30, 35, 43] Progressive spinal deformities ultimately require surgical stabilization. In the very young child with a paralytic deformity, bracing the trunk until it attains adequate height may be necessary before surgical fusion. If bracing does not control the spinal deformity, early fusion may be necessary. Laminectomy of the spine was shown to have no efficacy for return of function and was often associated with progressive spinal deformities.[35]

Other

Pulmonary compromise secondary to weak intercostal and abdominal musculature may be acute or become evident after multiple episodes of pneumonia.[1, 34, 53] Pneumonia is more frequent with high thoracic lesions. Urinary tract infections are common in patients with spinal cord injury. Gastrointestinal bleeding secondary to stress ulcers occurs in 10 per cent of patients. Deep venous thrombosis has been an uncommon complication. Decubiti often develop in patients immobilized with casts during the initial hospitalization. The neurologic status of the patient does not seem to affect the incidence of early decubiti. Decubiti presenting after the initial hospitalization occur in neurologically involved children.[1, 53] The latter decubiti are located at or below the previous injury and are difficult to treat. Death secondary to associated injuries in patients with thoracic and lumbar spinal injuries may be as high as 10 per cent.[1]

Fatigue Fractures of the Pars Interarticularis

Chronic hyperextension loading of the immature spine may result in fatigue of the pars interarticularis in the lower lumbar spine. This has been reported to occur in gymnastics, football (down linemen), weight lifting, karate, hurdling, pole vaulting, high jumping, hockey, and other jarring sports where repetitive hyperextension loading occurs.[31, 33, 52] Such fractures have also been reported in nonathletic individuals. Genetic family predisposition may be a factor in developing this entity. Unilateral or bilateral pars interarticularis defects may occur. Bilateral involvement may result in progressive spondylolisthesis.[33, 52]

Acute fractures of the pars interarticularis occur secondary to severe hyperextension trauma.[21, 40] Although few reports exist in the literature, such fractures usually occur in the lumbar spine with distraction of the anterior elements and shear or compression loading of the posterior elements. Nicoll believed that this rare lesion was always unstable and should be surgically repaired in the adult.[40] Whether this is true in the child is undocumented.

Clinical Findings

Hyperextension fatigue fractures may have an insidious onset with no specific traumatic incident remembered, or they may occur secondary to an identifiable traumatic incident.[31, 33, 52] The history is usually significant for some athletic participation that involves hyperextension loading of the spinal column. Patients with this problem usually have chronic aching low back pain aggravated by activities. Hyperextension of the spine tends to cause pain in athletes and its avoidance in the sport often relieves symptoms. Approximately 29 per cent of pars defects occurring in young athletes progress to significant spondylolisthesis.[52] In gymnasts the most common level involved is L5. Lesions in other athletically active individuals have been reported from L2 to L5.[31]

Radiographic Evaluation

Plain radiographs of the spine may initially fail to demonstrate a lesion, but subsequent radiographic evidence of a pars interarticularis fracture may appear after long-term follow-up.[52] Technetium bone scans in the acutely injured spine may demonstrate increased uptake in the posterior elements at a time when plain radiographs are normal. Subsequently the plain radiographs will demonstrate a fracture. Conversely, defects of the pars interarticularis that are present on plain roentgenograms may not demonstrate increased uptake on technetium bone scan. Such findings are believed to represent older lesions that are no longer actively undergoing repair.[52] CT scans have proved useful in demonstrating lesions that are neither recognizable on plain roentgenograms nor reactive on bone scan.[25, 37]

Treatment

A spectrum of successful treatments has been reported in patients with fatigue fractures in spondylolysis and spondylolisthesis. These include expectant observation, avoidance of painful activities—primarily repetitive hyperextension—while continuing sports activities, brace or cast immobilization of the spine, and surgical repair or fusion of the spinal defect. Conservative care in patients with spondylolysis should be the primary form of treatment. Immobilization of the spine by either casting or bracing is the most widely used initial treatment of a pars interarticularis defect. Frequent follow-up to document healing of the pars interarticularis defect is indicated.[33, 52] Even those patients with unsuccessful union of the pars interarticularis fracture frequently have subsiding symptoms, which allows the athlete to return successfully to the former sport.[33] Letts and associates reported a 50 per cent success rate in treating unilateral spondylolysis with cast immobilization, but no efficacy of casting bilateral spondylolysis or spondylolisthesis.[33] If the technetium bone scan is reactive, the pars interarticularis has active osteoblastic activity and may heal with more conservative measures. A nonreactive technetium bone scan in the face of an obvious pars interarticularis defect is interpreted as representing an atrophic nonunion. Although this may not rule out healing with conservative care, healing may be less likely to occur.[52] In these cases surgical grafting of the defect or fusion of the motion segment may be necessary. If the defect does not heal with conservative therapy and pain is debilitating to the individual, surgical repair of the pars interarticularis defect is indicated. Repair of the defect in the pars interarticularis in patients with spondylolysis or minimal degrees of slippage can be accomplished by bone grafting the defect or by fusion of the involved motion segment.[6] If a spondylolisthesis of greater than 50 per cent is present, surgical fusion of the involved motion segments should be considered. With a slip greater than 50 per cent, two motion segments should be fused to facilitate stabilization of the severely slipped segment. If the slip is less than 50 per cent, only one motion segment should be fused.[5, 27] Whether the use of instrumentation, with its higher complication rate, is warranted in children is questionable, since fusion rates of 90 per cent can be expected with posterior lateral fusions alone.[5, 7, 20, 33, 39, 46, 50]

References

1. Anderson, M. J., and Schutt, A. H.: Spinal injury in children: a review of 156 cases seen from 1950 through 1978. Mayo Clin. Proc. *55:*499–504, 1980.
2. Asher, M. A., and Jacobs, R. R.: Pediatric thoracolumbar spine trauma. *In* Bradford, D. S., and Hensinger, R. M. (eds.): The Pediatric Spine. New York, Thieme, Inc., 1985.
3. Aufdermaur, M.: Spinal injuries in juveniles: necropsy findings in twelve cases. J. Bone Joint Surg. *56B:*513–519, 1974.
4. Benner, B., Moiel, R., Dickson, J., and Harrington, P.: Instrumentation of the spine for fracture dislocations in children. Childs Brain *3:*249–255, 1977.
5. Boxall, D., Bradford, D. S., Winter, R. B., and Moe, J. H.: Management of severe spondylolisthesis in children and adolescents. J. Bone Joint Surg. *61A:*479–495, 1979.
6. Bradford, D. S., and Iza, J.: Repair of the defect in spondylolysis or minimal degrees of spondylolisthesis by segmental wire fixation and bone grafting. Spine *10:*673–679, 1985.
7. Bradford, D. S.: Spondylolysis and spondylolisthesis in children and adolescents: current concepts in management. *In* Bradford, D. S., and Hensinger, R. M. (eds.): The Pediatric Spine. New York, Thieme, Inc., 1985.
8. Bradford, D. S.: Treatment of severe spondylolisthesis: a combined approach for reduction and stabilization. Spine *4:*423, 1979.
9. Breig, A., and El-Nadi, A. F.: Biomechanics of the cervical spinal cord: relief of contact pressure on and overstretching of the spinal cord. Acta Radiol. (Diag.) *4:*602–624, 1966.
10. Burke, D. C.: Spinal cord trauma in children. Paraplegia *9:*1–14, 1971.
11. Burke, D. C.: Traumatic spinal paralysis in children. Paraplegia *11:*268, 276, 1974.
12. Calhoun, J., Allen, B. L., Jr., Ferguson, R. L., and Amparo, E.: Surface coil magnetic resonance imaging of the spine. American Academy of Orthopaedic Surgeons Annual Meeting Exhibit, Atlanta, GA, February, 1988.
13. Cheshire, D. J. E.: The paediatric syndrome of traumatic myelopathy without demonstrable vertebral injury. Paraplegia *15:*74–85, 1977–1978.
14. Crothers, B.: Injury of the spinal cord in breech extraction as an important cause of fetal death and of paraplegia in childhood. Am. J. Med. Sci. *165:*94, 1923.
15. Crothers, B.: The effect of breech extraction upon the central nervous system of the fetus. Med. Clin. North Am. *5:*1287, 1922.
16. Cullen, J. C.: Spinal lesions in battered babies. J. Bone Joint Surg. *57B:*364–366, 1975.
17. Dachling, P., and Wilberger, J. E.: Spinal cord injury without radiographic abnormalities in children. J. Neurosurg. *57:*114–119, 1982.

18. Dearolf, W. W., III, Betz, R. R., Vogel, L. C., et al.: Scoliosis in pediatric spinal cord-injured patients. J. Ped. Orthop. *10:*214–218, 1990.
19. Denis, F.: The three column spine and its significance in the classification of acute thoracolumbar spinal injuries. Spine *8:*817–831, 1983.
20. DeWald, R. L., Faut, M., Taddino, R. F., and Neuwirth, M. G.: Severe lumbosacral spondylolisthesis in adolescents: reduction and staged circumferential fusion. J. Bone Joint Surg. *63A:*619, 1981.
21. Ferguson, R. L., and Allen, B. L., Jr.: A mechanistic classification of thoracolumbar spine fractures. Clin. Orthop. *189:*77–88, 1984.
22. Forni, I.: Le fratturedel rachide nel bambino. Chir. Org. Movimento *31:*347–361, 1947.
23. Gelehrter, G.: Die Wirbel Korperbruche in Kindes and Jungendalter. Archiv Fur Orthopadische und Unfall-Chirurgie *49:*253–263, 1957.
24. Glasauer, F. E., and Cares, H. L.: Traumatic paraplegia in infancy. J. A. M. A. *219:*38–41, 1972.
25. Grogan, J. P., Hemminghytt, S., Williams, A. L., et al.: Spondylolysis studies with computed tomography. Radiology *145:*737–742, 1982.
26. Hachen, H. J.: Spinal cord injury in children and adolescents: diagnostic pitfalls and therapeutic considerations in the acute stage. Paraplegia *15:*55–64, 1977.
27. Harris, I. E., Weinstein, S. L.: Long-term follow-up of patients with grade-III and IV spondylolisthesis. J. Bone Joint Surg. *69A:*960–969, 1987.
28. Holdsworth, F.: Fractures, dislocations, and fracture-dislocations of the spine. J. Bone Joint Surg. *52A:*1534–1551, 1970.
29. Horal, J., Nachemson, A., and Scheller, S.: Clinical and radiological long term follow-up of vertebral fractures in children. Acta Orthop. Scand. *43:*491–503, 1972.
30. Hubbard, D. D.: Injuries of the spine in children and adolescents. Clin. Orthop. *112:*114–123, 1974.
31. Jackson, D. W., Wiltse, L. L., and Cirincione, R. J.: Spondylolysis in the female gymnast. Clin. Orthop. *117:*68–73, 1976.
32. LeBlanc, H. J., and Nadell, J.: Spinal cord injuries in children. Surg. Neurol. *2:*411–414, 1974.
33. Letts, M., Smallman, T., Afanasiev, R., and Gouw, G.: Fracture of the pars interarticularis in adolescent athletes: a clinical-biomechanical analysis. J. Ped. Orthop. *6:*40–46, 1986.
34. Leventhal, H. R.: Birth injuries of the spinal cord. J. Ped. *56:*447–453, 1960.
35. Mayfield, J. K., Erkkila, J. C., and Winter, R. B.: Spinal deformity subsequent to acquired childhood spinal cord injury. J. Bone Joint Surg. *63A:*1401–1411, 1981.
36. McAfee, P. C., Yuan, H. A., Fredrickson, B. E., and Lubicky, J. P.: The value of computed tomography in thoracolumbar fractures: an analysis of 100 consecutive cases and a new classification. J. Bone Joint Surg. *65A:*461–473, 1983.
37. McAfee, P. C., and Yuan, H. A.: Computed tomography in spondylolisthesis. Clin. Orthop. *166:*62–71, 1982.
38. Melzak, J.: Paraplegia among children. Lancet *2:*45–48, 1969.
39. Nachemson, A., and Wiltse, L. L.: Editorial comment: spondylolisthesis. Clin. Orthop. *117:*4, 1976.
40. Nicoll, E. A.: Fractures of the dorsolumbar spine. J. Bone Joint Surg. *31B:*376, 1949.
41. Pang, D., and Wilberger, J. E., Jr.: Spinal cord injury without radiographic abnormalities in children. J. Neurosurg. *57:*114–129, 1982.
42. Perey, O.: Fracture of the vertebral endplate in the lumbar spine. Acta Scand. Suppl., 1957.
43. Roaf, R.: Scoliosis secondary to paraplegia. Paraplegia *8:*42–47, 1970.
44. Rolander, S. D., and Blair, W. E.: Deformation and fracture of the lumbar vertebral endplate. Orthop. Clin. North Am. *6:*75, 1975.
45. Rolander, S. D.: Motion of the lumbar spine with special reference to the stabilizing effect of posterior fusion (thesis). Department of Orthopaedic Surgery, University of Gothenburg, Sweden, 1966.
46. Rombold, C.: Treatment of spondylolisthesis by posterior fusion, resection of pars interarticularis and prompt mobilization of the patient. J. Bone Joint Surg. *48A:*1282, 1966.
47. Scher, A. T.: Trauma of the spinal cord in children. S. Afr. Med. J. *50:*2023–2025, 1976.
48. Taylor, A.: The mechanism of injury to the spinal cord in the neck without damage to the vertebral column. J. Bone Joint Surg. *33B:*543–547, 1951.
49. Taylor, J. R.: Growth of human intervertebral discs and vertebral bodies. J. Anat. *120:*49–68, 1975.
50. Turner, R. H., and Bianco, A. J., Jr.: Spondylolysis and spondylolisthesis in children and teenagers. J. Bone Joint Surg. *53A:*1298, 1971.
51. White, A. A., and Panjabi, M. M.: Clinical Biomechanics of the Spine. Philadelphia, J. B. Lippincott Co., 1978.
52. Wiltse, L. L., Widdel, E. H., Jr., and Jackson, D. W.: Fatigue fracture: the basic lesion in isthmic spondylolisthesis. J. Bone Joint Surg. *57A:*17–22, 1975.
53. Yngve, D. A., Harris, W. P., Herndon, W. A., et al.: Spinal cord injury without osseous spine fracture. J. Ped. Orthop. *8:*153–159, 1988.

SECTION 3

ARTHRITIS AND DISC DISEASE IN THE ADULT

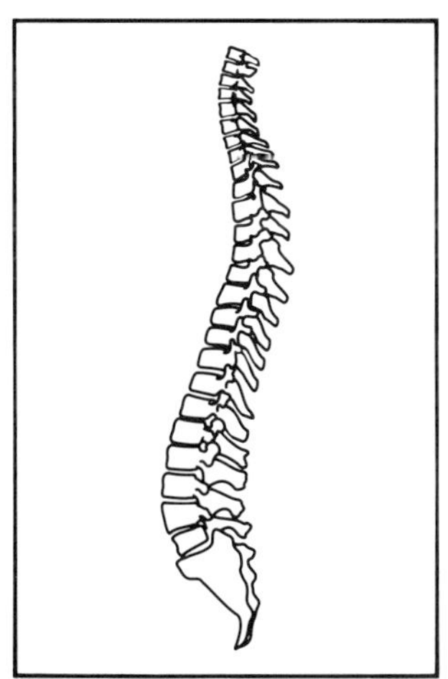

CHAPTER

18

ARTHRITIS OF THE SPINE

J. Michael Simpson, M.D.
Robert E. Booth, Jr., M.D.

True arthritides of the spine and sacroiliac joints are more prevalent than is commonly supposed. The differential diagnosis associated with such changes is extensive and may be confusing to the practicing orthopedist. The purpose of this chapter, in addition to presenting pertinent information about each disease entity, is to simplify the diagnostic process using ankylosing spondylitis as a role model of spinal arthropathy. The clinical and radiographic features differentiating each of these disease processes from ankylosing spondylitis are sufficiently distinctive to be helpful in diagnosis and treatment of spinal arthritis.

ANKYLOSING SPONDYLITIS

Ankylosing spondylitis is a seronegative spondyloarthropathy affecting both skeletal and extraskeletal tissues. It affects primarily the axial skeleton including ligaments and articulations of the pelvis and vertebral bodies. It was once believed to affect men predominantly; however, recent evidence suggests that women are affected equally but with less severe involvement. Eighty to ninety per cent of the patients are HLA-B27 positive. The incidence of ankylosing spondylitis in the general population has been estimated at 1 to 3 per 1000.[45]

Pathology

Cruickshank,[19] in postmortem studies looking at the manubriosternal joint and symphysis pubis, has developed a theory behind the pathologic series of changes seen in ankylosing spondylitis. An osteitis is seen initially that is localized to the joint margins. This is characterized by the presence of chronic inflammatory cells and granulation tissue. Bone tissue in the surrounding areas is osteoporotic secondary to an increase in osteoclastic activity. The subchondral bone and fibrocartilage are later replaced by fibrous tissue, with the joint surfaces showing corresponding changes in the form of erosion and degeneration. During the healing phase these fibrous tissues ossify, and in time lead to bony ankylosis.

Destructive lesions in the anterior spine encompass a spectrum of well-defined changes that have been documented both clinically and radiographically.[23, 31, 62] These anterior lesions may be classified as either localized or extensive forms of the disease process.

The Romanus lesion is an erosion of the anterior and anterolateral aspect of the vertebral rim at the vascular attachment site of the annulus fibrosus. This lesion represents an anterior spondylitis, which results in a focal osteitis as part of the inflammatory process of ankylosing spondylitis. Damage to these tissues subsequently results in a bony repair process, syndesmophyte formation, and ossification of the annulus fibrosus—the hallmark of ankylosing spondylitis. Osseous changes of this type in the thoracolumbar region yield the classic "bamboo spine." A second form of localized lesion is a vertebral rim defect where the avascular annulus is attached. This is believed to represent a traumatic lesion, since there is no evidence of primary focal osteitis occurring in the subchondral bone. Ossification of the apophyseal joints has also been observed. Inflammation localized to the capsule–bone interface presumably leads to ossification of this site in a fashion analogous to other lesions of the enthesis.

The first extensive destructive skeletal lesion in ankylosing spondylitis, described by Andersson, represents massive destruction of the discovertebral junction.[1] Both traumatic and inflammatory causes have been suggested as the source of these changes (Fig. 18–1). Wu and associates have suggested that the primary pathology lies in the intervertebral disc, which then initiates a chain of secondary events in the discovertebral junction and vertebral bone.[99] In a series of eight biopsy specimens evidence of fibrinoid necrosis in the intervertebral disc strongly implied that there was undue stress on these tissues. These findings are similar to the clinical suspicions of many suggesting that trauma and pseudarthrosis are the cause of the extensive discovertebral lesions in ankylosing spondylitis. Any inflammation represents a reaction to the trauma and tissue damage in that area.

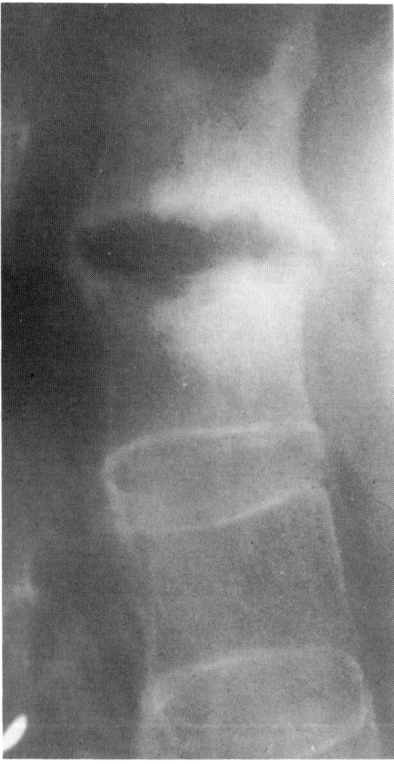

Figure 18–1. Andersson lesion: extensive central and peripheral destruction at the discovertebral junction. Both traumatic and inflammatory etiologies have been suggested.

Clinical Features

Ankylosing spondylitis typically occurs in the healthy young adult between the ages of 17 and 35. Sacroiliitis is usually the first manifestation of the disease. Symptoms including low back pain and unilateral or bilateral buttock, hip, and thigh pain are common and most often insidious in onset (70 to 80 per cent). A few patients may relate the onset to an episode of trauma. Pain mimicking sciatica may also be seen, although reflexes and muscle strength are preserved. The initial course of symptoms is marked by periods of remission lasting weeks to months. In women these symptoms are often attributed to gynecologic or renal problems common in this age group.

A key feature in the patient's history, and possibly the most diagnostic clue, is classical morning stiffness and pain of the low back. This pain typically improves with activity during the day and returns in the evening. Periods of rest seem to exacerbate these symptoms. Many patients awaken from sleep and feel the need to move around before returning to sleep.

Newton has described tests to detect sacroiliitis.[65] The first two are performed with the patient in the supine position. In the first test manual pressure is applied to each ilium in an anterior-to-posterior direction simultaneously. In the second test hands are applied to the ilia in a similar fashion but pressure is applied toward the midline. For the third test the patient is placed in the prone position and pressure is applied directly on the midportion of the sacrum in an anterior direction. When symptoms of pain localized to the sacroiliac, lumbosacral, buttock, or thigh areas are reproduced, the test is considered positive.

Involvement of the lumbar spine may produce many similar symptoms. Localized pain symptoms and referred pain to the buttock and posterior thigh are common. Palpable tenderness and paraspinal muscle can usually be elicited on examination during the early clinical course. With time, lumbar lordosis and motion are lost. The modified Schober test is the best clinical test to quantitate loss of lumbar motion.[49] In this test, points 10 cm above and 5 cm below the lumbosacral junction are identified and marked appropriately on the skin. The patient is asked to flex the spine maximally, and the distance between the marks is measured. The test is considered abnormal if this distance fails to expand by a distance of 6 cm (Fig. 18–2).

When the thoracic spine is involved pain may be localized to the costotransverse and costovertebral joints. Pain may also be referred to the chest wall or abdomen, mimicking other possible disease processes. With further involvement, the patient may describe stiffness or tightness of the chest wall and subjective difficulty in breathing. Limited chest expansion on examination is the most reliable clinical indicator of thoracic spine involvement and is evidence of disease affecting the costovertebral joints. In a normal adult man chest expansion measured at the nipple line should measure at least 5 cm.

The classically described physical findings in the thoracic and lumbar spine have come under scrutiny. In a study by Gran, the triad of reduced lateral mobility of the lumbar spine, reduced total spinal flexion of less than 40 degrees, and reduced total spinal extension of less than 20 degrees has been found to be a more sensitive and specific set of physical findings consistent with ankylosing spondylitis.[33] The presence of these findings increases the likelihood of ankylosing spondylitis 14-fold.

Symptoms of cervical spine involvement include pain, stiffness, and limited motion. The pain may be related directly to the neck or referred to the occiput, shoulders, or upper

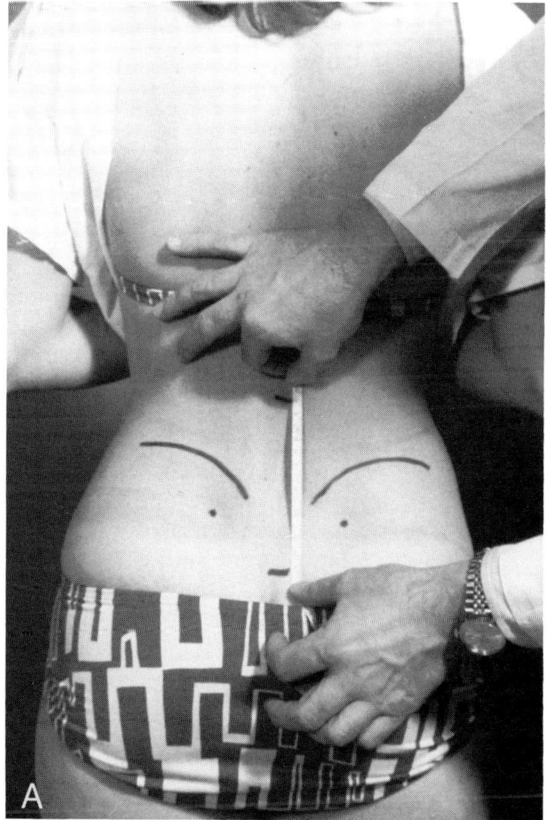

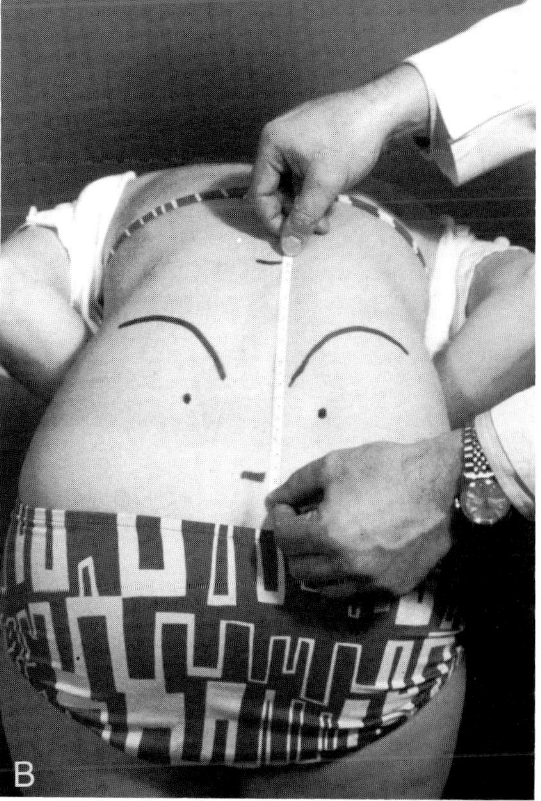

Figure 18–2. *A,* Modified Schober test: points 10 cm above and 5 cm below the lumbosacral junction are marked. *B,* The patient is then asked to maximally flex the spine and the distance is measured. The test is considered abnormal if the distance fails to expand by 6 cm.

chest regions. With more severe involvement, the pain and limited motion may progress to ankylosis. Kyphosis may be severe, limiting peripheral vision and ability to drive. Compensatory flexion contractures of the hips and knees may develop as the patient attempts to maintain an erect posture. As with the rheumatoid patient, atlantoaxial instability may also develop and require interval radiographic evaluation.

Twenty to thirty per cent of patients have synovitis of a peripheral joint, usually the hips, shoulders, knees, or wrists. This is especially true in the younger patient. Involvement is typically asymmetric.

There are several extraskeletal manifestations of ankylosing spondylitis that must be considered.[40] Among the most prominent and severe are recurrent iritis, aortitis, and carditis. Pulmonary involvement may rarely be seen.

Iritis is seen in 25 per cent of patients with ankylosing spondylitis. These attacks are usually unilateral, but recurrences may affect either eye (Fig. 18–3). The most common and severe cardiovascular abnormality in patients with ankylosing spondylitis is aortic valve insufficiency. Ten per cent of patients with the disease for more than 30 years have evidence of aortic regurgitation. Other earlier findings of cardiovascular involvement may include tachycardia, conduction defects, and pericarditis.

Pulmonary function is not significantly compromised by the limited motion of the costovertebral articulations; however, pulmonary fibrosis is occasionally seen in this patient population. The cause of development of these lesions is uncertain. Colonization of the lung with certain fungi, namely *aspergillus,* may be a causative agent.

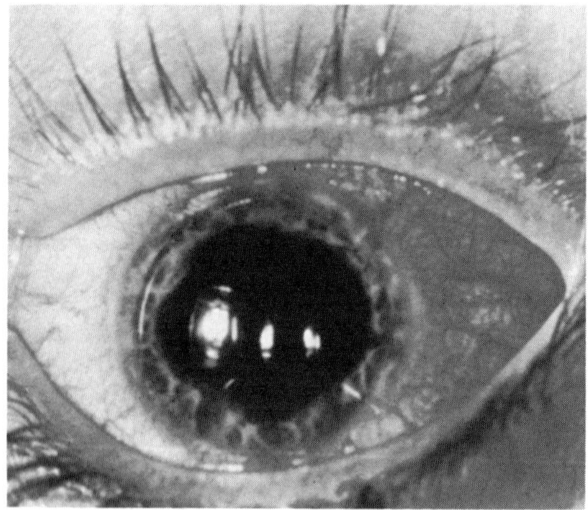

Figure 18–3. Recurrent episodes of acute iritis resulted in scarring and depigmentation of the iris and irregularity of the pupil.

Laboratory Tests

Laboratory studies are not diagnostic for ankylosing spondylitis and, with the exception of the erythrocyte sedimentation rate and HLA-B27 antigen, are not helpful. The HLA-B27 antigen has been found to be positive in 80 to 90 per cent of patients with ankylosing spondylitis whereas it is found in only 8 per cent of the general population. It is important to realize, however, that the risk of development of ankylosing spondylitis in individuals with this antigen is less than 2 per cent. First-degree relatives of HLA-B27 positive patients with ankylosing spondylitis have nearly a 20 per cent risk.[92] The erythrocyte sedimentation rate is elevated in approximately 80 per cent of patients, especially during the initial years of the disease process. It can also be elevated intermittently during periods of active disease but at other times remain normal.

Radiographic Features

In the absence of sufficient clinical or laboratory tests to confirm the diagnosis of ankylosing spondylitis, we must rely on its radiographic features. These may be detected approximately three to six months after the onset of the disease. These findings may seem complex, but by keeping the basic pathology in mind one can almost predict its subsequent radiographic representation. These changes include sites of osteoporosis secondary to osteitis; osteolysis and cyst formation due to fibrous tissue replacement of bone and cartilage; and ossification that leads to bony sclerosis and ankylosis. It should be remembered that these events tend to localize at the bone–ligament interface (enthesis) (Fig. 18–4).

The earliest radiographic findings almost invariably develop about the sacroiliac joints. The findings in the sacroiliac joints again reflect the pathologic sequence of events already described. These findings are characteristically symmetric bilaterally and include a patchy osteoporosis, ill-defined joint margins, and wid-

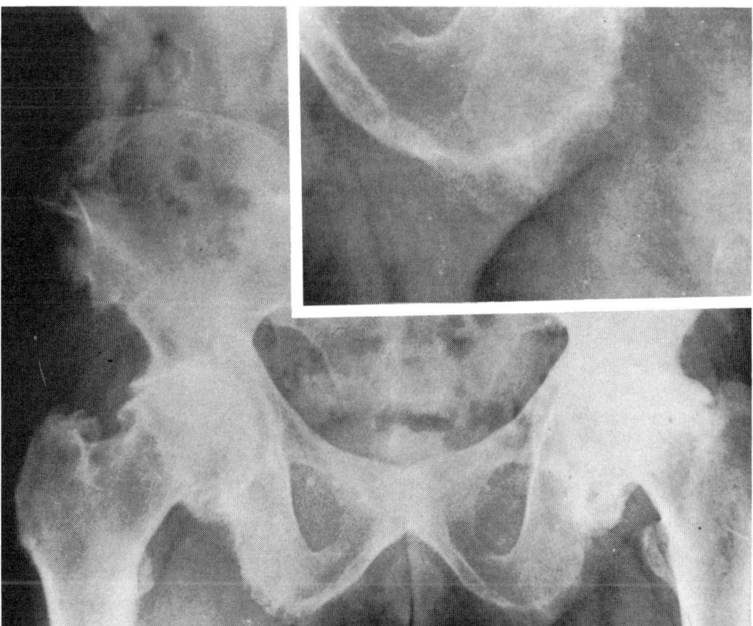

Figure 18–4. Entheses: general radiographic abnormalities in ankylosing spondylitis may include hyperostosis of the ilium and greater trochanter. Note the "whiskering" of the ilium.

ening of the joint space. Subchondral erosions develop as well, typically on the iliac side of the joint. These changes reflect the active inflammatory process of the disease. Purely subchondral sclerosis localized to the iliac side of the joint may be seen, representing the earliest phase of the ossification reaction. This patchy ossification then typically becomes widespread with irregular bridging of the joint, and frequently leads to complete obliteration of the joint (Fig. 18–5).

It is important that the bony changes in the spine secondary to ankylosing spondylitis be differentiated from other disease processes. Bone spur formation may result from osteoarthritis, hypermobility, Forestier's disease, ankylosing spondylitis, or other spondyloarthropathies. Each of these processes has characteristic radiographic features (Fig. 18–6). Osteophytes represent pathologic new bone formation at the attachment site of the spinal ligaments or intervertebral disc. These develop

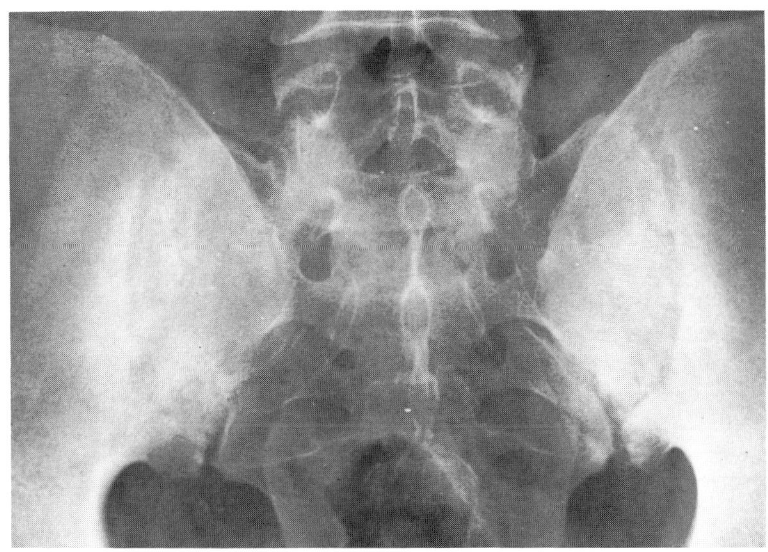

Figure 18–5. Advanced stage of sacroiliac involvement demonstrating extensive, symmetric, sclerotic changes on both the sacral and iliac portions of the joint. Focal areas of ankylosis are also seen.

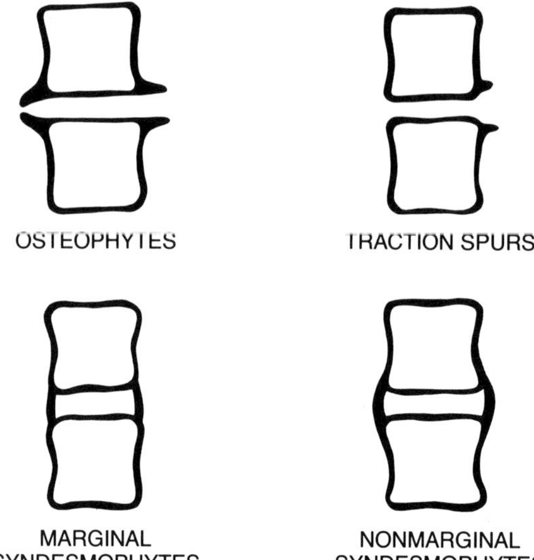

Figure 18–6. Diagrammatic representation of osteophytes, traction spurs, and marginal and nonmarginal syndesmophytes.

on the anterior and lateral surfaces of the vertebral body secondary to disc degeneration. These bone spurs have a typical horizontal orientation and are usually associated with significant narrowing of the joint space (Fig. 18–7). Macnab differentiates the traction spur from other osteophytes as they arise secondary to stress at the site of ligamentous attachment. These spurs are horizontally oriented as well and arise 2 mm away from the distal border of the anterior and lateral surfaces of the vertebral body. Their presence in the lumbar spine may denote segmental instability (Fig. 18–8). Marginal syndesmophytes are seen in ankylosing spondylitis and are represented by thin, vertically oriented ossification of the paravertebral region (Fig. 18–9). Nonmarginal syndesmophytes are typical of psoriatic arthritis and Reiter's syndrome and arise along the waist or midportion of the vertebral body, extending upward in a vertical fashion. They appear broader and coarser than those of ankylosing spondylitis (Fig. 18–10).

The earliest sign of change in the vertebral column in ankylosing spondylitis is a sharp squaring of the anterior portion of the vertebral body at the thoracolumbar junction. The anterior concavity of each vertebrae is lost, resulting in a square appearance (Fig. 18–11). Occasionally the Romanus lesion may be seen, represented by erosion and sclerosis localized to the upper or lower corner of the vertebrae. The reparative process eventually takes over, with sclerosis and syndesmophyte formation. This ossification process occurs beneath the anterior longitudinal ligament in the fibers of the annulus fibrosus at each level. The ossification is disposed in a vertical fashion, as opposed to the osteophytes of osteoarthritis, which extend radially or obliquely. The bamboo spine appearance eventually results (Fig. 18–12). The apophyseal joint later develops erosions, becomes narrow, and fuses. This

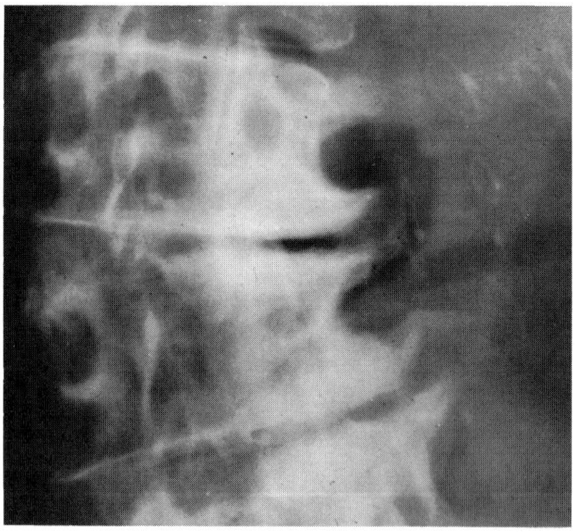

Figure 18–7. Extensive degenerative changes of the intervertebral disc associated with osteophyte formation. Note the horizontal orientation of the bone spurs and loss of disc height.

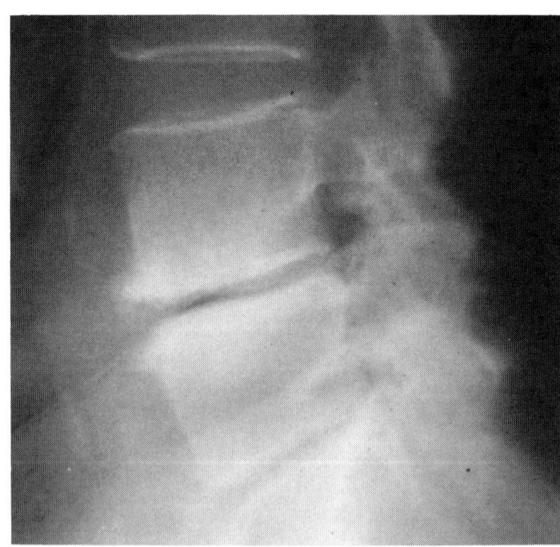

Figure 18–8. Traction spur: a horizontally directed bone spur arising 2 mm away from the disc space.

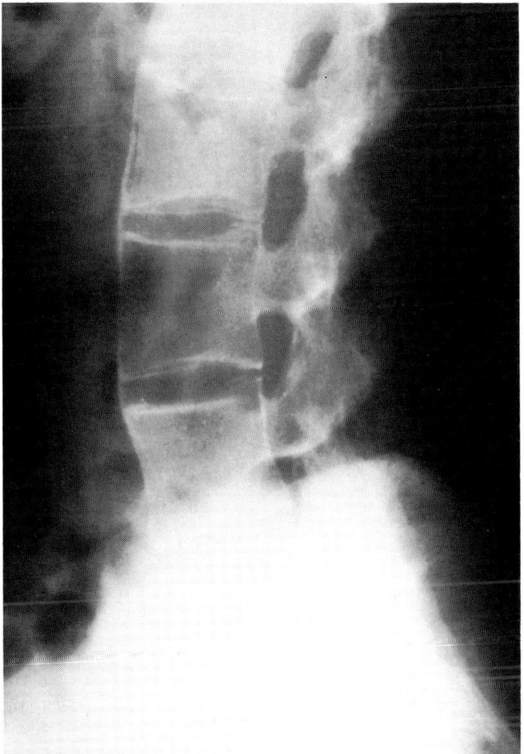

Figure 18–9. Lateral radiograph demonstrating typical marginal syndesmophytes. The ossification process occurs just beneath the anterior longitudinal ligament. Note the thin, vertical orientation of the syndesmophytes.

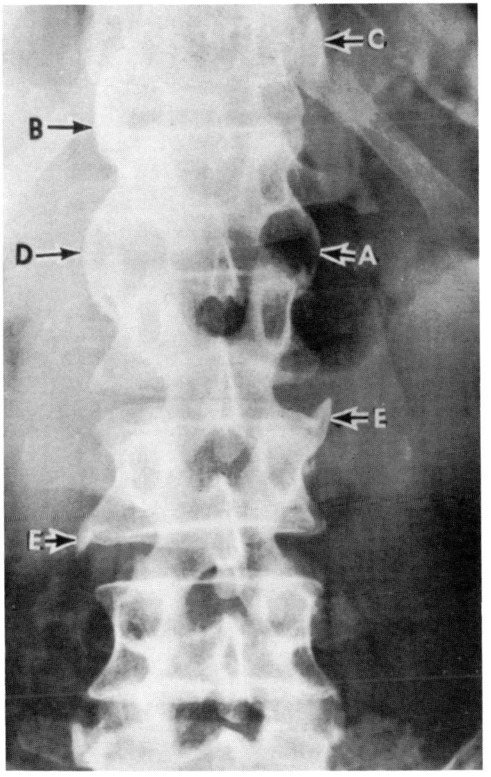

Figure 18–10. Nonmarginal syndesmophytes: vertically oriented, thick, bony bridges extend from the midportion of one vertebral body to another.

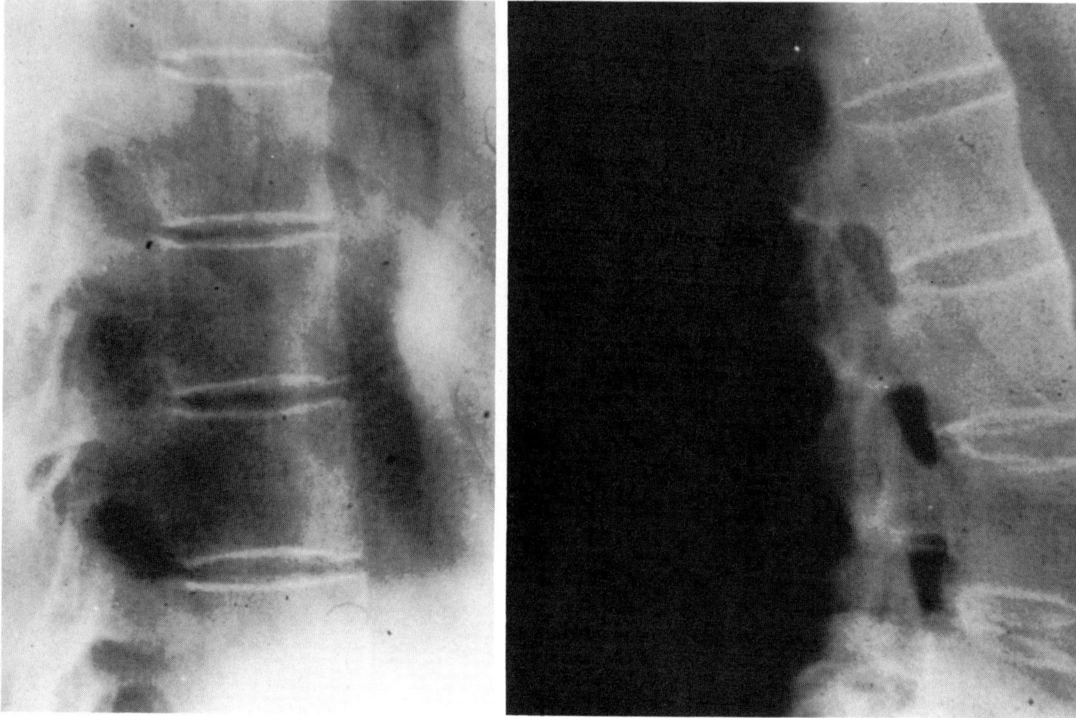

Figure 18–11. *Left,* Lateral radiograph of the thoracolumbar junction demonstrating squaring of the anterior portion of the vertebral body. This represents an early change secondary to a localized erosive osteitis. *Right,* In a different patient the reparative process is marked with syndesmophyte formation, representing ossification of the intervertebral disc.

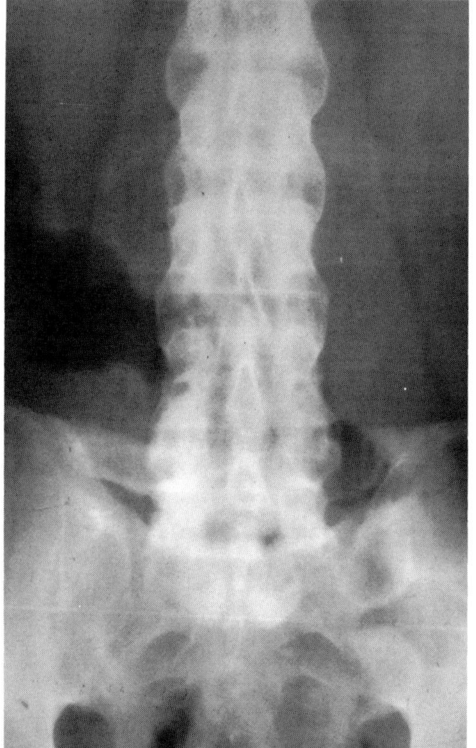

Figure 18–12. Frontal radiograph revealing extensive syndesmophyte formation extending upward in a vertical fashion from one vertebral body to the next, producing a "bamboo" appearance.

process tends to progress in a cephalad direction, involving the lumbar spine first, followed by the thoracic and cervical regions. Similar changes are seen in the thoracic region, many times resulting in a kyphotic deformity. Involvement of the cervical spine as well extends along the anterior aspect of the vertebral bodies, resulting in loss of the normal lordosis. In more severe cases a chin-on-chest type of deformity may result, with significant functional visual field impairment. Atlantoaxial instability, although not as common as in the rheumatoid patient, must be considered. Assessment for atlantoaxial instability is completed with flexion-extension views of the cervical spine. An atlantodental interval of more than 3 mm is considered abnormal in the adult.

Natural History

The natural history of ankylosing spondylitis is characterized by intermittent, active phases of the disease, producing symptoms and radiographic features already described. Involvement is typically initiated in the sacroiliac joints, followed by involvement of the thoracolumbar spine and subsequent upward extension into the thoracic and cervical regions. Between these periods of disease activity are periods of inactivity that may last months or years. As such, involvement of the cervical spine may occur over a period ranging from 5 to 30 years. Despite these extensive changes, most patients lead a reasonably normal life with average expectancy. In a study reviewing the natural history of the disease, Carette and associates found that 47 of 51 war veterans functioned well after a mean disease duration of 38 years despite the fact that nearly one half of these patients had severe restriction of spinal motion.[17] Furthermore, patients with only mild loss of spinal motion after 10 years failed to show evidence of progressive disease. The limiting factors in functional capacity appear most closely related to disease of the hips and extraskeletal manifestations of the disease. In Carette's study, early onset of peripheral joint involvement suggests a relatively bad prognosis. It was also found that if the hips were normal after 10 years, they do not become affected thereafter.[17]

Treatment

Conservative measures are the mainstay of treatment for patients with ankylosing spondylitis. Anti-inflammatory medications can be effective in diminishing the symptoms of pain and stiffness. Phenylbutazone and indomethacin appear more effective than aspirin in treating this condition.[32] Indomethacin has less serious side effects and therefore is generally considered the drug of choice. There has been no study to show that the natural history of the disease is altered with any form of medication; however, medication coupled with an exercise program to maintain motion and limit deformity is advocated.

Surgical intervention of the spine for patients with ankylosing spondylitis is uncommon; however, patients with severe deformity limiting their normal daily activity may require or be amenable to an extension osteotomy. The characteristic deformities as already described include a loss of lumbar lordosis, which may be associated with the excessive thoracic and cervical kyphosis. In the cervical region, atlantoaxial instability and atlanto-occipital disability present additional concerns to the surgeon.

In assessing the patient with ankylosing spondylitis, the primary site of deformity must be correctly recognized. Clinical and radiographic evaluation of the entire spine and hip joints is imperative to correctly address the patient's deformity surgically. Simmons believes that the most effective and reproducible method of measuring the deformity is the so called chin–brow to vertical angle.[84] This angle is measured from the brow to the chin to the vertical axis with the patient standing and hips and knees extended. The head is placed in the neutral or fixed position. In any patient with significant hip disease, surgical treatment of the hips must be addressed before spinal surgery.

Differential Diagnosis

Several other entities must be considered when patients present with a history of low back pain. A list of these conditions is presented in Table 18–1. Most of these will be discussed in abbreviated fashion, emphasizing the clinical and radiographic features distinguishing them from ankylosing spondylitis. The more common entities, including the seronegative spondyloarthropathies, rheumatoid arthritis, juvenile rheumatoid arthritis, and crystal-induced forms of arthritis, will be reviewed in more detail.

Table 18–1. RADIOGRAPHIC DIFFERENTIAL DIAGNOSIS OF SACROILIITIS

Ankylosing spondylitis
Enteropathic spondyloarthropathies
Ulcerative colitis
Crohn's disease
Whipple's disease
Reiter's syndrome
Psoriatic arthritis
Rheumatoid arthritis
Juvenile rheumatoid arthritis
Crystal-induced arthropathies
Gout
Calcium pyrophosphate crystal deposition disease
Diffuse idiopathic skeletal hyperostosis
Paraplegia
Osteitis condensans ilii
Fluorosis
Ochronosis
Behçet's syndrome
Neuropathic arthropathy
Paget's disease
Infection
Neoplasia
Osteoarthritis

Diffuse Idiopathic Skeletal Hyperostosis

Diffuse idiopathic skeletal hyperostosis (DISH) also known as Forestier's disease and ankylosing hyperostosis, is a relatively common disease affecting predominantly middle-aged and elderly men. It is often asymptomatic but may produce limited motion and discomfort. DISH is characterized radiographically by laminated new bone formation involving the anterior and lateral spinal ligaments of the thoracic, lumbar, and cervical spine without accompanying narrowing of the disc space, osteoporosis, or ankylosis (Fig. 18–13).[30, 89]

Specific criteria have been developed to differentiate DISH from either degenerative disc disease or ankylosing spondylitis.[75] These features include preservation of intervertebral disc height, ossification along the anterolateral aspect of at least four consecutive vertebral bodies, absence of apophyseal joint ankylosis

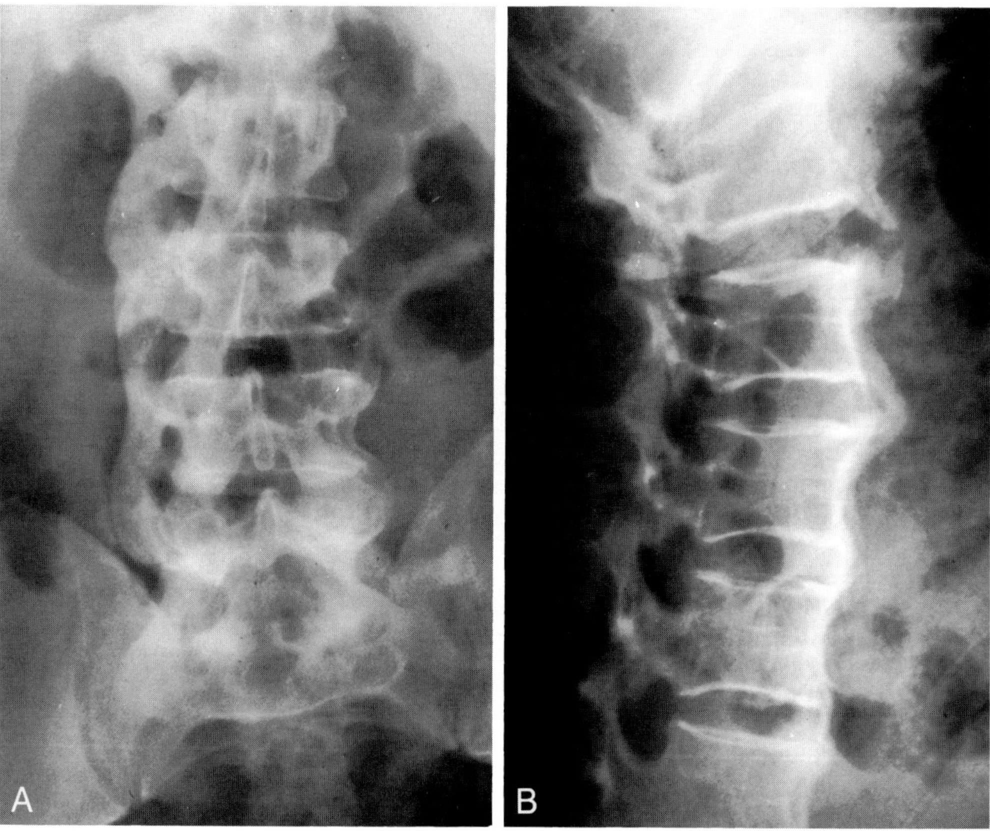

Figure 18–13. *A, B,* Forestier's disease: frontal and lateral radiographs of the lumbar region demonstrating "flowing mantles" of ossification without disc narrowing or osteoporosis. Note the preservation of the facet joints.

or sacroiliac joint erosions, sclerosis or fusion, and absence of vacuum phenomena or vertebral body marginal sclerosis. The thoracic spine is involved most often. It is interesting to note that the left side of the thoracic region is generally spared. These axial manifestations are often accompanied by similar peripheral changes at areas of musculotendinous and capsular insertions. Such diffuse radiographic findings suggest that this disorder represents a bone-forming diathesis rather than a localized disorder of the spine.

Paraplegia

Long-standing mechanical stress across the sacroiliac joint has been proposed as a mechanism of creating degenerative changes in the sacroiliac joints of paraplegics. The combined effect of osteoporosis and lack of muscular support for the spine and pelvis can lead to narrowing in the sacroiliac joints but is typically seen without erosions or ankylosis (Fig. 18–14). In a study of paraplegic men, such changes were noted in close to 30 per cent of the patients.[98]

Osteitis Condensans Ilii

Osteitis condensans ilii represents a lesion localized to the iliac side of the sacroiliac joint. It is characterized by a bilateral triangularly shaped area of sclerosis in the medial portion of the ilium.[66] Such changes are particularly common in postpartum women. The cause of this lesion is uncertain, but it has been postulated that it develops secondary to the mechanical strain placed on the joint during pregnancy. It should also be noted that there has been no direct association between the presence of this lesion and back pain. Therefore, in the presence of pain, other causes should be ruled out, including osteoid osteoma, osteoarthritis, or ankylosing spondylitis.

The radiographic features that differentiate osteitis condensans ilii from ankylosing spondylitis include preservation of the sacroiliac joint and sclerotic changes confined to the iliac side of the joint (Fig. 18–15).[88]

Fluorosis

Fluoride salts are used in industry in the production of several products, including insecticides. Chronic exposure to fluorides either from industry or through direct ingestion from drinking-water may result in fluorosis. In these instances fluorides are absorbed from the gut and form an insoluble precipitate with calcium, resulting in hypocalcemia. Clinically it is manifested by weight loss, weakness, anemia, osteosclerosis, progressive stiffness, and limited motion of the joints.[87] Evidence of osteosclerosis and formation of exostoses are usually first manifested in flat bones, especially the pelvis and jaw, and in the vertebrae. Severe

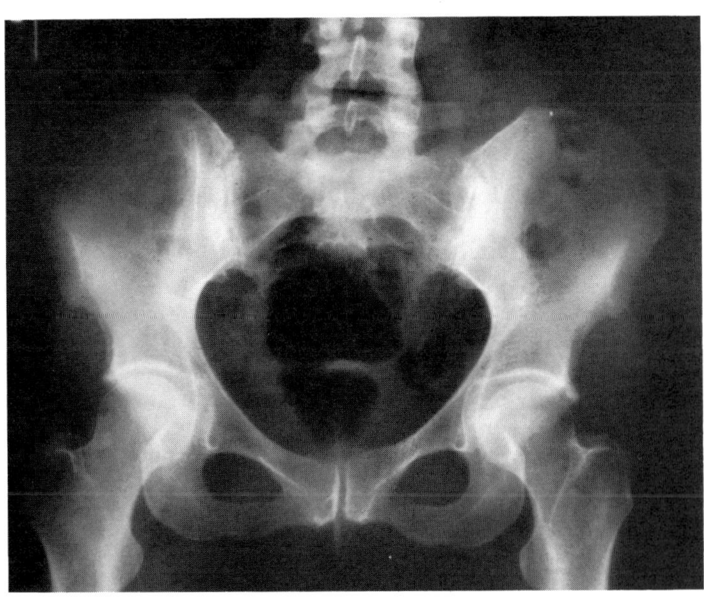

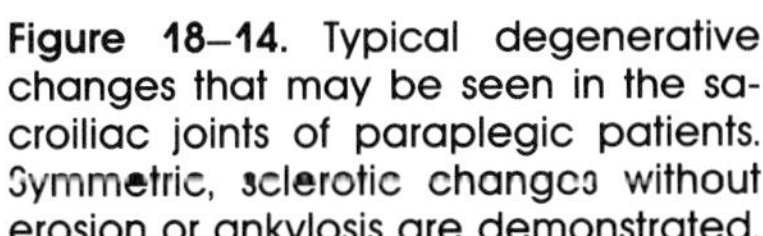
Figure 18–14. Typical degenerative changes that may be seen in the sacroiliac joints of paraplegic patients. Symmetric, sclerotic changes without erosion or ankylosis are demonstrated.

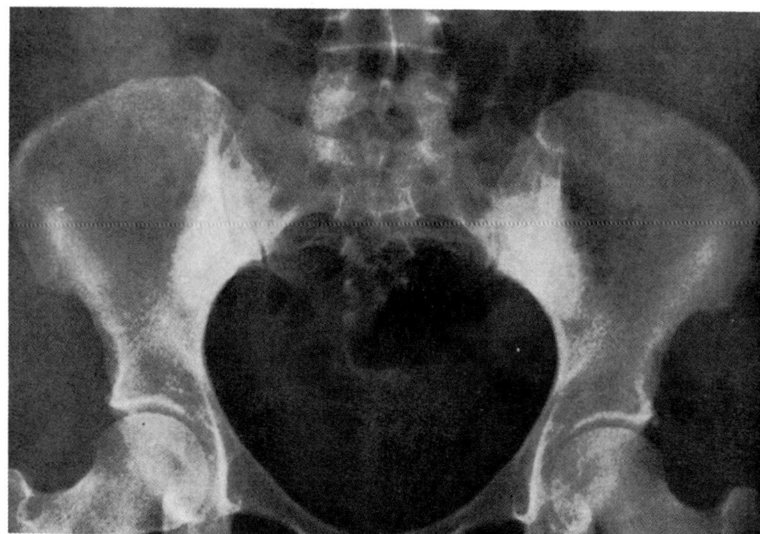

Figure 18–15. Osteitis condensans ilii: note the bilaterally symmetric triangular areas of sclerosis localized to the iliac side of the sacroiliac joint.

spinal involvement can result in ankylosis with mineralization of the spinal ligaments. The extensive and uniform nature of this osteosclerosis, coupled with eventual involvement of the appendicular skeleton and absence of erosions in the sacroiliac joints, are features that differentiate this process from ankylosing spondylitis (Fig. 18–16).

Ochronosis

Alkaptonuria is a rare disorder of tyrosine catabolism. Deficiency of the enzyme homogentisic acid oxidase leads to excretion of large amounts of homogentisic acid in the urine. Accumulation of oxidized homogentisic acid pigment in the connective tissue is known as ochronosis. After several years ochronosis produces a distinct form of degenerative arthritis.[68] This condition is probably transmitted by a single recessive autosomal gene.[42]

Clinically this condition often goes unrecognized until middle life, when degenerative joint disease appears. Ochronosis is detected earlier only if homogentisic acid is found in the urine. In the infant, once the urine is allowed to oxidize in the diaper, it will appear as a dark stain. Pigmentation of the ears, skin, and sclera are other early manifestations of ochronosis. Deposition of pigment in the intervertebral discs and articular cartilages of the lower joints also leads to symptoms of spondylosis and peripheral arthropathy. The clinical and radiographic findings associated with ochronosis are similar to those found in osteoarthritis.

Most patients with ochronosis past the age of 30 develop spondylosis. This often is the

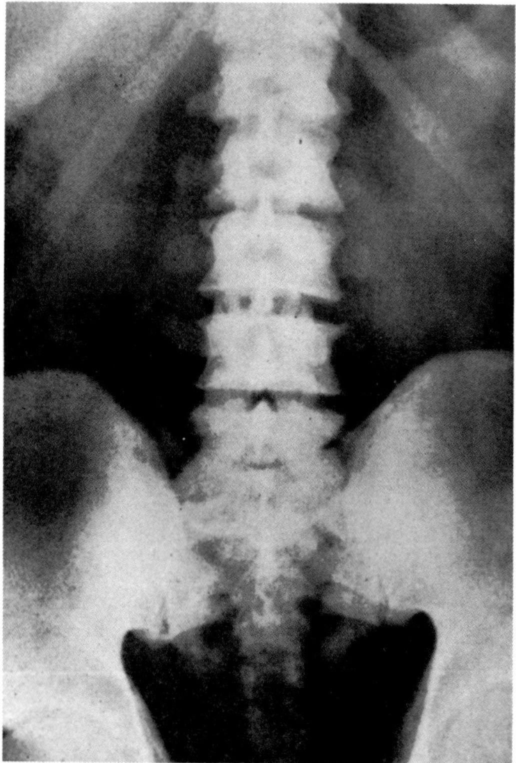

Figure 18–16. Fluorosis: dense osteosclerosis of the spine and pelvis.

first musculoskeletal manifestation of this disease. Stiffness is the usual primary complaint and is usually associated with some degree of discomfort. Examination of these patients reveals marked limitation of motion or even ankylosis in the lumbar and dorsal spine. Cervical spine involvement is also commonly seen radiographically but most of these patients maintain their motion in this region of the spine. The overall alignment of the spine in long-standing ochronosis is one of kyphosis and therefore may be confused with ankylosing spondylitis. It should be noted that many of these patients first have symptoms consistent with a herniated disc.[68] This may well be due to weakening of the annulus fibrosus with subsequent herniation.

The earliest radiographic changes in the spine of a patient with ochronosis include calcification and subsequent narrowing of the intervertebral discs. A study of these crystalline deposits has shown them to be hydroxyapatite. Such calcifications are not diagnostic of ochronosis, however, since they may be seen in hemochromatosis, pseudogout, and chronic respiratory paralytic poliomyelitis. Osteophytes tend to be relatively small in the early course of the disease but may be extensive in elderly patients. Osteoporosis of the vertebral bodies is also characteristic and tends to accentuate the calcified disc (Fig. 18–17).

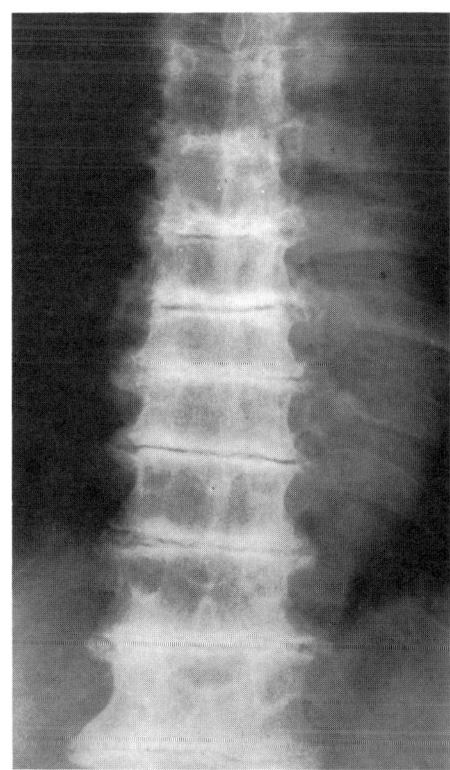

Figure 18–17. Ochronosis: frontal radiograph of the thoracic spine with extensive narrowing of the intervertebral discs. Calcification of the remaining disc, osteoporosis of the vertebral bodies, and osteophyte formation are all demonstrated.

Patients with ochronosis may be distinguished from those with ankylosing spondylitis by several radiographic features. In sharp contrast to ankylosing spondylitis in ochronosis, the sacroiliac joints are not fused but may show degenerative changes. In addition, the facet joints maintain their normal radiographic appearance, the lumbar vertebrae maintain their normal anterior concavity, and the bamboo appearance secondary to annular ossification does not appear.

Whipple's Disease

Whipple's disease is a rare disorder of unknown cause characterized by arthralgia, abdominal pain, diarrhea, progressive weight loss, and impaired intestinal absorption.[96] Low-grade fever, skin pigmentation, and peripheral lymphadenopathy are frequently seen.

Peripheral joint manifestations similar to those described in ulcerative colitis and Crohn's disease represent a prominent feature of Whipple's disease and have been reported in 65 to 90 per cent of cases. In approximately 50 per cent of these patients joint involvement antedates the development of intestinal disease. Arthritis is seen intermittently during the course of the disease and tends to have a migratory pattern. Involvement in any joint typically lasts for several days and only rarely leads to development of chronic or residual complaints. Involvement in the peripheral joints is typically bilateral but may occasionally manifest as monarticular disease. The knees, ankles, hands, hips, wrists, and elbows are most frequently involved.[41, 50, 79]

Sacroiliac involvement has been rarely reported in patients with Whipple's disease.[16, 41] In a report of 64 patients with Whipple's disease two were recorded as having bilateral sacroiliac fusion and another had unilateral fusion.[41] Nearly 20 per cent of the patients with Whipple's disease in this study were reported to have back pain yet failed to reveal any radiographic evidence of spondylitis.

In a more recent study, nearly one third of patients with Whipple's disease and evidence of arthritis displayed clinical or radiographic evidence of spinal involvement.[23] Such spondylitic changes occur with a much higher frequency than in the general population, yet in most cases they do not meet the criteria for ankylosing spondylitis.

Behçet's Syndrome

Behçet's syndrome is a multisystem disorder characterized by recurrent oral and genital ulcers and iritis.[5, 84] Other clinical manifestations include arthritis, thrombophlebitis, neurologic abnormalities, and skin lesions.[71]

Arthritis can be seen in approximately 50 per cent of patients and may precede, accompany, or follow the other symptoms of Behçet's syndrome. It most often involves the appendicular skeleton in a pattern similar to rheumatoid arthritis. The knees, elbows, and ankles are most commonly affected. The smaller joints of the hands and feet may also be involved. Skeletal involvement is typically polyarticular and asymmetric. These patients develop synovitis and effusions but rarely develop significant erosive changes. Sacroiliitis and spondylitis have been reported in patients with Behçet's syndrome. Whether this syndrome has some association with ankylosing spondylitis is also a matter of debate. In a report by Dilsen and associates, approximately 20 per cent of 106 patients with Behçet's syndrome had ankylosing spondylitis.[25] An additional 60 per cent of these patients had radiographic evidence of sacroiliitis. Both the ankylosing spondylitis and sacroiliitis were mild and not progressive. Other reports have not supported Dilsen's high incidence of spinal and sacroiliac involvement, however, and therefore the association of these symptoms with Behçet's syndrome remains unclear.[37, 70]

Neuropathic Arthropathy

Neuropathic joint disease (Charcot joints) is a form of chronic, progressive, and degenerative arthritis that may affect either peripheral or axial articulations. Charcot joints develop as a result of a disturbance in the normal sensory innervation of the joints and represent a complication of several neurologic disorders, including syringomyelia, paraplegia, peripheral neuropathy, diăbetes, and syphilitic tabes dorsalis.

The pathoetiology of such degenerative changes appears related to the loss of proprioceptive or pain sensation, leading to loss of sensory motor reflexes that normally protect the joint from the stresses of everyday motion. Chronic injury results in significant damage to the articular cartilage and subchondral fracture, which leads to significant deformity and instability. Pathologic findings are consistent with those seen in osteoarthritis.[36] Fibrillation and erosion of articular cartilage, loose body formation, and exuberant growth of marginal osteophytes are typically seen.

These patients have either pain or instability of the joint. Because of the neurologic impairment, however, pain is typically mild or moderate and generally inconsistent with the extensive physical findings. Such findings include effusions, deformity, instability, crepitation, and hypermobility. The large weight-bearing joints are usually affected in tabes dorsalis, and therefore such changes are typically seen in the hips, knees, and lumbar spine. In syringomyelia upper extremity changes are obviously more common. In diabetic neuropathy the foot and ankle represent the usual areas of involvement.

Vertebral neuroarthropathy is most often associated with tabes dorsalis but has also been described in syringomyelia and diabetes mellitus.[15, 21] The lumbar spine is most commonly affected in tabes dorsalis, but in more severe cases the thoracic and cervical regions also may be involved. In syringomyelia the cervical spine is most commonly affected. Patients with severe vertebral involvement may have symptoms of nerve root compression with either radicular pain or weakness in the lower extremity. Some patients may also complain of back pain, but the severity of this is generally not consistent with the extensive radiographic features. Deformity and instability may also be seen on clinical and radiographic examination. Radiographically, changes consistent with advanced spondylosis are seen and include osteophyte formation, facet hypertrophy, and vertebral body sclerosis.[76] Compression fractures also may be commonly seen (Fig. 18–18).

Initial treatment is usually conservative and may include rest, bracing, and anti-inflammatory medications. Intractable pain or weakness secondary to nerve root compression or evidence of spinal cord impingement serve as indications for surgery, however, particularly

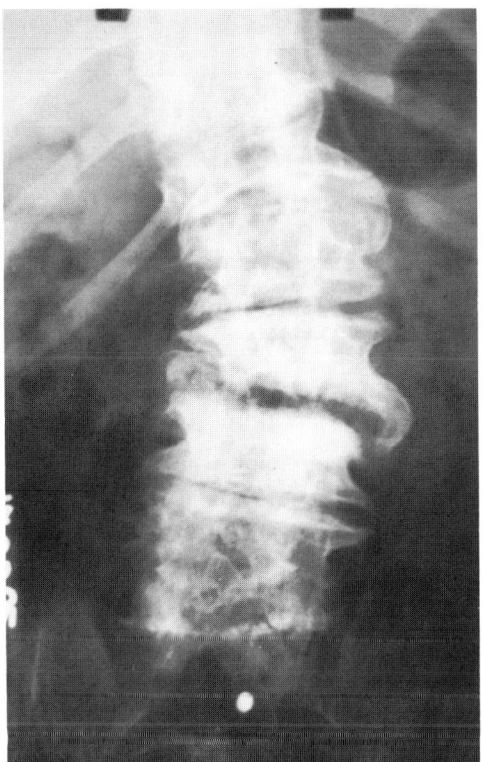

Figure 18–18. Charcot spine: advanced destructive changes in a patient with tabes dorsalis. Changes are consistent with extensive spondylosis, including osteophyte formation, vertebral body osteosclerosis, facet hypertrophy, deformity, and instability.

if these neurologic abnormalities are progressive.

Paget's Disease

Paget's disease is a chronic disturbance of the adult skeleton resulting in softening, enlargement, and bowing of the long bones with a disarranged osseous structure. The cause of this disorder remains unknown. Patients with Paget's disease may complain of low back pain but several features of this disease serve to easily differentiate it from ankylosing spondylitis. The onset of Paget's disease is typically in middle age and is associated with an elevated alkaline phosphatase during the active phases of the disease. These patients do not complain of stiffness in the spine and have normal lumbar motion and chest expansion.

The radiographic features of Paget's disease include diffuse, mottled, or linear areas of sclerosis with coarsened trabeculae and rarefaction. Such changes are commonly seen in the pelvis. There is no radiographic evidence of sacroiliitis because the joints are preserved (Fig. 18–19). Additionally, lack of syndesmophyte formation and squaring of the lumbar vertebral bodies are not seen in Paget's disease, which easily differentiates it from ankylosing spondylitis.

Infection and Neoplasia

Early in the course of ankylosing spondylitis unilateral sacroiliac involvement is not uncommon. Such changes upon initial evaluation may raise the possibility of infection. Other clinical features, including fever, excessive pain, or an elevated white blood cell count, tend to differentiate infection from ankylosing spondylitis. In the absence of such findings, follow-up radiographs at six to nine months typically show bilateral changes in the sacroiliac joints suggesting ankylosing spondylitis (Fig. 18–20).

The destructive lesions of the spine described in ankylosing spondylitis may also be confused with tumor. One must always consider these possibilities in patients with ankylosing spondylitis. Review of the patient's clinical presentation and examination, laboratory tests, and radiographs are necessary to determine the need for further investigative measures such as biopsy.

Osteoarthritis

Degenerative joint disease affecting the apophyseal and intervertebral joints of the lumbosacral spine is common. The typical clinical setting of an older patient with characteristic radiographic changes usually serves to differentiate this condition from inflammatory processes. Typical changes in the degenerative lumbar spine include disc narrowing and osteophyte formation. Because of the altered biomechanics of the intervertebral disc, the peripheral portion of the vertebral end plate takes on an increasing weight-bearing load with subsequent subchondral sclerosis. The facet joints also exhibit both hypertrophic and sclerotic changes.

ENTEROPATHIC SPONDYLOARTHROPATHIES

Spondylitis associated with both ulcerative colitis and Crohn's disease (regional enteritis) will be discussed.

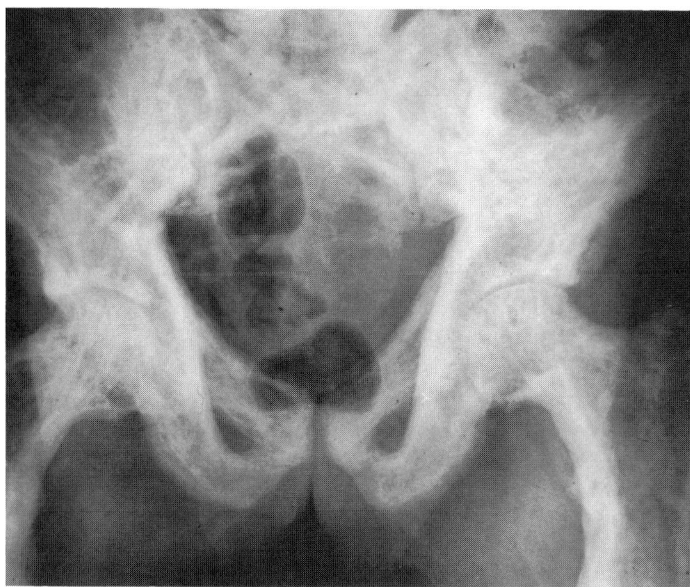

Figure 18–19. Diffuse, mottled appearance of the pelvis in a patient with Paget's disease. The sacroiliac joints are preserved.

Ulcerative colitis is common in the United States with prevalence rates of 40 to 100 per 100,000 population reported. Approximately 20 per cent of these patients develop either a peripheral arthropathy or spondylitis.[22, 60, 100] Crohn's disease or regional enteritis is a chronic granulomatous inflammatory disease capable of affecting both the small and large intestine. It affects patients during young adulthood with a prevalence of 20 to 40 per 100,000. The reported prevalence of spondylitis in patients with Crohn's disease ranges from 2 to 7 per cent.

Clinical Manifestations

Peripheral arthritis develops in approximately 15 per cent of both ulcerative colitis and Crohn's disease patients.[22, 60] This form of arthritis occurs with equal frequency in men and women and tends to occur either simultaneously with the colitis or closely follow the onset of the disease. Subsequent intermittent bouts of arthritis may accompany flare-ups of the intestinal disease. The peripheral form of arthritis is typically acute in onset and involves the large weight-bearing joints, with a predi-

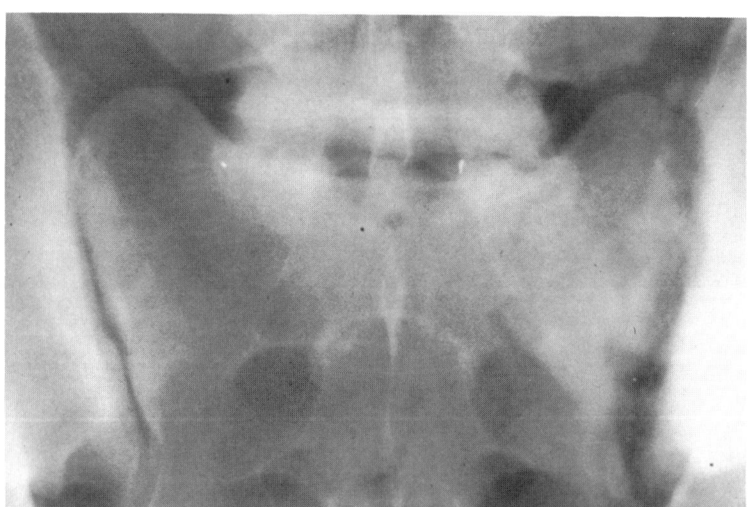

Figure 18–20. Unilateral widening and erosion of the sacroiliac joint in a patient with infection.

lection for the knees and ankles. A migratory pattern may be seen mimicking acute rheumatic fever. Joint involvement may or may not be symmetric and typically fails to produce significant clinical or radiographic evidence of permanent joint damage.

In patients with peripheral arthritis, tests for rheumatoid factor are typically negative, antistreptolysin titers (ASO) are normal, and no abnormalities of human lymphocyte antigens (HLA) have been found. Synovial fluid analysis reveals an inflammatory-type reactivity.

Spondylitis and sacroiliitis in either ulcerative colitis or regional enteritis follows a much different course from that of peripheral arthritis. The clinical and radiographic changes that occur here generally progress independently of the course of colitis, as opposed to peripheral involvement. There appear to be two forms of spondylitis that occur in patients with these inflammatory bowel diseases. The first is a relatively mild form and is often asymptomatic. These patients are HLA-B27 negative, and the onset of radiographic features or symptoms consistent with spondylitis often antedates the appearance of ulcerative colitis or regional enteritis. The second form displays features identical to those of classic idiopathic ankylosing spondylitis. The development of such changes appears related to the presence of the HLA-B27 antigen.[22, 61] Approximately 75 per cent of both ulcerative colitis and Crohn's disease patients who develop ankylosing spondylitis have been found to be HLA-B27 positive. These figures, in conjunction with the fact that relatives of these patients have a higher incidence of spondylitis or sacroiliitis, suggests that factors unrelated to the inflammation of Crohn's disease or ulcerative colitis are responsible for the development of these findings.

The clinical and radiographic findings are identical to those described for ankylosing spondylitis (Fig. 18–21). The spondylitis is generally progressive and, as indicated earlier, unrelated to the course of the bowel disease. Treatment for patients with either peripheral or spondylitic-type symptoms should be directed primarily at the underlying bowel disease. Peripheral joint symptoms can usually be managed adequately with a conservative regimen of rest, anti-inflammatory medications, and physical therapy. Successful treatment of the underlying disease process often ameliorates the symptoms of peripheral arthritis.

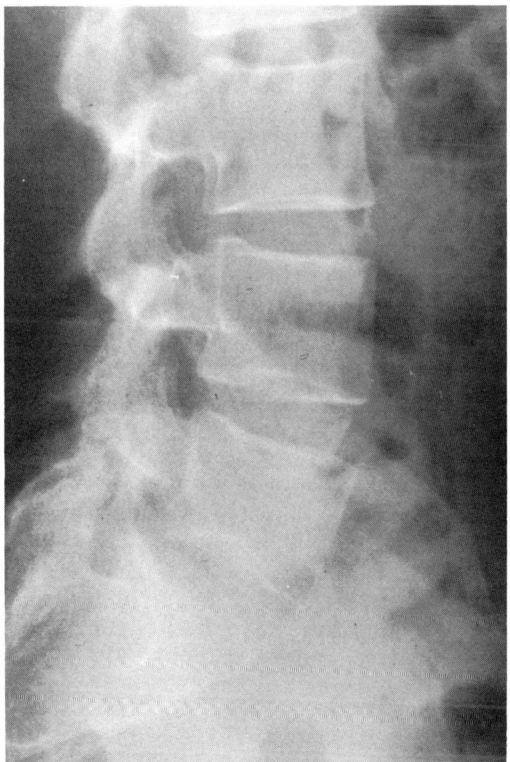

Figure 18–21. Enteropathic spondyloarthropathy: lateral radiograph of the lumbar spine demonstrating marginal syndesmophyte formation.

Treatment for spondylitis and sacroiliitis is similar to that outlined for ankylosing spondylitis. As opposed to the peripheral forms of arthritis, progressive spondylitis will not be affected by colectomy. These findings further support the completely different nature of these symptomatic processes.

REITER'S SYNDROME

Reiter's syndrome may be defined clinically by the presence of peripheral arthritis occurring with urethritis, conjunctivitis, and frequently mucocutaneous lesions. The occurrence of peripheral arthritis with two of the three nonarticular manifestations is the basis for clinical diagnosis. The American Rheumatism Association has developed new criteria for the disease. A comparative study of several spondyloarthropathies indicated that the most sensitive and specific variable for recognition of Reiter's syndrome is an episode of arthritis lasting at least one month after an episode of urethritis or cervicitis.[97]

The incidence and prevalence of this disease has been difficult to estimate because of several factors. It is believed that Reiter's syndrome is a relatively common rheumatic disease and in fact may be the most common cause of inflammatory arthropathy in young men. The development of arthritis in these patients may be related to the presence of the HLA-B27 antigen. Although only 3 per cent of patients with nonspecific urethritis develop arthritis, the risk appears to increase to nearly 20 per cent in the HLA-B27–positive population.

The diagnosis of Reiter's syndrome may be made at any age but is most often recognized during the third decade. Men are more commonly affected, but the condition is more difficult to diagnose in women. The sexually acquired form of the disease is almost always confined to men and is seen rarely in women. Postdysenteric forms of Reiter's syndrome probably have an equal sex distribution.

Etiology

The pathogenesis of Reiter's syndrome is probably determined by the interrelationship of environmental and genetic factors. Reiter's syndrome is considered by many investigators to be a postinfectious reactive form of arthritis. Postvenereal Reiter's syndrome is often considered the most common form of the disease, especially in the United States. These cases appear to be associated either with *Chlamydia* or *Ureaplasma* infection. This association has been disputed; however, evidence confirming the presence of synovial chlamydial antigen by immunoperoxidase and immunofluorescent techniques supports the belief that this organism may induce a reactive arthropathy.[39, 81]

Reiter's syndrome is also known to occur after outbreaks of bacillary dysentery secondary to *Shigella flexneri, Salmonella,* and *Yersinia enterocolitica,* although only 1 to 2 per cent of affected individuals will develop Reiter's syndrome. On a chronic basis these organisms may not cause obvious diarrhea, but can precipitate a recurrence of symptoms consistent with Reiter's syndrome without diarrhea.

The association of HLA-B27 antigen and development of Reiter's syndrome was first reported in 1973 by Brewerton and associates and subsequently reported by others.[9] It is generally believed to be present in approximately 60 to 85 per cent of patients. It has been suggested that non–HLA-B27–positive individuals with Reiter's syndrome are likely to have one of the other cross-reacting antigens, HLA-B217, Bw22, or Bw42, a finding that supports the theory that HLA-B27 or another cross-reacting antigen is relevant in the pathogenesis of the disease rather than a postulated immune response–linked gene.

Clinical Features

Reiter's syndrome is a systemic disorder. The two most common clinically evident features of the disease are polyarthritis and urethritis (or cervicitis); both are seen in over 90 per cent of patients.

The arthritis of Reiter's syndrome is asymmetric with a predilection for the large and small joints of the lower extremities, especially the knees and ankles. Upper extremity involvement, particularly of the shoulder and hand, is not infrequent. The typical patient presents with a knee effusion accompanied by involvement of the interphalangeal joints of the foot, producing a "sausage toe" or dactylitis. Accompanying symptoms of Achilles tendinitis, plantar fasciitis, back pain, chest wall pain, and other arthralgias are common. These represent forms of insertional tendinitis or enthesopathy. Heel pain ranks second to synovitis of the knee as the main musculoskeletal complaint.

Urinary tract symptoms are often a presenting feature of Reiter's syndrome. A mucopurulent discharge is often seen but with minimal symptoms of dysuria. In many cases it is unapparent to the patient, particularly in women. In a study by Paronen, 80 per cent of 334 patients exhibited some urogenital symptoms, most commonly in the form of urethritis.[72]

Ocular involvement consists primarily of a mild conjunctivitis, often bilateral, which typically resolves in a few days. The actual incidence of this symptom is not clear. During the course of the disease, uveitis may become a more significant problem, causing pain and possible serious debility. Acute iridocyclitis can occur early in the disease, but it is usually a late event.

The mucocutaneous manifestations of this disease, particularly the oral and genital ones, are frequently missed because of their painless and evanescent nature. The oral lesions resemble coalescing superficial ulcers with raised circinate margins. These are often clinically unapparent and disappear within a few days. Balanitis is the most common mucocutaneous lesion in men and may resemble the oral lesions described earlier or mimic hyperkeratotic psoriasiform lesions found on the soles, palms, trunk, or extremities. These lesions are painless. When present, cutaneous involvement is most common over the plantar surfaces of the feet. These lesions are called keratoderma blenorrhagicum and may be found elsewhere, including the toes, the palms of the hands, the glans penis, and possibly the shaft of the penis. In severe cases, the trunk and scalp may be involved, resulting in exfoliation. The typical course of events, however, involves a coalescence of vesicles, resulting in a hyperkeratotic crust lasting for days, weeks, or months. These may disappear or recur frequently. Nail involvement resembling psoriasiform lesions is also common, with brownish-yellow subungual hyperkeratosis that lifts the thickened and yellowed nail plate.

Symptoms of back pain may be seen with Reiter's syndrome. Sacroiliitis occurs, especially in long-standing or recurrent disease, with figures quoted as high as 80 per cent. A more reasonable figure is probably in the range of 20 to 30 per cent.[29, 51, 63, 67] In contrast to ankylosing spondylitis, sacroiliac involvement is frequently unilateral early in the disease. The patient with Reiter's syndrome should be questioned about back pain or stiffness and other symptoms suggestive of spondylitis. The typical history of back pain includes predominant morning stiffness that worsens with periods of rest and improves with exercise.

Late consequences of Reiter's syndrome are becoming increasingly apparent. Cardiac complications including aortic regurgitation and atrioventricular block are manifestations of mesaortitis.[20, 78] Although this is typically a late and uncommon feature of chronic Reiter's syndrome, it may be an early feature in the rare patient. Apical pulmonary fibrosis may develop in 5 per cent of patients but is clinically silent. As mentioned previously, progressive iridocyclitis with intra-articular hemorrhage, optic neuritis, and other problems may occur with Reiter's syndrome and possibly result in blindness.

Laboratory Findings

Laboratory findings in Reiter's syndrome include a mild leukocytosis, anemia, and a moderate increase in the erythrocyte sedimentation rate. Tests for rheumatoid factor and antinuclear antibodies are negative. HLA-B27 is found in 60 to 85 per cent of patients. Synovial fluid analysis is nonspecific, revealing a typically inflammatory type of reactivity.

Radiologic Findings

Radiographs are usually negative in the early stages of this disease. With progression of the disease, however, juxta-articular osteoporosis, joint space narrowing, and erosive changes may be seen.[77] Bone spur formation at the insertions of the Achilles and plantar fascia are commonly found. These may develop within a few weeks after the onset of symptoms.

Radiographic sacroiliitis is indistinguishable from that seen in ankylosing spondylitis but may be asymmetric or unilateral, especially early in the disease process. Oates and Young suggested that the incidence of sacroiliitis increases with time after the initial episode of symptoms.[67] It has also been found that the incidence of sacroiliitis is increased in patients with recurrent attacks of peripheral arthritis.

Spinal involvement in Reiter's syndrome, as in sacroiliitis, is less severe and extensive than in ankylosing spondylitis or colitic forms of the disease process. Although ankylosing spondylitis in colitic patients almost exclusively exhibits marginal, symmetric syndesmophyte formation, psoriatic and Reiter's patients exhibit both marginal and nonmarginal syndesmophytes in an asymmetric fashion. Additionally, although spinal involvement is progressive in an ascending fashion in both ankylosing spondylitis and colitis patients, spinal lesions in the psoriatic and Reiter's populations may have skip lesions with patchy asymmetric involvement of varying spinal segments.

Treatment

Reiter's syndrome is a chronic entity with no cure. Treatment remains controversial. The urethritis is self-limiting and is not affected by antibiotic therapy. The joint and soft tissue manifestations of the disease rarely respond to salicylates. Indomethacin, phenylbutazone, and other nonsteroidal anti-inflammatory agents are most effective and should be considered for initial therapy.

PSORIATIC ARTHRITIS

The association of arthritis with psoriasis was first noted during the latter part of the 19th century by Pierre Bazin.[4] It was not until 1964 that psoriatic arthritis was classified as a distinct and separate disease entity by the American Rheumatism Association. Although the definition of psoriatic arthritis is still debated, the most frequently accepted criteria are the presence of at least one patch of psoriasis in the presence of inflammatory arthritis and the absence of rheumatoid factor.

There is a much higher frequency of inflammatory arthritis in patients with psoriasis than in the general population. The frequency is between 5 and 10 per cent in most studies,[46] but may be higher in patients with severe cutaneous disease.

Etiology

The cause and pathogenesis of psoriatic arthritis remains unknown but probably involves genetic, immunologic, and environmental factors.

Experimentation and clinical studies suggest that psoriasis may have an immunologic basis.[38, 44] Increased levels of immunoglobulin A (IgA) immunoglobulins, circulating immune complexes, and the presence of antibodies against native collagens have been documented in the psoriatic patient population. The relationship of these factors to the presence or development of psoriatic arthritis is unknown, however. Additional information has suggested that cell-mediated immune responses may play a role in the development of psoriasis and psoriatic arthritis.[8]

Several studies have suggested a genetic component to the transmission or development of psoriasis in psoriatic arthritis.[28] Early studies identified an increase in the B13, B17, B27, and BW39 histocompatibility antigens in patients with psoriasis. More recent studies have shown an apparent link between the presence of CW6 and DRw7 and development of arthritis in the patient with psoriasis. The relationship remains unclear, however. Several environmental factors appear to play a role in the pathoetiology of psoriatic arthritis. Group A streptococci and staphylococcus appear to stimulate an abnormal humoral immune response in the psoriatic patient and may secondarily lead to the development of arthritic changes in the genetically predisposed patient.[64, 93] Trauma and vascular changes have also been cited as possible inciting events in the development of psoriasis and psoriatic arthritis.[6, 48]

Clinical Manifestations

The clinical manifestations of psoriatic arthritis are similar to those seen in Reiter's syndrome. The age of onset is similar, with the typical psoriatic skin lesions presenting in the third decade. Ten per cent of patients develop arthritis coincident with the skin disease. Usually, however, there is a lag phase of several months to several years before the onset of arthritis. The male-to-female ratio is approximately 1 to 1.[59]

The primary psoriatic skin lesions are papules or micropapules. These are characteristically covered with some sort of scale mimicking the keratodermia seen in Reiter's syndrome. These psoriatic lesions are well delineated from the unaffected surrounding skin. The scale tends to slough, and when intentionally removed leads to minute bleeding points, which is known as the Auspitz sign.

Mowl and Wright classified patients with psoriatic arthritis into five groups; however, the presentation and findings of these patients overlap significantly.[59] Most patients have initial involvement of the small joints of the hands and feet in an asymmetric fashion. The classic lesion affecting the distal interphalangeal joint produces a sausage digit, caused by inflammation of the joint and flexor tendon. Most of these patients will have nail manifestations in the form of pitting, onycholysis, or ridging. In a smaller percentage of patients distal interphalangeal joint involvement may be symmetric, mimicking rheumatoid arthritis. A negative rheumatoid factor and absence of subcutaneous nodules serve as useful distinguishing features.

In a study by Lambert and Wright, spondylitis was noted in 40 per cent of 130 patients with psoriatic arthritis. Twenty per cent were found to have sacroiliitis.[43] Spondylitis is the predominant clinical feature in only 5 per cent of psoriatic patients, however. It should be noted that HLA-B27 positivity is present in 60 to 80 per cent of patients with radiographic spondylitis and 40 to 80 per cent of patients with radiographic sacroiliitis, but it is found in only 20 per cent of the entire psoriatic arthritic population.[10] The sacroiliac and spine involvement is consistent with the findings described in Reiter's syndrome with asymmetric patchy type involvement. In its more severe form, however, it may resemble ankylosing spondylitis (Fig. 18–22).

It is increasingly appreciated that psoriatic arthritis is a systemic process. Eye inflammation appears to be the most frequent association and may be seen in 20 per cent of patients, most commonly in the form of conjunctivitis and iritis. Aortic insufficiency and upper-lobe pulmonary fibrosis have also been described, but their association is unproved.

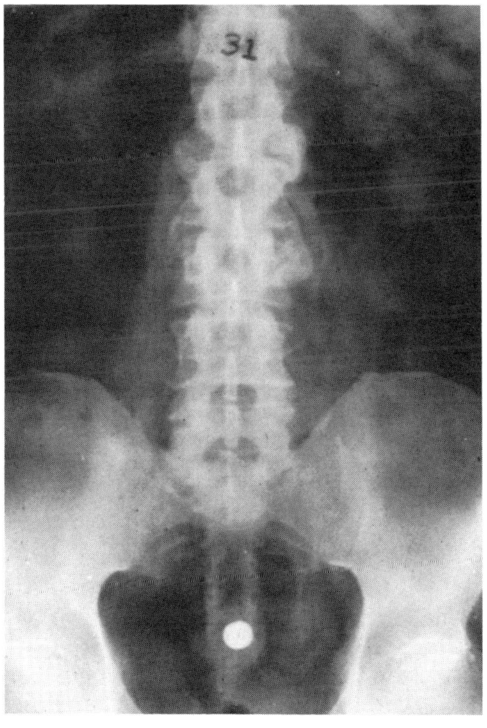

Figure 18–22. Psoriatic arthritis: frontal radiograph of the lumbar spine demonstrating nonmarginal syndesmophyte formation in a patchy distribution.

Laboratory Findings

Routine laboratory findings in psoriatic arthritis are nonspecific. Mild anemia and leukocytosis may be seen. The sedimentation rate is usually mildly elevated. Ten to twenty per cent of patients have an elevated uric acid level, which may be related to the rapid turnover of epidermal cells. Gout has often been reported in psoriatic arthritis patients.

Treatment

The initial management of psoriatic arthritis is similar to that of rheumatoid arthritis. Rest and physical modalities such as strengthening and range of motion are useful. Anti-inflammatory agents such as aspirin or nonsteroidal drugs may be used, although aspirin appears less effective.

RHEUMATOID ARTHRITIS

Rheumatoid arthritis is a systemic disorder of uncertain cause, manifested primarily by inflammatory arthritis of the smaller joints of the appendicular skeleton in a symmetric fashion. Involvement of the spine in long-standing rheumatoid disease is usually isolated to the cervical region. Systemic manifestations of the disease include hematologic, pulmonary, neurologic, and cardiovascular abnormalities.

Etiology

Susceptibility to rheumatoid arthritis may be influenced by a genetically determined immune response to some undetermined inciting agent. The histocompatibility antigen HLA-DRw4 has been found in 70 per cent of patients compared with an incidence of 28 per cent in the general population.[86] Researchers have demonstrated only a slight genetic predisposition, however, and current scientific opinions suggest that environmental factors far outweigh genetic factors in the development of rheumatoid arthritis.

Much work has been done to identify a virus or bacteria that may be responsible for triggering an immune response, but none has been identified. The current assumption is that synovial cells of patients with rheumatoid arthritis express a new antigen by an unknown mechanism. This chronic antigenic stimulus then triggers the body to produce rheumatoid factor, an immunoglobulin M (IgM) molecule directly against autologous immunoglobulin G (IgG). Approximately 75 to 80 per cent of patients with active rheumatoid disease are positive for IgM anti-IgG. The presence of rheumatoid factor alone in the synovial fluid will not produce rheumatoid arthritis, however. There is increasing evidence showing that immunologic mechanisms, including immune complex formation of antigen and antibodies followed by complement binding and polymorphonuclear cell infiltration, are important in the pathogenesis of rheumatoid arthritis.[34, 52, 90] Phagocytosis of the immune complex by polymorphonuclear cells results in the release of lysosomal enzymes capable of causing tissue damage. This same sequence of events may explain the pathogenesis of rheumatoid nodules and other systemic immune sequelae such as vasculitis.

Clinical Manifestations

In most patients the onset of rheumatoid arthritis is insidious. Prodromal symptoms of fatigue, joint stiffness, arthralgia, and myalgia may precede actual joint effusions. The small joints of the appendicular skeleton are typically involved in a symmetric fashion, especially the hands, wrists, and feet, but the large weight-bearing joints may be involved. Multiple joint involvement is typical, however, and one third of patients may have monarticular symptoms.

Examination of the patient reveals warmth, tenderness, and swelling of involved joints. Rheumatoid nodules may be found in 10 to 20 per cent of patients and most commonly are found on the extensor surface of the elbow. Muscle weakness and atrophy, diminished range of motion, contractures, and fixed deformities may develop and typically parallel the severity of the disease process. Swan-neck and boutonniere deformities may be seen in conjunction with volar subluxation and ulnar deviation of the fingers at the metacarpophalangeal joints. The course of the disease is generally progressive but may be marked early by periods of exacerbation and remission. Loss of motion, instability, and development of deformity are inevitable, however.

Rheumatoid spondylitis typically manifests in the cervical spine, but it may uncommonly involve the sacroiliac joints. Involvement of the thoracolumbar spine is extremely rare. Cervical spine involvement in the rheumatoid patient has been reported to be 25 to 95 per cent, depending on the particular study and diagnostic criteria.[7, 18, 54, 57, 73, 74] The pathologic changes in the cervical spine are identical to those that occur peripherally, as proved by biopsy.[3, 27] Types of cervical spine involvement seen, in decreasing order of frequency, include anterior atlantoaxial subluxation, atlantoaxial subluxation combined with subaxial subluxation, isolated subaxial subluxation, and superior migration of the odontoid (also known as basilar invagination or vertical atlantoaxial instability).

Anterior atlantoaxial subluxation is a result of severe erosive synovitis of the atlantoaxial and atlantodental articulations and tends to be more common in patients with severe peripheral rheumatoid arthritis. Conlon and associates reported a 25 per cent incidence of radiographic atlantoaxial subluxation in a hospital population of rheumatoid patients.[18] Radiographic progression has been reported to be approximately 40 per cent for anterior atlantoaxial subluxation, but development of neurologic symptoms is significantly less, ranging from 2 to 14 per cent.[85, 91, 95] Isolated vertical atlantoaxial instability is rare and more commonly is seen in association with anterior atlantoaxial instability. Significant risk factors for development of neurologic symptoms, as indicated by Weissman and associates, are an atlantodental distance of more than 9 mm and the presence of vertical atlantoaxial instability.[95]

The symptoms associated with atlantoaxial involvement result from a combination of factors. Localized mechanical pain secondary to the inflammatory and arthritic changes represents the most common complaint. Extremes of flexion-extension tend to exacerbate these symptoms, especially with advanced changes in the C1–C2 articulation. Neurologic dysfunction may manifest through compression of the brain stem, spinal cord, or peripheral nerve roots. Patients may complain of paresthesias and weakness in the upper and lower extremities and occasionally describe an electric shock sensation that traverses their entire body (Lhermitte's sign). Vertebral artery insufficiency may also be seen and is manifested by dizziness, headache, dysphagia, vertigo, visual disturbances, and nystagmus. Urinary retention or frequency can also be an important early warning sign of instability and should not be ignored.

Some authors believe that atlantoaxial subluxation is well tolerated by most rheumatoid patients without development of neurologic compromise; however, Matthews found that long track signs develop in nearly one third of patients with anterior C1–C2 subluxation and one half of those with vertical subluxation.[57]

Approximately 20 per cent of patients with rheumatoid arthritis may have radiographic manifestations of sacroiliac disease. It should be noted that this involvement is rarely symptomatic. The reasons for this are unclear but may be related to the severe nature of their peripheral involvement. Peripheral involvement in these patients may be unilateral or bilateral. Symptoms are more commonly seen in patients with long-standing disease of more than five years' duration.

Laboratory Tests

Rheumatoid factor is present in 70 to 80 per cent of patients with classic rheumatoid arthritis. Approximately 20 to 60 per cent of patients with active rheumatoid arthritis have a positive test for antinuclear antibody (ANA) factor. The erythrocyte sedimentation rate is usually increased to 30 mm per hour or above, and the hemoglobin is variably decreased, depending on the activity of the disease. Synovial fluid findings are nonspecific and typically are of the inflammatory type.

Radiographic Findings

Early in the course of the disease radiographic findings are nonspecific and limited to soft tissue swelling and possibly a mild periarticular osteopenia. These films are useful, however, and serve as a base line for evaluation of disease progression and treatment. With progression, narrowing of the joint spaces, marginal erosions, and severe subchondral osteoporosis may be appreciated, especially in the small joints of the appendicular skeleton.

Radiographic assessment of the cervical spine in the rheumatoid patient is necessary on an intermittent basis to assess atlantoaxial or subaxial instability. Atlantoaxial instability may occur in one of four forms. Anterior atlantoaxial instability is the most common, followed by lateral atlantoaxial subluxation, posterior atlantoaxial instability, and vertical migration of the odontoid.

Radiographically, anterior atlantoaxial instability is evidenced by an atlantodental distance of more than 3 mm on either lateral static or flexion-extension views of the cervical spine. This is measured from the posterior margin of the anterior ring of C1 to the anterior surface of the dens. Surgical stabilization, however, is not recommended in this patient population until an atlantodental interval of more than 9 mm develops or neurologic symptoms are manifested. Vertical migration of the odontoid may be evaluated by several methods. Chamberlain's line is drawn from the hard palate to the inner aspect of the posterior rim of the foramen magnum. The odontoid should not project more than 3 mm above this line, with more than 6 mm definitely being pathologic. Symptomatic basilar invagination typically requires significant protrusion. McGregor's line connects the posterior margin of the hard palate to the most caudal point of the occiput. The tip of the odontoid should not project more than 4.5 mm above of this line. Finally, McRae's line connects the front to the back of the foramen magnum. In the healthy patient the odontoid should not project beyond this point. Ranawat and associates devised another measurement technique to combat the difficulty in radiographically visualizing the hard palate.[74] On the lateral roentgenogram, the coronal axis of C1 is marked by connecting the anterior and posterior arches. A second vertical line is then drawn from the center of the sclerotic lines of C2 (pedicles) and extends up along the midaxis of the odontoid until it intersects the first line. A measurement of less than 13 mm is considered abnormal.

Lateral subluxation accounts for approximately 20 per cent of atlantoaxial subluxations and is more commonly found in patients with cord compression.[91] Overhang of the lateral mass of C1 or C2 of more than 2 mm on the anteroposterior open-mouth view is significant and evidence of instability.

Posterior atlantoaxial instability is rare and is usually associated with either fracture or erosion of the odontoid. In one series it accounted for 6.7 per cent of all atlantoaxial subluxations.[95] This is not a benign condition and may cause a myelopathy due to kinking of the posterior cord at the cervicomedullary junction.

Subaxial subluxations tend to be more subtle and may be located at multiple levels in the patient with rheumatoid arthritis, producing a step-ladder type of deformity. Such subluxation can be found in 10 to 20 per cent of patients with rheumatoid arthritis.[58, 82] Radiographic evidence of rheumatoid spondylitis in the subaxial portion of the cervical spine is marked by subluxation or dislocations, erosions, and disc narrowing. Such changes may result in neck pain, nerve root impingement secondary to foraminal stenosis, or myelopathy.

Different patterns of subaxial involvement have been described.[47] The most common of these is anterior subaxial subluxation. Subluxation may also occur above or below a previously performed fusion mass. Severe anterior spondylodiscitis as well as epidural rheumatoid granulations may be responsible for myelopathy.

As mentioned earlier, sacroiliac changes may be seen in approximately 20 per cent of patients with rheumatoid arthritis.[24, 53] In approximately two thirds of these patients involvement has been found to be bilateral, and typically consists of erosions without sclerosis. Ankylosis of the sacroiliac joints is unusual. It should be noted that changes in the sacroiliac joints are not an early feature of rheumatoid arthritis since most cases are seen in patients with long-standing disease. Patients with severe symptomatic involvement have often been found to be HLA-B27 positive.

JUVENILE RHEUMATOID ARTHRITIS

Juvenile rheumatoid arthritis (JRA) is a heterogeneous disease that continues to pose considerable diagnostic difficulty. Forty per cent of patients with juvenile rheumatoid arthritis are very young (1 to 3 years old) at the time of onset, but the disease may affect children at any age and tends to affect girls twice as often as boys.

JRA presents clinically in three distinct ways.[13, 14, 80] The polyarticular form is the most common and is seen in approximately 50 per cent of patients with JRA. Five or more joints are typically involved during the first six weeks of symptoms. The next most common presentation, seen in approximately 30 per cent of patients, is the mono- or pauciarticular form, involving one to four joints. The least common clinical presentation (20 per cent) is the systemic form of JRA, which may occur with or without initial arthritic complaints.

The polyarticular form of JRA affects primarily girls and involves five or more joints, with the knees, wrists, ankles, and elbows most commonly affected. The pattern of arthritis varies. It may be generalized, with symmetric involvement of multiple joints including the hands and feet mimicking the pattern seen in adult rheumatoid arthritis. Findings may be asymmetric, however, and have a migratory pattern, thus confusing JRA with other rheumatologic disorders.

The *systemic* form of JRA is characterized by daily remittent fever, adenopathy, splenomegaly, and an evanescent maculopapular rash involving the trunk and extremities. Symptoms of joint disease are often absent or mild, making the diagnosis of JRA difficult. Cardiac involvement in these patients may have serious, if not fatal, consequences. Myocarditis is the most serious consequence and may rapidly induce cardiac enlargement and subsequent heart failure. Pericarditis is more frequently seen than myocarditis, however, and is usually a benign manifestation that may tend to recur. The systemic form of JRA affects boys more than girls.

The pauciarticular form of JRA also affects girls more frequently. The onset of arthritis is usually insidious and is most often seen involving the knee. Joint pain is usually mild even in the presence of marked swelling and effusion. These patients, as well as those with polyarticular onset, are less likely to have systemic manifestations. Low-grade fever, rash, or lymphadenopathy and splenomegaly may occasionally be seen. The most potentially serious manifestation of this form of JRA is chronic iridocyclitis, which may be seen in 20 to 40 per cent of patients.

The clinical course of JRA is unpredictable and varies from complete remission to progressive disease. The course and prognosis for these patients have been categorized into various subgroups. Generally speaking, most patients with either the polyarticular form of JRA or systemic-onset JRA develop or maintain polyarthritic involvement manifested by flare-ups and remissions. Occasionally an unremitting and progressive downhill course may be seen. Most patients with pauciarticular-onset JRA have pauciarthritis with involvement of one to four joints, and some develop polyarthritis. The prognosis for these patients is good. Of the patients followed for as long as 15 years, complete remission occurred in approximately 50 per cent of patients, whereas 70 per cent regained normal function. The mortality rate in JRA is approximately 2 to 4 per cent. Systemic infections and amyloidosis are the most common causes of death.

Spondylitis of the cervical spine and sacroiliac disease are commonly seen in patients with JRA. Patients with polyarticular and systemic forms of the disease may develop significant pain and limited motion in the cervical spine early in the course of the disease, which is in contrast to the late onset of cervical spine findings in the adult form of rheumatoid arthritis. Cervical spine involvement has been reported in 66 per cent of patients with disease of at least 10 years' duration.[2] The results from long-standing cervical involvement may lead to significant loss of motion and ankylosis. Studies by Ansell have indicated that apophyseal joint changes, especially fusion, are the most common findings.[2] The incidence of fusion appears to increase at each level from a caudad to a cephalad direction. Patients who have onset of the disease in very early childhood experience abnormal development of the vertebral bodies. Atlantoaxial and subaxial subluxations characteristically seen in the adult rheumatoid arthritis patient are relatively uncommon in the JRA patient.

Sacroiliitis follows a course similar to that seen in the adult form of rheumatoid arthritis. Radiographic evidence of sacroiliitis has been reported in approximately 20 per cent of patients but is rarely symptomatic. Radiographic changes in the sacroiliac joints may range from ankylosis to mild erosive and sclerotic-type changes (Fig. 18–23). Changes in the thoracic or lumbar spine have not been noted.

Diagnosis

There is no single clinical or laboratory criterion specific to JRA. The diagnosis must be made on observation of the clinical picture and exclusion of other disease processes. Laboratory studies may show an elevated erythrocyte sedimentation rate and low-grade anemia, especially the acute phase of the disease process, except in the pauciarticular form of JRA. A significant leukocytosis, usually between 20,000 and 30,000, may be seen in the systemic form of JRA. The standard test for rheumatoid factor is generally negative. A subgroup of patients with the polyarticular form of JRA can have a positive rheumatoid factor (5 to 10 per cent). This is typically found

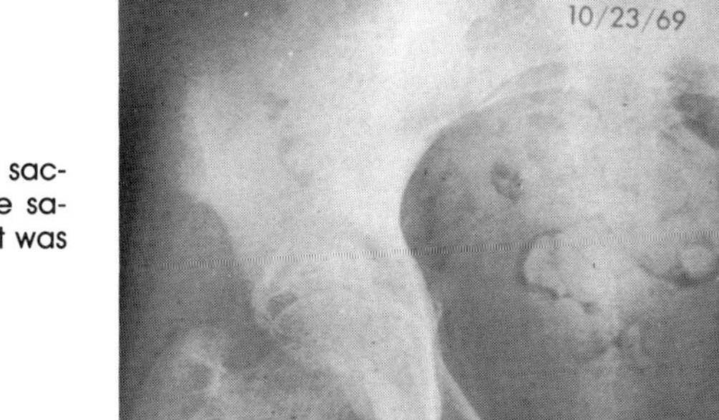

Figure 18–23. Juvenile rheumatoid sacroiliitis: complete obliteration of the sacroiliac joints bilaterally. The patient was never symptomatic.

in older children with severe disease. ANA tests may be positive in approximately 50 per cent of patients with the pauciarticular form of arthritis, but are generally negative in the systemic and polyarticular forms of JRA.

The radiographic features of JRA are nondiagnostic. Juxta-articular demineralization and soft-tissue swelling are typical findings early in the disease process. Periosteal proliferation and thickening may result from the inflammatory process.

CRYSTAL-INDUCED ARTHROPATHIES

Gout and pseudogout (calcium pyrophosphate crystal deposition disease) may be collectively termed crystal-induced arthropathies. Gouty arthropathy is the clinical expression of prolonged hyperuricemia. Hyperuricemia may result from increased uric acid production, diminished uric acid excretion, or a combination of both processes. Several enzymes identified in the synthetic pathway of uric acid may be responsible for many forms of primary gout. Excessive activity of phosphoribosylpyrophosphate (PRPP) synthetase has been described, resulting in enhanced production of the uric acid substrate PRPP. Such patients have onset of gouty arthritis at a relatively young age (often in the 20s) and often have uric acid nephrolithiasis and a family history of gout. Hypoxanthine-guanine-phosphoribosyl-transferase (HGPRTase) is an enzyme that catalyzes the conversion of intermediate products to purine ribonucleotides (PRN). PRNs inhibit uric acid production by a negative feedback mechanism. Therefore deficiencies in HGPRTase ultimately lead to increased production of uric acid. A complete lack of HGPRTase is seen in Lesch–Nyhan syndrome and is characterized by choreoathetosis, spasticity, mental retardation, and self-mutilation. Patients with glucose-6-phosphatase deficiency uniformly exhibit an increased concentration of PRPP, which is in turn responsible for accelerated production of uric acid. Deficiency of this enzyme is termed Type I (von Gierke) glycogen storage disease. This diagnosis should be considered in patients with atypical gout, such as young women. Xanthine oxidase (XO) is an enzyme that catalyzes the final steps of uric acid synthesis. There is no known genetic defect that produces excessive quantities of xanthine oxidase, but it should be noted that the drug allopurinol is useful in the treatment of hyperuricemia because it is a potent inhibitor of this enzyme.

Approximately 70 per cent of uric acid produced daily is excreted by the kidneys. In gout, decreased renal clearance of uric acid is common. A variety of pathologic and physiologic states are associated with abnormal renal excretion of uric acid. Included are diminished renal blood flow, drugs, hormones, renal tubular disorders, metal intoxications, toxemia of pregnancy, and hypertension.

Several pathogenic mechanisms for acute gouty synovitis have been proposed. Common to all is the presence of uric crystals in the synovium or joint space. A sufficient number of crystals in the joint space triggers an acute attack of gouty arthritis through a process that is not completely understood. Phagocytosis of crystals by leukocytes appears important and leads to the release of chemotactic proteins from the leukocytes themselves. Acute synovitis appears to develop when the crystal-containing leukocytes break down, releasing their lysosomal products into the synovial fluid. Activation of the kallikrein and complement systems also appears to play some role in the pathogenesis of acute gouty arthropathy, but their specific role remains unclear.

Clinical Manifestations

The typical manifestation of acute gouty arthritis is pain and swelling of the metatarsophalangeal joint of the great toe. This is seen in approximately 50 per cent of patients. Polyarticular involvement including the tarsals, ankle, wrists, and elbow may also be seen. In patients with severe established disease, attacks may also occur in the shoulder, hips, spine, and sacroiliac joints. The onset of these attacks is typically at night, when the patient is awakened by painful swelling in the involved joint. If untreated, gouty arthritis subsides over a period of two to six weeks. Between attacks (the intercritical period) the joints are entirely normal, a feature that may help differentiate gouty arthritis from rheumatoid arthritis. The duration of the intercritical period is variable but is typically about one year. As the disease progresses, the duration of each intercritical period shortens until persistent joint problems are present.

Tophaceous deposits are unique to gout, but

do not usually occur until several years after the onset of the disease. They represent deposits of uric acid crystals in the soft tissues around the joints, including cartilage, synovial membranes, and tendons. The rate of formation of these tophaceous deposits is a function of the severity and duration of the hyperuricemia. The classic locations of tophaceous formation is in the helix or antihelix of the ear, ulnar surface of the forearm, and Achilles tendon regions. They may be difficult to differentiate clinically from rheumatoid nodules, but microscopic examination of an aspirate will reveal typical monosodium urate crystals.

Finally, renal dysfunction occurs in up to 90 per cent of patients with gouty arthritis. Renal damage may be due to urate nephropathy secondary to deposition of monosodium urate crystals in the renal interstitial tissue. Obstructive uropathy may also result from collection of uric acid crystals in the collecting tubules or ureter.

Diagnosis of acute gouty arthritis can be made by identifying monosodium urate crystals in the synovial fluid or joint tissues. Urate crystals can be distinguished from calcium pyrophosphate by a polarizing light microscope. The uric acid crystals are negatively birefringent, needle-shaped structures.

Radiographic Findings

The radiographic findings most consistent with gout are well-defined punched out areas of bone lysis. These lesions are typically 5 mm or more in diameter and are most often observed in the head or base of the phalanges of the feet and hands. Martel noted a characteristic radiographic lesion in patients with gouty arthritis characterized by a bony erosion with a thin, shell-like rim of bone continuous with the adjacent bony contour, resulting in an overhanging margin.[55] Although such changes may be seen in other conditions, they are most characteristic of gout and are probably its most specific radiographic feature.

Radiographic findings in the spine are nonspecific and resemble spondylosis. Involvement of the sacroiliac joints is typified by sclerotic rimmed cystic lesions in the juxta-articular regions found in approximately 8 to 10 per cent of the patients with peripheral involvement of gouty arthritis.[94]

Treatment

Indomethacin or phenylbutazone are the most common drugs used for acute attacks of gouty arthritis. Colchicine has been used in the past, but is rarely used now because of associated nausea and diarrhea. Allopurinol and uricosuric agents are used for long-term management of gout and hyperuricemia.

CALCIUM PYROPHOSPHATE CRYSTAL DEPOSITION DISEASE (PSEUDOGOUT)

Calcium pyrophosphate crystal deposition (CPPD) disease is caused by the deposition of crystals of calcium pyrophosphate in the joints. The presence of these crystals in the joint space can lead to acute episodes of synovitis and on a chronic basis, may result in degenerative arthropathy. The pathoetiology of this disease is unknown, but in all likelihood it is similar to that already described for gout. CPPD disease has been associated with a number of other disorders, including hyperparathyroidism and hemosiderosis. These associations have not been helpful in delineating the mechanism of pyrophosphate deposition in these patients.

CPPD disease was first called pseudogout because patients have a typical picture of acute monoarticular arthritis, but it is now recognized that there are several variable clinical pictures of CPPD disease, only one of which is a pseudogout-like illness. Clinically, patients with CPPD disease are elderly, presenting in the middle or late decades. The male-to-female ratio is approximately 1.5 to 1.[69]

The most common clinical form of CPPD disease is pseudo-osteoarthritis with or without acute, superimposed synovitis. Women are the predominant sufferers The knees are the most commonly affected joint, followed by involvement of the wrist, metacarpophalangeal joints, hips, shoulders, elbows, and ankles. Involvement is typically symmetric, although the degenerative process may be further advanced unilaterally.

The pseudogout form of CPPD disease is also common and often involves the knee. Involvement is monarticular, resembling gout, and is marked by acute or subacute arthritic attacks lasting a few days to several weeks.

Other forms of CPPD disease include asymptomatic or lanthanic CPPD disease, pseudorheumatoid arthritis, and pseudoneuropathic joints. Lanthanic CPPD disease may be the most common form of this disease process. In one study 27 per cent of elderly volunteer subjects were found to have radiographic evidence of CPPD deposits on radiographic evaluation.[26] The pseudorheumatoid form accounts for approximately 5 per cent of patients with CPPD disease. These patients have multiple joint involvement with subacute attacks lasting for weeks to several months. They also have nonspecific symptoms of inflammation including morning stiffness and fatigue, often confusing them with rheumatoid patients. Severely destructive, neurotrophic-like arthropathy has been reported in patients with CPPD disease. This is seen in patients without neurologic abnormality and has been most commonly reported to occur in the knees. This is a rare manifestation of CPPD disease.

Evidence of CPPD disease may also be seen in the spine. Deposition of these crystals in the synovial line joints of the spine may occur but this remains difficult to diagnose. Patients with a long-standing history of CPPD disease may have radiographic evidence of calcium pyrophosphate crystal deposition in the intervertebral disc but remain asymptomatic. In a study by Bywaters and associates, six patients with idiopathic hemochromatosis were found to have radiographic evidence of chondrocalcinosis in the intervertebral discs.[12] None of these patients were symptomatic, although two had some associated degenerative changes. With more severe involvement of the spine, changes may be seen mimicking ankylosing spondylitis.

Diagnosis and Treatment

The diagnosis of CPPD disease depends on the identification of crystals in the synovial fluid. Polarizing light microscopy reveals rhomboid-shaped crystals, compared with the needle-shaped crystals seen in gout. In addition, these crystals exhibit a weekly positive birefringence, in contradistinction to those of gout.

The radiographic features of CPPD disease are helpful. Crystal deposition of calcium pyrophosphate in fibrocartilaginous structures,

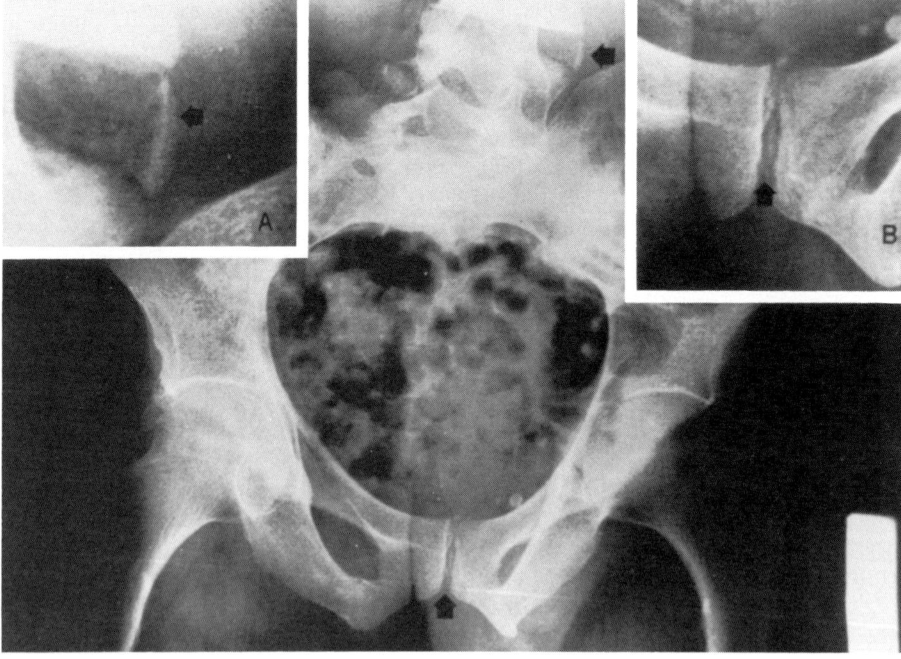

Figure 18–24. CPPD: deposition of calcium pyrophosphate crystals in *(A)* the annulus fibrosus and *(B)* fibrocartilaginous joint of the pubis symphysis.

hyaline cartilage, ligaments, and joint capsules may be striking. Presence of punctate, linear, or nodular calcifications localized to these areas of both the synovial and fibrocartilaginous joints is common (Fig. 18–24). The most common sites of crystal deposition include the menisci of the knee, the triangular fibrocartilaginous complex of the wrist, and the pubis symphysis. Radiographic screening of patients suspected to have chondrocalcinosis should include these areas.

There is currently no therapeutic treatment to halt the progressive deposition of crystals. Acute attacks of synovitis may be helped by aspiration and injection of intra-articular steroids. Oral nonsteroidal anti-inflammatory medications may also be effective. The management of chronic arthritis resulting from crystal deposition is similar to that of osteoarthritis.

References

1. Andersson, O.: Rontgenbilder vid Spondylarthritis ankylopoetica. Nord. Med. *14:*2000, 1937.
2. Ansell, B. M.: The cervical spine in post-pubertal patients with rheumatoid arthritis of juvenile onset. Ann. Rheum. Dis. *15:*40, 1956.
3. Ball, J., and Sharp, J.: Rheumatoid arthritis of the cervical spine. *In* Hill, A. G. S. (ed.): Modern Trends in Rheumatology. Vol. 2. New York, Appleton-Century-Crofts, 1971.
4. Bazin, P.: Lecons Theoriques et Cliniques sur les Affections cutanees de Nature Arthritique et Arthreux (Monograph). Paris, Delagaye, 1860.
5. Behcet, H.: Uber rezidivierende Apthose, durch ein virus verursachte Geschwure am Mund, am Auge und an den Genitalien. Dermatol. Wochenschr. *105:*1152, 1937.
6. Bieracki, R., Sadowska-Wroblewska, M., and Zabokrycki, J.: Acro-osteolysis in the course of ankylosing spondylitis. Rheumatologia *6:*163, 1968.
7. Bland, J. H.: Rheumatoid arthritis of the cervical spine. J. Rheumatol. *3:*319, 1974.
8. Braathen, L. R., Fynard, O., and Mellbye, O. J.: Predominance of cells with T-markers in the lymphocytic infiltrates of synovial tissue in psoriatic arthritis. Scand. J. Rheumatol. *8:*75, 1979.
9. Brewerton, D. A., Caffrey, M., Nicholls, A., et al.: Reiter's disease and HLA-B27. Lancet *2:*996, 1973.
10. Brewerton, D. A., Coffrey, M., and Nicholls, A.: HLA-B27 and the arthropathies associated with ulcerative colitis and psoriasis. Lancet *1:*956, 1974.
11. Bywaters, E. G. L., Dorling, J., and Sutor, J.: Ochronosis densification (abstract). Arthritis Rheum. Dis. *29:*563, 1970.
12. Bywaters, E. G. L., Hamilton, E. B. D., and Williams, R.: The spine in idiopathic hemochromatosis. Ann. Rheum. Dis. *30:*453, 1971.
13. Calabro, J.J., Holgerson, W. B., Sonpal, G. M., et al.: Juvenile rheumatoid arthritis: a general review and report of 100 patients observed for 15 years. Semin. Arthritis Rheum. *5:*257, 1976.
14. Calabro, J.J.: Juvenile rheumatoid arthritis: mode of onset as key to early diagnosis and management. Postgrad. Med. *70:*120, 1981.
15. Campbell, D. J., and Doyle, J. O.: Tabetic Charcot's spine: report of eight cases. Br. Med. J. *1:*1018, 1954.
16. Canoso, J. J., Saini, M., and Hermos, J. A.: Whipple's disease and ankylosing spondylitis: simultaneous occurrence in HLA-B27 positive males. J. Rheumatol. *5:*79, 1978.
17. Carette, S., Graham, D., Little, H., et al.: The natural disease course of ankylosing spondylitis. Arthritis Rheum. *26:*186, 1983.
18. Conlon, P. W., Isdale, I. C., and Rose, B. S.: Rheumatoid arthritis of 333 cases. Ann. Rheum. Dis. *25:*125, 1966.
19. Cruickshank, B.: Pathology of ankylosing spondylitis. Clin. Orthop. *74:*43, 1971.
20. Csonka, G. W., Litchfield, J. W., Oates, J. K., and Wilcox, R. R.: Cardiac lesions in Reiter's syndrome. Br. Med. J. *1:*243, 1961.
21. Culling, J.: Charcot's disease of the spine. Proc. R. Soc. Med. *67:*1026, 1974.
22. Dekker-Saeys, B. J., Meuwissen, S. G., Van Den Berg-Loonen, E. M., et al.: Prevalence of peripheral arthritis, sacroiliitis, and ankylosing spondylitis in patients suffering from inflammatory bowel disease. Ann. Rheum. Dis. *37:*33, 1978.
23. Dihlmann, W., and Delling, G.: Disco-vertebral destructive lesions (so-called Andersson lesions) associated with ankylosing spondylitis. Skeletal Radiol. *3:*10, 1978.
24. Dilsen, N., McEwen, C., Poppel, M., et al.: A comparative roentgenologic study of rheumatoid arthritis and rheumatoid (ankylosing) spondylitis. Arthritis Rheum. *5:*341, 1962.
25. Dilsen, N., Konice M., and Ovul, C.: Preliminary family study of Behçet's disease in Turkey. *In* Inaba, G. (ed.): Behçet's Disease. Tokyo, University of Tokyo Press, 1982, p. 103.
26. Ellman, M. H., and Levin, B.: Chondrocalcinosis in elderly persons. Arthritis Rheum. *18:*43, 1975.
27. Eulderink, F., and Meijers, K. A. E.: Pathology of the cervical spine in rheumatoid arthritis: controlled study of 44 spines. J. Pathol. *120:*91, 1976.
28. Farber, E. M., and Nall, M. L.: Genetics in psoriasis family study. *In* Farber, E. M., and Cox, A. J. (eds.): Psoriasis (Proceedings of the International Symposium, Stanford University). Stanford, Stanford University Press, 1971, p. 7.
29. Ford, D. K.: Arthritis and venereal urethritis. Br. J. Vener. Dis. *29:*123, 1953,
30. Forestier, J., and Lagier, R.: Ankylosing hyperostosis of the spine. Clin. Orthop. *74:*65, 1971.
31. Frank, P., and Gleeson, J. A.: Destructive vertebral lesions in ankylosing spondylitis. Br. J. Radiol. *48:*755, 1975.
32. Godfrey, R. G., Calabro, J. J., Mills, D., and Maltz, B. A.: A double blind crossover trial of aspirin, indomethacin and phenylbutazone in ankylosing spondylitis (abstract). Arthritis Rheum. *15:*110, 1972.
33. Gran, J. T.: An epidemiological survey of the signs and symptoms of ankylosing spondylitis. Clin. Rheum. Dis. *4:*161, 1985.

34. Gruhn, W. B., and McDuffie, F. C.: Studies of serum immunoglobulin binding to synovial fibroblast cultures from patients with rheumatoid arthritis. Arthritis Rheum. *23:*10, 1980.
35. Hanson, V., Kornreich, H., Bernstein, B., et al.: Prognosis of juvenile rheumatoid arthritis. Arthritis Rheum. (Suppl.) *20:*279, 1977.
36. Horwitz, T.: Bone and cartilage debris in the synovial membrane: its significance in the early diagnosis of neuroarthropathy. J. Bone Joint Surg. *30A:*579, 1948.
37. Jawad, A. S. M., and Goodwill, C. J.: Behçet's disease with erosive arthritis. Ann. Rheum. Dis. *45:*961, 1986.
38. Karsh, J., Espinoza, L. R., Dorval, G., et al.: Immune complexes in psoriasis with and without arthritis. J. Rheumatol. *5:*514, 1978.
39. Keat, A., Thomas, B., Dixey, J., et al.: Chlamydia trachomatis and reactive arthritis: the missing link. Lancet *1:*72, 1987.
40. Kellgren, J. H.: The epidemiology of rheumatic diseases. Ann. Rheum. Dis. *23:*109, 1964.
41. Kelly, J. J., and Weisiger, B. B.: The arthritis of Whipple's disease. Arthritis Rheum. *6:*615, 1963.
42. Knox, W. E.: Sir Archibald Garrold's inborn errors of metabolism. II. Alkaptonuria. Am. J. Hum. Genet. *10:*95, 1958.
43. Lambert, J. R., and Wright, V.: Psoriatic spondylitis: a clinical and radiological description of the spine in psoriatic arthritis. Q. J. Med. *46:*411, 1977.
44. Laurent, M. R., Ranayi, G. S., and Shepperd, P.: Circulating immune complexes, serum immunoglobulins, and acute phase proteins in psoriasis and psoriatic arthritis. Ann. Rheum. Dis. *40:*66, 1981.
45. Lawrence, J. S.: The prevalence of arthritis. Br. J. Clin. Pract. *17:*699, 1963.
46. Leczinsky, C. G.: The incidence of arthropathy in a ten year series of psoriasis cases. Acta Dermatol. Venereol. *28:*483, 1948.
47. Lipson, S. J.: Rheumatoid arthritis in the cervical spine. Clin. Orthop. *239:*121, 1989.
48. Lotz, M., Carsen, D. A., and Vaughn, J. H.: Substance P activation of rheumatoid synoviocytes: Neural pathway in pathogenesis of arthritis. Science *235:*893, 1987.
49. Macrae, I. F., and Wright, V.: Measurement of back movement. Ann. Rheum. Dis. *28:*584, 1969.
50. Maizel, H. M., Ruffin, J. M., and Dobbins, W. O., III: Whipple's disease: a review of 19 patients from one hospital and a review of the literature since 1950. Medicine *49:*175, 1970.
51. Marche, J.: L'atteinte des articulations sacroiliaques dans le-syndrome "dit" de Reiter. Rev. Rhum. *17:*449, 1950.
52. Marmion, B. P.: Infection, autoimmunity and rheumatoid arthritis. Clin. Rheum. Dis. *4:*565, 1978.
53. Martel, W., and Duff, I. F.: Pelvo-spondylitis in rheumatoid arthritis. Radiology *77:*744, 1961.
54. Martel, W., Duff, I. F., Preston, R. E., et al.: The cervical spine in rheumatoid arthritis: correlation of radiographic and clinical manifestations (abstract). Arthritis Rheum. *7:*326, 1964.
55. Martel, W.: The overhanging margin of bone: a roentgenologic manifestation of gout. Radiology *91:*755, 1968.
56. Mason, R. M., and Barnes, C. G.: Behçet's syndrome with arthritis. Ann. Rheum. Dis. *28:*95, 1969.
57. Mathews, J. A.: Atlantoaxial subluxation in rheumatoid arthritis. Ann. Rheum. Dis. *28:*260, 1969.
58. Meikle, J. A., and Wilkison, M.: Rheumatoid involvement of the cervical spine. Ann. Rheum. Dis. *30:*1541, 1971.
59. Moll, J. M. H., and Wright, V.: Psoriatic arthritis. Semin. Arthritis Rheum. *3:*55, 1973.
60. Moll, J. M.: Inflammatory bowel disease. Clin. Rheum. Dis. *11:*87, 1985.
61. Morris, R. I., Metzger, A. L., Bluestone, R., and Terasaki, P. I.: HLA-B27, a useful discriminator in the arthropathy of inflammatory bowel disease. N. Engl. J. Med. *290:*1117, 1974.
62. Murray, R. O., and Jacobsin, H. G.: The Radiology of Skeletal Disorders. London, Churchill Livingstone, 1981.
63. Murray, R. S., Oates, J. K., and Young, A. C.: Radiological changes in Reiter's syndrome and arthritis associated with urethritis. J. Fac. Radiol. (Lond.) *9:*37, 1958.
64. Mustakallio, K. K., and Lassus, A.: Staphylococcal alpha-antitoxin in psoriatic arthropathy. Br. J. Dermatol *76:*544, 1964.
65. Newton, D. R. L.: Discussion on the clinical and radiological aspects of sacroiliac disease. Proc. R. Soc. Med. *50:*850, 1957.
66. Numaguchi, Y.: Osteitis condensans ilii, including its resolution. Radiology *98:*1, 1971.
67. Oates, J. K., and Young, A. C.: Sacro-iliitis in Reiter's disease. Br. Med. J. *1:*1013, 1959.
68. O'Brien, W. M., LaDu, B. N., and Bunim, J. J.: Biomechanical, pathologic and clinical aspects of alcaptonuria, ochronosis and ochronotic arthropathy: review of world literature (1584–1962). Am. J. Med. *34:*813, 1963.
69. O'Duffy, J. D.: Clinical studies of acute pseudogout attacks. Arthritis Rheum. *19*(Suppl.):349, 1976.
70. O'Duffy, J. D., Lehner, T., and Barnes, C. G.: Summary of the third international conference on Behçet's disease. J. Rheumatol. *10:*154, 1983.
71. Oshima, Y., Shimizu, T., Yokohari, R., et al.: Clinical studies on Behçet's syndrome. Ann. Rheum. Dis. *22:*36, 1963.
72. Paronen, I.: Reiter's disease: a study of 344 cases observed in Finland. Acta Med. Scand. *131:*(Suppl. 212):1, 1948.
73. Pelici, P. O. M., Ranawat, S. C., Tsarairis, P., et al.: Progression of rheumatoid arthritis of the cervical spine. J. Bone Joint Surg. *63A:*342, 1981.
74. Ranawat, C. S., O'Leary, P., Pellici, P. M., et al.: Cervical spine fusion in rheumatoid arthritis. J. Bone Joint Surg. *61A:*1003, 1979.
75. Resnick, D., Shaul, S. R., and Robins, J. M.: Diffuse idiopathic skeletal hyperostosis (DISH): Forestier's disease with extraspinal manifestations. Radiology *115:*513, 1975.
76. Resnick, D., Niwayama, G., Goergen, T. G., et al.: Clinical, radiographic and pathologic abnormalities in calcium pyrophosphate dihydrate deposition disease (CPDD): pseudogout. Radiology *122:*1, 1977.
77. Reynolds, D. F., and Gonka, G. W.: Radiological aspects of Reiter's syndrome (venereal arthritis). J. Fac. Radiol. (Lond.) *9:*44, 1958.

78. Rodnan, G. P., Benedek, T. G., Shaver, J. A., and Fennell, R. M.: Reiter's syndrome and aortic insufficiency. JAMA *189:*889, 1964.
79. Rubinow, A., Canoso, J. J., Goldenberg, D. L., et al.: Arthritis in Whipple's disease. Isr. J. Med. Sci. *17:*445, 1981.
80. Schaller, J. G., and Wedgwood, R. J.: Is juvenile rheumatoid arthritis a single disease? A review. Pediatrics *50:*940, 1972.
81. Schumacher, H. R., Cherian, P. V., Sieck, M., and Clayburne, G.: Ultrastructural identification of chlamydial antigens in synovial membrane in acute Reiter's syndrome. Arthritis Rheum. *29:*531, 1986.
82. Sharp, J., and Purser, D. W.: Spontaneous atlanto-axial dislocation in ankylosing spondylitis and rheumatoid arthritis. Ann. Rheum. Dis. *20:*47, 1961.
83. Shimizu, T., Ehrlich, G. E., Inaba, G., and Hayashi, K.: Behçet disease. Semin. Arthritis Rheum. *8:*223–260, 1979.
84. Simmons, Z. H.: The surgical correction of flexion deformity of the cervical spine in ankylosing spondylitis. *In* Cervical Spine Research Society (eds.): The Cervical Spine. Philadelphia, J. B. Lippincott Co., 1989, p. 573.
85. Smith, P. H., Benn, R. T., and Sharp, J.: Natural history of rheumatoid cervical luxations. Ann. Rheum. Dis. *31:*431, 1972.
86. Stastny, P.: Association of the B-cell alloantigen DRw4 with rheumatoid arthritis. N. Engl. J. Med. *298:*869–871, 1978.
87. Steinberg, C. L., Gardner, D. E., Smith, F. A., and Hodge, H. C.: Comparison of rheumatoid (ankylosing) spondylitis and crippling fluorosis. Ann. Rheum. Dis. *14:*378, 1955.
88. Thompson, M.: Osteitis condensans ilii and its differentiation from ankylosing spondylitis. Ann. Rheum. Dis. *13:*147, 1954.
89. Utsinger, P. D., Resnick, D., and Shapiro, R.: Diffuse skeletal abnormalities in Forstier disease. Arch. Intern. Med. *136:*763, 1976.
90. Utsinger, P. D., Zvaifler, N. J., and Weiner, S. B.: Etiology of rheumatoid arthritis. *In* Utsinger, P. D., Zvaifler, N. J., and Ehrlich, G. E. (eds.): Rheumatoid Arthritis. Philadelphia, J. B. Lippincott Co., 1985, p. 21.
91. Van Beusekim, G. T.: The neurological syndrome associated with cervical luxations in rheumatoid arthritis. Acta Orthop. Belg. *58:*38, 1972.
92. van der Linden, S., Valkenburg, H., and Cats, A.: The risks of developing ankylosing spondylitis in HLA-B27 positive individuals: a family and population study. Br. J. Rheum. *22*(Suppl. 2):28, 1983.
93. Vasey, F. B., Deitz, C., Fenske, N. A., et al.: Possible involvement of group A streptococci in the pathogenesis of psoriatic arthritis. J. Rheumatol. *9:*719, 1982.
94. Vyhnanek, L., Lavicka, J., and Blahos, J.: Roentgenological findings in gout. Radiol. Clin. *29:*256, 1960.
95. Weissman, B. N. W., Aliabadi, P., Weinfeld, M. S., et al.: Prognostic features of atlantoaxial subluxation in rheumatoid arthritis patients. Radiology *144:*745, 1982.
96. Whipple, G. H.: A hitherto undescribed disease characterized anatomically by deposits of fat and fatty acids in the intestinal mesenteric lymphatic tissue. Bull. Johns Hopkins Hosp. *18:*302, 1907.
97. Willkens, R. F., Arnett, F. C., Bitter, T., et al.: Reiter's syndrome: evaluation of preliminary criteria for definite disease. Arthritis Rheum. *24:*844, 1981.
98. Wright, V., Catterall, R. D., and Cook, J. B.: Bone and joint changes in paraplegic men. Ann. Rheum. Dis. *24:*419, 1965.
99. Wu, P. C., Fang, D., Ho, E. K. W., and Leong, J. C. V.: The pathogenesis of extensive discovertebral destruction in ankylosing spondylitis. Clin. Orthop. *230:*154, 1988.
100. Zvaifler, N. J., and Martel, W.: Spondylitis and chronic ulcerative colitis. Arthritis Rheum. *3:*76, 1960.

CHAPTER

19

CERVICAL DISC DISEASE

Lawrence T. Kurz, M.D.
Frederick A. Simeone, M.D.
William H. Dillin, M.D.
Robert G. Watkins, M.D.
David P. Wesolowski, M.D.
Ay-Ming Wang, M.D.
Scott D. Boden, M.D.
Sam W. Wiesel, M.D.

THE DIFFERENTIAL DIAGNOSIS OF CERVICAL RADICULOPATHY

Lawrence T. Kurz, M.D.

Although the most common cause of a cervical radiculopathy is cervical disc disease, there are many other entities that have similar symptoms and signs. This section will compare and contrast the other disease states that should be considered in the differential diagnosis.

TUMORS

Both intraspinal and extraspinal tumors may give rise to symptoms that cause them to be confused with cervical radiculopathy. With cervical spine tumors, neural deficits may be secondary to structural changes in bone and soft tissues (vertebral body collapse, subluxation, kyphosis); direct compression from extension of the tumor mass itself; or to an inflammatory reaction consisting of edema, hemorrhage, adhesions, and scarring. Most malignant and some benign tumors, such as giant cell tumors and aneurysmal bone cysts, may be associated with large soft tissue masses and significant lytic destruction; however, they usually result in a myelopathy and major neurologic deficits. Most other benign tumors, such as osteoid osteoma, osteoblastoma, fibrous dysplasia, eosinophilic granuloma, and hemangioma, generally are not associated with large soft tissue masses or significant bony destruction, and thus usually do not cause neurologic symptoms.

A few benign tumors of the cervical spine may cause unilateral radiculopathy, however. Osteochondromas may undergo significant growth during adolescence. They usually originate from the posterior bony elements and are usually asymmetric. The asymmetry of their projection may cause unilateral impingement on a single cervical nerve root, usually within the spinal canal or foramen. Aneurysmal bony cyst, a lesion of adolescents and young adults, is typically associated with an expanding soft tissue mass, and may be associated with a myelopathy; however, its predilection for multiple spinal levels and asymmetry may sometimes result in unilateral nerve root impingement. Schwannomas are almost always asymmetric and frequently have radicular symptoms that worsen with maneuvers that increase intraspinal pressure. Although least likely to be found in the cervical region, spinal schwannomas are twice as common intradurally as extradurally. Their location, arising from the spinal nerve root, frequently causes them to compress the root at the foramen. Although early in their course they are likely to have localized root symptoms, they may grow large and cause significant compression, leading to a myelopathy. When associated with neurofibromatosis, the lesions may be multiple. Meningiomas most frequently occur in middle-aged women and, like schwannomas, are least likely to be found in the cervical region. Growth begins at the dorsal root, and thus symptoms of meningiomas may be clinically indistinguishable from those of schwannomas. Early in their course, radicular symptoms of both of these nerve tumors are more referable to sensory symptoms since the tumors originate from the sensory root.

Pain in the neck, shoulder, or arm is common with cervical spine tumors and is usually the primary and earliest symptom. Patients with tumors causing significant bony destruction most commonly complain of neck pain. The pain is frequently constant, and typically worse at night. Although rest pain is a particularly ominous symptom, implicating a tumor, destruction of cervical spine structures sufficient to cause instability may render the pain worse with neck movement and positioning. Posterior trapezius and shoulder pain may be secondary to irritation of posterior rami. Pain in a particular dermatomal distribution may follow from specific direct nerve root impingement. Schwannomas may cause localized erosion of bone easily documented as a foraminal enlargement on oblique roentgenograms, or computed or conventional tomography. Neck pain from significant bony destruction is usually detected by plain radiographs, although early detection may necessitate bone scanning.

Numerous extraspinal tumors may mimic or cause cervical radiculopathy. Tumors of the thyroid, upper esophagus, and pharynx may extend locally into the cervical spine. Apical carcinomas of the lung (Pancoast's tumors) may encroach on the brachial plexus or subclavian vessels. They may be difficult to detect on routine chest roentgenograms and may be visible on apical lordotic views only. Although they most commonly present with shoulder girdle pain and Horner's syndrome, Pancoast's tumors frequently are associated with profound unilateral upper extremity weakness. Shoulder weakness is seen almost as often as distal weakness, and the classic sensory deficit is in the ulnar nerve distribution. Paraplegia and long tract signs are also found. Nerve deficits are not always secondary to invasion of the brachial plexus. Epidural extension may also be seen because the tumor can compress the cervicothoracic nerve roots at the intervertebral foramina.

Primary or metastatic tumors of the clavicle, scapula, and proximal humerus usually cause pain in the region of the arm or shoulder girdle. Significant destruction of bony structures by aggressive lesions may cause weakness of the arm muscles through pain inhibition, joint instability, or a change in joint mechanics. Here again, upper extremity weakness and sensory disturbances may also be due to infiltration of the brachial plexus by soft tissue tumors or extension of the tumor mass from bony lesions.

Intracerebral tumors may cause symptoms and signs of cervical radiculopathy. Focal lesions in the contralateral parietal lobe may mimic root pain. Predominant loss of discriminative sensation and hyperreflexia are associated features.

Focal lesions of the cerebral hemisphere may produce monoparesis. The presence of hyperreflexia in the affected arm and subtle findings of hemiparesis are usually evident on examination and point to the correct localization.

FOCAL UPPER EXTREMITY ENTRAPMENT SYNDROMES

Peripheral nerves and blood vessels in the upper extremity may be compressed in predictable areas of disease, giving rise to upper extremity numbness, paresthesias, and sensory and motor loss. Although these radicular signs and symptoms may mimic radiculopathy due to cervical spine pathology, concomitant neck pain may be noncontributory, simply occurring simultaneously. Entrapments involving the median, ulnar, and radial nerves as well as the neurovascular structures in the thoracic outlet will be discussed.

Median Nerve

Pronator Syndrome

The median nerve may be compressed anywhere along its course, but it usually becomes compressed at defined levels. The most proximal level of compression may produce the "pronator syndrome." This is associated with pain in the proximal volar forearm, and sensory signs and symptoms in the radial 3½ digits of the hand. Weakness of all median nerve innervated muscles occurs since the compression is proximal to the branching of the anterior interosseous nerve. Augmentation of symptoms may give a clue as to the site of compression. Symptoms aggravated by flexion of the elbow against resistance between 90 and 135 degrees of flexion may be due to compression from the ligament of Struthers or the lacertus fibrosus. The ligament of Struthers may attach to an accessory bone, with the supracondylar process originating on the distal humeral shaft 5 cm proximal to the medial epicondyle. Both the ligament and the accessory bone may contribute to the compression. The lacertus fibrosus is a fascial investment from the bicipital tendon that fans out over the flexor muscles of the proximal forearm. Symptoms worsened by resistance to forced voluntary pronation of the forearm combined with simultaneous wrist flexion may indicate compression by the pronator teres muscle. This muscle may cause compression of the median nerve by hypertrophy, or a sharp aponeurotic edge of the deep head or reflected muscle fascia forming fibrous bands. Symptoms elicited by resisted flexion of the long-finger flexor digitorum superficialis muscle may be referable to compression from a deep tendinous aponeurotic arch of the muscle, underneath which the median nerve passes.

Sensory symptoms and signs of the pronator syndrome typically mimic a C6 and C7 radiculopathy with changes in the radial 3½ fingers. Although the pronator syndrome may affect the function of the median nerve innervated muscles in the C6 and C7 distribution (pronator teres and flexor carpi radialis), it will spare radial nerve innervated muscles in the C6 and C7 distribution (elbow, wrist, and finger extensors). In addition it may induce abnormalities in muscles innervated by the median nerve, but not in the C6 and C7 distribution (finger flexors and thenar muscles).

Anterior Interosseous Syndrome

Since the anterior interosseous nerve is essentially a motor branch of the median nerve, anterior interosseous syndrome is not characterized by sensory abnormalities. Pain in the proximal forearm is typically aggravated by exercise and abates with rest. Motor abnormalities are manifested as weakness, and are referable to those muscles innervated by this nerve (flexor pollicis longus, pronator quadratus, and flexor digitorum profundus of the index finger). This syndrome may mimic a C8 radiculopathy since this is the root through which they are all innervated. Other C8 innervated muscles unaffected by the anterior interosseous nerve syndrome include the flexor digitorum superficialis (median nerve proximal to anterior interosseous nerve) and the flexor carpi ulnaris and flexor digitorum profundus to the ring and little fingers (ulnar nerve). Electrodiagnostic evaluation may also be helpful in differentiating a C8 radiculopathy from this syndrome. The pathology is usually in the form of fascial bands on either the tendinous origin of the flexor digitorum superficialis or the deep head of the pronator teres.

Carpal Tunnel Syndrome

Compression of the median nerve in the carpal canal typically causes sensory symptoms. Night pain, paresthesias, and numbness in the hand and radial 3½ digits are common and are caused by a thickened transverse carpal ligament. The disease occurs most commonly in middle age and more frequently in women and those with occupations that require significant use and overuse of the hands and wrists. Symptoms may be referred proximally from the hand toward the forearm and even the elbow and may be reproduced or elicited by Phalen's or Tinel's tests. They may be relieved by splinting the wrist in a neutral position. Thenar muscle weakness and atrophy represent advanced disease. Sensory symptoms may mimic C6 and C7 radiculopathy, but no C6 or C7 muscles will demonstrate abnormalities since they are all innervated proximal to the carpal canal. Thenar motor weakness may mimic a T1 radiculopathy because of abnormalities of the opponens pollicis and the abductor pollicis brevis; however, other T1 innervated muscles will be normal, including the hypothenar muscles and the first dorsal interosseous (ulnar nerve).

Palmar Cutaneous Nerve

The palmar cutaneous nerve branch of the median nerve usually originates on the radial side of the nerve about 7 cm proximal to the proximal wrist flexion crease. It usually passes between the volar carpal ligament and the transverse carpal ligament to supply the thenar eminence with its sensation. Paresthesias or numbness in this distribution may occur if this sensory nerve is compressed as it pierces the antebrachial fascia or the volar carpal ligament. Sensory symptoms in the thenar eminence may mimic C6 radiculopathy, but no motor weakness will be present.

Ulnar Nerve

Cubital Tunnel Syndrome

The most common location of entrapment of the ulnar nerve is the elbow. Although there are various causes, they all share a common mechanism for the neuropathy—compression. The most typical symptom is aching pain on the medial aspect of the elbow, although radiation of the pain and paresthesias may migrate distally along the ulnar forearm and into the ulnar 1½ fingers. Symptoms are typically elicited either by percussion of the nerve behind the medial epicondyle or by acute, prolonged flexion of the elbow. Muscle atrophy frequently occurs even early in the course of the compression. The weakness is manifested in the muscles innervated by the ulnar nerve distal to the elbow (flexor carpi ulnaris, flexor digitorum profundus to the long and ring fingers, and the interossei and hypothenar muscles). All these muscles are innervated by the C8 and T1 nerve roots. However, since the sensory changes also occur in the distribution of the C8 and T1 roots, cubital tunnel syndrome may be difficult to differentiate from a C8 or T1 radiculopathy. Clinical tenderness and pain referable to the medial aspect of the elbow and electrodiagnostic studies demonstrating a significant conduction delay across the elbow may be useful in this regard. Furthermore, abnormalities in C8 or T1 innervated muscles that are not innervated by the ulnar nerve such as the flexor pollicis longus, the thenar muscles, and the index and long fingers flexors (median nerve) may signal a C8 or T1 radiculopathy rather than an ulnar nerve entrapment.

Guyon's Canal

The ulnar nerve may also be compressed at the wrist in Guyon's canal. Various causes include compression from a ganglion, repeated hypothenar trauma, or thrombosis of the ulnar artery. Compression at this level usually affects both the superficial and deep branches of the ulnar nerve. Therefore, sensory symptoms are referable to the volar aspect of the ulnar 1½ fingers. The dorsal aspect of these 1½ digits remains unaffected because that area of skin is supplied by the dorsal sensory branch of the ulnar nerve, which originates proximal to the wrist and does not transverse Guyon's canal. In Guyon's canal, the ulnar nerve splits into the deep and superficial branches. The deep branch is essentially all motor and the superficial branch is essentially all sensory. Therefore, motor symptoms, weakness, and atrophy are referable only to those muscles innervated by the deep branch of the ulnar nerve. These include the hypothenar muscles, the interossei, and the adductor pollicis. Since the sensory symptoms are in the C8 distribution and the abnormal muscles are innervated by T1 and C8, the syndrome may mimic a T1 and C8 radiculopathy. In this syndrome, however, sensation over the dorsum of the ulnar 1½ fingers is normal. In addition, median nerve innervated muscles in the T1 distribution (thenars) are normal.

Radial Nerve

The radial nerve is most commonly compressed at the elbow. Radial tunnel syndrome is a compression neuropathy of the radial nerve between the supinator muscle and the radial head. The typical culprit is the arcade of Frohse, a curved fibrous arch in the origin of the supinator muscle at the entrance to the radial tunnel. Other culprits may be fibrous or tendinous bands from the extensor carpi radialis brevis or a leash of vessels that supply the brachioradialis and extensor carpi radialis longus muscles. Just proximal to its entrance into the supinator muscle, the radial nerve gives motor branches to the brachioradialis, extensor carpi radialis longus and brevis, and supinator muscles, and then splits into a superficial sensory branch, which does not enter the radial tunnel, and the all-motor deep branch, the posterior interosseous nerve. The posterior interosseous nerve enters the supinator and later gives off motor branches to the muscles in the extensor compartment of the forearm. Because only the motor branch is compressed, sensory symptoms are rare, although aching over the site of compression is felt and may be elicited by full flexion of the elbow with the forearm in supination and the wrist neutral. The symptoms may also be aggravated by full flexion of the wrist with the forearm held in full pronation. Motor weakness is seen in those muscles supplied by the posterior interosseous nerve (extensor digitorum communis, extensor carpi ulnaris, abductor pollicis longus, and extensor pollicis longus), all of which are supplied by the C7 root. A C7 radiculopathy may be ruled out by noting no abnormalities in median innervated C7 muscles (flexor carpi radialis and pronator teres). In addition, the triceps (C7) muscle should be spared since it receives its radial nerve innervation in the upper arm, a significant distance proximal to the typical site of compression.

Thoracic Outlet Syndrome

Thoracic outlet syndrome (TOS) is multifactorial in its symptoms, clinical presentation, and anatomic pathology. The syndrome represents either vascular or neurologic symptomatology, or both, and pathology related to compression of the subclavian/axillary artery–vein complex or the lower two roots (C8, T1) of the brachial plexus. As they pass from the base of the neck through the axilla, these structures may be compressed by bony elements (cervical ribs, enlarged first thoracic rib, clavicle), muscles (scalenus anticus and pectoralis minor), or both. Vasomotor symptoms usually affect the radial side of the hand, whereas neurologic symptoms are usually located on the ulnar side of the hand.

Vascular TOS may be either arterial or venous.

Major Arterial TOS

Major arterial TOS is a rare disorder caused by subclavian artery compression with resultant aneurysm formation, more than 50 per cent of which is due to a cervical rib. Signs and symptoms of early aneurysm formation include asymmetric upper extremity pulses, supraclavicular bruit, distal upper extremity ischemic pain, muscle fatigue, or persistent unilateral Raynaud's phenomenon. Abrupt occurrence of paresthesias, pain, numbness, cyanosis, or ulceration may signal arterial emboli. Early resection of the aneurysm is obviously preferable to awaiting the appearance of emboli, which may require amputation.

Minor Arterial TOS

Minor arterial TOS is different from major arterial TOS in that to some degree it occurs in most people and is not associated with aneurysms or emboli. When the subclavian/axillary artery is compressed between the clavicle and pectoralis minor anteriorly and the first rib posteriorly, paresthesias, numbness, and arm weakness appear, probably secondary to nerve ischemia. Symptoms are usually elicited by elevation of the arm to the level of the shoulder with subsequent arterial compression and absence of distal pulses. Signs and symptoms usually appear within one minute and are reversible by lowering the height of the arm. Treatment of severe cases involves removal of the first rib, although most cases are treated by simple avoidance of the overhead position.

Venous TOS

Venous TOS is secondary to obstruction of the subclavian/axillary vein between the scalenus anticus muscle, the clavicle, and the first rib. Symptoms include swelling, pain, and cyanosis of the arm as well as exercise-induced fatigue. If positional, intermittent obstruction and symptoms tend to subside with rest; however, the syndrome is more likely to present with an acute thrombotic event. This syndrome is only rarely associated with cervical ribs. All three of these vascular syndromes may mimic a cervical radiculopathy, but they differ in a number of respects. In vascular TOS, no muscle weakness is seen at rest, and symptoms and signs of vascular obstruction (cyanosis, swelling, ulceration, diminished and asymmetric pulses) are usually clear (even if late) and may be positional. Furthermore, sensory symptoms and signs are frequently not in a specific dermatomal pattern, and there may be associated bony abnormalities.

True Neurogenic TOS

True neurogenic TOS is a rare entity that is almost invariably characterized by intrinsic hand muscle weakness and atrophy. The lateral thenar muscles are more severely affected than the interossei. Patients usually have a long history of sensory symptoms consisting of pain, paresthesias, and numbness in the medial arm, forearm, and hand, that is, cutaneous areas innervated by the lower trunk of the brachial plexus. Although roentgenograms almost invariably show a bony anomaly such as a rudimentary cervical rib or elongated C7 transverse process, the compression of the lower trunk is usually due to a taut, radiolucent band of tissue extending from the tip of the bony abnormality to the first rib. Neurogenic TOS differs significantly from arterial TOS since in neurogenic TOS the female-to-male ratio is 9:1 versus 1:1, and signs and symptoms are not usually affected by arm position.

Differentiation from other diagnoses is fairly easy since almost no other lesions produce changes in the median and ulnar nerve distribution and affect the median ones much more severely. Although sensory symptoms may mimic ulnar neuropathy, the sensory changes in the neurogenic TOS do not divide the ring finger in half as the ulnar neuropathy does. Sensory symptoms and lateral thenar wasting may mimic C8 and T1 radiculopathy, but ulnar innervated C8 and T1 muscles (interossei and hypothenars) are significantly less affected than the lateral thenars (median innervated C8 and T1 muscles). This is a hallmark of neurogenic TOS. The last major difference concerns carpal tunnel syndrome. Although lateral thenar wasting may be seen in carpal tunnel syndrome, it is uncommon, represents advanced disease, and is frequently seen in the elderly. In addition, patients with carpal tunnel syndrome have sensory symptoms and signs in the median nerve distribution, not the medial forearm and hand. And finally, if patients with carpal tunnel syndrome do have weakness, it is limited to the thenars and does not affect the other intrinsics.

BRACHIAL PLEXUS DISORDERS

Idiopathic Brachial Neuritis

The cause of idiopathic brachial neuritis is unknown. Typical features include unilateral neck and shoulder pain exacerbated by arm movements. Uually within two weeks the pain is followed by a profound but nonprogressive upper extremity weakness. The most common nerves affected include the axillary, long thoracic, and suprascapular nerves. Involvement of the musculocutaneous, radial, and median nerves is much less likely and the ulnar nerve is rarely affected. Muscle weakness most commonly is manifested in the shoulder abductors. There is usually a paucity of sensory findings. Electromyography (EMG) and nerve conduction studies are extremely useful in the differential diagnosis. Cervical radiculopathy should not be confused with idiopathic brachial neuritis. Because the lesions affect the proximal portions of the nerves in the brachial plexus, motor findings usually represent two or more roots and the sensory findings are frequently minimal.

Brachial Plexopathy

Patients with brachial plexopathy have significant pain beginning in the proximal shoulder area and radiating down the arm to the hand. The pain may be exacerbated by arm movement, and may be associated with sensory symptoms. EMG and nerve conduction studies are extremely helpful in localizing the specific site of pathology in the plexus. Causes of brachial plexopathy that, by history, are easily distinguishable from cervical radiculopathy include trauma (stretch, avulsion, gunshot wound, lacerations), postsurgical causes (transaxillary approach to first rib resection or sternal splitting procedures), and radiation treatment. Benign tumors (schwannomas) of the brachial plexus are rare and EMG is helpful in localizing the site of the lesion. In addition, the symptoms usually overlap at least two nerve roots. Malignant tumors of the brachial plexus usually present with shoulder and arm pain. Atrophy, weakness, and sensory changes in the distribution of the lower trunk (C8, T1) are the most common findings. Less likely is involvement of the entire plexus, and isolated involvement of the upper trunk (C5, C6) is distinctly unusual. Most tumors are metastatic and are from lung and breast carcinomas. Horner's syndrome and lymphedema and arm swelling due to infiltration of the lymphatic and venous system frequently occur.

SHOULDER DISEASE

Complaints caused by shoulder disease usually include some combination of pain, stiffness, instability, or weakness. Although these symptoms can mimic a proximal cervical radiculopathy, the signs on physical examination usually indicate a primary shoulder problem rather than a cervical radiculopathy. Although pain is usually experienced in the proximal arm and shoulder, tenderness may be elicited by manual palpation with rotator cuff tears, subacromial bursitis, adhesive capsulitis, degenerative disease of the acromioclavicular or glenohumeral joints, calcific tendinitis, and chronic instability or impingement. Tenderness over a specific, defined area of the shoulder is distinctly unusual with a cervical radiculopathy. Although stiffness is a common complaint, actual limitation to passive range of motion is the hallmark of adhesive capsulitis and is also frequently seen with most other shoulder disorders. Again, this sign is distinctly unusual in cervical radiculopathy.

Weakness usually clouds the differential diagnosis. Shoulder disease may produce proximal arm weakness due to pain or spasm but EMG and nerve conduction studies do not reveal denervation. The only significant cause of proximal arm weakness related to shoulder disease is a large rotator cuff tear, which can cause weakness of shoulder abduction. This can mimic a C5 radiculopathy simulating deltoid weakness. Other C5 root innervated muscles (biceps and pectoralis major) will be normal, however, although one must remember that the supraspinatus, which is usually torn with rotator cuff injuries, has its major innervation through C5. Sensory symptoms with shoulder disease are less frequent and signs are rare.

CERVICAL ANGINA

Cervical angina consists of cardiac ischemic symptoms referred to regions innervated by the C5–T1 nerve roots, thereby mimicking an acute cervical radiculopathy. Pain may radiate to the left shoulder or arm, accompanied by upper extremity numbness. Some fairly constant features of angina pectoris usually accompany the radicular symptoms. The pain of angina pectoris more frequently involves the chest and tends to be crushing or substernal. It is usually accentuated by exertion, diminished by nitrates, and unchanged by neck movement. Consideration of these factors allows differentiation between these two syndromes.

CONCLUSION

It is evident that cervical radiculopathy may be caused or mimicked by a host of disease entities. One must be cognizant of the differences between them and consider all the available data before attributing a cervical radiculopathy to its most common cause, cervical disc disease.

CERVICAL DISC DISEASE WITH RADICULOPATHY

Frederick A. Simeone, M.D.

This section refers to individuals who have radiating pain resulting from compression of cervical nerve roots by displaced cervical disc material at or near the vertebral foramen. It may be simplest to dispose of the most difficult problem relating to cervical disc disease quickly—axial or neck pain that may result from cervical disc degeneration. It is difficult to determine whether alterations in the cervical disc produce neck pain and, if so, which disc should be operated on to relieve such pain. Treatment of neck pain by cervical disc excision or decompression has a long and murky history. Many individuals who complain of axial pain have been subjected to disc excision, fusion, and even laminectomy with variable results. Patients believe the results are even worse if the neck pain is the result of an accident or compensable injury.[3]

Patients with neck pain may complain so bitterly that the surgeon feels compelled to perform some operative procedure to provide relief. These patients have normal neurologic examinations, and the only abnormality of any type is degeneration of the cervical discs demonstrated radiographically. For this reason, these discs may be attacked surgically. One must realize, however, that progressive radiographic degeneration of cervical discs must be considered a "normal" consequence of aging, and as individuals pass into their third, fourth, and fifth decades of life, radiographic abnormalities become increasingly common. There is no criterion to indicate whether an individual cervical disc is causing neck pain. In the past injection of the cervical disc at the time of discography with reproduction of the individual's axial pain was considered diagnostic. Subsequent investigations and the poor history of surgery in this condition has made this "disc distention" test of little use.

Subluxation of the cervical vertebrae is a painful condition. I use 4 mm or more as the "magic number." If vertebrae move radiographically on flexion and extension and the patient has pain, better results with fusion can be expected. In some instances, large midline disc herniations are associated with neck pain, but the reason for removal is usually decompression of the spinal cord, although gratifying results for relief of neck pain can occur in some instances.

In the absence of controlled studies that indicate whether cervical pain can be relieved by removal of degenerated discs, and specific studies that indicate which discs to remove, we are left with the concept that in most cases axial pain cannot be treated by operations on cervical discs. Consequently, the remainder of this discussion will consider radiating pain secondary to nerve root compression.

When the upper cervical nerve roots are affected, the principal point of radiation may be the neck. This applies to C3 and C4 radiculopathies because the sensory division of both of those spinal nerves incorporates the suboccipital region and root of the neck, with radiation as far out as the shoulder top. Fortunately, disc herniations affecting these nerve roots are relatively rare.

It may be best to begin the discussion by isolating the individual nerve roots. Radiculopathies above C2 are extremely unusual and rarely present a clinical problem.

C3 RADICULOPATHY

Primary disc pathology at C2–C3, which would affect the C3 nerve root, is extremely unusual. This interspace is minimally involved in neck flexion and extension and, therefore, acute and chronic protrusion of disc material with radiculopathy rarely occurs. The C3 nerve root radiates up the posterior aspect of the neck into the posterior suboccipital region and may affect the ear. The pain is extremely difficult to distinguish from muscle tension headache. There is no detectable motor involvement with complete section of the C3 nerve root. Numbness is difficult to detect because the patient rarely complains and only careful examination with a pin may discern diminished sensation in the above-mentioned areas.

C4 RADICULOPATHY

C4 radiculopathy is significantly more common and may be an unexplained cause of neck and shoulder pain. As with the C3 nerve root, there is no motor deficit. Although the C4 motor nerve root supplies the diaphragm, abnormalities of diaphragm function have not been detected on fluoroscopic studies in a few patients with known C4 radiculopathy. Numbness is rare, but if it occurs it may be appreciated at the root of the neck, extending approximately to the midshoulder, and posteriorly to the level of the scapula. As with other cervical radiculopathies, the pain may be aggravated by neck extension. This may be the only reliable clinical sign to indicate that the pain is of cervical nerve root origin.

EMG has not been valuable in the diagnosis of C4 radiculopathy. A combination of pain in the appropriate distribution, particularly when the pain is aggravated by neck extension, and clear-cut radiographic evidence of compression of the C4 nerve root is sufficient to substantiate the diagnosis. Because of the unusual nature of this specific nerve syndrome, preoperative water-soluble contrast myelography is recommended in most cases.

C5 RADICULOPATHY

The principal sensory distribution of this cervical nerve root is over the shoulder top to a point midway on the lateral aspect of the upper arm. This so-called "epaulet" pattern is highly specific for this nerve root. Patients often complain of numbness and localized shoulder pain that can be confused with mechanical or inflammatory derangements of the shoulder. The pain is not affected by internal or external rotation of the shoulder, however, nor is there tenderness in the glenohumeral fossa.

The principal motor distribution involves branches of the deltoid muscle. Patients may complain of difficulty in elevating the arm. Occasionally they lift the affected arm up with the healthy arm. Double simultaneous testing of the deltoid muscles by compression on the outstretched upper arms detects relatively minor degrees of weakness. Florid weakness of the deltoid muscle is disabling. Patients have difficulty feeding themselves, combing their hair, and putting on an overcoat. Because of the disabling nature of the weakness, a more aggressive approach to C5 nerve root lesions must be undertaken.

Additional muscles that may be involved in C5 root lesions, but are harder to test individually, include the supraspinatus, infraspinatus, and some of the flexor muscles at the elbow. The biceps reflex is inconsistently affected by C5 root compression.

C6 RADICULOPATHY

Herniations of the disc between C5 and C6 are the second most common radiculopathy encountered. The pain radiates across the top of the neck, along the biceps muscle, into the lateral aspect of the forearm, on the dorsal surface of the hand between the thumb and index finger, and finally through the tips of those fingers. Unlike the previously mentioned nerve roots, there is a reflex mediated by the C6 nerve root that makes earlier clinical detection by a truly objective test possible. Loss or diminution of the biceps reflex can occur early in the course of C6 nerve root compression syndrome. Biceps muscle weakness can be detected on examination before the patient is aware of such loss of strength. The pattern of numbness is highly variable but is usually below the elbow and down the dorsum of the hand over the thumb and index finger.[7]

Other muscles weakened by C6 nerve root lesions include the infraspinatus, serratus anterior, supinator, extensor pollicis, and extensor carpi radialis.

C7 RADICULOPATHY

Disc herniations at C6–C7 are the most common in the cervical region and consequently, C7 radiculopathy is a frequent occurrence. The patient complains of pain radiating across the back of the shoulder, across the triceps, then down the posterolateral aspect of the forearm, particularly to the middle finger.[2] Whereas C6 radiculopathies rarely involve the middle finger, C7 radiculopathies usually involve both the middle finger and the territory of C6, such as the thumb and index finger. Triceps reflex may be lost early. The triceps muscle is one of lesser importance in the functioning of the arm, despite its size. In many activities gravity can take over the function of the triceps muscle. Patients are usually amazed to learn how weak their triceps muscles are.

In some instances the pectoralis major muscle may be involved. Patients rarely complain of pectoralis muscle weakness, but atrophy may ensue after several months of C7 nerve root compression. Actual complaints of triceps muscle weakness occur under unusual circumstances, such as during the performance of pushups, backhand swings in tennis, and other activities that require forceful extension of the forearm at the elbow.

Additional muscles that can be affected in C7 root lesions include the pectoralis major, pronator, extensors of the wrist and fingers, latissimus dorsi, and possibly the supinator (in a manner indistinguishable from a C6 root lesion). Latissimus dorsi strength can be tested by having the patient cough vigorously while the examiner holds the bulky part of these muscles in each hand. The pectoralis muscle can be tested by forceful adduction of the humerus.

C8 RADICULOPATHY

Acute and chronic herniations of discs between C7 and T1 can affect the C8 nerve root. The principal sensory supply of this root is to the small finger of the hand and the medial half of the ring finger. The numbness can extend variably up the hand but is usually confined to below the wrist. Triceps, extensor carpi ulnaris, and wrist flexors may be involved, but these are indistinguishable from C7 lesions and are not useful diagnostically.

A significant motor function is supplied by the eighth cervical nerve root. This root supplies most of the small muscles of the hands, particularly the interossei. Consequently C8 radiculopathies are associated with difficulty in using the hand. Patients initially complain that they cannot hold a pencil, operate a spray bottle, or use a tool such as a hammer, which requires a strong grip, forcefully. Of all the cervical nerve roots, C8 compression is least likely to be associated with pain. Perhaps this results from the relatively large proportion of motor fibers to sensory fibers in this nerve root. Because the patient can have numbness of the ring and small finger associated with intrinsic hand muscle weakness without neck pain, C8 radiculopathies are often difficult to distinguish from ulnar neuropathy initially. EMG and nerve conduction velocity studies should differentiate between them. In older patients, however, slowing of the ulnar nerve across the elbow is seen commonly. EMG may demonstrate denervation of paraspinous muscles in a C8 distribution. It is usually possible to distinguish between the two with a combination of nerve conduction velocity studies, EMG, and water-soluble contrast myelography demonstrating the C8 nerve root. A more aggressive approach to this nerve root must be considered than to C7, for example, because of the disabling neurologic deficit that will become permanent if the condition goes untreated for a long interval. It would appear from our series that the C8 nerve root has the poorest prognosis for strength recovery.

The purpose of the above discussion was to mention specifics about each of the nerve roots. There are other muscles supplied by individual nerve roots, but routine testing of all these muscle groups usually does not add to the clinical and radiographic diagnosis. For this reason, a specific muscle group has been mentioned with each nerve root, because testing of this muscle is the most sensitive way to pick up early weakness in the distribution of each nerve root. There are, however, some generalities that should be considered in the history and diagnosis of patients with all cervical nerve root syndromes. These general symptoms will be discussed in a narrative fashion because they apply to all the above-mentioned nerve roots.

GENERAL SYMPTOMS OF ACUTE CERVICAL DISC HERNIATION

During the first phases of an acute disc herniation, the patient may be awakened frequently from a sound sleep because of neck pain. Some patients wake up three or four times a night. The most severely affected patients cannot sleep flat, but will try to sleep in a chair until the pain subsides. Even in the worst cases, the initial experience of constant pain during the day usually subsides. With rest and immobilization, these symptoms frequently improve. Night awakening is frequent, however, and lasts much longer during the acute phase. As the condition subsides, the patient may notice that he or she is able to sleep through the night. During the acute phase of any cervical disc herniation, the patient may find that it is more comfortable to keep the arm held over the head, particularly while in bed. Some patients maintain this posture even when awake. In the characteristic pose, the patient will rest the wrist or forearm on the top of the head, sometimes cocking the head away from the affected side.

Head position is important during acute disc herniation. Even mild degrees of extension may exacerbate the pain severely. In fact, it may be that mild degrees of neck extension during sleep are responsible for the nighttime awakening characteristic of patients with acute and subacute cervical disc herniations. During the examination, one may readily induce pain radiating down the arm into the fingers in a classic manner. Sometimes the pain is felt predominantly in the neck, but the paresthesias follow the course of the affected nerve root. The patient may reveal that extension of the neck and tilting the neck toward the pain are the least comfortable positions. If this has not been observed, however, this maneuver should be carried out by the examiner as a routine part of investigations of all patients who may have acute or subacute cervical disc herniations.[9]

Most patients soon learn that immobilization of the neck is comfortable. They may do this subconsciously by lying in bed, using a high-backed chair, or even applying some type of cervical immobilization. Their physician may apply a collar to produce some measure of relief. If the patient indicates that the collar has made the pain worse, it is probable that the collar is too high, causing the neck to be extended, thereby exacerbating the pain. Unfortunately cervical collars may be dispensed randomly. Clearly a standard collar is not acceptable for everyone. The distance between the chin and the manubrium of the sternum should be carefully examined when the collar is in place. The patient should be looking straight ahead or down when the collar is applied. If the neck is extended, the collar may worsen the pain.

Routine questioning about the maneuvers that make the pain worse should be part of every examination. If the patient says that looking overhead, extending the neck, and performing other activities requiring unusual positions of the neck exacerbate the pain, this favors cervical disc herniation as its cause. If the patient states that the pain is aggravated by arm movement, however, one may be dealing with an inflammatory or mechanical derangement of a joint rather than a disc problem in the neck.

Frozen shoulder can be associated with painful disc herniation at any level, but particularly with C5 and C6 radiculopathy. On examination the patient may have limited shoulder movement that could be attributed to deltoid muscle weakness secondary to C5 compression syndrome, for example. With further maneuvers, however, the examiner finds that the shoulder cannot be abducted both actively and passively beyond a certain point. The usual explanation is that the muscles and ligaments at the shoulder have become contracted because of disuse secondary to pain from the cervical radiculopathy. In some instances, the initial cervical radiculopathy may subside, but the frozen shoulder persists. Because most abduction maneuvers at the shoulder are painful, the patient continues to believe that he or she has residual pain from the original condition. Aggressive physical therapy to the shoulder may stretch the ligaments, and local anti-inflammatory treatment may prevent a recurrence.

The syndromes of each cervical nerve root compression are fairly well documented. Disc herniations affect the following nerve roots, in order of frequency, according to the classic study of Murphey and associates:[6]

1. C7 (393 cases).
2. C6 (171 cases).
3. C8 (50 cases).
4. C5 (26 cases).
5. T1 (4 cases).

Modern imaging has defined these lesions well. When there is empirical evidence of acute or chronic disc herniation on computed tomography (CT) or magnetic resonance (MR) scan, and this herniation is clearly associated with a foca neurologic deficit, CT or MR scan may be a stand-alone preoperative study. If there is no specific clinical syndrome that clearly isolates a nerve root, or if the radiographs do not indicate the cause for the patient's symptoms, water-soluble contrast myelography should be considered. This study most accurately demonstrates small compressive lesions of the cervical nerve roots. It is likely, however, that the next generation of scanners will make myelography obsolete.

UNUSUAL SYNDROMES THAT RESEMBLE CERVICAL RADICULOPATHY

Cervical radiculopathies may mimic some other entities, and these will be discussed briefly. A combination of electromyography and radiography can usually distinguish among them, but an occasional case can be difficult.

Motor Neuron Disease

It is possible for chronic cervical disc degeneration to affect many roots at once. Furthermore, it is possible for the motor portion of these nerve roots to be affected more than the sensory portion. If this occurs to a severe degree, the patient may have a painless loss of strength in the upper extremities, even associated with fasciculations.[4] Fasciculations are a late stage in the course of cervical nerve root compression syndrome. They are seen rarely even in the worse cases of cervical disc disease. A patient with a painless, spontaneous development of atrophy and fasciculations in the upper extremities is more likely to have a motor neuron disease, such as amyotrophic lateral sclerosis, than multilevel chronic cervical disc degeneration. EMG in motor neuron disease is usually diagnostic, particularly if the lower extremities are involved. Occasionally, however, myelography may be necessary to differentiate between the two. On rare occasions, EMG strongly suggests amyotrophic lateral sclerosis and the myelogram still shows multilevel cervical nerve root compression. It has been my experience that if such a combination is present, surgery is usually not effective, and the patient will eventually succumb to motor neuron disease.

Brachial Plexitis

Brachial plexitis is a specific clinical syndrome easy to confuse with cervical radiculopathy. Only a careful retrospective history, with some objective tests, can make the difference apparent.[8]

At the onset of brachial plexitis, the patient complains of severe pain principally involving the shoulder, although any part of the arm may be affected. After a few days of agonizing pain that does not respond to any measures, there is relief, followed in a few weeks by weakness and fasciculations of the involved muscle groups. This weakness may become advanced, but more often it subsides spontaneously and the lost strength is ultimately recovered.

EMG may demonstrate neurologic deficits in a brachial plexus distribution rather than in an individual nerve root distribution. Myelography is likely to be normal if the pain has indeed subsided so dramatically.

The precise cause of brachial plexitis has not been defined. Outbreaks have been reported among soldiers. Several members of the same family have been afflicted. Although it may follow a viral illness, no virus has been cultured acutely in patients with this syndrome.[5]

Occipital Neuralgia

Pain radiating up the posterior aspect of the head and across the suboccipital bone into the forehead has been seen with compression of the C2 and C3 nerve roots. This syndrome is frequently called occipital neuralgia because it involves compression of the greater occipital nerve, usually as it pierces the superior nuchal line on its way to the scalp. The occipital nerve can be blocked along the superior nuchal line at a point halfway between the inion and the mastoid tip. If this provides relief, the symptoms are probably not due to upper cervical nerve root compression.

Bursitis, Tendinitis, Adhesive Capsulitis

A variety of painful conditions may affect the shoulder and elbow joints. Sometimes these are interpreted as radiating pain, but careful examination should distinguish them. Point tenderness, pain with internal and external rotation of the shoulder, and pain initiated by arm movement rather than neck movement are typical. A careful history that emphasizes those types of activities that aggravate the pain, as well as a general examination of the shoulder joints should distinguish these conditions from cervical disc disease with radiculopathy. Limitation of shoulder movement and pain on abduction can follow an acute cervical radiculopathy, particularly one affecting the C5 and C6 spinal nerve roots. The history usually reveals that the painful abduction and limitation of motion are an epiphenomenon and that the initial pain more closely resembles a cervical radiculopathy.

Carpal Tunnel Syndrome

It is not infrequent to examine patients who have undergone unsuccessful resection of one or both transverse carpal ligaments in an effort to relieve numbness of the palms. I have seen the syndrome of uncomfortable palmar numbness, particularly in midline cervical disc herniations affecting the upper portion of the cervical spinal cord, especially C3 and C4. Although the mechanism is not fully explained, apparently this pattern of numbness, which is nondermatomal, can be associated with compression of either the posterior columns or the lateral spinal thalamic tracts. Although not specifically a cervical radiculopathy, and therefore not germane to this discussion, high spinal cord compression with palmar numbness deserves greater recognition to avoid unnecessary surgery. In carpal tunnel syndrome, the pattern of nighttime awakening with aggravation of the uncomfortable numbness is unique. Nerve conduction velocity studies of the median nerve should exclude carpal tunnel syndrome in patients with cervical disc lesions. In some instances, however, the results may be mildly abnormal and encourage the unwary surgeon to decompress the median nerve in the hand. Association of diffuse hyperreflexia and Hoffmann's signs with palmar numbness should further alert the surgeon to scan the upper cervical spine before attributing the numbness to median nerve compression.

Ulnar Neuropathy

Uncomfortable numbness in the ring and small finger is seen with both C8 radiculopathy and compression of the ulnar nerve. This may be associated with weakness of the intrinsic hand muscles. The numbness and weakness are the only presenting symptoms, and differentiation between ulnar neuropathy and C8 radiculopathy is difficult. The ulnar nerve may be entrapped at the elbow or in Guyon's canal at the wrist. Ulnar neuropathy at the elbow is generally aggravated by bending the arm at that joint. The ulnar nerve may be tender or thickened with scar tissue. Nerve conduction velocity studies of the ulnar nerve should differentiate between entrapment syndromes and cervical root compression.

Angina Pectoris

Cervical radiculopathy, particularly in the left arm, is more frequently confused with angina pectoris than vice versa. The pain in lower cervical root lesions, particularly C6 and C7, can radiate across the chest wall and down the arm. When this pain is aggravated by activity and relieved by rest, especially in a patient susceptible to vascular disease, cardiologic investigation is warranted. The pain is more diffuse and nonlocalized than in cervical radiculopathy, and a careful history should differentiate between the two.[1]

Sympathetic Nervous System–Mediated Pain

A variety of syndromes of arm pain may be mediated primarily by the sympathetic nervous system. These include reflex sympathetic dystrophy and shoulder–hand syndrome. They may be associated with peripheral nerve injuries or coronary artery disease. The pain is generally diffuse and poorly localized. It may be aggravated by light touch, such as rubbing a sleeve on some part of the upper extremity. The pain has been stereotyped despite the nature of the stimulus. It may be markedly aggravated by emotional stress. The hand may be swollen from disuse and the skin smooth and shiny. Clearly the precipitating stimuli to the pain involve contact with some part of the upper extremity and are not related to neck movement. Raynaud's syndrome, hyperhidrosis, mottling of the skin, and other neurovascular changes may corroborate the diagnosis. Diagnostic tests such as stellate ganglion block may be useful but they are generally not required in most cases.

RADIOLOGIC CONFIRMATION

Radiology of the cervical spine will be discussed elsewhere in this volume. I believe an epidemic of over-reading CT and MR scans of the cervical spine is affecting the clinical judgment of many spine surgeons. These radiographs may show disc herniations that do not compress the cervical nerve roots or the spinal cord, but their presence can lead to an unnecessary operation, particularly one considered "prophylactic." Until the community of spine surgeons is aware of exactly which abnormalities are clinically significant, strict criteria for surgery must be observed. I believe that the CT or MR scan can be stand-alone studies when there is a clear-cut cervical radiculopathy with neurologic deficit and an unequivocal radiographic finding that correlates with this deficit. In the absence of a perfect correlation, water-soluble contrast myelography remains the clearest way to demonstrate compression of a cervical nerve root in most cases. Unlike in the lumbar regions, symptomatic far-lateral cervical disc herniations are rare. The presence of a disc herniation alone, either laterally or centrally, does not suggest surgical treatment. In fact, after the fourth decade of life, such "bulges" and herniations are so common that they have little clinical significance.

EMG

EMG is rarely required to diagnose a specific cervical radiculopathy. In a typical case, EMG can help by detecting fibrillation in a specific pattern of muscles that relate to a single root. EMG is not required in the routine evaluation of cervical disc herniation. The study is important, however, when other disorders such as motor neuron disease, carpal tunnel syndrome, and brachial plexitis require differentiation.

CONCLUSION

The syndromes of cervical disc herniation with radiculopathy are stereotyped according to their root. Atypical histories or neurologic findings require careful investigation and more precise radiographic localization before surgery is considered. Knowledge of the specific root patterns of distribution of sensory and motor findings is necessary, and in most instances, the diagnosis can be made before radiographic confirmation.

References

1. Booth, R. D., and Rothman, R. H.: Cervical angina. Spine *1*:28–32, 1976.
2. Bucy, P. C., and Chenault, H.: Compression of the seventh cervical nerve root by herniation by an intervertebral disc. J.A.M.A. *126*:25–27, 1944.
3. Finneson, B.: Psycho-social considerations in low back pain. Presented at the meeting of the International Society for Study of the Lumbar Spine, Bermuda, June 1976.
4. Liversedge, L. A., Hutchinson, E. C., and Lyons, J. B.: Cervical spondylosis simulating motor neurone disease. Lancet *2*:652–659, 1953.
5. Magee, K. R., and DeJong, R. N.: Paralytic brachial neuritis. J.A.M.A. *174*:1258–1263, 1960.
6. Murphey, F., Simmons, J. C. H., and Brunson, B.: Ruptured cervical discs: 1939–1972. Clin. Neurosurg. *20*:9–17, 1973.
7. Semmes, R. E., and Murphey, F.: The syndrome of unilateral rupture of the sixth cervical intervertebral disk. J.A.M.A. *121*:1209–1214, 1943.
8. Spillane, J. D.: Localized neuritis of the shoulder girdle. Lancet *2*:532–535, 1943.
9. Spurling, R. G., and Bradford, F. K.: Neurologic aspects of herniated nucleus pulposus. J.A.M.A. *113*:2019–2022, 1939.

CLINICAL SYNDROMES IN CERVICAL MYELOPATHY

William H. Dillin, M.D.
Robert G. Watkins, M.D.

The diagnosis of disease is often easy, often difficult, often impossible.

PETER LATHAM
1789–1875

No other biology encountered in spinal surgery represents Latham's description of a disease continuum more appropriately than cervical myelopathy. Cervical myelopathy may masquerade in the most subtle and abstract of patient symptomatology or wield a profound gavel down upon the most basic of neurologic function. For the spinal surgeon, the crippling revelation of the wheelchair-bound patient binds him to Shakespeare's thoughts: "Past hope, past cure, past help!"[4] And why was this patient not discovered earlier? Is myelopathy hidden under the cover of a natural history that wanders? Is the penetration of its objective effects so delayed that we discover only the later states? Are the symptoms so tenuous and intangible at inception that patients cannot believe something so vague could be so real? We may be able to take comfort in the advice of physicians who have come before us, "a disease known is half cured."[4] Knowledge of myelopathy's diversity and suspicion of its presence may be our greatest allies.

Since myelopathy appears to span a diverse clinical spectrum, we could ask if there is a fixed pathology that might yield an explanation. Ono and associates autopsied the spinal cords of documented myelopathic patients and produced histologic evidence of "destruction of both gray matter and white matter and ascending and descending demyelinization above and below levels of spinal cord compression."[7, 50] They devised the anteroposterior (AP) compression ratio (the ratio of the AP to the lateral cord diameter) and effectively correlated it with the "most severe infarction of the cord."[7, 50] The concept of a compression ratio was further confirmed by autopsy specimens studied by Ogino and associates.[48]

This observation has been transferred from the morgue to the radiology suite. Computerized tomography myelography (CTM) depicted the pathology in cadaveric myelopathic specimens correlating the spinal cord transverse area and compression ratio morphology.[72]

Cross-sectional cord shapes were the basis of a study analyzing patients with myelopathy or radiculopathy classifying cord morphology by deformity: anterior cervical concavity, unilateral lateral deformity, bilateral lateral deformity, and flattened anterior surface.[72] The severity of symptoms correlated with the degree of spinal cord deformity; when analyzed in relationship to specific nerve root or spinal column involvement, these correlated to some degree.[72] A major issue in the study was the elimination of at least 40 per cent of all patients classified by this system because of other level involvement, and in a subgroup, the cord shape was undefinable or obliterated.[72]

Cervical spondylotic myelopathy has been demonstrated to be multisegmental in the patient over age 60 with an average of three lesions per individual.[30] These older patients exhibited dynamic canal stenosis in addition to the static process invoked by the aging spine.[30] Hayashi and associates concluded that the multisegmental lesions influenced the clinical presentation because there was poor correlation between neurologic level and maximum compressed level on CTM.[30] Clearly the suggestion of these data is the global nature of the process, making reduction to a single segmental analysis difficult in a significant proportion of patients.

Clinically, in an outcome study treating myelopathic patients, "neither the transverse area nor the compression ratio at the maximum compression level could be used to determine the pre-operative neurologic status."[25] Interestingly, the postoperative results were related to the restoration of cord morphology at the transverse area of maximum compression, with age at surgery and preoperative neurologic factors additional but less important considerations.[25] "The transverse area tended to decrease as multiplicity of involvement increased."[25] Sagittal images on MR scanning may ultimately describe this phenomenon in a more picturesque fashion. The presence of high signal intensity in the spinal cord on T2-weighted MR images correlated with poor outcomes in cervical cord compression, whether the patients were treated surgically or conservatively.[65]

Electric studies have become more prominently mentioned as factors related to diagnostic levels in myelopathy and prognosis. Some investigators have used evoked spinal cord potentials to correlate with the level of neurologic and radiologic severity of myelopathy.[60] Other investigators have suggested that outcome may be prognosticated from evoked spinal cord potentials and that local lesions fared better than the extensive lesions when confronted surgically.[61]

The neurologic picture may also be complicated by dynamic factors. Hukuda and associates produced experimental models that defined variations in spinal cord pathology at the site of compression when exposed to hypotension, hypertension, hyperflexion, hyperextension, and instability.[35] "The pathologic severity was proportional to the number of loadings. This study suggests that cervical spondylotic myelopathy might progress stepwise rather than linearly when these aggravating factors are loaded."[35]

Previous studies have pointed out the synergy between compression and ischemia in cervical spondylotic myelopathy in animal models.[32, 33]

The heterogeneity of these factors make the diagnosis of early myelopathy more difficult, but these are precisely the patients in whom treatment might be most efficacious. Ikeda and associates applied a quantification theory to the surgical results of myelopathic patients correlating results with the duration of the disease but not with the age of the patient.[37] It is tempting to conclude that duration is synonymous with damage.

DIAGNOSIS

Myelopathy due to cervical spondylosis was recognized in the 1950s as a clinical entity.[6, 11] Attributed to be the most common reason for spinal cord dysfunction in the more mature segment of the population, cervical spondylotic myelopathy has no pathognomonic symptom or physical sign.[62] Since no single neurologic exponent is unique to cervical myelopathy, the diagnosis must be established by affirmation of the associated clinical signs and symptoms, and exclusion of those clinical entities that may mimic the same. Phillips followed a group of

102 cases of cervical spondylotic myelopathy for ten years.[53] During this period, 23 additional cases of myelopathy associated with cervical spondylosis arose that graphically depicted other diagnoses associated with myelopathy, including desseminated sclerosis, motor neuron disease, subacute combined degeneration, syringomyelia, Arnold Chiari malformation, vertebrobasilar ischemia, peripheral neuritis, astrocytoma of the spinal cord, and cysts of the spinal cord.[53] Since cervical spondylosis is so common in patients over the age of 50, strict correlation is necessary to establish that an observed myelopathy is due to the degenerative process and not some other pathologic event.[9] In another clinical series with the established diagnosis of cervical spondylotic myelopathy, Veidlinger and associates pointed out that the heterogeneity of presentation of these patients often led to their misdiagnosis, and in this series, the other diagnoses considered included cerebral hemisphere disease, motor neuron disease, multiple sclerosis, poliomyelitis, Guillain-Barré syndrome, peripheral neuropathy, and arthritis. The exclusion of other disease processes is an important consideration in the establishment of cervical spondylosis as the pathologic source of a particular myelopathy.[69] Cervical spondylotic myelopathy is not simply a diagnosis of exclusion. On the affirmative side, myelopathy is a diagnosis structured on the typical history, and neurologic examination modeled on the physical signs pointing to cervical spine involvement and the objective studies interlinked to the pathology.

NATURAL HISTORY AND CLINICAL GRADES

But, as the world harmoniously confused: Where order in variety we see, And where, though all things differ, all agree.

ALEXANDER POPE
1688–1744.[4]

Approximately 40 years after the clinical description of myelopathy there is still no definable natural history. Cervical myelopathy almost makes a parody of chance; what we know is definable in the context of objective biology. What is missing is the prospective case with definable correlations.

One side of the equation of natural history describes an immutable biology. "The course of disease may be very prolonged. Long periods of non-progressive disability are the rule, and a few progressively deteriorating courses exceptional."[41] Lees and Turner conceded clinical exacerbations adding to neurologic deficit in patients with more than ten years of myelopathy, but emphasized the long periods of symptomatic hibernation between episodes.[41] Nurick supported this concept of an eternal clinical twilight, concluding that the amount of disability in cervical myelopathy was established early in the disease process, and in general did not progress significantly afterward.[46, 47]

Epstein's clinical review of 1355 patients with cervical spondylotic myelopathy determined in a conservative treatment group 36 per cent improvement, and 64 per cent nonimprovement. In the group that did not improve, 26 per cent deteriorated neurologically, the remainder remaining stable.[16]

Counterpoised are the ingredients of a different perspective. Clark and Robinson differed significantly in their evaluation of the natural history of myelopathy. Seventy-five per cent of their patients manifested symptoms that appeared in a series of episodes in which two thirds of these patients deteriorated and one third were unchanged.[11] Twenty per cent had the slow steady progression from the onset of symptomatology, whereas 5 per cent had rapid onset.[11] After onset of the clinical manifestations of cervical myelopathy, Clark and Robinson were unable to discover patients who reverted to a normal neurologic state, and discovered that it was uncommon for patients with neurologic deficits to undergo spontaneous regression.[11] Sixty-seven per cent of Symon and Lavender's patients displayed a linear relentless progression of neurologic dysfunction rather than episodic histories already described.[64] Perhaps there is some truth in a clinical plateau for cervical spondylotic myelopathy. Phillips was unable to demonstrate improvement in patients treated with symptoms for greater than two years.[9, 53] But there was clinical improvement in 50 per cent of patients with symptoms less than one year and 40 per cent in patients with between one and two years of symptoms.[9, 53] As in other areas of clinical medicine, the clear distinction of natural history is the basis against which all forms of intervention must be judged.

Attempts to grade myelopathy have focused on the overall effects of performance. Nurick concentrated on a grading system emphasizing consequences in gait abnormalities.[46, 47] His classification system involves a grading system of 0 to 5 with progressive disability for ambulation.[46, 47] Grade 0 exists when signs and symptoms are present but there is no evidence of cord involvement. Grade 1 depicts cord involvement but with a normal gait. Grade 2 demonstrates gait abnormalities but the ability to be employed. Grade 3 gait abnormality prevents employment. Grade 4 ambulation is only possible with assistance, and in Grade 5 the patient is unable to ambulate.[46, 47]

In an attempt to quantify the disability of myelopathy, the Japanese Orthopedic Association provided a scale concentrating on motor dysfunction of the upper extremity and the lower extremity, sensory deficit in the upper and lower extremity and over the trunk, and sphincter dysfunction.[34] This rating system not only allows for the more accurate assessment of postoperative recovery, but tends to describe the more global affects of myelopathy with additional potential involvements of the upper extremity and sphincters.[34]

PHYSICAL FINDINGS

The physical findings in cervical spondylytic myelopathy may vary considerably, depending on the exact level of compression, the degree of compression modified by aggravating factors, and the span of segments compressed in the cervical spinal cord. In general, motor neuron involvement may be characterized by conceiving of lower motor neuron involvement at the level of the clinically expressed lesion, with upper neuron involvement at levels below the site of clinical compression. Thus, the lower extremity involvement will represent the upper motor neuron configuration, while the upper extremities may be variable in terms of presentation, depending on the level and nature of compression. Clark proposed that the sensory findings in myelopathy usually encompass the preservation of touch, but the loss of pain and temperature, proprioception, and vibration below the level of the lesions.[10] He attributed these findings to the variation in the anatomic sites experiencing compression: the spinothalamic tract involving contralateral pain and temperature at several levels below the anatomic compression, posterior columns producing ipsilateral position and vibratory sense disturbance, and dorsal nerve root level producing dermatomal sensory loss in the upper extremity.[10] These factors are clearly influenced by the multiplicity of level and degree of compression.

Reflexes are generally hyperreflexic below the level of the anatomic lesion and hyporeflexic at the level of the anatomic lesion. Pathologic reflexes such as the presence of the Babinski reflex in the lower extremities and the Hoffmann reflex in the upper extremities characterize an upper motor neuron involvement in the cervical spine. In addition, clonus may be present in the lower extremities. Lhermitte's sign may be present when the patient flexes and extends the neck, producing a feeling of electric shock.

Distribution of these physical findings may vary considerably, as Lunsford and associates depicted in a clinical series.[47] Although a significant number of patients manifested hyperreflexia (87 per cent), only about one half had a Babinski, and less than one fifth had a Hoffmann reflex (13 per cent).[42] Fifty-eight per cent had motor weakness, 50 per cent had bladder dysfunction, but atrophy was rare (13 per cent).[42] Sensory levels could not be discretely defined in almost one half (41 per cent), and proprioception was disturbed in the lower and upper extremities in 39 per cent.[42] This series pointed to the absence of neck pain and the infrequency of clinical expression of Lhermitte's sign.[42]

CORD SYNDROMES

Crandall and Batsdorf classified patients into five groups based on dominant cord syndromes: (1) transverse lesions, with involvement of the appropriate neurologic tracts (corticospinal, spinothalamic, posterior columns) had severe spasticity and frequent sphincter involvement, and one third exhibited Lhermitte's symptom; (2) motor system lesions (anterior horn cells, corticospinal tract) showed spasticity, but relatively innocuous or absent sensory disturbance; (3) central cord syndrome had severe motor and sensory disturbances, with greater expression in the upper extremities (Lhermitte's phenomenon characterized this group); (4) Brown–Séquard syndrome had typical contralateral sensory deficits and ipsilateral motor deficits; and (5) brachalgia and cord syndrome demonstrated lower motor neuron–upper extremity involvement and upper motor neuron–lower extremity involvement. Radicular pain was the signature of this last group.[13]

Ferguson and Kaplan delineated four intermingled but defined clinical syndromes on the basis of neurologic malfunction due to spondylosis. These syndromes are: lateral or radicular syndrome, medial or spinal syndrome, combined medial/lateral syndrome, and a vascular syndrome.[21] The lateral or radicular syndrome is essentially an expression of nerve root pathology and the clinical presentation of symptoms that are the result of compressive factors.[21] In this classification, spinal cord dysfunction is absent.[21] The medial or spinal syndrome is a manifestation of the spinal cord abnormality. It has variable clinical signs that depend on the anatomic location of the pathologic factor and the severity of its effect on the cord.[21] Ferguson and Kaplan further cautioned that "the diagnosis of spondylotic or compressive myelopathy should not be made if the signs are purely pyramidal or purely sensory, as compression invariably has some effect on both the posterior and the lateral columns."[21] Clinical presentations limited to motor dysfunction with preservation of sensory perception have been documented, however, proposing isolated corticospinal tract abnormality associated with cervical spondylotic myelopathy.[14] The combined medial and lateral syndrome presents with evidence of both spinal cord and spinal nerve root symptomatology.[21] This syndrome shows an even greater heterogeneity of clinical symptoms and signs due to frequent nerve root dysfunction in the upper extremities, which are in conjunction with the upper motor neuron clinical examination in the lower extremities.[21] The vascular syndrome is composed of patients with acute-onset myelopathy in association with spondylosis when no other clear mechanism for the acute deterioration appears plausible.[21] Ferguson and Kaplan identified this category of patient with a sudden painless myelopathy in the absence of trauma, frequently associated with unimpressive myelograms in relation to the symptomatology, in whom the surgical results have been unrewarding.[21] Although Ferguson and Kaplan specified that many of these patients may have demonstrated minimal but insidious symptoms, the focus of presentation is dramatic acute worsening.[21]

GAIT

Gorter's 1976 review of cervical myelopathy concluded that cervical myelopathy usually presents initially as a subtle gait disturbance with a gradual deterioration.[28] He emphasized that spasticity and paretic dysfunction occur first, followed by numbness in the upper extremities and loss of fine motor movements.[28] Lunsford and associates series confirmed Gorter's statement that the lower extremity spasticity and gait disturbance generally occur earliest, followed by upper extremity involvement.[42] Clinical expression may vary from loss of balance, unsteadiness, stiffness with ambulation, and complaints of loss of power in the lower extremities. Myelopathic gait may appear somewhat broad-based with disruption of the smooth, rhythmic, normal function of gait replaced with a more hesitant and jerky motion.

BOWEL AND BLADDER SYMPTOMATOLOGY

Bowel and bladder dysfunction may occur in cervical myelopathy and are upper motor neuron manifestations. In the Lunsford series, 50 per cent of patients exhibited bowel and bladder dysfunction.[42] Bladder dysfunction was demonstrated in 15 per cent and bowel dysfunction in 18 per cent of a clinical series of 269 patients with myelopathy associated with cervical spondylosis.[34] In a clinical series involving patients over the age of 55 with cervical spondylotic myelopathy, 20 per cent of the patients exhibited bladder dysfunction with varying degrees of urinary retention.[20]

HAND

The term "myelopathy hand," coined by Ono and associates, focuses on the upper extremity involvement in myelopathy.[51] Myelopathy hand is defined as "loss of power of adduction and extension of the ulnar two or three fingers, and an inability to grip and release rapidly with these fingers."[51] The finger escape sign that shows the deficiency of adduction and/or extension can be distinguished from other causes (motor neuron disease or peripheral nerve entrapment syndrome) by normal active range of motion of the wrist.[51]

Ono and associates found that myelopathy hand was associated with spasticity in the lower extremities; the grading system they developed for the severity of hand involvement correlated with the performance of hand function (1 to 5).[51] Although no specific spinal level was diagnostic of myelopathy hand, its presence indicated dysfunction above the C6–C7 level.[51] Ono and associates stated, "in patients with marked spastic paraplegia and no signs of myelopathy hand, the responsible lesion is likely to be at or below the cervicodorsal junction."[51] Since myelopathy hand may be graded, careful search for its presence along with lower extremity spasticity may provide physical clues to early myelopathy.[51]

Hand involvement continues to draw attention in myelopathy. Good and associates reported a series of patients with cervical myelopathy (with compression between C3 and C5) in whom the main attribute was numbness in the hands.[27] In this group, decreased vibratory and position sense, stereoanesthesia, and diminished fine motions were present in the hands.[27] Although hyperreflexia was present in the upper extremities, only half were noted to have gait disorders and Babinski's reflex on examination. Atrophy of the hands was absent.[27] It should be realized that lesions in the foramen magnum area and a relative paucity of lower extremity symptoms often have similar hand symptoms.[27] Good and associates believed that focusing on the symptoms is key, since they may precede the onset of physical findings.[27] Less than 50 per cent of patients had the correct initial diagnosis, with attention diverted by other considerations, such as peripheral entrapment syndrome and neuropathy to explain the patients' complaints.[27]

In Epstein's series of patients over the age of 65 with cervical spondylotic myelopathy, 55 per cent of patients had the useless hand syndrome.[28] His clinical findings were associated with higher cervical spine cord involvement.[20]

In Yasuoka and associates' series of tumors at the foramen magnum, the initial examination was normal in about half of the patients.[73] "In this region are notable exceptions to the diagnostic rule that long tract signs or focal signs accurately identify the anatomic site of pathology."[73] The emphasis of this information is that the hand by symptom and physical examination must be conceptualized as the potential distal expression of the cervical spinal cord.

In contrast to the spastic hand with diminished pain sensation, Ibarra and associates characterized a myelopathy hand with wasting of the muscles—the amyotrophic type.[36] The precision of amyotropic type requires hand-muscle wasting, minimal sensory changes, hand-muscle weakness, no gait disorder, unilateral presentation, and, if bilateral, asymmetric presentation.[27] Other factors required are decreased AP diameter, lower cervical spondylosis, and reduced transectional cord area at C7 and below.[36] Two key factors are that muscle atrophy in the arms is confined to the ulnar side, and that patients responded to skull traction and surgery in six or seven cases.[36] An important factor in distinguishing this presentation caused by spondylotic disease rather than motor neuron disease is "if the distribution of the muscle atrophy corresponds to the spondylotic changes, and to the reduction of transsection area of the spinal cord."[36] In addition, myelopathy does not demonstrate neurogenic electromyographic abnormalities, or involve levels above the cord (face, tongue).[36]

UPPER EXTREMITY INVOLVEMENT

Phillips identified a subgroup of patients with cervical myelopathy and shoulder wasting and weakness.[54] The scapular and deltoid muscles were involved in 32 of the 40 cases because of myelopathies associated at the C3–C4 level, and only eight because of cervical radiculopathy at C4–C5 or C5–C6.[54] All patients with radiculopathy had pain, but only 25 per cent had myelopathy, 50 per cent had no sensory loss, and only six of 40 had deltoid area sensory loss.[54] It is interesting that in Epstein's series of patients over the age of 65 with cervical spondylotic myelopathy, 20 per cent had either unilateral or bilateral deltoid paralysis.[20]

COEXISTENT LUMBAR STENOSIS

We have focused on lower extremity spasticity in cervical spondylotic myelopathy, have identified clinical series in which patients had predominately upper extremity presentations, and have also identified a dearth of lower-extremity complaints on findings. Although spasticity is the most common issue in the lower extremities, other coexistent pathologies may present a confusing clinical picture. The biologic process of spondylosis is global, frequently affecting both the cervical and lumbar spine where motion is greatest. In a series of 214 patients, 13 per cent had symptoms in both the cervical and lumbar spine, and in this group, 64 per cent had spinal canal diameters below normal.[15] It is not surprising in the context of narrow spinal canals and spondylosis that both the cervical and lumbar spine could be symptomatic at the same time. In Epstein and associates' series of concomitant cervical and lumbar spinal stenosis, the combined pathology "resulted in the mixed and seemingly contradictory reflex picture of coincident upper and lower motor neuron dysfunction in the same patient."[19] They estimated that 5 per cent of patients with cervical stenosis also have lumbar stenosis.[19] Treatment directed to the cervical cord "often resulted in improvement in lumbar symptoms with resolution of pain, spasticity, and sensory deficits of myelopathic origin."[19] Latent symptoms of intermittent neurogenic claudication caused by lumbar stenosis were not affected by cervical decompression, however, and increased in severity.[19]

FALSE LOCALIZATION

In addition to the potential confusion resulting from coexistent pathology, cervical myelopathy may present at a painless and incorrectly localized sensory level. In a series of five cases, the cervical pathology (hard or soft disc with cord compression) was localized at the levels C3–C6, but all patients demonstrated sensory levels between T5 and T7.[63] The investigator speculated on the pathoanatomic mechanism, but the key issue is that the failure to demonstrate a satisfactory explanation for thoracic sensory deficit should invoke a consideration of cervical pathology as a possible cause.[63]

SUDDEN-ONSET MYELOPATHY

Although cervical myelopathy is generally considered a progressive, slowly developing process, there is a distinct segment of patients with acute symptomatology. Ferguson and Kaplan recognized a group with such presentation and labeled them vascular.[21] Criteria for inclusion in this group was the acute nature of the event, absence of obstruction on myelography, lack of pain, and failure to respond to surgery.[21] Vascular etiology predisposed an interruption in the competent supply of blood, via radicular spinal arteries to the anterior spinal artery, and thus the spinal cord. It has been proposed that "compression of one of these radicular spinal arteries at some point of its course or in the anterior spinal axis itself, by disc protrusions or bars, can produce ischemia of the spinal cord with zones of softening and necrosis, characteristic of cervical myelopathy."[58] Angiography (vertebral artery) has shown decreased filling of the radiculospinal arteries in cases of cervical myelopathy compared with controls.[58] The cord is most subject to compression in the lower cervical region and this represents the region of greatest vascular vulnerability on an anatomic basis.[52] Other investigators have cited a vascular lesion because of a discrepancy between level of compression and level of symptoms.[66] Clinically, the anterior spinal artery syndrome may have a variety of causes, but presents with sudden quadriparesis, and dissociation of sensory loss with preservation of vibration, position, and touch.[5] Traumatic causes have been proposed in children with spondylosis.[5] "Complete sensory and motor recovery from the anterior spinal artery syndrome after sprain of the cervical spine" has been observed.[24] The anterior spinal artery syndrome has multiple causes in which spondylosis is a rare but defined precipitant.[23] Perhaps the vulnerability to this syndrome is more prominent in those whose blood supply to the anterior two thirds of the spinal cord is derived from only one anterior radicular artery, as demonstrated in seven of 36 cadavers studied.[23]

Acute myelopathy may occur in the absence of fractures or dislocations of the cervical spine due to trauma. Out of a group of 200 patients admitted over a four-year period to a spinal cord injury unit, seven were identified with congenital narrowing of the spinal canal and showed no evidence of cervical spondylosis.[18] An additional 16 patients, comprising an older age group, featured typical cervical spondylotic changes.[18] In both groups there was a definite direct relationship between the small size of the spinal canal and the severity of the neurologic deficit.[18] No evidence of persistent myelographic impingement on the spinal cord was demonstrated in most of these patients.[18] In 16 of the 23 patients, the mechanism of injury was described as a fall and the hyperextension-induced central cord syndrome provides the most likely explanation.[18]

Radiographic analysis of patients with severe cord injuries but no bony architectural abnormalities (fracture or dislocations) showed cervical spondylosis in 96 per cent of patients.[57] This was in patients over the age of 40.[57] Falls accounted for over 50 per cent of the cases with minor degrees of presumed trauma.[57] Again, hyperextension was the presumed mechanism by which the spinal canal was dynamically narrowed, resulting in neurologic injury.[57] Cervical spondylosis was believed to narrow the canal premorbidly and the dynamics of hyperextension, precipitating a critical pathologic narrowing resulting in central cord syndrome.[57] In another series in which cervical spondylosis was associated with spinal cord injury, "most of the patients were partially or completely wheelchair dependent."[22]

Patients with congenital narrowing of the cervical canal (anterior posterior diameter less than 10 mm) and those with acquired narrowing appear to be vulnerable to acute spinal cord injury when exposed to sufficient force. The biomechanics of cord trauma has been studied by Raynor and Koplik who stated, "variations in the clinical syndromes are caused by exact magnitude and direction of the applied force of injury."[56] Since the neurologic injury may be permanent or irreversible, depending on the multiplicity of factors, efforts to identify the vulnerable individuals have been undertaken. Analyzing a group of patients with transient neurapraxia, Torg and associates determined that a spinal canal/body ratio of less than 0.80 on a lateral cervical spine roentgenogram is indicative of cervical spinal canal stenosis.[67] The relationship between cervical canal narrowing as defined by the spinal canal vertebral body ratio (Torg's ratio), and neurologic injury has not been correlated in a general population, however. This leads the investigators to conclude that individuals with ratios less than 0.80 "should not be precluded from further participation in contact sports whether or not they have had symptoms of cord neurapraxia."[68]

Watkins and Dillin proposed that multiple factors are involved in the decision-making process in patients with Torg ratios less than 0.80 rather than the absolute of the ratio itself.[70]

Spinal cord compression due to soft-disc herniation may also present as acute myelopathy and represents a group requiring acute surgical intervention.[55] In one series of 26 central disc herniations a disproportionate incidence of C3–C4 herniations was identified and the "impairment of posterior column function particularly in the upper limbs played a major part in producing disability."[49] O'Laoire and Thomas warned that acute disc herniations should be suspected in patients with myelopathy and "whose plain radiographs show congenital or spontaneous fusion, and in patients with previous history of cervical injury."[49]

Acute cervical spondylotic myelopathy can exist without an identifiable initiating event.[71]

STABILITY

Stability has been defined for the upper (C1–C2) and lower (C3–C7) aspects of the cervical spine.[2] In patients with critical narrowing of the cervical spinal canal secondary to spondylosis, retrolisthesis, or anterior listhesis of vertebrae, however, stiff segments may contribute to myelopathy on a dynamic basis.[8] In patients with documented cervical spondylotic myelopathy, those treated conservatively and possessing more cervical mobility appear to do worse than those with stiffer necks.[3] In this series, "the minimum AP diameter, minimum canal size, degree of subluxation, and the amount of posterior osteophytosis all had no predictive value."[3] Interestingly, static and dynamic anterior posterior canal diameters have been demonstrated to decrease with age, and the dynamic canal is much narrower than the static canal.[30] Dynamic factors appear to be empirically significant in the generation of myelopathic symptoms.

OTHER PATHOLOGIES

It is not our intention to belabor the multiple causes that lead to the final common expression of myelopathy. Although controversy swirls in relation to the outcome of surgical treatment, it is important to recognize that other pathologic entities may lead to spinal cord compression besides the spondylytic spur.

Although the spondylytic spurs commonly arise from the vertebral body area, posterior hypertrophy of the facets and lamina may cause compression.[17] Ossification of the ligamenta flavum has also been identified as a pathologic culprit.[39] Ossification of the posterior longitudinal ligament has been identified as an anterior compressive source in Asians with cervical cord compression.[1, 31, 38] Efforts have been directed at pointing out the occurrence of cervical myelopathy due to ossification of the posterior longitudinal ligament in non-Asians.[45] Finally, rheumatoid arthritis is commonly associated with subluxations of the atlantoaxial joint and the potential development of myelopathy.[43, 44, 59] Subaxial subluxations at single or multiple levels may produce myelopathy in rheumatoid arthritis.[29] Congenital block vertebrae may lead to hypermobility of the adjacent segment and compressive pathology.[40]

CONCLUSION

Cervical myelopathy is a graded process with variable clinical manifestations. Anatomic location of compression, ischemia, and dynamic factors also contribute to its spectrum. Perhaps the most important issue in myelopathy is that it is treatable and its early diagnosis enhances the pool of good results. This is precisely the time when vigorous suspicion and investigative histories are more salient features of the disease than the neurologic findings, however. Emphasis should be placed on obtaining histories of numbness and clumsiness in the hands, decreased fine motor movements, and subtle gait disorders. Suspicion of its clinical existence remains the single greatest element in the identification of early cervical spondylotic myelopathy. Only then can such vigilance "ring out old shapes of foul disease."[4]

References

1. Abe, H, Tsura, M, and Ito, T.: Anterior decompression for ossification of the posterior longitudinal ligament of the cervical spine. J. Neurosurg. *55:*108–116, 1981.
2. Bailey, R., et al.: The Cervical Spine. Philadelphia, J. B. Lippincott Co., 1983, pp 23–61.
3. Barnes, M. P., and Saunders, M.: The effect of cervical mobility on the natural history of cervical spondylotic myelopathy. J. Neurol. Neurosurg. Psychiatry *47:*17–20, 1984.
4. Bartlett's Familiar Quotations. Boston, Little, Brown & Co., 1980.
5. Blennow, G.: Anterior spinal artery syndrome. Pediatr. Neurosci. *13:*32–37, 1987.
6. Brain, W. R., Northfield, D. W., and Wilkinson, M.: The neurologic manifestations of cervical spondylosis. Brain *75:*187–225, 1952.
7. Bohlman, H., and Emery, S.: The pathophysiology of cervical spondylosis and myelopathy. Spine *13:*843 846, 1988.
8. Bohlman, H.: Cervical spondylosis with moderate to severe myelopathy. Spine *2:*151–162, 1977.
9. Campbell, A. M. G., and Phillips, D. G.: Cervical disk lesion with neurological disorder. Br. Med. J. *5197:*481–485, 1960.
10. Clark, C. R.: Cervical spondylotic myelopathy: history and physical findings. Spine *13:*847–849, 1988.
11. Clark, E., and Robinson, P. K.: Cervical myelopathy: a complication of cervical spondylosis. Brain *79:*483, 1956.
12. Commisse, G. E.: The Arteries and Veins of the Lumbar Spinal Cord from Birth. New York, Churchill Livingstone, 1975.
13. Crandall, P. H., and Batsdorf, U.: Cervical spondylotic myelopathy. J. Neurosurg. *25:*57–66, 1966.
14. Cusick, J., and Myklebust, B.: Isolated corticospinal tract abnormalities associated with segmental stenosis. Orthop. Trans. *11:*15, 1987.
15. Edwards, W., and Larocca, H.: The developmental segmental sagittal diameter in combined cervical and lumbar spondylosis. Spine *10:*42–49, 1985.
16. Epstein, J. A., and Epstein, W. E.: The surgical management of cervical spinal stenosis, spondylosis and myeloradiculopathy by means of the posterior approach. *In* The Cervical Spine Research Society: The Cervical Spine. 2nd ed. Philadelphia, J. B. Lippincott Co., 1989, pp. 625–643.
17. Epstein, J., Epstein, B., Lavine, L., et al.: Cervical myeloradiculopathy caused by arthrotic hypertrophy of the posterior facets and laminae. J. Neurosurg. *49:*387–392, 1978.
18. Epstein, N., Epstein, J., Benjamin, V., et al.: Traumatic myelopathy in patients with cervical spinal stenosis without fracture or dislocation. Spine *P5:*489–496, 1980.
19. Epstein, N., Epstein, J., Carras, R., et al.: Co-existing cervical and lumbar spinal stenosis: diagnosis and management. Neurosurgery *10:*489–496, 1984.
20. Epstein, N., Epstein, J., and Carras, R.: Cervical spondylostenosis and related disorders in patients over 65: current management and diagnostic techniques. Orthotransactions *11:*15, 1987.
21. Ferguson, R. J. L., and Kaplan, L. R.: Cervical spondylitic myelopathy. Neurol. Clin. *3:*373–382, 1985.
22. Foo, D.: Spinal cord injury in forty-four patients with cervical spondylosis. Paraplegia *24:*301–306, 1986.
23. Foo, D., and Rossier, A.: Anterior spinal artery syndrome and its natural history. Paraplegia *21:*1–10, 1983.
24. Foo, D., Rossier, A., and Cochran, T.: Complete sensory and motor recovery from anterior spinal artery syndrome after sprain of the cervical spine. Eur. Neurol. *23:*119–123, 1984.
25. Fujiwara, K., Yonenobu, K., Ebara, S., et al.: The prognosis of surgery for cervical compression myelopathy. J. Bone Joint Surg. *71B:*393–398, 1989.

26. Fujiwara, K., Yonenobu, K., and Hiroshima, K.: Morphometry of the cervical spinal cord and its relation to pathology in cases with compression myelopathy. Spine *13:*1212–1216, 1988.
27. Good, D., Couch, J., and Wacaster, L.: "Numb clumsy hands" and high cervical spondylosis. Surg. Neurol. *22:*285–291, 1984.
28. Gorter, K.: Influence of laminectomy on the course of cervical myelopathy. Acta Neurochir. *33:*265–281, 1976.
29. Halla, J., and Fallahi, S.: Cervical discovertebral destruction, subaxial subluxation and myelopathy in a patient with rheumatoid arthritis. Arthritis Rheum. *24:*944–947, 1981.
30. Hayashi, H., Okada, K., and Hashimoto, J.: Cervical spondylotic myelopathy in the aged patient. Spine *13:*618–625, 1988.
31. Hirabayashi, K., and Satomi, K.: Operative procedure and results of expansive open-door laminoplasty. Spine *13:*870–876, 1988.
32. Hoff, J., Nishimura, M., and Pitts, L.: The role of ischemia in the pathogenesis of cervical spondylotic myelopathy: a review and new microangiographic evidence. Spine *2:*100–108, 1977.
33. Hukuda, S., and Wilson, D.: Experimental cervical myelopathy: effects of compression and ischemia on the canine cervical cord. J. Neurosurg. *37:*631–652, 1972.
34. Hukuda, S., Mochizuki, T., Ogata, M., et al.: Operations for cervical spondylotic myelopathy. J. Bone Joint Surg. *67B:*609–615, 1985.
35. Hukuda, S., Ogata, M., and Katswura, A.: Experimental study on acute aggravating factors of cervical spondylotic myelopathy. Spine *13:*15–20, 1988.
36. Ibarra, S., Yonenobu, K., Fujiwara, K., et al.: Myelopathy hand characterized by muscle wasting. Spine *13:*785–791, 1988.
37. Ikeda, K., Wada, E., and Hosoe, H.: Numerical evaluation of symptoms in cervical myelopathy by quantification theory 111 (Hayashi). Spine *14:*1140–1143, 1989.
38. Kimura, I., Oh-Hama, M., and Shingu, H.: Cervical myelopathy treated by canal-expansive laminaplasty. J. Bone Joint Surg. *66A:*914–920, 1984.
39. Kubota, M., Baba, I., and Sumida, T.: Myelopathy due to the ossification of the ligamentum flavum of the cervical spine. Spine *6:*553–559, 1981.
40. Lee, C., and Weiss, A.: Isolated congenital cervical block vertebrae below the axis with neurological symptoms. Spine *6:*118–124, 1981.
41. Lees, F., and Turner, J. W. A.: Natural history and prognosis of cervical spondylosis. Br. Med. J. *2:*1607–1610, 1963.
42. Lunsford, L. D., Bissonette, D., and Zorub, D.: Anterior surgery for cervical disc disease. Part 2. J. Neurosurg. *53:*12–19, 1980.
43. Manz, H., Luessenhop, A., and Robertson, D.: Cervical myelopathy due to atlantoaxial and subaxial subluxation in rheumatoid arthritis. Arch. Pathol. Lab. Med. *107:*94–99, 1983.
44. Marks, J. S., and Sharp, J.: Rheumatoid cervical myelopathy. Q. J. Med. *199:*307–319, 1981.
45. McAfee, P., Regan, J., and Bohlman, H.: Cervical cord compression from ossification of the posterior longitudinal ligament in non-Orientals. J. Bone Joint Surg. *69B:*569–575, 1987.
46. Nurick, S.: The pathogenesis of the spinal cord disorder associated with cervical spondylosis. Brain *95:*87–100, 1972.
47. Nurick, S.: The natural history and the results of surgical treatment of the spinal cord disorder associated with cervical spondylosis. Brain *95:*101–108, 1972.
48. Ogino, H., Tada, K., Okada, K., et al.: Canal diameter, anteroposterior compression ratio, and spondylotic myelopathy of the cervical spine. Spine *8:*1–15, 1983.
49. O'Laoire, S., and Thomas, D.: Spinal cord compression due to prolapse of cervical intervertebral disc. J. Neurosurg. *59:*847–853, 1983.
50. Ono, K., Ota, H., Tada, K., and Yamamoto, T.: Cervical myelopathy secondary to multiple spondylotic protrusions: A clinicopathologic study. Spine *2:*109–125, 1977.
51. Ono, K., Ebara, S., Fiji, T., et al.: Myelopathy hand. J. Bone Joint Surg. *69B:*215–219, 1987.
52. Parke, W.: Correlative anatomy of cervical spondylotic myelopathy. Spine *13:*831–837, 1988.
53. Phillips, D. G.: Surgical treatment of myelopathy with cervical spondylosis. J. Neurol. Neurosurg. Psychiatry *36:*879–884, 1973.
54. Phillips, D. G.: The shoulder girdle disc. J. Neurol. Neurosurg. Psychiatry *39:*817–820, 1976.
55. Raynor, R.: Cervical cord compression secondary to acute disc protrusion in trauma. Spine *2:*39–43, 1977.
56. Raynor, R. B., and Koplik, B.: Cervical cord trauma: The relationship between clinical syndromes and force of injury. Spine *10:*193–197, 1985.
57. Regenbogen, V., Rogers, L., Atlas, S., et al.: Cervical spinal cord injuries in patients with cervical spondylosis. A.J.R. *146:*277–284, 1986.
58. Rovira, M., Torrent, O., and Ruscalleda, J.: Some aspects of the spinal cord circulation in cervical myelopathy. Neuroradiology *9:*209–214, 1975.
59. Santavirta, S., Slatis, P., and Kankaapaa, U.: Treatment of the cervical spine in rheumatoid arthritis. J. Bone Joint Surg. *70A:*658–667, 1988.
60. Satomi, K., Okuna, T., and Kenmotsu, K.: Level diagnosis of cervical myelopathy using evoked spinal cord potentials. Spine *13:*1217–1224, 1988.
61. Shinomiya, K., Okamoto, A., Matsuoka, T., et al.: 17th Annual Meeting Cervical Spine Research Society, December 1989.
62. Simeone, F. A., and Rothman, R. H.: Cervical disc disease. *In* Rothman, R. H., Simeone, F. A. (eds.): The Spine. Philadelphia, W. B. Saunders Co., 1982, pp 440–476.
63. Simmons, Z., Biller, J., and Beck, D.: Painless compressive cervical myelopathy with false localizing sensory findings. Spine *P9:*869–872, 1986.
64. Symon, L., and Lavender, P.: The surgical treatment of cervical spondylotic myelopathy. Neurology *17:*117–127, 1967.
65. Takahashi, M., Yamashita, Y., Sakamoto, Y., and Kojima, R.: Chronic cervical cord compression: clinical significance of increased signal intensity on MR images. Neuroradiology *173:*219–224, 1989.
66. Taylor, A. R.: Vascular factors in the myelopathy associated with cervical spondylosis. Neurology *14:*62–68, 1964.
67. Torg, J. S., Pavlov, H., Genuario, S. E., et al.: Neurapraxia of the cervical spinal cord with tran-

sient quadriplegia. J. Bone Joint Surg. *68A:*1354–1370, 1986.
68. Torg, J. S., Pavlov, H., and Warren, R.: The relationship of cervical spinal canal narrowing ("stenosis") to permanent neurologic injury to the athlete: an epidemiologic survey. Proceedings of Cervical Spine Research Society, 17th Annual Meeting, New Orleans, December, 1989.
69. Veidlinger, O. F., Colwill, J. C., Smyth, H. S., et al.: Cervical myelopathy and its relationship to cervical stenosis. Spine *6:*550–552, 1981.
70. Watkins, R., and Dillin, W.: Criteria for return to activity participation following cervical spine injuries. *In* Athletic Injuries to the Head, Neck and Face. 2nd ed. Chicago, Year Book Medical Publishers, 1990, pp. 132–166.
71. Wilberger, J., and Chadid, M.: Acute cervical spondylytic myelopathy. Neurosurgery *22:*145–146, 1988.
72. Yu, Y. L., DuBoulay, G. H., Stevens, J. M., et al.: Computer assisted myelography in cervical spondylotic myelopathy and radiculopathy. Brain *109:*259–278, 1986.
73. Yasuoka, S., Okazaki, H., and Daube, J.: Foramen magnun tumors, analysis of 57 cases of benign extramedullary tumors. J. Neurosurg. *49:*828–838, 1978.

RADIOLOGIC EVALUATION

David P. Wesolowski, M.D.
Ay-Ming Wang, M.D.

The recognition that cervical disc degeneration and consequent structural changes could lead to compression of neural elements and vasculature resulting in symptoms became widespread during the middle decades of this century.[5] Many reports dealing with the genetic, biochemical, and age-related factors involved in the cause of disc disease as well as several other reports dealing with the effects of developmental, traumatic, and psychosocial factors on the symptomatology have led to a much better understanding of the disease processes.[6, 9, 24, 26, 45, 50, 56, 59] Several authors observed that although acute cervical disc degeneration resulting in herniation of the nucleus pulposus and chronic disc degeneration resulting in spondylosis may be different manifestations of the same process, it is useful to distinguish between the two since the age of the patient, mode of onset of symptoms, and types of associated neurologic involvement may vary significantly.

The radiology of cervical disc disease evolved in response to the need to demonstrate the structural changes that occur and to correlate these changes with the patient's symptoms. The standard radiographic examination of the cervical spine is useful to display the bony relationships, the developmental anomalies, and some of the pathologic changes resulting in osteophyte formation and calcification; however, it was the development of myelography during the early years that first allowed demonstration of the neural involvement directly.[10, 25, 49] Technologic advances during the last decade, particularly the evolution of computerized imaging modalities, have resulted in the capability to demonstrate the structural changes that occur as a result of cervical disc disease with an unprecedented degree of precision and accuracy. In addition, the latest modality, magnetic resonance imaging (MRI), not only displays detailed spatial resolution but also provides information concerning the biochemical and pathophysiologic changes that often leads to a better understanding of the disease process.

These newer techniques combined with the standard radiographic examination and the various modifications of the myelogram are the main tools used in the radiology of cervical disc disease as the state of the art exists today. Which modalities are used and how they are sequenced depends on many factors. The clinical presentation of the patient, the experience of the physician, and even various economic and governmental regulatory policies that affect availability influence decision making.

This section will discuss the radiologic evaluation of the patient with cervical disc disease and present examples of the different techniques used. Discussion of the physical phenomena involved will be limited to what is believed necessary to properly tailor the evaluation to a particular patient.

TECHNICAL CONSIDERATIONS

Radiographic Examination

The radiographic examination of the cervical spine is a valuable first step in the radiologic evaluation of the patient with cervical disc disease, and when properly performed and interpreted, provides a cost-effective guide to tailoring the remainder of the evaluation. Current generation radiographic equipment uses smaller focal spot x-ray tubes and upright Bucky grids that, when combined with the newer rare-earth intensifying screens and film emulsions, result in much more detailed radiographs with less radiation dose to the patient than in the past. Higher kilovoltage–lower milliampere-second exposure techniques generally display longer scale contrast resolution, that is, more shades of gray, which is helpful when looking at soft tissues as well as fine bony details.

The examination should consist of AP, oblique, and lateral neutral-flexion-extension views of the entire cervical spine. The craniovertebral and cervicothoracic junctions should be demonstrated using open-mouth and "swimmer's" views as needed. The patient should be examined in a seated upright position whenever possible to assess the effects of weight bearing on the spatial relationships between contiguous segments as well as the regional curvatures. The upright position may result in a somewhat lower position of the shoulders, which enables a less obstructed lateral view of C7–T1 to be obtained. The target-film distance used must be consistent with the methods used to measure the sagittal and transverse diameters of the spinal canal.[12, 21, 41, 57, 64] A 72-inch target-film distance is used most often for the lateral views, resulting in a measurement of 13 mm as the lower limit of normal for the sagittal diameter of the cervical spinal canal.

Discography

The technique of discography described by Lindblom in 1948 consists of opacifying the nucleus pulposus by injecting radiopaque contrast media into the disc via a small-gauge needle inserted percutaneously.[33a] Although supporters of discography state that it can demonstrate abnormalities not seen on myelography, the true advantage of this technique may be the production of pain during the injection that reproduces the patient's symptoms.[50] Abnormal discograms may be seen in asymptomatic patients; therefore, since considerable discomfort is experienced by the patient during the procedure and there are serious potential complications, we do not recommend this technique as a routine radiologic imaging tool. Experienced physicians may want to use discography as a provocative clinical test in certain situations, however.

Myelography

The current technique of cervical myelography consists of injecting radiopaque contrast media into the subarachnoid space and maneuvering this material into the cervical region under fluoroscopic guidance with the patient secured to a fluoroscopic table that tilts 90 degrees in either direction. Fluoroscopic equipment designed primarily for myelography has biplane fluoroscopic capability; however, myelography can be satisfactorily performed using standard radiographic/fluoroscopic equipment. The flow characteristics and defects in the column of contrast medium are observed fluoroscopically and permanent images are recorded using spot-film techniques supplemented by standard radiographs when needed. Film-screen combinations should be chosen so as to maximize the visualization of the contrast media when operating within the kilovoltage range as determined by the absorption characteristics of the contrast medium used. Pantopaque, with its denser absorption characteristics, requires kilovoltage in the 90 to 110 kV range to penetrate the contrast column; as a result, par speed film-screen combinations (100 speed system) may be used that result in a spatial resolution of approximately 8 to 10 line pairs per millimeter (lp/mm). The absorption characteristics of the newer water-soluble contrast media are dependent on the concentration of iodine selected; in general, however, they appear much less dense than Pantopaque and require exposure techniques in the 60 to 90 kV range. With these lower exposures a rare-earth film screen combination (400 to 800 speed system) may be required with a slight diminution in the spatial resolution to approximately 4 to 5 lp/mm. Computerized techniques that enhance the contrast of fluoroscopic and radiographic images are being explored and may become widely used in the future.[54, 63]

There are several contrast media currently available for myelography. Pantopaque is an excellent contrast agent that may be used safely in most patients; however, its use for myelography has been associated with significant long-term complications including foreign-body granulomas and chronic adhesive arachnoiditis, often potentiated by certain iatrogenic factors such as bloody spinal tap and the administration of intrathecal steroid compounds.[4, 19, 33, 55] Long-term complications are virtually absent with the water-soluble contrast media; however, short-term side effects including seizure activity may occur, although much less frequently with iopamidol and iohexol than with metrizamide.[32, 34, 48] The incidence of serious side effects such as seizure activity is so rare with iopamidol and iohexol that myelography using these agents is routinely performed on an outpatient basis.[61] The contrast material may be instilled into the subarachnoid space by either lumbar or lateral C1–C2 puncture. The lateral cervical route allows direct injection of contrast media into the cervical spinal canal; as a result, lower concentrations and a lower total dose of iodine may be used. The lateral C1–C2 puncture is somewhat more painful and hazardous than lumbar puncture.[26, 39, 40] For these reasons we recommend a fluoroscopically guided lumbar puncture using a 22-gauge needle and 10 ml of contrast media in a 200 to 300 mg iodine per ml concentration, which nearly always yields satisfactory results. A split-dose technique for total columnar myelography has been described.[2] Gas myelography was never well suited to the demonstration of cervical disc disease.[12]

CT and CT Myelography

Detailed discussion of the physical phenomena involved and instrumentation used in the production of CT images is beyond the scope of this chapter; however, this information is available to those interested.[35] An understanding of certain factors is useful when this modality is contemplated in the evaluation of a particular patient, nonetheless.

A CT image is produced by passing a tightly collimated beam of x-rays produced in an x-ray tube through the patient's body, which absorbs or attenuates portions of the beam to varying degrees, depending on the initial intensity of the beam and the density of the structures encountered. The attenuated beam then produces flashes of light in detector crystals that are amplified and quantitated as electrical signals, which are manipulated by the computer to produce the resultant image. Since the detectors used in CT have a more linear response to radiation than the crystals of film emulsion, much smaller differences in the density of tissues may be perceived with CT than with radiographs. Also, the data can be manipulated by the computer to enhance the images and to reformat the images in multiple planes. Small structures, such as the cervical discs, require high levels of exposure (120 kV and 500 to 1000 MAS) and tightly collimated beams (1 to 2 mm) to be accurately displayed (Fig. 19–1). The time required to produce the images usually makes it impractical to study more than three segments during one examination. Precise clinical localization of the level of involvement is therefore important when CT is used to evaluate suspected cervical disc disease.

The lack of large amounts of epidural fat in the cervical region makes it difficult to perceive the posterior margins of the disc; as a result, pathologic changes are not as conspicuous as in the lumbar region. Intravenous infusion of contrast material during the procedure may help demonstrate disc herniations and free fragments more accurately.[52] The inability to remain motionless because of pain, distorted and angulated anatomy, and artifacts produced by thicker tissues in the lower cervical region limit the usefulness of CT in many patients.

A CT myelogram is a CT examination of the cervical spine after intrathecal instillation of water-soluble contrast media. The presence of water-soluble contrast media in the subarachnoid space greatly improves the value of the CT examination and can be performed either as an adjunct to standard myelography or as the primary procedure using lower dosages (3 to 5 ml) and lower concentrations (170 to 180 mg I/ml) of contrast. Using these lower doses of contrast media provides a safe method of studying patients on an outpatient basis; in one study of this technique using metrizamide,

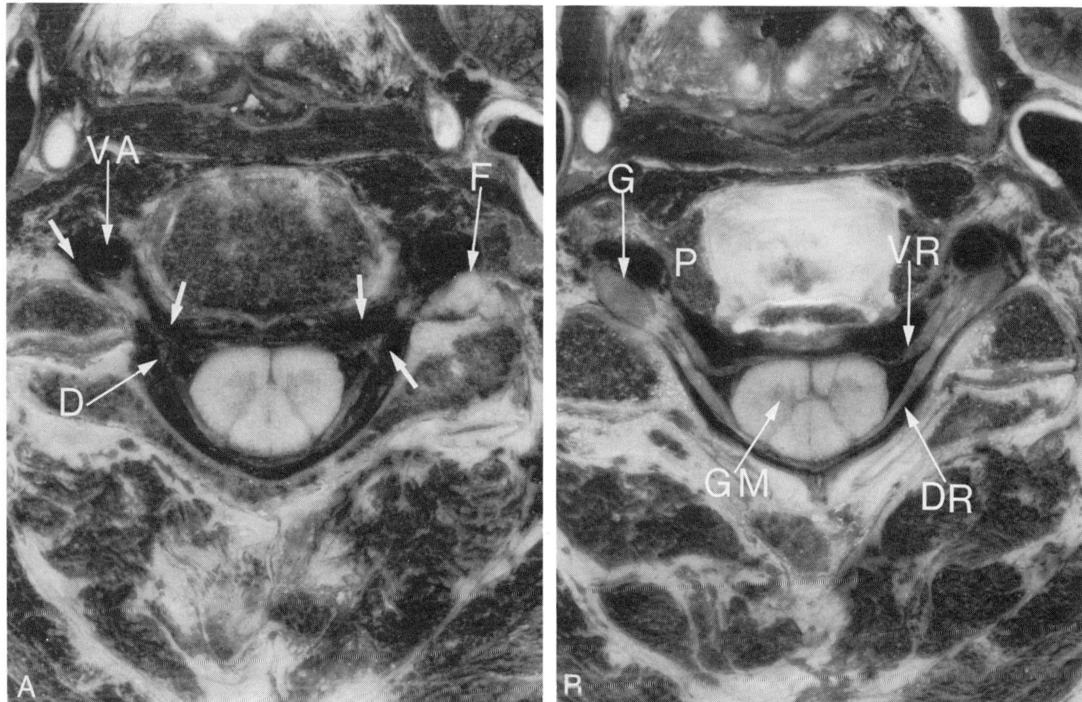

Figure 19–1. Comparative axial sections taken through a typical cervical segment at the level of the lower portion of the neural foramen. VA, vertebral artery; D, dura; DR, dorsal root; VR, ventral root; F, fat; G, ganglion; GM, gray matter; ID, intervertebral disc; P, uncinate process; HNP, herniated nucleus pulposus. *A,* A 1-mm thick anatomic section at the level of the lower margin of the C5 vertebral body. At this level the neural foramen contains mostly fat and prominent venous channels *(short arrows).* The rootlets emerge from the cord at this level but enter the neural foramen more inferiorly. Note that the vertebral arteries are surrounded by prominent venous channels, which results in an inhomogeneous signal intensity in this region on magnetic resonance imaging (MRI). *B,* A 1-mm anatomic section obtained 3 mm inferior to the section in *A.* Note the orientation of the ventral and dorsal roots. The dorsal root ganglion lies in the outer portions of the foramen, posterior to the vertebral artery and surrounding veins, within a little notch in the superior articular facet. Note the prominent venous channels within the foramina. The lateral portions of the discs are reinforced by the uncinate processes. The relationships of the ligamentum flavum to the posterolateral margins of the spinal cord can be seen.

Illustration continued on opposite page

which is more irritating than iopamidol or iohexol, approximately 90 per cent of patients remained asymptomatic after the procedure.[66] Although it has been demonstrated that the anatomy of the cervical neural foramina and contents may be shown well by conventional high-resolution CT, the addition of intrathecal contrast material allows the demonstration of swollen nerve roots and quantitative analysis of cord compression, which adds "specificity" to such findings that are useful when correlating structural changes with symptomatology (Fig. 19–1).[42, 43] Also, delayed CT myelography, which is performed 10 to 12 hours after administration of the contrast material, has been shown to demonstrate the cystic lesions within the spinal cord that are known to occur in association with long-standing cord compression. This additional information is useful when correlating structural changes with ambiguous clinical signs or lack of improvement after decompressive surgery.[28]

The accurate and often specific demonstration of extradural, intradural, and intramedullary lesions; ready availability; and good patient tolerance, even on an outpatient basis, are the main advantages of CT myelography. Relative disadvantages to be considered are the need to inject contrast medium and the use of ionizing radiation. It may not be possible to examine certain large patients (greater than 280 pounds) or patients with claustrophobia because of geometric or other design features of a particular CT scanner.

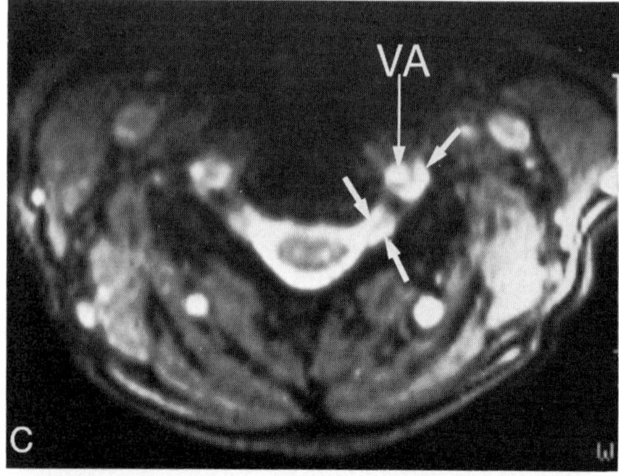

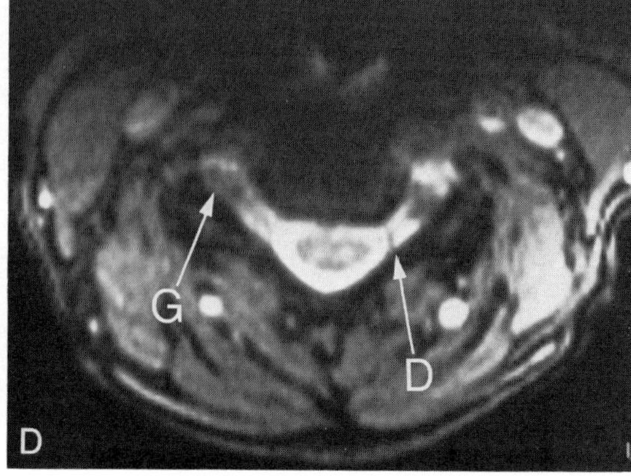

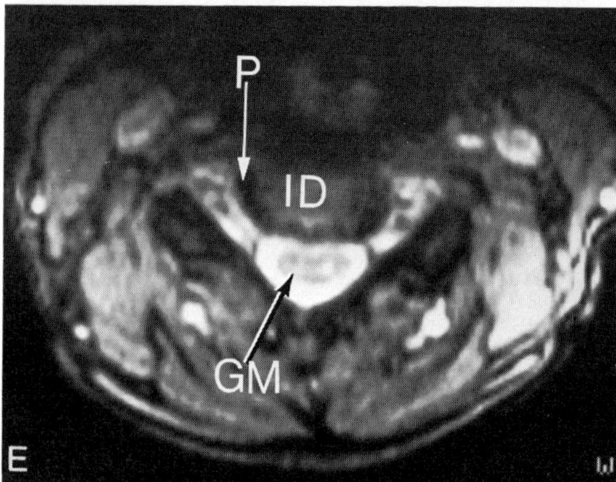

Figure 19–1 *Continued C* to *E*, Flow-compensated, T2-weighted, gradient-echo MRI scans taken through the C5–C6 neural foramina of a healthy volunteer. Overlapping 3-mm sections correspond to the anatomic levels shown in *A* and *B*. Note the good "myelogram effect" obtained by the high signal intensity produced by the cerebrospinal fluid (CSF). The flow compensation effects on this pulse sequence also result in bright signal from the blood within the epidural venous plexus and the veins surrounding the roots within the foramina and surrounding the vertebral arteries *(short arrows)*. Note the precise delineation of the gray matter within the spinal cord. The nerve roots and ganglia are somewhat indistinct because of the thickness of the sections, but are still identifiable. Note the hyperintense signal from the intervertebral disc and the lack of signal from the cortical bone. The bone marrow has an intermediate signal intensity.

MRI of the Spine

The nuclei of atoms containing odd numbers of protons (notably hydrogen), which normally behave as tiny spinning magnets randomly oriented in space, tend to align themselves with the magnetic lines of force when placed in a strong magnetic field. In this aligned state, the nuclei tend to precess, or "wobble," at a specific rate or frequency, termed Larmor frequency. This rate of revolution or frequency is approximately 42 million revolutions per second (42 MHz) at a magnetic strength of 1.0 tesla or 20,000 times the magnetic strength of the earth. When these nuclei are exposed to radiofrequency energy corresponding to the Larmor frequency, the orientation of the nuclei is perturbed or "tipped over." As the nuclei regain their aligned orientation, they emit a radio signal of exactly the same frequency. This phenomenon, termed nuclear magnetic resonance, has been used in analytical chemistry for several years and is the source of the radio signals analyzed in MRI. By setting up precisely specified magnetic field gradients, using precisely tuned radiofrequency signals, and precisely timing the phase relationships of the emitted radio signals, one can receive spatially encoded signals that can be used to produce exquisitely detailed anatomic images. The appearance of various tissues is a function of their chemical composition and their state of motion. The production and timing of the "echoes" or signals generated, compensation for motion, and certain geometric factors can be adjusted, which markedly changes the appearance of the resultant images. These complex sets of instructions, termed pulse sequences, may vary considerably, depending on the field strength of the magnet, and even between different magnets of the same strength. Much literature concerning these parameters exists, primarily written

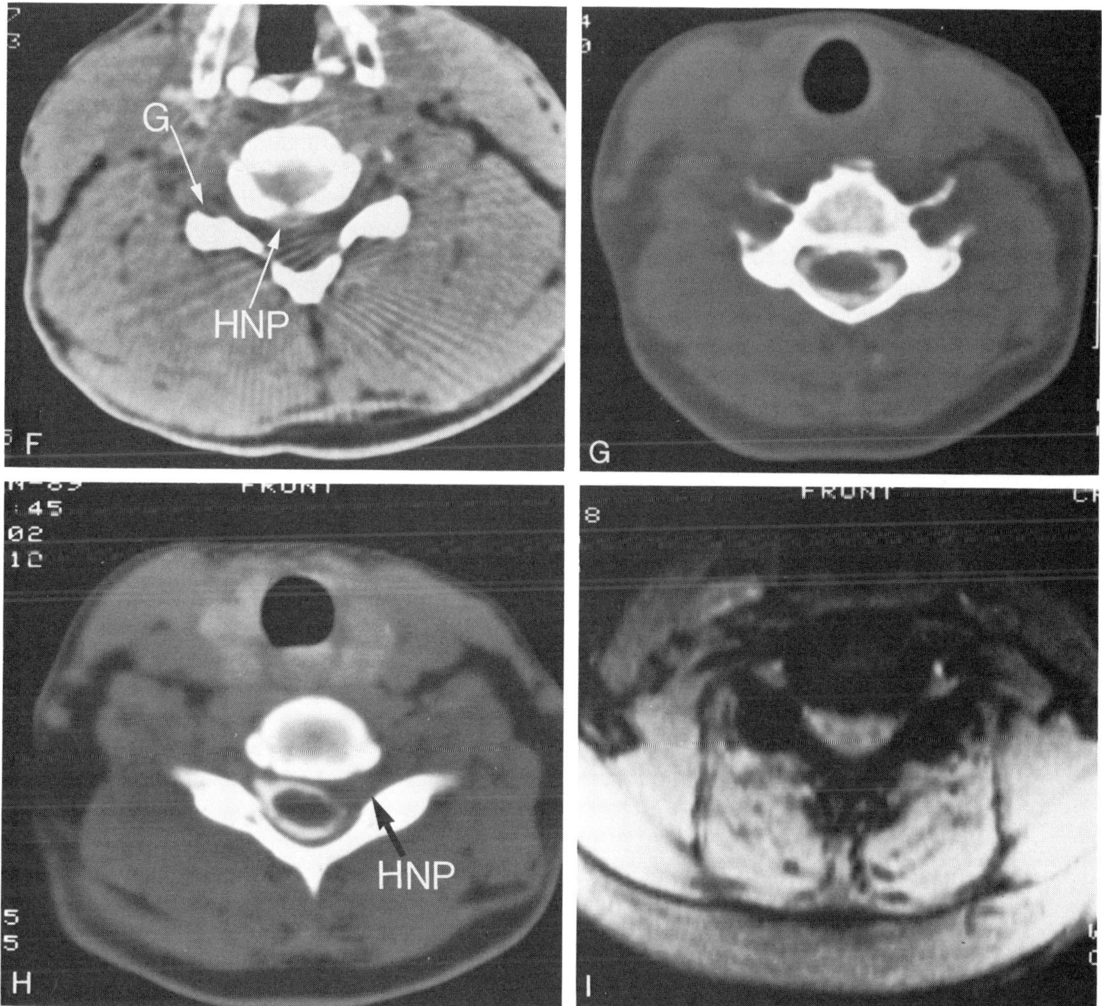

Figure 19–1 *Continued F,* High-resolution computed tomographic (CT) scan through the C5–C6 neural foramen; 125-kV, 1050-mAs, 2-mm slice thickness. Noncontrast CT demonstration of a moderately large central herniation of the C5–C6 intervertebral disc. Note the demonstration of the ganglia bilaterally. Streak artifacts obscure the visualization of the arachnoid sac and contents. *G, H,* CT myelogram demonstration of a large posterolateral disc herniation of the C6–C7 intervertebral disc and anterior and posterior spondylotic spurs near the upper margin of the C6 vertebral body. Moderate anterolateral compression of the arachnoid sac and cord as well as swelling of the ganglion on the left are demonstrated. Note the swollen dorsal and ventral nerve roots on the left, which are easily seen. The normal roots on the right side are barely visible. *I,* T2-weighted gradient-echo MRI scan obtained without flow compensation. Note the overall diminution of the signal intensity compared with the flow-compensated images shown above. Because of the diminished signal available, the slice thickness has been increased to 5 mm. Note the large circumferential spondylotic spur formation, which constricts the neural foramina. The cord is visible within the arachnoid sac and demonstrates considerable atrophy involving the posterolateral fiber tracks owing to long-standing canal stenosis. (*A* and *B* from Pech, P., Daniels, D. L., Williams, A. L., and Haughton, V. M.: The cervical neural foramina: correlation of microtomy and CT anatomy. Radiology *155:*143–146, 1985.)

for magnetic resonance physicists; however, the interested physician may obtain a working understanding of the physical phenomena from less intimidating publications.[62] Repetition time (TR), usually measured in seconds, and echo time (TE), usually measured in milliseconds, refer to the timing of the radio signals and largely determine the appearance of the image. Short TR and short TE result in T1-weighted images and long TR/long TE result in T2-weighted images. T1-weighted images, in which the cerebrospinal fluid (CSF) and cavities within the spinal cord appear dark, usually provide good spatial resolution; and T2-weighted images, in which the CSF, nucleus pulposus, and syrinx cavities appear white, help characterize the water content of normal and pathologic tissues. Spin-echo images, usually requiring 10 to 15 minutes to produce, contain more radio signal and therefore are more detailed. Gradient-echo sequences, which may be obtained much more rapidly, (usually 3 to 5 minutes) are somewhat less detailed but are not as susceptible to degradation by patient motion. Cardiac gating and other flow compensation techniques help limit the effects of physiologic motion, which is particularly important in the cervical region, where CSF pulsations may significantly degrade the image.

Routine magnetic resonance examination of the cervical spine consists of T1-weighted spin-echo images obtained in the sagittal plane; T2-weighted, spin-echo or gradient-echo, cardiac-gated images in the sagittal plane; and flow-compensated, T2-weighted, gradient echo images in the axial plane. A normal flow-compensated, T2-weighted, gradient-echo sequence in the axial plane correlated with anatomic sections is shown in Figure 19–1. Unlike the situation with imaging techniques using x-rays, where there are relatively few variables and fairly consistent results among various institutions and equipment manufacturers, there is considerable variability in the results obtained with MRI when comparing different institutions and equipment with unique characteristics. Reports of techniques to limit artifacts and optimize the examination of the cervical spine are useful in this regard.[7, 13, 14, 20, 23, 51] With optimal techniques, various aspects of the neurovascular anatomy can be emphasized and the normal physiologic changes that occur during maturation and aging of the intervertebral discs can be studied.[1, 15, 17, 22, 27, 60, 65] Bone marrow changes in the vertebral bodies and cystic degeneration within the spinal cord that accompany chronic disc degeneration can also be well demonstrated.[11, 18, 38, 58] Contrast media are usually not required with MRI, unlike CT; however, the intravenous administration of gadolinium-DTPA may help differentiate herniated free fragments from other epidural masses.

Whether one considers MRI of the cervical spine to be the preferred modality in the evaluation of cervical disc disease, as many do, it is clear that this technique is an extremely valuable addition in the diagnosis of cervical disc disease. Noninvasiveness, the ability to display spatial information in multiple planes, and the ability to characterize tissues more fully are the main advantages of this technique. Some of the disadvantages of MRI are that it is susceptible to motion artifacts and, depending on the field strength of the magnet, a complete examination requiring 45 to 60 minutes may not be tolerated by patients in severe pain. Other patient factors such as the presence of ferromagnetic surgical implants, large body habitus, and complex spine curvatures may also preclude use. Regional differences affecting availability of equipment and reimbursement policies of third-party payors are currently relative disadvantages in certain instances.

The results obtained by the radiologic and MRI evaluation of the patient with cervical disc disease are influenced by many factors. The myriad technical factors that determine the image quality of each of the modalities, as well as the experience of the physician interpreting the images, affect the level of certainty that accompanies the diagnoses made. The criteria used to confirm the accuracy of the resultant diagnosis may be influenced by the management decisions made; in this regard, reports of spontaneous regression and satisfactory conservative management of cervical disc herniation should be kept in mind.[16, 31] Several studies of the accuracy of the modalities used, either singly or in combination, report surgically confirmed cervical disc disease accurately diagnosed in as many as 90 per cent of patients with MRI and 92 per cent accuracy with the combination of water-soluble myelography followed by CT myelography. Lesser degrees of accuracy result when non–contrast-enhanced CT or myelography is used alone.[3, 8, 30, 37, 44]

ILLUSTRATIVE EXAMPLES

Acute Disc Degeneration/ Herniated Nucleus Pulposus

The terminology used to describe acute disc degeneration/herniation varies from one institution to another. For example, acute degeneration of a disc in which there is herniation of nuclear material through most but not all of the fibers of the annulus fibrosus, with intact Sharpey's fibers and an intact posterior longitudinal ligament, may be variously termed incomplete herniation, disc bulging, disc protrusion, disc prolapse, subligamentous herniation, "soft disc," and disc "slippage." Some institutions reserve the term herniation to describe only complete rupture of all the annular fibers, including Sharpey's fibers, by nuclear material. The institutions that termed the former situation herniation may use the term extruded disc to describe the latter. Herniated nuclear material no longer attached to the disc may be termed extruded disc by some and free fragment, extruded free fragment, or sequestered fragment by others. To avoid confusion within a particular institution, therefore, it is useful to clearly define the terminology used to describe the pathologic changes that is acceptable and understandable by all concerned. In this regard, it is desirable that there be personal consultation between the radiologist, surgeon, and other clinicians involved in management decisions, at which time the radiologic findings and clinical signs may be correlated.

Case 1: Acute degeneration resulting in incomplete herniation and central protrusion of the C5–C6 intervertebral disc.

The patient is a 40-year-old previously asymptomatic radiologist who awoke with moderately severe neck pain and stiffness and noted mild "heaviness" of both arms. Physical examination performed several days later revealed limited neck motion but was otherwise within normal limits. The patient refused surgery after a two-week course of conservative treatment with a soft cervical collar, during which time all symptoms resolved. The patient remains asymptomatic eight months after the onset of symptoms.

The radiographic examination of patients with acute cervical disc herniation may appear normal or reveal only subtle changes, depending on the amount of nuclear material extruded from the disc and the status of the remainder of the disc. The radiographic examination of this patient, shown in Figure 19–2*A* and *B*, revealed "classic" signs of acute disc degeneration characterized by loss of height of C5–C6 intervertebral disc space and straightening of the normal lordotic curvature. The AP projection demonstrates the closely opposed margins of the uncovertebral joints at the C5–C6 level resulting from the disc space narrowing, which is also well shown. T1-weighted sagittal and flow-compensated gradient-echo, axial MRI revealed localized compression of the anterior aspect of the arachnoid sac and cervical cord at the level of the C5–C6 intervertebral disc. Increased signal intensity identical with that of the nucleus pulposus is visible within the posterior margins of the C5–C6 intervertebral disc, which has a focally convex posterior margin and projects beyond the margin of the vertebral body. No definite disruption of Sharpy's fibers or the posterior longitudinal ligament is identified. These findings were interpreted as consistent with incomplete herniation of the C5–C6 intervertebral disc with a focal protrusion centrally.

Case 2: Acute disc degeneration of the C4–C5 and C5–C6 intervertebral discs with moderately large herniation, resulting in cord compression at C4–C5 and mild to moderate herniation with probable central protrusion at C5–C6.

The patient is a 45-year-old carpenter who experienced increasing neck pain and stiffness over several weeks and noted "heaviness" of the arms. No specific trauma could be recalled. Physical examination revealed limited neck motion with Lhermitte's sign present. Brisk tendon reflexes were noted bilaterally. Radiographic examination of the cervical spine (not shown) revealed mild diminution in the height of the C4–C5 intervertebral disc space. MR examination consisting of T1-weighted sagittal (Fig. 19–3*A*), T2-weighted sagittal (Fig. 19–3*B*), and flow-compensated gradient-echo axial (Fig. 19–3*C* and *D*) was performed. Herniated nucleus pulposus with bright signal intensity on the T2-weighted images is well demonstrated. Disruption of Sharpey's fibers along the posterior margin of the C4–C5 disc is also visible on the T1-weighted sagittal images. Increased signal consistent with nuclear

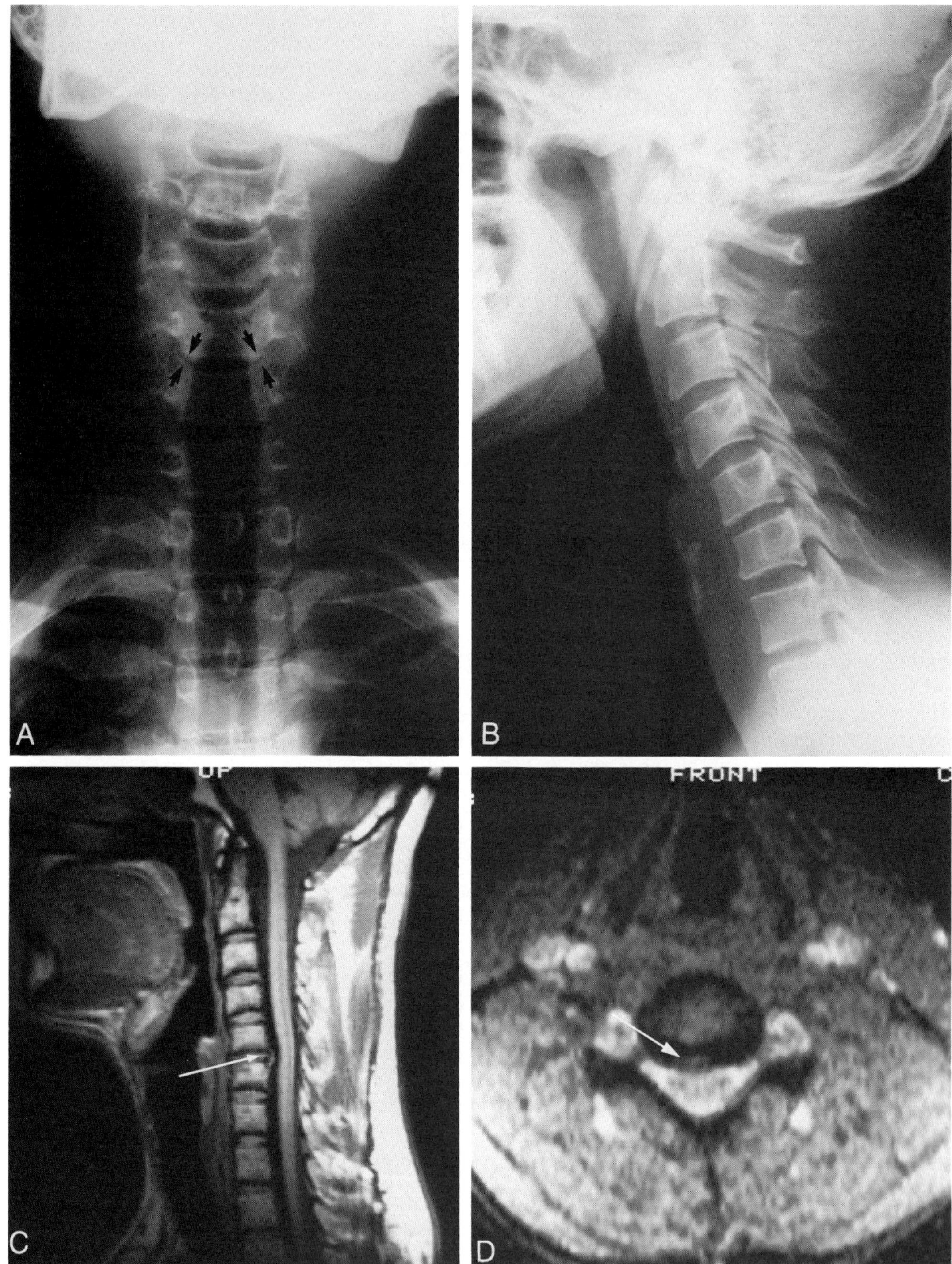

Figure 19–2. Case 1. *A, B,* Anteroposterior and lateral radiographs of the cervical spine showing narrowing of the C5–C6 intervertebral disc space and uncovertebral joints *(arrows). C,* A 4-mm thick, T1-weighted, sagittal MRI scan reveals small herniation of the C5–C6 intervertebral disc with mild distortion of the cervical cord. Mild irregularity of Sharpey's fibers is noted posteriorly *(arrow). D,* A 3-mm thick, flow-compensated, gradient-echo MRI scan demonstrates nuclear material projecting into the posterior margin of the disc *(arrow).*

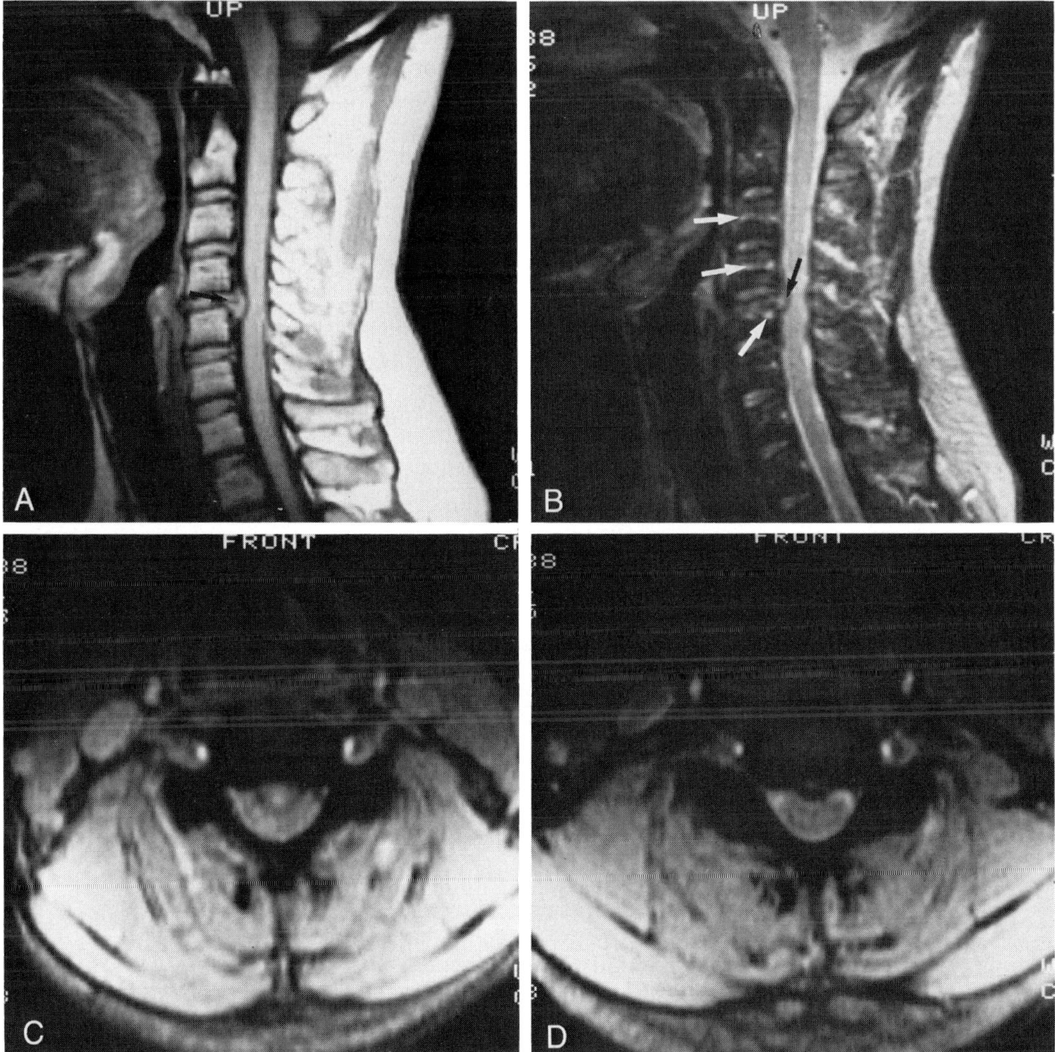

Figure 19–3. Case 2. Acute herniation of the C4–C5 and C5–C6 intervertebral discs with cord compression at C4–C5. *A,* T1-weighted sagittal MRI scan. Arrow points to disrupted Sharpey's fibers. *B,* T2-weighted sagittal MRI scan. An extruded fragment at the C4–C5 level has bright signal intensity *(black arrow).* Cardiac gating on this image limits the effects of pulsatile flow in the venous structures within the vertebral body; as a result, bright signal from the structures can be seen *(white arrows). C,* T2-weighted, gradient-echo axial image at the C4–C5 level. Bright signal is seen from the herniated nuclear material that projects beyond the margins of the disc. *D,* T2-weighted, gradient-echo axial image at the level of the C5–C6 disc. Herniated nuclear material with bright signal intensity distorts the posterior margin of the disc.

material is seen to project beyond the posterior margin of the C5–C6 disc; however, definite disruption of Sharpey's fibers is not well demonstrated. The patient underwent anterior discectomy and interbody fusion at C4–C5 and C5–C6, at which time extruded disc material was observed beneath the posterior longitudinal ligament at both levels. The patient has done well postoperatively and remains asymptomatic eight months after surgery.

Case 3: Acute degeneration of the C5–C6 disc with moderately large posterolateral herniation.

The patient is a 33-year-old physician's wife who experienced neck pain radiating into the right arm after she had painted the kitchen ceiling. Physical examination revealed limited neck motion and signs of a right C6 radiculopathy. Radiographic examination of the cervical spine revealed mild diminution in the height of the C5–C6 intervertebral disc space. Cervical myelography was performed using 10 ml of iohexol, 300 ml I/ml, instilled through a fluoroscopically guided lumbar puncture. A moderately large anterolateral defect on the contrast column was demonstrated on the frontal projection (Fig. 19–4*A*), and a "double density" at the level of C5–C6 was demonstrated on the lateral projection (Fig. 19–4*B*). CT examination immediately after the myelogram revealed findings consistent with a moderately large posterolateral herniation of the C5–C6 disc producing compression of the C6 root sleeve and distortion of the arachnoid sac and cord. The patient underwent anterior discectomy and interbody fusion at the C5–C6 level, at which time extruded disc material was found. The patient did well postoperatively and remains asymptomatic approximately ten months after surgery.

Case 4: Traumatic herniation with avulsion of cortical bone at the C5–C6 level with severe cord compression and quadriparesis.

The patient is a previously healthy, athletic, 38-year-old woman who experienced severe neck pain and weakness of all four extremities immediately after a skiing accident. The patient was brought to the emergency room, where a physical examination performed by the neurosurgeon revealed marked limitation of neck motion and quadriparesis. A cervical myelogram was performed on an emergent basis using 10 ml of iohexol, 300 ml I/ml (instilled through a fluoroscopically guided lumbar puncture). A complete block to rostral flow was noted at the C5–C6 level, with fusiform widening of the arachnoid sac and cord at the C5–C6 level demonstrated on the frontal projection (Fig. 19–5*A* and *B*). CT myelography performed immediately after the myelo-

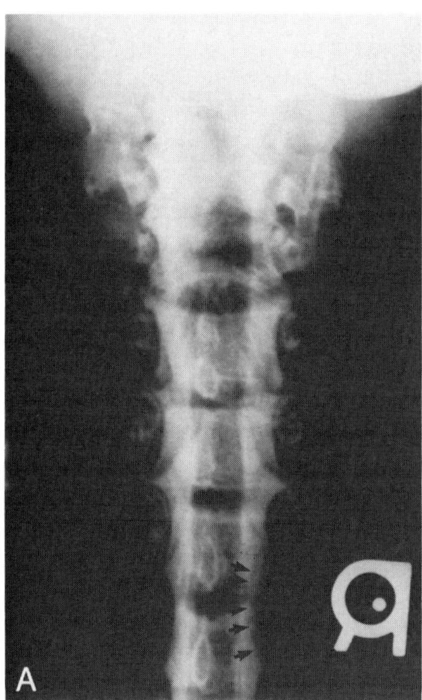

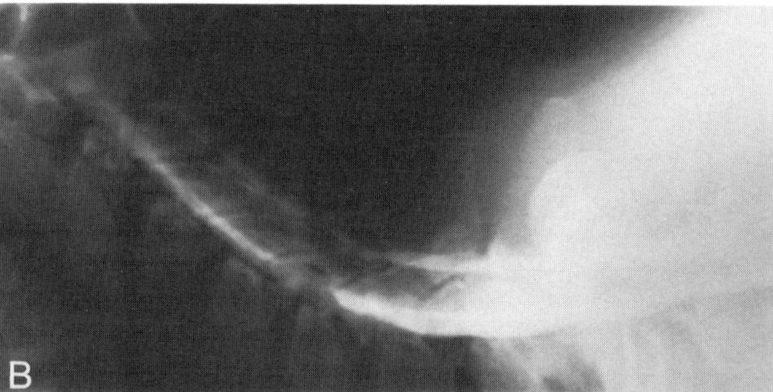

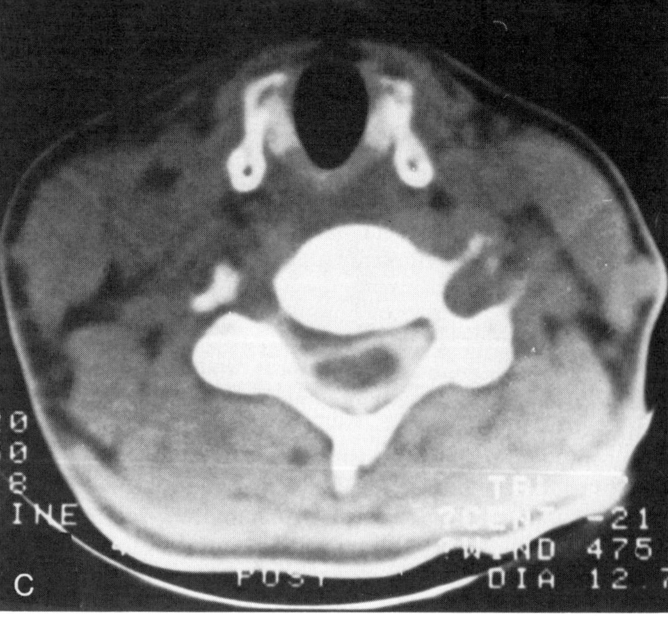

Figure 19–4. Case 3. *A, B,* Iohexol myelogram demonstrating anterolateral extradural defect at the C5–C6 level on the right *(small arrows). C,* CT myelogram. Moderately large disc herniation that distorts the anterolateral margin of the arachnoid sac and cord.

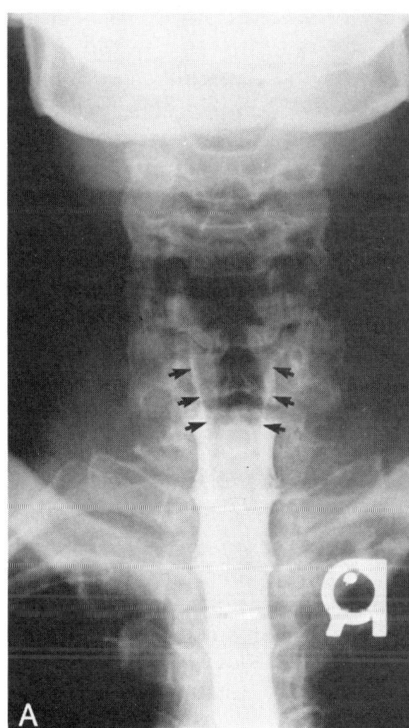

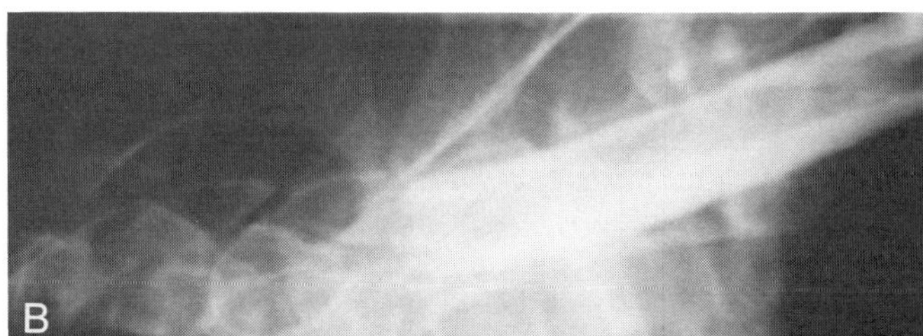

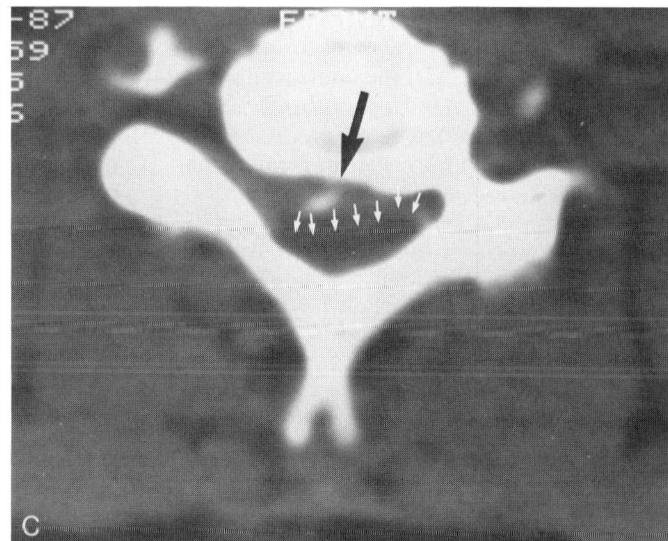

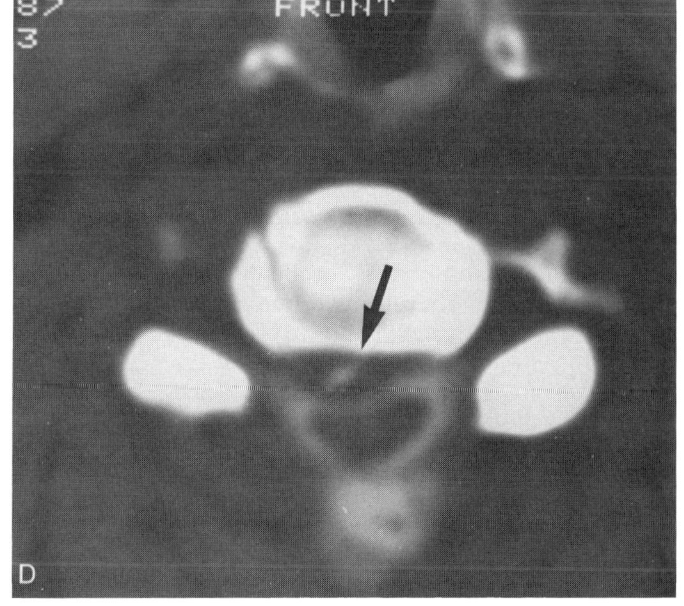

Figure 19–5. Case 4. *A, B,* Iohexol myelogram demonstrating a complete block to rostral flow at the C5–C6 level with fusiform widening of the arachnoid sac and cord on the frontal projection *(arrows). C,* CT myelogram demonstrates marked compression of the arachnoid sac with compression of the cord *(small white arrows).* Large posterolateral herniation of the C5–C6 disc is demonstrated with an avulsed fragment of bone visible *(black arrow). D,* Postoperative CT myelogram demonstrates adequate posterior decompression. A large herniation with avulsion fracture persists *(arrow).*

gram revealed a large central herniation of the C5–C6 disc resulting in severe compression of the arachnoid sac and cord (Fig. 19–5*C*). The patient experienced rapid progression of the neurologic deficit and became quadriplegic. Decompressive laminectomy was performed as quickly as possible. Quadriplegia persisted after surgery and a repeat CT examination performed approximately 24 hours after the first examination revealed adequate decompression posteriorly and the persistence of the large central herniation (Fig. 19–5*D*). The avulsed fragment of cortical bone that corresponds to a defect in the vertebral end plate has a density greater than the contrast material and is well demonstrated on both CT examinations. The patient has made gradual steady improvement postoperatively but is quadriparetic two years after surgery.

The neurosurgeon attributed the rapid deterioration in the neurologic status to acute "wedging" of the cord at the level of the complete block caused by continued leakage of spinal fluid through the needle defect in the lumbar region. When acute herniation resulting in a high-grade compressive myelopathy is suspected, one can avoid the possibility of acute "wedging" of the cord by performing MRI. If myelography must be performed, a lateral C1–C2 puncture should be employed.

COEXISTING ACUTE AND CHRONIC DISC DEGENERATION

Implicit in the concept that genetic, developmental, and other factors predispose certain patients to degenerative disc disease is the probability of multiple level involvement, which is frequently observed. Although many patients with multiple level involvement have changes in their later years that have obviously developed insidiously, a few patients have the degenerative process punctuated by an acute event that sometimes has confusing clinical manifestations. As a result, the radiologic demonstration of the structural changes and correlation with the clinical signs often presents an interesting challenge to the radiologist and surgeon.

Case 5: Acute central herniation of the C5–C6 intervertebral disc with spondylotic spur formation at C6–C7.

The patient is a 45-year-old car salesman with a history of chronic, intermittent, neck pain for several years. The patient experienced a somewhat more severe episode of neck pain persisting for two months and noted "heaviness" of the arms and legs. Physical examination revealed a mildly ataxic gait, brisk deep tendon reflexes, ankle clonus, and extensor plantar reflexes. Radiographic examination of the cervical spine revealed reversal of the lordotic curvature and spondylotic changes at the C6–C7 level with anterior and posterior spur formation. The sagittal diameter of the cervical spinal canal measured 13 mm at its narrowest point. The remainder of the segments were interpreted to be within normal limits; however, in retrospect, equivocal diminution in the height of the C5–C6 intervertebral disc space was present (Fig. 19–6*A*). The patient underwent cervical myelography using Pantopaque that revealed spondylotic compression of the C7 root sleeves bilaterally. A large central defect compressing the cord was demonstrated at the C5–C6 level (Fig. 19–6*B* and *C*). The patient underwent anterior discectomy and interbody fusion at the C5–C6 level, at which time a large extruded disc herniation was found. The patient did well postoperatively and remains asymptomatic four years after surgery.

This case demonstrates the importance of using high kilovolt techniques to adequately visualize the margins of the cord when performing Pantopaque myelography.

Case 6: Acute central herniation of the C4–C5 disc with resultant compressive myelopathy complicating preexisting spondylosis and moderate canal stenosis at C3–C4 and C5–C6.

The patient is a 55-year-old executive with a history of neck pain and stiffness for several years. The patient experienced acute neck pain and numbness and weakness of both arms and legs following a fall on an icy sidewalk. Physical examination revealed limited neck motion, slightly diminished sensation and strength in all four extremities, and brisk deep tendon reflexes. Radiographic examination of the cervical spine revealed chronic spondylotic changes at the C3–C4 and C5–C6 levels with large posterior osteophyte formation. The sagittal diameter of the spinal canal as measured from the tip of the large spondylotic spur at C5–C6 to the spinolaminar line was 11 mm. Mild diminution in the height of the C4–C5

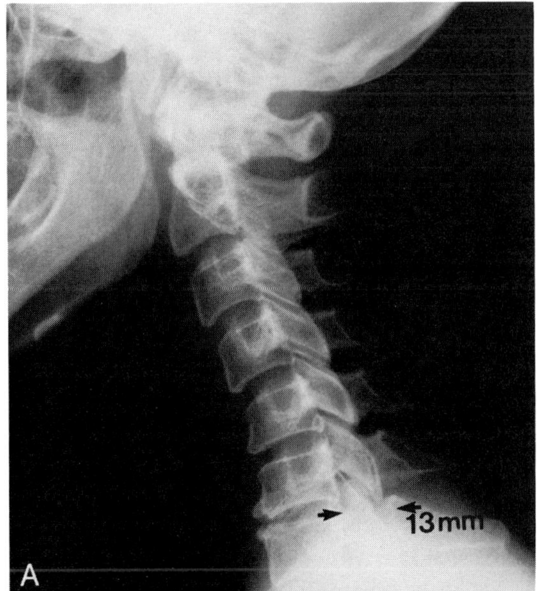

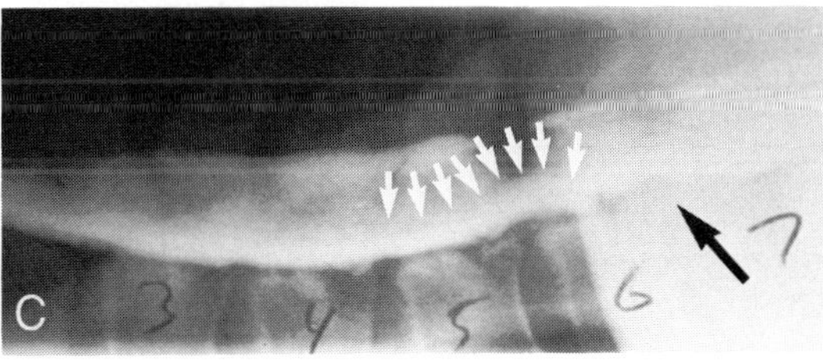

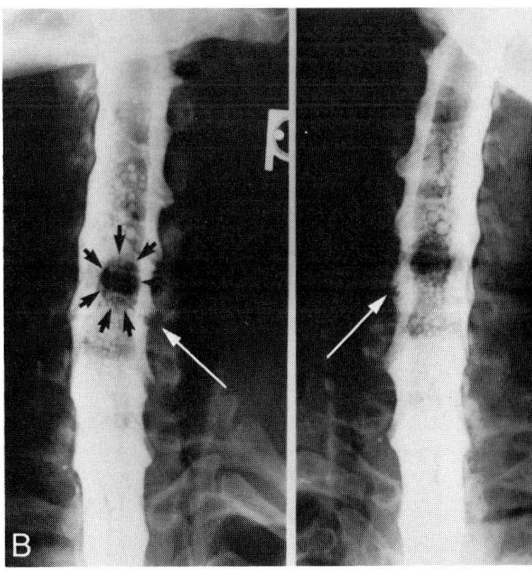

Figure 19–6. **Case 5.** *A,* Lateral radiograph of the cervical spine demonstrates moderate spondylotic changes at the C6–C7 level. Minimal diminution of the height of the C5–C6 interspace is noted. *B, C,* Pantopaque myelogram demonstrates an anterior defect secondary to spondylotic spur at the C6–C7 level *(black arrow).* Mild compression of the C7 root sleeves is noted bilaterally *(long white arrows).* A large central defect on the dye column is noted *(small black arrows),* compressing the anterior aspect of the spinal cord *(small white arrows).*

intervertebral disc space was noted (Fig. 19–7*A*). MR examination revealed a moderately large central herniation of the C4–C5 disc with moderate compression of the cervical cord at this level. Chronic spondylotic changes were noted at the C3–C4 and C5–C6 levels with evidence of mild cord compression. Fatty bone marrow changes of the vertebral bodies of C3 and C4 can be seen (Fig. 19–7*B*). The myelopathic signs resolved after decompressive laminectomy and the patient continues to do well approximately eight months after surgery.

Relatively asymptomatic patients with spondylosis and cervical canal stenosis may experience an acute myelopathy resulting from seemingly trivial hyperextension injuries, which may resolve with conservative treatment only. Acute central herniation resulting in myelopathy, which may also occur with relatively trivial trauma, as in this case, must be identified before management decisions are made.

Case 7: Acute posterolateral herniation of the C6–C7 disc with extrusion of a free fragment that became sequestered in the left C7 neural foramen in a patient with chronic spondylotic changes at the C5–C6 level and multiple breast masses resulting in abnormal mammography.

The patient is a 42-year-old female pathologist with a long history of intermittent neck pain radiating into the arms. She noted gradually increasing neck pain with radiating pain into the left arm that had recently become severe and unrelenting. Physical examination revealed marked limitation of neck motion due to pain and radicular signs suggesting multiple root involvement on the left. Breast examination revealed multiple palpable masses. Mammography revealed multiple cystic lesions within both breasts and a solid nodule containing discrete calcifications. Radiographic examination of the cervical spine revealed marked narrowing of the C5–C6 intervertebral disc with anterior and posterior spondylotic spur formation and kyphosis. Moderate narrowing of the C6–C7 intervertebral disc space was noted. No evidence of metastasis was identified. MR examination was technically

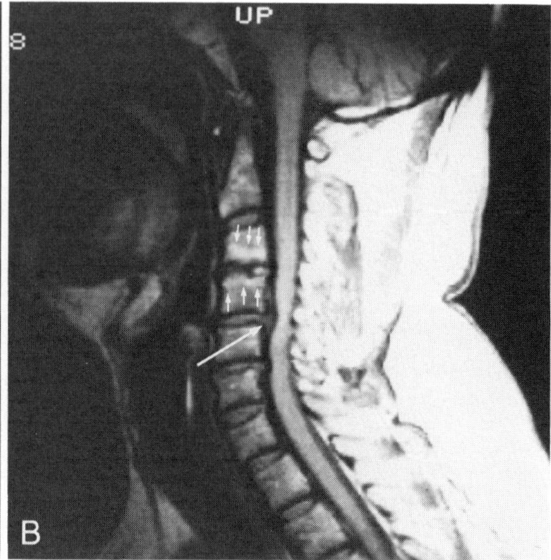

Figure 19–7. Case 6. *A,* Lateral radiograph demonstrating spondylotic changes at C3–C4 and C5–C6 with narrow anteroposterior diameter of the spinal canal *(arrows).* Reversal of the lordotic curvature and mild narrowing of the C4–C5 intervertebral disc is present. *B,* T1-weighted MRI scan in the sagittal plane demonstrates moderately large central herniation of the C4–C5 intervertebral disc with evidence of cord compression *(long arrow).* Spondylotic changes with distortion of the cord can be seen at C3–C4 and C5–C6. Note the fatty replacement of the bone marrow at C3 and C4 *(short arrows).*

less than optimal owing to the inability of the patient to remain motionless because of pain. A large mass with inconclusive signal characteristics could be seen filling the left C6–C7 neural foramen. Morphine sulfate administered intramuscularly resulted in satisfactory pain relief, and a second MRI was performed after intravenous administration of gadolinium-DTPA in an attempt to characterize the soft-tissue mass more fully (Fig. 19–8). T1-weighted sagittal and T1-weighted axial spin-echo images revealed an extruded fragment of disc material surrounded by intensely enhancing inflammatory tissue within the left C6–C7 neural foramen. Chronic degeneration of the C5–C6 disc with spondylotic spur formation and mild cord compression did not demonstrate enhancement. Anterior discectomy and interbody fusion was performed at the C6–C7 level and a large free fragment was removed. The patient was pain free after surgery and continues to do well one month postoperatively. A benign breast mass was removed under local anesthesia.

This case demonstrates the value of gadolinium-enhanced MRI in differentiating free fragments that are often surrounded by inflammatory tissue from neoplasms; most neoplasms tend to show uniform enhancement, whereas free fragments tend to appear as isointense structures surrounded by a halo of enhancement.

CHRONIC DISC DEGENERATION

Spondylosis

Although significant numbers of patients in their 90s reveal little or no evidence of cervical disc disease, most patients over the age of 50, although asymptomatic, have evidence of chronic cervical disc degeneration resulting in varying degrees of spondylotic change. A T2-weighted MRI demonstrating marked narrowing of the C5–C6 and C6–C7 intervertebral discs with moderate anterior spondylotic spur formation is shown in Figure 19–9. A capacious canal with ample room for the cervical cord is easily seen. This examination was performed on a 62-year-old member of our hospital's board of trustees who volunteered for the examination. She is an active woman whose only complaint is a somewhat diminished stature as she grows older.

Many patients with large posterior spondylotic spur formation, developmentally small

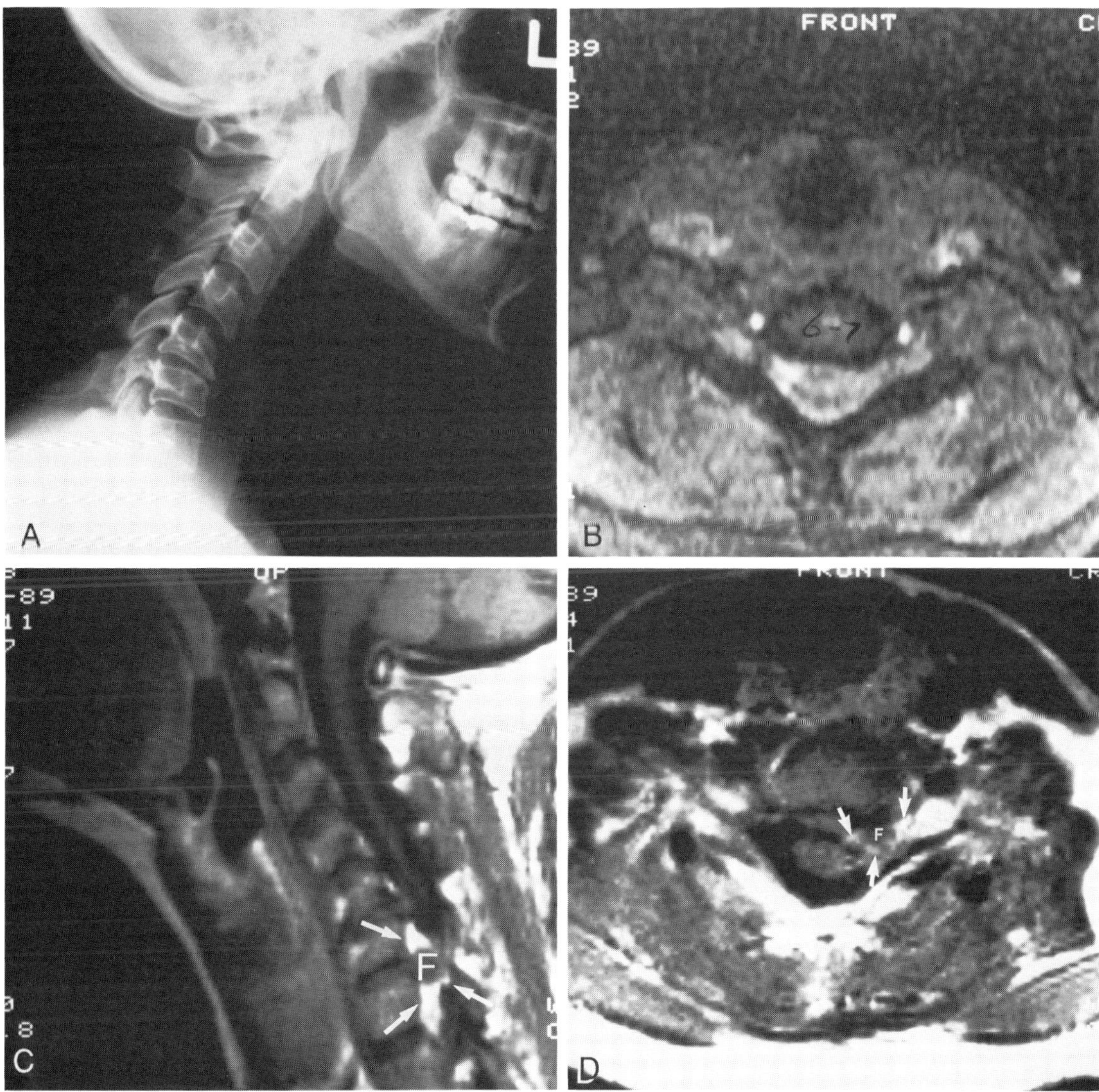

Figure 19–8. Acute herniation of the C6–C7 disc with extruded free fragment demonstrated by gadolinium-DTPA. *A*, Lateral radiograph of the cervical spine disclosing marked spondylotic change and reversal of the lordotic curvature at C5–C6. Moderate narrowing of the C6–C7 intervertebral disc space is seen. *B*, Gradient-echo MRI scan in the axial plane is degraded owing to patient motion. A soft tissue mass can be seen filling the left C7 neural foramen. *C, D*, T1-weighted sagittal and axial MRI examination after intravenous administration of gadolinium-DTPA demonstrates an extruded free fragment (F) outlined by bright signal representing enhancing inflammatory tissue *(arrows)*. A spondylotic spur at C5–C6 does not demonstrate enhancement.

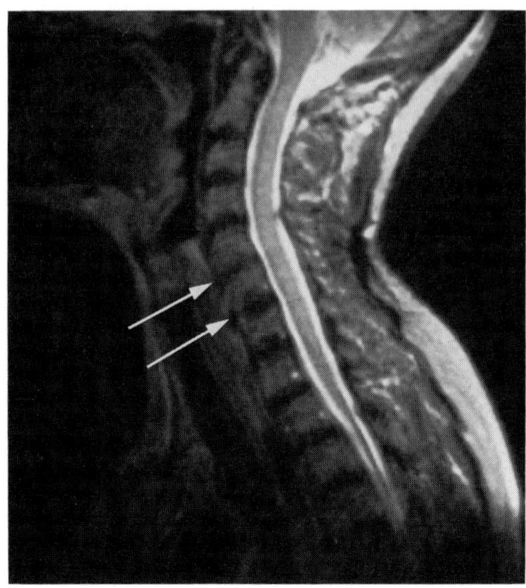

Figure 19–9. A flow-compensated, T2-weighted MRI scan in the sagittal plane demonstrates marked narrowing of the C5–C6 and C6–C7 intervertebral discs with anterior osteophyte formation *(arrows).*

cervical canals, hypertrophy of the ligamentum flavum, or concomitant degenerative changes in the apophyseal joints that result in degenerative listhesis may have a slowly progressive myelopathy or an acute myelopathy after relatively trivial trauma resulting from cord compression. Radiculopathy secondary to spondylotic compression of the neural foramina (see Fig. 19–1*F*) and vertebrobasilar insufficiency resulting from extrinsic compression of the vertebral arteries may also occur.

Multiple Level Involvement

The myelographic and MR appearance of multiple spondylotic ridges or "bars" associated with hypertrophy of the ligamentum flavum results in a "washboard" pattern. The resultant flattening of the cord produces a widened appearance on the frontal projection of the myelogram (Fig. 19–10*A*) and a "pinched" appearance in the lateral projections of the myelogram (Fig. 19–10*B*) and in the sagittal projection of the MRI (Fig. 19–10*C*).

Focal Compression of the Cord Secondary to Degenerative Listhesis

When cervical disc degeneration is associated with concomitant degenerative changes of the apophyseal joints, considerable listhesis may occur, resulting in focal constriction of the cervical canal, which can produce considerable compression of the cord. The radiographic assessment of the sagittal diameter of the cervical spinal canal is helpful when predicting the amount of cord compression (Fig. 19–11*A*). Flexion-extension views should also be obtained to assess the mobility of the affected segments. Patients with obvious high-grade lesions, particularly those that exhibit mobility, may not tolerate positioning maneuvers during myelography; as a result, MRI should be the procedure of choice, if available. MRI of this case demonstrates the focal constriction of the canal and resultant cord compression (Fig. 19–11*B* and *C*).

Acute Spondylotic Myelopathy

Patients with significant spondylotic compression and deformity of the cervical cord may remain relatively asymptomatic for long periods; however, they may develop acute quadriplegia after minor hyperextension injuries. MRI, which can demonstrate the structural changes and evaluate for parenchymal lesions within the cord such as contusion or hemorrhage, is the procedure of choice, if available. Figure 19–11*D* and *E* demonstrates a multiple-level cervical canal stenosis with moderate compression of the cervical cord at

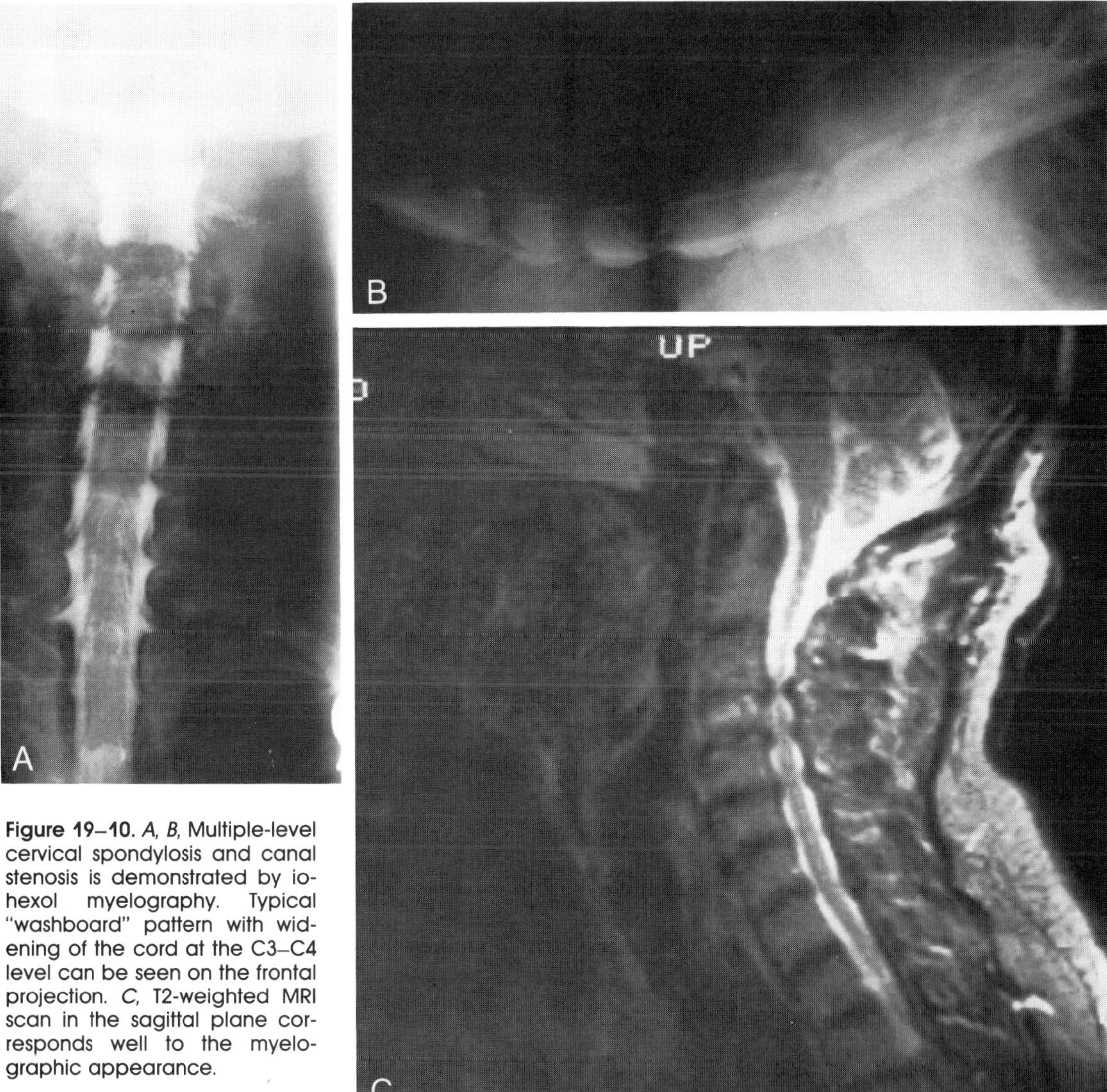

Figure 19–10. *A, B,* Multiple-level cervical spondylosis and canal stenosis is demonstrated by iohexol myelography. Typical "washboard" pattern with widening of the cord at the C3–C4 level can be seen on the frontal projection. *C,* T2-weighted MRI scan in the sagittal plane corresponds well to the myelographic appearance.

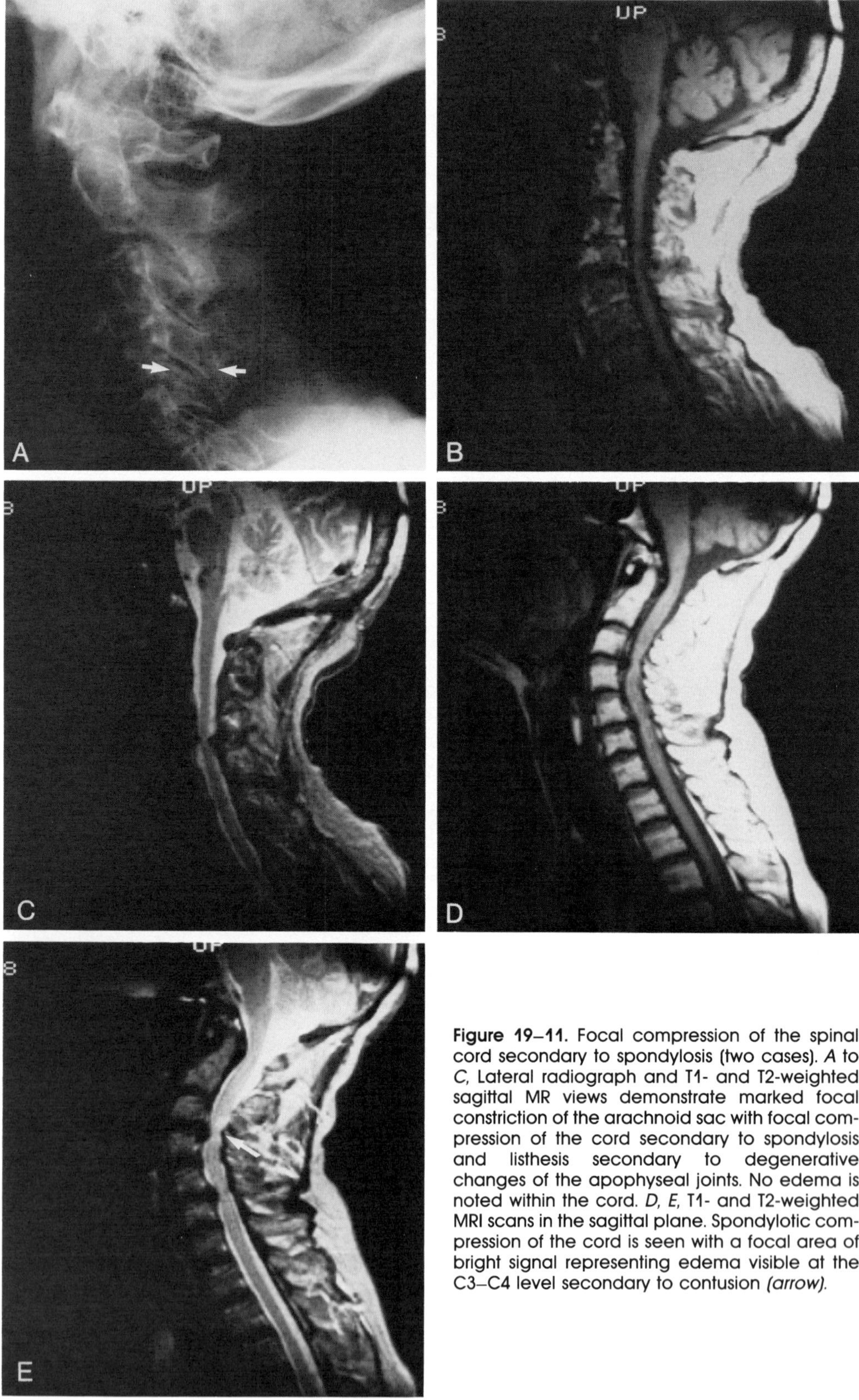

Figure 19–11. Focal compression of the spinal cord secondary to spondylosis (two cases). *A* to *C*, Lateral radiograph and T1- and T2-weighted sagittal MR views demonstrate marked focal constriction of the arachnoid sac with focal compression of the cord secondary to spondylosis and listhesis secondary to degenerative changes of the apophyseal joints. No edema is noted within the cord. *D*, *E*, T1- and T2-weighted MRI scans in the sagittal plane. Spondylotic compression of the cord is seen with a focal area of bright signal representing edema visible at the C3–C4 level secondary to contusion *(arrow)*.

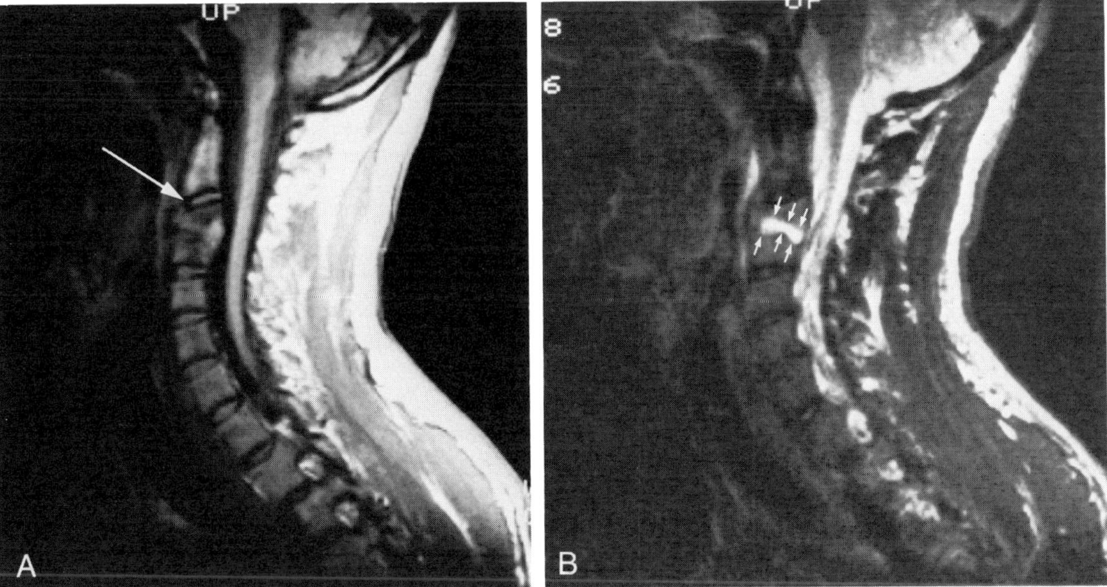

Figure 19–12. *A, B,* Disc space infection and vertebral osteomyelitis is demonstrated on T1- and T2-weighted MRI scans in the sagittal plane. Deformity of the body of C3 is shown *(long arrow)* on the T1-weighted sequence. Intense signal at the level of the disc space is demonstrated on the T2-weighted sequence *(short arrows).*

the C3–C4 level. Localized edema secondary to contusion exhibits bright signal intensity on the T2-weighted image.

DISC SPACE INFECTION

The diagnosis of disc space infection may be delayed, resulting in significantly increased morbidity.[44, 53] Radiographic and CT findings in disc space infection may be partially obscured by postsurgical changes or severe degenerative changes. In addition, patients on long-term hemodialysis, who are also at risk for disc space infection because of instrumentation, may exhibit noninfectious destruction of the disc space, which resembles infection, possibly secondary to deposition of crystals.[47] MRI of disc space infection has been shown to be accurate and highly specific and demonstrates high signal intensity at the level of the disc space on T2-weighted images.[35]

Figure 19–12*A* and *B* shows T1- and T2-weighted MR images obtained in a 28-year-old intravenous drug abuser who complained of neck pain for three weeks. He was treated with a soft cervical collar. The patient was involved in a motor vehicle accident, from which he experienced increased neck pain. Radiographic examination obtained in the emergency room disclosed compression deformities of C3 and C4 that suggested fracture, and CT suggested either compression fracture or disc space infection (images not shown). MRI was diagnostic in this case. CT-guided biopsy of the disc space yielded purulent material that contained staphylococcus.

We consider MRI to be the radiologic tool of choice in cases of suspected disc space infection.

References

1. Aguila, L. A., Piraino, D. W., Modic, M. T., et al.: The intranuclear cleft of the intervertebral disk: magnetic resonance imaging. Radiology *155:*155–158, 1985.
2. Alenghat, J. P., Kim, H. S., and Duda, E. E.: Cervical and lumbar metrizamide myelography: split-dose technique. Radiology *149:*852–853, 1983.
3. Badami, J. P., Norman, D., Barbaro, N. M., et al.: Metrizamide CT myelography in cervical myelopathy and radiculopathy: correlation with conventional myelography and surgical findings. A.J.R. *144:*675–680, 1985.
4. Bernat, J. L. Sadowsky, C. H., Vincent, F. M., et al.: Sclerosing spinal pachymeningitis. J. Neurol. Neurosurg. Psychiatry *39:*1124–1128, 1976.
5. Brain, W. R.: Some unsolved problems of cervical spondylosis. Br. Med. J. *1:*771–777, 1963.

6. Brain, W. R., Northfield, D., and Wilkinson, M.: The neurological manifestations of cervical spondylosis. Brain *75:*187–225, 1952.
7. Breger, R. K., Czervionke, L. F., Kass, E. G., et al.: Truncation artifact in MR images of the intervertebral disk. A.J.N.R. *9:*825–828, 1988.
8. Brown, B. M., Schwartz, R. H., Frank, E., et al.: Preoperative evaluation of cervical radiculopathy and myelopathy by surface-coil MR imaging. A.J.R. *151:*1205–1212, 1988.
9. Bull, J., El Gammal, T., and Popham, M.: A possible genetic factor in cervical spondylosis. Br. J. Radiol. *42:*9–16, 1969.
10. Camp, J. D.: Contrast myelography past and present. Radiology *54:*477–506, 1950.
11. Castillo, M., Quencer, R. M., Green, B. A., et al.: Syringomyelia as a consequence of compressive extramedullary lesions: postoperative clinical and radiological manifestations. A.J.R. *150:*391–396, 1988.
12. Christenson, P. C.: The radiologic study of the normal spine. Radiol. Clin. North Am. *15:*133–154, 1977.
13. Curtin, A. J., Chakeres, D. W., Bulas, R., et al.: MR imaging artifacts of the axial internal anatomy of the cervical spinal cord. A.J.N.R. *10:*19–26, 1989.
14. Czervionke, L. F., Czervioke, J. M., Daniels, D. L., et al.: Characteristic features of MR truncation artifacts. A.J.R. *151:*1219–1228, 1988.
15. Czervionke, L. F., Daniels, D. L., Ho, P. S., et al.: Cervical neural foramina: correlative anatomic and MR imaging study. Radiology *169:*753–759, 1988.
16. Daniels, D. L., Grogan, J. P., Johansen, J. G., et al.: Cervical radiculopathy: computed tomography and myelography compared. Radiology *151:*109–113, 1984.
17. Daniels, D. L., Hyde, J. S., Kneeland, J. B., et al.: The cervical nerves and foramina: local-coil MR imaging. A.J.N.R. *7:*129–133, 1986.
18. de Roos, A., Kressel, H., Spritzer, C., et al.: MR imaging of marrow changes adjacent to end plates in degenerative lumbar disk disease. A.J.R. *149:*531–534, 1987.
19. Dullerud, R., and Morland, T. J.: Adhesive arachnoiditis after lumbar radiculography with dimer-x and depo-medrol. Radiology *119:*153–155, 1976.
20. Enzmann, D. R., Rubin, J. B., and Wright, A.: Cervical spine MR imaging: generating high-signal CSF in sagittal and axial images. Radiology *163:*233–238, 1987.
21. Epstein, B. S., Epstein, J. A., and Jones, M. D.: Cervical spinal stenosis. Radiol. Clin. North Am. *15:*215–226, 1977.
22. Flannigan, B. D., Lufkin, R. B., McGlade, C., et al.: MR imaging of the cervical spine: Neurovascular anatomy. A.J.R. *148:*785–790, 1987.
23. Hedberg, M. C., Drayer, B. P., Flom, R. A., et al.: Gradient echo (grass) MR imaging in cervical radiculopathy. A.J.N.R. *9:*145–151, 1988.
24. Hendry, N. G.: The hydration of the nucleus pulposus and its relation to intervertebral disc derangement. J. Bone Joint Surg. *40B:*132–144, 1968.
25. Hesselink, J. R.: Spine imaging: history, achievements, remaining frontiers. A.J.R. *150:*1223–1229, 1988.
26. Hinck, V. C., and Sachdev, N. S.: Developmental stenosis of the cervical spinal canal. Brain *89:*27–41, 1966.
27. Ho, P. S., Yu, S., Sether, L. A., et al.: Progressive and regressive changes in the nucleus pulposus: part I. the neonate. Radiology *169:*87–91, 1988.
28. Jinkins, J. R., Bashir, R., Al-Mefty, O., et al.: Cystic necrosis of the spinal cord in compressive cervical myelopathy: demonstration by lopamidol CT-myelography. A.J.R. *147:*767–775, 1986.
29. Johansen, J. G., Orrison, W. W., and Amundsen, P.: Lateral C1-2 puncture for cervical myelography: part I: report of a complication. Radiology *146:*391–393, 1983.
30. Karnaze, M. G., Gado, M. H., Sartor, K. J., et al.: Comparison of MR and CT myelography in imaging the cervical and thoracic spine. A.J.N.R. *8:*983–989, 1987.
31. Laban, M. M.: Neck Pain. *In* Teninalli, J. E., Krome, R. L., and Ruiz, E. (eds.): Emergency Medicine: A Comprehensive Studyguide. 2nd ed. New York, McGraw-Hill Book Co., 1988, pp. 644–649.
32. Lamb, J. T.: Iohexol vs. iopamidol for myelography. Invest. Radiol. *20:*S37–S43, 1985.
33. Latchaw, R. E., Hirsch, W. L., Horton, J. A., et al.: Iohexol vs. metrizamide: study of efficacy and morbidity in cervical myelography. A.J.N.R. *6:*931–933, 1985.
33a. Lindblom, K.: Technique and results in myelography and disc puncture. Acta Radiol. Stockh. *34:*321, 1950.
34. Lipman, J. C., Wang, A. M., Brooks, M., et al.: Seizure after intrathecal administration of iopamidol. A.J.N.R. *9:*787–788, 1988.
35. Marshall, C.: The Physical Basis of Computed Tomography. St. Louis, Warren H. Green, 1982.
36. Modic, M. T., Feiglin, D. H., Piraino, D. W., et al.: Vertebral osteomyelitis: assessment using MR. Radiology *151:*157–166, 1985.
37. Modic, M. T., Masaryk, T. J., Mulopulos, G. P., et al.: Cervical radiculopathy: prospective evaluation with surface coil MR imaging, CT with metrizamide, and metrizamide myelography. Radiology *161:*753–759, 1986.
38. Modic, M. T., Steinberg, P. M., Ross, J. S., et al.: Degenerative disk disease: assessment of changes in vertebral body marrow with MR imaging. Radiology *166:*193–199, 1988.
39. Orrison, W. W., and Eldevik, O. P.: Lateral C1-2 puncture for cervical myelography: part III: historical, anatomic, and technical considerations. Radiology *146:*401–408, 1983.
40. Orrison, W. W., Sackett, J. F., and Amundsen, P.: Lateral C1-2 puncture for cervical myelography: part II: recognition of improper injection of contrast material. Radiology *146:*395–400, 1983.
41. Pavlov, H., Torg, J. S., Robie, B., et al.: Cervical spinal stenosis: determination with vertebral body ratio method. Radiology *164:*771–775, 1987.
42. Pech, P., Daniels, D. L., Williams, A. L., and Haughton, V. M.: The cervical neural foramina: correlation of microtomy and CT anatomy. Radiology *155:*143–146, 1985.
43. Penning, L., Wilmink, J. T., van Woerden, H. H., et al.: CT myelographic findings in degenerative disorders of the cervical spine: clinical significance. A.J.N.R. *7:*119–127, 1986.
44. Post, M. J., Quencer, R. M., Montalvo, B. M., et al.: Spinal infection: evaluation with MR imaging and intraoperative US. Radiology *169:*765–771, 1988.

45. Prusick, V. R., Samberg, L. C., and Wesolowski, D. P.: Klippel–Feil syndrome associated with spinal stenosis: a case report. J. Bone Joint Surg. *67:*161–164, 1985.
46. Quiles, M., Marchisello, J., and Tsairis, P.: Lumbar adhesive arachnoiditis. Spine *3:*45–50, 1978.
47. Rafto, S. E., Dalinka, M. K., Schiebler, M. L., et al.: Spondyloarthropathy of the cervical spine in long-term hemodialysis. Radiology *166:*201–204, 1988.
48. Ratcliff, G., Sandler, S., and Latchaw, R.: Cognitive and affective changes after myelography: a comparison of metrizamide and iohexol. A.J.R. *147:*777–781, 1986.
49. Resnick, D.: Degenerative diseases of the vertebral column. Radiology *156:*3–14, 1985.
50. Rothman, R., and Simeone, F.: The Spine. 2nd ed. Philadelphia, W. B. Saunders Co., 1982, pp. 216–233.
51. Rubin, J. B., and Enzmann, D. R.: Optimizing conventional MR imaging of the spine. Radiology *163:*777–783, 1987.
52. Russell, E. J., D'Angelo, C. M., Zimmerman, R. D., et al.: Cervical disk herniation: CT demonstration after contrast enhancement. Radiology *152:*703–712, 1984.
53. Sartoris, D. J., Moskowitz, P. S., and Kaufman, R. A.: Childhood diskitis: computed tomographic findings. Radiology *149:*701–707, 1983.
54. Sherry, R. G., and Anderson, R. E.: Real-time digitally subtracted fluoroscopy for cervical myelography. Radiology *151:*243–244, 1984.
55. Skalpe, I. O.: Adhesive arachnoiditis following lumbar myelography. Spine *3:*61–64, 1978.
56. Stoltmann, H. F., and Blackwood, W.: The role of the ligamenta flava in the pathogenesis of myelopathy in cervical spondylosis. Brain *87:*45–54, 1964.
57. Taveras, J. M., and Wood, E. H.: Diagnostic Neuroradiology. 2nd ed. Baltimore, Williams & Wilkins Co., 1976, pp. 1095–1100.
58. Teplick, J. G., and Haskin, M. E.: Spontaneous regression of herniated nucleus pulposus. A.J.N.R. *6:*331–335, 1985.
59. Teresi, L. M., Lufkin, R. B., Reicher, M. A., et al.: Asymptomatic degenerative disk disease and spondylosis of the cervical spine: MR imaging. Radiology *164:*83–88, 1987.
60. VanDyke, C., Ross, J. S., Tkach, J., et al.: Gradient-echo MR imaging of the cervical spine: evaluation of extradural disease. A.J.N.R. *10:*627–632, 1989.
61. Vezina, J. L., Fontaine, S., and Laperriere, J.: Outpatient myelography with fine-needle technique: an appraisal. A.J.N.R. *10:*615–617, 1989.
62. Wehrli, F. W.: Principles of magnetic resonance. *In* Stark, D. D., and Bradley, W. G., Jr. (eds.): Magnetic Resonance Imaging. St. Louis, C.V. Mosby Co., 1988, pp. 3–23.
63. Yang, P. J., Seeley, G. W., Carmody, R. F., et al.: Conventional vs computed radiography: evaluation of myelography. A.J.N.R. *9:*165–168, 1988.
64. Yousefzadeh, D. K., El-Khoury, G. Y., and Smith, W. L.: Normal sagittal diameter and variation in the pediatric cervical spine. Radiology *144:*319–325, 1982.
65. Yu, S., Haughton, V. M., Ho, P. S., et al.: Progressive and regressive changes in the nucleus pulposus: part II. the adult. Radiology *169:*93–97, 1988.
66. Zinreich, S. J., Wang, H., Updike, M. L., et al.: CT myelography for outpatients: an inpatient/outpatient pilot study to assess methodology. Radiology *157:*387–390, 1985.

CONSERVATIVE TREATMENT

Scott D. Boden, M.D.
Sam W. Wiesel, M.D.

All patients with neck pain, excluding those with fractures, dislocations, or cervical myelopathy, should be given an initial period of conservative therapy. There are many noninvasive treatment modalities available; unfortunately, most of them are based on empiricism and tradition. Although there are few prospective, randomized, double-blind studies for conservative treatment of lumbar disc disease, even less scientifically valid data exist for cervical disc disease.[1] Each treatment in popular use today is surrounded by conflicting claims for its indication and efficacy. Therefore, treatments prescribed should at least be safe, inexpensive, and have a reasonable chance of effective results.

The goals of noninvasive treatment of cervical disc disease are to return the patient to normal activity rapidly with the least diagnostic and therapeutic expense, and, most of all, to do no harm. The purpose of this section is to present several of the more common therapeutic modalities along with the available scientific evidence for and against their use. In addition, a strategy for conservative management of cervical disc disease will be outlined. The treatment protocol presented here has been empirically developed by us; other temporal sequences for the various treatment modalities may also be effective.

NONOPERATIVE TREATMENT MODALITIES

As stated earlier, most patients with pain from cervical disc disease achieve some relief from a conscientious program of conservative care. The multitude of treatment tools are based on empiricism and tradition. The following section will discuss the rationale behind the use of some of the more common therapeutic measures.

Immobilization

The cornerstone of conservative therapy is immobilization of the cervical spine.[15] The goal of immobilization is to rest the neck to facilitate healing of torn or attenuated soft tissues. In patients with an exacerbation of chronic symptoms, the purpose of immobilization is to reduce any inflammation in the supporting soft tissues and around the nerve roots.

Immobilization can be best achieved by use of a soft cervical collar that holds the head in a neutral or slightly flexed position. The collar must fit properly; if the neck is held in hyperextension the patient is often uncomfortable and will not derive any benefit from its use. Acutely, the collar should be worn 24 hours a day, until the pain subsides. The amount of immobilization required varies for each patient and should be guided by improvement of symptoms. Once acute symptoms have improved, the ideal long-term immobilization is strong paracervical musculature. Therefore, excessive external immobilization that will cause atrophy of these muscles should be avoided.

In addition to the soft collar, other devices such as plastic collars and metal braces are available to achieve immobilization. In our experience, these are more burdensome to the patient than soft collars and are less effective in the relief of pain. Furthermore, when the rigid devices are used for a prolonged period, they may lead to marked soft tissue atrophy and stiffness, which are not generally found with use of the soft collar.

Another component of immobilization is bed rest. The benefits are not only the relief of axial compressive forces on the cervical spine, but also the limitation of other daily activities that exacerbate the problem. Bed rest with cervical support is a viable option acutely for extremely severe pain, or for patients who would not otherwise comply with limitation of physical activities.

Drug Therapy

Anti-inflammatory medications are used because it is believed that inflammation in the soft tissues is a major contributor to pain production in the cervical spine. This is especially true for those patients with symptoms secondary to cervical disc herniation. The resulting arm pain is due not only to mechanical pressure from the ruptured disc, but also to inflammation around the involved nerve roots.

None of the vast spectrum of anti-inflammatory drugs has been proved superior. Accordingly, the usual treatment plan is to begin the patient on adequate doses of aspirin, which is effective and inexpensive. If the response is not satisfactory, other agents such as naproxen, ibuprofen, or indomethacin are tried. It should be stressed that anti-inflammatory agents are used in conjunction with immobilization; they do not replace adequate rest.

Analgesic medication is also important during the acute phase of an episode of neck pain. Most patients respond to the equivalent of 30 to 60 mg of codeine every four to six hours. If stronger analgesia is required, they should be monitored closely and admitted to the hospital for observation. Patients with peptic ulcer disease should not be treated with conventional anti-inflammatory agents. Some salicylates are now available with a pH-sensitive coating that prevents digestion in the stomach and duodenum.

Muscle relaxants are another useful class of medication in the conservative treatment of cervical disc disease. Painful muscle spasm may frequently be a significant contributor to pain after injury to any of the tissues in the cervical spine. Spasm leads to ischemia, which causes a further increase in pain. A muscle relaxant can frequently break the muscle spasm–pain cycle and allow an increased range of motion in the cervical spine. Methocarbamol or carisoprodol in adequate doses are the drugs commonly used. Diazepam (Valium) is not recommended for use in these patients as a muscle relaxant because it is also a psychologic depressant, and many neck-pain patients may already have some degree of clinical depression.

Traction

Although cervical traction has been used for many years, current opinions regarding its effectiveness are variable. Although some studies have suggested that traction is a valuable clinical therapy, others have concluded that it is either ineffective or potentially harmful in an acutely injured cervical spine.[2, 9, 10, 16] Certainly traction should never be prescribed unless roentgenograms have been reviewed for fracture, tumor, and infection. Traction is still an empirical form of therapy and should be employed only when more conservative treatment is not effective.

Cervical traction is contraindicated in several situations, including malignancy, cord compression, infection, osteoporosis, and rheumatoid arthritis. It is also commonly believed that when there is a frank herniated disc either in the midline or laterally, traction should not be considered.

Cervical traction may be administered in several ways: mechanical or manual, continuous or intermittent, and sitting or supine. Many believe that manual traction is preferable because of the interaction between the therapist and patient and the potential for individually varying the traction. We prefer a home traction device with minimal weights (5 to 10 pounds) pulling in slight flexion. Since there is evidence that at least 25 pounds are necessary to actually distract the cervical vertebrae, the major benefit of low-weight traction is probably from the immobilization.[13] There is no uniform idea of how traction actually works and no valid scientific evidence that traction alone is effective.

Trigger Point Injection

Many patients complain of localized tender points in the paravertebral area. The object of a trigger-point injection is to decrease the inflammation in a specific anatomic area. The more localized the trigger point, the more effective is this form of therapy. Injections may be repeated at intervals of one to three weeks. There have been no true randomized clinical trials to study the efficacy of this modality in the cervical spine, but the injections empirically seem to work well for both neck pain and brachialgia in some patients.

Epidural Steroids

A large component of cervical radiculopathy is often related to secondary inflammation of the involved nerve root. Reduction of the edema and the local inflammatory response theoretically should help to relieve symptoms. Cervical epidural injections of a local anesthetic and steroid may provide some pain relief. This procedure requires experience and technical competence and is not without complications, however. Although some have had limited success with this technique, we do not use cervical epidural injections.

Exercises

After a patient's acute symptoms have resolved and there is no significant pain or spasm, an exercise regimen is recommended. The exercises should be directed at strengthening the paravertebral musculature rather than at increasing the range of motion. Motion will generally return with the disappearance of pain.

We suggest that isometric exercises be performed once each day with increasing repetitions. It should be appreciated that there are no scientific studies demonstrating that isometric or any type of exercises will reduce the frequency or duration of recurrent neck pain episodes. Empirically, exercise regimens do appear to have a positive psychologic effect and give the patient an active part in the treatment program.

Physical Therapy Modalities

Other unproved modalities are safer and may achieve relief in some patients. Moist heat, transcutaneous electrical nerve stimulation (TENS), and ultrasound may be effective. Scientific data supporting these modalities is scant; however, they are safe, relatively inexpensive, and worthy of a brief trial in refractory patients. In addition, patient education about sleeping with the neck in a neutral position; avoiding automobile travel during the acute injury phase; and customizing work areas to avoid extreme neck flexion, extension, or rotation is worthwhile.

Manipulation

Manipulation of the cervical spine should be approached carefully. There is no real scientific evidence that manipulation is effective in the treatment of acute or chronic neck disorders. There have been tragic complications associated with the use of cervical manipulation.[12] It is our belief that the hazards are too great to warrant its use and that manipulation at this time has no place in the treatment of cervical spine disorders.

NONOPERATIVE TREATMENT PROTOCOL

After a cervical myelopathy has been ruled out, the remainder of neck pain patients—an overwhelming majority—should be started on a course of conservative (nonoperative) management (Fig. 19–13). Initially, a specific diagnosis, whether it be a herniated disc or neck strain, is not required, since the entire group is treated in the same fashion.

Immobilization is the mainstay of therapy in both acute episodes and exacerbations in patients with chronic cervical disc disease.[3] A soft felt collar should fit properly and will usually provide comfort for the patient; it should initially be worn continuously, day and night. The patient must understand that the neck is especially unprotected from awkward positions and movements during sleep and that the collar is important. The other major component of the initial treatment program is drug therapy. Anti-inflammatory drugs, analgesics, and muscle relaxants usually increase patient comfort and should supplement immobilization. Medication is not a substitute for proper immobilization.

Most patients respond to this approach of immobilization and pharmacotherapy in the first ten days. Those who do improve should be encouraged to gradually increase their activities and begin a program of exercises directed at strengthening the paravertebral musculature rather than at increasing the range of motion. The patient is then weaned off the soft collar over the subsequent two to three weeks. Unimproved patients should continue with immobilization and anti-inflammatory medication.

If there is not a significant improvement in symptoms after three to four weeks, a local injection into the area of maximal tenderness in the paravertebral musculature and trapezii should be considered. Marked relief of symptoms is often achieved dramatically by infiltration of these trigger points with a combination of 3 to 5 ml of lidocaine (Xylocaine) and 10 mg of a corticosteroid preparation. If the trigger-point injection is not successful at four to five weeks after the onset of symptoms, a trial of cervical traction may be instituted. A home traction device with minimal weights is preferred.

The patient should be treated conservatively for up to six weeks. Most cervical spine patients get better. If the initial conservative treatment regimen fails, symptomatic patients may be separated into two groups. The first consists of patients with neck pain as a predominant complaint, with or without interscapular radiation; the second of those who complain primarily of arm pain (brachialgia).

Neck Pain

If no symptomatic improvement in neck pain is achieved after six weeks of conservative therapy, further studies including lateral flexion-extension roentgenograms, a bone scan, and a medical evaluation must be obtained to assess the cervical spine for instability, arthritis, tumor, and infection. Roentgenograms before this point are not usually helpful because of the lack of significant differences between symptomatic and asymptomatic patients.[6, 7] A thorough medical examination may also reveal problems missed in the early stages of neck pain evaluation. If the above work-up is negative, the patient should have a complete psychosocial evaluation and receive treatment when appropriate for depression or substance dependence, which are frequently seen in association with neck pain.

If the psychosocial evaluation proves normal, the patient is considered to have chronic neck pain. These patients require encourage-

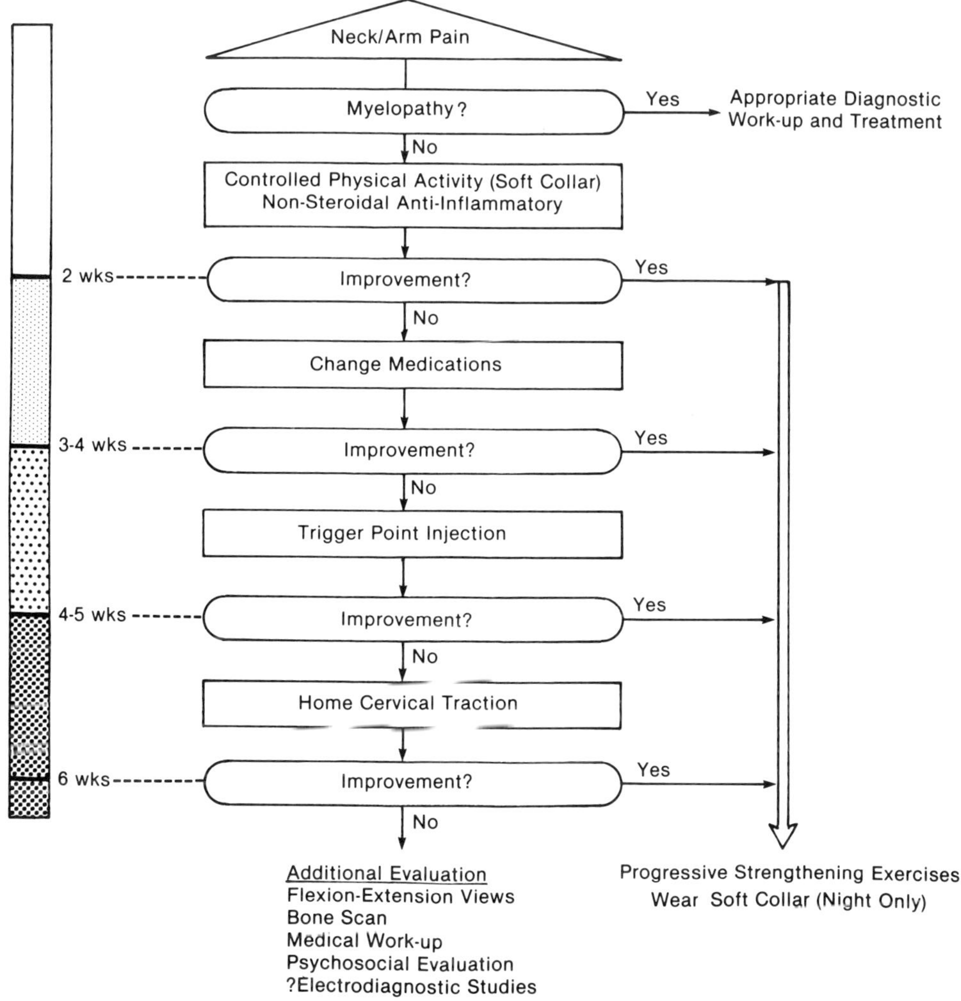

Figure 19–13. Treatment for neck pain: flow chart.

ment, patience, and education. They especially need to be detoxified from narcotic drugs and placed on an exercise regimen. Many respond to antidepressant drugs such as amitryptyline (Elavil). Regardless, these patients need to be periodically reevaluated to avoid missing any new problems.

It is occasionally difficult to distinguish patients who have a true neck problem from those who either use their neck as an excuse to stay out of work and collect compensation or contemplate litigation. The outcome of treatment of cervical disc disease has been shown to be adversely affected by litigation.[5] Frequently with hyperextension neck injuries, there are no objective findings to substantiate the subjective complaints. The best solution to this dilemma in the compensation setting is to recommend an independent medical examination early in the treatment course.

Brachialgia

The patients with predominantly arm pain (brachialgia) may have symptoms due to mechanical pressure from a herniated disc and secondary inflammation of the involved nerve roots.[14] Extrinsic pressure on the vascular structures or peripheral nerves is the most likely imitator of brachialgia and must be ruled out. Pathology in the chest and shoulder must also be considered. Otherwise, if there is unequivocal evidence of nerve root compression (neurologic deficit, positive EMG, and positive myelogram or MRI) consistent with the physical findings, surgical decompression should be considered. Some studies suggest that patients with radicular symptoms do better with surgery.[4] Although conservative management of patients with radicular symptoms has shown that this problem rarely progresses to cervical myelopathy, persistent symptoms are common.[11]

CONCLUSION

Unlike acute lumbar disc disease, which is usually self-limiting, at least one third of the cervical disc disease patients have persistent pain.[8] The role of conservative therapy in this disease is strengthened by some studies that suggest that operative intervention may not provide any long-term advantages over nonoperative management.[4, 5] Much of the evidence for conservative treatment is empirical, however, and there are no data to suggest that any of the conservative modalities influence the natural history of cervical disc disease other than alleviating acute symptoms.[8]

The authors maintain that all patients with an exacerbation of cervical disc disease should have up to six weeks of conservative therapy in the absence of myelopathy. The specific temporal sequence for use of the various conservative modalities may be variable. A conscientious program of a soft cervical collar and anti-inflammatory medications is recommended, occasionally followed by trigger-point injections or home traction if necessary. This regimen has been effective empirically in treating most patients with exacerbations of cervical disc disease.

References

1. Block, R: Methodology in clinical back pain trials. Spine *12*:430–432, 1987.
2. British Association of Physical Medicine: Pain in the neck and arm: a multicentre trial of the effects of physiotherapy. Br. Med. J. *1*:253, 1966.
3. DePalma, A. F., and Rothman, R. H.: The Intervertebral Disc. Philadelphia, W. B. Saunders Co., 1970.
4. DePalma, A. F., Rothman, R. H., Levitt, R. L., et al.: The natural history of severe cervical disc degeneration. Acta Orthop. Scand. *43*:392–396, 1972.
5. Dillin, W., Booth, R., Cuckler, J., et al.: Cervical radiculopathy: a review. Spine *11*:988–991, 1986.
6. Friedenberg, Z. B., and Miller, W. T.: Degenerative disease of the cervical spine. J. Bone Joint Surg. *45A*:1171–1178, 1963.
7. Gore, D. R., Sepic, S. B., and Gardner, G. M.: Roentgenographic findings of the cervical spine in asymptomatic people. Spine *11*:521–524, 1986.
8. Gore, D. R., Sepic, S. B., Gardner, G. M., et al.: Neck pain: a long-term follow-up of 205 patients. Spine *12*:1–5, 1987.
9. Greenfield, J., and Ilfeld, F. W.: Acute cervical strain. Clin. Orthop. *122*:196–200, 1977.
10. Harris, W.: Cervical traction: review of the literature and treatment guidelines. Physical Therapy *57*:8, 1977.
11. Lees, F., and Turner, J. W.: Natural history and prognosis of cervical spondylosis. Br. Med. J. *2*:1607–1610, 1963.
12. Livingston, M. C. P.: Spinal manipulation causing injury (a three year study). Clin. Orthop. *81*:82–86, 1971.
13. Rath, W. W.: Cervical traction: a clinical perspective. Orthop. Rev. *13*:430–449, 1984.
14. Rothman, R. H., and Marvel, J. P.: The acute cervical disc. Clin. Orthop. *129*:59–68, 1975.
15. Rothman, R. H., and Simeone, F.: The Spine. 2nd ed. Philadelphia, W. B. Saunders Co., 1982.
16. Zhongda, L.: A study of the effect of manipulative treatment on 158 cases of cervical syndrome. J. Tradit. Chin. Med. *7*:205–208, 1987.

CHAPTER

20

SURGICAL MANAGEMENT OF CERVICAL DISC DISEASE

Harry N. Herkowitz, M.D.
Frederick A. Simeone, M.D.
Kalman D. Blumberg, M.D.
William H. Dillin, M.D.

Perhaps no other area of spine surgery has been subject to such a diversity of approaches as that of the surgical management of cervical radiculopathy and myelopathy. Factors including (1) soft disc as opposed to spondylotic spurs (hard disc) as the cause of neural compression; (2) the location, i.e., central versus posterolateral; and (3) radiculopathy versus myelopathy influence the surgical approach. Support can be found in the orthopedic and neurosurgical literature for the use of posterior laminectomy, laminotomy-foraminotomy, laminaplasty, anterior fusion, and anterior discectomy without fusion for the surgical management of radiculopathy and myelopathy in the cervical spine. The purpose of this chapter is to identify the surgical approaches, indications, techniques, results, and complications so that the reader can formulate a logical approach to the surgical management of these conditions.

The indications for surgery are based on several factors: (1) the length and severity of pain, (2) the presence of a neurologic deficit, and (3) a confirmatory radiographic study such as myelography, myelography combined with computed tomography (CT) or magnetic resonance imaging (MRI) *correlating* with the clinical findings.

It is essential for the surgeon to understand the natural history of cervical radiculopathy and myelopathy so that a rational decision for the timing of surgical intervention can be rendered.

SURGICAL MANAGEMENT OF CERVICAL RADICULOPATHY: ANTERIOR FUSION

Harry N. Herkowitz, M. D.

The natural history of cervical spondylosis has been elucidated by several authors. In 1963 Lees and Turner reported on 51 patients with cervical spondylosis followed for two to 19 years.[49] Of these, 45 per cent had one episode without recurrence, 30 per cent had intermittent symptoms, and 25 per cent had persistent symptoms. This shows that some patients do not improve with time or other conservative measures. A study of the results of treatment coupled with a detailed examination of the disease pattern led Lees and Turner to conclude that wearing a collar often relieves symptoms, but that any or no treatment will often give the same ultimate results.

A study of the natural history of cervical spondylosis in patients without significant radicular disease was made by DePalma and colleagues, who reported on 229 patients treated conservatively.[21] At the end of three months, 29 per cent had complete relief, 49 per cent had partial relief, and 22 per cent had no relief. The group of patients with no relief were followed for one year, and those who declined surgery were then followed for five years. Of this group, 45 per cent obtained a satisfactory and 55 per cent an unsatisfactory result; 25 per cent of the latter were unable to resume their previous jobs. It was found that litigation and hyperextension injuries had the poorest results. In addition, there was an initial period of rapid improvement followed by a very slow progress in most of the patients in all groups. Thus, the authors concluded that cervical disc degeneration is a chronic disease that may produce significant pain and result in incapacity over a long period.

In a study by Gore and associates, 205 patients with neck pain were followed for ten years.[28] These authors reported that 79 per cent of their patients had decreased pain; 43 per cent of these had no pain but 32 per cent of the study group had moderate or severe pain. It was found that those patients with initial significant and severe pain had significant pain at the study's end. In other words, those with the most severe involvement appeared not to improve. In addition, those with radicular pain, especially bilateral radicular pain, did the worst.

It can be seen from these long-term studies of cervical spondylosis that a certain subset of patients do not respond to conservative treatment.

ANTERIOR FUSION

Disc degeneration is a normal aging phenomenon of the cervical spine. Cadaver studies have shown progressive deterioration with age.[73] Disc degeneration often initiates further changes in the adjacent vertebrae, including facet joint arthritis, osteophyte formation along the posterior and anterior vertebral body borders, thickening of the ligamentum flavum, and degeneration of the uncovertebral joints (joints of Luschka) (Fig. 20–1).[73] It can be seen from the anatomy of the neuroforamen that degenerative changes at the facet joint or uncus may lead to nerve root impingement (Fig. 20–2). The chosen surgical approach must take into account the cause of nerve root impingement both to provide decompression and to prevent further deterioration. This was the impetus for the development of anterior cervical fusion, which was initially described by Robinson and Smith in 1955.[69] The benefits of this approach were that (1) further formation of anterior and posterior spurs would no longer occur, (2) spurs already present would regress from stability provided by the fusion, and (3) by distraction of the disc space, buckling of the ligamentum flavum would be reduced and the neuroforamen would be enlarged, resulting in decompression of the nerve root. Various configurations of cervical grafts have been developed over the years; the horseshoe-shaped graft of Robinson and colleagues (Fig. 20–3),[69, 70] the dowel graft developed by Cloward,[17] the iliac strut graft of Bailey and Badgley,[5] and the keystone graft of Simmons and Bhalla.[77] Grafting for multiple level vertebrectomies utilizes iliac crest or fibula strut grafts. White and Hirsch biomechanically studied the various graft configurations and concluded that the Robinson graft is the strongest.[83] This graft configuration is preferred by the author of this section of the chapter.

INDICATIONS FOR SURGERY

The indications for surgery in cervical radiculopathy are as follows:

1. Persistent or recurrent arm pain not responsive to a trial of conservative treatment (three months).
2. Progressive neurologic deficit.
3. Static neurologic deficit associated with radicular pain.
4. A confirmatory imaging study, myelography with CT or MRI, consistent with clinical findings.

The anterior approach to the cervical spine can be from the left or right. The advantages of the left-sided approach are comfort for a right-handed surgeon and less risk of injury to the recurrent laryngeal nerve. On the left side

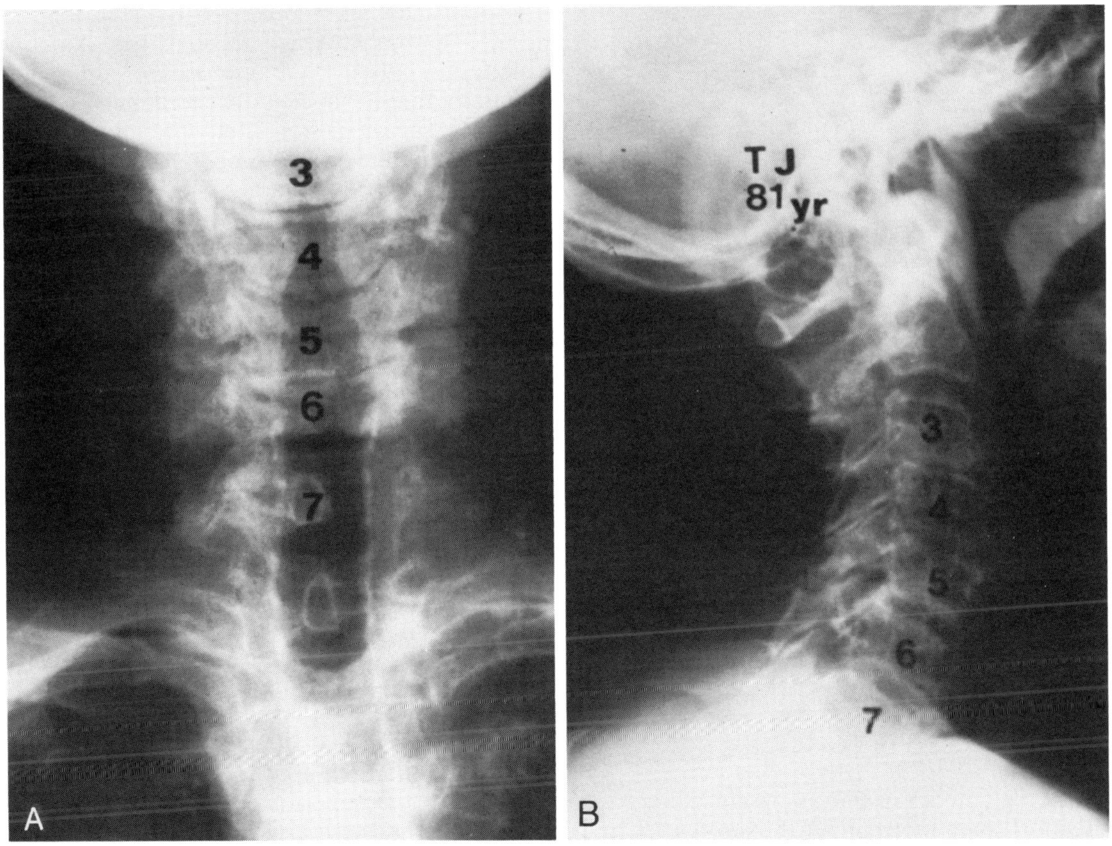

Figure 20–1. *A, B,* Anteroposterior and lateral cervical spine x-ray films demonstrating the typical appearance of cervical osteoarthritis with disc narrowing, spurring of the vertebral border, erosion of the facet joints, and hypertrophy of the uncovertebral joints.

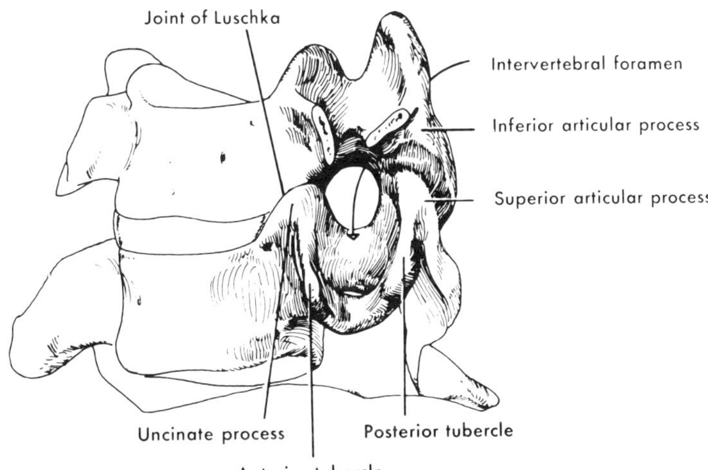

Figure 20–2. Anatomic borders of the neurocanal.

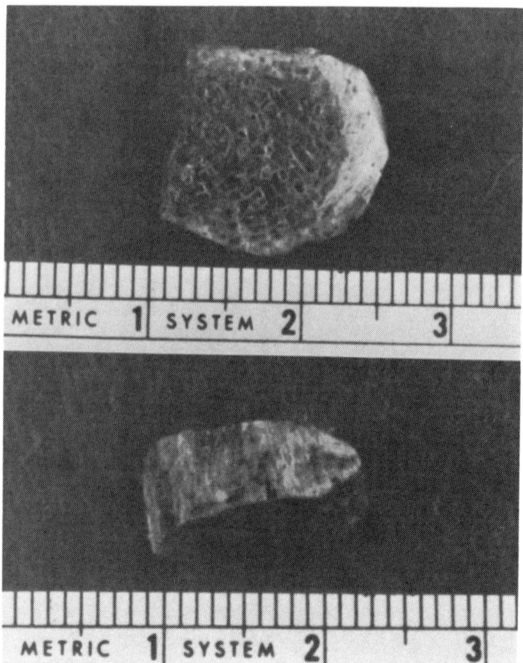

Figure 20–3. Robinson horseshoe graft.

the nerve enters the thorax within the carotid sheath. It then loops under the aortic arch and ascends into the neck beside the trachea and esophagus. On the right side, however, it may leave the carotid sheath at a higher level, crossing anteriorly behind the thyroid, thus leaving itself more susceptible to injury if the incision is on the right (Fig. 20–4).[78] The disadvantage of the left-sided approach for a lesion at the cervicothoracic junction is possible laceration of the thoracic duct, since the duct ascends lateral to the esophagus and lies on the prevertebral fascia at this level. It loops over the subclavian artery at the first thoracic vertebra and enters the subclavian vein.

The incision may be transverse or longitudinal, following the anterior border of the sternocleidomastoid muscle. Knowledge of the anatomic landmarks is helpful for placement of the skin incision. Generally, the hyoid bone is at the level of C3, the thyroid cartilage at C4–C5, and the cricoid cartilage at C6 (Fig. 20–5). The transverse incision is preferred for a one- or two-level fusion, while the longitudinal approach is best for three or more levels. At the cervicothoracic junction, the longitudinal incision may be preferred, since inadvertent injury to the inferior thyroid vessels can be managed more readily through a longitudinal approach. Once through the skin and platysma muscles, the approach proceeds medial to the sternocleidomastoid muscle. The carotid sheath is retracted laterally and the esophagus and trachea medially, using handheld blunt retractors. The superior and inferior thyroid vessels, which traverse from the carotid artery to the midline structures, may limit the extent to which this plane can be opened and may have to be divided. The vertebral bodies and discs can be identified by palpation in the midline. Once the prevertebral fascia and longus colli muscles have been dissected away from the vertebral bodies, a spinal needle should be inserted into the appropriate disc space and lateral radiographs of the cervical spine obtained to identify accurately the surgical level(s).

After significant disc material is removed, a small intervertebral body spreader is placed to allow careful distraction of the disc space. Disc remnant and cartilage end plates are removed back to the posterior longitudinal ligament, which if intact is not incised. If a rent in the ligament is noted it is resected. A micronervehook is then used to probe the posterior border of the superior and inferior vertebrae for any sequestered disc fragments. Removal of posterior osteophytes is not routinely necessary, since resorption often occurs with a solid bony fusion.[18, 61–63, 70] In addition, a small spinal canal carries the danger of iatrogenically producing increased neurologic deficit by contusing the spinal cord.[5] When compression by an osteophyte is thought to cause significant neurologic problems, a more generous resection of the vertebral bodies should be carried out, allowing direct visualization of the osteophyte so that excessive manipulation of the spinal cord can be avoided.

The disc space (height and depth) is measured and the graft harvested from iliac crest. To avoid resorption, the graft should measure a minimum of 5 mm high.[7] It should be recessed 1 to 2 mm posterior to the anterior cortex (Fig. 20–6). Before the graft is inserted, holes should be made through the end plates to bleeding subchondral bone. Although all cartilage should be removed, the entire bony end plate should not be completely removed. Distraction of the disc space is performed via manual traction by the anesthesiologist, or tong traction when deformity is being corrected with a long strut graft. Stability can be

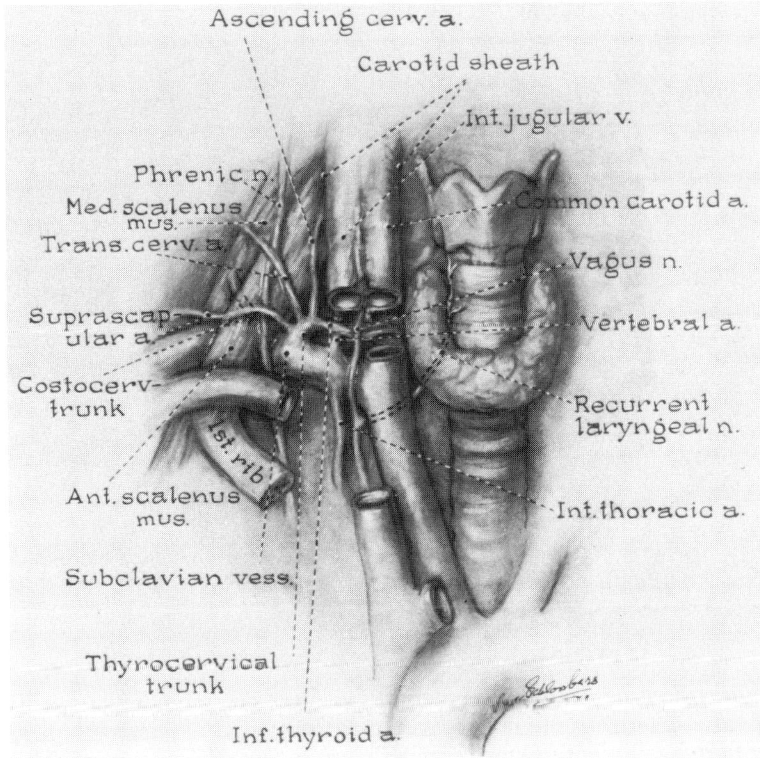

Figure 20–4. Arteries and nerves at the base of the neck on the right side. The right recurrent laryngeal nerve arises from the vagus at the level of the subclavian artery, loops beneath it, and ascends between the trachea and esophagus. The nerve can recur above the level of the subclavian artery and be injured in an approach to the middle cervical spine from the right side.

verified before closure by gentle rotation of the patient's head with the traction removed.

Postoperatively, the patient should be placed in a firm cervical collar. The orthosis can usually be discontinued by six weeks, but a longer period may be necessary if fusion has not been demonstrated radiographically at follow-up.

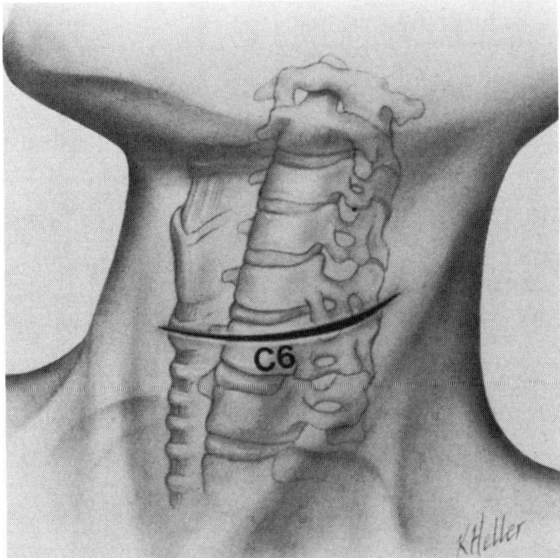

Figure 20–5. Superficial landmarks are helpful in placing the skin incision. The hyoid bone is at the level of C3, the thyroid cartilage is at C4–C5, and the cricoid is opposite C6.

COMPLICATIONS

Complications can be divided into those occurring at the graft site and those occurring at the neck.

The most common postoperative problems are transient sore throat, hoarseness, or difficulty in swallowing.[13, 36, 84] However, serious complications can arise as a result of the surgical approach. Perforating injuries to carotid and vertebral vessels, as well as the esophagus and trachea, are rarely reported but can be life-threatening.[57] The risk of injury may be decreased by use of dull retractors.

Although the recurrent laryngeal nerve is at greater risk when the neck is approached from the right side, many right handed surgeons find this approach more comfortable. Injury to the nerve may be transient or permanent;[13] it is the single largest neurologic complication in more than 36,000 cases reviewed in a 1982

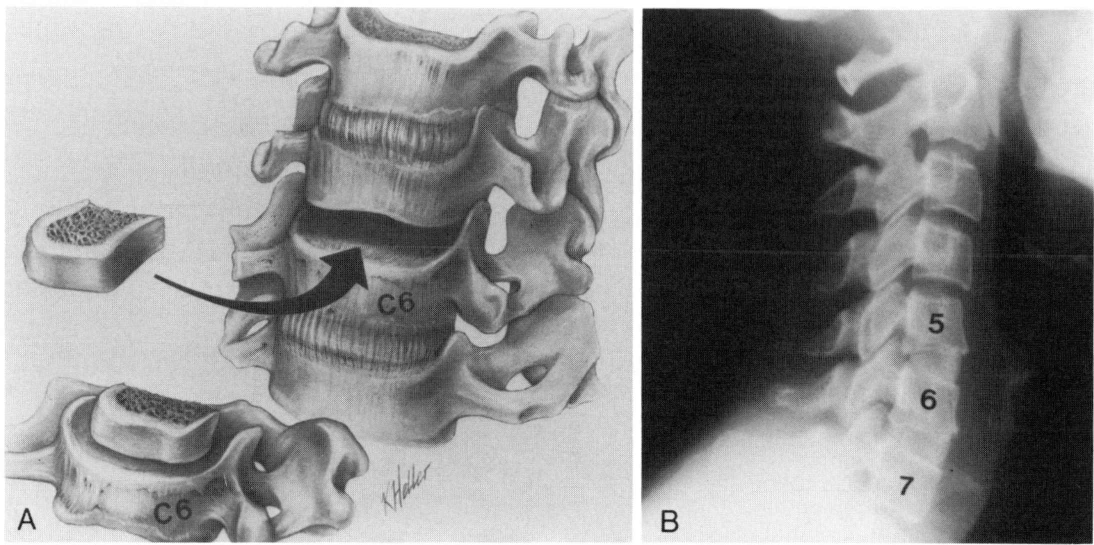

Figure 20–6. *A*, The graft harvested from the iliac crest is measured for height and depth (generally 15 mm × 7 mm). It should be recessed 2 mm posteriorly to the anterior cortex. Holes should be made through the end plates before the bone graft is inserted. *B*, Lateral x-ray film showing the correct graft placement.

report.[26] A thorough knowledge of the surgical anatomy helps to minimize this complication.

Perhaps the most feared complication is that of permanent spinal cord or nerve injury. Flynn, reporting on the experience of a large group of neurosurgeons, described 311 neurologic complications out of 36,657 cases.[26] Significant permanent radiculomyelopathy or myelopathy was noted in 100 of these patients. Other reports of cord damage are documented in the literature.[6, 46, 84]

Graft extrusion or resorption can occur with any of the grafting techniques.[66, 67, 86] If the graft completely extrudes, it should be replaced to avoid esophageal damage.

The occurrence of pseudarthrosis is inversely proportional to the number of levels fused.[18, 71] Although some investigators reported better results with a solid union, others could find no correlation between a pseudarthrosis and surgical outcome.[21, 67] Careful patient reevaluation is required before considering anterior revision or posterior fusion.

Complications at the donor site also commonly occur and include hematoma, infection, lateral femoral cutaneous nerve injury, muscle herniation, and persistent pain over the iliac crest. Although frequently reported, these usually do not cause permanent disability.[47, 66, 74, 77, 84] Careful attention to placement of the incision, and meticulous hemostasis with placement of the drain before closure, help minimize some of the risks.

The results of multiple series of anterior fusions have been satisfactory in over 90 per cent of patients.[7, 17, 18, 21, 22, 29, 34, 69–71, 77, 82, 85, 86] It is helpful, however, to review the results for single- versus multiple-level fusions, and nerve root compression due to spondylosis (hard disc) versus soft disc herniation.

The results as well as the problems associated with the surgical treatment of multiple-level cervical radiculopathy differ from those of single-level disease.

In a series reported by Robinson and associates of 55 patients who had undergone anterior fusion with the horseshoe bone graft, the results were inversely proportional to the number of levels fused.[70] For a one-level fusion, 94 per cent had a satisfactory result, as opposed to 73 per cent for a two-level fusion and only 50 per cent satisfactory results for a three-level fusion.

Simmons and Bhalla reported 68 patients who had undergone anterior fusion with a keystone graft.[77] Poor results were noted in three patients, all of whom had undergone multiple-level anterior fusion.

The reasons for poorer results in multilevel fusions have been related to two factors: (1) the greater severity of multiple-level disease and (2) failure of fusion of the bone graft to the adjacent vertebrae, which is inversely proportional to the number of levels fused. Connolly and associates demonstrated a pseudarthrosis rate of 15 per cent of one- to two-level fusions and 46 per cent for three-level fusions with the Cloward graft.[18] This was substantiated by White and colleagues, who reported an 80 per cent union rate for one-level fusions, as opposed to 66 per cent for multiple-level fusions.[82] In addition, when union occurred, 73 per cent of the patients had excellent to good results, as opposed to 53 per cent when union did not occur.[82]

Although most authors described better results when bony union occurs, a review by DePalma and associates of 229 patients who had undergone anterior cervical fusion with Robinson horseshoe grafts found no statistical difference in the results whether or not bony union had occurred.[21] Pseudarthrosis or nonunion was found in 22 of 58 levels fused (37 per cent). Satisfactory results, however, were reported in 92 per cent of patients undergoing anterior fusion. This can be explained by the fact that even though bony union does not occur, a stable fibrous union does. Second, removal of the degenerative disc alleviates some of the mechanical pressure on the nerve roots. Third, distraction of the disc space and neuroforamen occurs even though much of the initial height of the vertebral interspace gained by the bone graft is lost. Another factor that may contribute to the success of multiple-level fusion may be the policy of fusing each level demonstrating nerve root compression. Williams and colleagues reported 76 per cent excellent and good results when surgery was performed at all levels demonstrating myelographic defects, while such results fell to 54 per cent when only selected levels were operated on.[86] The clinical examination of patients with multiple-level radiculopathy often does not demonstrate hypesthesia or neurologic loss in a specific dermatome. Therefore, it is important to decompress each level exhibiting nerve root compression on the confirmatory study to ensure adequate decompression.

A comparative study of anterior fusion, laminectomy, and laminaplasty for multiple-level cervical spondylosis reported significantly better results for anterior fusion compared with laminectomy, and slightly better results compared with laminaplasty.[34] For anterior fusion the percentage of excellent to good results was 92 per cent, for laminectomy 66 per cent, and for laminaplasty 86 per cent. Although pseudarthrosis occurred at 37 per cent of the levels fused anteriorly, the results were not affected. The problems associated with laminectomy were the development of cervical kyphosis in four of 12 patients, and subluxation at 13 of 38 operated levels (Fig. 20–7). For the laminaplasty group the complications were "closing" of the laminaplasty door in two of 15 patients (Fig. 20–8).

Unlike the surgical management of a lumbar disc herniation, the operative approach to cervical soft disc herniation has remained controversial. Published series utilizing posterior and anterior approaches have demonstrated similar results.[4, 24, 29, 33, 75] Henderson and associates described the results in 846 patients undergoing posterolateral foraminotomy for nerve root compression due to soft disc herniation and cervical spondylosis.[33] They reported a 96 per cent success rate, but 14 per cent of this group required repeat surgery the reasons for which were not defined within the article. Lunsford

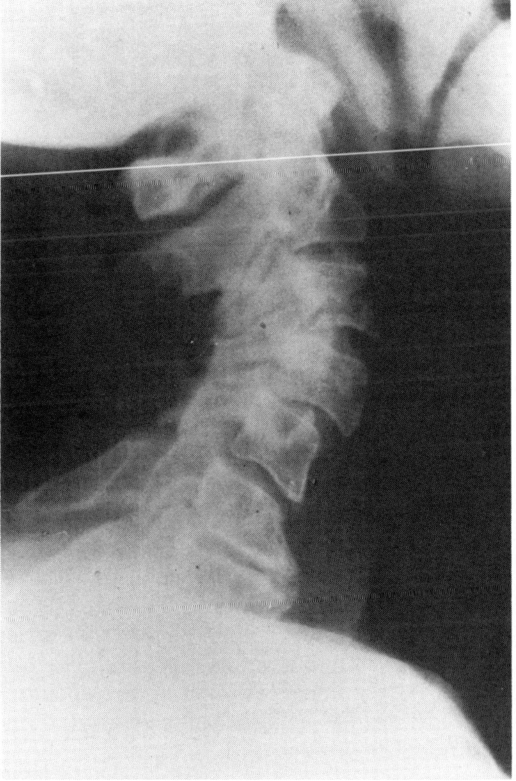

Figure 20–7. Lateral roentgenogram demonstrating the multiple-level cervical subluxations that may develop after decompressive cervical laminectomy.

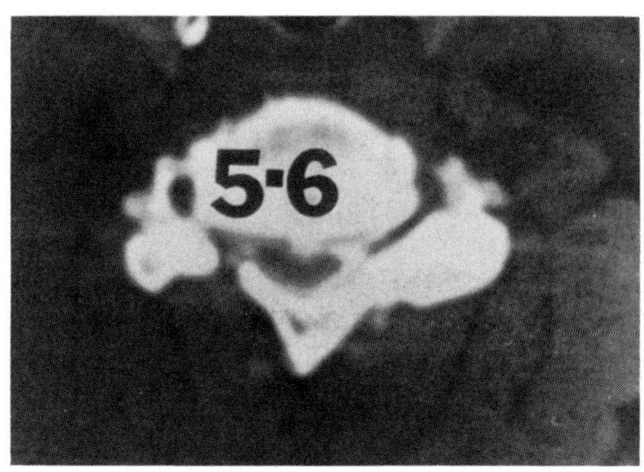

Figure 20–8. Closing of the hinge after laminaplasty with recurrence of cord compression.

and associates published their series of 295 surgical cases of cervical nerve root compression, of which 101 were classified as soft disc herniations while 194 cases were nerve root compression due to cervical spondylosis.[51] The success rates were 87 and 83 per cent, respectively. Dillin and Simeone reported 50 patients who had undergone posterolateral foraminotomy for soft disc herniation; all had myelographically proved lesions.[23] The range of follow-up was one to six years and they reported a 96 per cent success rate.

Aronson described 88 cases of soft cervical disc herniation treated by anterior discectomy and fusion.[4] He noted a success rate of 100 per cent but did not document the criteria for success, and also the follow-up was incomplete. Gore and Sepic reported 146 patients who underwent anterior cervical discectomy and fusion and noted a 96 per cent improvement rate.[29] Twenty-five per cent of the 146 were classified as soft disc herniations; the etiology in the remainder was spondylotic spurs causing nerve root compression.

The decision to perform an anterior discectomy and fusion or a posterior laminotomy-foraminotomy for a patient with a posterolateral soft disc herniation cannot be determined by a review of the previously published series, for the following reasons: (1) the patient demographics cannot be compared from series to series; (2) previous series include the results of surgical treatment for spondylotic radiculopathy (hard disc) as well for soft disc herniation; (3) surgical technique differs among authors, and therefore a comparison of anterior fusion and posterior laminotomy among series is not valid; (4) the criteria for a successful result differ from series to series, and thus comparisons cannot be made; and (5) in most series patient follow-up is incomplete and of inadequate length to evaluate the success or failure of a surgical procedure.

The following prospective study is reported to assist the reader in deciding which approach to use in the surgical management of a soft disc herniation.

Forty-four consecutive patients with the clinical diagnosis of cervical radiculopathy or myelopathy with a soft cervical disc herniation confirmed by myelography or myelography with CT or MRI at one intervertebral disc level form the basis of this study.[37] The disc herniations were classified into two types. Type I were posterolateral herniations defined by unilateral nerve root and dural sac compression (Fig. 20–9). Type II were central herniations with midline compression of the dural sac with or without nerve root compression (Fig. 20–10). Surgical evaluation was undertaken after an adequate trial of conservative therapy had failed (three months) or symptoms or signs worsened during treatment. For patients with Type I herniations (posterolateral), the surgical procedure alternated between anterior discectomy and fusion (Robinson horseshoe graft)[69] and cervical laminectomy-foraminotomy as described by Dillin and Simeone and Rothman and Simeone.[23, 74]

Patients with Type II herniations were treated by anterior fusion only, since the prevailing literature cannot justify the posterior laminectomy approach.[6, 15, 16, 20, 22, 23, 36, 63, 69, 70, 74, 85]

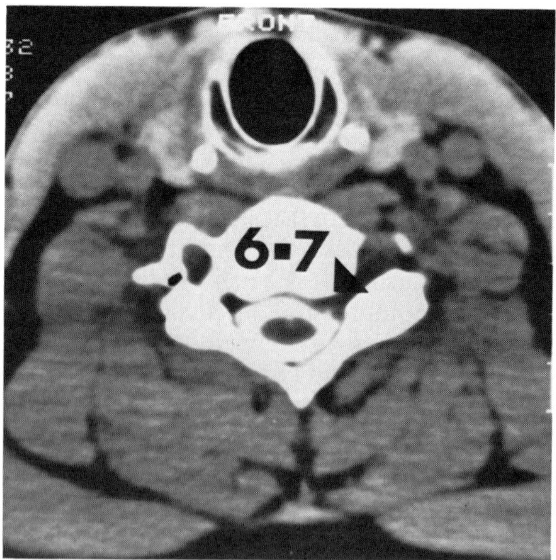

Figure 20–9. Myelogram with CT follow-up demonstrating posterolateral soft disc herniation (*arrowhead*).

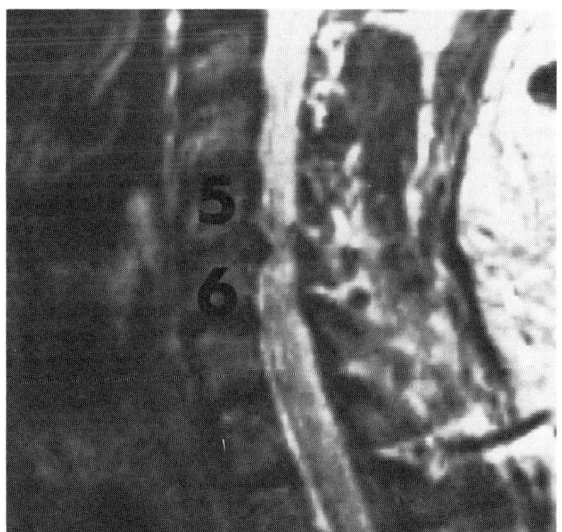

Figure 20–10. MRI scan demonstrating central cervical disc herniation at C5–C6.

The results were graded as *excellent* (complete relief of pain and weakness), *good* (improvement in pain and weakness requiring occasional analgesics without life style restrictions), *fair* (improvement in pain and weakness requiring analgesics with life style restrictions), and *poor* (no improvement over preoperative symptoms and signs). Statistical analysis utilizing the Fischer exact test was used to determine the significance of the results.

There were 44 patients, 27 male and 17 female. The age range was 21 to 56 years with a mean of 41 years. The follow-up was 1.6 to 8.2 years with a mean of 4.2 years. Table 20–1 lists the level of herniation for each group. The Type I group (posterolateral herniation) consisted of 33 patients, 19 male and 14 female. The clinical pattern in all patients with Type I herniation consisted of neck and/or unilateral radiculopathy of a sensory and/or motor component. Of the 33 patients with Type I herniations, anterior cervical fusion (Robinson technique) was performed in 17 patients, 10 males and seven females. The age range was 26 to 52 years (mean of 43 years). Sixteen of the 33 Type I patients underwent a laminotomy-foraminotomy: nine males and seven females with an age range of 21 to 50 years (mean of 39 years).

Table 20–1. STATISTICAL ANALYSIS USING FISCHER EXACT TEST FOR RESULTS OF TYPE I HERNIATION COMPARING ANTERIOR FUSION WITH POSTERIOR LAMINOTOMY-FORAMINOTOMY (33 PATIENTS) (P <.175)

Results	Anterior Fusion (No. of Patients)	Laminotomy (No. of Patients)
Excellent-good	16	12
Fair-poor	1	4

The Type II group (central disc herniation) consisted of 11 patients, eight males and three females with a mean age of 40 years (range 29 to 46 years). The clinical pattern in these 11 consisted of myelopathy in seven patients, categorized as Nurick I in four and Nurick II in three. The remaining four patients complained of axial symptoms (neck and interscapular pain) and "burning or shooting" sensations down the arms (bilateral in three, unilateral in one). The surgical procedure performed in patients with Type II herniations was an anterior discectomy and fusion (Robinson horseshoe graft).

The results for patients with a posterolateral disc herniation (Type I, 33 patients) were excellent in 17, good in 11, fair in four, and poor in one. This represents a 96 per cent improvement rate (excellent-good-fair [E-G-F]) and an 85 per cent excellent-good (E-G) result. For the 17 patients who had undergone anterior fusion in this group, the results were excellent in 11, good in five, and fair in one (E-G-F, 100 per cent; E-G, 94 per cent). Of the 16 patients who had undergone laminotomy-foraminotomy, there were excellent results in six, good results in six, fair results in three, and poor results in 1 (E-G-F, 93 per cent; E-G, 75 per cent). Table 20–1 shows the statistical analysis utilizing the Fischer Exact Test. In this test the excellent-good results for anterior fusion and laminotomy-foraminotomy were compared with the fair-poor results in each group. Although the results were not statistically significant to a P value less than .175, a definite trend was present for better results when an anterior discectomy and fusion was performed rather than a laminotomy-foraminotomy.

For patients with a Type II herniation, excellent results were noted in six, good results in four, and fair results in one (E-G-F, 100 per cent; E-G, 91 per cent).

The complications in this series for anterior fusion were pseudarthrosis in two patients with a good and fair result, respectively. One patient had iliac graft site pain for three weeks. Hoarseness present for four weeks was noted in another and partial slippage of the graft in another; in the latter further surgery was not required and the patient was categorized as a good result.

The complications noted in the laminotomy group consisted of two patients with persistent serous drainage, lasting three weeks in one and four weeks in the other without evidence of infection.

ANTERIOR DISCECTOMY WITHOUT FUSION

Anterior discectomy without fusion developed as an alternative to fusion based on the premise that if successful results of anterior fusion occur in the face of pseudarthrosis, discectomy can be performed without fusion. Several studies have advocated anterior cervical discectomy without fusion, reporting success rates similar to those with fusion.[41, 48, 56, 72] This procedure defeats the principles of anterior fusion, which are based on neuroforamen distraction and reduction of buckling of the ligamentum flavum. In addition, by its very nature this surgery is designed to create a pseudarthrosis, which may lead to a less satisfactory result. The series reported to date have limited clinical follow-up study and poor roentgenographic correlation to determine the development of instability or kyphotic angulation. This procedure should not be performed until better follow-up studies are available.

References

1. Abitol, J. J., and Garfin, S.: Surgical management of cervical disc disease: anterior cervical fusion. Semin. Spine Surg. *1*:233–238, 1989.
2. Adams, C., and Logue, U.: Studies in cervical spondylotic myelopathy. Brain *94*:569–586, 1971.
3. Arima, T.: Post laminectomy malalignments of the cervical spine. J. Brain Nerve Trauma (Jpn.) *1*:71–78, 1969.
4. Aronson, N.: The management of soft cervical disc protrusions using the Smith Robinson approach. Clin. Neurosurg. *20*:253–258, 1973.
5. Bailey, R. W., and Badgley, C. E.: Stabilization of the cervical spine by anterior fusion. J. Bone Joint Surg. *42A*:565–594, 1960.
6. Bohlman, H.: Cervical spondylosis with moderate to severe myelopathy. Spine *2*:151–162, 1977.
7. Bohlman, H.: Degenerative arthrosis of the lower cervical spine. *In* Evarts, C. M. (ed.): Surgery of the Musculoskeletal System. Vol. 2. New York, Churchill Livingstone, 1983, pp. 25–35.
8. Boni, M., Cherubino, P., Denaro, U., and Benazzo, F.: Multiple subtotal somatectomy. Spine *9*:358–362, 1984.
9. Brain, R. W., Northfield, D., and Wilkinson, M.: The neurologic manifestations of cervical spondylosis. Brain *75*:187–225, 1952.
10. Brain, L., and Wilkinson, M.: Cervical spondylosis and other disorders of the cervical spine. Philadelphia, W. B. Saunders Co., 1967, p. 226.
11. Breig, A., Turnbull, I., and Hassler, O.: Effects of mechanical stresses on the spinal cord in cervical spondylosis. J. Neurosurg. *25*:45, 1966.
12. Brodsky, A.: Management of radiculopathy secondary to acute cervical disc degeneration and spondylosis by the posterior approach. *In* Cervical Spine Research Society (eds.): The Cervical Spine. Philadelphia, J. B. Lippincott Co., 1983, pp. 395–402.
13. Bulgar, R., Rejowski, J., and Beatty, R.: Vocal cord paralysis associated with anterior cervical fusion: considerations for prevention and treatment. J. Neurosurg. *62*:657–661, 1985.
14. Callahan, R., Johnson, R., Margolis, R., et al.: Cervical facet fusion for control of instability following laminectomy. J. Bone Joint Surg. *59A*:991–1002, 1977.
15. Clark, C.: Indications and surgical management of cervical myelopathy. Semin. Spine Surg. *1*:254–261, 1989.
16. Clarke, E., and Robinson, P.: Cervical myelopathy: a complication of cervical spondylosis. Brain *79*:483, 1956.
17. Cloward, R. B.: The anterior approach for ruptured cervical discs. J. Neurosurg. *15*:602, 1958.
18. Connolly, E. S., Seymour, R. J., and Adams, J. E.: Clinical evaluation of anterior cervical fusion for degenerative cervical disc disease. J. Neurosurg. *23*:431–437, 1965.
19. Crandall, P., and Batzdorf, U.: Cervical spondylotic myelopathy. J. Neurosurg. *25*:57–66, 1966.
20. Crandall, P., and Gregonius, F.: Long-term follow-up of cervical spondylotic myelopathy. Spine *2*:139–146, 1977.
21. DePalma, A., Rothman, R., Lewinnnek, G., et al.: Anterior interbody fusion for severe cervical disc degeneration. Surg. Gynecol. Obstet. *134*:755–758, 1972.
22. Dillin, W., Booth, R., Cuckler, J., et al.: Cervical radiculopathy: a review. Spine *11*:988–991, 1986.
23. Dillin, W., and Simeone, F. A.: Treatment of cervical disc disease. Selection of operative approaches. Contemp. Neurosurg. *8*:1–6, 1986.
24. Epstein, J., and Janin, Y.: Management of cervical spondylotic myeloradiculopathy by the posterior approach. *In* Cervical Spine Research Society (eds.): The Cervical Spine. Philadelphia, J. B. Lippincott Co., 1983, pp. 402–410.
25. Epstein, J., Janin, Y., Carras, R., and Lavine, L.: A comparative study of the treatment of cervical spondylotic myeloradiculopathy. Acta Neurochir. *61*:89–104, 1982.
26. Flynn, T. B.: Neurologic complications of anterior fusion. Spine 7:536–539, 1982.
27. Gooding, M., Wilson, C., and Hoff, J.: Experimental cervical myelopathy. J. Neurosurg. *43*:9–17, 1975.
28. Gore, D., Sepic, S., Gardner, G., and Murray, M.: Neck pain: a long-term follow-up of 205 patients. Spine *12*:1–5, 1987.

29. Gore, D., and Sepic, S.: Anterior cervical fusion for degenerated or protruded discs. Spine *9*:667–671, 1984.
30. Gregorius, F. K., Estin, T. E., and Crandall, P. H.: Cervical spondylotic radiculopathy and myelopathy. Arch Neurol. *33*:618–625, 1976.
31. Grisoli, F., Graziani, N., Fabrizi, A. P., et al.: Anterior discectomy without fusion for treatment of cervical lateral soft disc extrusion: a follow-up of 120 cases. Neurosurgery *24*:853–859, 1989.
32. Haft, H., and Shenkin, H. A.: Surgical end results of cervical ridge and disc problems. J.A.M.A. *186*:312–315, 1963.
33. Henderson, C., Hennessy, R., Shuey, H., and Shackelford, E.: Posterior-lateral foraminotomy as an exclusive operative technique for cervical radiculopathy: a review of 846 consecutively operated cases. Neurosurgery *13*:504–511, 1983.
34. Herkowitz, H. N.: A comparison of anterior cervical fusion, cervical laminectomy and cervical laminaplasty for the surgical management of multiple level spondylotic radiculopathy. Spine *13*:774–780, 1988.
35. Herkowitz, H. N.: Cervical laminaplasty: its role in the treatment of cervical radiculopathy. J. Spinal Dis. *1*:179–188, 1988.
36. Herkowitz, H. N.: The surgical management of cervical spondylotic radiculopathy and myelopathy. Clin. Orthop. *239*:94–108, 1989.
37. Herkowitz, H. N., Kurz, L. T., and Overholt, D. P.: The surgical management of cervical soft disc herniation: a comparison between the anterior and posterior approach. Spine *15*:1026–1030, 1990.
38. Hirabayashi, K., Miyakawa, J., Satomi, K., et al.: Operative results and post-operative progression of ossification among patients with ossification of cervical posterior longitudinal ligaments. Spine *6*:354–364, 1981.
39. Hirabayashi, K., Watanabe, K., Wakano, K., et al.: Expansive open-door laminoplasty for cervical spinal stenotic myelopathy. Spine *8*:693–699, 1983.
40. Hukuda, S., Mochizuki, T., Ogata, M., et al.: Operations for cervical spondylotic myelopathy. J. Bone Joint Surg. *67B*:609–615, 1985.
41. Hunter, L., Braunstein, E., and Bailey, R.: Radiographic changes following anterior cervical fusion. Spine *5*:399–401, 1980.
42. Ishida, Y., Suzuki, K., Ohmori, K., et al.: Critical analysis of extensive cervical laminectomy. Neurosurgery *24*:215–222, 1989.
43. Itoh, T., and Tsuji, H.: Technical improvements and results of laminaplasty for compressive myelopathy in the cervical spine. Spine *10*:729–736, 1985.
44. Kimura, I., Oh-Hama, M., and Shingu, H.: Cervical myelopathy treated by canal-expansive laminaplasty. J. Bone Joint Surg. *66A*:914–920, 1984.
45. Kozak, J., Hanson, G., Rose, J., et al.: Anterior discectomy, microscopic decompression and fusion: a treatment for cervical spondylotic radiculopathy. J. Spinal Dis. *2*:43–46, 1989.
46. Kraus, F. R., and Stauffer, E. S.: Spinal cord injury as a complication of elective anterior cervical fusion. Clin. Orthop. *112*:130–141, 1975.
47. Kurz, L. T., Garfin, S. R., and Booth, R.: Harvesting autogenous iliac bone graft: a review of complications and techniques. Spine *14*:1324–1331, 1990.
48. Laoire, S., and Thomas, D.: Spinal cord compression due to prolapse of cervical intervertebral disc: treatment of 26 cases by discectomy without interbody bone graft. J. Neurosurg. *59*:847–853, 1983.
49. Lees, F., and Turner, J. W.: Natural history and prognosis of cervical spondylosis. Br. Med. J. *5373*:1607–1610, 1963.
50. Lonstein, J.: Post-laminectomy Kyphosis, Spinal Deformities and Neurologic Dysfunction. New York, Raven Press, 1978, pp. 53–63.
51. Lunsford, L., Bissonette, D., Jannetha, P., et al.: Anterior surgery for cervical disc disease: treatment of lateral cervical disc herniation in 253 cases. J. Neurosurg. *53*:1–11, 1980.
52. Lunsford, L., Bissonette, D., and Zorub, D.: Anterior surgery for cervical disc disease: treatment of cervical spondylotic myelopathy in 32 cases. J. Neurosurg. *53*:12–19, 1980.
53. Manabe, S., and Tateishi, A.: Epidural migration of extruded cervical disc and its surgical treatment. Spine *11*:873–878, 1986.
54. Mann, K., Khosla, V., and Gulati, D.: Cervical spondylotic myelopathy treated by single stage multilevel anterior decompression. J. Neurosurg. *60*:81–87, 1984.
55. Munroe, I.: The importance of the sagittal diameters of the cervical spinal canal in relation to spondylosis and myelopathy. J. Bone Joint Surg. *56B*:30, 1974.
56. Murphy, M., and Gadd, M.: Anterior cervical discectomy without interbody bone graft. J. Neurosurg. *37*:71–74, 1972.
57. Newhouse, K., Lindsey, R., Clark, C., et al.: Esophageal perforation following anterior cervical spine surgery. Spine *14*:1051–1056, 1989.
58. Nurick, S.: The natural history and the results of surgical treatment of the spinal cord disorder associated with cervical spondylosis. Brain *95*:101–108, 1972.
59. Nurick, S.: The pathogenesis of the spinal cord disorder associated with cervical spondylosis. Brain *95*:87, 1972.
60. Oiwa, T., Hirabayshi, K., Mitsuyoshi, U., and Ohira, T.: Experimental study of post-laminectomy deterioration of cervical spondylotic myelopathy. Spine *10*:717–721, 1985.
61. Penning, L., and VanDer Zwaag, P.: Biomechanical aspects of spondylotic myelopathy. Acta Radiol. *5*:1090, 1966.
62. Perry, S., and Nickel, V. L.: Total cervical spine fusion for neck paralysis. J. Bone Joint Surg. *41A*:37–60, 1959.
63. Phillips, D. G.: Surgical treatment of myelopathy with cervical spondylosis. J. Neurol. Neurosurg. Psychiatry *36*:879–884, 1973.
64. Raynor, R.: Anterior or posterior approach to the cervical spine: an anatomical and radiographic evaluation and comparison. Neurosurgery *12*:7–13, 1983.
65. Raynor, R., Pugh, J., and Shapiro, I.: Cervical facetectomy and its effect on spine strength. J. Neurosurg. *63*:278–282, 1985.
66. Riley, L.: Anterior cervical spine surgery. *In* AAOS Instructional Course Lectures. Vol. XXVII. St. Louis, C. V. Mosby Co., 1978, pp. 154–158.
67. Riley, L., Robinson, R., Johnson, K., and Walker, A.: The results of anterior interbody fusion of the cervical spine. J. Neurosurg. *30*:127, 1969.
68. Robinson, R., Afeiche, N., Dunn, E., and Northrup, B.: Cervical spondylotic myelopathy. Spine *2*:89–99, 1977.

69. Robinson, R. A., and Smith, G. W.: Anterolateral cervical disc removal and interbody fusion for cervical disc syndrome. Bull. Johns Hopkins Hosp. *96*:223–224, 1955.
70. Robinson, R., Walker, A., and Ferlic, D.: The results of anterior interbody fusion of the cervical spine. J. Bone Joint Surg. *44A*:1569–1587, 1962.
71. Robinson, R. A., and Smith, G. W.: The treatment of certain spine disorders by anterior removal of the intervertebral disc and interbody fusion. J. Bone Joint Surg. *40A*:607, 1958.
72. Rosenorn, J., Hansen, E., and Rosenorn, M.: Anterior cervical discectomy with and without fusion. J. Neurosurg. *59*:252–255, 1983.
73. Rothman, R., and Rashbaum, R.: Pathogenesis of signs and symptoms of cervical disc degeneration. *In* AAOS Instructional Course Lectures. Vol. XXVII. St. Louis, C. V. Mosby Co., 1978, pp. 203–215.
74. Rothman, R. H., and Simeone, F. A.: Cervical Disc Disease. *In* Rothman, R. H., and Simeone, F. A. (eds.): The Spine. 2nd ed. Vol. 1. Philadelphia, W. B. Saunders Co., 1982, pp. 440–499.
75. Scoville, W., Dohrmann, G., and Corkill, G.: Late results of cervical disc surgery. J. Neurosurg. *45*:203–210, 1976.
76. Sim, F. H., Suien, H. J., Bickel, W. H., and Janes, J. M.: Swan neck deformity following extensive cervical laminectomy. J. Bone Joint Surg. *56A*:564–580, 1974.
77. Simmons, E., and Bhalla, S.: Anterior cervical discectomy and fusion. J. Bone Joint Surg. *51B*:225–237, 1969.
78. Southwick, W. O., and Robinson, R. A.: Surgical approaches to the vertebral bodies in the cervical and lumbar regions. J. Bone Joint Surg. *39A*:631–644, 1957.
79. Tachdjian, M., and Matson, D.: Orthopedic aspects of intraspinal tumor in infants and children. J. Bone Joint Surg. *47A*:223, 1965.
80. Tsuji, H.: Laminaplasty for patients with compressive myelopathy due to so-called spinal canal stenosis in cervical and thoracic regions. Spine *7*:28–34, 1982.
81. Verbeist, H.: The management of cervical spondylosis. Clin. Neurosurg. *20*:262–294, 1973.
82. White, A., Southwick, W., DePonte, R., et al.: Relief of pain by anterior cervical spine fusion for spondylosis. J. Bone Joint Surg. *55A*:525–534, 1973.
83. White, A., and Hirsch, C.: An experimental study of the immediate load-bearing capacity of some commonly used iliac bone grafts. Acta Orthop. Scand. *42*:482–490, 1971.
84. Whitecloud, T.: Complications of anterior cervical fusion. *In* Instructional Course Lectures. Vol. XXVII. St. Louis, C. V. Mosby Co., 1978, pp. 223–227.
85. Whitecloud, T.: Management of radiculopathy and myelopathy by the anterior approach. *In* Cervical Spine Research Society (eds.): The Cervical Spine. Philadelphia, J. B. Lippincott Co., 1983, pp. 411–424.
86. Williams, J., Allen, M., and Harkess, J.: Late results of cervical discectomy and interbody fusion: some factors influencing the results. J. Bone Joint Surg. *50A*:277–286, 1968.
87. Wolf, B., Khilnani, M., and Malis, L.: The sagittal diameter of the bony cervical canal and its significance in cervical spondylosis. J. Mt. Sinai Hosp. *23*:283–292, 1956.
88. Yonenobu, K., Fuji, T., Ono, K., et al.: Choice of surgical treatment for multisegmental cervical spondylotic myelopathy. Spine *10*:710–716, 1985.

SURGICAL MANAGEMENT OF CERVICAL RADICULOPATHY: POSTERIOR APPROACH

Frederick A. Simeone, M. D.

The diagnosis of cervical disc disease with radiculopathy is very specific. Localized pain pattern, associated with reflex, motor, and sensory deficits, and definitive radiographic findings, are necessary before consideration of surgical treatment. The failure of nonoperative surgery or the rapid development of neurologic deficit encourages operative decisions.

The cervical spine can be approached anteriorly or posteriorly. Many factors contribute to the individual surgeon's choice of operation in a given patient. Factors influencing this decision reflect peculiarities among surgeons as well as the specific nature of the disease to be treated. An individual surgeon's training, familiarity with each technique, previous favorable or unfavorable experiences with a certain operation, and his general concept of pathologic mechanisms that he has treated all contribute to the choice. Surgeons seem to fall into one of two camps: those who believe that the signs and symptoms should be treated specifically and those who believe that the correction of radiographic abnormalities remains the principal goal of surgery. As long as spine surgeons view their goals differently, controversies about surgical technique are bound to continue. A competent spine surgeon is able to perform all approaches safely and in this way can offer patients the advantages of modern surgical technology. The author finds himself in the camp that favors treatment of symptoms and neurologic findings over radiographic abnormalities.

Anterior surgery plays a role in the treatment of all forms of cervical spine pathology. We believe anterior surgery is the treatment of choice in the following disorders:

1. Midline soft disc herniation with symptomatic myelopathy at one or several levels.
2. Midline hard disc protrusion at one or two levels.
3. Disc herniation with bilateral radiculopathy at the same level.
4. Resection of a disease process in the vertebral body.

The posterior approach is used for

1. Unilateral radiculopathy at one or more levels (posterior foraminotomy).
2. Cervical myelopathy with spinal cord compression at three or more levels (posterior laminectomy with or without laminaplasty).
3. Spinal cord compression secondary to degenerative subluxation (posterior laminectomy with facet joint fusion).
4. Spinal cord compression secondary to congenital spinal stenosis or acquired stenosis from posterior compression (e.g., ligamentum flavum).

The clinical syndromes of cervical disc disease and radiographic abnormalities are discussed elsewhere and no attempt is made to review these in great detail here. It may be worthwhile, however, to cite some of the author's preferences. Nonoperative therapy (a term I prefer to "conservative") should be maintained as long as there is evidence of progressive improvement in pain and minor neurologic deficit. More advanced neurologic deficit, particularly if there is disabling loss of function, should be treated promptly. I am particularly aggressive with C5 lesions (because loss of deltoid function can be devastating) and C8 lesions (in which loss of intrinsic hand function can destroy the individual's working life). Fortunately, radiculopathy secondary to herniated cervical discs more frequently affects the C6 and C7 roots; weakness in the latter often progresses unnoticed. Nonoperative treatment of neck pain is the principal mode of therapy, and unless there is obvious evidence of substantial motion of the cervical spine on flexion and extension films (greater than 3 mm), surgery is not recommended. Most statistical series of cervical spine disc disease have shown that neck pain responds poorly to treatment. In Williams' series, only 27 per cent of patients with neck pain responded to therapy.[5]

Radiographic abnormalities are discussed elsewhere. It is important to realize that the understanding of MRI has not reached the level of sophistication seen with myelography, CT, and postmyelography CT. Computer-assisted myelography is complementary to water-soluble contrast myelography, and the merits of one supplement the limitations of the other. As we gain experience with MRI, the significance of "abnormalities" must be evaluated in the light of symptoms and signs. At present, a full understanding of the role of certain MRI changes with reference to symptoms or neurologic findings has not yet been delineated, so that if there is any doubt, further investigations must be performed before surgery.

TECHNIQUE: POSTERIOR NERVE ROOT DECOMPRESSION (FORAMINOTOMY)

The patient is carefully intubated and placed in a kneeling position with the head flexed and held in a Mayfield pinholder headrest. The operating table is tilted so that the cervical spine is roughly parallel to the floor. This allows for partial collapse of epidural veins yet frees the surgeon from concern over air embolism. No signs or symptoms of air embolism have ever occurred in this position in the author's series.

The appropriate spinal level is identified by inserting a needle through the skin to a spinous process. Radiographs are taken while the neck is being prepared. An incision, ordinarily about 3 cm long, covering the two spinous processes between which the offending disc lies is carried down to the laminae, which are held in place with a Taylor retractor. With a thin Schlesinger rongeur, a circular defect is made approximately 8 mm in diameter, half of which is on the superior lamina and the other half on the inferior lamina. This laterally placed laminotomy forms the circular portion of the "keyhole." Using magnification, either in the form of three-power loupes or with the operating microscope (this is the surgeon's choice), a high-speed air drill with a diamond tip is used to thin the bone over the nerve root. Because the nerve root leaves between the two laminae, the drilling straddles the facet joint. A superior- and inferior-most extension of the drilling process goes from pedicle to pedicle. It is possible to drill into the pedicle at this point if one proceeds too far superiorly or inferiorly.

Ultimately, as the drilling progresses, it becomes obvious that the laminae have thinned and that the roof of the foramen is now delicate. At this point, even though the lateral-most extension of the foraminotomy may not be completed, it is wise to chip off the thin layer of remaining bone over the nerve root with an angled curet. In so doing, one avoids mechanical and thermal injury to the underlying nerve root. As the bone is chipped away, one can appreciate the fact that the nerve root is tight up against the inferior surface of the facet joint. It may be necessary to drill farther in order to make the residual bone thinner, or to carry the foraminotomy out more laterally. The lateral extent of the foraminotomy is determined by passing a thin-angled instrument, such as a Woodson elevator or a fine dental pick, out of the foramen. If the instrument can slip comfortably between the tissues around the nerve root and bony foramen, the foraminotomy is complete; if, on the other hand, any resistance is felt, more foraminotomy is necessary. Nerve roots should be loose both laterally and medially. Fine instruments should pass easily around the shoulder and axilla of the nerve root as well as out laterally, as previously described.

At this point the operation is complete if the patient has hard disc pathology. By stopping the operation at this point, it is not necessary to remove a cuff of veins and other extraneous soft tissue that actually cover the dura over the nerve root. The author agrees that it is not necessary to remove this tissue in order to achieve a decompression. However, he had one patient with a large soft cervical disc herniation in whom cervical decompression was obviously not enough. Pain persisted in the immediate postoperative period, and a few days after the foraminotomy an anterior discectomy was necessary to totally decompress the root and achieve a satisfactory result. For this reason, in patients with soft disc pathology, I now remove the vascular cuff over the dura and inspect the nerve roots directly. Under magnification, one can see that the nerve root's dural sheath is divided into ventral and dorsal sections. With the Rosen knife or the microsurgical Penfield dissector, it is possible to reach under the ventral root and palpate the disc bulge. If the bulge is substantial and soft, the annulus is cut with a No. 11 scalpel blade, care being taken not to involve the dura of the nerve root sheath, which can be substantially thinned when under pressure.

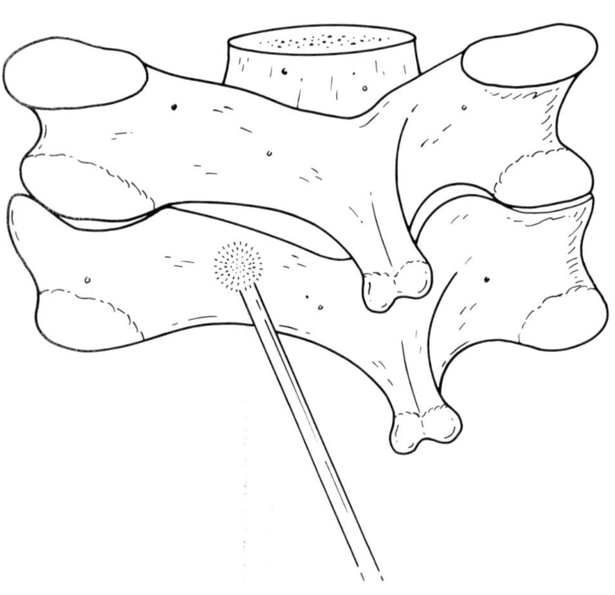

Figure 20–11. A diamond burr begins keyhole laminotomy. The bone is thinned until it can be chipped away with a fine curette. Decompression is carried laterally until the root is free.

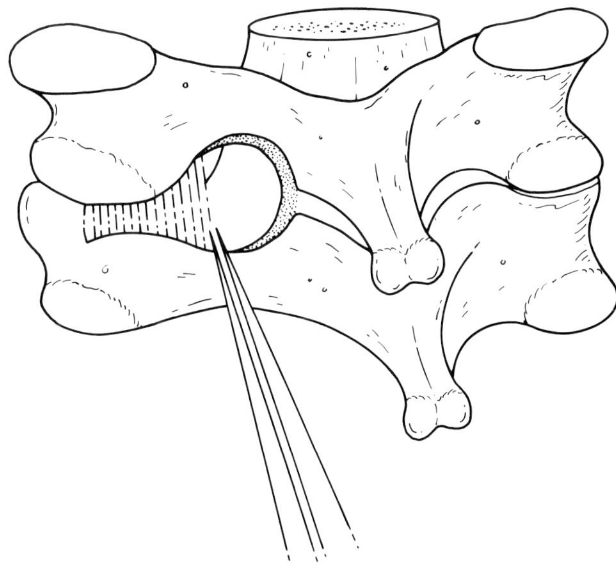

Figure 20–12. Many authors believe this procedure can be discontinued after bony decompression (Henderson). Here, epidural venous cuff is being cauterized before its removal.

Incision of the annulus is usually associated with extrusion of disc material. If this does not occur, the Rosen knife can be placed under the ventral portion of the nerve root, and disc material can be expressed through the opening in the annulus fibrosus. The decision whether to incise the annulus over the shoulder of the root or in the axilla depends on the apex of the bulging disc. In some instances this maneuver can yield substantial portions of disc material, sometimes fragmented into larger chunks. In other instances, particularly with chronically degenerated soft discs, the yield is disappointing. A long, straight hemostat may be used to enter the interspace, but the space itself is generally too narrow to accept any ordinary disc (pituitary) rongeur. When the nerve root is compressed from one below and the annulus fibrosus is relatively flat, one can easily demonstrate marked "looseness" in the mobility of the root when it is palpated in all directions. At this point the operation is generally complete. If no soft disc material is found or expressed, the results are still excellent because the decompressive procedure is the definitive operation.

The nerve root is covered with a small portion of fat and the paraspinous muscles are approximated. A two-layer skin closure with a running subcuticular suture of 4-0 nylon maintains the skin together until the first postoperative office visit, which may be three to four

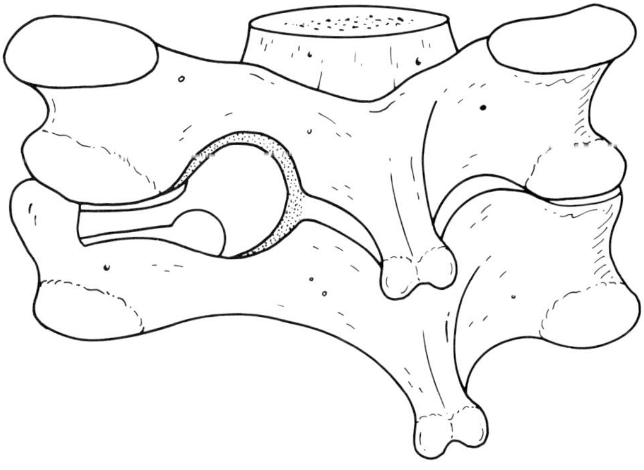

Figure 20–13. The dura over the nerve root is exposed to allow visualization of the floor of the canal.

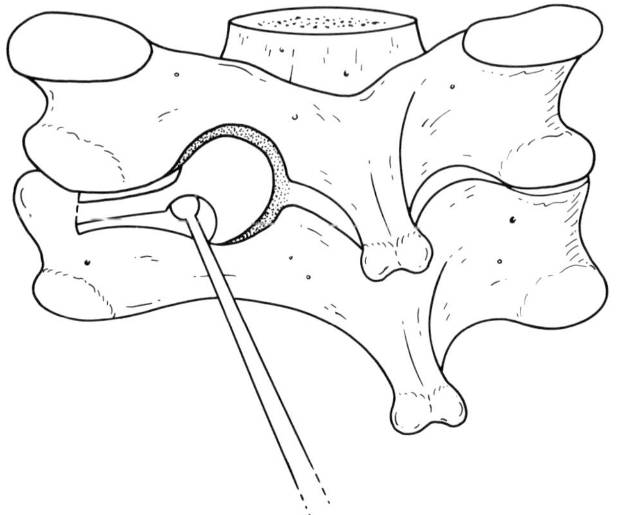

Figure 20–14. With a small Rosen knife, or other fine dissecting instrument, the anterior canal is palpated, and the disc fragment, if present, can be expressed by downward pressure. Disc fragments can be removed with a fine, long hemostat.

weeks after surgery. Henderson and colleagues described a similar operation without advocating an attempt to remove soft disc material.[1]

RESULTS

The author is extremely circumspect in operating on patients who are involved in compensation claims, or who believe that their surgical problem is the result of an injury for which there is ongoing litigation. These patients are rarely treated surgically unless they are developing disabling neurologic deficits. This is because other statistical series and the author's experience show that results for pain relief are poor in patients involved in compensation and litigation claims. If the purpose of the operation is to relieve pain, and the results are no better than those from nonsurgical care, it stands to reason that these patients should not undergo surgery unless there is a progressive and disabling neurologic deficit. Other categories of patients treated more cautiously include those involved in chronic use of self-administered narcotics. Many patients have continuing pain after technically successful surgery because they have never overcome the addiction that was present preoperatively. Patients who take self-administered narcotics are often unaware that their pain can be cycled by narcotic administration. These patients should be weaned from narcotics and their pain syndrome should be evaluated periodically. Similarly, patients with a long history of preexisting depression should be treated with greater conservatism, because experience shows that chronic depressive patients relinquish their symptoms very slowly. Surgery should be performed if they are disabled and under maximal treatment for chronic depressive illness.

In Rothman and Simeone's group of patients, 98 per cent followed one to eight years after surgery reported good to excellent results in terms of return to outside work or housework, freedom from taking analgesic medication, ability to sleep through the night, and ability to become involved in other physical activities.[2]

Among the patients who complained after surgery, CT scans continued to show disc bulging, but they nonetheless ultimately made spontaneous recovery (with the exception of one who required anterior discectomy to decompress the nerve root adequately). In this series, good to excellent results could be expected despite the patient's age, the degree of initial neurologic deficit, and the severity of pain.[2]

Most large series of patients with cervical disc herniation reported similarly good results.[3, 5] Henderson and colleagues' report of 96 per cent excellent results in a series of 846 patients with posterior decompression and no disc removal is truly impressive!

COMPLICATIONS

The complications rate in patients with posterior nerve root decompressions is very low. It includes failure to operate at the correct level, nerve root injury, and inadequate foraminotomy. These problems become less common as surgeons develop their technique. Careful intraoperative radiographs, magnification, and repeated palpation for nerve root "looseness" are necessary. Other complications of posterior disc surgery are extremely rare. In general, patients recover from surgery without arm pain and can be discharged on the second postoperative day without a collar. This freedom from complications and rapid return to normal activity compares favorably with anterior disc surgery in which reported results for arm pain relief are approximately the same. However, with the anterior approach the following complications have been reported: spinal cord injury, nerve root injury, espophageal perforation, recurrent laryngeal nerve injury, thoracic duct injury, Horner's syndrome, airway obstruction, and bone graft mishaps.[4]

CONCLUSION

The author believes that for both hard and soft cervical disc disease with radiculopathy the posterior approach offers the advantages of safety, quick recovery, significantly fewer complications, and a single incision without the necessity for a cervical collar. The excellent success rate of both anterior and posterior approaches in this disease is gratifying in patients not involved in compensation, litigation, or other psychologic problems. Patients with symptomatic spinal cord compression from soft or hard disc material anteriorly at one or two levels are best treated by anterior disc excision and fusion.

Spine surgeons should be able to perform all operative procedures well and with confidence. They must carefully review the current literature and modify their approach according to the results of many conscientious investigators. Because most patients with cervical disc disease and radiculopathy feel improved shortly after surgery, surgeons cannot ignore the long-term effects of the operation or the continued progression of the disease. Nevertheless, they are obliged to perform the simplest procedure that gives the most viable results. The author's experience favors a combination of anterior and posterior approaches for the varieties of chronic disc degeneration.

References

1. Henderson, C. M., Hennessy, R. G., Shuey, H. M., Jr., and Shackelford, E. G.: Posterior-lateral foraminotomy as an exclusive operative technique for cervical radiculopathy: a review of 846 consecutively operated cases. Neurosurgery *13*:504, 1983.
2. Rothman, R. H., and Simeone, F. A.: The Spine. 2nd ed. Philadelphia, W. B. Saunders Co., 1982.
3. Scoville, W. B., Dohrmann, G. J., and Corkill, G.: Late results of cervical disc surgery. J. Neurosurg. *45*:203, 1976.
4. Whitecloud, T.: Complications of anterior cervical fusion. Instr. Course Lect. *27*, 1978.
5. Williams, R. W.: Microcervical foraminotomy. Spine *8*:711, 1983.

INDICATIONS FOR SURGERY IN CERVICAL MYELOPATHY: ANTERIOR VERSUS POSTERIOR APPROACH

Kalman D. Blumberg, M.D.
Frederick A. Simeone, M.D.

Consideration of surgical indications for a disease process, or any type of treatment for any disease, is predicated on an understanding of that disease's natural history. Likewise, risk:benefit ratio determines which particular type of treatment or operative procedure is chosen. The history, physical examination, and radiologic work-up must all correlate to confirm the diagnosis of cervical spondylotic myelopathy (CSM), and these factors are discussed elsewhere in this book. Once the proper diagnosis is assured, patient selection for surgery can proceed on the basis of the natural history of the disease and treatment results.

NATURAL HISTORY

In a review of the natural history of CSM, it becomes readily apparent that there is a lack of studies available in which patients received no treatment. Review of a group of untreated patients would of course be the ideal comparative setting for the determination of proper treatment. Most studies include patients who were treated conservatively with a collar, and rarely is more information given to the reader. This section will group together these patients with those reported as having received no treatment for CSM, to permit some comparison of operative treatment in order to determine indications for surgery.

Numerous reports describe the course of CSM and the effects of treatment on this disease. Clarke and Robinson's report of 120 patients with CSM provides the first careful examination of the disease's natural history, describing the disease's course in these patients before the onset of therapy, either operative or nonoperative.[5] Before Clarke and Robinson's paper, literature reports on CSM included cases of acute cervical disc herniations. This caused confusion in regard to natural history and therapy. Clarke and Robinson eliminated from consideration acute disc herniations as the cause of myelopathy. Of their 120 patients, 75 per cent underwent a course defined by episodes of worsening symptoms and signs. Two thirds of this 75 per cent showed ongoing deterioration between the acute clinical episodes. The remaining one third showed stabilization between the episodes of acute clinical deterioration. These periods of stability lasted from a few weeks to several years. Twenty per cent of the 120 patients showed a slow steady progression without periods of remission. The remaining 5 per cent were characterized by rapid onset and progression of signs and symptoms to a point of stabilization. Deaths related direclty to CSM occurred in 5 per cent of the patients, being due to pulmonary or urinary infection. Clarke and Robinson's study revealed a number of possible courses. Most underwent an episodic but unpredictable pathway. A minority of patients underwent a relentless progression of symptoms. Clarke and Robinson concluded that although a patient's course may be slow, the prognosis is poor, and noted that true improvement is rare. They felt it was possible that a patient who reports improvement may actually be more successfully coping with the disability. If clinical progression has discontinued, this may also be interpreted as improvement. They noted spontaneous regression in only two patients with predominantly sensory complaints. Neck, bladder, and sensory findings tended to be more transient than motor complaints. Upper extremity difficulties tended to be sensory in nature and lower extremity difficulties to be motor. Age was not correlated with CSM progression.

In 1963 Lees and Turner reported 95 patients with cervical spondylosis, 44 of whom presented with myelopathy.[22] Only eleven of these 44 went without treatment to genuinely reflect the natural history. The 44 CSM patients were split into groups with more or less than ten years of follow-up. Both groups showed an episodic course similar to that of Clarke and Robinson's patients. Lees and Turner felt that the periods between episodes of worsening were marked by a static or improving nature. They reported that in patients with symptoms lasting longer than ten years, the episodes of worsening were often shorter than one year. Of patients followed for less than ten years, 50 per cent showed episodes of worsening lasting longer than one year. The authors did not characterize the periods of static or improving symptomatology, but did categorize their myelopathic patients into those with mild, moderate, and severe disability (Table 20–2). Patients were classified into these groups on the basis of the maximal degree of disability reached at the time of their worst symptoms. None of the patients in the mild disability group recovered to the point of no disability. One of the moderately disabled and seven of 25 severely disabled patients improved by one category of disability. Ob-

Table 20–2. LEES AND TURNER CLASSIFICATION

Degree	
Mild	Symptoms in hands and arms, producing some incapacity but not preventing ordinary everyday activity
Moderate	Considerable difficulty in using hands or legs, sufficient to affect performance of everyday tasks and to cause slowness in walking or disturbance of balance
Severe	Patient can hardly walk or needs sticks or crutches, and at time of worst symptoms is unable to walk and often confined to bed, chair, or house

From Lees, F., and Turner, J. W. A.: Natural history and prognosis of cervical spondylosis. Br. Med. J. *2*:1607–1610, 1963.

viously none of these patients worsened during follow-up, because the groups were defined according to the worst level of disability reached during the course of the disease. Lees and Turner provided follow-up information to describe improvement or subsequent stasis, but no specific information about patients' episodic course before reaching their worst disability. We are not told the natural history of the patients that presented with a certain level of disability, e.g., mild, and then progressed to moderate or severe disability during the course of conservative treatment. Ten patients died during follow-up, but only two deaths could be attributed to complications of CSM.

Lees and Turner concluded that CSM is a disease in which "long periods of nonprogressive disability are the rule, and a progressively deteriorating course is exceptional." They classified CSM as a relatively benign condition with good prognosis, although none of their patients, even those treated with cervical immobilization, were completely relieved of their disability. Only eight of 44 patients improved by one degree of disability. No information was provided as to how many patients progressed in degree of disability during follow-up. There was no correlation between age of onset and prognosis. Therefore, Lees and Turner described only the natural history of CSM after maximal neurologic deficit is reached. This period in the natural history is characterized by rare improvement and never by complete resolution of myelopathy.

Nurick's 1972 reports are often considered with others on the natural history of CSM.[25, 26] In reality, all Nurick's 91 patients received treatment for their myelopathy. Of the 91 patients in the study, only 37 received conservative therapy, average follow-up for these being 31 months. Of the 37 patients treated conservatively, 12 worsened and eight improved by at least one grade (Table 20–3). The remaining were either lost to follow-up or unchanged. Forty-five patients were treated with laminectomy, and although a larger percentage improved with this treatment, no statistical difference was found between conservative care and laminectomy. Nurick found age to be the major predictor of how well patients with CSM will do with any form of treatment. Radiologic findings of cord compression were correlated with severity of paraparesis at the time of admission, but were not found to have an effect on the subsequent course of the myelopathy. Nurick found, as did Lees and Turner, that CSM is a benign, nonprogressive condition. He also concluded that surgical treatment should be undertaken only in patients with progressive disability, especially those over 60 years old.

Table 20–3. NURICK CLASSIFICATION

Grade	
1	Signs of spinal cord disease but no difficulty in walking
2	Slight difficulty walking but does not prevent full-time employment
3	Difficulty in walking that prevents full-time employment or the ability to do all housework, but is not so severe as to require someone else's help to walk
4	Ability to walk only with someone else's help or with the aid of a frame
5	Chairbound or bedridden

From Phillips, D. G.: Surgical treatment of myelopathy with cervical spondylosis. J. Neurol. Neurosurg. Psychiatry *36:*879–884, 1973.

Symon and Lavender reported surgical treatment by laminectomy in 48 patients with proved CSM.[32] Their surgical results are discussed later in this chapter. They also reported on their patients' course before operation. Unlike the above-discussed authors, Symon and Lavender stated that 66 per cent of their patients had a progressive downhill course before surgery. This figure was less than 20 per cent for Clarke and Robinson, and only a few of Lees and Turner's patients gradually deteriorated over many years. Symon and Lavender's high estimate of the number of patients with progressive disability is unreliable as an indicator of natural history. These patients may have come to surgery before a plateau in their clinical course. The often-mentioned disparity between Symon and Lavender's patient population and that of other authors[21] may not exist, especially with the limited information and follow-up available.

Phillips in 1973 reported the results of 102 cases of CSM treated with collar, laminectomy, or anterior decompression with Cloward graft fusion.[28] Patient selection led to collar and anterior surgery treatment in the milder cases of CSM, laminectomy being performed in older patients with more severe disability. Collar treatment resulted in an improvement rate of 37 per cent. The length of time over which patients had reported symptomatology was correlated with the outcome of treatment. Collar therapy resulted in improvement in 54 per cent of those with a symptom duration of less than one year and 40 per cent of those with symptoms lasting one to two years; no patients improved with collar treatment when symptoms had been present for longer than two years.

The above reports are the most commonly reviewed literature for the natural history of CSM. A closer look and some mathematics reveals that we base our impression of the natural history of CSM on approximately 270 patients, over 200 of whom were described before 1970. No two studies in the group use the same classification of clinical disability to describe these patients, so there is no way to compare them accurately.

Although we are at a disadvantage in understanding with confidence the natural history of CSM, there is a distillate of common information. Age at presentation and duration of disease before treatment were shown to be important factors affecting prognosis. Increased age at presentation is associated with poorer results. If the symptoms of myelopathy have been present for more than one year, the chances of improvement are significantly reduced. Certainly these elements may be dependent on each other, and authors have only recently been able to estimate their relative importance.

Other common ground between these natural history reviews may suggest a relatively benign course for CSM, but this is not borne out by the information. Very few of the patients in these studies went on to reverse their myelopathy with conservative or no care. It is possible, as suggested by Clarke and Robinson, that subjectively reported improvement may actually be a plateau with lack of progression or the patient growing more able to live with the disability. In most patients the myelopathy seems to have a stepwise course with poorly defined periods of nonprogression between episodes of acute worsening. A minority of patients present with progression that continues onward to severe disability. The factors initiating progression are unknown. Hypotheses include moderate to severe acute trauma or possibly a type of microtrauma causing continual cord ischemia or mechanical damage. In any event, CSM cannot be considered a benign disease by today's standards of evaluation. It is true that not all CSM patients end up in a wheelchair, but it is also true that the vast majority have some continued disability, commonly in gait, motor strength, or hand function, if conservative treatment is selected. Caution and close observation should be the rule when conservative care of the myelopathic patient is chosen.

The alternative to conservative care obviously is surgery. Many procedures have been described in the treatment of CSM and are grouped into anterior and posterior approaches. Below we examine the results of posterior surgery, including laminectomy and laminaplasty.

Operative Treatment

Cervical Laminectomy

Symon and Lavender, as mentioned previously, described the surgical treatment of 48 cases of CSM.[32] The procedures all included laminectomy, with seven patients receiving durotomy. An additional seven underwent section of the dentate ligaments, and two had spondylotic bar resection from this posterior approach. The cases were classified in a fashion similar to that of Lees and Turner,[22] except that they were grouped at the time of admission for surgery and not at their worst clinical presentation (Table 20–4). A preponderance of severely disabled patients is represented owing to the selection process for surgery. Minimum follow-up was 12 months. Fifty-two per cent improved by one category, 18 per cent improved by two categories (total 70 per cent improvement), 25 per cent were unchanged, and 5 per cent worsened by one category. The greatest improvement was in patients with the most disability. One patient died perioperatively.

Table 20–4. SYMON AND LAVENDER CLASSIFICATION

Grade	
Mild	Same as Lees and Turner classification (Table 20–2)
Moderate	Same as Lees and Turner classification (Table 20–2)
Severe	Nonbedridden: cannot work but can get about indoors
Severe	Bedridden: confined to bed with substantial limb weakness or ataxia, unable to stand or walk unsupported

From Symon, L., and Lavender, P.: The surgical treatment of cervical spondylotic myelopathy. Neurology *17*:117–127, 1967.

As pointed out by Rogers, the dentate ligaments were thought by Kahn and others to hold the cord in an anterior position so that after laminectomy it was unable to shift posteriorly away from anterior impingement.[30] Many authors reported the results of durotomy and dentate ligament resection to decompress the myelopathic cord.[9, 13, 14, 32] Reid studied the relative motion of the cervical spine, dura, and cord in flexion extension movements and found that the cord did not move in relation to the dura.[29] He disproved the theory that mobilization of the dura without dentate ligament resection causes continued tethering of the cord anteriorly.

Rogers briefly reviewed thirty-three patients treated surgically for CSM.[30] He performed complete C1 to T1 laminectomy, durotomy, and dentate ligament resection. Rogers' maximal follow-up was six years and he reported encouraging results without specific findings. He cited the common occurrence of cervical spondylosis in association with congenital narrowing of the cervical canal producing myelopathy and believed that surgery should be performed at any sign of cord involvement in association with cervical spondylosis.

Jenkins[19] reported five patients with long-term follow-up from a group of patients first reported by Rogers.[30] Complete cervical laminectomy had been performed 12 to 17 years before Jenkins' review. All the patients were improved neurologically after surgery. This neural improvement accompanied by full mobility had been sustained without deterioration during the follow-up period. There was no deformity of the cervical spine due to laminectomy.

Gorter reported his patients with CSM who had received either a limited laminectomy or a complete laminectomy from C2 to T1 without durotomy.[13] He found no significant difference between these two procedures in terms of improvement of clinical status, but noted that younger patients improved more than older patients. It was also apparent that the shorter the history of symptoms, the better was the result of decompression. Gorter concluded that patients should be considered for surgery soon after symptoms of myelopathy appear if conservative therapy fails. If a limited area of cord compression is present, a limited laminectomy should be performed. Total laminectomy should be reserved for patients with evidence of widespread cervical cord compression. Gorter also felt that if there was no cerebrospinal fluid (CSF) block, anterior surgery was indicated rather than laminectomy.

In studying deformity and instability after laminectomy, Mikawa and colleagues found that in 64 patients who had undergone cervical laminectomy, 14 per cent showed deformity of the spine and 36 per cent demonstrated altered curvature from the preoperative type of curvature.[24] No neurologic findings could be attributed to this radiographic result. Deformity occurred only in patients with ossification of the posterior longitudinal ligament (OPLL), not in CSM patients. Studies also showed that severe deformity can occur in children undergoing cervical laminectomy.[1, 19, 23, 31, 38]

Epstein reviewed the surgical management of CSM by the posterior approach.[11] He noted that durotomy and dentate ligament resection have been minimized or eliminated from practice. In reporting an 80 to 85 per cent improvement and stabilization rate with laminectomy and foraminotomy, he addressed many points not well developed in earlier discussions of CSM. Epstein reiterated the need for adequate patient selection to ensure good surgical results. History and physical examination must be correlated with the proper radiologic studies to guarantee a confident diagnosis of CSM. The diagnosis of common similar disorders producing myelopathy must be eliminated. The presence of cervical spondylosis without concomitant development of cervical stenosis will most likely not produce a myelopathic picture, and therefore accurate measurements must be made of the preexisting sagittal canal diameter. The anatomic association of congenital anteroposterior canal narrowing has been shown to be almost a prerequisite for making the diagnosis of myelopathy due to cervical spondylosis.[12, 16, 27, 34] Epstein reminded us of the 10 per cent association of lumbar spinal stenosis and cervical spondylosis. The coexistence of lumbar stenosis must be considered in treatment planning. The presence of diabetes and alcoholism can add further neuropathy and myelopathy to the clinical picture. The risks of surgical complications of wound healing and infection are present in these patients. Epstein also pointed out the need for a stable neurologic picture preoperatively to avoid the often-associated poor surgical results.

Laminaplasty has generally been developed by the Japanese for treating OPLL but has also been used for patients with cervical spondylosis. Tsuji described this procedure in a group of patients, most of whom had OPLL.[33] Significant is his finding that leaving the posterior structures with laminaplasty led to a postoperative decrease in cervical range of motion; this was not accompanied by pain or cervical deformity. The lamina hinge may undergo fusion or in some other way limit motion. Other studies have shown an immediate loss of cervical extension with this procedure before spontaneous fusion.

The development of laminectomy and laminoplasty to treat CSM therefore raises some new considerations beyond those arising strictly from conservative care. The risks of laminectomy have to be considered during patient selection. Procedures such as durotomy, dentate ligament resection, and osteophyte removal from the posterior approach have for the most part been abandoned. There is significant risk of neurologic damage and poor clinical results with these additions to laminectomy. Postlaminectomy deformity, as noted above, has been well documented in skeletally immature individuals and OPLL patients. Range of motion in CSM patients after laminectomy has been shown to decrease, this phenomenon being even more apparent after laminaplasty.[33] Some studies documented reversal of cervical lordosis or subluxations less than 2 mm, but none reviewed here have documented worsening myelopathy postlaminectomy as a result of these curvature changes. As noted later in this chapter, some authors have reported neurologic deterioration after posterior surgery for CSM in long-term follow-up.

The results of laminectomy have not been universally good, but some patient groups have shown more improvement than others. The younger, less neurologically involved adult patient with a short duration of disease will reach the greatest level of improvement. This does not mean that surgery is hopeless in the older patient with severe neurologic impairment; such a patient may in fact improve a greater amount relative to the initial condition than less involved patients. As emphasized by Epstein, proper diagnosis of CSM and other diseases that may add to the myelopathy is crucial.[11]

Anterior Cervical Fusion

Multiple techniques are available for anterior decompression and fusion of the cervical spine. Although the approach is the same, fusion techniques include Cloward, Smith-Robinson, and corpectomy with strut grafting. As noted by Whitecloud in his review of anterior surgery for CSM, surgeon preference remains the guide in the choice of approach to decompression and fusion.[36] Bohlman reported 17 patients with CSM of Nurick Grade 3 or greater (see Table 20–3) treated by anterior cervical fusion with Smith-Robinson–type grafting without anterior decompression.[3] Sixteen of the 17 improved their degree of CSM by one or more Nurick grades; one patient with Grade 5 disability failed to improve; no loss of function was noted in any patient. One nonunion and one delayed union occurred without compromise of surgical result. One patient later required posterior decompression for continued posterior tract findings.

Zhang and colleagues reported 121 patients with CSM treated by anterior cervical discectomy and Smith-Robinson–type interbody fusion.[39] Surgery was indicated in patients who had failed conservative therapy, with evidence of blockage on myelography. Poor medical condition or advanced age contraindicated surgery. Pre- and postoperative function was graded by Okamato's scale, which is based mostly on gait. Most patients had three or more disc spaces fused. Autografts and allografts were used; 85 per cent of the autografts fused but only 50 per cent of the allografts. This is significant, since 80 per cent of the patients with bone union had good results whereas only 22 per cent of those with absorbed grafts had good results. Ninety per cent of the 121 patients were improved and 72 per cent resumed work. Unlike the outcome in other studies, severe myelopathy did not necessarily lead to a poor postoperative result, and therefore severe paralysis was not a contraindication to surgery. Only two patients required reoperation for failed anterior surgery. Removal of anterior osteophytes was not addressed. Preoperative duration of symptoms and age at onset was not examined in relationship to clinical results.

Anterior osteophytectomy has been a controversial point since the first anterior cervical fusions for spondylotic disease were performed. Inherent risks of manipulation of an already compromised cord became evident when some patients did not improve or worsened after anterior surgery. Many surgeons chose to simply clear the disc space and fuse the segments. This provides a stable environment, allowing remodeling and regression of the osteophytes. Other surgeons chose to remove these osteophytes, hoping for a better return of function. Kadoya and associates reported the use of an operating microscope, significantly reducing the risk of neural damage during osteophytectomy.[20] Using the Nurick grading system, these authors classified 43 myelopathic patients pre- and postoperatively: 91 per cent showed improvement and no patients worsened; 9 per cent remained unchanged. These results equal any reported for the surgical treatment of CSM. It is interesting that Kadoya and associates also reported a series of ten patients treated with anterior decompression without fusion of the interspaces. In six patients there was an immediate postoperative painful radiculopathy, presumably due to collapse of the intervertebral foramen. Avoiding this collapse is an advantage of inserting a bone graft for fusion. Improvement of the myelopathy was not influenced by fusion or nonfusion. Two patients had pseudarthrosis after attempted fusion. This was thought to contribute to a course of improvement with subsequent deterioration in one of these patients. Kadoya and associates concluded that anterior osteophyte removal was safe with the use of an operating microscope and that fusion with autologous bone was a necessary adjunct to the procedure.

Yang and colleagues reported 214 cases of anterior cervical fusion apparently without osteophyte removal as per the Smith-Robinson technique.[37] Their patients had an average of 3.1 levels fused. The nonunion rate of the grafts was 37 per cent, rather higher than in many other studies. Lack of radiographic union did not affect the clinical results of surgery. Nearly 90 per cent of all patients showed some improvement. Results were dependent on the duration of symptoms.

More recently, surgeons have begun approaching the spondylotic cervical spine with anterior vertebral body resection, osteophyte removal, and strut graft fusion. This procedure allows complete removal of anterior cord impingement and creation of a stable spine. Advantages over Smith-Robinson type of grafting are easier osteophyte resection and possibly lessened risk of neurologic damage. Subtotal somatectomy, as described by Boni and associates, involves removal of a gutter of contiguous vertebral bodies approximately 15 mm wide at a depth to the posterior longitudinal ligament.[4] An iliac crest tricortical graft, or a graft from another donor site, is placed as a strut by keying it into the superior and inferior unresected vertebral bodies. Boni and associates reported 29 CSM patients who had a follow-up of six months to 13 years after having undergone subtotal somatectomy. Cases were classified postoperatively as good, moderate, or poor on the basis of motor strength, gait, and patient satisfaction. Of these 29 patients, 51 per cent were classified as good, 47 per cent as moderate, and 2 per cent as poor; therefore, over 90 per cent were improved. There were no nonunions, but in long-term follow-up the mobile segments above and below the fusion were found to degenerate or become hypermobile. There were no symptoms related to these adjacent level findings. Similar adjacent level changes would be expected with any fusion technique.

Hanai and colleagues reported 30 CSM patients who underwent the same operation as that of Boni.[15] Follow-up averaged three years. Pre- and postoperative clinical grading was performed according to the Japanese Orthopaedic Association (JOA) score (Table 20–5). All patients improved without deterioration during follow-up. The mean preoperative JOA score was 8.9 and mean postoperative score 13.9. No statistical analysis was performed. Postoperative range of motion of the cervical spine was decreased by one third to one half of preoperative range. No patients reported cervical pain after fusion, no pseudarthrosis was noted, and no adjacent level degeneration was found.

Bernard and Whitecloud reported 21 patients with CSM treated with subtotal vertebrectomy and fusion with autogenous fibula strut grafting.[2] Follow-up averaged 32 months. Sixteen of 21 patients improved in terms of the Nurick grading system, three were unimproved, and two improved but later deteriorated. There were no nonunions of the grafts and one graft dislodged postoperatively. Patients with symptoms of less than one year's duration and preoperative Nurick grades 1, 2, or 3 showed the most improvement. Higher-grade disability and long-term disability were associated with a poorer outcome. Surgical treatment in these severely affected patients should be undertaken with realistic expectations of disease arrest rather than reversal. Bernard and Whitecloud considered fibula to be a better source of donor material than iliac crest because of equal fusion rate and superior biomechanical properties.

Table 20–5. JAPANESE ORTHOPAEDIC ASSOCIATION CLASSIFICATION

	Grade
I. Motor Function: Arms	
Unable to feed oneself with chopsticks or a spoon	0
Able to feed oneself with a spoon but not with chopsticks	1
Able to use chopsticks	2
Slightly clumsy in using chopsticks	3
Normal	4
II. Motor Function: Legs	
Unable to walk by any means	0
Unable to walk without a cane or other support on the level	1
Able to walk independently on the level but needs support on stairs	2
Slightly clumsy in walking	3
Normal	4
III. Sensation	
Arms: definitely impaired	0
slightly impaired or subjectively numb	1
normal	2
Trunk: 0 to 2 as above	
Legs: 0 to 2 as above	
IV. Bladder Function	
Incontinent	0
Great difficulty	1
Slight difficulty	2
Normal	3
Total for Normal Patient	*17*

From Hukuda, S., Mochizuki, T., Ogata, M., et al.: Operations for cervical spondylotic myelopathy. A comparison of the results of anterior and posterior procedures. J. Bone Joint Surg. *67B*:609–615, 1985.

The advent of anterior surgery has probably raised even more questions and considerations than posterior surgery. Removal of the anterior osteophytes through the anterior approach has many proponents. Some feel that the osteophytes will remodel and waste away when the motion segment is stabilized. This has been shown to occur, but the clinical significance of this phenomenon in relation to the risk of osteophyte removal has not been determined. Current authors continue to avoid osteophyte removal and simply clear the disc space, while others have added osteophyte removal to the standard Smith-Robinson procedure. The more bone resected to perform the procedure, the easier it is to resect the osteophytes safely. However, there is a point at which so much bone is resected that the bed for graft placement is compromised. This leads to an increased rate of kyphosis and possibly nonunion. If the vertebral end plate is removed as in the Cloward procedure structural stability is lost, possibly leading to kyphosis at healing. The nonunion rate of the grafts is directly proportional to the number of levels fused. When three or more levels are fused anteriorly, the nonunion rate may jump from less than 10 to over 30 per cent. The use of a postoperative halo-vest may increase the union rate but may also be inappropriate in some CSM patients. Some authors have correlated graft nonunion not only with deformity of the spine but also with neurologic sequelae. It would seem that in severely involved elderly patients with multilevel disease, the risks of managing them in a halo and being forced to use poor-quality donor site bone graft would outweigh the advantages of anterior surgery. Although allograft is a possible donor source, most studies that have described the use of allograft bone for fusions in the cervical spine have shown a higher nonunion rate. However, in patients without increased risk of graft nonunion, such as younger adults with less than three-level involvement, anterior cervical fusion offers a reliable prognosis for excellent recovery. Younger adults with more extensive disease may also be appropriately managed with anterior cervical fusion, possibly incorporating a halo. Subtotal vertebrectomy is still under investigation. Recent studies have reported little or no nonunions with both iliac crest and fibular grafts. Even so, the removal of such a large amount of anterior support is more destabilizing than any other anterior procedure. If the long strut graft fails to heal, disaster could result. We must wait for more studies with longer follow-up before this approach to relieving CSM is wholeheartedly adopted.

An additional consideration with anterior fusion is adjacent level deterioration. As in deformity after laminectomy, adjacent unfused level deterioration has not yet been shown to have neurologic sequelae. It can easily be postulated that in CSM patients with congenital stenosis, deterioration of the levels adjacent to the fused segments will lead to myelopathy when followed over the long term. Hypermobility as a compensatory response to the fused segment may eventually lead to enough spondylosis to become clinically significant.

It can be seen that anterior cervical fusion, although shown to be efficacious in the treatment of CSM, involves many important considerations. Some patients may not be good candidates for this type of surgery. It will require comparative studies to try to determine which patients should be selected for a certain type of treatment.

Comparative Studies

Many studies compare the results of posterior and anterior surgery in the treatment of CSM. Phillips graded his patients' clinical status before and after surgical treatment using Nurick's classification.[28] Laminectomy in 24 patients resulted in improvement in 38 per cent, no change in 38 per cent, and worsening in 24 per cent. Patients whose symptoms had lasted less than one year showed 67 per cent improvement; duration of one to two years showed 25 per cent improvement and longer than two years 20 per cent improvement. Sixty-five patients underwent anterior cervical decompression and fusion with the Cloward technique; 57 per cent improved in clinical grade, 29 per cent were unchanged, and 14 per cent worsened. Duration of symptoms also affected the clinical results in patients receiving the Cloward operation. Of those with symptom duration of less than one year, 86 per cent were improved; 85 per cent with symptoms for one to two years were improved; and 33 per cent of those with symptoms lasting longer than two years were improved. Follow-up was a minimum of two years. Phillips concluded that the anterior approach with thorough decompression and Cloward interbody fusion was superior to laminectomy or conservative management, and furthermore that laminectomy should be reserved for patients with narrow canals and multiple constrictions. He also pointed out that the longer the duration of symptoms preoperatively, the worse are the results of surgery. Phillips believed that undue persistence of conservative management in patients with more than very mild myelopathy ran the risk of a poor result.

Many variations on the laminectomy theme have been studied, including laminectomy with durotomy, dentate ligament resection, osteophyte resection, and limited or partial foraminotomies. Gorter reviewed the literature in 1976, comparing results of anterior fusion versus total laminectomy versus laminectomy with durotomy and dentate ligament division.[13] Anterior surgery gave the overall best results, with 33.4 per cent of patients cured, 40 per cent improved, 18.7 per cent unchanged, and 6.9 per cent worsened. Total laminectomy averaged 17.2 per cent cured, 53.1 per cent improved, 18.2 per cent unchanged, and 7.5 per cent worsened. The more extensive laminectomy, durotomy, and dentate ligament resection resulted in the worst results with 10.4 per cent cured, 47.4 per cent improved, 22.7 per cent unchanged, and 14.8 per cent worsened. Gorter also reviewed conservative treatment: no patients were cured without surgery, 49.3 per cent improved, 35.9 per cent remained the same, and 14.8 per cent worsened.

Guidetti and Fortuna studied the variations of laminectomy and how these fared against anterior cervical fusion with osteophyte resection.[14] They found the anterior approach to provide better improvement, with 51 per cent good or very good results and 31 per cent fair results. This compared favorably with laminectomy and variations of laminectomy, the best results of which were found in laminectomy and foraminotomy, with 42 per cent good or very good and 36 per cent fair results. Additional surgery beyond laminectomy, such as dentate ligament resection, osteophyte resection, and extended laminectomy from C1 to T1, all yielded lesser results. This may be due to more severe myelopathy in the patients with these extensive operations. Guidetti and Fortuna also found the disease duration to markedly affect the result of surgery. Patients with disease for less than six months had 51 per cent good or very good results. Patients with greater than 12 months' duration of symptoms had 16 per cent good or very good results. Age was also found to correlate with success: the older the patient, the worse the results. The authors also mentioned that these two factors were in effect at the same time in that older patients with short duration of disease had better results than older patients with longer disease duration (38 per cent versus 12 per cent good or very good results). In addition to these two coexistent factors, Guidetti and Fortuna found the preexisting severity of disease to be of prognostic value: the worse the patient's condition at the time of surgery, the less likely was that patient to have a good result. The conclusion when all the factors are measured in terms of results is "that age and the severity of the clinical syndrome are less important factors than the duration of the disease and the type of operation performed; it means that an appropriate operation performed at an early stage can yield an excellent result even in an elderly patient with severe cord damage."[14] Guidetti and Fortuna concluded that in diffuse spondylosis with narrowing of the canal, extended laminectomy with or without foraminotomy is indicated. In patients with disease over fewer levels (one or two), anterior osteophyte resection and fusion are appropriate.

Crandall and Gregorius compared 55 patients, 26 treated with anterior cervical fusion and 29 treated with laminectomy and additional dural grafting.[9] On long-term follow-up, these authors found a tendency toward improvement in the anterior cervical fusion patients and a tendency toward late deterioration in patients treated with laminectomy. Early results were similar in both groups. This late worsening in laminectomy patients occurred as long after surgery as eight years after a plateau had been reached. Again, preoperative duration of symptoms for longer than 12 months was correlated with a poorer outcome. Preoperative sphincter disturbance was similarly associated with poor clinical outcome. Long-term deterioration was found to be associated with pseudomeningocele formation, retained arch of C3, and degeneration of a disc space adjacent to a fused level. The causes of late deterioration in laminectomy patients could be avoided by removing all levels involved in the disease process and avoiding intentional durotomy. Therefore, this study should not be used as evidence of long-term failure of laminectomy in the treatment of CSM.

In 1985 Hukuda and colleagues published the results of six different operations, three posterior and three anterior.[18] In 191 CSM patients there were 151 anterior, 25 posterior, and 15 combined procedures. The patients' clinical syndromes were categorized as per Crandall and Batzdorf's classification system, which places patients into one of five categories: transverse lesions, motor syndrome, central cord syndrome, brachialgia, and Brown-Séquard syndrome.[8] The patients were categorized pre- and postoperatively. The JOA clinical grading scale was also used (Table 20–5). The anterior operations performed included the Cloward, Smith-Robinson, and subtotal vertebrectomy procedures. The posterior operations included laminectomy, french-window laminaplasty, and french-window laminectomy. The french-window procedures differ from standard posterior procedures in that the posterior structures are split down the midline instead of bilaterally at the lamina-lateral mass junction. Although a small number of posterior procedures were performed, the authors do discuss the considerations for procedure selection. Radiologic findings were the major factors in determining the surgical approach. When myelography showed one- or two-level involvement, the Cloward or Smith-Robinson procedures were performed. Subtotal spondylectomy was performed when two or three levels were involved and there was an associated narrow canal. When three or more levels were involved and there was no gross instability, one of the posterior approaches was selected. Through this selection and classification process, patients tended to be grouped as follows: (1) anterior procedures were usually performed in patients with a milder clinical grade (JOA) of brachialgia or central cord and (2) posterior procedures were commonly performed in patients with severe clinical grade (JOA) and transverse lesions. Therefore the posterior procedures were performed in patients with severe myelopathy, and the anterior procedures in those with milder myelopathy. Patients were followed for one to 12 years.

Remarkably, Hukuda and colleagues found that the posterior procedures returned the patients with severe myelopathy to a level equal to that in the anterior procedures performed in the milder myelopathy patients. No one anterior procedure was shown to work better than the others. The same was true for the three posterior procedures. Degree of preoperative disability, age, and preoperative duration of symptoms were again shown to affect the final results. Recurrence of symptoms was found in 5 per cent of the anterior and 10.5 per cent of the posterior procedures. Reasons for recurrence of myelopathy included post-laminectomy instability, degeneration of adjacent levels in fusion patients, and failure to perform posterior procedures in high-grade developmental stenosis. The authors concluded that operative selection is a major factor in determining success. They thought that disease limited to one or two levels should be approached anteriorly, and more extensive disease posteriorly. No one anterior or posterior procedure was significantly more successful, and the authors currently use laminaplasty and Smith-Robinson techniques. The type, severity, and duration of myelopathy were the most important preoperative associated factors in determining final outcome. The authors felt that operative intervention should not be withheld in elderly patients and should not be delayed after conservative treatment has failed.

Herkowitz retrospectively reviewed a series of 45 patients with radicular symptoms due to cervical spondylosis who received one of three procedures: anterior cervical fusion, laminaplasty, or laminectomy.[17] The presence of myelopathy was not addressed. Nonetheless, Herkowitz points out many interesting findings: good to excellent results in 92 per cent of the anterior cervical fusion group, 86 per cent of the laminaplasty group, and only 66 per cent of the laminectomy group. The anterior cervical fusion patients did not undergo osteophyte resection. The patients also had at least three levels of clinical involvement. The nonunion rate for the anterior cervical fusion group was 37 per cent. Although this is a large number of nonhealing grafts, Herkowitz found at a minimum of two years' follow-up that the presence of a nonunion was not related to a lesser clinical result. The literature reports mixed results as far as a correlation between nonunion and clinical results in anterior cervical fusion patients. Herkowitz pointed out that Connolly and associates[7] and White and associates[35] both reported increased nonunion with greater levels of fusion. White and associates reported lesser results with more levels and greater nonunion rate. DePalma and colleagues found no relationship of clinical results to the nonunion rate.[10] Herkowitz also reported that three patients who received laminectomy developed cervical kyphosis eight to 24 months after surgery. This has been a rare occurrence so far in older patients with cervical spondylotic disease. Possibly a more aggressive foraminotomy was performed in this group of patients with radicular symptoms than is commonly performed in patients with myelopathy. This may have led to greater postoperative instability. Herkowitz concluded that anterior cervical fusion was the procedure of choice for multiple-level cervical radiculopathy Laminaplasty should be used in patients with congenital canal narrowing or in whom anterior surgery has failed. Laminectomy should be employed for failed laminaplasty patients or those with bony ankylosis due to other disease processes.

Caution should be exercised in considering these comparative studies. None are prospective randomized in format. They each represent combined retrospective reviews of the different types of procedures that happen to have been performed at the same institution. Only Hukuda and colleagues acknowledged this fact, concluding that patient selection for a particular procedure determines the successful outcome and resolution of the myelopathy. Anterior surgery resulted in better improvement in all the studies, but the lack of sufficient clinical grading and randomization significantly dim the light on these comparisons. Significant factors relating to quality of outcome can be identified from these studies, including age at onset, duration of disease before surgery, and severity and type of myelopathy. Possibly, as pointed out by Guidetti and Fortuna, duration of disease and operative approach are the most important predictive factors.

Surgical Indications

The determination of indications for surgery in CSM is based on the disease's natural history and the results of surgical treatment. The significant papers on the natural history have been reviewed but do not provide a clear view. The hope of obtaining additional natural history data is remote, considering the relatively aggressive nature of the modern approach to this disease process. In general, it can be stated that CSM is an intermittently progressive disease process without significant chance of reversal without treatment. Conservative therapy rarely resolves the myelopathy. Once patients have presented with the signs and symptoms of CSM, most have some degree of permanent disability and many progress at some time. The nature of this progression has been poorly described in the literature. Because postoperative progression is rare with modern techniques, and the natural history is characterized by intermittent progression, surgery is indicated in any patient who shows progression of the myelopathy There is a low chance of symptom resolution with conservative treatment, and therefore any patient with moderate or severe myelopathy is a candidate for surgery. A patient with mild signs of myelopathy but with unacceptable compromise of the activities of daily living is also a good candidate for decompressive surgery. Advanced age and symptom severity are prognostic indicators of a poor outcome but not contradications to surgery. Certainly an older patient with mild to moderate CSM will benefit from surgery. The patient with severe disability from CSM has more to gain from surgery than the patient with relatively mild disease. Duration of disease is perhaps a relative contraindication to decompressive surgery in that patients with more than one year of symptomatology have a markedly poorer postoperative outcome. Surgery in the severely involved patient should not be withheld for this reason, but the prognosis should be understood by both surgeon and patient. The importance of the duration of disease bespeaks the need for early surgical treatment of the myelopathic patient.

Surgical results continue to improve. Both posterior and anterior surgery have been reported to lead to marked improvement in the myelopathy associated with cervical spondylosis. In the absence of prospective randomized trials comparing these two approaches, we cannot definitively state the preferred choice of surgical treatment. Posterior surgery has shown promising results in cases in which anterior surgery has a high risk of a poorer outcome. In patients with multilevel involvement, i.e., greater than three levels of cord compression, cervical laminectomy may be the procedure of choice. Elderly patients with poor bone quality, especially considering the bone graft donor site, may also have a better outcome with posterior surgery. In the younger patient with fewer levels of involvement, anterior surgery can be predictably and safely performed.

There are many variations to the anterior and posterior approaches. Durotomy, dentate ligament resection, and osteophyte removal have not been shown to improve the results of posterior surgery. Laminectomy and laminaplasty have demonstrated equal results overall. Laminectomy with foraminotomy for myelopathy with radiculopathy is a proved adjunct to posterior surgery. The possibility of posterior surgery with additional facet joint fusion with or without instrumentation has not been evaluated in this group of patients. This may eliminate some of the common complaints of postoperative deformity and instability associated with posterior surgery.

Osteophyte resection has been performed safely for anterior cervical fusion. This provides immediate cord decompression, especially when the height of the disc space can be reconstituted with an appropriate anterior graft. Some authors continue to avoid the possibility of cord damage by not removing the osteophytes, providing stabilization of the interspace in the expectation that the osteophytes will resolve. The Smith-Robinson type of iliac crest graft is presently the most widely used fusion technique. Some continue to use the Cloward graft, citing the advantage of more accessibility for osteophyte removal. The anterior subtotal vertebrectomy with strut grafting continues to be evaluated to determine the proper indications for its use.

The future holds the greatest challenge for physicians treating this interesting disease process. A standard for comparison of patients and treatment modalities in the form of a universal grading scale for CSM would perhaps advance our knowledge the most. Prospective randomized trials will be the only method by which many controversies can be settled.

References

1. Arima, T.: Changes in the cervical spine after laminectomy. Brain Nerve Injury *1*:17–78, 1969.
2. Bernard, T. N., and Whitecloud, T. S.: Cervical spondylotic myelopathy and myeloradiculopathy anterior decompression and stabilization with autogenous fibula strut graft. *221*:149–160, 1987.
3. Bohlman, H. H.: Cervical spondylosis with moderate to severe myelopathy: a report of seventeen cases treated by Robinson anterior cervical discectomy and fusion. Spine *2*:151–162, 1977.
4. Boni, M., Cherubino, P., Denaro, V., and Benazzo, F.: Multiple subtotal somatectomy technique and evaluation of a series of 38 cases. Spine *9*:358–362, 1984.
5. Clarke, E., and Robinson, P. K.: Cervical myelopathy. A complication of cervical spondylosis. Brain *79*:483–510, 1956.
6. Concha, S., and McQueen, J. D.: Anterior cervical fusions for spondylotic myelopathy: a preliminary report. Spine *2*:147–151, 1977.
7. Connolly, E. S., Seymour, R. J., and Adams, J. E.: Clinical evaluation of anterior cervical fusion for degenerative disc disease. J. Neurosurg. *23*:431–437, 1965.
8. Crandall, P. H., and Batzdorf, U.: Cervical spondylotic myelopathy. J. Neurosurg. *25*:57–66, 1966.
9. Crandall, P. H., and Gregorius, F. K.: Long-term followup of surgical treatment of cervical spondylotic myelopathy. Spine *2*:139–146, 1977.
10. DePalma, A. F., Rothman, R. H., Lewinnek, G. E., et al.: Anterior interbody fusion for severe cervical disc degeneration. Surg. Gynecol. Obstet. *134*:755–758, 1972.
11. Epstein, J. A.: The surgical management of cervical spinal stenosis, spondylosis, and myeloradiculopathy by means of the posterior approach. Spine *13*:864–869, 1988.

12. Fujiwara, K., Yonenobu, K., Hiroshima, K., et al.: Morphometry of the cervical spinal cord and its relation to pathology in cases with compression myelopathy. Spine *13*:1212–1216, 1988.
13. Gorter, K.: Influence of laminectomy on the course of cervical myelopathy. Acta Neurochir. *33*:265–281, 1976.
14. Guidetti, B., and Fortuna, A.: Long-term results of surgical treatment of myelopathy due to cervical spondylosis. J. Neurosurg. *30*:714–721, 1969.
15. Hanai, K., Fujiyoshi, F., and Kamei, K.: Subtotal vertebrectomy and spinal fusion for cervical spondylotic myelopathy. Spine *11*:310–315, 1986.
16. Hayashi, H., Okada, K., Hashimoto, J., et al.: Cervical spondylotic myelopathy in the aged patient. A radiologic evaluation of the aging changes in the cervical spine and etiologic factors of myelopathy. Spine *13*:618–625, 1988.
17. Herkowitz, H. N.: A comparison of anterior cervical fusion, cervical laminectomy, and cervical laminoplasty for the surgical management of multiple level spondylotic radiculopathy. Spine *13*:774–780, 1988.
18. Hukuda, S., Mochizuki, T., Ogata, M., et al.: Operations for cervical spondylotic myelopathy. A comparison of the results of anterior and posterior procedures. J. Bone Joint Surg. *67B*:609–615, 1985.
19. Jenkins, D. H. R.: Extensive cervical laminectomy: long-term results. Br. J. Surg. *60*:852–854, 1973.
20. Kadoya, S., Nakamura, T., and Kwak, R.: A microsurgical anterior osteophytectomy for cervical spondylotic myelopathy. Spine *9*:437–441, 1984.
21. Larocca, H.: Cervical spondylotic myelopathy: natural history. Spine *13*:854–855, 1988.
22. Lees, F., and Turner, J. W. A.: Natural history and prognosis of cervical spondylosis. Br. Med. J. *2*:1607–1610, 1963.
23. Lonstein, J. E.: Post-laminectomy kyphosis. Clin. Orthop. *128*:93–100, 1977.
24. Mikawa, Y., Shikata, J., and Yamamuro, T.: Spinal deformity and instability after multilevel cervical laminectomy. Spine *12*:6–11, 1987.
25. Nurick, S.: The pathogenesis of the spinal cord disorder associated with cervical spondylosis. Brain *96*:87–100, 1972.
26. Nurick, S.: The natural history and the results of surgical treatment of the spinal cord disorder associated with cervical spondylosis. Brain *95*:101–108, 1972.
27. Ogino, H., Tada, K., Okada, K., et al.: Canal diameter, anteroposterior compression ratio, and spondylotic myelopathy of the cervical spine. Spine *8*:1–15, 1983.
28. Phillips, D. G.: Surgical treatment of myelopathy with cervical spondylosis. J. Neurol. Neurosurg. Psychiatry *36*:879–884, 1973.
29. Reid, J. D.: Effects of flexion-extension movements of the head and spine upon the spinal cord and nerve roots. J. Neurol. Neurosurg. Psychiatry *23*:214–221, 1960.
30. Rogers, L.: The surgical treatment of cervical spondylotic myelopathy. J. Bone Joint Surg. *43*:3–6, 1961.
31. Sim, F. H., Svien, H. J., and Bickell, W. H.: Swan-neck deformity following extensive cervical laminectomy. J. Bone Joint Surg. *56A*:564–580, 1974.
32. Symon, L., and Lavender, P.: The surgical treatment of cervical spondylotic myelopathy. Neurology *17*:117–127, 1967.
33. Tsuji, H.: Laminoplasty for patients with compressive myelopathy due to so-called spinal canal stenosis in cervical and thoracic regions. Spine *7*:28–34, 1982.
34. Veidlinger, O. F., Colwill, J. C., Smyth, H. S., and Turner, D.: Cervical myelopathy and its relationship to cervical stenosis. Spine *6*:550–552, 1981.
35. White, A., Southwick, W., DePonte, R., et al.: Relief of pain by anterior cervical spine fusion for spondylosis. J. Bone Joint Surg. *55A*:525–534, 1973.
36. Whitecloud, T. S.: Anterior surgery for cervical spondylotic myelopathy: Smith-Robinson, Cloward, and vertebrectomy. Spine *13*:861–863, 1988.
37. Yang, K. C., Lu, X. S., Cai, Q. L., et al.: Cervical spondylotic myelopathy treated by anterior multilevel decompression and fusion. Clin. Orthop. *221*:161–164, 1987.
38. Yasuoka, S., Peterson, H. A., and MacCarty, C. S.: Incidence of spinal column deformity after multilevel laminectomy in children and adults. J. Neurosurg. *57*:441–445, 1982.
39. Zhang, Z. H., Yin, H., Yang, K., et al.: Anterior intervertebral disc excision and bone grafting in cervical spondylotic myelopathy. Spine *8*:16–19, 1983.

SURGICAL MANAGEMENT OF CERVICAL MYELOPATHY: LAMINECTOMY

Frederick A. Simeone, M.D.
William H. Dillin, M.D.

The space available for the spinal cord can be increased by cervical laminectomy. This technique is the definitive treatment for disorders that compress the spinal cord posteriorly, such as thickened laminae or a congenitally small spinal canal. Laminectomy is frequently used to decompress the spinal cord when the source of compression is anteriorly placed. Ideally, the source of compression in such instances should be excised through an anterior approach. Sometimes, however, an extensive anterior operation is inordinately complicated, and cervical laminectomy can be an alternative. In extensive ossification of the posterior longitudinal ligament, ideal treatment involves removal of the ligament and anterior decompression of the cord. This, however, may involve resection of several cervical vertebral bodies, and then removal of the ligament itself, which may be adherent to the surrounding dura. If patients undergo this procedure without complications, they are faced with a long interval of disability and inconvenience in a halo apparatus while fusion of the graft and vertebral body replacement develops. Consequently, in parts of the world where symptomatic posterior longitudinal ligament disease is common, there has been a gradual return to cervical laminectomy as the treatment of choice.[8]

Generally speaking, single-level, anteriorly placed lesions about the intervertebral disc that compress the spinal cord should be removed anteriorly. Multilevel cervical disc disorders may be treated with laminectomy, even though better anatomic decompression can be effected anteriorly. The question revolves about the relative morbidity of, e.g., a four-level anterior disc excision and fusion, compared with the much less traumatic four-level cervical laminectomy.

This discussion continues elsewhere. The purpose of this section is to discuss the authors' surgical technique for the performance of multilevel laminectomy. The author favors laminaplasty in certain instances, but the specific technique of laminoplasty is discussed in another chapter.

ANESTHETIC TECHNIQUES

Patients who have spinal cord compression secondary to cervical disc degeneration, and therefore are undergoing cervical laminectomy, must be considered at risk for any inordinate neck hyperextension. It is known that under the effects of neuromuscular blocking agents and general anesthesia, the neck can be hyperextended to a greater degree than can be achieved voluntarily. It is possible during induction to hyperextend the neck and produce spinal cord compression in the face of a "tight" spinal canal. Consequently, the authors insist on fiberoptic intubation in an awake patient whose neurologic status after the tube is in place can be rechecked before final positioning.

INTRAOPERATIVE NEUROPHYSIOLOGIC MONITORING

The authors have not as yet made a definitive decision regarding their role of intraoperative monitoring in patients undergoing cervical laminectomy for spinal cord compression. At the time of this writing, all patients with spinal cord compression are monitored throughout the operation by continuous sensory evoked response measurement. Stimulating points are usually on the posterior tibial, median, or ulnar nerves. Recording points are from the upper cervical spine and scalp representation of the sensory cerebral cortex. Patients are also monitored preoperatively. From an anatomic viewpoint this technique measures conduction in the posterior columns of the spinal cord. During the operation, one frequently sees an improvement in response amplitude and latency after the laminae are removed. It is rare, however, to see a degradation of these parameters that can be explained in an intraoperative event. During the past few years in which we have used this monitoring routinely, we have rarely had to alter the operative procedure because of change in the sensory evoked response. This has led us to question the actual value of this monitoring technique and its associated expenses. It would appear that motor evoked response monitoring may be a more efficient way of determining subtle changes in spinal cord compression. So far, however, a practical method for measuring motor evoked responses in an operating room setting has not evolved at Pennsylvania Hospital, although the technique is being developed elsewhere.

POSITIONING

The patient is positioned in a face-down, semikneeling position with the chin moderately flexed. When the chin is flexed at 45 degrees, for example, the posterior aspect of the neck can be parallel to the ground, and the body, from the shoulders down, is angulated so as to reduce venous pressure in the cervical spine. At the time of surgery there is a significant lack of venous engorgement, yet the veins do bleed, and air embolus has never been a consideration in or complication of this procedure. We believe this method of positioning to be far superior to sitting the patient up because of the absence of air embolism, the greater control of blood pressure, and the ability to alter the tilt of the table during the operation, depending on the needs of the operating surgeon or the patient's cardiovascular status.

SURGICAL TECHNIQUE

Once the posterior aspect of the neck has been properly prepared, the spinous processes are exposed, and when there is a multilevel cervical laminectomy it is usually possible to feel the second cervical vertebra and thereby appropriately count the spinous processes with the aid of preoperative radiographs of the cervical spine. If there is any doubt, intraoperative radiographs should be taken. At this point the surgeon may wish to remove the spinous processes of the lamina to be excised, although if he is not certain whether he wishes to perform an open-door laminaplasty, they should be kept intact. Some surgeons find it easier to manipulate the cervical lamina with the spinous processes removed.

Drilling is begun with a 3.0-mm round cutting burr. Some surgeons prefer a diamond burr, although this can generate significant heat and may actually be more dangerous than the sharper-cutting, more aggressive 3.0-m round cutting burr. The drilling procedure is performed with constant irrigation. The surgeon must wear magnifying loupes to allow him to visualize the inner cortex, which is generally the stopping point of the drilling procedure.

Two troughs are drilled, beginning with the lower lamina to be excised and extending upward. The exact drill site may be difficult to determine by ordinary visual landmarks. The lamina ordinarily widens slightly as it forms the superior portion of the facet joint. An ideal cervical laminectomy should be carried out just lateral to the dural margin so that most of the drilling and rongeuring procedure is over the lateral CSF-containing space of the spinal canal (Figs. 20–15, 20–16).

As the drilling progresses from lamina to lamina, the surgeon becomes more confident of drilling through the outer cortex, through cancellous bone, but does not drill through the inner cortex of the lamina. Very often, the

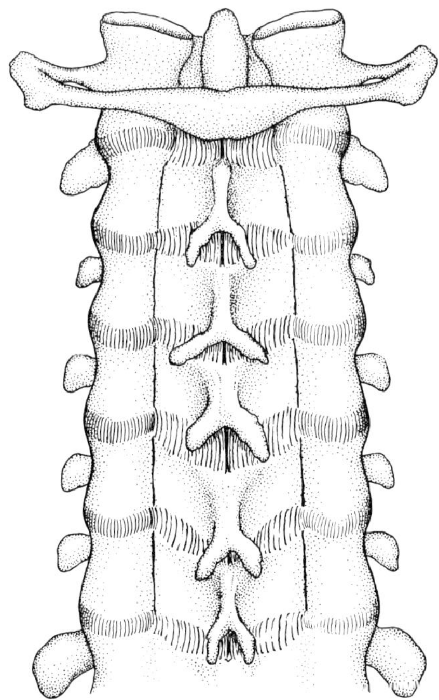

Figure 20–15. Operative view of the cervical spine. The vertical line on each side of the laminae indicates the drilling paths for creation of the troughs.

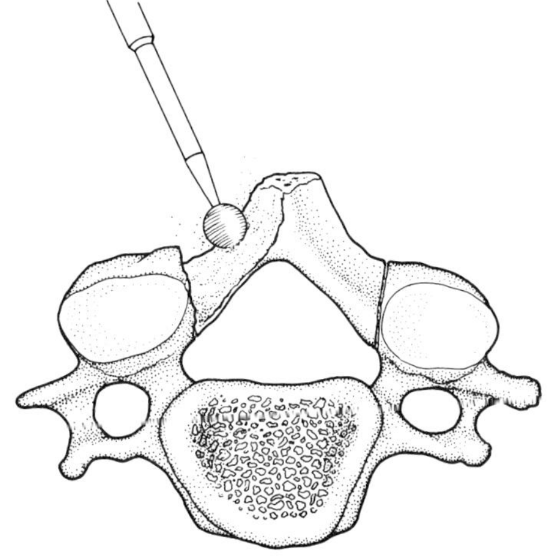

Figure 20–16. The vertical line on the laminae on the right shows the location of the trough. This lies just medial to the facet joint. On the left the laminae are being thinned by the cutting burr. This maneuver ordinarily is not necessary unless the laminae are too thick to perform the procedure safely as described.

ligamentum flavum is exposed, indicating that the surgeon has gone through the ventral cortex of the lamina. Too aggressive drilling at this point can cause a dural tear, but because the drilling is lateral to the spinal cord, damage to that structure is not likely. Posteriorly deviated nerve roots may be in the path of the drill, so care must be taken at this point in the procedure. On two occasions, when the dura has been entered over a nerve root, in the author's experience (FAS) the patient has only noted some numbness and never a motor deficit, apparently because the dorsal root is closest to the dura and therefore most vulnerable.

After both troughs are drilled, the thinned lamina is now delicate enough to be excised with the smallest (1-mm) Spurling-Kerrison rongeur. This instrument will carry the trough through the inner table of the lamina and remove the ligamentum flavum as well. When the two troughs have been completed, the ligamentum flavum attaching the block of lamina to be removed must also be excised. With a towel clip, the loose spinous process is lifted away from the dura, and the remaining ligamentum flavum is cut with a curved No. 12 scalpel blade or with fine scissors. When this is completed, it is possible to remove the block of excised vertebrae, still attached by the ligamentum flavum (Fig. 20–17). When the procedure is properly carried out, the lateral margins of the dura are visible but the facet joints are left intact (Fig. 20–18). Meticulous hemostasis must be achieved because there may be bleeding from the lateral epidural veins, which is managed readily with bipolar cautery.

As discussed in another chapter, this can be carried out on one side and then hinged on the other side, rather than rongeured through the other trough, so that an open-door laminaplasty can be made. In our experience, however, postoperative instability does not occur in adults whose preoperative radiographs did not demonstrate subluxation. Mikawa and associates in 64 patients who had undergone multilevel cervical laminectomy made extensive evaluation of spinal deformity and stability.[5] They reported that no adult patient required further operation for spinal deformity or instability. They did have two patients under 20 years of age who developed significant spinal deformity, and this procedure therefore is not recommended for juveniles. This con-

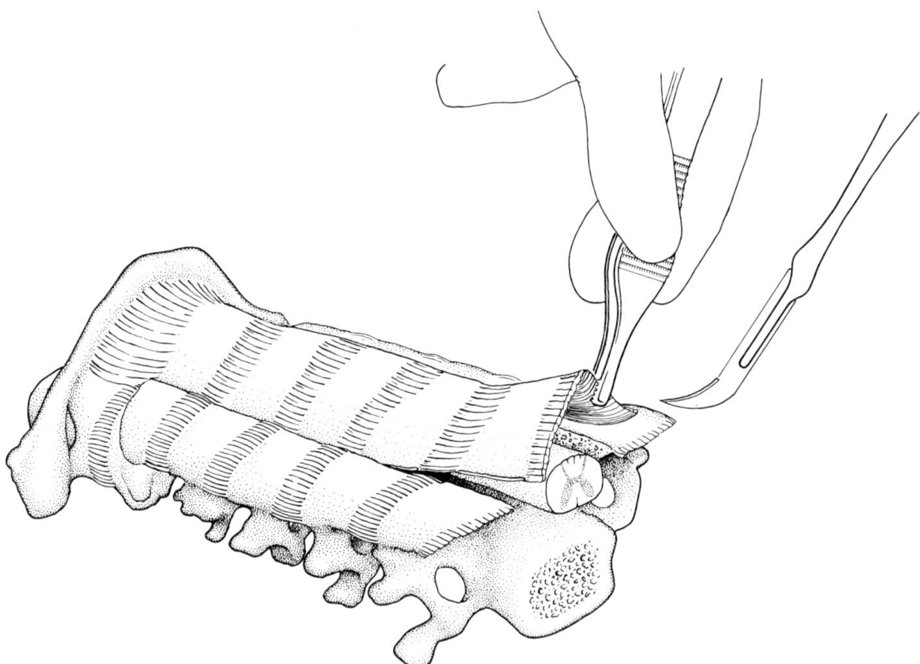

Figure 20–17. The spinous processes have been removed. Troughs have been cut on either side. The remaining block of cervical laminae connected by their ligamentum flavum are lifted and a curved scalpel is used to incise the residual ligament.

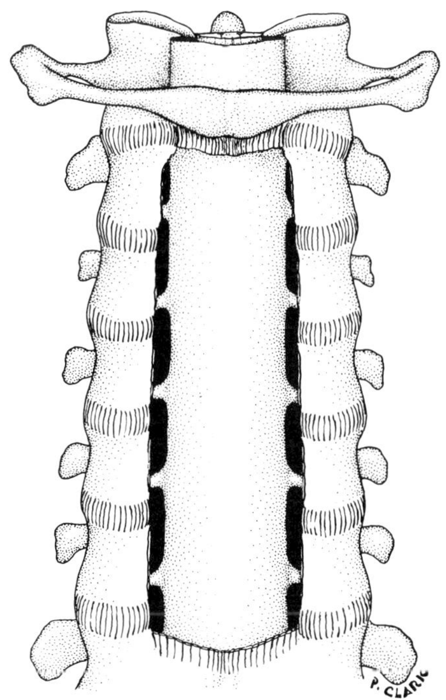
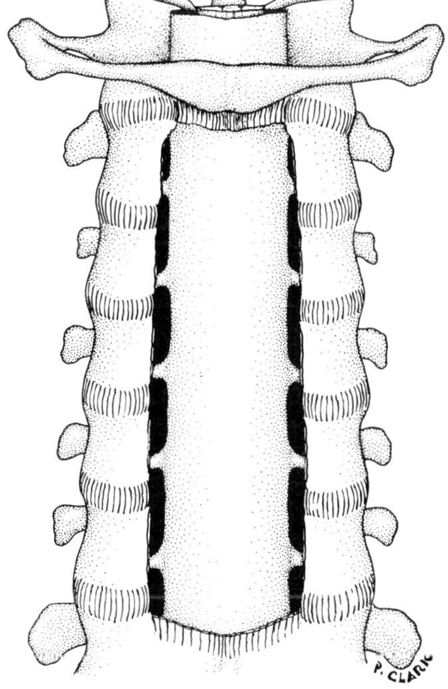

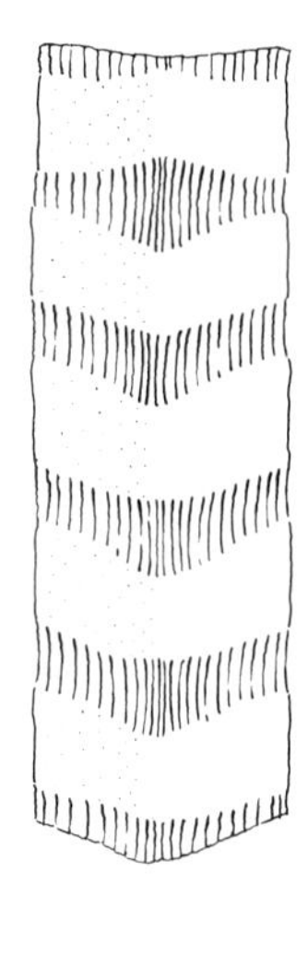

Figure 20–18. *Left,* The decompressed dura after removal of the cervical laminae. *Right,* A block of five cervical laminae, with spinous processes removed, connected by ligamentum flavum.

firmed the work of Arima, who noted cervical deformity in young patients after cervical laminectomy, but not in older patients with chronic disc degeneration.[1] Yasuoko and colleagues nicely demonstrated the responses of the cervical spine to multilevel laminectomy in children and adults.[7]

Meticulous closure of the incision is important. The paraspinous muscles must be approximated tightly. The skin is usually closed in two layers, and the authors have used a running subcuticular suture that is left in place for several weeks and removed at the first routine postoperative visit.

POSTOPERATIVE CARE

Currently, patients are observed in a neurologic intensive care unit overnight. This is primarily to detect any postoperative hematoma or other cause of worsening neurologic deficit. In our experience, this has not happened, and no patient has had to return to the operating room for these reasons. Consequently, we are currently reevaluating the role of intensive care admission for this operative procedure. An analysis of patients going to intensive care after cervical laminectomy indicated that among 13 patients studied carefully after cervical laminectomy, none actually benefited from such a stay.[6] "Benefit" was defined as some form of therapy initiated for such serious complications as hypotension, arrhythmia, angina, hematoma, respiratory difficulties, or neurologic deterioration, or more than one therapy begun for lesser problems such as acute hypertension, acute tachycardia, acute bradycardia, and hypovolemia. Our impression is similar, and it is not likely that intensive care unit monitoring is cost effective.

Patients are ordinarily discharged with a soft cervical collar to be worn for comfort, particularly when riding in a car.

CONCLUSION

In the past, cervical laminectomy was criticized because some patients experienced worsening of neurologic deficit after surgery. This was in the days when the laminectomy was performed entirely with a rongeur. The action of a rongeur requires that a portion of the instrument is placed under the lamina, and therefore spinal cord compression is possible during the several rongeur bites necessary to perform an extensive laminectomy (Fig. 20–

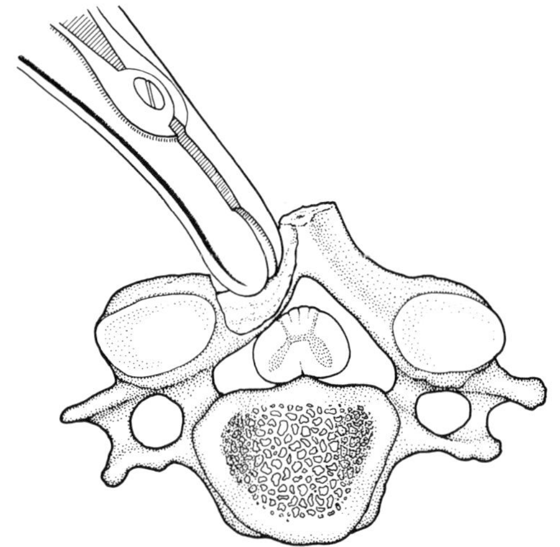

Figure 20–19. This indicates some of the pitfalls of removal of compressed cervical laminae by the ordinary rongeur technique. Thinned laminae can be pushed up against the cord, or the jaws of the rongeur themselves can injure the spinal cord if interposed under the laminae. With the trough-drilling technique, all dissection is carried laterally, not over the spinal cord itself.

19). The general development of better high-speed air drills with a variety of surgical burrs has replaced the rongeuring technique, and during the past few years air drill laminectomy has become more widely used throughout the world. Since this development, the incidence of postoperative neurologic deficit after laminectomy has been reduced.

Another criticism of cervical laminectomy has been aimed at the development of postoperative deformity, but as previously indicated, this deformity is not associated with neurologic deficit, nor does it require subsequent operations. Herkowitz compared a group of patients who had undergone anterior fusion, cervical laminectomy, or cervical laminaplasty.[3,4] He concluded that open-door laminaplasty should be considered an alternative to anterior fusion when three or more levels are involved. He also considered laminaplasty preferable in patients with developmental cervical stenosis and those with failed anterior neck surgery. We generally agree with this concept and recognize that anterior surgery often directly attacks the problem and that immediate and long-term results may be better with successful anterior cervical spine surgery. Nevertheless, in many patients, resection of vertebral bodies, multilevel fusions, and the use of a postoperative halo apparatus may preclude such surgery.

The authors believe that competent spinal surgeons should be capable of performing both anterior and posterior cervical spine surgery with delicacy and confidence, and that they should tailor the operation not to their surgical preferences, but to the safest and most efficient way of relieving compression on the cervical spinal cord.

References

1. Arima, T.: Changes in the cervical spine after laminectomy (in Japanese). Brain Nerve Injury *1*:17–78, 1969.
2. Cattell, H. S., and Clark, G. I., Jr.: Cervical kyphosis and instability following multiple laminectomies in children. J. Bone Joint Surg. *49A*:713–720, 1967.
3. Herkowitz, H. N.: A comparison of anterior cervical fusion, cervical laminectomy, and cervical laminoplasty for the surgical management of multiple level spondylotic radiculopathy. Spine *13*:774–780, 1988.
4. Herkowitz, H. N.: The surgical management of cervical spondylotic radiculopathy and myelopathy. Clin. Orthop. *239*:94–108, 1989.
5. Mikawa, Y., Shikata, J., and Yamamuro, T.: Spinal deformity and instability after multilevel cervical laminectomy. Spine *12*:6–11, 1987.
6. Teplick, R., Caldera, D. L., Gilbert, J. P., and Cullen, D. J.: Benefit of elective intensive care admission after certain operations. Anesth. Analg. *62*:572–577, 1983.
7. Yasuoka, S., Peterson, H. A., and Laws, E. R.: Pathogenesis and prophylaxis of postlaminectomy deformity of the spine after multi-level laminectomy: difference between children and adults. Neurosurgery *9*:145–152, 1981.
8. Yoshhiro, I., Suzuki, K., Ohmori, K., et al.: Critical analysis of extensive cervical laminectomy. Spine *12*:6–11, 1987.

CERVICAL LAMINAPLASTY

Harry N. Herkowitz, M.D.

The surgical treatment for multilevel cervical myelopathy and radiculopathy has historically been confined to anterior cervical fusion or cervical laminectomy.

In patients who have multiple-level disease, the neurologic picture is such that identification of one specific level for surgical intervention is often not possible. Figure 20–20 shows the typical myelographic appearance of a patient with bilateral myeloradiculopathy. The myelogram reveals five-level disease with spondylytic transverse bars and bilateral nerve root compression at each level. Bilateral laminectomy would require five-level decompression with foraminotomy, while fusion anteriorly would require multilevel grafting.

Raynor and colleagues showed that in order to decompress the cervical nerve roots adequately, 30 to 50 per cent of the respective facet joint must be removed.[65] In patients with multilevel bilateral nerve root compression, this would result in facet removal bilaterally at each cervical level, leading to a loss of mechanical support. It should also be remembered that the osteoarthritic facet joints do not provide the support similar to the normal facet joints that were used in the experimental models.

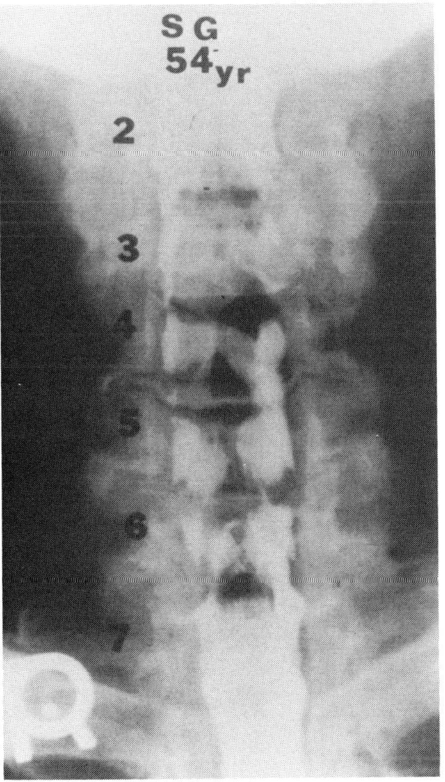

Figure 20–20. Anteroposterior myelogram demonstrating multilevel nerve root compression due to severe cervical spondylosis.

Several factors contribute to the development of cervical kyphosis or swan-neck deformity, the most important being lack of mechanical support and the age of the patient.[50, 60] Children have the highest incidence owing to their ligamentous laxity and underdeveloped cervical vertebrae.[50] Tachdjian and Matson reported a 40 per cent incidence of cervical kyphosis in 115 children.[79] Other factors involved in producing a postoperative cervical deformity are neuromuscular disease contributing to weakening of the muscular support of the cervical spine, and radiation therapy.[79]

In the elderly age group undergoing multilevel cervical laminectomy, lack of mechanical support and poor muscular tone are the most common causes for the development of cervical deformity. Yonenobu and associates reported the occurrence of neurologic deterioration after extensive cervical laminectomy for spondylosis in four of 22 patients.[88] The cause was the development of instability and cervical kyphosis after the extensive decompression. Late neurologic regression after extensive laminectomy for cervical myelopathy was reported by Crandall and Gregorius, who noted deterioration in 60 per cent of patients undergoing cervical laminectomy as opposed to 20 per cent undergoing anterior cervical fusion.[20]

Besides decompression laminectomy, another option for patients with multilevel nerve compression is anterior fusion. The procedures are broken down into those that remove the involved vertebrae and disc as a block[7, 8] and those that remove the disc at each level and replace it with a bone graft.[5, 17, 66–70] For elderly patients with three- or four-level nerve compression, this requires prolonged operating time under general anesthesia (Fig. 20–22). In

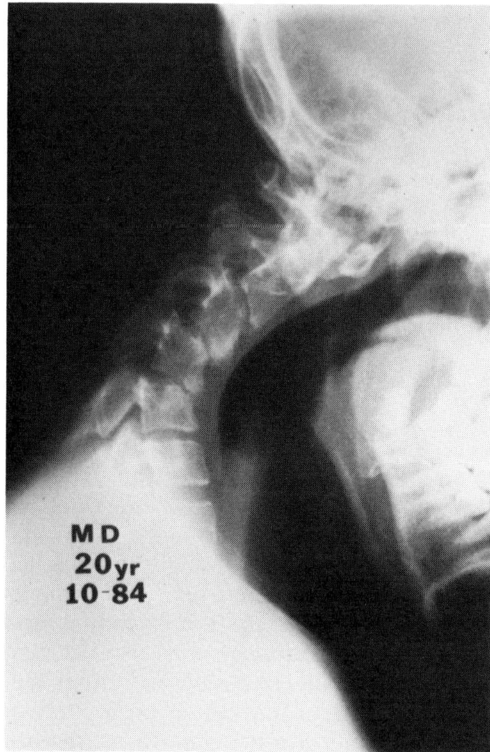

Figure 20–21. Lateral cervical spine radiograph in this 20-year-old male shows a severe swan-neck deformity that occurred after extensive cervical laminectomy.

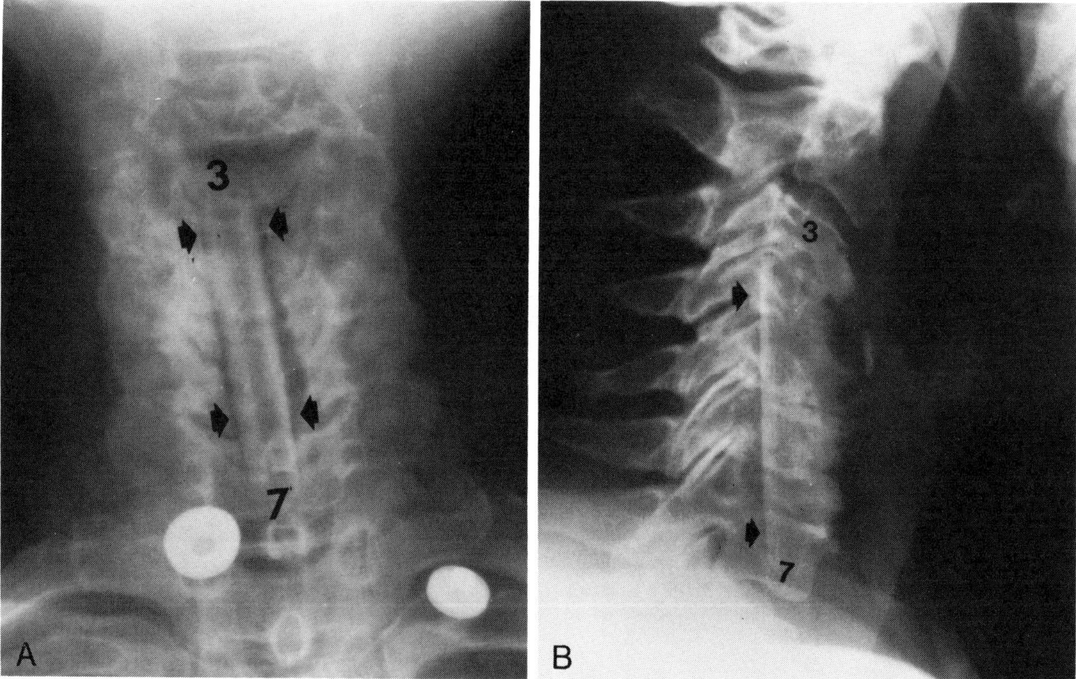

Figure 20–22. *A, B,* Lateral x-ray films demonstrating a fibular strut graft in place (*arrows*) after multilevel vertebrectomy for spondylotic myelopathy.

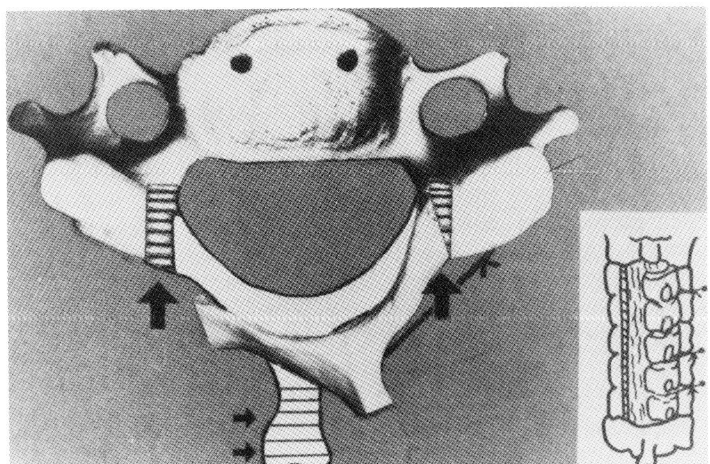

Figure 20–23. Schematic of expansive open-door laminaplasty.

addition, there is a potential risk of precipitating carotid artery ischemia or esophageal injury from prolonged retraction during surgery.

The use of a single strut graft to span three or four levels carries the risk of dislodgment, graft breakage, or collapse due to the osteopenia in elderly patients. Postoperative use of the halo-vest in this age group also carries with it the risk of infection and patient intolerance.[8]

Cervical laminaplasty is a decompressive procedure of the cervical spine developed by the Japanese in response to the high incidence of postlaminectomy deformity seen after extensive cervical laminectomy for myelopathy due to cervical spinal stenosis, spondylosis, or ossification of the posterior longitudinal ligament.[39] This procedure was originally described in 1972 by Hattori, who developed the expansive lamina-Z-plasty.[39] Because of technical problems, this procedure did not gain popularity until it was modified by Hirabayashi in 1977 as the "expansive open door laminaplasty" (Fig. 20–23).[39] The indications for this procedure, according to Hirabayashi, are myelopathy due to (1) cervical spinal stenosis (12 mm or less) (Fig. 20–24), (2) continuous-type ossification of the posterior longitudinal ligament, or (3) multiple-level (four or more) spondylosis. This procedure has also been employed for patients with cervical radiculopathy due to multisegmental (three or more) cervical spondylosis or cervical spinal stenosis.[35]

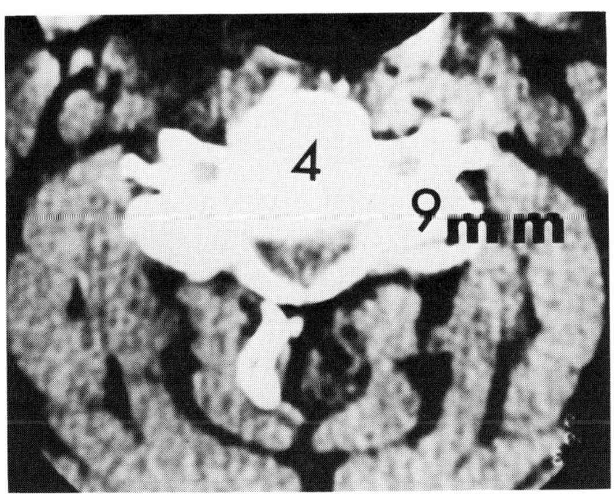

Figure 20–24. CT–myelogram demonstrating severe cervical stenosis (4 mm) at the C4 level.

SURGICAL TECHNIQUE

Step 1. The patient is positioned head down on a horseshoe head rest with the neck in a neutral or slightly flexed position.

Step 2. After exposure two bony gutters are made with a high-speed burr from the upper to the lower vertebrae involved. This should be performed just medial to the facet joint and pedicle (for example, with stenosis at C3–C4, C4–C5, and C5–C6, the bony gutter is developed through C3 superiorly and C6 inferiorly). On the side exhibiting the greatest narrowing or the side with the most significant radiculopathy, the burr should go to the inner cortex and break through at one segment. On the opposite side the burr is used to go through the outer cortex. It may be necessary to burr to the inner cortex, but *not* through it. Next, a 1-mm Kerrison punch is used to remove the inner cortex from top to bottom on the side for which the lamina is to be elevated (Fig. 20–25). In patients with significant radiculopathy, foraminotomies are performed at each segment (Fig. 20–26).

Step 3. Nonabsorbable sutures are passed through the base of the spinous processes at each segment. The tips of the spinous processes are removed at each level and fashioned into small strips for later use. Gently, pressure is put along the spinous processes until the lamina begins to give way. It is essential to make sure adhesions are not present between the dural sac and the undersurface of the lamina. A Penfield elevator is used to eliminate such adhesions (Fig. 20–27). The amount of laminar elevation should be 10 to 15 mm. Kimura and associates showed that a laminar elevation of 10 mm will expand the sagittal diameter of the spinal canal by 4 to 5 mm (Fig. 20–28).[44]

Step 4. Once the expansion is performed, the sutures within the spinous processes are secured into the facet capsules at each segment. The bone previously removed is placed in the trough on the hinged side. A thin layer of fat is removed from the subcutaneous tissue

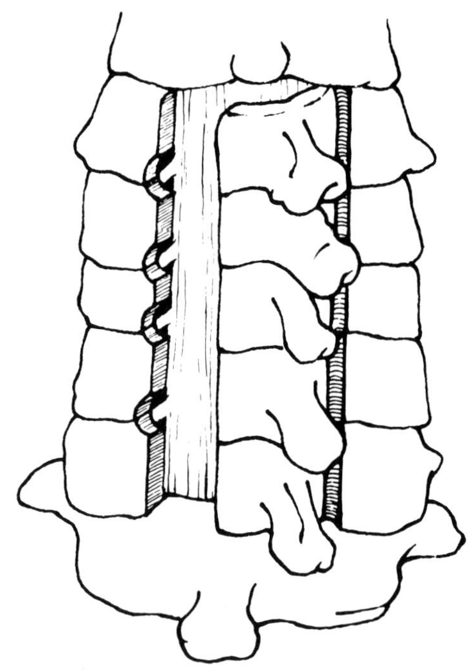

Figure 20–26. Schematic demonstrating foraminotomies made along the open-door side at each level.

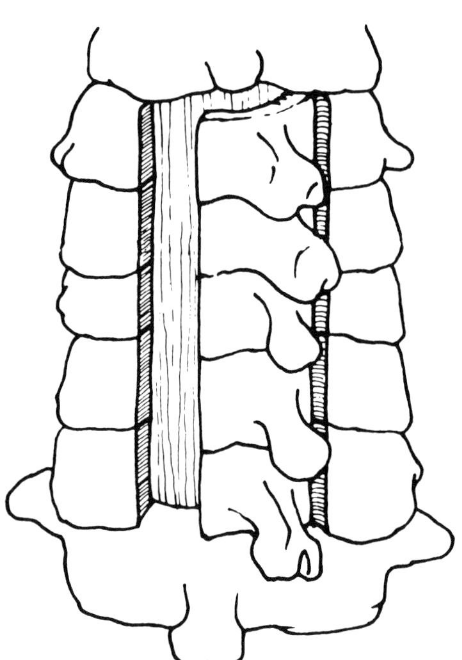

Figure 20–25. Schematic demonstrating the opening made for laminaplasty.

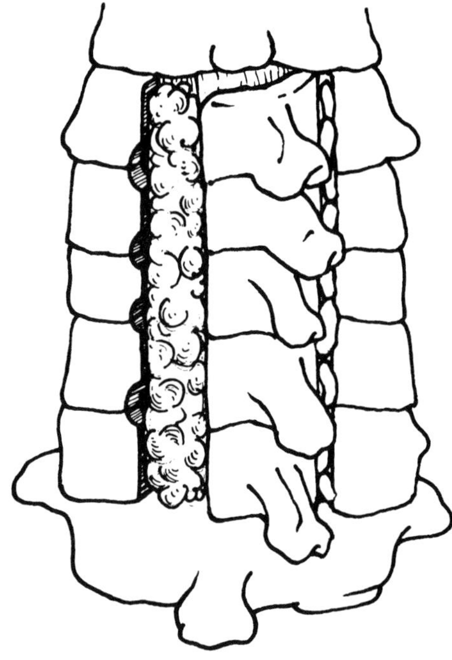

Figure 20–27. Schematic showing a free fat graft applied over the exposed dura. Note the bone graft placed along the hinged side after the lamina is manually opened. At this stage the sutures have usually been placed through the spinous processes.

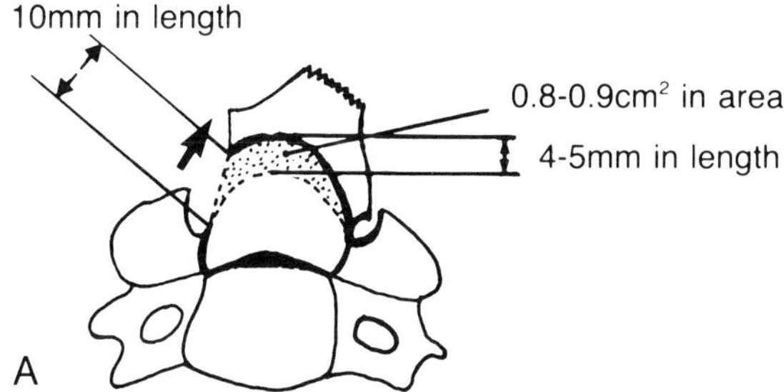

Widening of the Canal	Recovery Rate (%)
0.0–1.0 mm	34
1.0–2.0	62
2.0–3.0	65
3.0–4.0	72
4.0–5.0	81
5.0–6.0	60
6.0–7.0	62
7.0–8.0	57

B

Figure 20–28. *A, B,* The distance that the laminae are evaluated on the opened side is correlated with the extent of spinal canal enlargement. (From Kimura, I., Oh-Hama, M., and Shingu, H.: Cervical myelopathy treated by canal-expansive laminoplasty. J. Bone Joint Surg. *66A:*914–920, 1984.)

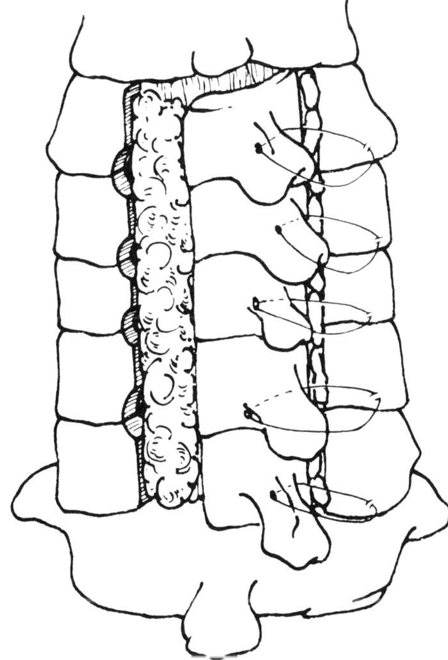

Figure 20–29. Schematic showing completed laminaplasty.

and placed over the exposed dura. If fat is not available, a Gelfoam pad is used (Fig. 20–29).

Step 5. The patient is maintained in a Minerva brace for six weeks postoperatively.

The results of this procedure for myelopathy demonstrate significant improvement in neurologic function in the reported series.[38–40, 43, 44] Hirabayashi correlated the clinical recovery rate with the amount of widening of the sagittal diameter of the spinal canal, demonstrating best results with a canal expansion of 4 to 5 mm (Table 20–6).[39]

Table 20–6. THE RELATIONSHIP BETWEEN AP DIAMETER WIDENING OF THE SPINAL CANAL AND THE CLINICAL RECOVERY RATE

Widening of the Canal (mm)	Recovery Rate (%)
0.0–1.0	34
1.0–2.0	62
2.0–3.0	65
3.0–4.0	72
4.0–5.0	81
5.0–6.0	60
6.0–7.0	62
7.0–8.0	57

From Hirabayashi, K.: Expensive open-door laminoplasty for cervical spinal stenotic myelopathy. Spine *8:*697, 1983.

The results of this procedure performed in patients with multilevel spondylotic radiculopathy demonstrate significant relief of radicular pain in most individuals.[34] In addition, patients with bilateral radiculopathy fared as well as those with unilateral radiculopathy.

The complications of this procedure appear to be limited to loss of canal expansion from "closing of the door" (Fig. 20–30). With suturing of the lamina to the facet, this can

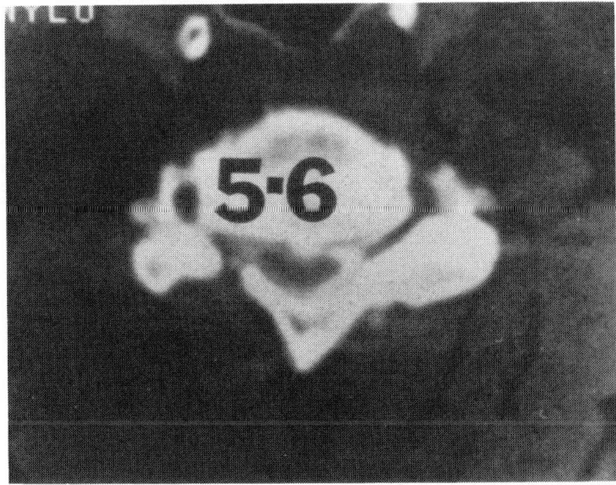

Figure 20–30. Myelogram–CT scan demonstrating closing of the laminaplasty door.

usually be prevented. Another problem that can be associated with the laminaplasty procedure is loss of cervical motion, especially rotation and lateral flexion. This is due to bony ankylosis that occurs along the hinge side of the laminaplasty.

In summary, the open-door laminaplasty procedure provides an effective alternative to anterior fusion or laminectomy for myelopathy or radiculopathy due to (1) multiple-level (three or more) cervical spinal stenosis or (2) multiple-level (three or more) cervical spondylosis with spinal cord and/or nerve root compression proved by myelography, myelography with CT, or MRI.

References

1. Abitol, J. J., and Garfin, S.: Surgical management of cervical disc disease: anterior cervical fusion. Semin. Spine Surg. *1*:233–238, 1989.
2. Adams, C., and Logue, U.: Studies in cervical spondylotic myelopathy. Brain *94*:569–586, 1971.
3. Arima, T.: Post laminectomy malalignments of the cervical spine. J. Brain Nerve Trauma (Jpn.) *1*:71–78, 1969.
4. Aronson, N.: The management of soft cervical disc protrusions using the Smith-Robinson approach. Clin. Neurosurg. *20*:253–259, 1973.
5. Bailey, R., and Bagley, C.: Stabilization of the cervical spine by anterior fusion. J. Bone Joint Surg. *42A*:565–594, 1960.
6. Bohlman, H.: Cervical spondylosis with moderate to severe myelopathy. Spine *2*:151–162, 1977.
7. Bohlman, H.: Degenerative arthrosis of the lower cervical spine. *In* Evarts, C. M. (ed.): Surgery of the Musculoskeletal System. Vol. 2. New York, Churchill Livingstone, 1983, pp. 25–35.
8. Boni, M., Cherubino, P., Denaro, U., and Benazzo, F.: Multiple subtotal somatectomy. Spine *9*:358–362, 1984.
9. Brain, R. W., Northfield, D., and Wilkinson, M.: The neurologic manifestations of cervical spondylosis. Brain *75*:187–225, 1952.
10. Brain, L., and Wilkinson, M.: Cervical Spondylosis and Other Disorders of the Cervical Spine. Philadelphia, W. B. Saunders Co., 1967, p. 226.
11. Breig, A., Turnbull, I., and Hassler, O.: Effects of mechanical stresses on the spinal cord in cervical spondylosis. J. Neurosurg. *25*:45, 1966.
12. Brodsky, A.: Management of radiculopathy secondary to acute cervical disc degeneration and spondylosis by the posterior approach. *In* Cervical Spine Research Society (eds.): The Cervical Spine. Philadelphia, J. B. Lippincott Co., 1983, pp. 395–402.
13. Bulgar, R., Rejowski, J., and Beatty, R.: Vocal cord paralysis associated with anterior cervical fusion: considerations for prevention and treatment. J. Neurosurg. *62*:657–661, 1985.
14. Callahan, R., Johnson, R., Margolis, R., et al.: Cervical facet fusion for control of instability following laminectomy. J. Bone Joint Surg. *59A*:991–1002, 1977.
15. Clark, C.: Indications and surgical management of cervical myelopathy. Semin. Spine Surg. *1*:254–261, 1989.
16. Clarke, E., and Robinson, P.: Cervical myelopathy: a complication of cervical spondylosis. Brain *79*:483, 1956.
17. Cloward, R. B.: The anterior approach for ruptured cervical discs. J. Neurosurg. *15*:602, 1958.
18. Connolly, E. S., Seymour, R. J., and Adams, J. E.: Clinical evaluation of anterior cervical fusion for degenerative cervical disc disease. J. Neurosurg. *23*:431–437, 1965.
19. Crandall, P., and Batzdorf, U.: Cervical spondylotic myelopathy. J. Neurosurg. *25*:57–66, 1966.
20. Crandall, P., and Gregorius, F.: Long-term follow-up of cervical spondylotic myelopathy. Spine *2*:139–146, 1977.
21. DePalma, A., Rothman, R., Lewinnnek, G., et al.: Anterior interbody fusion for severe cervical disc degeneration. Surg. Gynecol. Obstet. *134*:755, 758, 1972.
22. Dillin, W., Booth, R., Cuckler, J., et al.: Cervical radiculopathy: a review. Spine *11*:988–991, 1986.
23. Dillin, W., and Simeone, F. A.: Treatment of cervical disc disease. Selection of operative approaches. Contemp. Neurosurg. *8*:1–6, 1986.
24. Epstein, J., and Janin, Y.: Management of cervical spondylotic myeloradiculopathy by the posterior approach. *In* Cervical Spine Research Society (eds.): The Cervical Spine. Philadelphia, J. B. Lippincott Co., 1983, pp. 402–410.
25. Epstein, J., Janin, Y., Carras, R., and Lavine, L.: A comparative study of the treatment of cervical spondylotic myeloradiculopathy. Acta Neurochir. *61*:89–104, 1982.
26. Flynn, T. B.: Neurologic complications of anterior fusion. Spine *7*:536–539, 1982.
27. Gooding, M., Wilson, C., and Hoff, J.: Experimental cervical myelopathy. J. Neurosurg. *43*:9–17, 1975.
28. Gore, D., Sepic, S., Gardner, G., and Murray, M.: Neck pain: a long-term follow-up of 205 patients. Spine *12*:1–5, 1987.
29. Gore, D., and Sepic, S.: Anterior cervical fusion for degenerated or protruded discs. Spine *9*:667–671, 1984.
30. Gregorius, F. K., Estin, T. E., and Crandall, P. H.: Cervical spondylotic radiculopathy and myelopathy. Arch. Neurol. *33*:618–625, 1976.
31. Grisol, F., Graziani, N., Fabrizi, A. P., et al.: Anterior discectomy without fusion for treatment of cervical lateral soft disc extrusion: a follow-up of 120 cases. Neurosurgery *24*:853–859, 1989.
32. Haft, H., and Shenkin, H. A.: Surgical end results of cervical ridge and disc problems. J.A.M.A. *186*:312–315, 1963.
33. Henderson, C., Hennessy, R., Shuey, H., and Shackelford, E.: Posterior-lateral foraminotomy as an exclusive operative technique for cervical radiculopathy: a review of 846 consecutively operated cases. Neurosurgery *13*:504–511, 1983.
34. Herkowitz, H. N.: A comparison of anterior cervical fusion, cervical laminectomy and cervical laminaplasty for the surgical management of multiple level spondylotic radiculopathy. Spine *13*:774–780, 1988.
35. Herkowitz, H. N.: Cervical laminaplasty: its role in

the treatment of cervical radiculopathy. J. Spinal Dis. *1*:179–188, 1988.

36. Herkowitz, H. N.: The surgical management of cervical spondylotic radiculopathy and myelopathy. Clin. Orthop. *239*:94–108, 1989.
37. Herkowitz, H. N., Kurz, L. T., and Overholt, D. P.: The surgical management of cervical soft disc herniation: a comparison between the anterior and posterior approach. Spine *15*:1026–1030, 1990.
38. Hirabayashi, K., Miyakawa, J., Satomi, K., et al.: Operative results and postoperative progression of ossification among patients with ossification of cervical posterior longitudinal ligaments. Spine *6*:354–364, 1981.
39. Hirabayashi, K., Watanabe, K., Wakano, K., et al.: Expansive open-door laminoplasty for cervical spinal stenotic myelopathy. Spine *8*:693–699, 1983.
40. Hukuda, S., Mochizuki, T., Ogata, M., et al.: Operations for cervical spondylotic myelopathy. J. Bone Joint Surg. *67B*:609–615, 1985.
41. Hunter, L., Braunstein, E., and Bailey, R.: Radiographic changes following anterior cervical fusion. Spine *5*:399–401, 1980.
42. Ishida, Y., Suzuki, K., Ohmori, K., et al.: Critical analysis of extensive cervical laminectomy. Neurosurgery *24*:215–222, 1989.
43. Itoh, T., and Tsuji, H.: Technical improvements and results of laminaplasty for compressive myelopathy in the cervical spine. Spine *10*:729–736, 1985.
44. Kimura, I., Oh-Hama, M., and Shingu, H.: Cervical myelopathy treated by canal-expansive laminaplasty. J. Bone Joint Surg. *66A*:914–920, 1984.
45. Kozak, J., Hansen, G., Rose, J., et al.: Anterior discectomy, microscopic decompression and fusion: a treatment for cervical spondylotic radiculopathy. J. Spinal Dis. *2*:43–46, 1989.
46. Kraus, F. R., and Stauffer, E. S.: Spinal cord injury as a complication of elective anterior cervical fusion. Clin. Orthop. *112*:130–141, 1975.
47. Kurz, L. T., Garfin, S. R., and Booth, R.: Harvesting autogenous iliac bone graft: a review of complications and techniques. Spine *14*:1324–1331, 1990.
48. Laoire, S., and Thomas, D.: Spinal cord compression due to prolapse of cervical intervertebral disc: treatment of 26 cases by discectomy without interbody bone graft. J. Neurosurg. *59*:847–853, 1983.
49. Lees, F., and Turner, J.: Natural history and prognosis of cervical spondylosis. Br. Med. J. *5373*:1607–1610, 1963.
50. Lonstein, J.: Post-laminectomy Kyphosis, Spinal Deformities and Neurologic Dysfunction. New York, Raven Press, 1978, pp. 53–63.
51. Lunsford, L., Bissonette, D., Jannetha, P., et al.: Anterior surgery for cervical disc disease: treatment of lateral cervical disc herniation in 253 cases. J. Neurosurg. *53*:1–11, 1980.
52. Lunsford, L., Bissonette, D., and Zorub, D.: Anterior surgery for cervical disc disease: treatment of cervical spondylotic myelopathy in 32 cases. J. Neurosurg. *53*:12–19, 1980.
53. Manabe, S., and Tateishi, A.: Epidural migration of extruded cervical disc and its surgical treatment. Spine *11*:873–878, 1986.
54. Mann, K., Khosla, V., and Gulati, D.: Cervical spondylotic myelopathy treated by single stage multilevel anterior decompression. J. Neurosurg. *60*:81–87, 1984.
55. Munroe, I.: The importance of the sagittal diameters of the cervical spinal canal in relation to spondylosis and myelopathy. J. Bone Joint Surg. *56B*:30, 1974.
56. Murphy, M., and Gadd, M.: Anterior cervical discectomy without interbody bone graft. J. Neurosurg. *37*:71–74, 1972.
57. Newhouse, K., Lindsey, R., Clark, C., et al.: Esophageal perforation following anterior cervical spine surgery. Spine *14*:1051–1056, 1989.
58. Nurick, S.: The natural history and the results of surgical treatment of the spinal cord disorder associated with cervical spondylosis. Brain *95*:101–108, 1972.
59. Nurick, S.: The pathogenesis of the spinal cord disorder associated with cervical spondylosis. Brain *95*:87, 1972.
60. Oiwa, T., Hirabayshi, K., Mitsuyoshi, U., and Ohira, T.: Experimental study of post-laminectomy deterioration of cervical spondylotic myelopathy. Spine *10*:717–721, 1985.
61. Penning, L., and VanDer Zwaag, P.: Biomechanical aspects of spondylotic myelopathy. Acta Radiol. *5*:1090, 1966.
62. Perry, S., and Nickel, V. L.: Total cervical spine fusion for neck paralysis. J. Bone Joint Surg. *41A*:37–60, 1959.
63. Phillips, D. G.: Surgical treatment of myelopathy with cervical spondylosis. J. Neurol. Neurosurg. Pyschiatry *36*:879–884, 1973.
64. Raynor, R.: Anterior or posterior approach to the cervical spine: an anatomical and radiographic evaluation and comparison. Neurosurgery *12*:7–13, 1983.
65. Raynor, R., Pugh, J., and Shapiro, I.: Cervical facetectomy and its effect on spine strength. J. Neurosurg. *63*:278–282, 1985.
66. Riley, L.: Anterior Cervical Spine Surgery. *In* AAOS Instructional Course Lectures. Vol. XXVII. St. Louis, C. V. Mosby Co., 1978, pp. 154–158.
67. Riley, L., Robinson, R., Johnson, K., and Walker, A.: The results of anterior interbody fusion of the cervical spine. J. Neurosurg. *30*:127, 1969.
68. Robinson, R., Afeiche, N., Dunn, E., and Northrup, B.: Cervical spondylotic myelopathy. Spine *2*:89–99, 1977.
69. Robinson, R. A., and Smith, G. W.: Anterolateral cervical disc removal and interbody fusion for cervical disc syndrome. Bull. Johns Hopkins Hosp. *96*:223–224, 1955.
70. Robinson, R., Walker, A., and Ferlic, D.: The results of anterior interbody fusion of the cervical spine. J. Bone Joint Surg. *44A*:1569–1587, 1962.
71. Robinson, R. A., and Smith, G. W.: The treatment of certain spine disorders by anterior removal of the intervertebral disc and interbody fusion. J. Bone Joint Surg. *40A*:607, 1958.
72. Rosenorn, J., Hansen, E., and Rosenorn, M.: Anterior cervical discectomy with and without fusion. J. Neurosurg. *59*:252–255, 1983.
73. Rothman, R., and Rashbaum, R.: Pathogenesis of signs and symptoms of cervical disc degeneration. *In* AAOS Instructional Course Lectures. Vol. XXVII. St. Louis, C. V. Mosby Co., 1978, pp. 203–215.
74. Rothman, R. H., and Simeone, F.: Cervical disc disease. *In* Rothman, R. H., and Simeone, F. A. (eds.): The Spine. 2nd ed. Vol. 1. Philadelphia, W. B. Saunders Co., 1982, pp. 440–499.

75. Scoville, W., Dohrmann, G., and Corkill, G.: Late results of cervical disc surgery. J. Neurosurg. *45*:203–210, 1976.
76. Sim, F. H., Suien, H. J., Bickel, W. H., and Janes, J. M.: Swan neck deformity following extensive cervical laminectomy. J. Bone Joint Surg. *56A*:564–580, 1974.
77. Simmons, E., and Bhalla, S.: Anterior cervical discectomy and fusion. J. Bone Joint Surg. *51B*:225–237, 1969.
78. Southwick, W. O., and Robinson, R. A.: Surgical approaches to the vertebral bodies in the cervical and lumbar regions. J. Bone Joint Surg. *39A*:631–644, 1957.
79. Tachdjian, M., and Matson, D.: Orthopedic aspects of intraspinal tumor in infants and children. J. Bone Joint Surg. *47A*:223, 1965.
80. Tsuji, H.: Laminaplasty for patients with compressive myelopathy due to so-called spinal canal stenosis in cervical and thoracic regions. Spine *7*:28–34, 1982.
81. Verbeist, H.: The management of cervical spondylosis. Clin. Neurosurg. *20*:262–294, 1973.
82. White, A., Southwick, W., DePonte, R., et al.: Relief of pain by anterior cervical spine fusion for spondylosis. J. Bone Joint Surg. *55A*:525–534, 1973.
83. White, A., and Hirsch, C.: An experimental study of the immediate load-bearing capacity of some commonly used iliac bone grafts. Acta Orthop. Scand. *42*:482–490, 1971.
84. Whitecloud, T.: Complications of anterior cervical fusion. *In* Instructional Course Lectures. Vol. XXVII. St. Louis, C. V. Mosby Co., 1978, pp. 223–237.
85. Whitecloud, T.: Management of radiculopathy and myelopathy by the anterior approach. *In* Cervical Spine Research Society (ed.): The Cervical Spine. Philadelphia, J. B. Lippincott Co., 1983, pp. 411–424.
86. Williams, J., Allen, M., and Harkess, J.: Late results of cervical discectomy and interbody fusion: some factors influencing the results. J. Bone Joint Surg. *50A*:277–286, 1968.
87. Wolf, B., Khilnani, M., and Malis, L.: The sagittal diameter of the bony cervical canal and its significance in cervical spondylosis. J. Mt. Sinai Hosp. *23*:283–292, 1956.
88. Yonenobu, K., Fuji, T., Ono, K., et al.: Choice of surgical treatment for multisegmental cervical spondylotic myelopathy. Spine *10*:710–716, 1985.

CHAPTER

21

OSSIFICATION OF THE POSTERIOR LONGITUDINAL LIGAMENT

Kazuhiko Satomi, M.D.
Kiyoshi Hirabayashi, M.D.

Ossification of the posterior longitudinal ligament (OPLL) appears as an abnormal radiopacity along the posterior margins of the vertebral bodies on lateral views of the roentgenogram. The pathogenesis of OPLL has not yet been clarified, but severe myelopathy or radiculopathy may be elicited by OPLL, which is much more common among Japanese and other Orientals than whites.[2–5, 17, 19, 27, 28, 40] OPLL has been found at a similar rate on roentgenograms taken before World War II.[40]

The first report on cervical compressive myelopathy due to OPLL was made by Key in 1838.[16] Tsukimoto was the first to describe OPLL in Japan, using autopsy findings in 1960, and Onji and associates clinically reviewed 18 cases of OPLL in 1967.[28, 38] Since then, many reports on this disease have been published in Japan.[36, 43]

OPLL of the cervical spine will be reviewed here. OPLL of the thoracic spine and lumbar spine is less frequent and has different roentgenographic characteristics, pathology, and treatment.

INCIDENCE

In eastern Asiatic countries including Japan, OPLL is observed in approximately 2 to 3 per cent of the cervical roentgenograms from outpatients, compared with 0.2 per cent at the Mayo Clinic and 0.6 per cent in Hawaii.[39] The incidence is 1.7 per cent in Italy.[14]

It is not unexpected that roentgenographic evidence of ossification is found much more frequently in the adult cervical spine, since OPLL does not always cause clinical signs and symptoms. The incidence of asymptomatic ossification showed a roughly linear progression with advancing age: 11 per cent of healthy individuals in the sixth decade of life had roentgenologic changes suggestive of ossification.[25]

ETIOLOGY

The cause of OPLL remains obscure. Results of routine laboratory examination are almost within normal range; however, a decrease of Ca resorption in the small intestine is reported in OPLL.[12]

Studies of the family histories of patients with OPLL revealed the possibility of an autosomal dominant inheritance.[42] It was suggested that the incidence of OPLL among family members of second-order kinship to the patient is about 30 per cent, which is 15 times the general incidence.[40]

It has been suggested that patients with OPLL had a tendency to develop generalized hyperostosis of the spinal ligaments, such as diffuse idiopathic skeletal hyperostosis (DISH), because ankylosing spinal hyperostosis (ASH) was observed in 23.9 to 30 per cent of patients with OPLL and ankylosing spondylitis was observed in 2.0 per cent.[20, 26, 31, 39]

Many authors reported a high incidence of diabetes mellitus among patients with OPLL.[39] Glucose tolerance tests in 535 patients resulted in identification of 152 (28 per cent) diabetic and 95 (18 per cent) borderline diabetics, whereas the incidence of OPLL in diabetic patients was 16 per cent.[14] A high incidence of OPLL has also been reported in other hormonal disorders, such as acromegaly and hypoparathyroidism.

ROENTGENOGRAPHIC FINDINGS AND CLASSIFICATION

The early changes of OPLL are inconspicuous on lateral films of the cervical spine. Roentgenographically, OPLL of the cervical spine is classified as segmental type, with OPLL behind each vertebral body; continuous with OPLL over several vertebrae; mixed, with both segmental and continuous lesions; and localized, with OPLL over the intervertebral disc space (Fig. 21–1). The segmental and localized types of OPLL are sometimes difficult to define on lateral films of the cervical spine.

It has been reported that the segmental type of OPLL was noted in 39.0 per cent of patients, the continuous type in 27.3 per cent, the mixed type in 29.2 per cent, and the localized type in 7.5 per cent of patients.[39]

OPLL is most frequently observed at the C4, C5, and C6 levels on the lateral films. The peak of OPLL thickness is often seen at the same levels. The average number of vertebral bodies involved was 3.1 in the accumulated series.[39]

Narrowing of the spinal canal due to the ossified mass is calculated as a ratio of the maximal thickness of OPLL to the anteroposterior diameter of the spinal canal on lateral views. The narrowing ratio is higher in the mixed and continuous types than in the segmental and localized types of OPLL.

X-ray surveys of the thoracic and lumbar spine and the pelvis are necessary for patients with OPLL, because various ligaments in these areas occasionally show ossification.[26] Yanagi and associates reported that the incidence of ossification of the yellow ligament (OYL) in the thoracic spine was 13 per cent in patients with cervical OPLL.[43] Patients who have OPLL, OYL, or both in the thoracic spine combined with cervical OPLL have more severe disabilities than patients with cervical OPLL alone.

Computed tomography (CT) is particularly helpful to show not only the existence of OPLL but also the thickness, lateral extension, and shape of OPLL, and the extent the spinal canal is narrowed by OPLL (Fig. 21–2).[17, 41] Authors classified OPLL seen on CT into three types—square, mushroom, and hill—at the level of the most narrowed spinal canal.

PATHOLOGIC CHANGES

The posterior longitudinal ligament (PLL) consists of deep and superficial layers and connects continuously to the vertebral bodies and the intervertebral discs by fibrous tissue in the midline portion of the ligaments. The lateral portion of the PLL connects only to the upper and lower margins of the vertebral bodies.

Pathohistologically, ossification generally begins in the portion of the PLL fibrously connected to the vertebral body, where the stress converges by the cervical motion. Rapid growth of OPLL is not explained by this theory, however. Hyperplasia of PLL is believed to exist, but has not yet been proven by clinical findings.[42] The ossified mass of OPLL consists mainly of lamellar bone, with some irregular woven bone surrounding the fibrocartilage and an area of calcified cartilage. Enchondral ossification plays a key role in the formation of OPLL.

In autopsy cases with OPLL, the spinal cords were extremely compressed anteriorly as a result of the condition.[8, 9, 22, 29] The total amount of neural tissue was remarkably decreased. Intensive damage was seen in the gray matter compared with the white matter. The most seriously damaged parts of the spinal cord showed tissue necrosis and cavity formation extending from the central parts of the gray matter to the ventral parts of the posterior

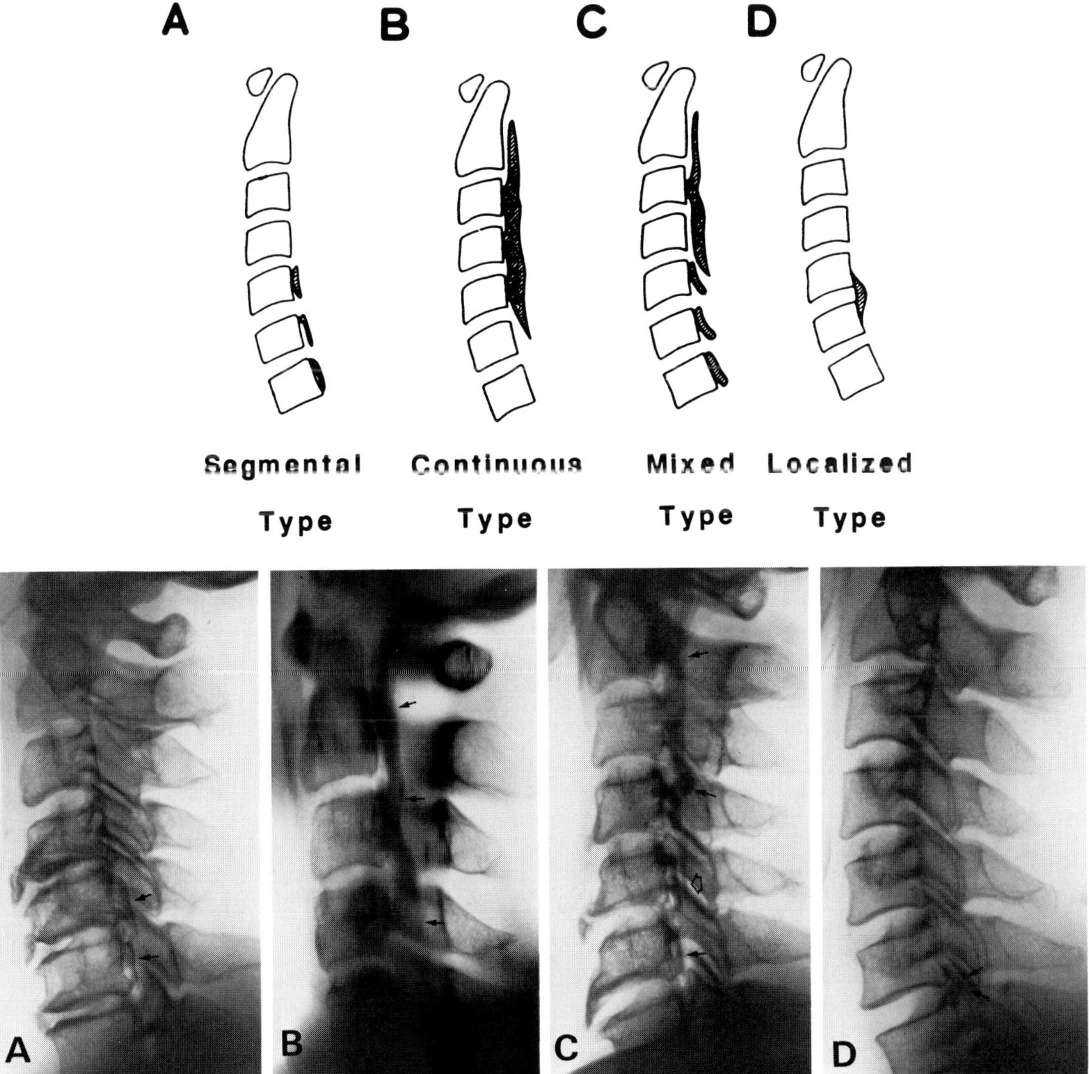

Figure 21–1. *A* to *D*, Schematic presentation and roentgenogram of each type of OPLL. Arrows show OPLL, and the open arrow indicates ossification of dura. (Top portion from Hirabayashi, K., Satomi, K., and Sasaki, T.: Ossification of the posterior longitudinal ligament in the cervical spine. *In* Cervical Spine Research Society Editorial Committee (eds.): The Cervical Spine. 2nd ed. Philadelphia, J. B. Lippincott Co., 1989, p. 679.)

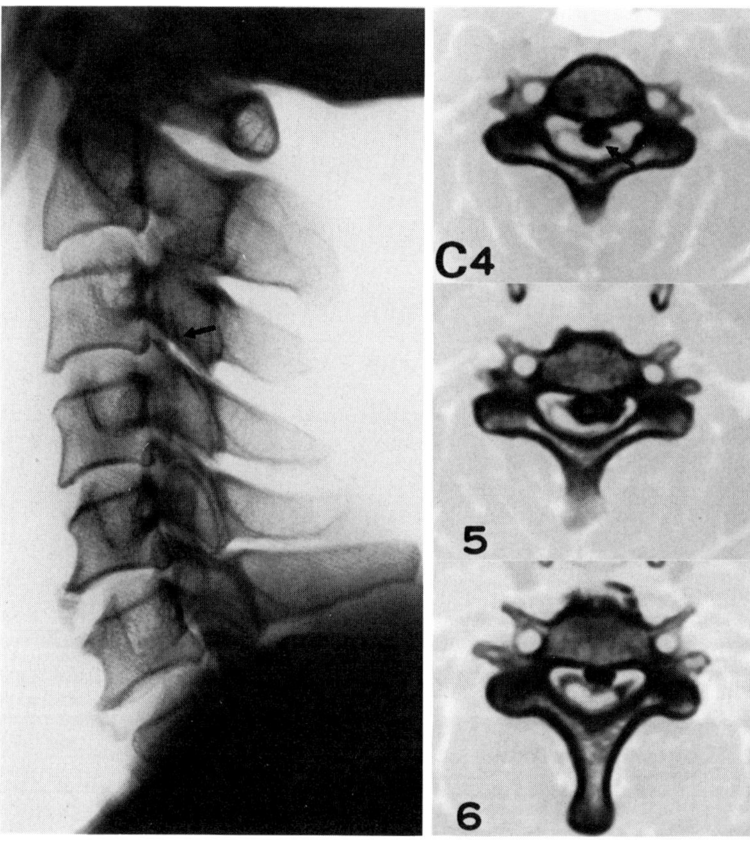

Figure 21–2. Myelogram and CT myelogram of the mixed type of OPLL in a 52-year-old female. Ossification of dura *(arrow)* and flattening of the spinal cord are well observed on CT myelogram.

columns (Fig. 21–3).[33] The horn cells were reduced in both number and size. Demyelinization was observed extensively in the white matter. These distributions of degeneration may be caused by ischemia or venous stasis in the boundary areas of the anterior and posterior spinal artery tributaries in the spinal cord.[22]

Relatively good spinal cord function was preserved before death, however. Thus, stability of the cervical spine provided by OPLL acts as a protective mechanism against damage to the spinal cord, and the spinal cord also has a high degree of tolerance to slowly increasing mechanical pressure with OPLL, until 50 to 60 per cent of the anteroposterior diameter of the spinal canal is occupied. In subclinical patients with severe OPLL in whom the spinal cords are compressed to a critical degree, however, mild traumatic forces may readily cause complete tetraplegia.[30]

CLINICAL SYMPTOMS

It is widely recognized that almost all patients with OPLL have only mild subjective complaints, such as neck pain and numbness in the hand, and do not have disturbances in the activity of daily living (ADL).[24] Spastic gait disturbance and clumsiness of the fingers were recognized objectively in 15 and 10 per cent of them, respectively, however (Table 21–1). The average age of onset of the initial symptoms was 51.2 years in men and 48.9 years in women, respectively.[39]

Severity of cervical myelopathy is described using an evaluating score proposed by the Japanese Orthopaedic Association (JOA). This score has 17 points in all, consisting of four points for motor dysfunction of the upper and lower extremities, respectively; two points for sensory dysfunction of the upper and lower extremities and trunk, respectively; and three points for bladder dysfunction (Table 21–2). JOA scores less than seven generally indicate severe myelopathy; scores between eight and 12 indicate moderate myelopathy; and scores over 13 indicate mild myelopathy.

An acute development or aggravation of tetraparesis after a minor trauma, such as slipping, was noticed in 20.6 per cent of the registered cases.[39]

Table 21–1. INITIAL SYMPTOMS OF OPLL

Symptom	Frequency (%)
Neck pain	41.9
Pain or dysesthesia in upper extremities	47.7
Motor dysfunction in upper extremities	10.4
Dysesthesia in lower extremities	19.0
Motor dysfunctions in lower extremities	15.4
Bladder disturbance	1.0

Total number of patients: 2162 (accumulated cases). From Hirabayashi, K., Satomi, K., and Sasaki, T.: Ossification of the posterior longitudinal ligament in the cervical spine. *In* Cervical Spine Research Society Editorial Committee (eds.): The Cervical Spine. 2nd ed. Philadelphia, J. B. Lippincott Co., 1989, p. 681.

Table 21–2. CRITERIA FOR EVALUATION OF THE OPERATIVE RESULTS OF PATIENTS WITH CERVICAL MYELOPATHY BY THE JAPANESE ORTHOPAEDIC ASSOCIATION (JOA SCORE)

I. Upper extremity function
  0. Impossible to eat with either chopsticks or spoon
  1. Possible to eat with spoon, but not with chopsticks
  2. Possible to eat with chopsticks, but inadequate
  3. Possible to eat with chopsticks, but awkward
  4. Normal

II. Lower extremity function
  0. Impossible to walk
  1. Need cane or aid on flat ground
  2. Need cane or aid only on stairs
  3. Possible to walk without cane or aid, but slow
  4. Normal

III. Sensory
  A. Upper extremity
    0. Apparent sensory loss
    1. Minimal sensory loss
    2. Normal
  B. Lower extremity, same as A
  C. Trunk, same as A

IV. Bladder function
  0. Complete retention
  1. Severe disturbance
    (1) Inadequate evacuation of the bladder
    (2) Straining
    (3) Dribbling of urine
  2. Mild disturbance
    (1) Urinary frequency
    (2) Urinary hesitancy
  3. Normal

Total 17 points.

Recovery rate = $\dfrac{\text{postoperative condition}^* - \text{preoperative condition}^*}{17 - \text{preoperative condition}^*} \times 100$ (*signifies summated JOA score)

From Hirabayashi, K., Satomi, K., and Sasaki, T.: Ossification of the posterior longitudinal ligament in the cervical spine. *In* Cervical Spine Research Society Editorial Committee (eds.): The Cervical Spine. 2nd ed. Philadelphia, J. B. Lippincott Co., 1989, p. 681.

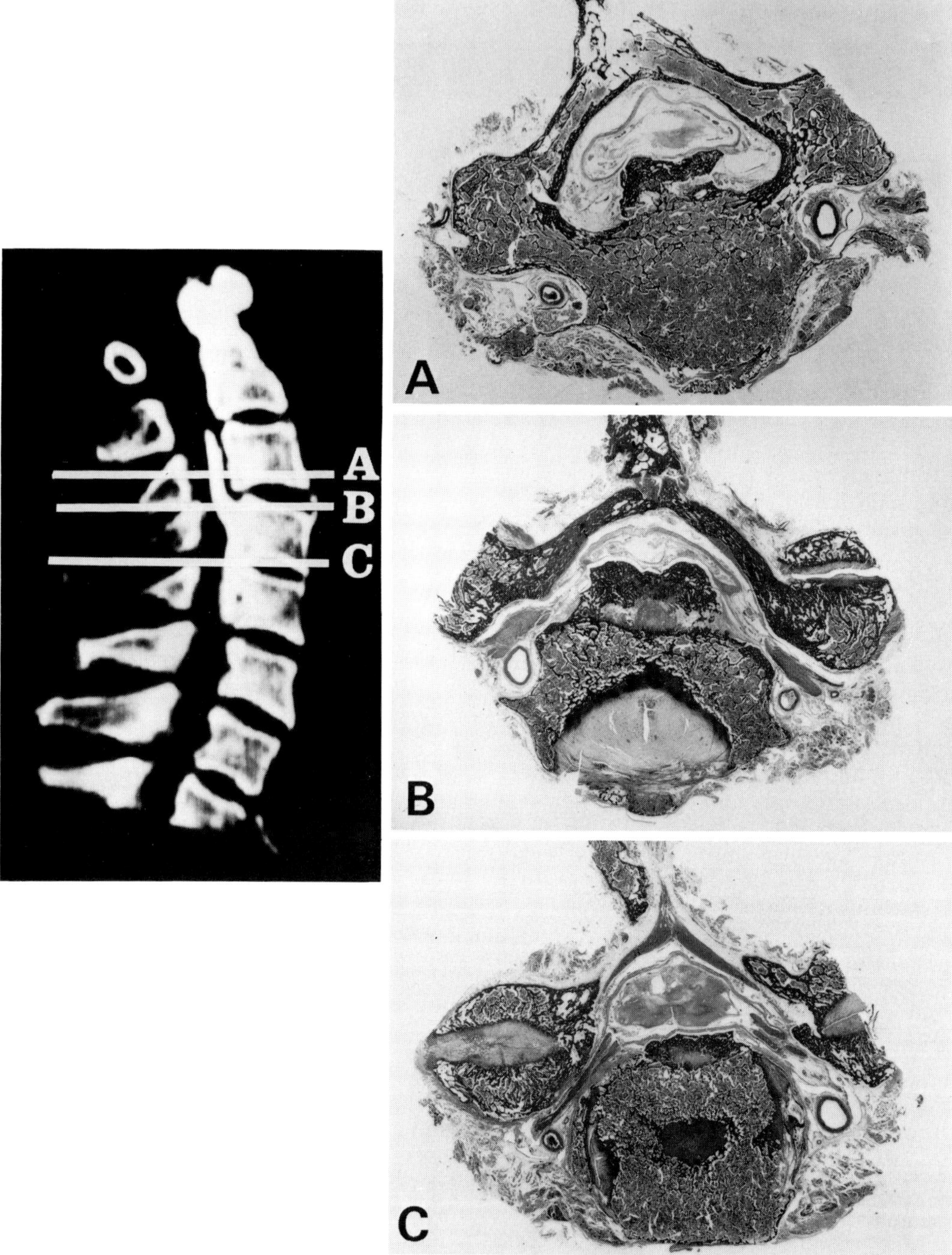

Figure 21–3. *A* to *C*, Horizontal cross section of a specimen autopsied from a case of continuous OPLL in a 74-year-old male. Pathohistologic view (H & E) shows maturated ossification of the ligament and marked damage of the spinal cord. (From Hirabayashi, K., Satomi, K., and Sasaki, T.: Ossification of the posterior longitudinal ligament in the cervical spine. *In* Cervical Spine Research Society Editorial Committee (eds.): The Cervical Spine. 2nd ed. Philadelphia, J. B. Lippincott Co., 1989, p. 680.)

DIAGNOSIS

Plain Film Examination

OPLL can be diagnosed on plain lateral roentgenograms of the cervical spine in patients with myeloradiculopathy. Although the continuous and mixed types of OPLL are generally easily diagnosed, the segmental and localized types of OPLL are sometimes apt to be overlooked (see Fig. 21–1).

Tomography and Plain CT

Tomography is important for the demonstration of small foci of ossification and is indispensable for visualization of the detailed outline of the ossified mass in most cases. CT scanning is most useful for determining the configuration of the ossification in the horizontal cross-section of the spinal canal (see Fig. 21–2).[15, 17, 41] OPLL at the lower cervical levels, which otherwise may be masked by the massive shadows of the shoulder girdles, can be detected by CT scanning with ease. Attention also should be paid to the possibility of a silent OPLL in any patient with myeloradiculopathy of unknown origin, and any patient in whom OPLL is suspected should be examined by tomography and CT scanning.

Myelography and CT after Myelography

Although myelography using water-soluble contrast media sometimes shows complete obstruction to the flow of the contrast medium in severe OPLL, it does not generally show distinct obstruction to the flow of contrast medium, because contrast media pass around OPLL bilaterally. CT after myelography (CTM) does show the flattening of the spinal cord by compression due to OPLL (see Fig. 21–2). It is said that the greater the flattening of the spinal cord, the lower the recovery from clinical symptoms after decompressive surgery.

Magnetic Resonance Imaging

Magnetic resonance imaging (MRI) is not effective to diagnose OPLL because of its low signal, but it does show the pathology of the spinal cord (Fig. 21–4).[7, 18]

Electrophysiologic Examination

Electromyography and motor and sensory nerve conduction studies do not play a large

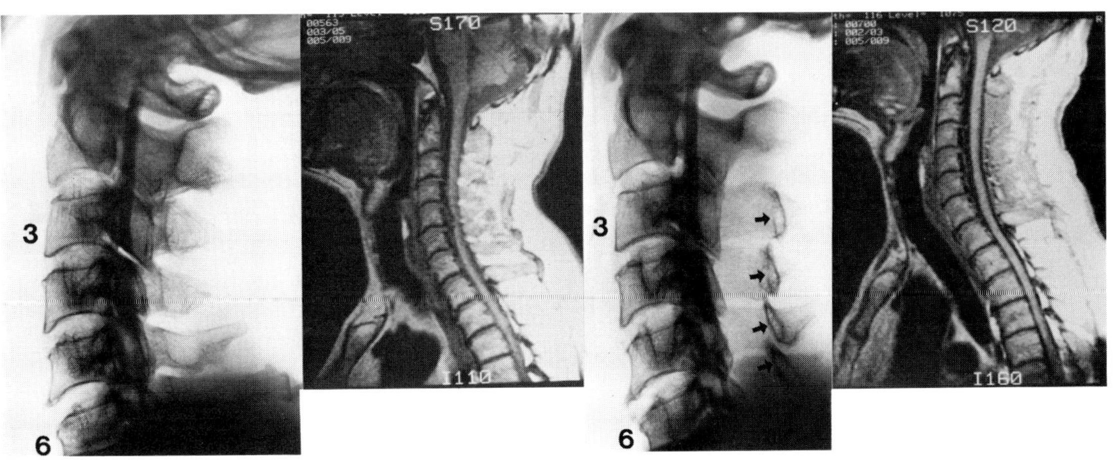

Figure 21–4. OPLLs are shown as low-signal shadows on T1-weighted MRI (TR 500, TE 20). The cervical cord compressed by OPLL anteriorly is decompressed by expansive open-door laminaplasty between C3 and C7.

part in diagnosing the level of spinal lesion in patients with myelopathy due to OPLL. Study of evoked potentials due to median nerve or spinal cord stimulation is effective to diagnose the main spinal lesion in OPLL (Fig. 21–5).[35, 44] Authors reported that the level diagnostic rates of primary lesion in cervical myelopathy determined using evoked potentials were 94.7 per cent in posterior recordings and 74.1 per cent in anterior recordings intraoperatively.[35]

TREATMENT

Conservative Treatment

Conservative treatment for OPLL with myeloradiculopathy consists of continuous skull traction using a halo brace, bed rest with halter traction, and application of a neck brace. Such conservative treatment eliminates dynamic irritating factors, but almost all patients with severe myelopathy cannot be treated sufficiently by conservative therapy.

After more than five years of follow-up, 54.8 per cent of patients with OPLL who were treated conservatively for mild disturbances of ADL showed no change, 26.7 per cent showed improvement, and 18.5 per cent showed aggravation of symptoms.[14]

Surgical Treatment

Surgery in patients with OPLL is indicated in those who have six to 12 points on the JOA score (Table 21–2). This decision should consider patient age. Even if their myelopathy is not as severe, surgery may be indicated when patients are relatively young and have severe

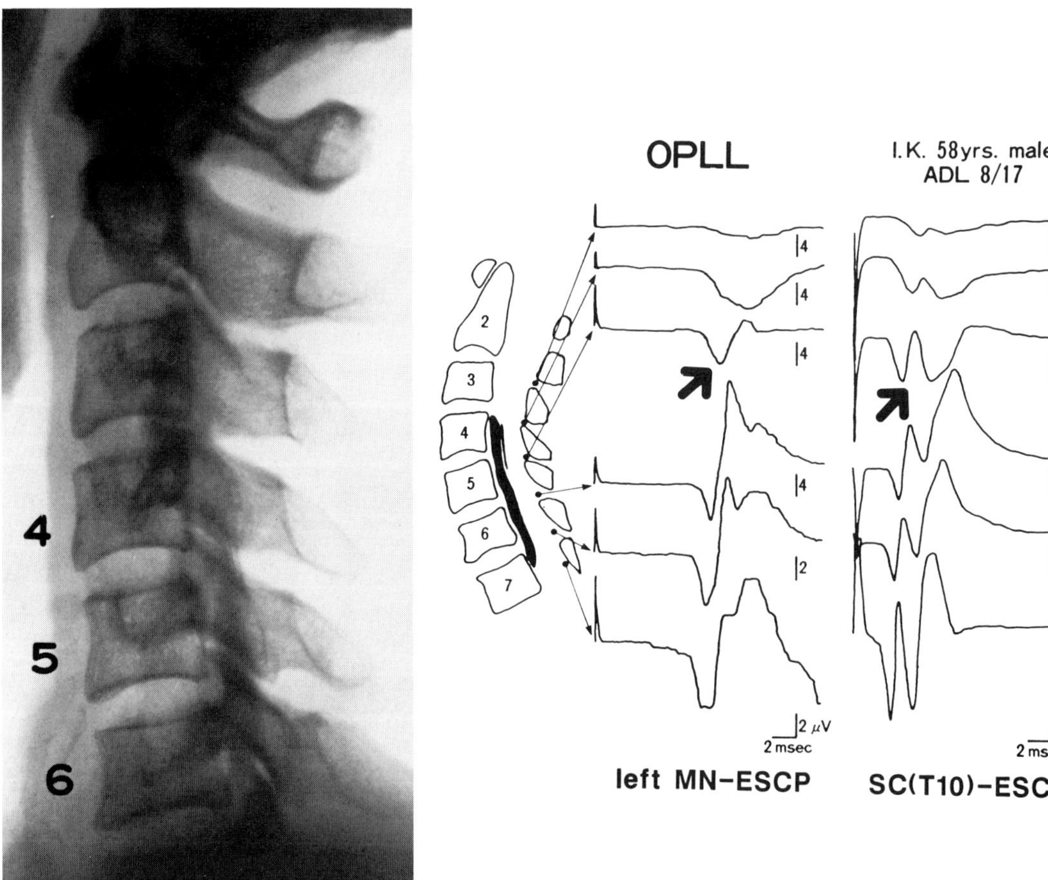

Figure 21–5. Level diagnosis by evoked spinal cord potentials on OPLL. Positivization of potentials is observed at the C4–C5 spinal level on both ESCPs *(arrows)*, and the main lesion in the cervical cord is diagnosed at the C4–C5 level.

spinal stenosis. Patients with radiculopathy who complain of unendurable pain radiating to the upper arm are sometimes operated on as well, if conservative treatment is not effective.

Choice of Operative Methods

Anterior Decompressive Surgery. In the most radical type of operation, the ossified ligaments compressing the spinal cord and causing neurologic symptoms are extirpated or floated anteriorly to obtain anterior decompression.[6] In the segmental and localized types of OPLL below the C3–C4 level, anterior decompression followed by vertebral body fusion is routinely selected when fewer than three disc levels are affected (Fig. 21–6*A, B*).[1, 7, 32, 42]

Anterior interbody fusion without decompression is sometimes effective in cases in which instability exists at the intervertebral space between OPLL, such as in the mixed type of OPLL.[37]

Posterior Decompressive Surgery. In posterior decompressive surgery the spinal cord compressed by OPLL is expected to be decompressed by the posterior shift of the spinal cord.[23] In the continuous type of OPLL, extensive laminectomy and expansive laminaplasty for posterior decompression have been performed.[21] Posterior decompression is performed as far as one level below and above the stenotic site. Nerve root decompression can also be achieved at the open side. Although posterior surgery is not true decompressive surgery for the spinal cord compressed by OPLL anteriorly, it is considered a much safer and easier procedure in the severely deteriorated spinal cord compared with anterior surgery.[2, 28]

Combined Posterior and Anterior Decompressive Surgery. In the case of mixed OPLL, which has locally prominent ossified masses, we have performed a two-stage combined operation when necessary. The first operation, posterior decompression, is performed to provide space posteriorly for compressed spinal cord shifting. Anterior decompression is performed three to six weeks later. This combined posteroanterior operation is probably safer than the anteroposterior procedure.[1, 34]

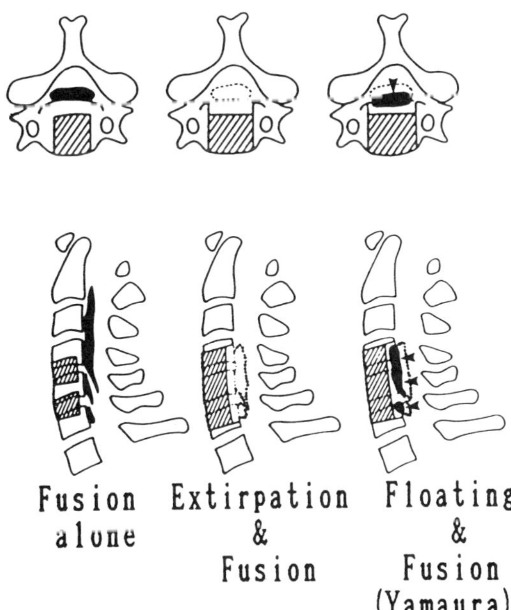

Figure 21–6. Schematic presentation of anterior surgical procedures on OPLL. (From Hirabayashi, K., Satomi, K., and Sasaki, T.: Ossification of the posterior longitudinal ligament in the cervical spine. *In* Cervical Spine Research Society Editorial Committee (eds.): The Cervical Spine. 2nd ed. Philadelphia, J. B. Lippincott Co., 1989, p. 682.)

Operative Technique

Anterior Approach. Cervical spines are exposed anteriorly using the conventional method. Ossified posterior longitudinal ligaments, sometimes with ossified dura, are extirpated or floated, followed by vertebral body fusion with fibula strut after two to three vertebral bodies are resected using an air drill (Fig. 21–7).

This operative procedure produces particularly good results for patients with clumsiness of the fingers, severe intrinsic muscle atrophy caused by lesions of the anterior horn cells, or both, but sometimes causes neurologic complications in the vulnerable spinal cord.

Posterior Approach. In 1968 Kirita introduced a new cervical laminectomy procedure as a safer posterior decompressive method for the compressed spinal cord.[21] It consisted of simultaneous middorsal division of the laminae and excision of the laminae bilaterally after thinning the laminae with an air drill. Oyama and Hattori first devised expansive lamina Z-plasty to prevent postlaminectomy invasion of the laminectomy membrane in 1972 (Fig. 21–8)[29a]; however, this procedure has not been accepted because of the technical difficulties

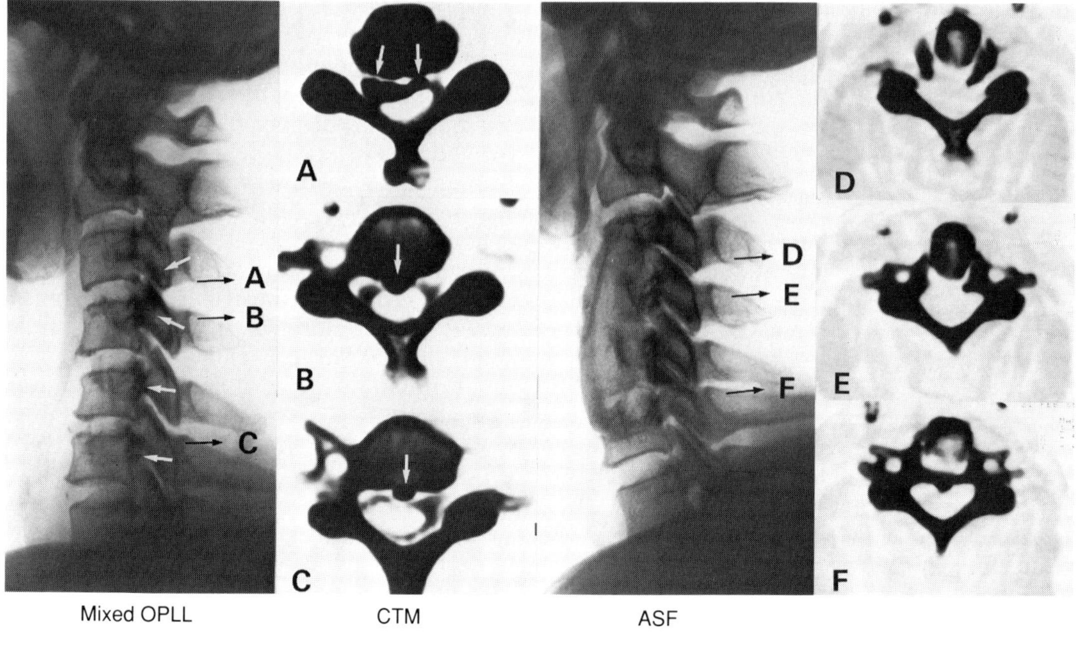

Figure 21–7. Pre- and postoperative x-ray and CT scan of OPLL treated by anterior decompression in a 52-year-old male.

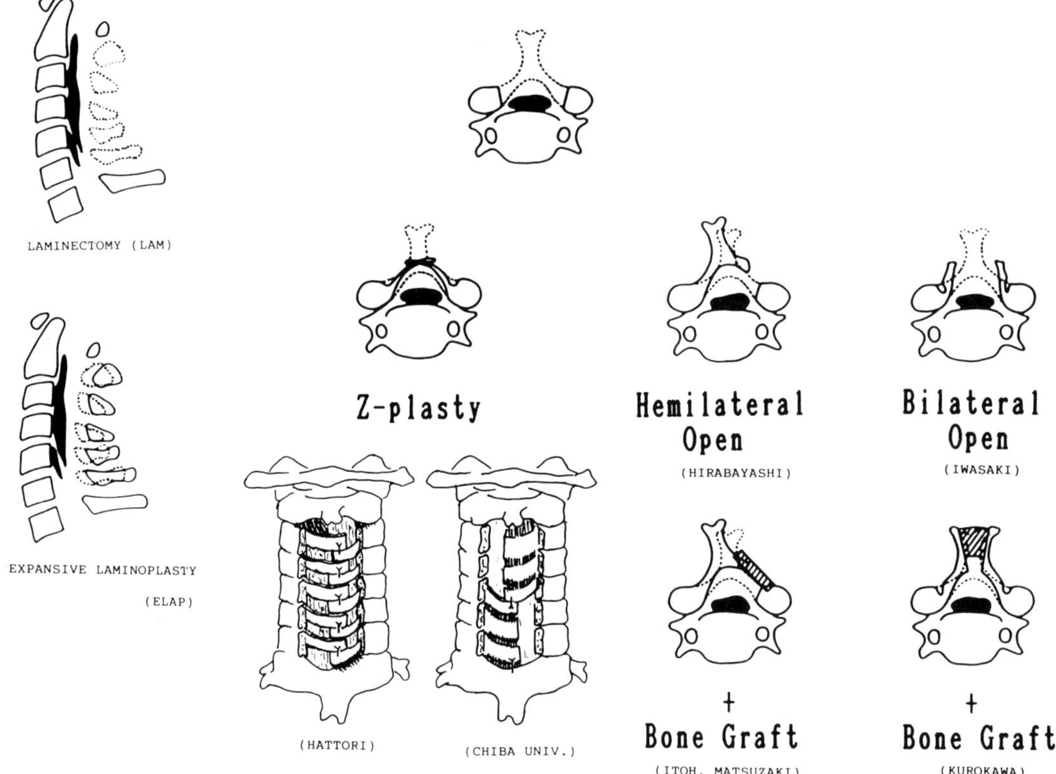

Figure 21–8. Schematic presentation of posterior surgical procedures. Various modifications of expansive laminaplasties are shown.

of the operation. Thus, Hirabayashi devised an open-door expansive laminaplasty for posterior decompression because he had observed dural tube pulsation before resection of the laminae as a whole.[10, 11] This method allows widening of the stenotic spinal canal without the structural loss caused by laminectomy (Fig. 21–9), in which postoperative malalignment, instability, and fragility of the spine to neck trauma may occur. Since then many modifications of laminaplasty have been devised in Japan, such as Itoh's, using wiring; Matsuzaki's, using iliac bone graft; and Kurokawa's, using midlongitudinal bone graft (see Fig. 21–8).[40]

Expansive Open-Door Laminaplasty. ***Operative Procedures.*** The operative procedure is as follows (Fig. 21–10):[11]

1. After the spinal processes and laminae are exposed subperiosteally between one level below and one above the lamina of the stenotic site, the spinous processes are partially resected to be shortened.
2. A bony gutter is drilled laterally and the thinned border of the laminae is excised.
3. Another bony gutter is drilled at the contralateral laminae.
4. Sutures for preventing the laminar door from being closed are stitched around each facet of the hinged side.
5. The spinous processes and laminae are pushed laterally, as if to open a door.
6. The bases of the spinous processes are sutured to keep the laminar door open using the threads stitched in the fourth procedure.

The patient is kept in bed for two days postoperatively, and ambulates using a cervical brace for three months.

Results. Operative results were calculated from the recovery rate using JOA score (see Table 21–2). A recovery rate over 75 per cent is considered an excellent operative result; over 50 per cent is good; over 25 per cent is slightly good; and less than 25 per cent is unchanged or fair.

The operative results in 107 cases of OPLL

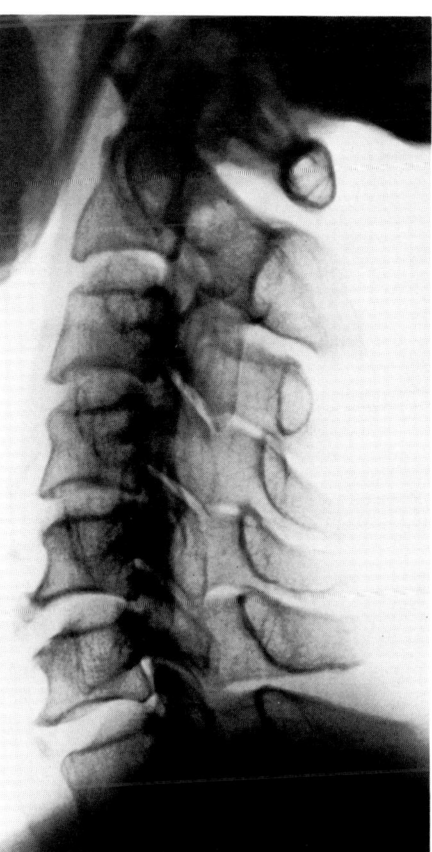

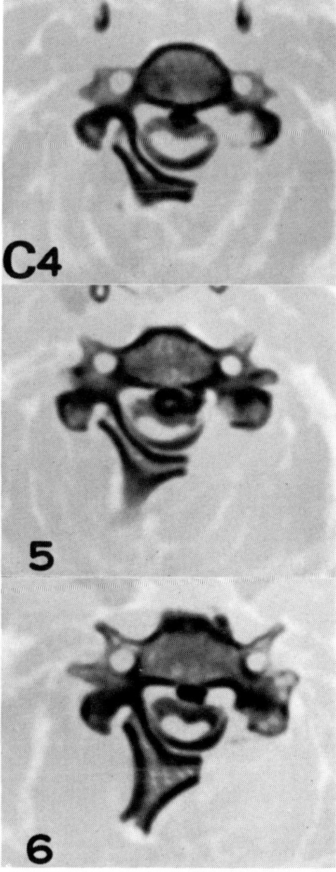

Figure 21–9. Postoperative x-ray and CT myelogram of OPLL treated by expansive open-door laminaplasty from C3 to C7 (Hirabayashi). Posterior shift of the spinal cord and recovery of the metrizamide ring around the spinal cord are observed on CT myelogram (same case as in Fig. 21–2).

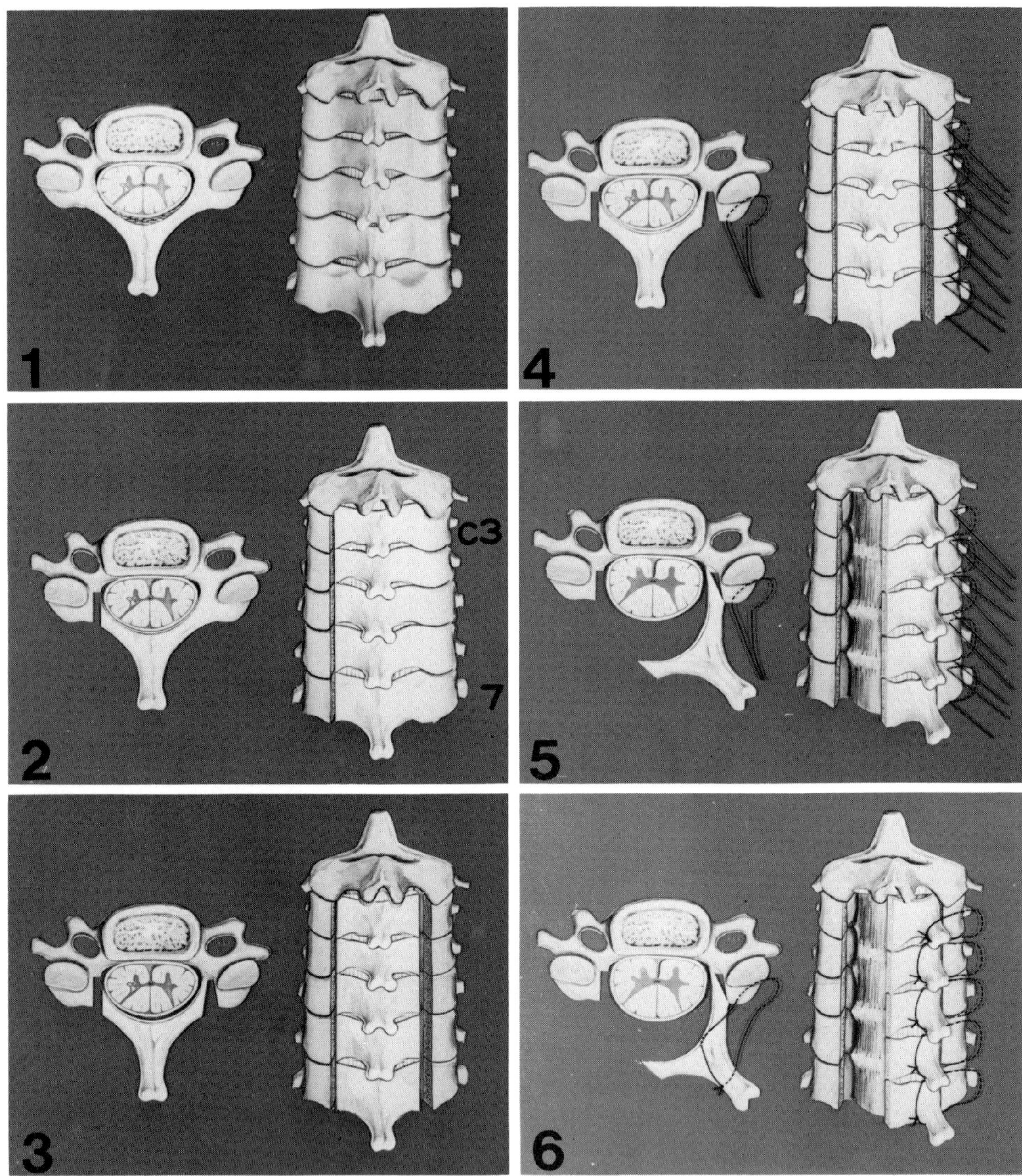

Figure 21–10. Schematic presentation of expansive open-door laminaplasty (Hirabayashi). (From Hirabayashi, K., Satomi, K., and Sasaki, T.: Ossification of the posterior longitudinal ligament in the cervical spine. *In* Cervical Spine Research Society Editorial Committee (eds.): The Cervical Spine. 2nd ed. Philadelphia, J. B. Lippincott Co., 1989, p. 688.)

treated with various procedures have been reported. The average JOA score was 8.3 preoperatively and 13.2 postoperatively. The average rate of recovery was 58.3 per cent and satisfactory improvement in over 50 per cent of recovery rates was obtained in 71 per cent of the patients operated. Comparing the results with operative methods shows that patients treated by expansive open-door laminaplasty had the highest recovery rate (62.2 per cent), although there the indications for operative methods differed for each case (Table 21–3).[13]

Complications. Closure of the opened laminae is one of the complications of open-door laminaplasty. It is possible to keep the canal open successfully by adding stay sutures, which are fastened between and around the bases of the spinous processes, deep muscles, and capsules around the facets in the position of an open door (see Fig. 21–10).

Other complications are transient muscle paraparesis of the shoulder girdle and severe neck pain, resulting from the tethering effect of the nerve roots of C5 or C6 and disjointing of the hinge. Disjointing of the hinge occurs easily in floating laminae and is followed by closure of the laminar door.[11] To prevent this complication, it is important that the hinge side of the bony gutter be drilled after completing resection of the medial side of the bony gutter at the open side (see Fig. 21–10). The hinge stability should be checked frequently by pushing the spinous processes.[11] Although there is no way to prevent complications resulting from the tethering effect of the nerve roots, spontaneous recovery can be expected in most cases.

Significance. Open-door laminaplasty for posterior decompression of the spinal cord has the following advantages:

Table 21–3. OPERATIVE RESULTS FOR OPLL

	No. of Cases	Recovery Rate (%)
Laminectomy (LAM)	28	53.4
Expansive laminaplasty (ELP)	54	62.8
Anterior spinal fusion (ASF)	16	57.7
LAM / ELP } and ASF	9	53.1
Total	107	

From Hirabayashi, K., Satomi, K., and Sasaki, T.: Ossification of the posterior longitudinal ligament in the cervical spine. *In* Cervical Spine Research Society Editorial Committee (eds.): The Cervical Spine. 2nd ed. Philadelphia, J. B. Lippincott Co., 1989, p. 689.

1. The operative technique is relatively easier and safer than others.
2. Postoperative supportability is better than laminectomy.
3. Postoperative dynamic factor can be eliminated, because the range of motion of the preoperative cervical spine has been reduced to 50 per cent by ankylosing of the bony gutter on the hinge side.

In the continuous and mixed types of OPLL, the ossified ligaments may be biologically stimulated by the operative procedure, which may accelerate the postoperative growth of OPLL, as shown by the higher incidence of postoperative growth of OPLL compared with nonoperative cases. The structural weakness caused by laminectomy may evoke postoperative growth of OPLL as a compensatory process. This is shown by the fact that the incidence of the postoperative growth of OPLL in the laminectomy group was higher than that in the laminectomy group—especially the incidence of transverse growth. The mobility at the intervertebral space between the OPLL may also cause postoperative growth of OPLL, shown by the fact that development from the mixed to the continuous type of OPLL was observed with elimination of mobility at the involved disc space, whereas pseudarthrosis-like thickening is seen at the mobile disc space.

Combined Approach. Anterior decompression by excision of OPLL followed by interbody fusion is applied three to six weeks after expansive open-door laminaplasty (Fig. 21–11).[34]

Factors Influencing Operative Results of OPLL

After observations of these cases, it was concluded that the operative results of surgery for OPLL were influenced by preoperative factors such as disability of ADL, duration of the myelopathic symptoms, age of the patient, onset with or without trauma, stenotic condition of the spinal canal, and kyphotic curvature of the spine. Better operative results could not have been obtained in the patients over 65 years old; those with severe disability of ADL (less than seven points on JOA score); those with myelopathy for more than two years preoperatively; those with traumatic onset; and

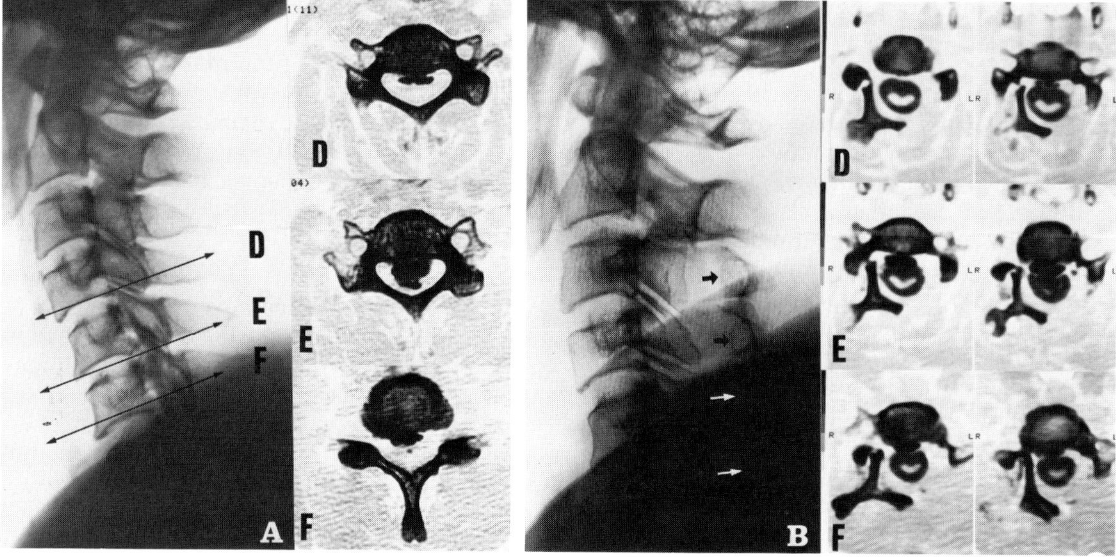

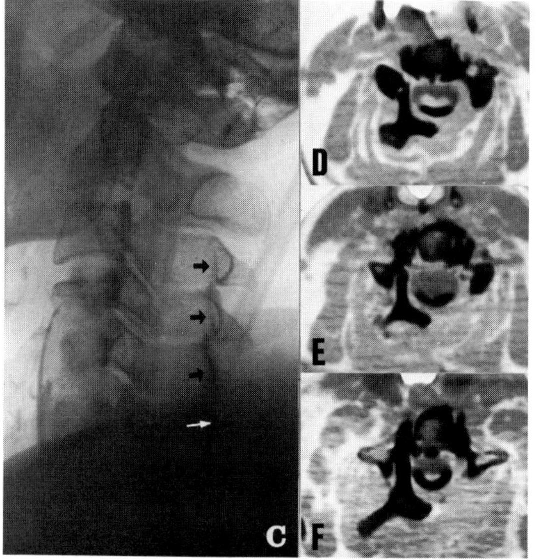

Figure 21–11. Roentgenogram and CT scan of OPLL in a 57-year-old female who was treated by combined staged decompressive surgeries. OPLL between C4 and C7 *(A)* is widely occupied in the spinal canal on CT. Posterior shift of the spinal cord is observed on CT myelogram after expansive laminoplasty (ELP) from C3 to C7 *(B)*. Three weeks later anterior decompression by extirpation of OPLL followed by anterior spinal fusion (ASF) between C4 and C7 is performed *(C)*, and flattening of the spinal cord is recovered on CT myelogram.

those with severe stenosis of the spinal canal (more than 60 per cent on rate of stenosis) and kyphotic curvature of the spine.

OPLL sometimes grows in either a longitudinal or transverse direction, although growth in the continuous and mixed types is more frequent than in the segmental type, which also influenced the long-term outcome. After more than five years of follow-up, the overall incidences of longitudinal and transverse growth of OPLL were reported as 24 per cent and 11 per cent respectively in the 338 nonoperative cases, and as 28 per cent and 24 per cent respectively in the 295 operative cases.[14] In our series, incidences of postoperative growth of the continuous and mixed types of OPLL was 89 per cent in the laminectomized group, 34 per cent in those with laminaplasty, and 20 per cent in the anterior spinal fusion group (Table 21–4). A comparison between the laminectomized group and laminaplastied group found a significant difference in trans-

Table 21–4. INCIDENCE OF POSTOPERATIVE GROWTH OF OPLL (CONTINUOUS AND MIXED TYPE)

LAM	16/18 cases (89%)
ELP	12/35 cases (34%)
ASF	1/5 cases (20%)
LAM and ASF	2/4 cases (50%)
ELP and ASF	0/4 cases (0%)

From Hirabayashi, K., Satomi, K., and Sasaki, T.: Ossification of the posterior longitudinal ligament in the cervical spine. *In* Cervical Spine Research Society Editorial Committee (eds.): The Cervical Spine. 2nd ed. Philadelphia, J. B. Lippincott Co., 1989, p. 689. ASF, anterior spinal fusion; ELP, expansive laminoplasty; LAM, laminectomy.

verse growth but not in longitudinal growth. Thus, the frequency of OPLL without growth was three to four times higher in the laminaplastied patients than in laminectomized patients, although the follow-up time of each group was different. Progression to the final stage of ossification, such as from the mixed type to the continuous type of OPLL, was frequently observed in cases of OPLL with growth in laminaplastied patients.

References

1. Abe, H., Tsuru, M., Ito, T., et al.: Anterior decompression for ossification of the posterior longitudinal ligament of the cervical spine. J. Neurosurg. *55:*108–116, 1981.
2. Bakay, L., Cares, H. L., and Smith, R. J.: Ossification in the region of the posterior longitudinal ligament as a cause of cervical myelopathy. J. Neurol. Neurosurg. Psychiatry *33:*263–268, 1970.
3. Dietemann, J. L., Dirheimer, Y., Babin, E., et al.: Ossification of the posterior longitudinal ligament (Japanese disease), a radiological study in 12 cases. J. Neuroradiol. *12:*212–222, 1985.
4. Firooznia, H., Rafii, M., Golimbu, C., et al.: Computed tomography of calcification and ossification of posterior longitudinal ligament of the spine. J. Comput. Tomogr. *8:*317–324, 1984.
5. Gui, L., Merlini, L., Savini, R., and Davidovits, P.: Cervical myelopathy due to ossification of the posterior longitudinal ligament. Ital. J. Orthop. Traumatol. *9:*269–280, 1983.
6. Hanai, K., Inouye, Y., Kawai, K., et al.: Anterior decompression for myelopathy resulting from ossification of the posterior longitudinal ligament. J. Bone Joint Surg. *64B:*561–564, 1982.
7. Harsh, G. R., IV, Sypert, G. W., Weinstein, P. R., et al.: Cervical spine stenosis to ossification of the posterior longitudinal ligament. J. Neurosurg. *67:*349–357, 1987.
8. Hashizume, Y.: Pathological studies on the ossification of the posterior longitudinal ligament (OPLL). Acta. Pathol. Jpn. *30:*255–273, 1980.
9. Hashizume, Y., Iijima, S., Kishimoto, H., and Yanagi, T.: Pathology of spinal cord lesions caused by ossification of the posterior longitudinal ligament. Acta Neuropathol. *63:*123–130, 1984.
10. Hirabayashi, K., Miyakawa, J., Satami, K., et al.: Operative results and postoperative progression of ossification among patients with cervical posterior longitudinal ligament. Spine *6:*354–364, 1981.
11. Hirabayashi, K., and Satomi, K.: Operative procedure and results of expansive open-door laminaplasty. Spine *13:*870–876, 1988.
12. Hosino, Y., Kurokawa, T., Iizuka, T., et al.: Calcium metabolism in OPLL. Seikeigeka Mook (Jpn) *50:*146–151, 1987.
13. Ichimura, S., Hirabayashi, K., Satomi, K., et al.: Results of surgical treatment for cervical myelopathy caused by ossification of the posterior longitudinal ligament. Rinshouseikei (Jpn) *23:*555–562, 1988.
14. Japanese Ministry of Public Health and Welfare: Investigation Committee Reports on OPLL. Tokyo, 1981–1985.
15. Kadoya, S., Nakamura, T., and Tada, A.: Neuroradiology of ossification of the posterior longitudinal spinal ligament: comparative studies with computer tomography. Neuroradiology *16:*357–358, 1978.
16. Key, C. A.: Paraplegia depending on disease of the ligaments of the spine. Guys Hosp. Rep. *3:*17–34, 1838.
17. Klara, M., and McDonnell, D. E.: Ossification of the posterior longitudinal ligament in caucasians: diagnosis and surgical intervention. Neurosurgery *19:*212–217, 1986.
18. McAfee, P. C., Regan, J. J., and Bohlman, H. H.: Cervical cord compression from ossification of the posterior longitudinal ligament in non-orientals. J. Bone Joint Surg. *69B:*569–575, 1987.
19. Minagi, H., and Gronner, A. T.: Calcification of the posterior longitudinal ligament: a cause of cervical myelopathy. Am. J. Roentgenol. *105:*365–369, 1969.
20. Mitsui, H., Sonozaki, H., Juji, T., et al.: Ankylosing spinal hyperostosis (ASH) and ossification of the posterior longitudinal ligament (OPLL). Arch. Orthop. Traumat. Surg. *94:*21–23, 1979.
21. Miyazaki, K., and Kirita, Y.: Extensive simultaneous multisegment laminectomy for myelopathy due to the ossification of the posterior longitudinal ligament in the cervical region. Spine *11:*531–542, 1986.
22. Murakami, N., Muroga, T., and Sobue, I.: Cervical myelopathy due to ossification of the posterior longitudinal ligament: a clinicopathologic study. Arch. Neurol. *35:*33–36, 1978.
23. Nagashima, C.: Cervical myelopathy due to ossification of the posterior longitudinal ligament. J. Neurosurg. *37:*653–660, 1972.
24. Nakanishi, T., Mannen, T., and Tokoyura, Y.: Asymptomatic ossification of the posterior longitudinal ligament of the cervical spine: incidence and roentgenographic findings. J. Neurol. Sci. *19:*375–381, 1973.
25. Nakanishi, T., Mannen, T., Tokoyura, Y., et al.: Symptomatic ossification of the cervical spine. Neurology *24:*1139–1143, 1974.

26. Ohtsuka, K., Terayama, K., Yanagihara, M., et al.: An epidemiological survey on ossification of ligaments in the cervical and thoracic spine in individuals over 50 years of age. J. Jpn. Orthop. Assoc. *60:*1087–1098, 1986.
27. Okamoto, Y., and Yasuma, T.: Ossification of the posterior longitudinal ligament of cervical spine with or without myelopathy. J. Jpn. Orthop. Assoc. *40:*1349–1360, 1967.
28. Onji, Y., Akiyama, H., Shimomura, Y., et al.: Posterior paravertebral ossification causing cervical myelopathy: a report of eighteen cases. J. Bone Joint Surg. *49A:*1314–1328, 1967.
29. Ono, K., Ota, H., Tada, K., et al.: Ossified posterior longitudinal ligament, a clinicopathologic study. Spine *2:*126–138, 1977.
29a. Oyama, M., Hattori, S., Moriwaki, N., et al.: A new method of cervical laminectomy. Chubuseisaisi (Jpn) *16*:792–794, 1973.
30. Pouchot, J., Watts, C. S., Esdaile, J. M., and Hill, R. O.: Sudden quadriplegia complicating ossification longitudinal ligament and diffuse idiopathic skeletal hyperostosis. Arthritis Rheum. *30:*1069–1072, 1987.
31. Resnick, D., Guerra, J., Jr., Robinson, C. A., and Vint, V. C.: Association of diffuse idiopathic skeletal hyperostosis (DISH) and calcification and ossification of the posterior longitudinal ligament. Am. J. Roentgenol. *131:*1049–1053, 1978.
32. Sakou, T., Miyazaki, A., Tomimura, K., et al.: Ossification of the posterior longitudinal ligament of the cervical spine: subtotal vertebrectomy as a treatment. Clin. Orthop. *140:*58–65, 1979.
33. Sasaki, T., Shiobara, H., Ogawa, K., et al.: An autopsy report of OPLL. *In* Japanese Ministry of Public Health and Welfare: Investigation Committee Reports on OPLL. (Jpn) Tokyo, 1980, pp. 127–130.
34. Satomi, K., Hirabayashi, K., Itoh, Y., et al.: Two-staged posterior and anterior decompressive surgery for cervical myelopathy with narrowed spinal canal. Seikeigeka (Jpn) *28:*1617–1626, 1977.
35. Satomi, K., Okuma, T., Kenmotsu, K., et al.: Level diagnosis of cervical myelopathy using evoked spinal cord potentials. Spine *13:*1217–1224, 1988.
36. Terayama, K.: The ossification of the cervical posterior longitudinal ligament. J. Jpn. Orthop. Assoc. *50:*415–442, 1976.
37. Tominaga, S.: The effects of intervertebral fusion in patients with myelopathy due to ossification of the posterior longitudinal ligament of the cervical spine. Int. Orthop. *4:*183–191, 1980.
38. Tsukimoto, H.: A case report: autopsy of syndrome of compression of spinal cord owing to ossification within spinal canal of cervical spine. Nippon Geka Hokan (Jpn) *29:*1003–1007, 1960.
39. Tsuyama, N., Terayama, K., Ohtani, K., et al.: The ossification of the posterior longitudinal ligament of the spine (OPLL). J. Jpn. Orthop. Assoc. *55:*425–440, 1981.
40. Tsuyama, N.: Ossification of the posterior longitudinal ligament of the spine. Clin. Orthop. *184:*71–84, 1984.
41. Yamamoto, I., Kageyama, N., Nakamura, K., et al.: Computed tomography in ossification of the posterior longitudinal ligament in the cervical spine. Surg. Neurol. *12:*414–418, 1979.
42. Yamaura, I.: Pathogenesis and treatment of the ossification of the posterior longitudinal ligament. J. Jpn. Orthop. Assoc. *63:*355–369, 1989.
43. Yanagi, T., Kato, H., Yamamura, Y., et al.: Ossification of spinal ligaments. Rinsho Sinkei (Jpn) *12:*571–577, 1972.
44. Yu, Y. L., Leong, J. C. Y., Fang, D., et al.: Cervical myelopathy due to ossification of the posterior longitudinal ligament. Brain *111:*769–783, 1988.

CHAPTER

22

THORACIC DISC DISEASE

Bradford L. Currier, M.D.
Frank J. Eismont, M.D.
Barth A. Green, M.D.

Thoracic disc herniation is an uncommon condition that, in the past, was difficult to diagnose. The many different presenting symptoms often delay diagnosis. Surgery generally is regarded as the treatment of choice for a symptomatic herniated thoracic disc to prevent the sequelae of cord compression. The prognosis associated with decompression by laminectomy, previously dismal, has improved dramatically with the advent of techniques for disc excision without cord manipulation. Advances in imaging technology are revolutionizing the diagnosis of thoracic disc disease and may improve the prognosis further.

HISTORICAL BACKGROUND

Key wrote the first report, in 1838, of a herniated thoracic disc causing spinal cord injury.[40] Middleton and Teacher reported the second case 73 years later.[55] The first recorded surgical procedure on a patient with a herniated thoracic disc was performed by Adson in 1922.[49] In their classic 1934 monograph on ruptured intervertebral discs, Mixter and Barr described four cases of thoracic disc herniation; two of the three patients treated surgically were rendered paraplegic, emphasizing the challenge to management of the disease.[56] In the ensuing years a number of reports helped to define the disease and to document that treatment by laminectomy is unpredictable and exceedingly risky.[1, 8, 26, 28, 33, 36, 41, 47, 49, 61, 74, 76, 77]

The costotransversectomy approach was introduced by Ménard in 1900; the slight modification of it by Capener was shown to be effective in Pott's disease.[15, 54] At Alexander's suggestion, Hulme was the first to use this approach in the management of a herniated thoracic disc.[4, 36] In 1960 Hulme reported his experience in six patients treated by costotransversectomy and demonstrated that it was a safer, more effective approach than laminectomy.[36] In a review of 49 cases reported in the literature, 82 per cent of the patients improved, 14 per cent were unchanged, and only 4 per cent were made worse by the procedure.[6]

Hodgson and Stock popularized the anterior approach to the spine for the treatment of Pott's disease.[35] In 1958, Crafoord and associates reported the first transthoracic procedure on the spine for a herniated disc.[20] They performed a "fenestration" or windowing of the disc without any attempt at disc removal or cord decompression. The one patient described in their paper did well. Simultaneous reports by Perot and Munro and Ransohoff and associates in 1969 established transthoracic spinal cord decompression as a viable alternative to costotransversectomy.[62, 63]

The posterolateral approach was described

by Carson and associates in 1971 and was modified by Patterson and Arbit in 1978.[16, 60]

All the approaches have undergone minor modifications, including the application of microsurgical techniques.[46, 69, 71] Each technique has advantages and disadvantages, and all but laminectomy are currently acceptable.

Over the past two years, numerous investigators have reported on the use of magnetic resonance imaging (MRI) to diagnose herniated thoracic discs.[12, 17, 29, 66] MRI seems likely to replace myelography as the standard for the diagnosis of this condition in the near future. Because MRI is rapid, noninvasive, and increasingly available, this undoubtedly will decrease delay in diagnosis, leading to earlier treatment and perhaps improved prognosis. The new challenge will be to avoid overdiagnosis and unnecessary operations on asymptomatic lesions.[81]

INCIDENCE

Because of the difficulty in making the diagnosis, herniated thoracic discs probably are more common than reported. Thoracic disc excision accounts for 0.22 to 1.8 per cent of all operations performed on herniated discs.[1, 8, 48, 49, 58, 59, 71, 77] Logue reported an incidence of 4 per cent but believed that selection bias had exaggerated the true incidence.[47] Carson and associates believed that the true prevalence of patients who have neurologic abnormalities from a protruded thoracic disc is one per million per year.[16] Many cases must be either unrecognized or asymptomatic.

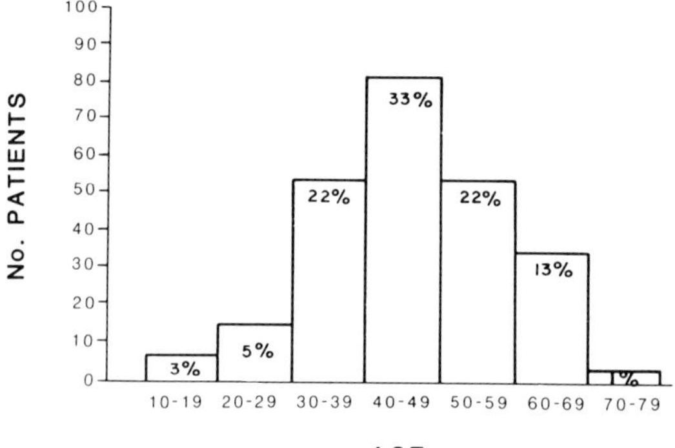

Figure 22–1. Distribution of 238 cases of thoracic disc herniation according to age. (From Arce, C. A., and Dohrmann, G. J.: Herniated thoracic discs. Neurol. Clin. *3*:383–392, 1985.)

In a group of 270 patients undergoing computed tomography (CT) of the thorax for suspected malignancy, Ryan and associates found four (1.5 per cent) who had asymptomatic calcified herniated thoracic discs.[68] A cadaver study by Haley and Perry showed that 11 per cent of unselected autopsies reveal protruded thoracic discs; two of 99 specimens in their series had discs protruding 4 to 7 mm into the canal.[32] With the advent of MRI, the diagnosis is being made much more frequently. Ross and associates diagnosed 20 cases (16 confirmed) by MRI in a two-year period.[66] This contrasts with the report by Love and Kiefer in 1949 of 17 cases seen over 26 years.[48]

PATIENT PROFILE

The typical patient is a man about 50 years of age. In a review of 288 cases reported in the literature, Arce and Dohrmann found a slight male preponderance (1.5:1).[6] Eighty per cent of the patients were in their fourth to sixth decades; 33 per cent were in their fifth decade (Fig. 22–1). Cases have been reported in patients as young as age 11 years and as old as 75 years.[13, 16, 59]

CLINICAL PRESENTATION

There is extreme variation in the clinical presentation of patients with a herniated thoracic disc. This explains why no clear-cut syndrome has been identified. The signs and symptoms depend on location of herniation in the sagittal as well as the transverse plane, size of the lesion, duration of compression, degree of vascular compromise, size of the bony canal, and health of the spinal cord.

In general, the condition is dynamic and the symptoms progress.[33] Tovi and Strang outlined the usual chronologic progression, which begins with pain followed by sensory disturbances, weakness, and finally bowel and bladder dysfunction.[77] Arce and Dohrmann confirmed this pattern in their review of the literature: of 179 patients who described their initial symptom, 57 per cent reported pain, 24 per cent reported sensory disturbance, 17 per cent noted motor weakness, and 2 per cent described bladder dysfunction (Table 22–1).[6] By the time of presentation, 90 per cent of the patients had signs and symptoms of cord com-

Table 22–1. INITIAL SYMPTOMS OF PROTRUDED THORACIC DISC

Initial Symptom	Number of Patients	Per cent
Pain	102	57
Sensory	42	24
Motor	31	17
Bladder	4	2

From Arce, C. A., and Dohrmann, G. J.: Herniated thoracic disks. Neurol. Clin. *3*:383–392, 1985.

pression, 61 per cent had both motor and sensory complaints, and 30 per cent had bowel or bladder dysfunction (Table 22–2). The duration of symptoms before presentation varied from hours to 16 years in one series.[49]

The pain can be midline, unilateral, or bilateral, depending on the location of the herniation. In some cases, there may be no pain. Coughing and sneezing may aggravate the pain, as with herniated discs in the cervical and lumbar regions. With herniation of the T1 disc, the pain may be in the neck and upper extremity, simulating a cervical disc problem and causing upper extremity numbness, intrinsic muscle weakness, and Horner's syndrome.[1, 31, 60]

When the herniation is in the midthoracic spine, radiation of pain into the chest or abdomen can simulate cardiac or abdominal disease, clouding an already complex clinical picture. In the four cases reported by Epstein, one underwent an unnecessary thoracotomy for excision of a pericardial cyst and in another hysterectomy and salpingo-oophorectomy were performed; a third patient almost underwent an abdominal exploration for endometriosis before the true cause of her symptoms was identified.[26] Pain from a lower thoracic disc herniation may radiate to the groin, simulating ureteral calculi or renal disease.[75] Herniated discs at the lowest thoracic levels can impinge on the cauda equina as well as on the distal spinal cord, causing lower extremity pain and mimicking a herniated lumbar disc. On physical examination, flexion of the neck may induce back or root pain with lesions below the midthoracic level.[16] A thorough neurologic examination is mandatory, and the examiner should pay close attention to long tract signs and other evidence of myelopathy.

Table 22–2. PRESENTING SYMPTOMS OF THORACIC DISC HERNIATION

	Number of Patients	Per cent
Motor and sensory	131	61
Brown-Séquard syndrome	18	9
Sensory symptoms only	33	15
Motor symptoms only	13	6
Radicular pain only	20	9
Bladder or sphincter	65	30

From Arce, C. A., and Dohrmann, G. J.: Herniated thoracic disks. Neurol. Clin. *3*:383–392, 1985.

Some investigators believe that the occurrence of pronounced sensory changes with relatively minor motor deficits is highly suggestive of a herniated thoracic disc.[16, 42] Sensory disturbances, motor weakness, sphincter dysfunction, and gait abnormalities should direct the examiner's attention to the nervous system as the source of the problem.

LEVEL AND CLASSIFICATION OF HERNIATION

Three fourths of the cases occur between T8 and L1; the peak is at T11–T12, where 26 per cent of herniations occur (Fig. 22–2).[6] Herniations are distinctly uncommon in the upper thoracic spine.[6, 31, 60] Haley and Perry found a similar distribution in their cadaver study of 99 spines and theorized that the increased incidence in the thoracolumbar area is due to the greater degree of motion in this region.[32] The reason that the incidence at T11–T12 is greater than that at T12–L1 (9 per cent) may be the facet orientation. Malmivaara and associates believed that the frontally oriented facets in the upper thoracolumbar region have less torsional resistance than the sagitally oriented facets at T12–L1; therefore, the T11–T12 disc is exposed to greater stress and has a higher likelihood of degeneration.[52]

Herniated thoracic discs can be classified by location or by symptoms. Most authors describe the location of the herniation as central, centrolateral, or lateral, and roughly 70 per cent of the cases are either central or centrolateral.[6] Abbott and Retter classified cases by symptoms and reported that lateral protrusions cause root compression and patients have radicular pain and minimal or no signs of cord compression.[1] Patients with herniation of central discs in the upper and middle thoracic spine have myelopathy. Protrusions at T11 and T12 compress the conus and cauda equina and

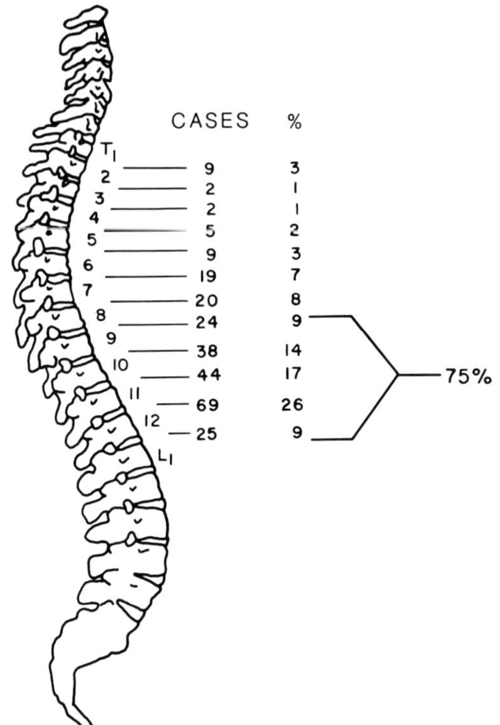

Figure 22–2. Levels of thoracic disc protrusion in 258 cases. (From Arce, C. A., and Dohrmann, G. J.: Herniated thoracic discs. Neurol. Clin. *3*:383–392, 1985.)

may cause pain referred to the lower limbs and sphincter disturbance.

Few cases of intradural herniation of thoracic discs have been reported, suggesting that the incidence is low.[27, 28, 37, 38, 49, 60, 77] In Love and Schorn's series of 61 cases, however, there were seven in which the disc had eroded through the anterior dura, an incidence of 11 per cent.[49]

The exact incidence of multiple-level herniations is not known.[1, 12, 19, 74] Arseni and Nash reviewed the literature in 1960 and found multiple herniations in only four of the 106 cases reported.[8] A report by Bohlman and Zdeblick suggests that the incidence may be much higher than previously recognized, however.[12] Of their 19 patients, three (16 per cent) had herniations at two levels. The sensitivity of MRI may be partially responsible for this increased frequency.[29, 66] Ross and associates reported that three (23 per cent) of 13 patients diagnosed by MRI had multiple-level involvement.[66] This is similar to the findings in Haley and Perry's autopsy study, in which two of seven patients had more than one protruded disc.[32]

Van Landingham suggested an association between Scheuermann's disease and multiple-level herniation, but a report by Lesoin and associates of six cases of single-level herniations in patients with Scheuermann's disease makes it unlikely that there is a significant association.[45, 79]

CAUSE

The role of trauma in the cause of herniated thoracic discs is controversial. A history of trauma can be elicited in 14 to 63 per cent of patients.[11, 12] The mean incidence in ten random series was 34 per cent. In some patients the causal relationship is undeniable; in others, trauma may have been an aggravating factor or purely coincidental. The degree of trauma reported as responsible for the herniation ranges from minor twisting strains and chiropractic manipulation to major falls or motor vehicle accidents.[43]

Most authors favor degenerative processes as the major causative factor in the development of a herniation.[6, 32, 49] This theory is supported by the higher incidence of herniation in the thoracolumbar spine, where greater degenerative changes take place.[75]

Several authors have suggested an association between Scheuermann's disease and herniated thoracic discs.[12, 45, 79] The primary pathogenetic process in the disease or secondary disc degeneration may be the factors promoting herniation.

PATHOGENESIS

The pathogenesis of neurologic compromise secondary to herniated thoracic discs is believed to be a combination of direct neural compression and vascular insufficiency.[8, 47, 49, 55, 60] Middleton and Teacher suggested this in a case report as early as 1911.[55] Severe back pain developed while this patient was lifting a heavy object. Approximately 20 hours later, he felt a sudden severe pain shoot from his chest to his feet and he became almost completely paraplegic. He died 16 days later from urosepsis. The autopsy revealed a herniated thoracic disc opposite a section of cord that was compressed, degenerated, and hemorrhagic. A thrombosed vessel was found in the section of cord showing the most hemorrhage.

Several anatomic features make the thoracic cord vulnerable to manipulation and trauma.[60] The thoracic spinal canal is small, and most of its available space is occupied by the cord. The blood supply to the cord is tenuous in this region, especially in the "critical zone" of T4–T9.[23] In addition, thoracic disc protrusions are more common centrally than laterally, are often calcified, and may adhere to or penetrate the dura.[6, 34, 47, 49, 50, 62, 77]

The theory of direct compression causing neural compromise is supported by Logue's report of a patient who died after a 14-month course of progressive paraplegia.[47] The autopsy showed extreme distortion of the cord, but the anterior spinal artery and vein were patent and showed no evidence of damage.

Kahn suggested that, in addition to direct anterior compression by the herniated disc, the dentate ligaments may resist posterior displacement of the cord, leading to traction and distortion of neural structures.[39]

Vascular insufficiency has been the explanation for unusual cases such as those with transitory paresis and instances in which the segmental level of involvement was higher than expected from the location of the herniated disc.[8, 49] Significant neural deficits may be caused by herniations that appear too small to cause significant compression. This theory also helps explain cases that show no improvement after complete decompression as well as those that have an abrupt onset of paraplegia in the presence of a chronic calcified disc. The theory is supported by cases in which the disc herniation has been shown to cause anterior spinal artery thrombosis.[47]

Doppman and Girton performed an angiographic study of the effect of laminectomy in the presence of acute anterior epidural masses.[24] They found that when decompression restored normal arteriovenous hemodynamics, the animals were neurologically intact despite significant cord distortion. When either the artery or the vein remained obstructed, however, the animals remained paraplegic.

DIFFERENTIAL DIAGNOSIS

Love and Schorn reported that before myelography the correct diagnosis was made in 13 of 61 patients and was considered in the differential diagnosis in only seven others; even after myelography, the correct diagnosis was made preoperatively in only 56 per cent of patients.[49] With greater awareness of the diagnosis and the improved imaging techniques now available, the correct diagnosis should be made before operation in almost all cases. The list of other conditions to consider is long, however, and patients require thorough preoperative investigation.

The differential diagnosis of back pain includes spinal tumors and infections, ankylosing spondylitis, fractures, intercostal neuralgia, herpes zoster, and cervical and lumbar herniated discs. Diseases of the thoracic and abdominal viscera may have a similar presentation. Neurosis is another possibility. The differential diagnosis of myelopathy includes demyelinating and degenerative processes of the central nervous system such as multiple sclerosis and amyotrophic lateral sclerosis.[21, 65] Intraspinal tumors, brain tumors, and cerebrovascular accidents also should be considered.[6, 49]

In patients who have a neurologic deficit and radiographic evidence of Scheuermann's disease, the differential diagnosis includes an extradural cyst or compression from an angular kyphosis.[45, 67] In the series by Lesoin and associates, the mean age of the patients who had a herniated thoracic disc in association with Scheuermann's disease was 44 years, similar to the population without Scheuermann's disease.[45] This is in contrast to a mean age of 17 years in three patients in whom neurologic compromise developed secondary to bony cord compression at the apex of the kyphosis.[67]

NATURAL HISTORY

There are no long-term reports of untreated adults with herniated thoracic discs. The natural history of the disorder is one of progression, and nearly all patients eventually undergo operation for progressive neurologic deficit or unremitting pain.[41, 49] The most characteristic chronologic progression of symptoms is pain followed by sensory disturbance, weakness, and bowel and bladder dysfunction.[77] The course can be extremely variable, however, and it is unknown whether neurologic signs or symptoms ever would have developed in patients operated on for pain alone. Some patients might have improved spontaneously if not subjected to surgical treatment.

Arseni and Nash described two general patterns for the time course of symptoms.[8] The first, which occurs in younger patients with a history of trauma, is backache that can be followed by a rapidly evolving myelopathy. In the second pattern, which occurs in patients past middle age who have degenerative disc disease without any significant trauma, signs and symptoms of cord compression develop slowly and progressively.

Tovi and Strang found that when the first symptom to develop was unilateral, the course tended to be one of slow progression with periods of stabilization and occasional slight remissions.[77] Rapid, irreversible progression generally was noted in cases with a bilateral onset.

Calcification of the disc in children is considered to be a painful but self-limited process, with eventual resolution of the pain and resorption of the calcified deposit. It generally occurs in the cervical spine. About half of the cases are preceded by a history of either trauma (30 per cent) or upper respiratory infection.[14, 73] The natural history of herniated, calcified thoracic discs in children was reviewed by Nicolau and associates.[57] The course was similar to cases without herniation: the patients improved spontaneously and the calcified fragment resorbed. The progression is not always benign, however. Two cases in children have been reported in which myelopathy from cord compression developed and required operation.[50, 61]

Disc calcification in adults is different from that in children. The thoracolumbar spine is the most frequent site of calcification, and the condition generally is asymptomatic unless herniation of the disc occurs.[14] The deposits may accelerate degeneration by interfering in the biomechanics and nutrition of the disc.[14, 80] Disc calcification is found on routine radiographs in 4 to 6 per cent of patients without disc herniation compared with up to 70 per cent of those with disc prolapse.[14, 47] The natural history of disc herniation in the adult has not been conclusively shown to be altered by disc calcification.

DIAGNOSTIC EVALUATION

Spine Radiographs

Plain radiographs of the spine generally are helpful only if they demonstrate disc calcification. The calcified disc is not always the one that is herniated, but the association at least suggests the diagnosis.[9, 49] Detection of a cal-

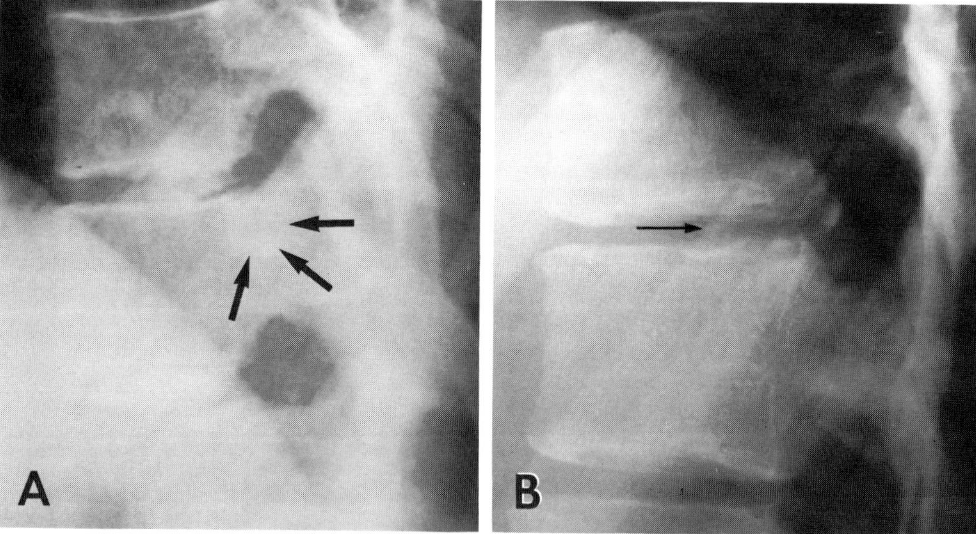

Figure 22–3. Plain radiographs are pathognomonic of herniated discs only when calcification is seen within the spinal canal. *A,* A large calcified disc within the canal is nearly obscured by overlying ribs (see Figs. 22–7 and 22–8 for CT and MRI scans of the same patient). *B,* A tiny nidus of calcium is visible in the canal posterior to the narrowed 11th interspace. (*B,* From Baker, H. L., Jr., Love, J. G., and Uihlein, A.: Roentgenologic features of protruded thoracic intervertebral disks. Radiology *84:*1059–1065, 1965. By permission of The Radiological Society of North America.)

cified disc in the canal is pathognomonic of disc herniation.[9, 46, 47, 69] Baker and associates identified two radiographic patterns of calcification (Fig. 22–3).[9] One consisted of extensive calcification posteriorly in the interspace and bulging into the canal. The other pattern, which is subtle and often overlooked initially, is a small nidus just posterior to the narrowed interspace. Studies of adult lumbar discs have shown that the deposits may be calcium pyrophosphate dihydrate or calcium hydroxyapatite.[14, 80] The clinical significance of the different radiographic patterns or chemical compositions has not been determined.

The proposed association between Scheuermann's disease and herniated thoracic discs has been discussed above. A patient found to have kyphosis with vertebral body wedging and end plate irregularity in association with back pain or a neurologic deficit should undergo other studies to rule out a herniated disc. Other radiographic findings, such as narrowing and hypertrophic changes, are nonspecific and are not helpful in the diagnosis.[9, 47, 49]

Myelography

The thoracic spine is difficult to image by myelography because of the thoracic kyphosis and superimposition of mediastinal structures. Myelography alone is diagnostic in only 56 per cent of cases and has a false-negative rate of 8 per cent.[9, 49] A complete block is found in 10 to 15 per cent of cases.[9, 77] Myelography is performed by pooling water-soluble contrast agent in the lumbosacral canal, removing the spinal needle, and placing the patient supine so that the contrast agent will pool in the dependent thoracic kyphosis.[17] Use of both anteroposterior and lateral films is essential. A herniated disc appears as a central filling defect at the level of the disc space (Fig. 22–4). Central protrusions produce discrete oval or round filling defects. In large protrusions, a complete block occurs with a blunt, convex, leading edge.[9, 47] Lateral discs produce triangular or semicircular indentations with displacement of the cord to the opposite side (Fig. 22–5).[9] Spinal fluid evaluation at the time of myelography is nonspecific.[33] The protein content is increased in less than 50 per cent of patients and helps only to focus attention on the central nervous system. It generally is in the range of 50 to 100 mg/dl but may be greater than 400 mg/dl.[49] Currently myelography is most helpful in localizing lesions to allow directed CT and in preparation for operation.[2, 12]

Computed Tomography

Enhanced CT after myelography with a water-soluble contrast agent is an extremely valuable technique and has been the diagnostic standard in recent years (Fig. 22–6).[5, 7, 12, 17, 66] When combined with standard myelography, CT not only improves sensitivity and accuracy but also can detect intradural penetration of the disc.[7]

CT alone may be helpful when the disc is calcified (Fig. 22–7) but it is impractical to image the entire thoracic spine and it is not as sensitive as CT with intrathecal injection of a contrast agent.[34] The criterion for diagnosis of a herniated disc by CT is a focal extension of the disc beyond the posterior aspect of the vertebral body with spinal cord compression or displacement.[66]

Magnetic Resonance Imaging

MRI is revolutionizing the diagnostic evaluation of thoracic disc disease, although the technique is still being refined. Some centers rely on it almost exclusively, but others still perform myelography and CT when operation is being considered.[12, 17, 29] MRI is a rapid, noninvasive, outpatient procedure that does not use ionizing radiation and causes no morbidity. It is a sensitive, specific technique that makes it easy to obtain sagittal sections of the entire thoracic spine.[17, 29, 66] The findings on MRI are similar to those of myelography and CT, but it is necessary to use information from sagittal T1- and T2-weighted and axial T1-weighted images to achieve similar sensitivity (Fig. 22–8).[66]

MRI is a highly technical procedure, and the evaluation of herniated thoracic discs has not yet been standardized. To a great degree the expertise of the radiologist and the design of the scanner will determine the accuracy of the test. There are pitfalls of MRI, such as partial volume averaging (due to the relatively large section thickness), the cerebrospinal fluid flow-void sign (regions of low signal intensity within the fluid due to its pulsatile motion),

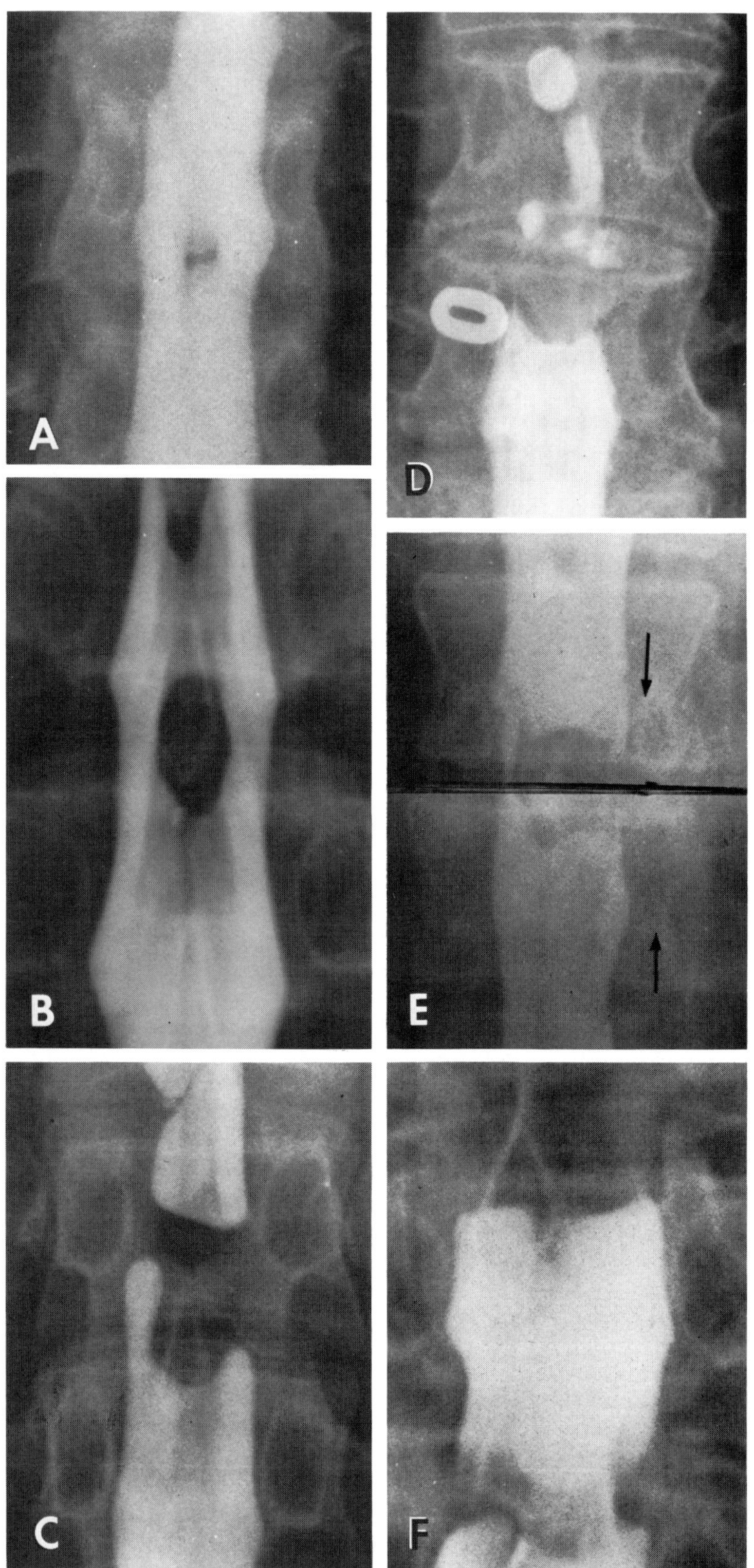

Figure 22–4. Oval filling defects in opaque column of iophendylate (Pantopaque) myelogram resulting from central protruded thoracic discs. Note the midline position of the spinal cord in all cases. *A,* A tiny protrusion is visible at the T9 interspace. *B,* A small protrusion at T12. *C,* A moderately large slightly obstructing protrusion at T12. *D,* A large, severely obstructing protrusion at T12. *E,* The upper margin was outlined only when oil flowed caudally. *F,* A completely obstructing protrusion at T12. Note the blunt, convex leading edge of the column. (From Baker, H. L., Jr., Love, J. G., and Uihlein, A.: Roentgenologic features of protruded thoracic intervertebral disks. Radiology *84:* 1059–1065, 1965. By permission of The Radiological Society of North America.)

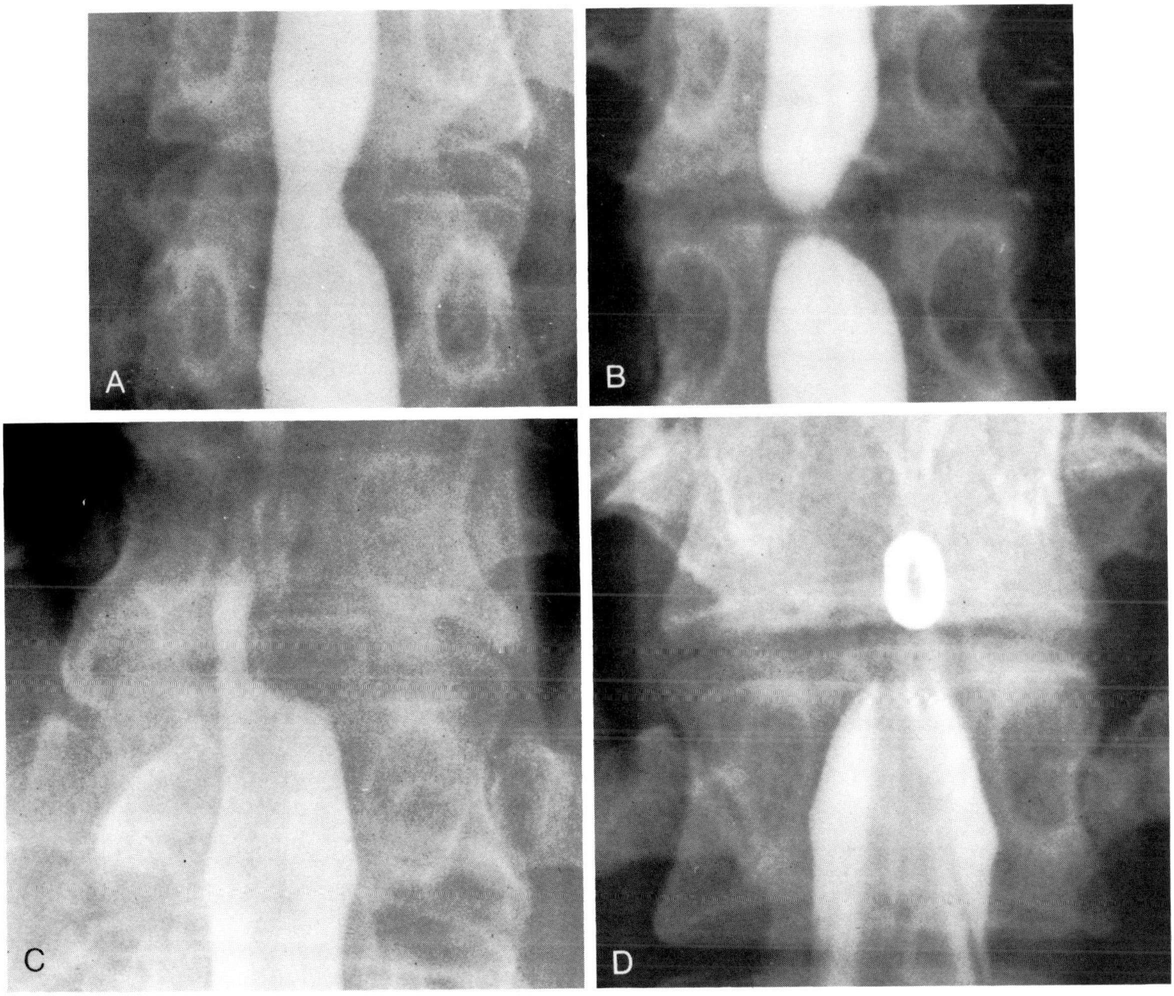

Figure 22–5. Filling defects in opaque column of iophendylate (Pantopaque) myelogram resulting from a lateral protruded thoracic disc. Note the lateral displacement of the spinal cord in several cases. *A,* A small lateral protrusion at T11. *B,* A moderately large, slightly obstructing protrusion at T10. *C,* A large obstructing protrusion at T9. *D,* A completely obstructing protrusion at T10. Note the pointing of the column and deviation of the spinal cord to the left. (From Baker, H. L., Jr., Love, J. G., and Uihlein, A.: Roentgenologic features of protruded thoracic intervertebral disks. Radiology *84:*1059–1065, 1965. By permission of The Radiological Society of North America.)

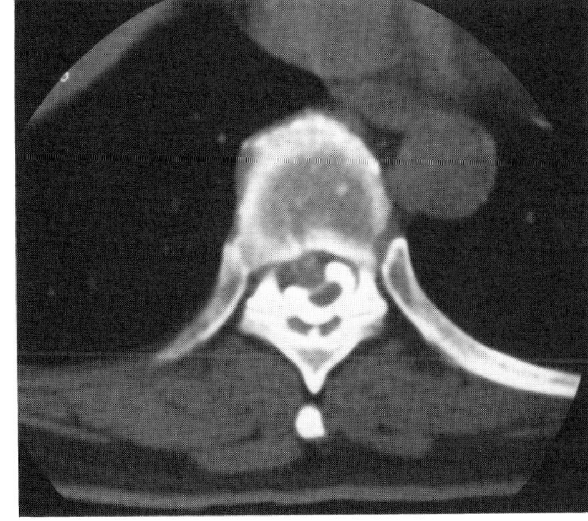

Figure 22–6. Postmyelography CT scan, showing a large, right, centrolateral herniated disc at T8–T9.

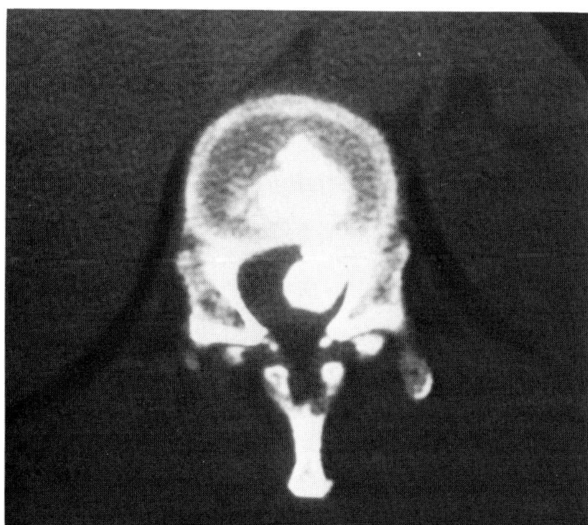

Figure 22–7. CT scan showing calcification of a centrolateral herniated thoracic disc.

signal dropout from calcified discs, chemical shift artifacts from marrow fat, and mismapped signal from cardiac motion.[17, 25, 66] These limitations are likely to be overcome in the near future but, at the present, MRI scans must be interpreted cautiously.

TREATMENT

There are anecdotal reports of patients improving without operation; however, the natural history of this disorder generally mandates surgical treatment.[82] Some believe that if the protrusion is far lateral with nerve root compression only the situation is not urgent and the decision to operate should be based on the degree of pain.[26] There have been reports of lateral lesions causing severe neurologic deficits from compression of a major medullary feeder vessel, however.[53] Small herniations also should be respected. Abrupt, severe, and irreversible deficits can occur, and therefore some investigators have concluded that there is no relationship between the size of the herniation and the gravity of the clinical picture.[41, 46]

Most authors recommend early decompression. If the patient comes for treatment late, however, favorable results are still possible despite significant delays and the presence of major neurologic deficits.[12] A less aggressive approach may be taken in children because the natural history of the disorder appears to be different.[57]

The surgical management of this disorder has evolved in recent years. Laminectomy with disc excision was the benchmark approach 30 years ago but has been abandoned because of the risk of neurologic deterioration (Fig. 22–9). Since the introduction of alternative techniques of decompression, Ravichandran and Frankel have noted a significant decrease in admissions to spinal cord injury centers of patients with paralysis after treatment of herniated thoracic discs.[64] In a review of 135 cases,

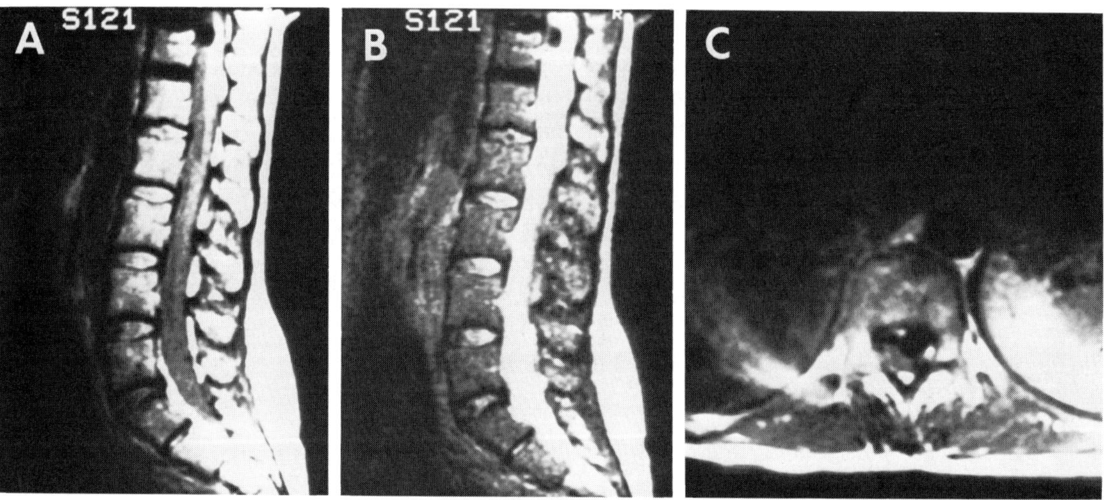

Figure 22–8. MRI scan of the patient in Figure 22–7 showing a large, calcified, herniated thoracic disc at T11–T12. *A,* T1-weighted sagittal image. *B,* T2-weighted sagittal image. *C,* T1-weighted axial image.

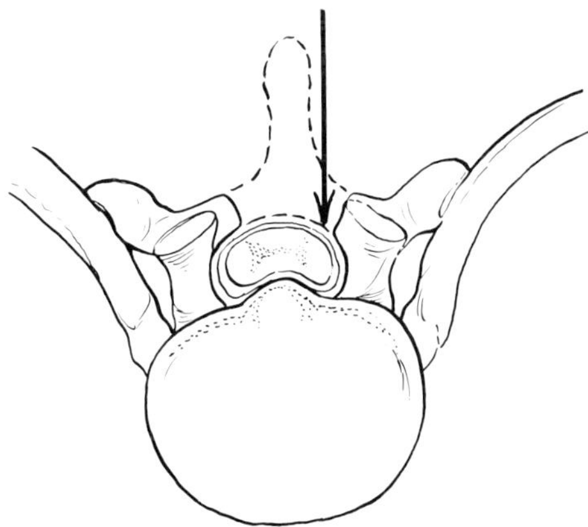

Figure 22–9. Attempted decompression by laminectomy would require manipulation of the cord and a high risk of neurologic deterioration.

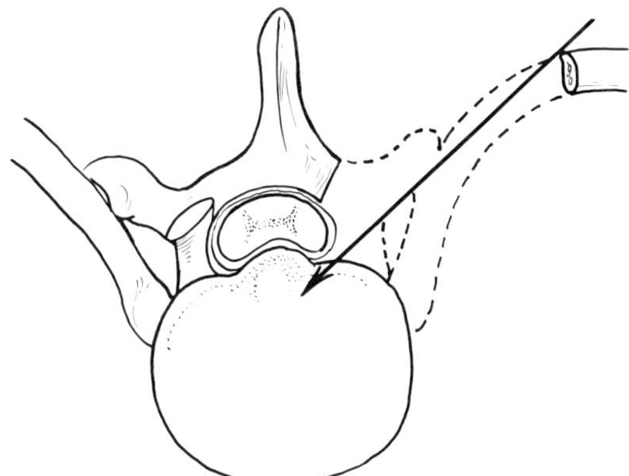

Figure 22–10. Decompression by costotransversectomy is possible without manipulation of the cord.

Arce and Dohrmann found that, after laminectomy, 58 per cent were improved, 10 per cent were unchanged, 28 per cent were worse, and 4 per cent died.[6] There is also evidence that patients who do not improve or who are made worse by laminectomy are less likely to be helped by later anterior decompression.[21] The best results are obtained in patients who have lateral lesions above T10–T11, who have minimal neurologic deficits, and who are operated on early after the onset of symptoms.[26, 47, 49, 62, 77] Although laminectomy is still occasionally advocated for lateral lesions, most authors think that the procedure is contraindicated.[31, 74]

Singounas and Karvounis described good results in patients treated by decompressive laminectomy alone without attempted disc removal.[72] Others have described disastrous results with this technique, however.[28, 47] Studies in animals have found consistent neurologic deterioration after decompressive laminectomy for anterior epidural masses.[10, 24]

Costotransversectomy is an effective technique for managing herniated thoracic discs (Fig. 22–10). Disc excision is carried out through a paramedian incision with the patient prone.[36] The paraspinal muscles are either retracted medially or split transversely.[11, 36] The posterior portion of each rib on the side of the herniated disc is excised, and the pleura is mobilized and reflected anterolaterally. The transverse processes and remaining head and neck of each excised rib are then removed. The intervertebral foramen is located by tracing the intercostal nerve medially. The foramen is enlarged by partial removal of the corresponding pedicles, and the dural sac is exposed. A cavity is created in the posterior aspect of the bodies and disc, allowing gentle removal of disc fragments through the defect without manipulation of the spinal cord.[11, 18, 30, 36]

Transthoracic spinal cord decompression has been shown to be a viable alternative to costotransversectomy (Fig. 22–11).[62, 63] The advantages include a more direct approach to the lesion and better visualization, facilitating excision of central herniations and those with intradural penetration. The disadvantages of the procedure include the potential complications associated with a thoracotomy.

Although many complications after thoracotomy for other disorders have been described, few have been reported as occurring after discectomy.[3, 4, 6, 12, 21, 62, 63] The results of

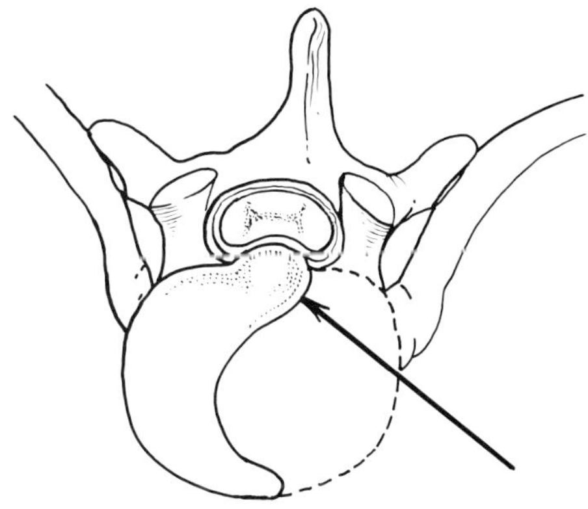

Figure 22–11. Transthoracic decompression allows the most direct approach to the lesion without manipulation of the spinal cord.

transthoracic decompression are similar to those of costotransversectomy. In 53 cases collected from the literature, 52 patients improved, one was unchanged, and none was worse. Bohlman and Zdeblick reported the outcome in 19 patients treated by either costotransversectomy or transthoracic decompression.[12] The two poor outcomes in their series were in cases treated by costotransversectomy. They concluded that the transthoracic approach with its superior exposure was the preferred procedure.

Some authors recommend preoperative angiography to determine the location of the artery of Adamkiewicz and other major medullary feeder vessels.[27, 51, 59, 62, 63] If such a vessel is found at the level of the disc herniation, the spine could be approached from the opposite side. By carefully avoiding dissection in the neural foramina, however, this problem can be obviated without the need for an arteriogram. There is generally abundant collateral circulation in the region of the neural foramina that provides blood flow to the cord even with ligation of the artery of Adamkiewicz.[22, 23, 44] We routinely ligate the segmental vessels adjacent to the herniated disc midway between the foramina and the aorta and have not observed any untoward effects (Fig. 22–12).[21]

The patient is placed in the lateral decubitus position. A lateral prolapse is best approached from the ipsilateral side; a midline herniation may be approached from either side. In the upper or midthoracic spine, the right side has the advantage of avoiding the great vessels and the heart. There also is statistically less risk to the artery of Adamkiewicz because this vessel is on the left in approximately 80 per cent of the patients.[23] When the herniation is in the lower thoracic spine, a left thoracotomy is preferred because it is easier to mobilize the aorta than the vena cava and the liver does not crowd the field.[12, 62]

The level of rib resection is chosen to give the most direct access to the affected disc (Fig. 22–12*A*). A horizontal line drawn on a chest radiograph from the disc space to the chest wall will intersect the rib that should be resected. This is generally one to two ribs above the affected disc in the middle and lower thoracic spine.[27] In the upper thoracic spine the exposure is limited somewhat by the scapula, and it is generally necessary to excise the fifth or sixth rib and then work cranially.

The recommended extent of bone and disc removal varies from a relatively small trough in the posterior aspect of the disc to complete discectomy with partial corpectomy of the adjacent bodies (Fig. 22–12*B*).[12, 21, 27, 62, 69] We think that the latter approach is safer because it provides the greatest degree of visualization and allows complete discectomy without disturbing the foraminal vessels. In either case, great care is taken to perform the decompression without any manipulation of or pressure on the spinal cord.

Fusion is indicated when stability is compromised by the decompression and in cases associated with Scheuermann's disease.[12] When only a small amount of bone and disc is excised, fusion generally is not recommended.[12, 27, 62, 69] Conversely, with complete discectomy, fusion is mandatory (Fig. 22–12*C*). In addition to providing stability, fusion may limit local pain secondary to motion of the degenerated segment. Recurrence of thoracic disc herniation has not been reported, but complete discectomy and fusion theoretically is the best way to prevent this complication.

At the conclusion of the procedure, a chest tube is placed and attached to water-seal suction. If a fusion has been performed, a thoracolumbosacral orthosis brace should be used.

Otani and associates described a modification of the transthoracic procedure in which the pleura is dissected away from the chest wall after rib excision.[59] This allows the approach to be entirely extrapleural. Their results are similar to those in other series of transthoracic decompressions. The advantage of the technique is the avoidance of a chest tube postoperatively. Claims of a lower incidence of pulmonary complications may be more theoretic than real because few such complications have been reported.

A posterolateral approach was described by Carson and associates in 1971 (Fig. 22–13).[16] They performed a complete laminectomy of the vertebrae adjacent to the herniated disc combined with a medial facetectomy and excision of the transverse process. A T-shaped incision through the erector muscle of the spine then allowed an oblique approach to the anterior epidural space. Patterson and Arbit modified the approach in 1978 to include removal of the facet and pedicle of the vertebra caudal to the protruded disc through a straight midline incision.[60] The central portion of the disc then is removed by creating a cavity. The protruded material is excised by reduction of

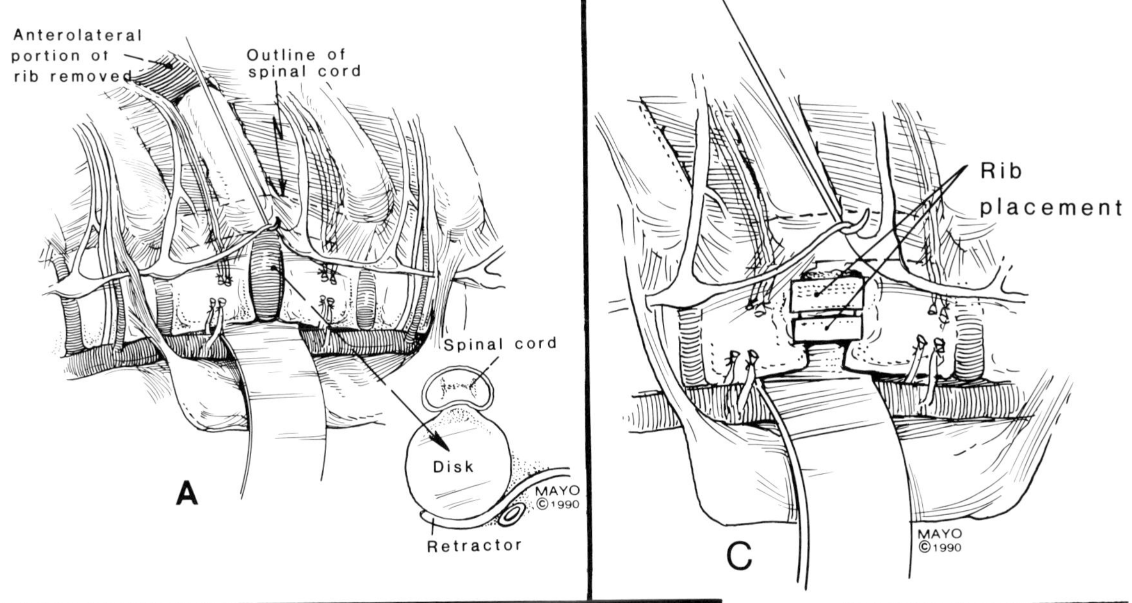

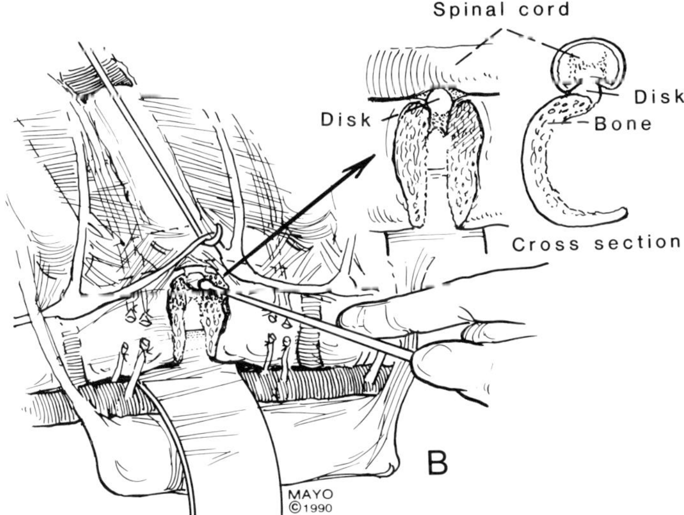

Figure 22–12. *A,* Exposure provided by a transthoracic approach. The great vessels are mobilized by ligation of the segmental vessels midway between the aorta and the neural foramina. A malleable retractor may be placed for protection of the great vessels. *B,* Complete discectomy and partial corpectomy of adjacent vertebral bodies provides excellent visualization and allows complete decompression without disturbance of the collateral vessels within the neural foramina. *C,* Fusion is indicated when stability is compromised by the decompression. (By permission of Mayo Foundation.)

disc and bone into the cavity before removal. After anterior decompression, a complete laminectomy can be performed.

Lesoin and associates described a slightly more extensive exposure in which the transverse process, articular facets, and portions of the adjacent pedicles are removed.[46] They reported good results with this technique. The extent of bone removal requires that a fusion be performed, and the authors recommended unilateral Harrington rod instrumentation. Spinal deformity has been reported to occur after posterolateral decompression without fusion.[76] Of the 45 cases reported in the literature, the patients were improved in 40 (89 per cent), unchanged in three, and worse in one; one patient died.[6] Some claim that intradural disc herniation can be dealt with much more easily with this approach than with any other; however, approaching anterior dural erosion by this technique would require some degree of manipulation of the cord.[70]

Except for laminectomy, all the techniques described are reasonable approaches to herniated thoracic discs. Perhaps the most rational way to manage the problem is to select the approach best suited to the disease present. Posterolateral techniques are ideal for lateral

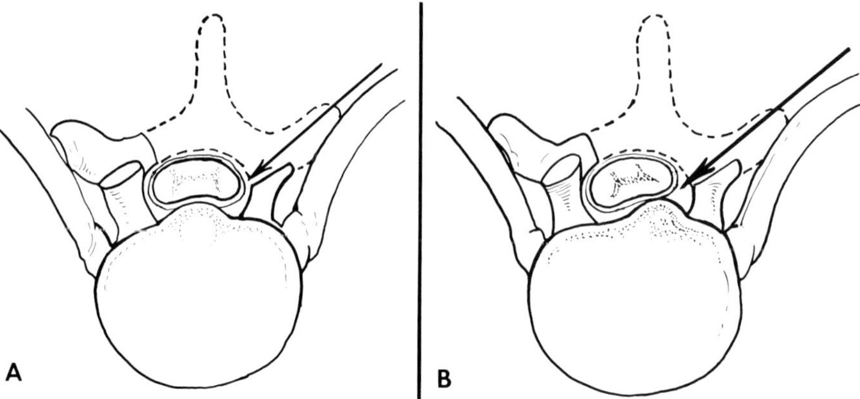

Figure 22–13. Posterolateral decompression. *A*, Removal of a central herniation would require some manipulation of the cord. *B*, Lateral herniations may be approached by this technique without manipulation of the cord.

lesions and may be the best choice for herniated discs with coexistent stenosis.[78] The transthoracic approach permits the best visualization for central lesions. Upper thoracic central lesions, which are more difficult to approach through the chest, may be managed best by costotransversectomy.

CONCLUSION

Herniated thoracic discs are uncommon lesions that usually affect middle-aged patients and cause many symptoms. In general, the natural history of the disorder is progression, often starting with pain followed sequentially by sensory, motor, gait, and sphincter disturbances. There is no clear-cut clinical syndrome. Many patients complain only of pain; others present with painless myelopathy.

Most herniations occur in the lower thoracic region, and central protrusions are more common than lateral ones. Multiple herniations and intradural penetration are uncommon. In most cases the cause is a degenerative process, but a history of trauma can be elicited in approximately one third of the cases. An association with Scheuermann's disease has been suggested by several authors. The pathogenesis of neurologic compromise is believed to be a combination of direct neural compression and vascular insufficiency. The differential diagnosis is long and requires careful consideration. Radiologic evaluation is essential for the diagnosis, but plain films are helpful only if disc calcification is present. The standard is CT and myelography, but MRI is likely to replace this procedure in the near future.

Laminectomy is no longer indicated for treatment of this disorder because of a high risk of neurologic deterioration and the fact that it may compromise the results of later anterior decompression. Discectomy may be carried out by a costotransversectomy, thoracotomy, or posterolateral technique. The approach chosen should be based on the location of the herniation and the experience of the surgeon. Arthrodesis should be performed whenever decompression causes instability or in cases of Scheuermann's disease and may prove to be beneficial in all cases.

The prognosis of herniated thoracic discs treated surgically is favorable and early operative intervention is advised. The techniques are exacting, however, and still carry a significant risk of neurologic deterioration.

References

1. Abbott, K. H., and Retter, R. H.: Protrusions of thoracic intervertebral disks. Neurology *6:*1–10, 1956.
2. Alberico, A. M., Sahni, K. S., Hall, J. A., Jr., and Young, H. F.: High thoracic disc herniation. Neurosurgery *19:*449–451, 1986.
3. Albrand, O. W., and Corkill, G.: Thoracic disc herniation: treatment and prognosis. Spine *4:*41–46, 1979.
4. Alexander, G. L.: Cited by Hulme, A.[36]
5. Alvarez, O., Roque, C. T., and Pampati, M.: Multilevel thoracic disk herniations: CT and MR studies. J. Comput. Assist. Tomogr. *12:*649–652, 1988.
6. Arce, C. A., and Dohrmann, G. J.: Herniated thoracic disks. Neurol. Clin. *3:*383–392, 1985.

7. Arce, C. A., and Dohrmann, G. J.: Thoracic disc herniation: improved diagnosis with computed tomographic scanning and a review of the literature. Surg. Neurol. *23:*356–361, 1985.
8. Arseni, C., and Nash, F.: Thoracic intervertebral disc protrusion: a clinical study. J. Neurosurg. *17:*418–430, 1960.
9. Baker, H. L., Jr., Love, J. G., and Uihlein, A.: Roentgenologic features of protruded thoracic intervertebral disks. Radiology *84:*1059–1065, 1965.
10. Bennett, M. H., and McCallum, J. E.: Experimental decompression of spinal cord. Surg. Neurol. *8:*63–67, 1977.
11. Benson, M. K. D., and Byrnes, D. P.: The clinical syndromes and surgical treatment of thoracic intervertebral disc prolapse. J. Bone Joint Surg. *57B:*471–477, 1975.
12. Bohlman, H. H., and Zdeblick, T. A.: Anterior excision of herniated thoracic discs. J. Bone Joint Surg. *70A:*1038–1047, 1988.
13. Brennan, M., Perrin, J. C. S., Canady, A., and Wesolowski, D.: Paraparesis in a child with a herniated thoracic disc. Arch. Phys. Med. Rehabil. *68:*806–808, 1987.
14. Bullough, P. G., and Boachie-Adjei, O.: Atlas of Spinal Diseases. Philadelphia, J. B. Lippincott Co., 1988.
15. Capener, N.: The evolution of lateral rachotomy. J. Bone Joint Surg. *36B:*173–179, 1954.
16. Carson, J., Gumpert, J., and Jefferson, A.: Diagnosis and treatment of thoracic intervertebral disc protrusions. J. Neurol. Neurosurg. Psychiatry *34:*68–77, 1971.
17. Chambers, A. A.: Thoracic disk herniation. Semin. Roentgenol. *23:*111–117, 1988.
18. Chesterman, P. J.: Spastic paraplegia caused by sequestrated thoracic intervertebral disc. Proc. R. Soc. Med. *57:*87–88, 1964.
19. Chin, L. S., Black, K. L., and Hoff, J. T.: Multiple thoracic disc herniations: case report. J. Neurosurg. *66:*290–292, 1987.
20. Crafoord, C., Hiertonn, T., Lindblom, K., and Olsson, S.-E.: Spinal cord compression caused by a protruded thoracic disc: report of a case treated with antero-lateral fenestration of the disc. Acta Orthop. Scand. *28:*103–107, 1958.
21. Currier, B. L., Eismont, F. J., and Green, B.: Transthoracic disc excision and fusion for central herniated thoracic discs. Orthop. Trans. *14:*636, 1990.
22. Di Chiro, G., Fried, L. C., and Doppman, J. L.: Experimental spinal cord angiography. Br. J. Radiol. *43:*19–30, 1970.
23. Dommisse, G. F.: The blood supply of the spinal cord: a critical vascular zone in spinal surgery. J. Bone Joint Surg. *56B:*225–235, 1974.
24. Doppman, J. L., and Girton, M.: Angiographic study of the effect of laminectomy in the presence of acute anterior epidural masses. J. Neurosurg. *45:*195–202, 1976.
25. Enzmann, D. R., Griffin, C., and Rubin, J. B.: Potential false-negative MR images of the thoracic spine in disk disease with switching of phase- and frequency-encoding gradients. Radiology *165:*635–637, 1987.
26. Epstein, J. A.: The syndrome of herniation of the lower thoracic intervertebral discs with nerve root and spinal cord compression: a presentation of four cases with a review of the literature, methods of diagnosis and treatment. J. Neurosurg. *11:*525–538, 1954.
27. Fidler, M. W., and Goedhart, Z. D.: Excision of prolapse of thoracic intervertebral disc: a transthoracic technique. J. Bone Joint Surg. *66B:*518–522, 1984.
28. Fisher, R. G.: Protrusions of thoracic disc: the factor of herniation through the dura mater. J. Neurosurg. *22:*591–593, 1965.
29. Francavilla, T. L., Powers, A., Dina, T., and Rizzoli, H. V.: MR imaging of thoracic disk herniations. J. Comput. Assist. Tomogr. *11:*1062–1065, 1987.
30. Garrido, E.: Modified costotransversectomy: A surgical approach to ventrally placed lesions in the thoracic spinal canal. Surg. Neurol. *13:*109–113, 1980.
31. Gelch, M. M.: Herniated thoracic disc at T1–2 level associated with Horner's syndrome: case report. J. Neurosurg. *48:*128–130, 1978.
32. Haley, J. C., and Perry, J. H.: Protrusions of intervertebral discs: study of their distribution, characteristics and effects on the nervous system. Am. J. Surg. *80:*394–404, 1950.
33. Hawk, W. A.: Spinal compression caused by ecchondrosis of the intervertebral fibrocartilage: with a review of the recent literature. Brain *59:*204–224, 1936.
34. Hochman, M. S., Pena, C., and Ramirez, R.: Calcified herniated thoracic disc diagnosed by computerized tomography: case report. J. Neurosurg. *52:*722–723, 1980.
35. Hodgson, A. R., and Stock, F. E.: Anterior spinal fusion: a preliminary communication on the radical treatment of Pott's disease and Pott's paraplegia. Br. J. Surg. *44:*266–275, 1956.
36. Hulme, A.: The surgical approach to thoracic intervertebral disc protrusions. J. Neurol. Neurosurg. Psychiatry *23:*133–137, 1960.
37. Isla, A., Roda, J. M., Bencosme, J., et al.: Intradural herniated dorsal disc: case report and review of the literature. Neurosurgery *22:*737–738, 1988.
38. Jefferson, A.: The treatment of thoracic intervertebral disc protrusions. Clin. Neurol. Neurosurg. *78:*1–9, 1975.
39. Kahn, E. A.: The role of the dentate ligaments in spinal cord compression and the syndrome of lateral sclerosis. J. Neurosurg. *4:*191–199, 1947.
40. Key, C. A.: On paraplegia: depending on disease of the ligaments of the spine. Guys Hosp. Rep. *3:*17–34, 1838.
41. Kite, W. C., Jr., Whitfield, R. D., and Campbell, E.: The thoracic herniated intervertebral disc syndrome. J. Neurosurg. *14:*61–67, 1957.
42. Kuhlendahl, H.: Der thorakale Bandscheibenprolaps als extramedullärer Spinaltumor und in seinen Beziehungen zu internen Organsyndromen. Ärztl. Wochnschr. *6:*154–157, 1951.
43. Lanska, D. J., Lanska, M. J., Fenstermaker, R., et al.: Thoracic disk herniation associated with chiropractic spinal manipulation (letter to the editor). Arch. Neurol. *44:*996–997, 1987.
44. Lazorthes, G., Gouaze, A., Zadeh, J. O., et al.: Arterial vascularization of the spinal cord: recent studies of the anastomotic substitution pathways. J. Neurosurg. *35:*253–262, 1971.
45. Lesoin, F., Leys, D., Rousseaux, M., et al.: Thoracic

disk herniation and Scheuermann's disease. Eur. Neurol. *26:*145–152, 1987.
46. Lesoin, F., Rousseaux, M., Autricque, A., et al.: Thoracic disc herniations: evolution in the approach and indications. Acta Neurochir. (Wien) *80:*30–34, 1986.
47. Logue, V.: Thoracic intervertebral disc prolapse with spinal cord compression. J. Neurol. Neurosurg. Psychiatry *15:*227–241, 1952.
48. Love, J. G., and Kiefer, E. J.: Root pain and paraplegia due to protrusions of thoracic intervertebral disks. J. Neurosurg. *7:*62–69, 1950.
49. Love, J. G., and Schorn, V. G.: Thoracic-disk protrusions. J.A.M.A. *191:*627–631, 1965.
50. MacCartee, C. C., Jr., Griffin, P. P., and Byrd, E. B.: Ruptured calcified thoracic disc in a child: report of a case. J. Bone Joint Surg. *54A:*1272–1274, 1972.
51. Maiman, D. J., Larson, S. J., Luck, E., and El-Ghatit, A.: Lateral extracavitary approach to the spine for thoracic disc herniation: report of 23 cases. Neurosurgery *14:*178–182, 1984.
52. Malmivaara, A., Videman, T., Kuosma, E., and Troup, J. D. G.: Facet joint orientation, facet and costovertebral joint osteoarthrosis, disc degeneration, vertebral body osteophytosis, and Schmorl's nodes in the thoracolumbar junctional region of cadaveric spines. Spine *12:*458–463, 1987.
53. Mansour, H., Hammoud, F., and Vlahovitch, B.: Syndrome de Brown Sequard par hernie discale foraminale et calcifiée, responsable d'une compression directe de l'artère d'Adamkiewicz. Neurochirurgie *33:*478–481, 1987.
54. Ménard, V.: Étude pratique sur le mal de Pott. Paris, Masson et Cie, 1900.
55. Middleton, G. S., and Teacher, J. H.: Injury of the spinal cord due to rupture of an intervertebral disc during muscular effort. Glasgow Med. J. *76:*1–6, 1911.
56. Mixter, W. J., and Barr, J. S.: Rupture of the intervertebral disc with involvement of the spinal canal. N. Engl. J. Med. *211:*210–214, 1934.
57. Nicolau, A., Diard, F., Darrigade, J. M., et al.: Hernie postérieure d'un disque calcifié chez l'enfant: a propos de 2 observations. J. Radiol. *66:*683–688, 1985.
58. Otani, K., Manzoku, S., Shibasaki, K., and Monachi, S.: The surgical treatment of thoracic and thoracolumbar disc lesions using the anterior approach: report of six cases. Spine *2:*266–275, 1977.
59. Otani, K., Yoshida, M., Fujii, E., et al.: Thoracic disc herniation: surgical treatment in 23 patients. Spine *13:*1262–1267, 1988.
60. Patterson, R. H., Jr., and Arbit, E.: A surgical approach through the pedicle to protruded thoracic discs. J. Neurosurg. *48:*768–772, 1978.
61. Peck, F. C., Jr.: A calcified thoracic intervertebral disk with herniation and spinal cord compression in a child: case report. J. Neurosurg. *14:*105–109, 1957.
62. Perot, P. H., Jr., and Munro, D. D.: Transthoracic removal of midline thoracic disc protrusions causing spinal cord compression. J. Neurosurg. *31:*452–458, 1969.
63. Ransohoff, J., Spencer, F., Siew, F., and Gage, L., Jr.: Case reports and technical notes: transthoracic removal of thoracic disc; report of three cases. J. Neurosurg. *31:*459–461, 1969.
64. Ravichandran, G., and Frankel, H. L.: Paraplegia due to intervertebral disc lesions: a review of 57 operated cases. Paraplegia *19:*133–139, 1981.
65. Roosen, N., Dietrich, U., Nicola, N., et al.: Case report: MR imaging of calcified herniated thoracic disk. J. Comput. Assist. Tomogr. *11:*733–735, 1987.
66. Ross, J. S., Perez-Reyes, N., Masaryk, T. J., et al.: Thoracic disk herniation: MR imaging. Radiology *165:*511–515, 1987.
67. Ryan, M. D., and Taylor, T. K. F.: Acute spinal cord compression in Scheuermann's disease. J. Bone Joint Surg. *64B:*409–412, 1982.
68. Ryan, R. W., Lally, J. F., and Kozic, Z.: Asymptomatic calcified herniated thoracic disks: CT recognition. A.J.N.R. *9:*363–366, 1988.
69. Safdari, H., and Baker, R. L., II: Microsurgical anatomy and related techniques to an anterolateral transthoracic approach to thoracic disc herniations. Surg. Neurol. *23:*589–593, 1985.
70. Sekhar, L. N., and Jannetta, P. J.: Thoracic disc herniation: operative approaches and results. Neurosurgery *12:*303–305, 1983.
71. Signorini, G., Baldini, M., Vivenza, C., et al.: Surgical treatment of thoracic disc protrusion. Acta Neurochir. (Wien) *49:*245–254, 1979.
72. Singounas, E. G., and Karvounis, P. C.: Thoracic disc protrusion (analysis of 8 cases). Acta Neurochir. *39:*251–258, 1977.
73. Sonnabend, D. H., Taylor, T. K. F., and Chapman, G. K.: Intervertebral disc calcification syndromes in children. J. Bone Joint Surg. *64B:*25–31, 1982.
74. Svien, H. J., and Karavitis, A. L.: Multiple protrusions of intervertebral disks in the upper thoracic region: report of case. Proc. Staff. Meet. Mayo Clin. *29:*375–378, 1954.
75. Tahmouresie, A.: Herniated thoracic intervertebral disc—an unusual presentation: case report. Neurosurgery *7:*623–625, 1980.
76. Terry, A. F., McSweeney, T., and Jones, H. W. F.: Paraplegia as a sequela to dorsal disc prolapse. Paraplegia *19:*111–117, 1981.
77. Tovi, D., and Strang, R. R.: Thoracic intervertebral disk protrusions. Acta Chir. Scand. Suppl. *267:*6–41, 1960.
78. Ungersböck, K., Perneczky, A., and Korn, A.: Thoracic vertebrostenosis combined with thoracic disc herniation: case report and review of the literature. Spine *12:*612–615, 1987.
79. Van Landingham, J. H.: Herniation of thoracic intervertebral discs with spinal cord compression in kyphosis dorsalis juvenilis (Scheuermann's disease): case report. J. Neurosurg. *11:*327–329, 1954.
80. Weinberger, A., and Myers, A. R.: Intervertebral disk calcification in adults: a review. Semin. Arthritis Rheum. *8:*69–75, 1978.
81. Williams, M. P., and Cherryman, G. R.: Thoracic disk herniation: MR imaging (letter to the editor). Radiology *167:*874–875, 1988.
82. Williams, R.: Complete protrusion of a calcified nucleus pulposus in the thoracic spine: report of a case. J. Bone Joint Surg. *36B:*597–600, 1954.

CHAPTER

23

LUMBAR DISC DISEASE

Ronald J. Wisneski, M.D.
Steven R. Garfin, M.D.
Richard H. Rothman, M.D., Ph.D.

Back pain has plagued humans for many thousands of years. There are descriptions of lumbago and sciatica in the Bible and in the writings of Hippocrates. Despite the long history of awareness of this problem, a reasonable and scientific explanation of the source of low back and leg pain did not emerge until 1934 with the publication of the classic paper by Mixter and Barr.[184] These investigators, for the first time, delineated prolapse of the intervertebral disc as the etiologic agent in the production of these symptoms. It is commonly acknowledged today that derangements of the intervertebral disc represent the great majority of cases of back pain and sciatica.

Human disease assumes importance as a cause of either death or disability. Degenerative disease of the spine for all intents and purposes is a nonlethal entity, and its priority must rest on determination of its prevalence in the population and its impact on this population in terms of pain and disability.

THE PATIENT POPULATION

The frequently ill-defined and multifaceted causes of postural low back and leg pain have prevented accurate evaluation of the epidemiology of low back pain syndromes. Estimates have been made, but these reported figures have been derived primarily from the industrial compensation setting.

In Sweden, each member of the National Health Insurance, in order to receive compensation, reports his or her illnesses by telephone to a central bureau. Thus, excellent statistics are readily available in terms of population analysis. Back pain has been reported in 53 per cent of persons engaged in light physical activity and in 64 per cent of those involved in heavy labor.[124]

The disability of endemic proportions resulting from a painful low back can be better appreciated in terms of its economic impact. Benn and Wood[17] reviewed various medical National Insurance statistics in the United Kingdom and found that more than 13 million days were lost annually owing to a painful back. This ranked third behind chronic and acute pulmonary disease and atherosclerotic coronary vessel disease and was responsible for more working time lost than labor strikes in the United Kingdom in 1970.

Nachemson[196] estimated that at some time during our adult life 80 per cent of us will experience back pain to a significant extent. An extensive investigation by Horal[123] showed that low back pain of a significant degree begins in the younger age groups with a mean age of onset of 35 years. Kelsey[141, 142] found a similar age onset in males with low back pain due to disc disease, but noted that females averaged nearly a decade of delay in the development of significant symptoms. In Horal's study of the individuals complaining of low back pain, only 35 per cent developed sciatica. After subsidence of the original attack of low back pain, 90 per cent had a future recurrence.

Although Kelsey found that males underwent surgery for low back pain and sciatica due to disc disease significantly more often than females, the male predominance was not as evident in the overall sample of low back pain sufferers. Furthermore, there were no racial differences in the incidence of low back pain and sciatica due to disc disease.

Kelsey and White,[139] as well as others,[123] have summarized the scope of the low back problem in the United States. They pointed out that, among chronic conditions, impairments of the back and spine are the most frequent cause of activity limitation in persons under 45 years of age. These impairments rank third after heart conditions and arthritis and rheumatism in persons 45 to 64 years of age. In Rowe's ten-year industrial study,[225] he indicated that 35 per cent of sedentary workers and 45 per cent of heavy laborers visited the medical department with complaints of back pain. Furthermore, four hours per person per year were lost because of low back pain, this figure being second only to hours lost from upper respiratory tract infections. Other investigators[246] have pointed out that the longer patients are absent from work the greater is the likelihood that they will remain disabled and never return to productive employment. In McGill's study,[177] absenteeism of greater than one year because of a low back disorder reduced the probability of return to work to only 25 per cent, and after two years of absence, the likelihood of working again was negligible.

There is a wide range of reports of low back pain without definite diagnosis. In Dillane and colleagues' study,[64] performed in a primary care setting, no specific cause was identified with 79 per cent of first attacks of low back pain in men and 89 per cent in women. Waddell[253] performed a prospective clinical review of 900 patients sent to a back clinic servicing the west of Scotland. In 97 per cent of the patients the major presenting complaint was low back pain. Seventy per cent complained of leg pain as well. In this group 47 per cent of the leg pain was in a referred pattern and 23 per cent was true radicular pain. Of the entire group, 153 (one sixth) were found to have clearly identifiable causes for their back pain such as tumors, infection, osteoporotic fractures, post-traumatic fractures, and spondylolisthesis. Only 3 per cent of the patients with low back pain presenting to Waddell's clinic were found to have extraspinal causes for their complaints such as retroperitoneal or pelvic pathosis, hip disease, peripheral vascular disease, or primary neurologic disorders. Excluding these patients, Waddell and others[17, 225] found that in most cases in which a definite diagnosis is possible, the pain is attributed to disorders involving the lumbar intervertebral discs and facet joints.

Bell and Rothman[15] summarized the enormity of the clinical problem of sciatica as it relates to lumbar disc degeneration. Sciatica is a common ailment with a large economic impact, both on the individual and on industry.[196] Prevalence data indicate that 4.8 per cent of men and 2.5 per cent of women beyond the age of 35 will experience sciatica. The average age of onset of the first sciatic attack is approximately 37 years, with an antecedent initial event of low back pain in 76 per cent of these patients approximately a decade earlier. It is important to remember that the prognosis for the patient who develops severe, unilateral sciatica from a herniated disc is not gloomy. Hakelius[104] reported that 75 per cent of such patients improved 10 to 30 days from the onset of symptoms, and only 19 per cent eventually became surgical candidates.

An even more optimistic conservative response rate was reported by Saal and Saal.[227] In their retrospective cohort study, only six of 58 patients undergoing an aggressive physical rehabilitation program for treatment of herniated discs required surgery, and four of the six had concomitant spinal stenosis.

NATURAL HISTORY

Intelligent treatment of lumbar disc degeneration must be predicated on a thorough knowledge of the natural history of the disorder. If this information is not available to treating physicians and to patients, they will be unable to honestly and effectively make the decisions necessary for the management of this disorder. All too often, decisions for or against surgical intervention are based on distorted concepts of disc disease.

Back pain can be expected to precede the onset of radicular symptoms by approximately six to ten years.[259] The initial low back pain episode is usually of acute onset, whereas subsequent recurrences[101, 259] tend to surface insidiously. The radicular component often originates insidiously and recurs in a similar fashion.[259]

A group of 583 patients were studied at the Karolinska Institute after their first attack of sciatica. Surgery was undertaken in 28 per cent of the group, and patients who had undergone surgery, as well as those who had not, were followed for an average of seven years.[104] The results of this study indicated that the acute episodes of sciatica ran a relatively brief course in most cases, regardless of whether the treatment was conservative or surgical. However, the subacute or chronic symptoms secondary to disc degeneration, although less dramatic, were prolonged and had a profound effect on the patients' lives. At the end of the follow-up period, approximately 15 per cent of the conservatively treated group continued to have a reduced work capacity and restricted leisure activities, and reported regular sleep disturbances. Twenty per cent of the conservatively treated group continued to have pronounced residual sciatica.

Weber[259, 260] conducted a carefully controlled, well-documented prospective study of 280 patients with low lumbar disc herniations. All herniations were myelographically proved. All patients initially received 14 days of conservative management in the hospital (a luxury that today's health care system no longer affords). At the completion of this regimen, the study group with relative indications for surgery were assigned randomly into either a nonoperative or a surgical treatment group. Those who improved were dropped from the study. Those with a sphincter disorder or progressive neurologic deficit were treated surgically and dropped from the study. At the one-year follow-up examination of the randomized study group, surgery was found to be superior to the conservative regimen in regard to relief of low back pain and the radicular component of the pain caused by the disc herniation. After four years, however, the nonoperatively treated group improved. Although the tendency toward better results following surgery prevailed, the differences in the success of treatment were no longer significant. Similar long-term studies of nonoperative treatment by other authors[209] also observed the longer morbidity involved, the slow but definite improvement realized, and the acceptable though perhaps less than ideal results.

It is important to note that in Weber's study there was no loss of quality of surgical results over a three-month period of observation. Therefore, in the absence of urgent indications for surgery (cauda equina syndrome or a progressive neurologic deficit), one can allow some time to pass (three months) in case the symptoms resolve spontaneously, sparing many patients a needless operation. Beyond a 12-month period from the onset of leg pain, however, the quality of surgical results definitely deteriorates.

In general, an encouraging picture is found when one examines the natural history of low back pain. Only a small percentage of afflicted patients have symptoms that persist beyond two weeks (Table 23–1).[62] What is equally apparent, however, is that recurrence rates can be high, even after complete resolution of symptoms. In the occupational setting 60 per cent of patients have recurrent symptoms within one year, with a lessening risk of recurrence after two years.[260] Recurrent sciatica occurs in 10 per cent of men and 14 per cent of women.[20] Sciatica clearly tends to have a more protracted course, but at least 50 per cent of patients recover in one month.[7]

Disability from lumbar disc disease must be considered in terms of back and leg pain with its attendant limitation of function. Although neurologic deficits, including motor weakness, are helpful diagnostically, they are not necessarily compelling surgical factors because residual weakness is not markedly different in patients treated surgically and those treated nonoperatively.[104] Bowel or bladder dysfunc-

Table 23–1. PREVALENCE OF BACK PAIN AND SCIATICA IN THE ENTIRE ADULT POPULATION

Characteristic	Prevalence (%)
Any low back pain	60 to 80
Ever any low back pain persisting at least 2 weeks	14
Low back pain persisting at least 2 weeks at a given time (point prevalence)	7
Back pain with features of sciatica lasting at least 2 weeks	1.6
Lumbar spine surgery	1 to 2

Reproduced, with permission, from Deyo R. A., Loeser, J., and Bigos, S.: Herniated lumbar intervertebral disc. Ann. Intern. Med. *112*:598–603, 1990.

tion affects a relatively small percentage of patients, but assumes greater significance in terms of surgical urgency.

With this background the treating physician and the patient must make their decision regarding the role of surgery. If, after careful diagnostic evaluation, (1) a firm diagnosis can be established, (2) a course of conservative treatment has failed, and (3) the treating surgeon feels that operative intervention would, with a reasonable degree of certainty, shorten the disease process, surgery can or should be recommended.

ALGORITHMIC DECISION MAKING IN SPINAL DISORDERS

The task of the clinician who approaches the patient with low back pain is to return that

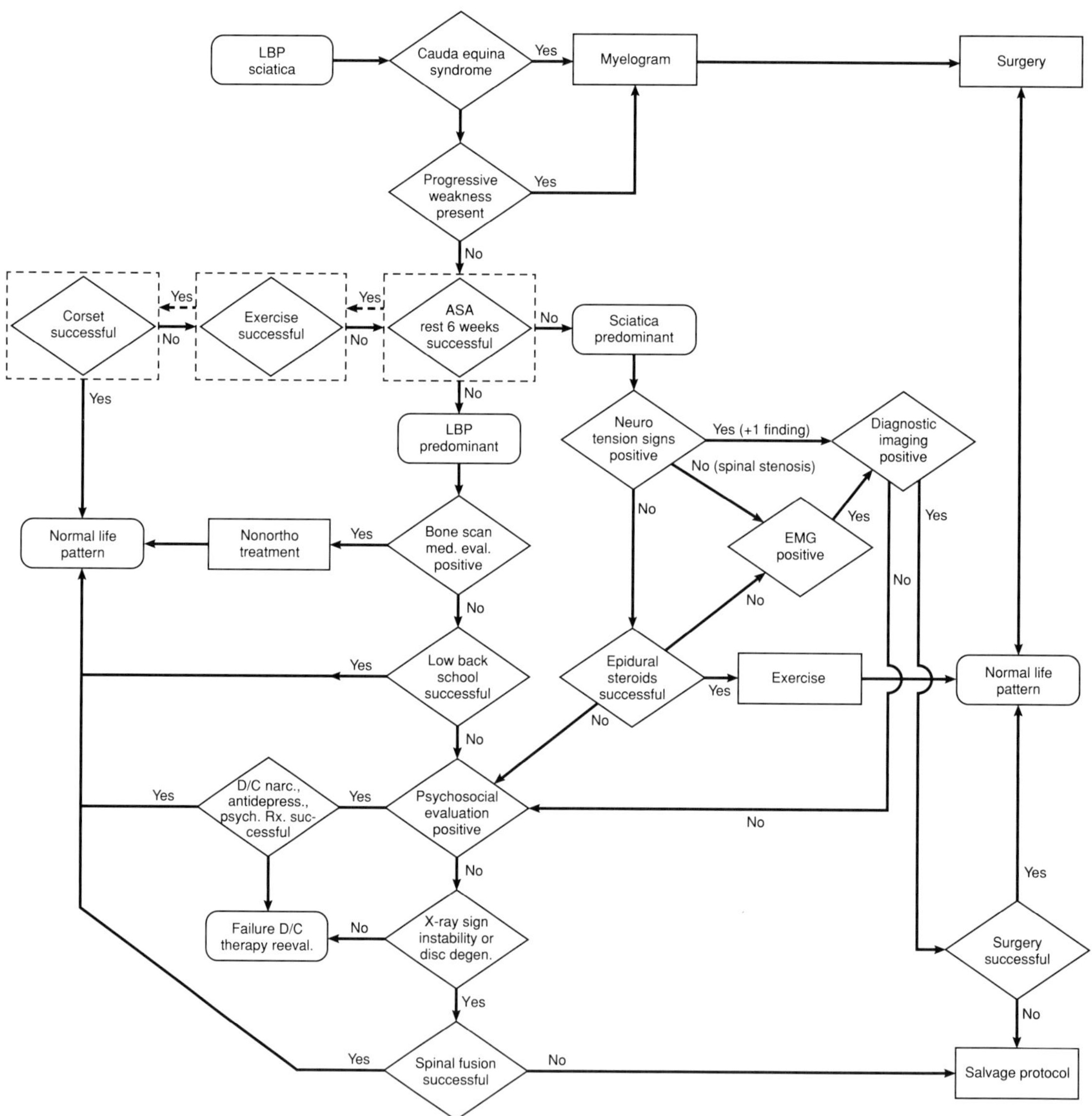

Figure 23–1. Pennsylvania Plan Algorithm for evaluation of low back and leg pain. The flow and decision points are based primarily on available knowledge of the natural history of low back and leg pain as related to degenerative conditions of the spine.

individual as promptly as possible to a normal functional existence. The ability to achieve that idealized goal is dependent, not so much on technical excellence in the operating room, as on the precision and accuracy of the decision-making process.

In an effort to help practitioners improve their decision-making capabilities, we have developed a systematized approach to patients presenting with low back pain and sciatica in combination, or alone.

The plan outlined (Fig. 23–1) is derived not only from careful evaluation of therapeutic successes, but also, and probably of greater significance, from evaluation of the genesis of the patients who have failed to respond to operative measures of treatment, the so-called "failed back surgery syndrome." By relying heavily on these clinical data, we have been able to devise a format and approach that has optimized our therapeutic effort, basing our decisions on well-delineated rules rather than on emotion and intuition.

Webster defined an algorithm as "a set of rules for solving a particular problem within a finite number of steps." This is in effect an organized pattern of decision making and thought processes that we have found useful in approaching the problem of lumbar disc disease. Since first submitting the disc-degeneration algorithm for publication in 1979,[120] and since its subsequent revision in 1985,[277] we have made several changes in its organization. These primarily relate to increased experience in the area of spinal stenosis; the use of the computed tomographic (CT) and magnetic resonance imaging (MRI) scans, which have to a large extent negated the diagnostic value of the epidural venogram; and the withdrawal of our previous recommendation for the use of radiofrequency facet rhizotomy. With regard to the latter, we no longer believe that denervation of the facet joint using a percutaneous radiofrequency rhizolysis technique has more than a transient placebo effect.[127] There are no controlled studies demonstrating any long term efficacy of this procedure.

The teaching of algorithmic decision making for low back disorders is by no means a unique concept in spine care. Mooney[187] designed an algorithm for selecting treatments for common degenerative problems. Simmons[233] designed an algorithm for the evaluation, diagnosis, and treatment of difficult back problems, especially in patients with workmen's compensation injuries. Chapter 48 deals with the inherent complexity of the patient who presents after one or more failed spine operations. As reported by Rothman and Bernini,[223] an algorithm for salvage surgery of the lumbar spine provides for prompt recognition and treatment of those problems that are surgically remediable, such as recurrent disc herniation or spinal stenosis. Careful adherence to this salvage algorithm will prevent the physician from advising the failed back patient with arachnoiditis, for example, to undergo yet another futile surgical experience. Spengler,[239] in constructing his algorithm for chronic low back pain, advocated the team approach; in his study only 3 per cent of patients fulfilled criteria for surgical intervention. Behavior modification programs enabled approximately 25 to 40 per cent of patients to return to work. These programs, although expensive, are cost effective in the long term. At the University of Washington, cost effectiveness is felt to have been achieved if one patient out of 20 returns to work.

QUEBEC TASK FORCE ON SPINAL DISORDERS

In 1983 the Institute for Workers' Health and Safety in the Province of Quebec, Canada, received a request from the Quebec Workers' Health and Safety Commission to undertake clinical research on the problem of spinal disorders occurring in the workplace. The mandates of the task force that was created were as follows: (1) to develop and test a typology for the various treatments utilized in a variety of spinal conditions found in injured workers (develop matrices for the evaluation of both diagnostic and therapeutic measures), (2) to evaluate the effectiveness of physical therapy in the course of different stages of these disorders, (3) to determine the causes of the differences in duration of treatment between one institution and another for identical conditions, and (4) to make recommendations designed to improve the quality of treatment for injured workers with spinal disorders.[241]

To deal with the first mandate, the Task Force developed a classification of spinal disorders based on simple clinical criteria that represent most cases seen in practice (Table 23–2). Although these classifications are dif-

Table 23–2. EPIDEMIOLOGY: RISK FACTORS FOR LOW BACK PAIN BASED ON A LARGE POPULATION STUDY

Type of Factor	Known Risk Factors	Factors Not Associated With Low Back Pain
Constitutional	Age	Sex
	Physical fitness	Weight
	Abdominal muscle strength	Height
	Flexor/extensor balance	Davenport index
	Muscular insufficiency	
Postural/structural	Severe scoliosis	Lordosis
	Some congenital abnormalities	Disc space narrowing
	Narrowed spinal canal	Schmorl's nodes
	Spondylolisthesis	Spina bifida occulta
	Fractures	Osteophytes
	Multilevel degenerative disc disease	Transitional anomalies
	Spondyloarthropathies	Facet arthropathy
		Facet tropism
Environmental	Smoking	
Occupational	Heavy lifting	
	Twisting	
	Bending	
	Stooping	
	Floor surface conditions	
	Prolonged sitting	
	Vibration (vehicular and nonvehicular)	
Psychosocial	Anxiety	Psychoses
	Depression	Most neuroses
	Hypochondriasis	
	Somatization	
	Work dissatisfaction	
	Stress	
	Hysteria	
Recreational	Golf	Snowmobiling
	Tennis	Downhill skiing
	Football	Ice hockey
	Gymnastics	Baseball
	Jogging	Other sports
	Cross-country skiing	
Other	Multiple births	
	Possible genetic clustering	
Radiographic signs with equal prevalence in symptomatic and asymptomatic patients		
Disc space narrowing, osteophytes, facet arthropathy, facet tropism, Schmorl's nodes, spina bifida occulta, lumbarization, sacralization		

From Frymoyer, J. W., Pope, M. H., Castanza, M. C., et al.: Epidemiologic studies of low back pain. Spine *5*:419, 1980.

ferent from the more common diagnoses in present use, it was suggested that a uniform system such as this created a means of resolving confusion. This is particularly the case when dealing with low back pain, in which it often is not possible to identify the exact anatomic source of the symptoms.

For each class of symptoms, the value of certain diagnostic and therapeutic measures, based on a review of the literature, was given one of the following ranks: (1) supported by randomized control studies, (2) supported by nonrandomized control studies, (3) not supported by data but in common practice, (4) not supported by data and not in common practice, and (5) contraindicated on the basis of scientific evidence. In order to develop a matrix for or ranking of each diagnostic and therapeutic measure, ten literature data banks were searched and 721 abstract articles were found, which in turn were considered relevant up to December, 1985. After each of these articles was evaluated, 252 were rejected, leaving 469 publications describing diagnostic and treatment guidelines, which were then ranked.

After compiling the above data, the Task Force proposed an algorithm for the early management of spinal disorders that spans the first three months after initial presentation. Timing for specific evaluation and treatment steps based on our current understanding of the natural history of the disease process was a critical element within the management guideline proposed. This algorithm illustrates the fact that most cases in both the acute (less than seven days) and subacute (seven days to seven weeks) presentations improve in one month. Treatment can be limited to bed rest (no longer than two days), but may be longer for more severe symptoms.

For patients who do not improve after four weeks of conservative therapy, it is necessary to reevaluate them completely, perform a thorough history and physical examination, and obtain lumbar spine radiographs, as well as the erythrocyte sedimentation rate (ESR). The latter is obtained to rule out an occult inflammatory process. Appropriate conservative treatment should be continued, and consideration should be given to obtaining a medical or neurologic consultation at this time if the patient has not improved.

For patients who are tending toward chronicity (symptoms longer than three months in duration), it was suggested that they be evaluated by a multidisciplinary team familiar with the medical, emotional, and rehabilitation concerns resulting from chronic pain and disability.

A decision-making algorithm for specialized diagnostic testing and for surgical interventions was not presented. It was clearly stated, however, that studies such as myelography and discography are contraindicated in the early phases of patient treatment when there is no evidence of a neurologic deficit and no history of severe trauma. Similarly, surgical intervention was believed to be contraindicated, except for verified radicular compression and spinal stenosis.

The report also encouraged physicians to be familiar with the condition and circumstances within the workplace where the patient was injured. Lastly, acknowledgement of the inadequacies of the current scientific literature and recommendations for future research were described.

As the research concluded, "work-related spinal disorders account for such a high percentage of worker absenteeism and institutional compensatory costs, it is important to identify ways to ameliorate this problem." Readers are encouraged to review the Quebec Task Force publication[241] in its entirety as an aid in accomplishing this goal.

TREATMENT GOALS

The goals that we initially set for ourselves in the management of this population of patients with low back pain and sciatica from lumbar disc degeneration are as follows: (1) prompt return to normal function, (2) low cost to society, (3) minimizing of ineffectual surgery, and (4) efficient use of diagnostic studies.

For the first of these, total relief of pain is not always an attainable goal. However, even in persons in whom pain cannot be completely eradicated, we believe that return to a fruitful endeavor must be sought. In this regard the algorithm has a few exit points. Most involve a return to a normal life style, without restrictions. However, an exit also must be made if the work-up is completed, if there is no evidence of serious or treatable disease, and if pain persists. This is an important step for the patient and physician, accepting that not all back pain will resolve, or be "cured," and that some failures will occur.

Nachemson[194] stated that in 80 per cent of patients with low back pain, no objective cause for the pain can be found after a thorough examination. Furthermore, new information dealing with educational, ergonomic, psychiatric, and other treatment modalities will constitute the data base for a new form of therapy: early, gradual, biomechanically controlled return to activity and work. In our offices, we have seen numerous persons who have refrained from work, recreation, or their household function simply because increased activity produced mild pain. In the mind of these persons, any pain was a signal that they were causing harm to their spine. It is critical, therefore, that we, as physicians, reassure patients that a diagnosis of lumbar disc disease does not herald the onset of a progressive crippling disorder, that disc disease by itself is a normal pattern of aging, and that the usual clinical course is one of gradual improvement. These few words of reassurance may serve to avoid any addition to a patient's psychologic disability. Waddell[254] suggested that we must change our whole approach to low back disorders and recognize the need to consider the psychologic and social, as well as the physical, aspects. He pointed out in proposing his biopsychosocial model of low back disease that the physician must be both healer and counselor. Furthermore, "the patient's role must correspondingly change from passive recipient of treatment to a more active sharing of responsibility for his or her own progress."

The second goal is to have available a treatment format that will make therapy available at a tolerable and minimal cost to society. In a disease that has the tremendous prevalence and economic impact that we see with low back pain, it is vital that the individual and society as a whole be able to readily afford the necessary modalities of diagnosis and therapy. In this day of the $500 CT scan and the $5,000 surgical endeavor, we must be careful to refrain from unnecessary and ineffectual measures.

The third goal is to minimize ineffectual surgery. Surgical intervention that is premature, and thus by definition unnecessary or ineffectual in attaining the desired goals, has been a terrible burden to the spinal surgeon and the luckless patient. To emphasize this point, one need only look at the review published by Aitken and Bradford in 1947.[2] They investigated 169 surgical cases from the files of a large national compensation carrier between 1940 and 1944 and found that only 17 per cent of the results were good and 45 per cent were judged poor or "bad." The review showed that discs were removed at levels that did not correlate with the neurologic examination or the myelogram. Extensive laminectomies were performed for single-level disc disease. Postoperative roentgenograms demonstrated laminectomies performed at the wrong levels. One seventh of the patients were operated on within two months of the first episode of lumbar pain. In another one seventh of the patients, there was ample preoperative evidence of a psychoneurotic disorder. The mortality rate in the 169 cases was 3 per cent. Complications such as postoperative footdrop developed in six patients and paralysis of the quadriceps muscles in three. Fortunately, as modern series have been reported, the results have become better than in this startling account. A major review[132] summarizing the experience in over 13,000 operations performed by 35 investigators for lumbar disc degeneration was published in 1961. Unfortunately, it is often difficult to compare findings from one series with those in the next, but two terms and factors are equivocal. The first of these is complete relief of pain, which was achieved in only 46 per cent of cases, a mark quite short of an ideal goal. The second factor, complete failure of pain relief, is rather constant at 10 per cent. We recount these data not out of historical interest alone but also as a caution for those who are willing to relax their preoperative indications for patients undergoing chemonucleolysis, percutaneous discectomy, or internal fixation procedures for lumbar disc disease, lest they succeed in creating another generation of failed back surgery cripples. We should not let our zest for technology outweigh reasoning that is based on sound scientific principles that have been subjected to the scrutiny of prospective, randomized, controlled clinical study. In a review[87] of 800 patients selected for lumbar spine surgery using the disc-degeneration algorithm, 270 had primary degenerative disc disease that led to a lumbar laminectomy or discectomy during a five-year time frame. After a minimum of six months of postoperative follow-up study, a standardized questionnaire was used to assess patients' satisfaction with their operative procedures. The results demonstrated that with the correct patient selection there was a high rate (90 or 95 per cent) of satisfaction in the patient and a 90 to 95 per cent chance of reducing leg pain. It is also important to note that 80 to 85 per cent of patients reported a significant diminution of back pain. Needless to say, these excellent results justify our continued espousal of the use of the algorithm. We strongly believe that when conservative treatment has failed and the patient has a pathosis that will lend itself to surgical intervention, one should not procrastinate too long. We know that surgical therapy undertaken for sciatica becomes considerably less effective when delayed for more than three months and is almost worthless when one to two years have gone by.[237] The reasons for this are still unclear, but present research into the pathophysiology of nerve root compression may provide the answers. There is an optimal time for surgical intervention, and this must be clearly understood.

The final and most important goal in today's medical world is the efficient and precise use of diagnostic studies. Now that we are surrounded by the availability of CT, MRI, psychologic profiles, and numerous consultants, each with their own battery of tests, we must resist our own impulses to use every test available and our patients' often insistent demands for the "latest study." There is a proper time and indication for each of these diagnostic measures. The decision making can in fact be made more difficult and less accurate when excessive amounts of data are made available too early in the treatment process.

Striving to achieve these goals will in turn facilitate our ultimate goal of excellence in managing our patients with symptomatic lumbar disc disease in all its manifestations. A wise physician once said that in order to achieve excellence in the art and science of medicine, a physician needs to practice the five "A"s: availability, affability, ability, appreciating the plight of the patient, and affordability.

THE ALGORITHM

As we begin outlining our management protocol, we find that disorders such as degenerative disc disease, osteoarthritis of the zygopophyseal joints, herniated intervertebral discs, fractures, muscular strain and ligamentous sprain injuries, and spondylolisthesis can be diagnosed as distinct entities. Often, these few conditions may not be associated with distinct symptoms, but it is clear that they constitute a significant portion of distinct diagnostic entities in the overall clinical problem of the differential diagnosis of low back pain and sciatica.

One of the key prerequisites for any physician treating a patient with low back pain is, therefore, a knowledge of the pathophysiology of these disorders. Physicians concerned with treating such a patient must seek to expand their knowledge of the fundamental processes occurring during disc degeneration, and not confine efforts to channeling patients through the algorithm for the purpose of the simple extirpation of protruding intervertebral discs. Physicians who do this succumb to the myopia of the technician. It is the purpose of the algorithm to widen our field of interest and place some of the disease processes that can be productive of low back pain and sciatica in clear perspective.

PATIENT EVALUATION

Beginning with the broad range of patients who present to our offices with low back pain, with or without sciatica, the keystone of clinical diagnosis remains the history and physical examination. The history should allow one to develop a precise subjective assessment of the patient's pain syndrome. The patient should be asked to describe the character (C) of the pain, whether it be sharp, dull, aching, burning, or dysthetic. He or she should describe the location (L) of the pain. Exacerbating (E) and ameliorating (A) phenomena should be defined; it is particularly important to differentiate back pain that is mechanical in nature from pain that is nonmechanical and present at rest. Any pattern of radiation (R) should be defined; in this regard it is important to differentiate referred (sclerotomal) from true radicular (neurotomal) radiation of the pain. The patient should be questioned for any particular time relationships (TR) that the pain syndrome exhibits. Pain that intensifies at night and keeps the patient from obtaining a sound sleep should often alert one to the possibility of a neoplastic condition. Lastly, in performing a thorough review of systems, one should question the patient specifically as to any associated phenomena (AP) that may exist in addition to the pain. We specifically question the patient with regard to the presence or absence of numbness, paresthesias, weakness, a sense of instability in the lower extremities, stiffness, change in bowel or bladder habits, and constitutional symptoms such as fever, chills, and weight loss. Any change in the patient's appetite, exercise tolerance, sleep habits, or pattern of social and sexual activity may give a clue to an underlying malignancy, but much more frequently indicates an underlying depressive disorder. It is also important to obtain any history of trauma along with the precise details of the mechanism of injury. Notice by the acronym capitals in parentheses that they conveniently combine to produce the mnemonic CLEAR TRAP, a convenient memory device that we routinely teach to our medical students and residents.

In performing the physical examination one should orient the differential diagnosis to distinguishing between intraspinal and extraspinal causes of the pain. Intraspinal causes may be secondary to intradural (intramedullary, extramedullary) or extradural (epidural, foraminal, paraspinal) pathologic conditions. Extraspinal causes similarly can be divided into intrapelvic and extrapelvic pathoses. In this regard, it is important to examine the abdomen and perform a rectal examination, if the patient has not had a recent examination, and also to consider early gynecologic consultation, if the

Table 23–3. ETIOLOGIES OF RADICULAR LEG PAIN AND SEGMENTAL SENSORY DISTURBANCES: AN ANATOMIC CLASSIFICATION

Myelogenic
- Spinal cord tumor
  - Ependymoma
  - Astrocytoma
  - Hemangioblastoma
- Multiple sclerosis

Root
- Spondylogenic
  - Prolapsed disc
  - Spinal stenosis
  - Foraminal stenosis/lateral recess syndrome
  - Spondyloarthropathies
  - Achondroplasia
  - Metabolic: Paget's disease, osteoporosis, extramedullary hematopoiesis
  - Bone lesions: chordoma, chondrosarcoma, aneurysmal bone cyst, osteoma, osteogenic sarcoma, eosinophilic granuloma, other bone tumors, sacral cyst
  - Infectious: osteomyelitis, discitis
- Pyogenic
- Nonpyogenic (tuberculous, fungal)
- Nonbony tumors
  - Neurofibroma/schwannoma
  - Meningioma
  - Ependymoma
  - Lipoma
  - Metastasis (breast, lung, thyroid, prostate, renal cell, multiple myeloma)
- Infection/inflammation
  - Herpes
  - Syphilis
  - Arachnoiditis
- Trauma
  - Fracture-dislocation
  - Epidural hematoma
- Miscellaneous
  - Subarachnoid hemorrhage
  - Aneurysm
  - Perineural root cyst
  - Extradural meningeal root cyst

Plexus
- Abdominal tumor
- Endometriosis
- Appendiceal abscess/retroperitoneal infection
- Retroperitoneal hematoma
- Pelvic fracture

Peripheral
- Diabetes mellitus
- Trauma
  - Intramuscular injection
  - Posterior dislocated femur
  - Inferior gluteal artery aneurysm
- Entrapment
  - Meralgia paresthetica
  - Obturator syndrome
  - Piriformis syndrome
  - Common peroneal palsy
  - Tarsal tunnel syndrome
- Wartenberg's neuritis
- Tumor

Miscellaneous
- Primary sciatica

From Couldwell W. T., and Weiss, M. H.: Leg radicular pain and sensory disturbance. The differential diagnosis. Spine *2*:671, 1988.

examination of a female patient leads one to suspect a pathologic pelvic condition.

In the process of performing a physical examination, we scrupulously observe the patient to detect any nonorganic physical signs. We use Waddell and colleagues'[256] standardized group of tests, specifically performing simulation tests; distraction tests; tests to detect tenderness that is superficial; nonanatomic, regional motor, or sensory deficit tests; as well as tests of patterns of overreaction to the examiner's maneuvers. If three or more of these nonorganic signs are present, it is often necessary to perform a more detailed psychosocial history taking and examination in order to fully appreciate how patients' interactions with their environment may be impacting on their disease process or its presentation.

CLINICAL SYNDROME OF LUMBAR DISC DISEASE

Lumbar disc degeneration is the most common cause of back and leg pain. It is a multifaceted syndrome and must be recognized as such if the diagnosis is to be correct and the treatment effective. One sees with disturbing regularity missed diagnoses of herniated lumbar discs that present in an atypical fashion unfamiliar to the practitioner. It is equally precarious, however, to polarize one's thinking at the opposite extreme and attribute all cases of back and leg pain to abnormalities of the intervertebral disc. A wide variety of vascular, infectious, and space-occupying lesions can mimic the herniated lumbar disc (Table 23–3). An attempt will be made to outline the classic picture of the lumbar disc syndrome, as well as the more common variants. The algorithm approach presented is based on a knowledge of the natural history of degenerative disc disease, an awareness of its relatively benign course, and an acceptance that perhaps initially some more severe disorders may be missed. However, these are rare and should be detected by appropriate history taking and physical examination, along with the passage of a little time.

It is important from the outset to recognize that the clinical syndromes discussed represent manifestations of the sequential spectrum of degeneration that affects the "three joint complex."[77] That is, the clinical presentation ranging from backache with and without referred pain through radicular pain to neurogenic claudication is a reflection of the totality of degeneration of the intervertebral disc and the facet joints. Furthermore, symptoms can be conveyed over well-defined but often simultaneously stimulated pain pathways (the sinuvertebral nerves to the annulus and theca, the spinal nerves, and the medial and lateral branches of the posterior rami). Systematic analysis of these pathways will allow a more exact therapeutic solution.

History

Back Pain

Most patients with degenerative disc disease in the lumbar spine have low back pain as the earliest symptom. Spangfort's[238] computerized analysis of 2504 disc operations demonstrated a mean duration of low back pain of 5.6 years before surgery, and this temporal disability preceded the onset of complaints of leg pain by nearly two years. This is similar to the results of Garfin and colleagues[87] in an analysis of the Pennsylvania Plan Algorithm for treating patients. Weber's excellent prospective study[260] of lumbar disc herniation suggested that in more than 90 per cent of patients studied there were nearly ten years of episodic low back pain before the insidious onset of a radicular component. Often the patient recalls that after periods of demanding physical activity or of seemingly benign but prolonged postures, pain appears in the lumbosacral area. The pain may last a few days and usually subsides with limitation of activity and bed rest. The pain pattern at this time is mechanical in nature in the sense that it is made worse by standing, lifting, and prolonged sitting and is relieved by rest.

It is the authors' feeling that pain at this stage is due to early degeneration of the annulus fibrosus and desiccation of the nucleus pulposus. Since the nucleus no longer functions as a perfect gel with viscoelastic properties, it will transmit forces in a nonlinear and asymmetric fashion (Fig. 23–2).[152]

Disc degeneration, with its dorsally situated sinovertebral sensory nerve involvement, may be implicated in this pain syndrome. The initial onset of low back pain in the late 20s and early 30s coincides with the obliteration of vascular

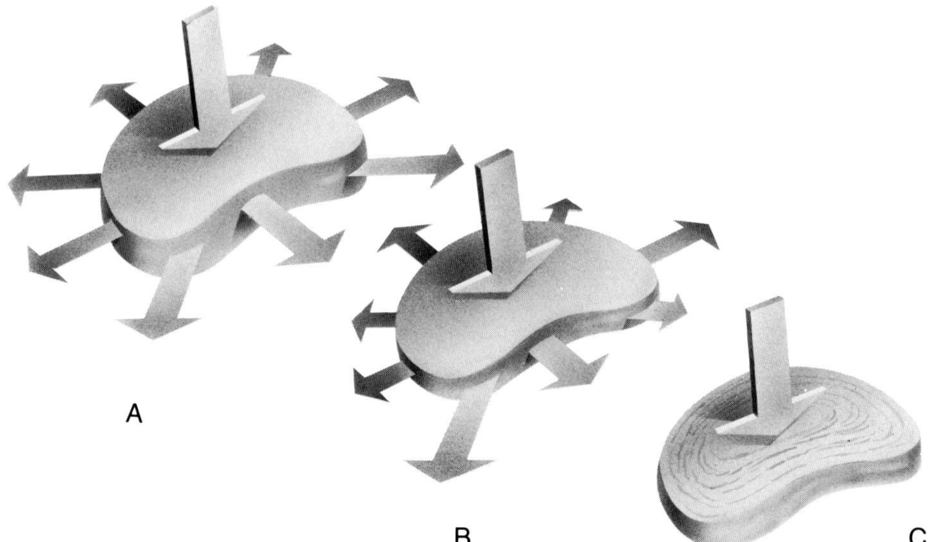

Figure 23–2. Distribution of forces in the normal and abnormal disc. *A*, When the disc functions normally, as in the early decades of life, the nucleus distributes the forces of compression and tension equally to all parts of the annulus. *B*, With degeneration, the nucleus no longer functions as a perfect gel and the forces transmitted to the annulus are unequal. *C*, With advanced degeneration of the nucleus, the distribution of forces to the annulus from within is completely lost since the nucleus now acts as a solid rather than a liquid. For this reason, disc herniation is unusual in the elderly.

supply to the nucleus pulposus in all but the most peripheral aspects of the annulus fibrosus. The subsequent age-related defective diffusion mechanism at the vertebral end plate–annular interface[33, 168] provides a basis for the loss of structural integrity of the disc at this time in the axial skeleton's aging process. The mechanical intensification and relief seen in this clinical syndrome can also be attributed to disc degeneration and easily understood in light of Nachemson's[191, 193] landmark in vivo determination of disc pressure in various postures (Fig. 23–3).

It should be reemphasized that at this early stage, disc degeneration cannot be clearly differentiated from certain other commonly referred to (but also poorly understood or defined) causes of low back pain such as neural arch defects, postural strain, and unstable lumbosacral mechanisms.

With the passage of time, these painful episodes may become more frequent and intense and may lead to more disability. Between acute episodes of back pain, the patient may describe a sense of stiffness, weakness, or instability that is present at a low, but noticeable level. These may be manifestations of adverse motion segment (vertebral body, disc, and facet joint) behavior alterations.[152] Defined changes do occur in disc geometry, in annular structural integrity, and in the way the disc nucleus is pressurized prior to load. Discogenic pain usually has the mechanical quality of being accentuated with prolonged sitting and standing. There is a clinical correlation of increased load with increased symptoms. An

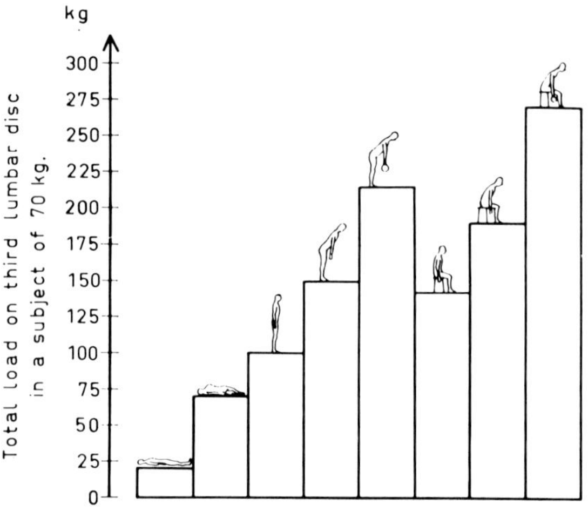

Figure 23–3. The total load on the third lumbar disc in a subject weighing 70 kg. (From Nachemson, A.: In vivo discometry in lumbar discs with irregular nucleograms. Acta Orthop. Scand. *36*:426, 1965. © 1965 Munksgaard International Publishers Ltd., Copenhagen, Denmark.)

intermittent character of the pain is also characteristic of disc degeneration. One should be wary when the patient states that from the onset the pain has been unrelenting and progressive, as this suggests an infectious or neoplastic state.

Injury is frequently noted by the patient at some time during the clinical course. In many instances, some spine pain was present before the injury. Weber's study[259] revealed precipitating events for the first episode of low back pain in 55 per cent of patients who eventually developed disc herniations. The trauma reported, however, ranged from a falling episode and lifting and heavy work activity to nothing more serious than an abrupt movement. It is interesting that these incidents of pain often occur during the early hours of the day after an extended recumbent position in sleep, when the turgor and hydration of the nucleus pulposus is at its maximum (Fig. 23–4).[193]

Our current concepts of the pathophysiology of symptomatic disc disease show trauma to be a precipitating, rather than a causative, factor. Jayson and colleagues[131] subjected 78 cadaver intervertebral discs to discography and roentgenographically classified their nuclear morphology. When these were subjected to compressive loads, bursting most commonly occurred into the adjacent vertebral bodies and not posteriorly. When nuclear herniation was realized posterolaterally and directly posterior, it occurred in discs that were previously noted to have posterolateral, direct posterior, or degenerative nuclear morphology. While the discs were subject to compressive forces only, the premorbid nuclear and annular status is of major importance.

Excessive stress applied to a young, healthy spine will fracture the osseous elements of the vertebra before the disc ruptures. When disc herniation occurs in young spines not yet subject to disc degeneration, the herniation will also likely follow areas of premorbid structural weakness. This often occurs into residual indentations in the cartilaginous end plate that remains as a result of notochord or embryologic vascular regression, yielding Schmorl's nodes.[219] One other premorbid area of relative structural weakness that persists is at the interface between the cartilaginous end plate and the ossified portion of the vertebral body. In adolescents this leads to ring apophyses, subluxations, and neural element compromise if it occurs posteriorly,[136] or to anterior Schmorl's nodes or a limbus vertebra if the separation is anterior.

Referred Pain

When certain of the mesodermal structures, such as ligaments, periosteum, joint capsule, and annulus, are subjected to abnormal stimuli, such as excessive stretching or injection of hypertonic saline, a deep, ill-defined, dull, aching discomfort is noted that may be referred into the areas of the lumbosacral joint, sacroiliac joint, buttocks, or legs (Fig. 23–5).[138, 189] The pattern of referral is to the area designated the sclerotome, which has the same embryonic origin as the mesodermal tissues stimulated. While this peripheral pathway can explain the referred pattern, the individual variations encountered must include consideration of central neural pathways. Kellgren[138] concluded that the referred distribution of pain depends

Experimental flow of fluid in autopsy discs.

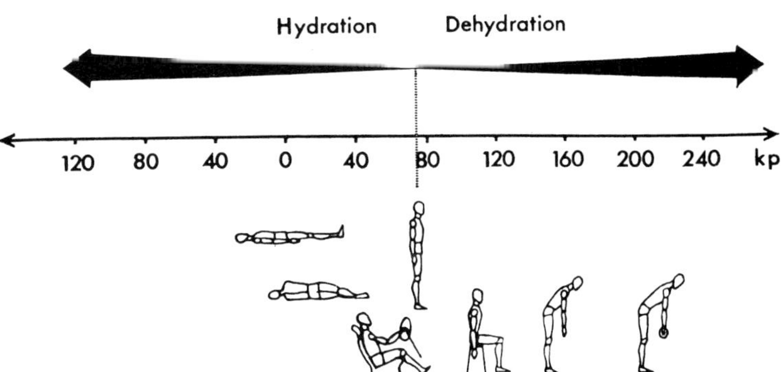

Figure 23–4. Theoretical calculation on the hydration-dehydration points, as obtained experimentally by Kramer, combined with the findings of intradiscal pressure measurements by Nachemson. (From Nachemson, A.: Toward a better understanding of low-back pain: a review of the mechanics of the lumbar disc. Rheumatol. Rehabil. *14*:129, 1975.)

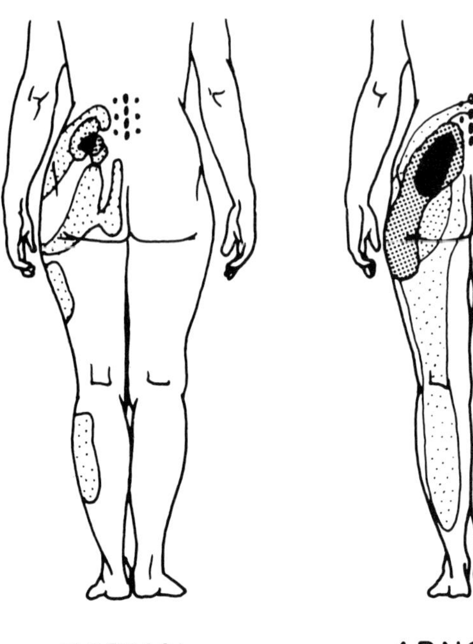

Figure 23–5. Pain referral pattern for asymptomatic and symptomatic subjects. This confirms that the pain referral pattern from stimulation of the lumbar facet joint is in the typical locations of lumbago. (From Mooney, V., and Robertson, J.: The facet syndrome. Clin. Orthop. *115*:149, 1976.)

not only on segmental innervation, but also on the severity of pain and the extent to which an individual is cognizant of the stimulated components of the axial skeleton.

Pain of this type can often present concurrently with radicular pain from nerve root compression or inflammation. The deeper, boring pain is classically attributed to a distribution along myotome and sclerotomes, and the sharper and better localized superficial pain is conveyed along the dermatomes.[71] The two may be easily confused. Moreover, sympathetic dystrophic signs and symptoms due to nerve root encroachment can further confuse the presentation, since the causalgia may exist with or without the more classic complaints associated with radiculopathy.[18]

Radicular Symptoms

Pressure on an inflamed nerve root by a disc fragment, bulging annulus, or compromised lateral recess may produce pain and motor and/or sensory signs and symptoms in the lower extremities. It had been first suggested by Smyth and Wright in 1958[235] and later demonstrated by MacNab[165] that normal, nonirritated nerve roots subjected to compression will produce paresthesias and functional changes, whereas nerves that are inflamed will also yield a painful response to the manipulation.

The etiologic role of mechanical tension on the nerve root yielding radicular pain is generally accepted, but whether there is damage to the intrinsic structure of the neural tissue, its accompanying vasculature, or both is uncertain.[190] The inflammatory component of the radicular syndrome is of obvious significance, but the causative agents are uncertain. With the evolution of annular rents, the avascular nucleus pulposus may evoke an autoimmune response and act as a causative factor.[21, 201] This has been theorized because of observations of the susceptibility of nerve roots to inflammatory agents and an enhanced immune cellular response to homogenized disc material in both animals and humans.[22, 73] As yet, no specific immunoglobulins have been found in disc tissue removed at the time of surgery.

The interaction of mechanical and inflammatory components yielding signs and symptoms of the various lumbar disc syndromes is important, but specific information concerning the dynamics of that interaction is only beginning to evolve.

The patient often describes a sharp, lancinating pain, usually starting in the hip or proximal portion of the thigh and ultimately progressing distally in a dermatome pattern.

The L5 and S1 spinal nerves are most frequently involved, reflecting the fact that the greater number of disc herniations occur at L4–L5 and L5–S1.[215, 238] While the onset of leg pain may be insidious, or extremely rapid and dramatic and associated with a tearing or snapping sensation in the spine, the former presentation is more usual for both the first sciatic attack and those that precipitated the surgical intervention.[259]

At the time of onset of the sciatica the back pain may suddenly abate. The pathoanatomic explanation of this is probably that once the annulus has ruptured, it is no longer placed under tension and there is no longer a stimulus for pain in the lower back.

When the sciatic pain is acute, the patient or family of the patient may note that he or she is listing, usually away from the side of the sciatica. Occasionally, if the disc herniation is axillary or central in position, the patient may list toward the side of the sciatica. These maneuvers tend to decrease tension on the compromised nerve root.

The pain is frequently made worse by any activity that increases intraspinal and intradiscal pressures such as the Valsalva maneuver, coughing, sneezing, and bearing down during defecation. These also correlate with Nachemson's in vivo disc pressure studies.

Patients may be aware of a marked limitation of motion in the spine, and often state that their back is "locked." This is particularly true in adolescents with disc herniations.[29, 34] In extreme cases the pain may prevent any stress from being placed on the back or leg, and patients may lie helpless on the floor or in bed with the feeling that they are "paralyzed." In reality the limiting factor is pain. In high disc lesions affecting the upper lumbar spinal nerves, the pain may be isolated to the area of the knee, and patients may protest vigorously that the difficulty is confined only to the knee joint and may discourage any examination of the lumbar spine. When the clinical course has progressed to motor weakness involving the quadriceps muscle, patients may complain of buckling of the knee in addition to the knee pain, which makes the situation still more confusing.

Motor Symptoms

Infrequently, the patient may present with lower extremity weakness, which may be disabling but occur without symptomatology or clinically appreciated sphincter disturbances. This is particularly true in lesions affecting the fourth and fifth spinal nerve roots.

If the fifth lumbar nerve is compromised, the patient may note weakness on dorsiflexion of the foot and toes, and occasionally a complete footdrop. The hip abductors may likewise be affected, yielding an abductor lurch with an associated positive Trendelenburg sign. Hakelius and Hindmarsh[105] found an equal number of disc herniations in patients with isolated dorsiflexion weakness compared with patients who also had other neurologic signs. Nonetheless, a *relatively painless* monoradicular or particularly multiradicular paresis must suggest the possibility of a metabolic or infectious neuropathy, or space-occupying lesion of the cord, although a disc herniation or stenosis might also cause this.

Disc Syndromes

Sciatic Pain. It is not uncommon with the acute extrusion of a disc fragment against a nerve root to have the sudden onset of sciatica without concomitant back pain. The diagnosis of discogenic disease is suggested by accentuation of this leg pain by the Valsalva maneuver, an activity that increases intradiscal pressure, cerebrospinal fluid (CSF) pressure (and therefore, perhaps, spinal nerve root size), and neural irritation. This, of course, would not be present in leg pain caused by pathologic conditions of the joints of the lower extremities, or more peripheral lesions of the sciatic nerve itself. Although the patient may be free of back pain, there may be a marked list, muscle spasm, and limitation of motion in the lumbar spine. This is particularly true of lateral lumbar disc herniations.[1] The limited lumbar mobility is not purely a defensive and learned reaction to discogenic and radicular pain, but may be a manifestation of the pathophysiology of the "disease" process. Fidler and colleagues[81] found in biopsies of the multifidus muscles from patients with positive root signs, studied to differentiate slow fibers (low levels of myosin-ATPase activity), which primarily function in a postural role, from fast fibers, which function more dynamically, that there was a higher ratio of slow to fast fibers than normally found. The cross-sectional area of the fast fibers was also increased. These findings, different from the pattern usually found in normal individuals, were interpreted as reflecting a selective injury to fast fiber motor neurons, as a result of either ischemia or mechanical injury, in the anterior root of the involved spinal nerve.

It should be pointed out that in certain individuals, isolated areas of pain in the lower extremities are noted rather than the typical pattern of dermatome involvement. The primary complaint may be pain of, or at, the knee, calf, ankle, or heel (Fig. 23–6). In studying pain and spinal root lesions, Friis and colleagues[84] found that approximately 10 per cent of patients with L5 or S1 lesions, in particular, had asymptomatic areas between painful foci. The unwary examiner who fails to instruct the patient to completely undress and who does not perform a meticulously thorough examination can obviously be led astray in these instances.

Back Pain Alone. It has been pointed out that most patients with discogenic pain have intermittent episodes of back pain at the onset of their clinical course. Most of these individuals proceed through the entire natural history of their "disease" and never experience sciatica. During acute exacerbation the back pain will be accentuated by the Valsalva maneuver, and there are findings in the lumbar area typical of degenerative disc disease. This group of patients rarely develop a surgical lesion. The treating physician must rule out other causes of back pain, such as tumor, infection, and intra-abdominal disease, before this diagnostic category (degenerating or degenerative disc disease) is utilized.

Neurogenic Claudication. With increased awareness of this syndrome,[74, 273] first appreciated by Verbiest[251] in 1954, many more patients are benefiting from a correct diagnosis of the cause of their leg pain. Vague leg pain, dysesthesias, and paresthesias distributed over the anterior and posterior thighs and calves, often not in a single pure dermatomal pattern, are brought on by spinal postures that mechanically compromise the neural canal and the neural foramina.

The clinical presentation is well documented.[73, 275] Patients of either sex, usually not before their fifth decade, first appreciate vague

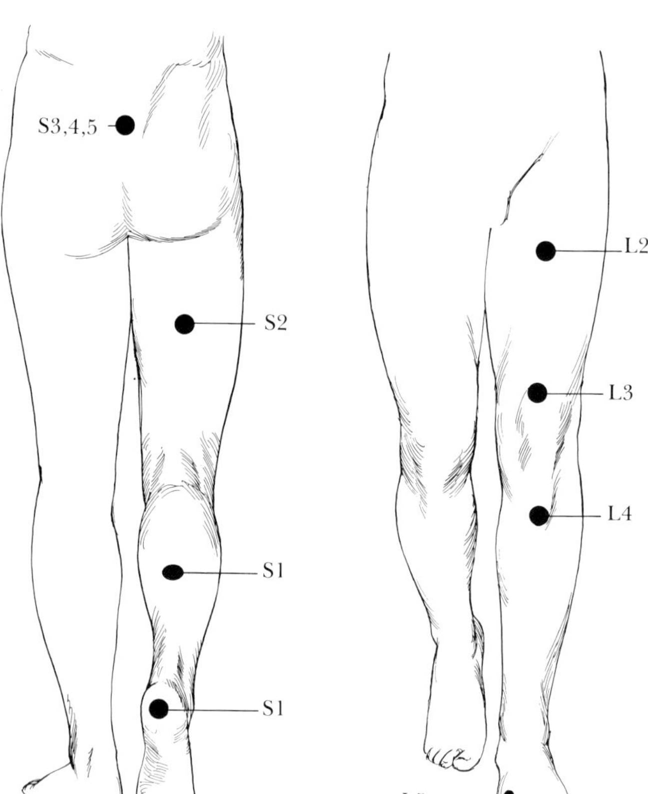

Figure 23–6. Pain may radiate to small, isolated, specific areas along the course of a dermatome.

pains, dysesthesia, and paresthesias with ambulation and will obtain some relief of their symptoms by sitting or assuming a supine posture. The increased lordotic stance with walking and particularly walking down grades increases the complaints. This symptomatic relationship to posture has been verified with the "bicycle test" of van Gelderen,[69] in which claudication symptoms are not produced while on a bicycle in a flexed position, bent over the handlebars, since there is a reduction of the lumbar lordosis and a subsequent increase in the central sagittal and foraminal dimensions of the canal. In contrast, muscle claudication symptoms will be produced with ambulation up grades or bicycling sitting straight up or extended. The absence of pulses below the hips and rubor and pallor changes with elevation are classic for vascular claudication, but not neurogenic claudication. In cases in which the diagnosis is uncertain, vascular flow studies and/or arteriography may be necessary.

With the maturation of the syndrome, symptoms at rest occur, and muscle weakness and atrophy and asymmetric reflex changes may then be appreciated, but as long as the symptoms are only aggravated dynamically, abnormal neurologic findings may appear only after stressing the patient.

The clinical syndrome has been associated with lumbar spinal stenosis and nerve root entrapment syndromes. An internationally accepted classification of the anatomic syndrome (Fig. 23–7) has been defined, and the production of symptoms has been attributed to those changes occurring locally, segmentally, or generalized in affecting osseous and soft tissue. It is, however, important to realize that structural changes in the spinal and foraminal canals exaggerated with posture are, as noted by Verbiest,[252] "conditions, but not absolute determinants of intermittent claudication." Indeed, the symptoms manifested may vary significantly among patients with similar pathomorphologic changes owing to the temporal framework within which the neural compression has occurred, the individual susceptibility of the nerves involved, and the unique functional demands and pain tolerance of the patient. A more detailed discussion can be found in Chapter 25.

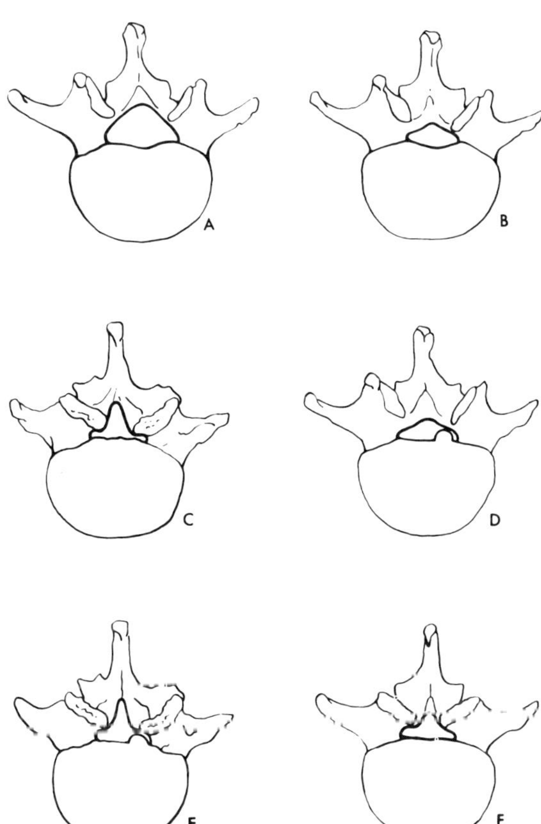

Figure 23–7. Types of lumbar spinal stenosis. *A*, Normal canal. *B*, Congenital/developmental stenosis. *C*, Degenerative stenosis. *D*, Congenital/developmental stenosis with disc herniation. *E*, Degenerative stenosis with disc herniation. *F*, Congenital/developmental stenosis with superimposed degenerative stenosis. (From Arnoldi, C. C., Brodsky, A. E., Cauchoix, J., et al.: Lumbar spinal stenosis and nerve root entrapment syndromes. Clin. Orthop. *115*:4, 1976.)

Cauda Equina Syndrome. Occasionally, a large midline disc herniation may compress several roots of the cauda equina. Raaf[215] reported an incidence of 2 per cent in 624 patients with protruded discs. Spangfort[238] reported 1.2 per cent in 2500 cases. His review of the literature found a total incidence of approximately 2.4 per cent. He further found no noticeable differences in sex distribution or age. Lower lumbar discs were the most common levels of offending herniations, but there is a significantly larger number of high lumbar herniations leading to this problem than seen in other disc syndromes. Peyser and Harari[212] reviewed the literature and found an extremely high occurrence (11 of 17 cases) of cauda equina syndrome when there was an intradural rupture of the intervertebral disc. These herniations occur predominantly in the high lumbar areas and fortunately represent only 0.2 per cent of all disc herniations.

If the lesion reaches a large size it may mimic an intraspinal tumor, particularly if it has been slowly progressing. Often, back or perianal pain will predominate, and radicular symptoms may be masked or minimal. Difficulty with urination, including either frequency or overflow incontinence, may develop relatively early. In males a recent history of impotence may be elicited. If leg pain develops, this may be followed by numbness of the feet and difficulty in walking. Large midline disc lesions, which ordinarily produce complete myelographic blocks when associated with these symptoms, compress several spinal nerve roots. When compromised, the centrally placed sacral fibers to the lower abdominal viscera produce symptoms that characterize cauda equina compression. Perianal numbness, saddle dysesthesia, and a loss of the anal reflex or diminished rectal tone characterize an advanced cauda equina syndrome. Sensory deficit is usual, and frequently involves the lower sacral roots.

Confusion as to the exact diagnosis may arise if the lesion is incomplete or slowly evolving. It has been reported presenting as a lower motor neuron lesion, or more frequently with abnormal radicular signs and normal or upper motor neuron lesion activity.[172] This latter lesion can be explained only on a vascular basis, but the specific mechanism in these cases is purely speculative.

The significance of this entity is that it must be considered a reason for prompt surgical intervention since spontaneous neurologic recovery has not been observed.[149] If incontinence is present, only prompt surgery can offer a chance to lessen the hazards of possible future urinary drainage problems. Similarly, sudden severe paresis or paraplegia merits prompt and generous decompression. When the symptoms are florid, a careful preoperative myelogram or MRI scan for level identification should be performed on an emergency basis (Fig. 23–8).

Bladder Symptoms

Disc protrusions may present as an abnormality of bowel and bladder function in pa-

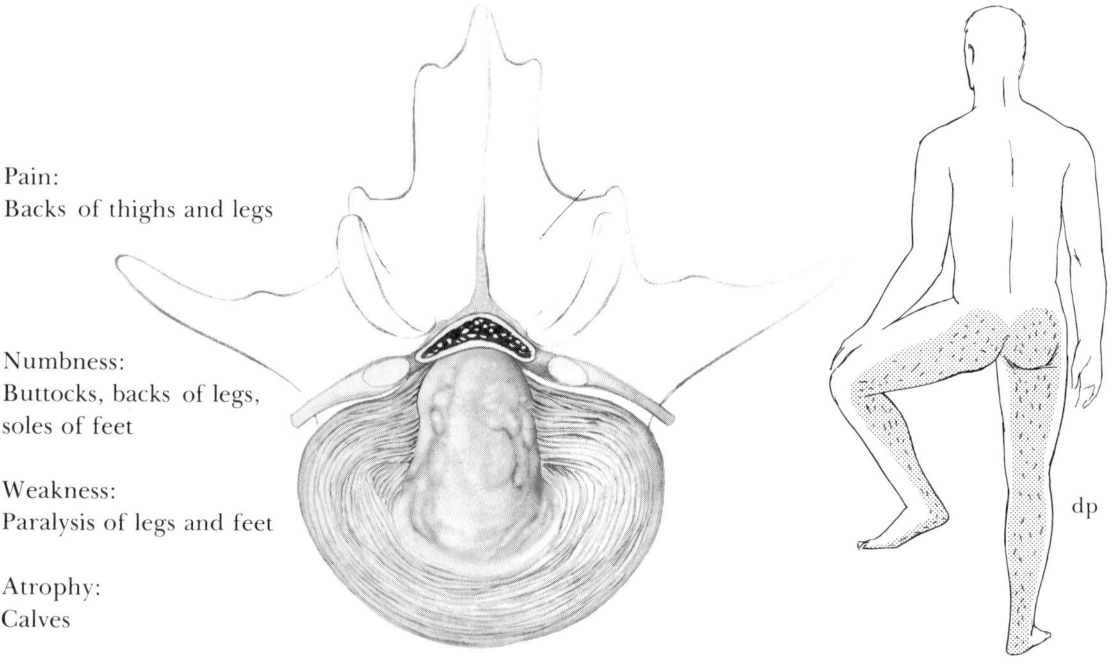

Figure 23–8. Massive herniation at the level of the third, fourth, or fifth disc may cause severe compression of the cauda equina. Pain is confined chiefly to the buttocks and the back of the thighs and legs. Numbness is widespread from the buttocks to the soles of the feet. Motor weakness or loss is present in the legs and feet with loss of muscle mass in the calves. The bladder and bowels can be paralyzed. (From DePalma, A. F., and Rothman, R. H.: The Intervertebral Disc. Philadelphia, W. B. Saunders Co., 1970.)

tients with minimal or absent back pain and sciatica. It has been well documented by Emmett and Love[72] and Ross and Jackson[222] that disc disease should be ruled out in young or middle-aged patients who develop urinary retention, vesical irritability, or incontinence. This is particularly true in the absence of infection or other pelvic abnormalities.

Four syndromes have been described in regard to bladder abnormalities caused by disc derangement: (1) total urinary retention; (2) chronic, long-standing, partial retention; (3) vesicular irritability; and (4) loss of desire to void, associated with an unawareness of the necessity to void. Jones and Moore[133] considered that the uninhibited type of neuropathic bladder dysfunction, without loss of bladder sensation, represents an incipient stage of an evolving neurogenic bladder disorder due to increasing involvement of the sacral roots.

Sharr and colleagues[232] emphasized the occurrence of bladder dysfunction with spinal stenosis. While the same neuropathic bladder disorders were encountered in patients with disc herniation, the intermittency of symptoms was emphasized, thus adding another facet to the weakness, dysesthesia, and paresthesias already associated with intermittent neurogenic claudication. If these symptoms, particularly in their more subtle forms, are not specifically sought, they will often be overlooked. Cystoscopy and a cystometrogram, in conjunction with radiographic assessment, are most helpful in obtaining a definite diagnosis. These clinical syndromes are unlikely to occur with monoradicular involvement.

Physical Examination

Inspection

Limitation of spine motion is usually noted during the symptomatic phase of lumbar disc disease. The range of motion should be noted not only in forward flexion but also in extension. The examiner must not equate flexion of the hips with flexion of the lumbar spine. Attention should be directed toward whether reversal of the normal lumbar lordosis occurs. It has been previously noted that even in patients who have only sciatica, marked restriction of motion may be present in the lumbar spine.

When acute sciatica is present, the patient may list away from the side of the sciatica, producing a "sciatic scoliosis" (Fig. 23–9). When the disc herniation is lateral to the nerve root, the patient may deviate the back away from the side of the irritated nerve in an attempt to draw the nerve root away from the disc fragment. This is dramatically demonstrated with extreme lateral disc herniations in that efforts at lateral bending to the side of the lesion markedly exaggerate the patient's pain and paresthesias.[9, 74]

When the herniation is in an axillary position, medial to the nerve root, the patient may list toward the side of the lesion in an effort to decompress the nerve root.

The gait and stance of patients with acute disc syndrome also are often characteristic. The patient usually holds the painful leg in a flexed position and is reluctant to place the foot flat, directly on the floor. Presumably, flexion of the leg relaxes the spinal nerve roots and is an involuntary effort at decompression of the root. When walking, the patient has an antalgic gait, putting as little weight as possible on the extremity and quickly transferring weight to the unaffected side. Gait disturbances, as well as significant loss of lumbar motility, are fairly common with disc herniations, particularly in adolescents.[1]

Loss of normal lumbar lordosis and paravertebral muscle spasm also are usually seen during the acute phase of the disease. These abnormalities may be appreciated on inspection, particularly the contracted mass of the paravertebral muscles when the spasm is extreme. Occasionally, in less acute situations, the muscle spasm can be elicited only when the patient is stressed by prolonged standing or forward flexion of the spine. Muscle spasm may on occasion be appreciated only unilaterally, which may indicate an extreme lateral disc protrusion.[74]

Palpation and Percussion

Palpation of the lumbar spine in the midline may elicit pain at the level of the symptomatic degenerative disc. This sign, however, is vague and inconclusive. It is not unusual to find tenderness laterally along the iliac crest and iliolumbar ligament, and/or over the sacroiliac joint. In many instances this tenderness does not reflect disease in these lateral areas, but rather hyperesthesia from nerve root irritation. Often, no tenderness is elicited with palpation of the lumbar spine.

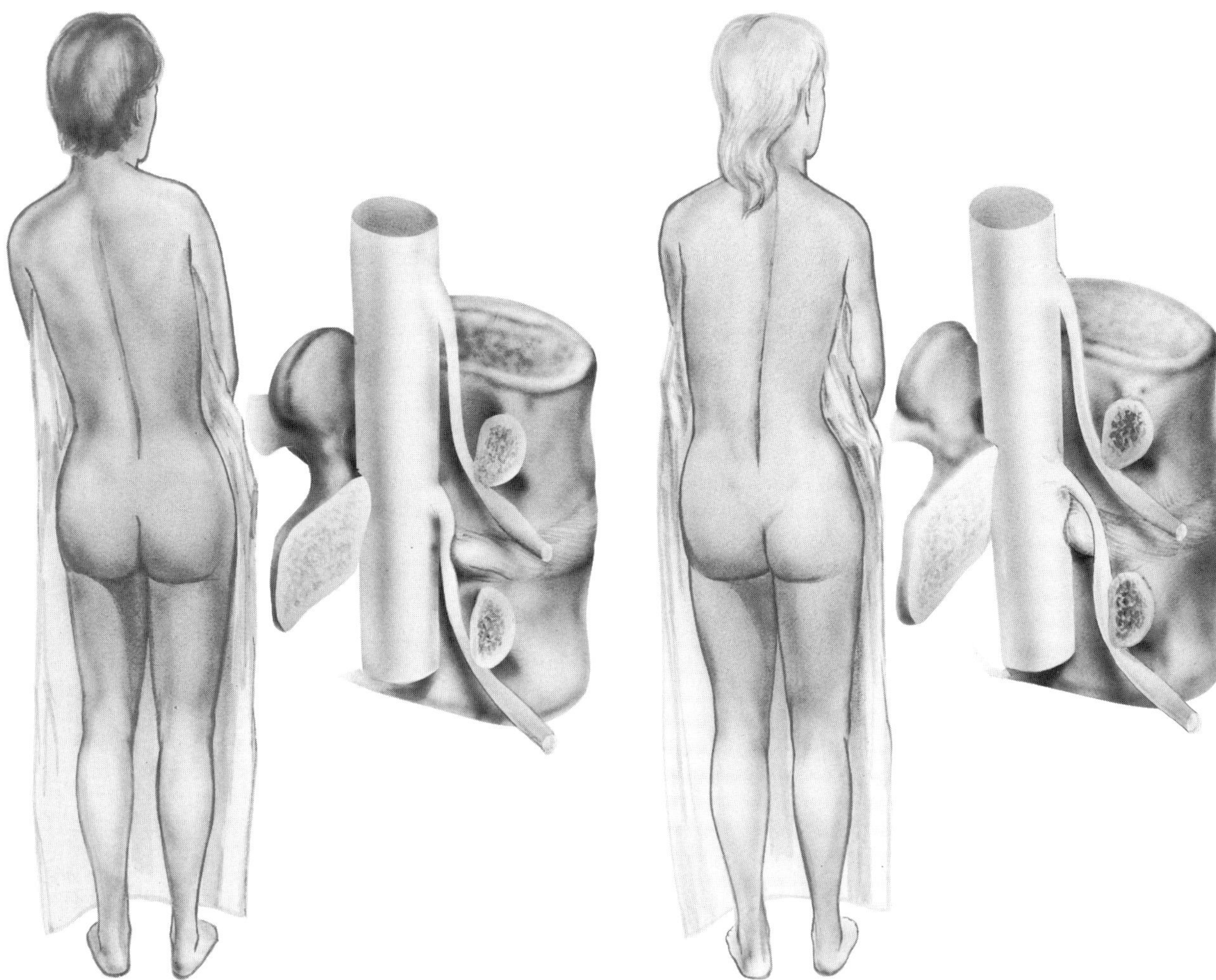

Figure 23–9. *A*, Herniation of the disc lateral to the nerve root. This usually produces a sciatic list away from the side of the irritated nerve root. *B*, Herniation of the disc medial to the nerve root and in an axillary position. This may produce a sciatic list toward the side of the irritated nerve root.

When spasm is present, palpation will reveal significant firmness in the contracted muscle mass. This may be tender on firm palpation. In less marked cases of paravertebral muscle spasm, palpation should not be directed over the muscle belly but should start in the midline with pressure exerted laterally in order to appreciate more subtle differences in muscle tone.

Percussion of the lumbar spine either may elicit local pain or, more significantly, may reproduce sciatica when nerve root compression is present. As with many of the previously noted findings, it is suggestive but not pathognomonic of herniated discs. Severe pain with palpation, including withdrawal and knee buckling, may also be associated with an underlying tumor, infection, or pathologic fracture. Alternatively, it may be a manifestation of a functional disorder (symptom magnification).[256]

Palpation should also be performed in the sciatic notch, along the course of the sciatic nerve itself. Hyperesthesia along the nerve is often found, and local tumors of the nerve may also be discovered in this manner.

The presence of tender motor points (Fig. 23–10) in the lower extremity is of some diagnostic and prognostic importance. These tender motor points represent the main neuromuscular junction in the involved muscle groups. They are fairly constant in their anatomic position from patient to patient. Diagnostically, it has been found that all patients

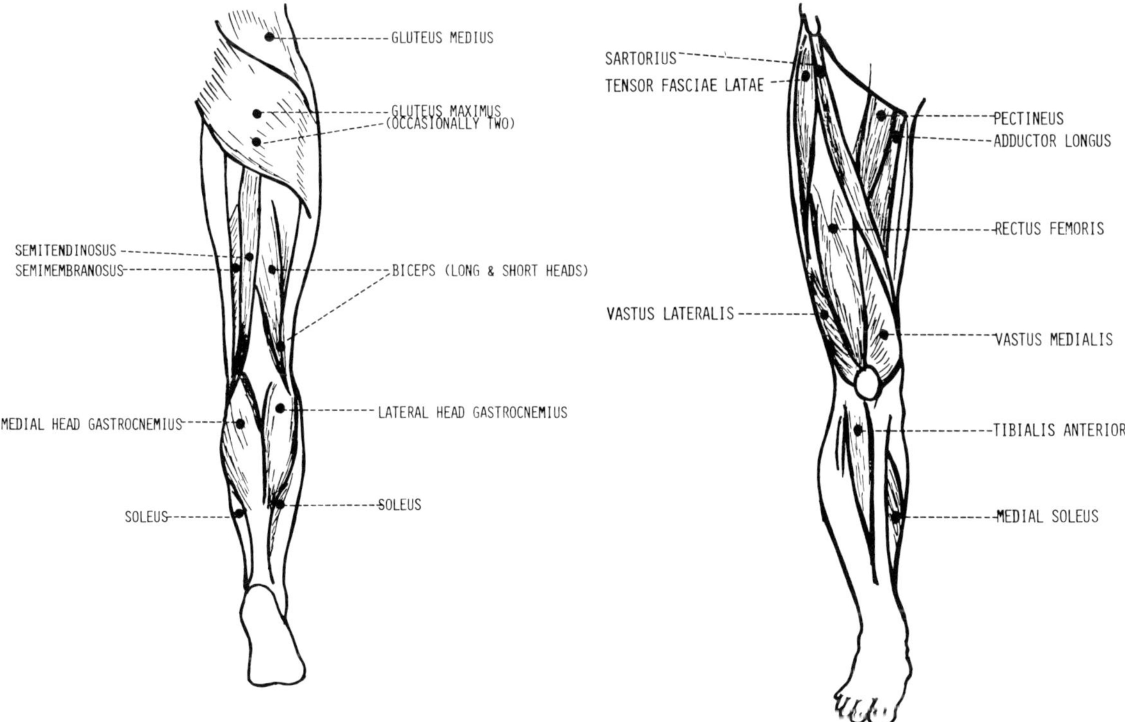

Figure 23–10. Motor points of the lower extremities. (From Gunn, C. C., Chir, B., and Milbrant, W. E.: Tenderness at motor points: a diagnostic and prognostic aid for low-back injury. J. Bone Joint Surg. *58A*:815, 1976.)

with signs and symptoms of a radiculopathy have tender motor points in the myotome corresponding to the probable segmental level of nerve root involvement.

Prognostically, in the absence of radicular signs, back pain patients with tender motor points remain disabled nearly three times as long as those without tenderness. If a radiculopathy is present with the back pain, the disability is nearly four times as long. Frequently, this tenderness, particularly when it is in the calf, has been misinterpreted as a thrombophlebitis.

Neurologic Examination

A meticulous neurologic examination often, but not always, yields objective evidence of nerve root compression. It suggests the level of disc herniation but is not conclusive in this regard. The two most common levels of disc herniation are L4–L5 and L5–S1. The L3–L4 disc level is the next most common. Disc herniations at L5–S1 usually compromise the first sacral nerve root (Fig. 23–11). In a similar fashion, a disc herniation at L4–L5 most often compresses the fifth lumbar root (Fig. 23–12), while a herniation at L3–L4 more frequently involves the fourth lumbar root (Table 23–4). However, owing to variation in root configuration and the position of the herniation itself, disc herniation, particularly at L4–L5, not only

Table 23–4. NERVE ROOT PATTERNS

L4 Nerve Root
1. Pain and numbness: L4 dermatome, posterolateral aspect of thigh, across patella, anteromedial aspect of leg
2. Weakness and atrophy: weak extension of knee and quadriceps muscle atrophy
3. Reflex: depression of patellar reflex

L5 Nerve Root
1. Pain and numbness: L5 dermatome, posterior aspect of thigh, anterolateral aspect of leg, medial aspect of foot and great toe
2. Weakness and atrophy: weak dorsiflexion of foot and toes and atrophy of anterior compartment of leg
3. Reflex: none, or absent posterior tibial tendon reflex

S1 Nerve Root
1. Pain and numbness: S1 dermatome, posterior aspect of thigh, posterior aspect of leg, posterolateral aspect of foot, lateral toes
2. Weakness and atrophy: weak plantar flexion of foot and toes and atrophy of posterior compartment of leg
3. Reflex: depression of Achilles reflex

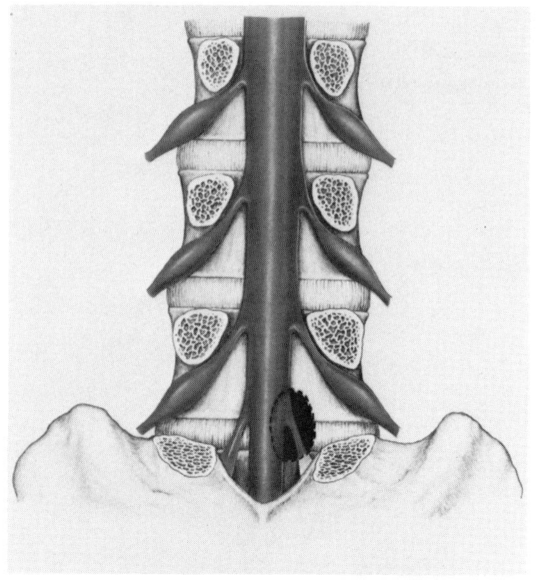

Figure 23–11. A right L5–S1 posterolateral disc herniation. The symptoms would be primarily related to the S1 nerve root on the right. (From Stambough, J. L., and Booth, R. E.: Complications in spine surgery as a consequence of anatomic variations. *In* Garfin, S. R. (ed.): Complications of Spine Surgery. Baltimore, Williams & Wilkins Co., 1989, pp. 89–109.)

can affect the fifth lumbar nerve, but also may involve the first sacral nerve (Figs. 23–12, 23–13). In extreme lateral herniations, the nerve exiting at the same level of the disc is involved; that is, with an L4–L5 disc herniation, the L4 nerve root would be compressed on its course out of the neural foramen at that level (Fig. 23–14). The pattern of neurologic involvement is frequently more confusing when, in addition to a disc herniation, there is a superimposed facet arthritis with lateral encroachment of the foramina (Figs. 23–15, 23–16). Functional or anatomic variations may also occur to alter the presumed level in a significant number of patients.

For this reason, even though the neurologic picture is well defined, radiographic confirmation should be obtained to further localize the level of the lesion when surgery is indicated.

Compression of the motor fibers of the nerve root results in weakness or paralysis of the muscle group in its distribution. Associated

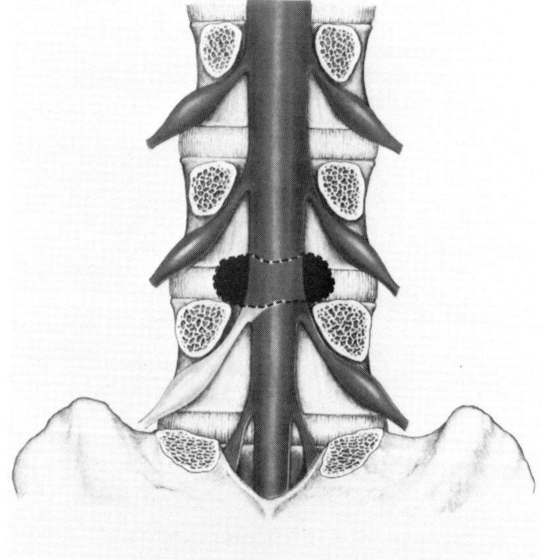

Figure 23–12. A central L4–L5 disc herniation deviated more toward the right. The symptoms would primarily involve the L5 nerve root on the right *(shaded)*. However, a large disc could lead to left-sided symptoms as well as involvement of the sacral roots. (From Stambough, J. L., and Booth, R. E.: Complications in spine surgery as a consequence of anatomic variations. *In* Garfin, S. R. (ed.): Complications of Spine Surgery. Baltimore, Williams & Wilkins Co., 1989, pp. 89–109.)

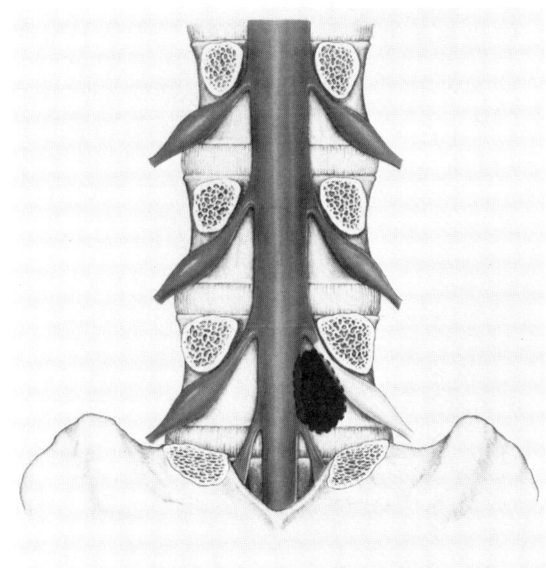

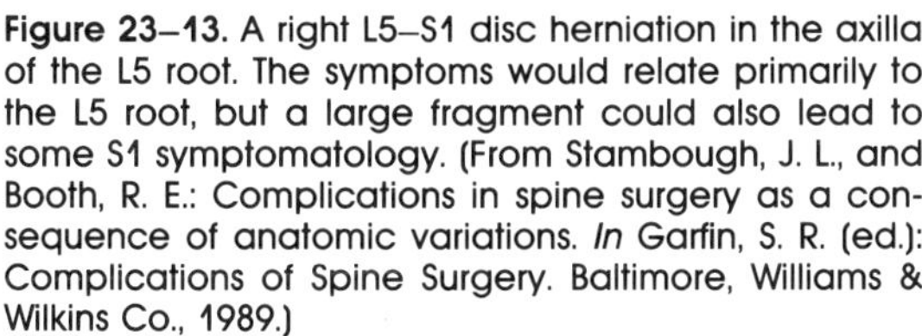

Figure 23–13. A right L5–S1 disc herniation in the axilla of the L5 root. The symptoms would relate primarily to the L5 root, but a large fragment could also lead to some S1 symptomatology. (From Stambough, J. L., and Booth, R. E.: Complications in spine surgery as a consequence of anatomic variations. *In* Garfin, S. R. (ed.): Complications of Spine Surgery. Baltimore, Williams & Wilkins Co., 1989.)

loss of tone and mass of the muscle belly (atrophy) may also be seen, particularly if the compression is prolonged. Usually a group of muscles, rather than a particular one, is involved. The patient may not be aware of this weakness until the loss is rather profound. With compression of the first sacral nerve root, because of the power in the gastric soleus muscle, little motor involvement is noted other than an occasional weakness in flexion of the foot and great toe. With compromise of the fifth lumbar nerve root, weakness primarily of the great toe extensor hallucis longus muscle (Fig. 23–17), other toe extensors, and less often the evertors and dorsiflexors of the foot, is noted. With compression of the fourth or third lumbar nerve root, the quadriceps muscle is frequently affected, the patient noting in the knee weakness of extension and perhaps instability. Atrophy may be prominent. This weakness often manifests itself by difficulty in going upstairs on the affected leg. An L2 or L3 radiculopathy often involves iliopsoas (hip flexion) weakness.

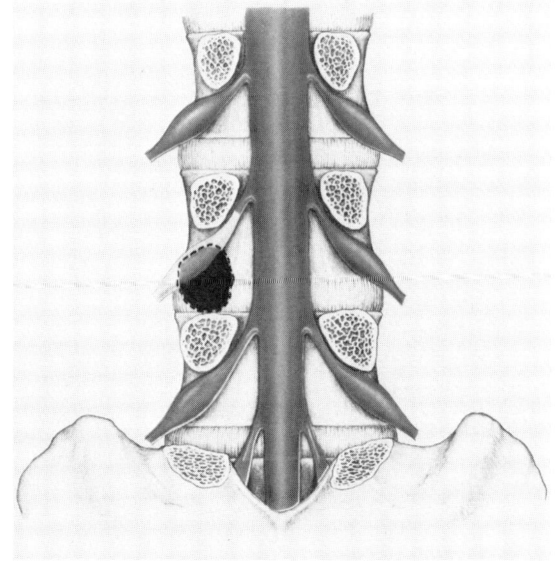

Figure 23–14. An extreme lateral L4–L5 disc herniation involving primarily the L4 root *(shaded)*. Classically, L4–L5 disc herniations lead to L5 nerve root involvement. (From Stambough, J. L., and Booth, R. E.: Complications in spine surgery as a consequence of anatomic variations. *In* Garfin, S. R. (ed.): Complications of Spine Surgery. Baltimore, Williams & Wilkins Co., 1989.)

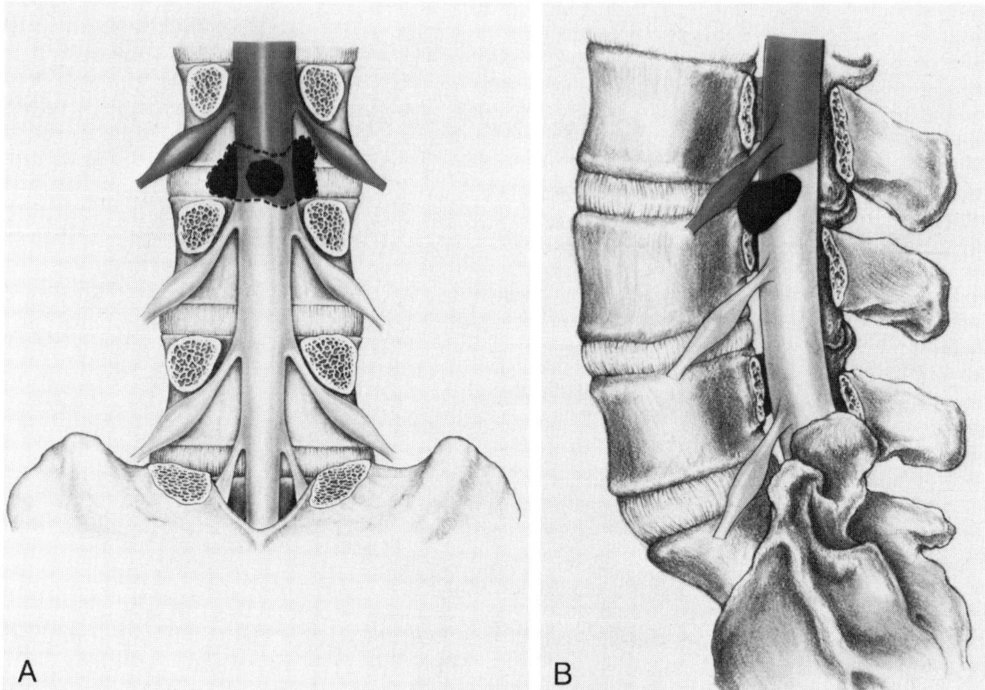

Figure 23–15. A central disc herniation at L3–L4. All the roots caudal to the herniation *(shaded)* could develop signs and symptoms related to this one-level herniation. *A*, Anterior projection. *B*, Lateral projection. (From Stambough, J. L., and Booth, R. E.: Complications in spine surgery as a consequence of anatomic variations. *In* Garfin, S. R. (ed.): Complications of Spine Surgery. Baltimore, Williams & Wilkins Co., 1989.)

One must keep in mind that motor weakness may be a manifestation of a metabolic or peripheral neuropathy, such as diabetes. Clinically, the differentiation can be made since the paresis associated with compromise of the fifth lumbar nerve frequently spares the tibialis anterior, whereas in diabetic peroneal neuropathy, this muscle is usually involved. Further-

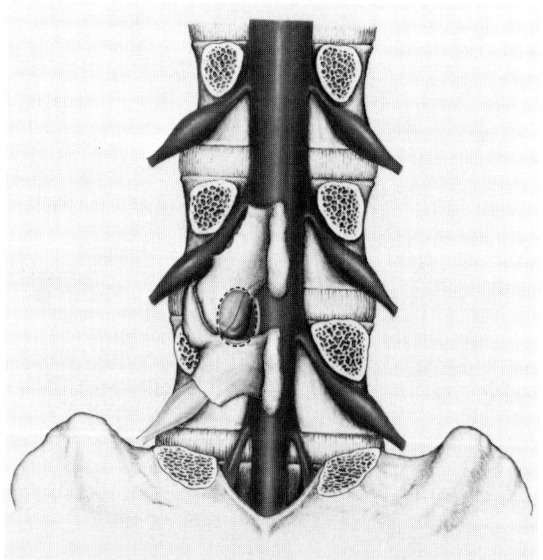

Figure 23–16. A combination of disc herniation with lateral recess stenosis. The circled cutaway demonstrates the disc herniation deviating the nerve root. The L5 root *(shaded)* would be primarily involved. A simple disc excision, however, may not completely relieve the symptoms. (From Stambough, J. L., and Booth, R. E.: Complications in spine surgery as a consequence of anatomic variations. *In* Garfin, S. R. (ed.): Complications of Spine Surgery. Baltimore, Williams & Wilkins Co., 1989, pp. 89–109.)

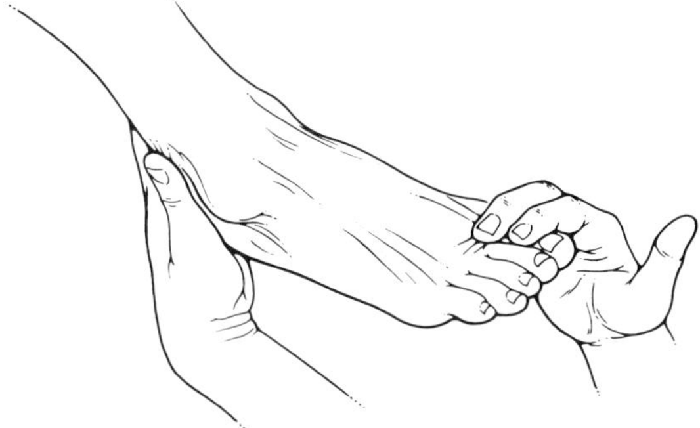

Figure 23–17. To test the strength of the extensor hallucis longus muscle, manual resistance is applied to the great toe during active dorsiflexion. (From Garfin, S. R.: Acquired spinal stenosis: making the diagnosis in the elderly. J. Musculoskel. Med. *4(1)*:64, 1987.)

more, the presence of a Trendelenburg sign due to gluteus medius denervation resulting from a fifth lumbar radiculopathy is not present with diabetic peroneal neuropathy (Fig. 23–18).

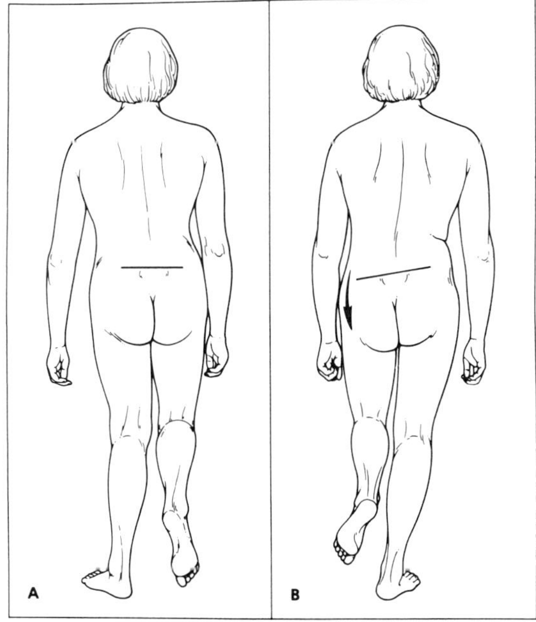

Figure 23–18. Example of a positive Trendelenburg sign. *A*, Normally, when one leg is raised, the pelvis remains horizontal. The pelvis is balanced by the abductor muscles (gluteus medius and minimus) on the side where the leg remains on the ground. *B*, A positive Trendelenburg sign is seen when the iliac crest on the side where the leg is raised falls. This implies that the contralateral abductor muscles are weak. These muscles are primarily innervated by the L5 nerve root.

Sensory Changes

The pattern of sensory involvement when nerve root compression is present usually follows the dermatome of the affected nerve root. However, this has been shown to be a nonspecific finding, which is often more helpful in spinal cord injury than in determining disc disease status. The sensory pattern of the thigh and buttocks is less specific than that in the leg and the foot. With compression of the fourth lumbar nerve root, sensory abnormalities may be noted in the anteromedial aspect of the leg. With compromise of the fifth lumbar nerve root, sensory abnormalities may be noted in the anterolateral portion of the leg and along the medial aspect of the foot to the great toe. S1 radiculopathy usually involves sensory changes in the posterior aspect of the calf and lateral aspect of the foot (Fig. 23–19).

Reflex Changes

The deep tendon reflexes are frequently altered in nerve root compression syndromes. The Achilles reflex is diminished or absent with compression of the first sacral nerve root. Hakelius and Hindmarsh[105] noted that the incidence of disc herniation among patients when the Achilles reflex was absent was higher than among those in whom this reflex was simply diminished. Compression of the fifth lumbar nerve root most commonly causes no reflex change, but on occasion a diminution in the posterior tibial reflex can be elicited. It is important to note, however, that the absence of this reflex must be asymmetric to have any clinical significance. Involvement of the fourth lumbar nerve root and/or the third may result in a decrease or absence of a patellar tendon reflex; however, it is not uncommon to find a lateral L4–L5 disc herniation resulting in this patellar tendon abnormality.[105]

At the actual eliciting of the reflexes, it is suggested that several tendon taps should be performed in order to assess the true amplitude of a response. Frequently, one may actually be able to fatigue a reflex response when the involved reflex arc is compromised owing to disc herniation.

One should remember that many etiologic factors other than disc herniation can produce abnormalities of the deep tendon reflexes. Indeed, on a statistical basis, absence of the Achilles reflex in particular is more often a

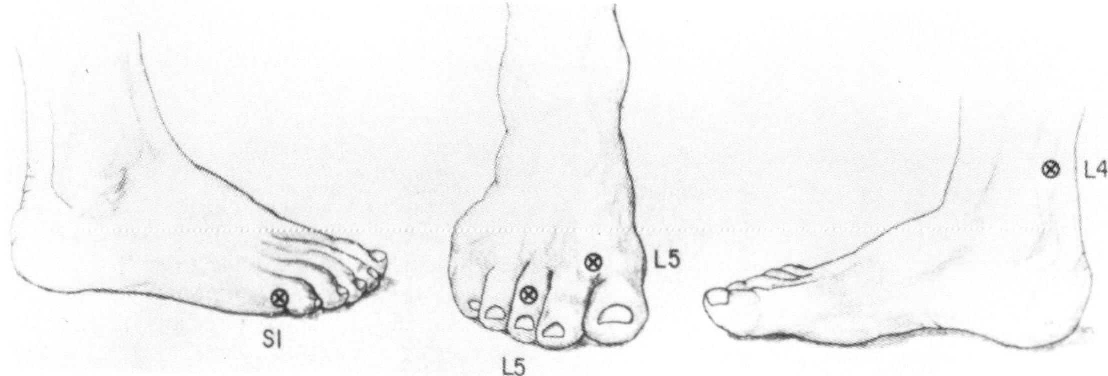

Figure 23–19. Discrete areas of nerve root sensory supply. These areas are consistently depicted as being nerve root specific on all dermatomal diagrams. (From Weise, M. D., Garfin, S. R., Gelberman, R. H., et al.: Lower extremity sensibility testing in patients with herniated lumbar intervertebral discs. J. Bone Joint Surg. *67A*:1220, 1985.)

concomitant of advanced age than of a radiculopathy.

Straight Leg Raising (SLR) Test and Its Variants

There are several maneuvers that tighten the sciatic nerve and in doing so further compress an inflamed nerve root against a herniated lumbar disc. An excellent comprehensive review of the so-called "tension signs" in lumbar disc prolapse has been presented by Scham and Taylor.[229] With the straight leg raising (SLR) maneuver, the L5 and S1 nerve roots move 2 to 6 mm at the level of the foramina. Whether this is a true sliding movement of the nerve or passive deformation of the nerve within the neural canal and foramina[31] is debatable. What is of importance, however, is that when the SLR test is per-

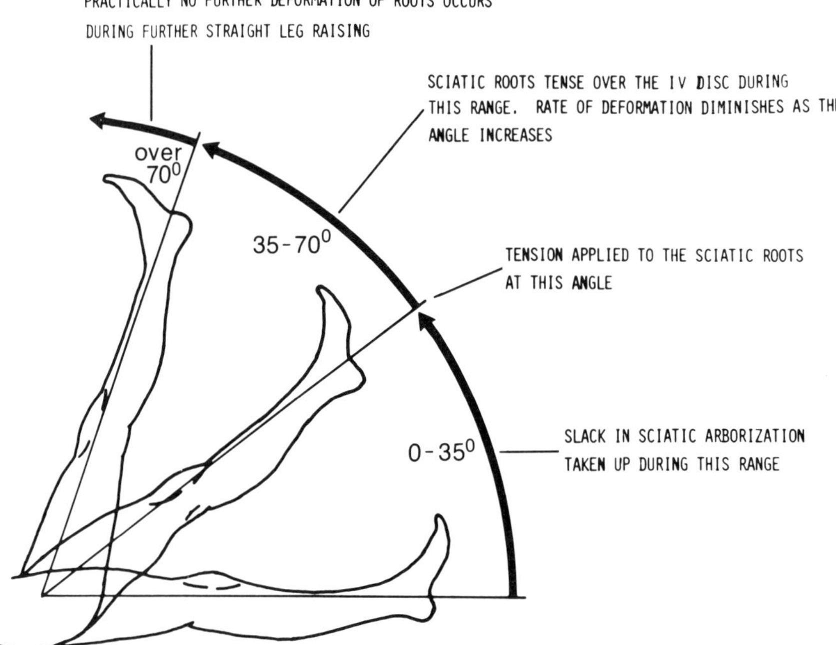

Figure 23–20. The dynamics of the straight leg raising (SLR) test. (Modified from Fahrni, W. H.: Observations on straight leg raising, with special reference to nerve root adhesions. Can. J. Surg. *9*:44, 1966. Reprinted by permission of the publisher.)

formed in a patient with a three-dimensionally *compromised* canal or foramen (more often asymmetric) and an *inflamed* nerve root, the involved nerve is subject to a tensile or compressive force (or both) to which it cannot accommodate without producing radicular symptoms. The L4 nerve root moves a lesser distance, and the more proximal roots show little motion with this maneuver. Thus, the SLR test is of most importance and value in lesions of the fifth lumbar and first sacral nerve roots.

In an analysis of the dynamics of the SLR test it was noted that tension is realized within the nerve roots contributing to the sciatic nerve at 35 to 70 degrees of elevation from the supine position. Since deformation after 70 degrees of elevation occurs in the sciatic nerve distal to the neural foramina, any radicular pain precipitated at this elevation should not be attributed to the sequela of degenerative disc disease (Fig. 23–20).

In a review of 2000 patients with surgically proved disc herniations, the SLR sign was positive in 90 per cent.[238] Younger patients were shown to have a marked propensity for limitation in the SLR test, although the test itself is not pathognomonic.[238] However, a negative test essentially excludes, with great probability, the presence of a herniated disc in young individuals. After the age of 30, a negative SLR test may occur in the presence of a herniated disc (Fig. 23–21). It is often negative in spinal stenosis.

The SLR test is classically described as being performed with the patient supine with the head flat or on a low pillow. One of the examiner's hands is placed on the ilium to stabilize the pelvis, and the other hand slowly elevates the leg by the heel with the knee straight. The patient should be asked whether this produces leg pain. However, the authors routinely perform this maneuver with the patient sitting (seated SLR). While examining the foot or knee, the hip can be flexed and the knee extended, achieving the same postural result and tension on the nerve as in the supine position. Attention should be paid to hip extension by the patient during this maneuver, as this is "protective" and indicative of a positive test. Only when leg pain or radicular symptoms are produced are these tests considered positive. Back pain alone is not a positive finding.

Many variations of this test have been described. The knee may first be flexed to 90 degrees and the hip then flexed to 90 degrees. Next, the knee is gradually extended. If this maneuver produces leg pain, the test is considered positive. Both this test and the SLR test have been attributed to Lasègue. A variation of the SLR test has been described in which, following hip flexion with the knee extended, the foot is dorsiflexed. This not only may produce an exacerbation of the pain in the SLR test, but also could reproduce radicular pain when the conventional SLR test is negative.

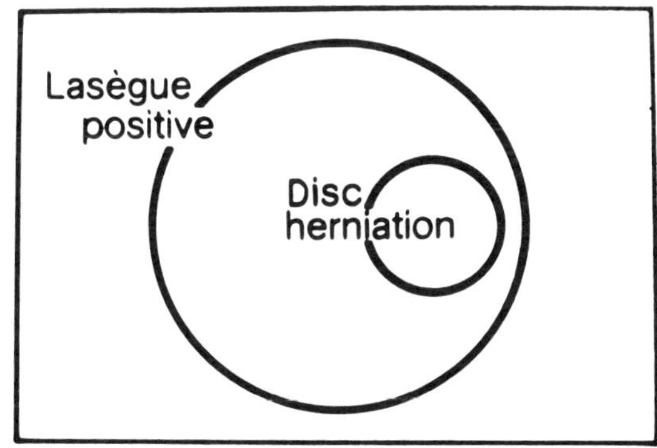

Age: under 30 years

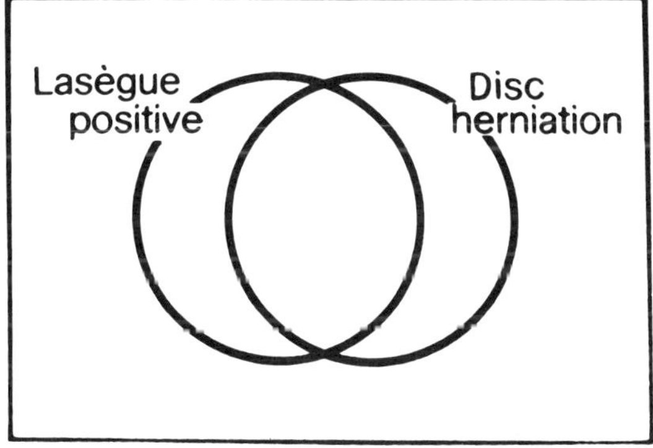

Age: over 30 years

Figure 23–21 These Venn diagrams illustrate the marked propensity for a positive Lasègue test (SLR) with disc herniation in the young. Over the age of 30 the propensity decreases, although the specificity increases for this test in disc herniation. (From Spangfort, E.: Lasègue's sign in patients with lumbar disc herniation. Acta Orthop. Scand. *42*:459, 1971. © 1971 Munksgaard International Publishers Ltd., Copenhagen, Denmark.)

MacNab[163] stated that the most reliable test of spinal nerve root tension is the bowstring sign, another manifestation of the SLR test. The SLR test is performed as usual until pain is elicited. At this point, however, the knee is flexed, which usually significantly reduces symptoms. Finger pressure is then applied to the popliteal space (over the terminal aspect of the sciatic nerve). Reestablishment of the painful radicular symptom is a positive sign of root tension from disc herniation.

Medial rotation of the hip joint can also apply tension to the sacral plexus in the supine position. It has been reported that sciatic pain can be reproduced when medial hip rotation is performed at the pain-free limits of the SLR test.

The contralateral SLR test is performed in the same manner as the SLR test, except that the nonpainful leg is raised. If this produces the sciatica in the opposite extremity, the test is considered positive. This is very suggestive of a herniated disc, particularly one with a free fragment. Ninety-seven per cent of patients who undergo laminectomies and have a positive crossed-SLR test have surgically confirmed disc herniations. The prolapse is often large, but not in the usual lateral pattern. At surgery the disc is often noted medial to the nerve root in the axilla (Fig. 23–22).

It should be noted that when the roots of the femoral nerve are involved, they are tensed not by the SLR test but by the reverse SLR test, i.e., by hip extension and knee flexion. This is usually performed while the patient is prone or laterally with the unaffected side down. As with the SLR test, there is a contralateral femoral traction sign.[68] In these cases

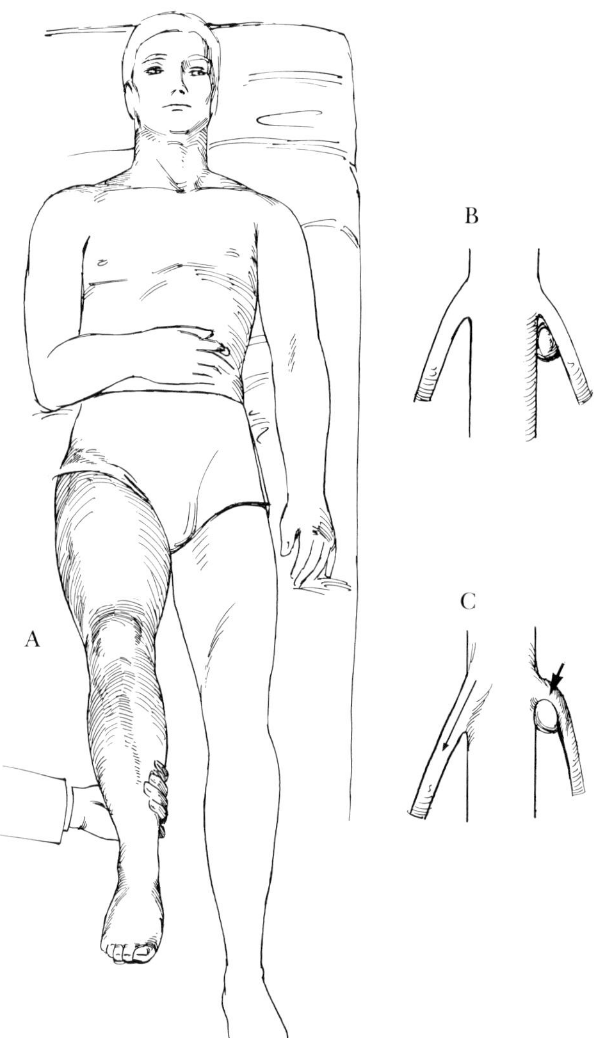

Figure 23–22. Movement of nerve roots when the leg on the opposite side is raised. *A*, When the leg is raised on the unaffected side, the roots on the opposite side slide slightly downward and toward the midline. *B*, In the presence of a disc lesion, particularly in an axillary location, this movement *(C)* increases the root tension. (From DePalma, A. F., and Rothman, R. H.: The Intervertebral Disc. Philadelphia, W. B. Saunders Co., 1970.)

the pain reproduction is usually in the anterior or lateral aspect of the groin, thigh, knee, and/or leg.

Peripheral Vascular Examination

No examination of a patient with back or leg pain can be considered complete without evaluation of the peripheral circulation. Examination of the posterior tibial and dorsalis pedis arterial pulses should be performed, as well as routine examination of the skin temperature and inspection for the presence of atrophic changes, as seen with ischemic disease.

In addition to the peripheral vascular examination, several other clinical findings, coupled with the history, usually help differentiate vascular claudication from intermittent neurogenic claudication. In cases in which the history and physical findings could be compatible with both types of claudication, quantitative studies of the arterial system and consultation with a vascular surgeon are indicated.

Hip Joint Examination

One can usually differentiate intra-articular hip disease from symptomatic degenerative disc disease. Limitation of range of motion of the hip, particularly in rotation, along with groin discomfort, is most indicative of hip disease. Furthermore, with examination of the hip, coincident hip flexion and knee extension should not elicit any tension signs, which implicates nerve root tension.

It is of interest, however, that evidence of degenerative hip disease was found in 10 per cent of approximately 400 patients suffering from low back pain. In the older patient with spinal stenosis, it is not uncommon to have radiographic, and perhaps clinical, evidence of both degenerative disease of a hip and concomitant spinal stenosis. Both areas may require surgical treatment.

Abdominal and Rectal Examination

Many intra-abdominal and retroperitoneal abnormalities can result in back and referred leg pain. A careful history as well as thorough palpation of the abdomen, together with rectal and pelvic examinations, may disclose lesions that lead to a nonspinal diagnosis.

Treatment Considerations: Cauda Equina Syndrome

In considering patients who present with a low back pain syndrome, with or without sciatica, it can be assumed that most will have symptoms attributable to lumbar disc degeneration. Provided that these patients have not previously been treated, we recommend that an overwhelming number should be instructed to begin a course of nonoperative, conditioning exercise therapy. Only the patient with a frank cauda equina syndrome or unequivocal progressive motor weakness should proceed along a more rapid line of radiologic evaluation and possible surgery.

The cauda equina syndrome has been described as a complex of low back pain, bilateral sciatica, saddle anesthesia or dysesthesia, and motor weakness in the lower extremities that may progress to paraplegia with bowel and bladder incontinence.[57] Kostuik and colleagues,[149] in a retrospective review of 31 patients with a cauda equina syndrome secondary to a herniated disc, identified two modes of presentation. The first group (ten patients) had an acute onset of symptoms with heightened severity, and had a poorer prognosis after decompression, especially for bladder function deficits. The second group had a more insidious onset of symptoms. All patients in this latter group had urinary retention preoperatively. Seventy-seven per cent regained clinically normal voiding patterns postoperatively, but follow-up cystometric studies were not performed. Twenty-seven per cent of patients had sexual dysfunction of varying degrees. Ninety per cent of these regained normal motor function after decompression. Trauma played an inciting role in four patients, three of whom had undergone chiropractic manipulation of the spine.

The average time from onset of symptoms was 1.1 days (range six hours to two days) in the acute-onset group and 3.3 days (range one day to several weeks) in the second group. Patients with acute urinary retention were operated on early. There was no correlation of these times with return of function, but the authors concluded that early surgery should be performed. However, it does not have to occur within six hours, as had been previously recommended.

Low Back Pain and/or Sciatica

The early stage of treatment of all other low back complaints related to lumbar disc disease (other than a cauda equina syndrome or progressive motor weakness) is a waiting game. With the passage of time, salicylates (or other anti-inflammatories) and bed rest are the therapies that have proved safest and most effective. We advise an initial period of treatment along these lines for up to six weeks. In our experience, emergency surgical intervention is justified in only a few patients a year. However, in the face of a frank cauda equina syndrome or truly progressive motor weakness, equivocation and procrastination are not warranted and a vigorous recommendation for definitive diagnostic imaging is indicated. In these instances, myelography, MRI, and/or CT are almost always clearly positive and should be promptly followed by surgical decompression; since tumors can present with a similar clinical picture, we do not recommend unenhanced CT to obtain the diagnosis in this setting. One can almost always expect dramatic resolution of pain, if not of motor deficit, with a prompt return to normal life patterns. Even in these patients, one might argue that evidence substantiating this aggressive surgical posture is not adequate, but for now our recommendations remain as stated.

Profound or progressive motor weakness requires more judgment in terms of urgency as a criterion for surgical intervention. Owing to their functional importance, acute complete paralysis of the quadriceps muscle and acute complete paralysis of the dorsiflexors of the foot are indications for surgical decompression of the involved spinal nerves. The more prolonged the pressure on the spinal nerve and the more intense the compression, the less likely is the return of function. However, this guideline is not absolute.

Independent of surgery, return of motor function can be anticipated.[259, 260] In Weber's excellent prospective study,[260] the degree of residual paresis was similar in the surgically and conservatively treated groups after three years. However, with acute profound motor weakness, decompression should be considered as soon as possible. When lesser degrees of motor weakness are present, judgment must be exercised as to when surgery should be recommended. If the weakness is mild to moderate and compatible with adequate function of the extremity, a period of observation and nonoperative treatment is indicated. This is particularly true in subacute and chronic situations. However, if the motor weakness is progressive in nature and becomes significant in terms of function, surgical intervention becomes more important.

Sensory and reflex changes are helpful in terms of diagnosis, but are not in themselves indications for surgical intervention and are of no prognostic value in predicting the ultimate outcome of the disease, or the location of the herniated disc.[259, 263] Weber found sensory dysfunction in nearly 46 per cent of his total series of patients after four years. The abnormalities encountered either existed before treatment or developed subsequent to surgical or nonoperative management. It is interesting to note that no patient was disabled because of sensory deficits. Similarly, a diminution or loss of reflex in the face of lessening pain is not an indication for urgent surgery.

Initial Nonoperative Treatment Options

Deyo[59] evaluated the statistical validity of 59 articles in the literature dealing with various forms of nonoperative treatment for low back pain. Isometric flexion exercises, each of three drugs, one traction method, and certain manipulations were supported by single studies of reasonable validity. Overt problems in evaluating many of the studies dealing with this subject included failure to (a) randomize subjects, (b) blind observers, (c) measure compliance, and (d) adequately describe cointerventions.

On the basis of this relative dearth of scientific evidence of the efficacy of various types of nonoperative therapy, our approach to treatment has been developed partly out of empiricism and cost effectiveness, and partly in relation to the aforementioned goals of the algorithm.

Bed Rest

There is general agreement that bed rest is an important element of therapy for acute episodes of back pain, with or without accompanying radicular signs and symptoms.[268] The optimal duration of bed rest, however, remains debatable. Treatment schedules vary widely, ranging from two days to six weeks.[61, 214, 225]

Regardless of the period of bed rest or sedentary activity prescribed, it is important to remember that time spent devoid of any substantial physical activity can lead to "disease of disuse" manifested as muscle atrophy, joint stiffness, osteoporosis of disuse, and psychologic effects. Many authors believe that these negative effects need to be minimized in order to avert the development of a chronic pain syndrome, and point out that deconditioning effects from overprescription of bed rest simply serve to prolong the rehabilitation process.

There are few comparative reports in the literature dealing with bed rest and its efficacy in comparison with other therapies for back pain. Gilbert and colleagues[93] compared bed rest with physiotherapy and educational programs. The results of this study favored early mobilization over bed rest and suggested that passive physiotherapy and educational programs were doing more harm than good. The recommended duration of prescribed bed rest in this study was four days.

Wiesel and colleagues[269] conducted a random study on the efficacy of bed rest for acute low back pain in 980 military basic combat trainees. All the patients had back pain, but none had a significant radicular component in their symptom complex. One group of patients, kept on complete bed rest, returned to full duty 50 per cent faster and experienced 60 per cent less pain than a second group of patients who were retained on an ambulatory status. A more recent controlled trial of the efficacy of bed rest was presented by Deyo and colleagues.[61] These investigators compared the effects of two days' and seven days' rest on patients with acute low back pain. Out of the multitude of variables assessed, the only statistically significant difference involved the conclusion that two days of bed rest was just as effective as seven days; the group that was kept at rest for two days, however, lost significantly less time from work. This study has laid the foundation for our ability to assure patients that a graduated program of steadily increasing activity will not, in most cases, have an adverse effect on the natural history of an isolated episode of low back pain.

Scientific Foundation of Bed Rest. Nachemson[192] established in vivo data verifying that in the L3 intervertebral disc, pressure can be significantly reduced in the supine posture. In comparison with the sitting position, an 86 per cent decrease in intradiscal pressure can result from assuming a supine posture in a semi-Fowler's position. Andersson and colleagues[6] demonstrated a reduction of dorsal and abdominal muscle activity as a more horizontal position is assumed. Assuming the validity of the hypothesis that increasing pressure on the disc leads to increasing symptoms in the lumbar spine, bed rest would seem to be the rational first line in conservative management. An additional conceptual benefit to be derived from bed rest, particularly in the case of an acute soft disc herniation with associated nerve root inflammation, is the reduction in the inflammatory component of the patient's pain provided by (short-term) immobilization.

On the basis of the studies presented above, the current trend in treating acute low back pain is toward shorter periods of recumbency. To date, however, no study has been published exclusively dealing with the ideal duration of bed rest in treating sciatica. Few patients can tolerate prolonged recumbency, particularly those with acute symptoms of sciatica who are accustomed to an active, vigorous life style. It is our current recommendation to individualize the duration of bed rest to each patient and combine this with other clinically useful treatment measures, including reassurance, an optimistic discussion of the natural history of the problem, education, and scientifically based recommendations for controlling symptoms by modification of postural factors that can mechanically affect the stress on the lumbar spine. For example, patients should be aware that although recumbency decreases intradiscal pressure to its minimal level, the standing posture provides an approximately 80 per cent reduction in disc pressure compared with sitting. It therefore seems rational to recommend avoidance of sitting and to allow patients who are improving to gradually increase their standing and walking activity, as opposed to maintaining complete, debilitating bed rest for extended periods. We also prescribe and give instructions in the proper use of non-narcotic analgesics for pain relief.

Bed rest can be accomplished most effectively at home, where the patient is comfortable in familiar surroundings and is cared for by family members or friends. Hospitalization, however, may be justified in the setting of severe, nonmechanical pain when a tumor or infectious process is suspected, or for a patient who presents with a profound neurologic deficit in which close monitoring is necessary to rule out progressive deterioration. In a patient with a clinically diagnosed disc herniation and sciatica who is improving, expectations for a resumption of regular activities should be clearly explained. It may be unrealistic to expect a patient with a frank disc herniation to return to full activities in less than one month. Compromise on this point is frequently sought by patients, but in the long run may not be in their benefit. It should be pointed out to the patient that operative intervention in itself requires a prolonged period of rehabilitation and that strict adherence to a graduated activity program may avoid the need for surgery.

When a disc herniation is the cause of patients' impairment, it is also important to advise them that reversion to additional periods of bed rest may be necessary throughout the treatment program as a first aid measure for effecting a gradual reduction in the overall intensity and frequency of the symptom complex. Such discussion should include an admission of our inability, on the basis of available basic science and clinical information, to preselect those patients with a disc herniation (leading to sciatica) who will ultimately improve to the point at which surgery is no longer a consideration.

Drug Therapy

The intelligent use of drug therapy is an important part of the treatment of lumbar disc disease. Five categories of pharmacologic agents have been suggested as potentially useful: analgesics, anti-inflammatory agents, oral steroids, muscle relaxants, and antidepressants.

Oral Drug Therapy

Analgesic and Anti-inflammatory Agents. The judicious use of analgesics is of great importance during the acute phase of low back pain and sciatica. It is a rare patient who requires hospitalization for pain control. When this is the case, however, a straight dosage regimen of narcotic pain relievers for a period of 24 to 48 hours should be considered as opposed to p.r.n. prescriptions. This in turn relieves the patient of the anxiety that often accompanies waiting for nurses to obtain pain medication. When pain is severe and incapacitating and the patient is hospitalized, an intramuscular dose of morphine sulfate (0.1 to 0.2 mg per kg every four hours) or codeine (30 to 60 mg every four hours) or other narcotic medications can produce adequate pain relief. Constipation, respiratory depression, and altered mental status are frequent side effects when narcotics are required; dosages should be adjusted accordingly. We do not prescribe narcotic analgesics for chronic back pain owing to the high potential for addiction and oversedation, which are both counterproductive to the rehabilitation process.

Most cases are amenable to outpatient treatment. In this circumstance, the prescription of aspirin, acetaminophen, and nonsteroidal anti-inflammatory agents has a rational basis in the acute phase of managing patients with low back pain and sciatica. Occasionally, one to two weeks of oral narcotic medication (e.g., acetaminophen with 30 mg codeine) may be useful. Some authors[110] advise that the first step in treating acute back pain is a trial of acetaminophen because no studies have conclusively shown that nonsteroidal anti-inflammatories are superior in this setting. Acetaminophen has both antipyretic and analgesic properties. Unlike aspirin, gastric side effects are minimal. Of all of the analgesic drugs, salicylates are the ones most commonly prescribed, least costly, and most thoroughly studied. Salicylates act by inhibiting migration of polymorphonuclear leukocytes and inhibiting prostaglandin synthesis. Their analgesic effects work through both the peripheral and central nervous systems. Small doses of aspirin in the range of 325 to 650 mg are sufficient for both antipyretic and analgesic action. Serum levels of 290 to 300 μg per ml must be maintained if salicylates are to have an anti-inflammatory effect. For the average adult, these serum levels require a starting regimen of 12 to 16 tablets per day in divided doses taken along with meals, or antacids. Elderly patients may benefit from a lower dosage. Buffered or enteric coated preparations may help decrease gastrointestinal distress. Administration of salicylates can increase the prothrombin time, and their use in patients already taking anticoagulants should be avoided or allowed with great caution.

Nonsteroidal anti-inflammatory drugs (NSAIDs) can be divided into six groups: indoles, such as indomethacin, sulindac, and tolmetin sodium; pyrazolone derivatives, such as phenylbutazone; propionic acids (fenoprofen, ibuprofen, naproxen, flurbiprofen, and ketoprofen); oxicams (piroxicam); phenylacetic acids (diclofenac); and anthranilic acid derivatives (meclofenamate and mefenamic acid). None of these medications has been proved superior to aspirin alone in equipotent dosage regimens.[59]

If pain does not improve with acetaminophen or aspirin, the choice of NSAID should be based on the pharmacology of each agent, compliance factors, familiarity with the side effects of the medication, and the age and overall medical status of the patient. Medications that can increase compliance by virtue of a long serum half-life maintained on a once-or-twice-a-day dosage regimen include piroxicam, naproxen, and sulindac. When cost control is a consideration, salicylate derivatives and ibuprofen are available over the counter or can be prescribed to decrease patient expense. In the patient who has active gastritis or peptic ulcer disease, consideration should be given to using nonacetylated salicylates and adding antacids or sucralfate for cytoprotection of the gastric mucosa. As a group, NSAIDs need to be administered cautiously in elderly patients with impaired renal function. In patients whose back pain is based on a seronegative spondyloarthropathy, such as Reiter's syndrome, ankylosing spondylitis, psoriatic arthritis, or the arthritis associated with inflammatory bowel disease, long-term NSAID therapy may be indicated. Routine monitoring of renal, hepatic, and hematologic parameters is necessary.

Piroxicam was compared with placebo in one trial of acute low back pain without radicular involvement.[4] Improvement was noted in both groups, but the piroxicam-treated patients experienced greater pain relief, required less analgesia, and returned to work earlier. Unfortunately, a control group using a strictly analgesic medication without inflammatory properties, such as acetaminophen, was not utilized.

Kellett[137] reviewed the drug literature dealing with the acute treatment of soft tissue injuries and concluded that NSAIDs should be restricted to the first three days after injury. His conclusion was derived from the dearth of firm scientific evidence in the literature demonstrating the efficacy of these medications weighed against the potential for side effects of varying severity. When anti-inflammatory agents are used in treating back pain and sciatica for longer periods, the justification centers around the contention that an inflammatory reaction contributes to the pathogenesis of the various degenerative disc syndromes. Naylor and colleagues[201] demonstrated that humeral autoimmunity can occur in response to an immune system challenge by nucleus pulposus antigen. McCarron and colleagues,[176] likewise, demonstrated marked local inflammatory changes in the epidural space after canine injection of autologous homogenized disc material. MacNab[163] showed intraoperatively that nerve roots that are compressed by disc material and are inflamed are painful when compressed; roots that were not inflamed or otherwise chronically irritated produced non-painful paresthesia upon intraoperative stimulation.

The role of inflammation in back pain caused by disorders other than inflammatory arthritis and sciatica is less clear. Empirically it seems that when osteoarthritic disease affects the facet joints, some degree of inflammation results. Similarly, changes may be present in acutely and chronically traumatized muscles, ligaments, tendons, and synovia.

Oral Steroids. Oral corticosteroids have been demonstrated to improve the symptoms and signs associated with a herniated disc. Dexamethasone is the most commonly used agent reported.[101] The results of three studies[101, 104, 249] indicated that dexamethasone administered orally in a short-term tapering dosage regimen is a relatively safe form of therapy for lumbar radiculopathy secondary to herniated nucleus pulposus. When this form of treatment is used, prophylaxis against a Cushing ulcer should include concomitant treatment using either sucralfate or an H_2 receptor blocker. Long-term effects such as avascular necrosis are difficult to assess, but should be considered if these agents are used on a routine basis.

Muscle Relaxants. The authors infrequently use muscle relaxants. Methocarbamol and carisoprodol are commonly used for this purpose. Either of these drugs can cause drowsiness, which may be their main beneficial effect; being sedentary is thereby made more tolerable. Muscle spasm may result from secondary protective reflex phenomena or direct trauma. In patients with spasms severe enough to warrant therapy with antispasmodic medications, we recommend cyclobenzaprine or baclofen. The latter agent has demonstrated superiority over placebo in the management of back pain.[49] Diazepam should not be used because of its physiologic depressing effects and addiction potential.

Antidepressants. Chemical mediators and inhibitors of pain have been studied in relation to chronic low back pain. Endogenous opiate systems have been demonstrated to be responsible for stimulation-produced analgesia. Patients with chronic low back pain frequently show the sleep disturbances and mood depression thought to be associated with serotonin depression in the brain.[129] A trial of tricyclic antidepressant therapy is warranted in patients with chronic low back pain manifesting clinical signs of depression including one or more of the following:[129] (1) severe anhedonia and lack of reactivity of mood to usually pleasurable stimuli, (2) sleep disturbance (particularly middle and terminal insomnia), (3) diurnal variations of symptoms (morning being worse than evening), (4) marked psychomotor retardation or agitation, (5) excessive or inappropriate guilt, and (6) severe anorexia or weight loss. Previous success with antidepressant treatment also portends a heightened probability of improvement with reinstitution of such medications.

Many clinical studies[1, 213, 257] have demonstrated the superiority of tricyclic antidepressants over a placebo. A response in terms of the patient's mood and sleep habits can usually be expected after 10 to 14 days of treatment. The dosage required to obtain relief is usually less than that necessary for treating a major reactive or psychotic depressive disorder. Additionally, at low doses these drugs may affect peripheral nerve membranes, thereby also helping decrease pain on a cellular basis (separate from central nervous system effects). In patients who manifest major abnormalities in thought content, cognitive skills, affect, mood, and behavior, psychiatric consultation is advisable.

Injection Therapy

Trigger Point Injections. Localized tender areas, or trigger points, in the paravertebral musculature are found in many individuals with acute and chronic low back pain. Garvey and colleagues[88] performed a prospective randomized double-blind study of trigger point injection therapy. Results, although not statistically significant, indicated that the control group who received only a vapocoolant spray showed the greatest improvement, followed in decreasing order of effectiveness by pressure from the plastic needle guard, dry needlestick, steroid/lidocaine injection, and lidocaine injection alone. The conclusion from this study is that local injection of medication may not be the determining factor for success when injections are used for local pain relief. Perhaps a mechanism similar to that reported with acupuncture is operative.

Epidural Steroids. Evans[75] in 1930 was the first to popularize the use of epidural injections for treating sciatica. He reported a 60 per cent rate of improvement in 40 patients with chronic sciatica; however, this was an uncontrolled study and no differences were noted in patients treated with either physiologic saline or local anesthetic. Dilke and colleagues[63] in 1973 conducted a double-blind, controlled, randomized prospective study in 100 patients and found a significant improvement in the epidural steroid groups compared with a controlled, dry-needle group, both initially and at three months. The overall success rate was 45 per cent, which compares poorly with higher success rates reported in other studies in which follow-up, as well as the duration from the time of onset of symptoms, was short. The latter fact has produced a strong impression in the literature that the more favorable results are observed in early or acute cases. Adding credence to this is the study of Cuckler and associates,[43] which concluded that epidural steroids have no value in the treatment of lumbar radicular pain. This study preselected only those patients with radiographically defined lesions who had been treated with two weeks of bed rest before injection was considered. Patients were randomized to either a steroid and local anesthetic or local anesthetic alone group. Only one injection was administered and results were evaluated after 24 hours. Many physicians are currently recommending a series of three injections, usually given at one-week intervals.

White[265] reviewed 300 consecutive patients treated with epidural steroid injections and observed 82 per cent relief for a duration of one day, 50 per cent relief for two weeks, and 16 per cent for two months.

Since open trials[36, 92] suggest that some patients can benefit, at least temporarily, the authors presently recommend their use to patients with radicular syndromes who are not responding to therapy, who have incomplete symptom resolution, or in whom surgical intervention is not considered a treatment option at the time. We emphasize to all patients who elect to undergo injection that it is only one part of their overall treatment plan, and explain that if there is a positive response to the injection, it may be temporary.

The complication rate when the injection is competently performed is extremely low.[54, 76, 279] Approximately 10 per cent of patients experience a temporary exacerbation of pain. More serious complications are rare and include the following: immediate—(1) high spinal anesthesia, (2) intravascular injection, and (3) hypotension from sympathetic blockade; delayed—(1) 24 to 48 hours of increased symptoms, (2) spinal headache (less than 1 per cent), (3) neural damage or radicular symptoms, and (4) systemic effects.

Facet Joint Injections and Denervation. Numerous studies indicate that the facet joint may be a clinically important source of back and referred leg pain.[76] This observation, in turn, has been supported experimentally by producing pain through the injection of hypertonic saline into the facet joint, which in turn can be blocked with lidocaine.[161] The postganglionic posterior primary ramus branch of the spinal nerve supplies afferent sensory input from the articular cartilage synovium and capsule of the diarthrodial facet joint. Each facet joint is innervated by branches from two spinal levels. The posterior primary ramus is also responsible for innervation of the dorsal musculature and ligaments.[25]

There are multiple techniques for disrupting the innervation to the facet joint. At the time of surgery, stripping of the paraspinal muscles from the facet joints produces iatrogenic denervation. Percutaneous transection has been performed by some authors, phenol blocks can be used, direct injection under fluoroscopic control has been reported to be beneficial as both a diagnostic and therapeutic maneuver, and lastly radiofrequency facet rhizotomy has been used to create controlled thermal coagulation and resultant permanent denervation. Unfortunately, none of the studies in the literature have adequate controls, randomization, or independent evaluation.[127, 217] Proper prospective, randomized, double-blind studies are needed to prove any long-term beneficial effect of facet joint injection or radiofrequency denervation that lasts beyond the natural history of the disease, as well as any exclusive effect that exceeds the expected outcome of a noninvasive rehabilitation program for the treatment of localized mechanical low back pain.

Exercise Therapy

Historical Background. Williams[271] in 1937 suggested that back and leg pain were the direct result of compression of the nerve in the area of the intervertebral foramina and created a program of flexion exercises for his patients in order to effect foraminal decompression. Kendall and Jenkins,[144] in a well-designed study, evaluated the effects of three different types of exercises in 42 patients with long-standing low back pain. The regimens included lumbar extension, mobilizing flexion, and isometric flexion exercises. After three months, a larger percentage of the patients improved in the isometric group. Davies and colleagues,[51] in a similar study, compared the effects of short-wave diathermy alone with short-wave therapy and either hyperextension or isometric flexion exercises. In this study, none of the patients in the extension group were made worse and pain worsened in 70 per cent of the flexion and control groups. Cady and associates[38] conducted a study in 1970 for the Los Angeles County Health Service documenting the effectiveness of a fitness program for firefighters in promoting increases in physical work capacity, spinal flexibility, and decreases in disabling injuries and workmen's compensation costs. In 1985 a follow-up study by Cady and associates[39] revealed that back injuries were ten times higher for the least fit group of firefighters compared with those with a high level of fitness, as determined by measuring aerobic endurance capacity, isometric strength of selected muscle groups, total spine flexibility, diastolic blood pressure at a heart rate of 160 beats per minute, and heart rate two minutes after standardized bicycle exercise. They concluded that fitness and conditioning are useful preventive measures for addressing the problem of low back pain.

There is general agreement among physicians that exercise exerts a positive impact on many aspects of health in addition to low back pain, yet 40 per cent of American adults remain entirely sedentary.[221] Society's current emphasis on health and longevity, as well as the epidemic of low back pain, has resulted in a large outpouring of research dealing with the potential benefits of exercise (see Table 23–1). Jackson and Brown[125] summarized the purported benefits of exercise in the care of patients with low back pain. It has been suggested that there are multiple mechanisms for pain reduction through various regimens of exercise. Williams,[271] as already mentioned, believed that foraminal decompression through flexion exercises can reduce nerve root compression. A more current rationale for flexion exercises revolves around the potential protective effect of strong abdominal muscles protecting the lumbar discs from excessive loads.[13] Some authors discredit this concept, pointing to the fact that a flexion moment induced on the lumbar spine clearly increases intradiscal pressure.[197]

Extension exercises, when used for pain relief, are hypothesized to produce a shift of nuclear material away from the posterior rim of the annulus and thereby decrease nociceptive input from the annulus fibrosus that is pathologic, or reduce disc material that has already protruded through an annular tear. Evidence regarding this hypothesis is contradictory.[148, 150, 231] Kramer[150] demonstrated that there are pressure-dependent fluid shifts in the intervertebral disc. In a more recent study, Korenko and associates[148] were not able to demonstrate any detectable changes on postexercise CT scans or any positional differences in the MR images of the lumbar spine when a prospective comparison of McKenzie extension exercises was made with a nonexercise control group. Others, however, have noted that the McKenzie exercises may be a provocative test for prognosis in treating acute herniated discs. Kopp and associates,[147] in a retrospective study, reported that 97 per cent of patients achieving normal lumbar extension responded to nonoperative treatment, whereas only 6 per cent in the group undergoing surgery had normal extension preoperatively.

The role of muscular weakness in low back pain and its treatment through strengthening exercises have substantial support.[208] Decreased trunk strength can commonly be found in patients with chronic low back pain on the basis of isometric or isokinetic testing.[50] In a normal situation, the spinal extensors are stronger than the abdominal flexors. DeVries,[58] utilizing electromyographic measurement of trunk extensor activity during various postural activities, demonstrated the more easy fatigability of the erector spinae group in patients who complained of back pain, compared with normal controls. Endurance, therefore, appears to be a key contributing factor in the pathogenesis of low back pain when it is due to muscular insufficiency.

Whether specific flexion or extension programs are helpful in reducing mechanical stress on the disc or facet joints has not yet been conclusively proved. It seems reasonable, however, to conclude that extension may aggravate the complaints of patients who have severe osteoarthritic involvement of the facet joint. Extension may also increase symptoms in patients with degenerative lumbar spinal stenosis due to a deleterious effect on the cross-sectional area available for the nerve roots when the spine assumes a hyperlordotic posture.

That aerobic capacity has a beneficial effect on injury protection is well documented.[39] For patients with low back pain, aerobic exercises should, in general, be of "low" impact and straight ahead (brisk walking, swimming, cross-country ski machines, bicycling). Jogging need not be discouraged if it is tolerated by the patient. More vigorous aerobic activity, such as aerobic dance and high-intensity racket sports, may produce excessive torsional stresses that can propagate disc injuries or back pain.

Reports that exercise can stabilize hypermobile segments in the lumbosacral spine, or result in postural improvements, are currently lacking in confirmation. The beneficial effects are probably primarily related to endorphin release and increase in muscle strength and perhaps blood flow.

Types of Exercise. The various types of exercises can be grouped according to the following categories: (1) range of motion and stretching, (2) isometric, (3) isotonic, (4) isokinetic, (5) aerobic, and (6) recreational.

Range of Motion and Stretching. Range of motion or stretching exercises can be one of three types: (1) passive stretching, in which a therapist causes movement in the patient; (2) active assistive, where the patient and therapist participate together in the stretching activity; and (3) active, in which the patient alone performs the stretching maneuver.

Extension stretching of the lumbar spine may be beneficial by producing shifts in intradiscal pressure and relaxation of neuromeningeal tethering phenomena. Hyperextension stretching has been advocated by Cyriax[45] and McKenzie[178] in order to increase mobility of the spine and restore the normal lumbar lordosis, along with facilitating a shift of nuclear material in the disc and strengthening of the erector spinae. Shah[231] and others demonstrated a slight shift in the nucleus pulposus toward an anterior direction with compressive loading; Korenko and associates,[148] on the other hand, were unable to show detectable changes on CT or MR images obtained after exercise. It is the author's (RJW) belief that the beneficial effect of extension posturing of the spine results in decreased neuromeningeal tension on a nerve root that is being compressed by anteriorly situated disc material; however, this hypothesis remains to be proved. Extension exercises may increase pain in patients with spinal stenosis, particularly in those with lateral recess stenosis, since lordotic posturing of the spine often aggravates nerve root compression.

Flexion stretching has many strong advocates. Starting with the classic study of Williams,[271] which reported a beneficial effect from increasing the cross-sectional area of the neural foramina and thereby reducing nerve compression, further rationales for the use of Williams' flexion exercises now exist. Stretching of hip flexors and back extensors, strengthening of abdominal musculature, increase of intra-abdominal pressure, and reduction of stress on the disc, as well as promotion of facet joint and disc nutrition, have all been suggested as potential beneficial effects.

Flexion exercises may be used in an isometric fashion to strengthen abdominal musculature. They often are beneficial in promoting relief of symptoms of spinal stenosis, but frequently are not helpful in the patient with an acute prolapsed disc.

We do not consider rotational stretching to be advantageous in the management of acute low back pain. In this regard, Farfan and colleagues[78] showed the potentially injurious effect of rotational forces in the pathogenesis of disc disease.

Isometric Exercise. When isometric muscle contraction occurs, no lengthening or shortening of muscle fibers is present and joints are not actively moved. Isometric exercise programs have been shown to be associated with the least amount of stress across joints,[182] and are easy and safe to perform in patients with symptomatic low back pain. A study by Manniche and colleagues[166] showed that more intensive isometric exercise results in greater improvement in patients with low back pain. In this study, 105 chronic low back pain patients were randomized to one of three groups. The first group received heat and massage, with mainly isometric exercises repeated ten times for one hour in eight sessions spanning a one-month interval. The second and third groups performed the same exercises during 30 sessions for a three-month interval; however, the third group exercised twice as long (90 versus 45 minutes). The rates of improvement were 19, 42, and 74 per cent, respectively. The authors concluded that intensive exercise carried out for a longer time will counteract the conditioning effects of muscular fatigue and tenderness that are often encountered in the process of rehabilitating patients with chronic musculoskeletal pain.

Isometric strengthening of weak erector spinae muscles can be accomplished through an extension exercise in which the patient is placed at the edge of a treatment table and positioned in 45 degrees of trunk flexion. He or she is then asked to perform an isotonic contraction to the neutral position against the force of gravity, and hold this position.

Isometric quadriceps, gluteal, hamstring, and upper extremity exercises, when performed on a regular basis, can also result in increased muscular strength and should be recommended in terms of a more global approach to fitness as the patient improves.

Isotonic Exercise. In patients performing an isotonic contraction, there is either lengthening (eccentric) or shortening (concentric) movement of muscle fibers while the adjacent joint is put through a range of motion. Additional force across the joint also occurs when a counterforce (free weight, machine) is added. Isotonic strengthening programs facilitate mobility as well as providing strength gains.

Since the medical literature is replete with reports emphasizing the strength deficit seen in the spinal extensors in patients with chronic low back pain,[174, 175] isotonic trunk strengthening with various machines has been gaining increasing popularity. Most commercially available machines provide isotonic exercise through weights that in turn exert the same force throughout the dynamic range of motion.

Isokinetic Exercise. In contrast, there is a proliferation of isokinetic strengthening equipment that requires a dynamometer device limiting the speed to a preset level. Isokinetic exercise maintains speed while allowing the production of torque around the central axis, which eliminates the effect of acceleration on energy production. The usefulness of isokinetic devices in a low back strengthening program is still a subject of debate. At the present time, it appears that the isokinetic device is a useful means of quantitating trunk flexor and extensor strength with reasonable reproducibility. These machines can also be used to test the endurance of individual muscle groups—endurance being defined as the ability to perform repetitive motions. Isokinetic exercise places more force across the joints and muscles than isometric or isotonic exercise and may increase pain in patients with inflammatory arthritis or osteoporosis. Isotonic exercise has been demonstrated to increase strength as much as isokinetic exercise when rehabilitating quadriceps deficiencies.[52] A comparison of back muscle extensor strengthening programs is not available at the present time.

Aerobic Exercise. Aerobic exercise can increase muscle strength as well as endurance. In Cady and associates'[38] study of firefighters who had a previous episode of back pain, none of the most aerobically fit subjects had recurrences, whereas one third of the least fit experienced at least one recurrence. Many methods of measuring aerobic fitness are currently in use, including measurement of the maximal rate of oxygen consumption (VO_2 max) and estimating endurance on a bicycle ergometer or treadmill. Patients entering into an aerobic endurance program should be screened for significant cardiovascular risk factors.[107] Improvements in VO_2 max may result from participation in activities such as brisk walking, swimming, and stationary bicycling. In situations in which minimal stress on the back is advisable, upper body ergometer arm crank machines can be used.

A secondary benefit to be derived from aerobic activity is an increase in endorphin levels.[8, 11] Multiple studies have demonstrated an increase in beta-endorphin in the serum of both trained athletes and normal nonathletes during strenuous aerobic exercise activity. Endorphins may play a key role in individual sensitivity to noxious stimuli. Furthermore, it is postulated that aerobically fit individuals have an increased subjective sense of well-being and thereby recover more promptly from minor episodes of low back pain.[159] Further research studies of aerobic exercise alone or in combination with stretching and strengthening protocols are likely to result in a broadened knowledge of the potential benefits of exercise in the treatment of low back pain and sciatica.

In summary, there are multiple philosophies extolling the beneficial effects of specific types of exercise for treating lumbar disc disease in all its manifestations. Contradictory reports abound. It is clear, however, that fitness creates an overall protective effect on the spine. A properly designed graduated program of exercise activities, based on a thorough understanding of the natural history and pathogenesis of the disease process being treated, is useful for many patients. The goals of such treatment should be to relieve pain, strengthen weak muscles, and improve overall fitness. It is rational to conclude that such treatment, in conjunction with other therapies, will diminish or eliminate the negative effects of excessive passive treatment of the patient.

Orthotics and Postural Devices

Numerous external support orthoses are currently used to treat low back pain and sciatica. According to Deyo,[59] there are no rigorous trials available supporting their efficacy. The potential beneficial effects of external spinal bracing include limiting movement, altering intra-abdominal pressure, modifying muscle action, and producing warmth. Fidler and Plasmans[82] conducted a study comparing the effects of a canvas corset with those of posterior steel supports, the Raney flexion jacket, a Baycast jacket, and a Baycast spica incorporating the left thigh. Flexion-extension films were obtained of the volunteers in each group, and the results indicated that the canvas corset reduced the mean angular movement at each lumbar motion segment, including the lumbosacral junction, to two thirds of normal. The Raney and Baycast jackets reduced angular motion in the middle of the lumbar spine to one third of normal. The Baycast spica was the most effective in restricting angular movements below the third lumbar vertebra, and especially at the L4–L5 and L5–S1 levels. Nachemson and Morris[198] demonstrated a 25 per cent decrease in intradiscal pressure in normal standing subjects wearing an inflatable corset. Hadler and colleagues[102] pointed out that prolonged use of braces or corsets may cause diffuse atrophy of the muscles that support the lumbar spine. Grew and Deane[100] demonstrated that external bracing results in increased local skin temperature, as would be expected. The increase in local regional blood flow may in turn be beneficial in relieving inflammation and promoting increased regional blood flow. In this article, the authors emphasized that bracing should always be employed in the context of other therapies such as an active exercise program.

In a survey performed by the American Academy of Orthopaedic Surgeons Subcommittee on Orthotics, Perry[211] pointed out that bracing is a common adjunct to treatment of low back pain. Results indicated that 85 per cent of physicians used back supports to treat back pain.

Our current recommendation is that in both the acute and subacute phases of low back pain, braces of one form or another may be helpful in more rapidly mobilizing a patient after a period of rest has resulted in reduction of symptoms. In this circumstance, the brace is thought to function both as an external reminder to minimize bending and twisting stress on the low back area and in the capacity of a mildly immobilizing device. Patients are encouraged to wean themselves rapidly from any dependency on the brace as their symptoms subside, certainly within six weeks.

In the case of acute pars stress fractures or mechanical back pain from already present spondylolytic and spondylolisthetic deformity, we advocate a trial of bracing with a thermoplastic antilordotic low back brace. Micheli and associates[183] reported their experience with such a device in the treatment of 31 young athletes. Twenty-eight of the 31 followed for an average of 15 months improved in response to antilordotic bracing. Best results were obtained in spondylolysis. Therapy for discogenic back pain with the brace was effective in only 50 per cent of patients. These braces were used full time for three to six months in conjunction with flexibility and muscle-strengthening exercises.

Physical Therapy

Heat, cold, massage, ultrasonography, and cold laser treatments have all been advocated in the treatment of acute and chronic low back pain syndromes. Firm scientific evidence of the efficacy of these treatments is lacking. In general, their use beyond two to four weeks is not necessary or useful on a routine basis.[134]

It is often not useful to administer heat during the first 72 hours after a severe soft tissue injury.[137, 158] Heat treatment may increase local blood flow and result in increased edema, hemorrhage, and other components of the local inflammatory response.

Cryotherapy, with local applications of ice to an area of acutely injured soft tissue, has a rational foundation in terms of the ability of cold temperatures to decrease regional blood flow. It has also been suggested that the cooling effect can produce a topical form of anesthesia.[134] However, neither heat nor cold has been demonstrated to have any significant metabolic effects on structures deep to the layer of insulating subcutaneous fat.

Ultrasonography and other forms of short wave diathermy are believed to produce increased heat below the subcutaneous fat layer.[158] The use of ultrasound has been associated with increases in regional blood flow, tissue metabolism, and vascular permeability. Low-power or laser treatment has demonstrated favorable results when used to treat patients with neck and back pain in one uncontrolled study.[14] The exact mechanism of action of such treatment has not been elucidated.

Massage has been described as an "addictively good" treatment when used to relieve musculoskeletal pain. Reports of its efficacy are based on empirical observations, and controlled studies are again lacking.

With these, as with other passive modalities, it is important to appreciate the high frequency of the "hands on" placebo effect and emphasize to the patient that although such therapies may produce patient comfort, there is no proven direct beneficial effect in terms of hastening the resolution of an acute episode or preventing recurrences. It needs to be emphasized that in 90 per cent of back pain patients problems resolve spontaneously in two to three months in the face of almost all, as well as no, treatment.

Traction

Traction methods remain a traditional treatment for lumbar disc disease in many clinics. A wide variety of methods are in routine use throughout the United States, including manual traction, autotraction,[156] gravity lumbar reduction, inversion therapy, and 90-90 traction. Traction can be applied intermittently or continuously. The theoretical basis for the use of traction involves the concept that a distraction force can physiologically unload the spine by causing widening of a disc space, with resultant decrease in intradiscal pressure.[214] Experimentally, Nachemson and Elfstrom[197] showed that a 30-kg traction force applied in a supine position reduces intradiscal pressure by 25 per cent at the L3 level. A force of at least 25 per cent of the patient's body weight is necessary to alter the disc space. The hypothesis that traction can produce a beneficial effect in relieving nerve root compression was examined by Natchev and Valentino[199] with CT scans. Observable changes in the size and shape of herniated discs occurred in six of 17 patients examined during autotraction.

Clinically, Weber[261] was not able to show any significant effect due to traction treatment in patients with herniated discs. He compared sham traction with one third body weight.

There are few studies comparing the various methods of traction. Weber and colleagues[262] compared autotraction to passive bed traction and found no statistically significant difference between them. Burton[37] has been one of the most vocal advocates of the gravity lumbar reduction form of traction therapy. In this method, the patient is hung from a torso sling on a tilting bed or frame at an angle of 35 to 90 degrees from the horizontal. A 70 per cent success rate in treating acute contained discs has been reported; however, after discharge from in-hospital treatment for a period of approximately eight days, gravity traction is continued at home for one hour twice a day for six to 12 months. In this report, as in most other studies,[206] major flaws exist in the shape of poorly defined outcome measures, concomitant variables, limited statistics, and inadequate or absent control groups.

The extreme opposite of the gravity lumbar reduction method is inversion therapy.[202] Using this technique, the patient hangs upside down from boots or other supportive devices. This therapy is not without substantial risk in that it has been documented to produce changes in blood pressure and heart rate, and adversely affect intraocular hemodynamics.[12, 145] Clinical trials supporting its efficacy are nonexistent and its use is discouraged by the authors.

The technique of 90-90 traction failed to produce any demonstrable improvement in patients receiving such treatment for sciatica.[154, 261] When 90-90 traction treatment is compared with an individualized exercise program, patients receiving active exercise treatment for back pain and sciatica improved to a greater degree.[249]

In summary, the use of conventional or alternative forms of traction is not supported by rigorous studies. All the studies reported above can be criticized because of major design flaws. In studies that compare alternative forms of traction, superiority of one form over another is not demonstrated.[65]

Spinal Manipulation

Methods of manipulation vary widely among chiropractors, physiotherapists, osteopathic physicians, and orthopedic surgeons. The techniques are equally divergent, with a force range encompassing gentle repetitive range of motion movements in an active assisted fashion to high-velocity flexion and rotation thrust motions produced by the manipulator on a totally passive patient.[204] In chiropractic methods, the foundation for manipulating the spine often centers on the concept that subluxation of the vertebral elements produces low back pain and also contributes to a variety of other ills. Scientific documentation of this global concept is lacking.[44] Serious complications occurring as a direct result of spinal manipulation, including acute disc ruptures, cauda equina syndrome, vertebral basilar insufficiency, and spinal column fracture, have been reported.[47, 86] Advocates of manipulation point to studies demonstrating its efficacy in providing short-term pain relief in patients with acute back pain. Hochler and colleagues' study[118] demonstrated greater pain relief after initial treatment with manipulation than after local massage. No statistically significant difference was detected at the end of three weeks of treatment, however. The attrition rate was 27 per cent and randomization occurred after a rigorous preselection process. Farrell and Twomey[79] studied passive manipulation as compared with diathermy and isometric abdominal exercises. No statistically significant difference was noted at the three-week examination. Patients in short-term manipulation fared better.

Aside from the issue of efficacy, the question of the cost:benefit ratio is clearly present when one considers the study of Breen.[30] He found on reviewing 1598 patients receiving chiropractic care in Great Britain that an average of seven visits was necessary over approximately 4½ weeks in order to effect relief in subjects responding to manipulative therapy. Maintenance therapy was required for approximately one third of the patients responding. It seems that although manipulation may speed recovery in acute cases of low back pain, it does not affect the long-term prognosis. When effective, the relief may be short-lived in up to one third. Additional research is needed to address the issues of standardization of techniques, cost:benefit ratio, and a more complete understanding of the physiologic and biomechanical effects of manipulation itself.

It is the authors' opinion that since this type of therapy is totally passive, it should not routinely be used alone without a more active rehabilitation program. Its continuance on a regular basis past a three-week interval is not supported by controlled studies in the medical literature.

Counter-irritation Techniques

Transcutaneous electrical nerve stimulation (TENS), acupuncture, self-hypnosis, and biofeedback have all been advocated as potentially useful in decreasing low back pain perception. Central to the mechanism of action is Melzack and Wall's theory[179] of the gate control mechanism of pain perception. This theory, in essence, suggests that afferent, nociceptive pain input transmitted along slow-conducting, poorly myelinated sensory fibers can be blocked by overloading the fast-conducting, highly myelinated sensory fibers. Richardson and associates' study[220] of functional low back pain patients reported a 40 per cent response rate. In many of the responders, however, a gradual reduction in the efficacy of this treatment occurred over a two-month period.

Some studies[90, 180, 181] point toward acupuncture reducing both acute and chronic low back pain. There are no controlled studies demonstrating its superiority over other forms of treatment. Biofeedback has been used to teach specific muscle control as an aid in breaking the pain-spasm-pain cycle. This methodology has been used to correct postural problems identified from electromyographic scanning procedures.[67] Biofeedback for paraspinal muscle reeducation lacks a sound theoretical or clinical basis.

Pregnancy and Low Back Pain

Kelsey and colleagues,[143] in an epidemiologic study, found that multiple pregnancies resulting in live births were a factor predisposing to herniated discs. LaBan and associates,[153] in reviewing 49,760 deliveries, found an incidence of only one per 10,000.

Fast and colleagues[80] studied the problem of low back pain in pregnancy. In this study, 200 patients were interviewed within 24 to 36 hours after labor. Results of the interview demonstrated that 56 per cent suffered from low back pain during pregnancy. The percentage of Caucasians was statistically higher than that of Hispanics in the back pain group. No incidence correlations were identified when examining patients' age and weight gain, the baby's weight, the number of previous pregnancies, or the number of previous children. Pain radiated to the lower extremities in 45.5 per cent. Most patients started suffering from back pain between the fifth and seventh months of pregnancy.

Several theories currently exist to explain the occurrence of low back pain during pregnancy. These include increased lumbar lordosis, ligamentous laxity caused by either pelvic muscular insufficiency or the effects of the hormone relaxin,[245] which is secreted by the corpus luteum and prepares the pelvis to accommodate the fetus during pregnancy and delivery. In addition, there is firm scientific evidence of ischemic effects on the aorta, vena cava, and potentially the lumbosacral plexus in response to the pressure changes induced by the gravid uterus. However, there is no firm substantiation of a causal effect that directly proves any of these theories.

Therapeutic tools available during pregnancy are limited. For the most part, one must depend on rest, postural counseling, occasional use of a supporting corset, and the tincture of time.

Medication should be prescribed in conjunction with the obstetrician. Confirmation of the diagnosis is also somewhat hampered by the need to limit the use of radiography during the first trimester of pregnancy. In the authors' experience, most sciatica rapidly improves after labor and delivery, and the standard measures already discussed are applicable.

Back Pain Versus Sciatica

If the initial battery of therapeutic measures has failed and six to eight weeks have passed, it is advisable to divide these patients into two groups, the first those with predominant sciatica and thc sccond those in whom low back pain is the major complaint. In patients in whom low back pain is the predominant and persisting symptom despite six weeks of treatment, we advise a technetium bone scan and a complete medical evaluation. In patients in whom sciatica is the predominant and persisting symptom, we escalate our evaluation and treatment to determine whether surgery is a useful option.

The pathways along the algorithm can go in either dierection, and if regression occurs, with exacerbation of symptoms, one can resort to more stringent nonoperative measures. Most patients with acute low back pain proceed along the improvement pathway, returning to a normal life pattern within two months of the onset of symptoms. Our personal experience has led us to be cautious in responding to inquiries about the failure of therapy and the necessity for operative intervention when dealing with sciatica. We have found that only about 20 per cent or less of patients with a firm diagnosis of an acute disc herniation ultimately seek surgery when followed over a period of years. This finding is in agreement with several reports in the literature.

Sciatica Predominant

Surgical Considerations in Sciatica

If the various nonsurgical therapies available are unsuccessful in relieving the leg pain, surgery should be considered.

Hakelius[104] retrospectively evaluated the results (pain relief) in 583 patients with unilateral L5 or S1 sciatica. Almost all the patients (93 per cent) had been treated for two months with rest and a corset brace. In the group of patients with myelographically proved disc herniations, more of the surgically treated group did well (81 per cent versus 52 per cent) in the first few months after surgery than a comparable group of nonoperatively treated patients. At six months, however, there was no significant difference between the two groups. At three months of follow-up the surgically treated group still fared better than the unoperated patients (88 per cent versus 73 per cent asymptomatic). This difference, however, was not statistically significant at six months of follow-up. Hakelius succeeded in following 526 of his original patient group for an average of seven years and four months. At that time, the nonoperatively managed group reported more low back pain (71 per cent versus 48 per cent), greater residual sciatica (61 per cent versus 44 per cent), more recurrences of significant sciatic discomfort (20 per cent versus 10 per cent), and more time lost from work.

This study effectively demonstrates that in most cases acute sciatica is a transient and self-limited condition that resolves satisfactorily regardless of whether the method of treatment is surgical or conservative. Surgical intervention, however, seems to offer a better long-term prognosis for the patient's subjective complaints of low back pain, residual sciatica, and frequency of recurrences.

The problem patients who do not meet the criteria for early surgical intervention and are not responding promptly to therapy are the subject of another classic prospective study performed in Oslo, Norway, by Weber.[259] A total of 126 patients with myelographic and clinical evidence of a herniated lumbar disc were randomly assigned to either a surgical or a nonsurgical group. Both groups have been followed for 10 years. The results of treatment (related to their leg pain complaints) at the end of one year in the nonoperated group revealed that 60 per cent were improved and 40 per cent unimproved.

Compared with the nonoperatively treated group, surgery clearly improved the quality of the result during the first year. Of those who underwent operations, 92 per cent had improvement in leg pain, and only 8 per cent remained unimproved. When these two groups were evaluated at the end of four years, however, the differences were not statistically significant; 90 per cent of the operated group as compared with 85 per cent of the nonoperatively treated group reported satisfactory results. Thus, the results of surgery are clearly better than those of nonoperative treatment in the early phases of sciatica, but it is equally obvious that if one chooses to wait some surgery can be avoided.

Weber[260] reported the ten year follow-up in the same two groups of patients, with only minimal attrition, stating that only minor changes took place during the last six years of observation. This suggests that four years is a sufficient follow-up time for final evaluation of these patients.

It has become evident through examination of these data that the final surgery result is not prejudiced by a three-month period of delay before surgery.[237] During these three months, many patients with disc herniations spontaneously improve and do not request operative intervention. Those who fail to respond by the end of three months can then undergo surgical intervention, with no sacrifice in expected quality of result. We believe that it is important to understand this time sequence; there is little reason to rush a patient with typical sciatica complaints to surgery during the first few weeks of symptoms.

It would be ideal if we could predict at the onset which patients will respond to nonoperative treatment. If this identification were made, surgery could be recommended for the appropriate patients. Unfortunately, this is not possible, and therefore observation is advised for all patients except those who meet the previously listed criteria for immediate surgery.

Although a measure of delay does not prejudice the outcome, results will clearly be worse if an inordinate delay is allowed. In persons who continue with symptoms for longer than one year, the results of surgical intervention are not as good in relieving leg pain as in patients who undergo surgery within three months from the onset of sciatica. It is not clear whether this is attributable to neurologic damage, intraneural fibrosis, or altered behavior patterns.

An area of persistent controversy is the relative urgency of surgical intervention in the face of muscle weakness. Muscular weakness per se is not regarded as an absolute indication for surgery, since it has been demonstrated that return of muscle power is not influenced by the timing of surgical intervention except in the most severe progressive situations. Certainly, progressive paralysis is an indication for surgical decompression, but this is not the usual situation. Moderate degrees of motor weakness allow for the usual period of observation and decision making. Recovery of strength is common in both operated and nonoperated patients.[260] In Weber's study,[260] muscle weakness was observed in 64 patients, of whom 32 had surgery and 31 had nonoperative treatment. One patient was excluded because of lack of cooperation. At follow-up evaluation at one year, the restitution of muscle strength was equal in both treatment groups. The improvement of muscle strength continued during the next three years of observation. At the four-year follow-up interval, muscle weakness was present in 20 patients. Only 5 patients had muscle weakness, equally distributed in both treatment groups, at the time of the final examination at ten years.

It was interesting that sensory dysfunction was still demonstrable in more than 35 per cent of the patients ten years after treatment. Abolished reflexes and positive tension signs were also equally distributed in the two treatment groups at the 10-year follow-up.

Tension Sign Positive

With the above knowledge of the medical history of sciatica in hand, our next decision making is centered around the continued demonstration of a positive tension sign. An SLR test (Lasègue's sign) is considered positive if it produces a radiating type of pain in the sciatic distribution, or femoral distribution, when the femoral stretch test is performed.[237] Young persons with disc herniations at the L4 or L5 level essentially all demonstrate a positive SLR test if significant nerve root compression is produced by the herniation. Scham and Taylor[229] described the many variations of this test and observed that the crossed Lasègue sign, in which elevation of the opposite or painless extremity reproduces the sciatica in the opposite leg, surpasses any other single sign in the diagnosis of disc herniation, if it is present. It is more specific and less sensitive than the ipsilateral Lasègue sign.

If the tension sign is positive, we proceed to diagnostic imaging in this group of patients with leg pain. The added finding of a neurologic deficit in the neurotomal distribution of the radicular pain further reinforces the decision to proceed with definitive radiographic imaging. Statistically, the best predictive factors in an attempt to find a disc protrusion are a well-defined neurologic deficit, a positive SLR test, and positive myelographic, CT, or MRI results. If all three factors are present, exploration will almost always reveal a significant disc herniation. In the absence of one of these factors, surgery may still be productive, and if two of the three factors are absent, more than half the patients will have no demonstrable pathologic condition.

Considerations in Radiologic Evaluation of Low Back Pain and Sciatica

Diagnostic imaging of the lumbosacral spine and pelvis may yield important information regarding the integrity of bony and ligamentous support structures, as well as the alignment of the vertebral column, patency of the spinal canal, and presence of pathology. The imaging data synthesized, along with the patient's subjective complaints and objective physical examination findings, allow the examining physician to arrive at a presumptive diagnosis and outline a rational plan of management.

Routine Radiography. In the atraumatic setting, it is generally agreed that lumbosacral spine radiographs are often unnecessary, particularly at the time of an initial office visit. Liang and Komaroff[160] compared the benefits, risks, and costs of obtaining a radiograph of the lumbar spine at the time of an initial office visit with obtaining it only if the patient fails to improve after an initial eight-week period of therapy. They concluded that the favorable natural history of low back pain does not justify routine radiography at the time of an initial evaluation.

Scavone and colleagues[228] estimated that 7 million lumbar radiographs (at a cost of 500 million dollars) are taken annually in the United States. They calculated that only one in eight of the studies taken provides any valuable diagnostic information.

Table 23–2, adapted from the epidemiologic work of Frymoyer and colleagues,[85] illustrates that relatively few postural/structural diagnoses are detectable by plain radiographic examination alone. This study suggests that most of the commonly observed roentgenographic abnormalities such as disc space narrowing, spinal osteophytes, facet arthropathy, facet tropism, Schmorl's nodes, lumbarization, sacralization, and spina bifida occulta occur with equal prevalence in symptomatic and asymptomatic individuals.

Deyo and Diehl[60] suggested the following guidelines for considering the urgency factor in ordering plain radiographs: patients over age 50, history of serious trauma, known cancer, night pain, pain at rest, unexplained weight loss, drug or alcohol abuse, treatment with corticosteroids, temperature above 38°C, or a clinical history and examination that raise a suspicion of ankylosing spondylitis or demonstrate a neuromotor deficit.

Advanced Spinal Imaging. In today's era of sophisticated imaging technology there is no single "gold standard" imaging tool that allows precise, accurate, cost-effective, low-morbidity, and three-dimensional characterization of the broad spectrum of conditions represented as lumbar disc disease and mimicking disorders.

In the recent past it has been true that myelography with or without postmyelographic multiplanar CT most closely approximated a "gold standard" test.

The now classic study of Hirsch and Nachemson[116] demonstrated that a well-trained surgeon can expect a 95 per cent operative confirmation of pathology when a patient has a positive water-soluble contrast myelogram combined with correlative tension signs and objective neurologic findings. This study was performed with oil-based contrast myelography (Pantopaque). A double-blind study[114] comparing two forms of water-soluble contrast myelography demonstrated that iohexol is superior to metrizamide in terms of the frequency of adverse reactions. Iohexol remains the agent of choice for optimal contrast filling of the lumbar root sheaths.

Because spinal nerves do not fill throughout their length even with water-soluble contrast media, CT and MRI are helpful and, in fact, have replaced myelography. This is particularly true in many cases in which the suspected pathology lies beyond the area defined by the contrast medium. Other advantages of CT and MRI include increased patient comfort due to the noninvasive nature of the procedures, less radiation exposure, and ease of outpatient performance.[186] MRI also offers the possibility of continuous sagittal plane imaging of the thoracolumbar junction, and superior visualization of soft tissue structures such as the conus medullaris and the spinal cord, disc, and both intra- and extramedullary soft tissue tumors within the spinal canal. Many investigators regard MRI as the study of choice in diagnosing vertebral osteomyelitis,[185] as well as disc herniation.[16, 171, 186]

It is of utmost clinical importance to note those studies in the literature that have examined the specificity of all three of these imaging tools in asymptomatic groups of patients. This point deserves emphasis particularly when surgical decision making is at hand. There needs to be strict correlation between clinical findings and the significance attached to observed abnormalities on myelographic, CT, or MRI images.

Hitselberger and Witten[117] reviewed 300 oil-based contrast myelograms performed in patients being evaluated for posterior cranial fossa disease who did not have back or leg complaints, and found that 24 per cent of the lumbar films revealed evidence of disc abnormalities ("false-positives"). Likewise, Wiesel and associates[267] demonstrated a 35 per cent incidence of asymptomatic abnormal readings and root compression in a group of 52 asymptomatic volunteers. Nineteen per cent of the individuals in their study in the under-40 age group demonstrated herniated discs. In patients over age 40, 50 per cent had findings that appeared abnormal. Boden and colleagues[23] performed a similar study with MRI and documented a 28 per cent incidence of abnormalities in asymptomatic persons.

Other studies have also compared the relative accuracy of the various imaging modalities. In the largest study of its kind reported to date, Bell and colleagues[15, 16] compared high-resolution CT images with metrizamide myelography and found the myelogram to be more accurate in the diagnosis of both herniated discs and spinal stenosis when the imaging results were compared with surgical findings. The authors of this study found that metrizamide myelography supersedes the accuracy of CT in diagnosing herniated discs (83 per cent versus 72 per cent) and is slightly, but not significantly, more accurate in the global picture of spinal stenosis (93 per cent versus 89 per cent). Critics of this study point out that only 5-mm-thick slides, each 4 mm apart, were used for the CT evaluations. It is likely that if more sophisticated CT formats are used and the examinations are monitored by a radiologist who has discussed the case beforehand with the treating physician, the diagnostic accuracy and corresponding clinical utility will increase.

Modic and associates[186] examined the diagnostic accuracy of MRI, metrizamide myelography, and CT and concluded that the use of multiple diagnostic tests improves the overall accuracy. Interstudy comparison data from the report of Modic and associates suggested that MRI was more accurate than metrizamide myelography (82.3 per cent versus 71.4 per cent) and was equal to CT (82.3 per cent versus 83 per cent) in diagnosing herniated discs and spinal stenosis. Combining the data from two separate tests, the confidence limits increased, as did the diagnostic accuracy. The combination of MRI and CT was equal in diagnostic accuracy to the combination of CT and metrizamide myelography (92.5 per cent versus 89.4 per cent). Since the former combination is totally noninvasive, it is an obvious advantage to the patient.

MRI technology itself is still in a rapidly expanding phase of evolution. It has demonstrated clinical utility in differentiating between the various types of disc herniations (i.e., prolapsed, protrusion, extrusion, and sequestration).[171] This feature carries with it potential prognostic significance in considering the likelihood of a patient's responding to nonoperative treatment, chemonucleolysis,[27, 170] or percutaneous discectomy.

Manipulation of the MRI signals is also of use for considering the differential features of a recurrent herniated disc and epidural fibrosis in a patient who has undergone previous back surgery.[35] Studies using gadolinium-DTPA[53] suggested that this intravenously administered ferromagnetic contrast material is of substantial use in differentiating between recurrent herniations and epidural fibrosis, as well as for more detailed evaluation of spinal neoplasms.

In considering all the above data, it is clearly important to reemphasize that any test has its own inherent false-negative and false-positive rates. In some clinical cases, the accuracy of decision making will be enhanced by ordering more than one test, or by combining the individual characteristics of separate tests (e.g., intrathecally enhanced, multiplanar CT). Ultimately, however, each piece of information obtained from imaging studies needs to be combined with the analysis of subjective historical details and objective examination findings in developing the highest degree of certainty in clinical diagnosis, and in making recommendations surrounding the advantages, disadvantages, and risks involved in surgical treatment of lumbar disc disease.

In keeping with our final goal of the algorithm, a major effort should be made to use efficiently and precisely the available diagnostic studies that can unequivocally document the presence or absence of pathosis amenable to surgical intervention. The ideal study is one tailored to the diagnostic requirements of the individual patient. As such, a "shotgun" approach to spinal imaging is decried and the studies ordered should provide the clinician with an expedient answer, have the greatest sensitivity and specificity ratios, and in turn have a low patient morbidity factor.

In today's world of fast-paced medical technologic expansion, there is no single diagnostic test that meets all these requirements. Imaging tests are best planned after thorough consideration of the clinical records, including previous diagnostic testing. In general, it is wise to enlist the cooperation of the radiologist who will be administering or monitoring the imaging, since unmonitored examinations may be technically inadequate or provide less than optimal visualization of the pathologic process.

A more detailed comparison and explanation of the roles of water-soluble myelography, unenhanced and intravenously enhanced CT (IV-CT), intrathecally enhanced CT (myelo-CT), and unenhanced and IV-enhanced MRI will be found elsewhere in this book. Pantopaque and air myelography as well as epidural venography and epidurography are no longer in routine use in North America.

Recurrent Episodes of Sciatica

Certain individuals, after an initial successful course of treatment, have recurrent sciatica that becomes incapacitating. There may be a complete absence of symptoms between the acute episodes, or low-grade sciatica may continue to a greater or lesser extent. If the recurrent episodes are not disabling, and if the intensity of the symptoms is within the patient's tolerance, persistent nonoperative therapy is indicated. However, if the frequency and intensity of the attacks are severe enough to interfere with the individual's ability to follow gainful employment and enjoy normal activities of daily living, surgery should be considered.

Personality Factors

Care must be taken to evaluate the emotional stability of patients and their reaction to pain. A person who continues to have minor symptoms despite appropriate therapy but who manifests an overwhelming emotional reaction to this pain, particularly if an element of hostility is present, usually does poorly after surgery.

However, it is emphasized that this admonition is not made in order to differentiate the "functional" from the "organic" back pain patient. It would be naive to overlook the reciprocal interaction between the patient's somatic and emotional state. Rather, effective management of this disabling episode of pain may rest on coincident psychotherapeutic support, carefully monitored antidepressant medication, or both.[169]

An efficient and rapid psychiatric assessment[278] can be elicited using the following points of subjectivity:

1. Has the patient's pain precipitated adverse mood changes? (That is, are the patient's "spirits down?")
2. Has there been an onset of vegetative behavioral changes (appetite alterations, sleep disturbances, and diminution in libido)?
3. Has the pain created problems at home or work?
4. Has the patient demonstrated an appropriate response to management thus far?

The use of the MMPI Conversion 5 profile, as demonstrated by Hanvick,[108] its modified form,[276] or the pain drawing screening test introduced by Ransford and colleagues[216] may shed some light on the psychiatric factors involved. In and of themselves, however, these ancillary studies are more a temporal indication of the patient's focus on the intensity or fear of pain, rather than a statement about the etiology of that pain.[40, 188]

If there is any uncertainty over the emotional stability of the patient, psychiatric consultation is mandatory. This is not to say that all patients with emotional problems, particularly those with long-standing pain, should be denied surgical relief. It has been well demonstrated that long-standing pain leads to depression, even in basically stable individuals, and that depression sometimes lifts after the pain is alleviated. In general, it is a good rule of thumb to treat the emotional factors before rendering a surgical decision. More often than not, intolerable pain becomes tolerable once depression has lifted.

In most instances when surgery is undertaken for the relief of sciatic pain, its effectiveness will depend on the discovery and relief of pressure on the neural elements. Ideally, every operative procedure undertaken to relieve sciatica would reveal mechanical compromise of the nerve roots. This occasionally is not the case, and in these instances surgery will often fail. One might assume that failure to discover mechanical compression is due to one of two factors, either an inadequate exploration or a nonmechanical cause of the sciatica. The former factor may be remedied by more thorough exploration (pre- and/or intraoperative) and more complete understanding of the pathologic condition. The nonmechanical sciatica is best appreciated by an analysis of those factors present in the preoperative evaluation that correlate with the presence or absence of demonstrable nerve root compression. The most thorough study in this regard is that of Hirsch.[115] In a review of some 3000 low back operations he found that the most significant preoperative factors in the determination of mechanical spinal nerve compression were (1) a well-defined neurologic deficit, (2) a positive myelogram, and (3) a positive SLR test. Today, CT and MRI have helped improve the accuracy of diagnosis and the effectiveness of surgical planning. When all these factors are present, surgery usually uncovers mechanical compression and is followed by a good result. If one or more of these factors is absent, much deliberation should take place before surgery is undertaken. This is not to say that one should not recommend surgery in the absence of a neurologic deficit or tension sign, but that careful evaluation of these cases should be undertaken.

The authors have modified these guidelines as follows. In order to predict mechanical root compression, the patient must have (1) either a positive tension sign or a neurologic deficit and (2) a correlative finding on radiographic studies (CT, MRI, myelography). It would be most unusual to undertake exploration without radiographic confirmation of root compression. False-negative results are becoming increasingly rare.

Selection of the Operation

The surgical treatment of low back disorders has followed three major trends in the 20th century. After the descriptions by Dandy,[47a] and later Mixter and Barr,[184] of ruptured discs leading to clinical symptoms of low back pain, and surgery alleviating those complaints, most symptoms of low back pain were thought to be due to degenerative or herniated discs. Following Mixter and Barr's report, laminectomy and discectomy became the standard treatment for the care of almost all low back disorders when nonoperative measures failed.

However, back pain frequently persisted, despite removal of the disc, and new concepts were developed, suggesting that herniated discs were not the sole cause of low back pain. This led to the concept of anatomic variation or instability as the reason for lingering pain. This in turn led to recommendations for the addition of fusion after laminectomies and discectomies.[48, 91, 96, 113, 234, 243, 266, 272] In the mid-1900s fusion became the standard treatment for back pain, even if discectomy was not performed. Later, Hirsch,[115] Nachemson and Elfstrom,[197] and DePalma and Rothman[55, 57] questioned the value of routine fusions in the treatment of low back disorders. After these studies, attention was turned more to the radicular or leg pain component of the complaints, with focus on the identification of discrete disc herniation, than instabilities as the cause of back pain. This led once again to laminectomy and discectomy as the primary treatment of low back disorders, but again with attention focused on the symptoms and signs of radiculopathy. It was clear that back pain, per se, was not treated as well by surgical means. Currently, indications for fusions vary. The literature is replete with articles demonstrating a high success rate for the treatment of radiculopathy, and consistently less good results when back pain becomes the focus of surgical attention.

Acute Disc Herniation

In most individuals with acute disc herniations the primary compelling symptom that leads to surgery is sciatica. Although the patient may have had many years of troublesome but tolerable back pain, the leg symptoms ultimately lead toward surgery. In individuals such as this, limited laminectomy with excision of the herniated material is the procedure of choice. The approach may be limited, and in cases with a wide interlaminar space, little or no bone need be removed. It is essential that the nerve root be completely explored, well out through the foramen, and be free of all external pressure and tension at the termination of the procedure.

Chronic Disc Degeneration and Spinal Stenosis

Back Pain Only. Most individuals with chronic disc degeneration and back pain can be managed effectively with nonoperative treatment. The authors strongly advocate a nonsurgical treatment of patients with disc degeneration and back pain only. The rationale for this is that disc degeneration often becomes a diffuse process throughout the entire lumbar spine. It often is extremely difficult to determine with certainty which of the several levels may be the source of the pain. Occasionally an individual develops severe incapacitating back pain that is intractable to medical therapy and is clearly limited to one or two disc spaces. These individuals may obtain relief through arthrodesis of the spine. We prefer a bilateral spine fusion across the affected levels, although discectomies and interbody fusions have a number of advocates. Discography may have some value in defining this level symptomatically in carefully selected patients. In the authors' large, multicentered experiences, fusion for low back pain is rarely performed. If fusions are performed, bone graft should not be placed in the midline over the lamina, as this may lead to thickening of the lamina with the possible late formation of spinal stenosis (see Fig. 23–31).

Back and Leg Pain. Patients with chronic disc degeneration present with a wide variety of ratios of back to leg pain. One extreme is the patient with florid sciatica and negligible back pain. This individual requires decompression only, if it can be accomplished without creation of instability during the operation. If a strong component of back pain is present, stabilization at the same time may be considered, with a bilateral lateral spinal fusion incorporating the degenerated levels. This combined procedure of decompression and fusion is also indicated if iatrogenic instability is created or if demonstrable radiographic instability is evident.

The type of pathologic condition present dictates the extent and type of decompression required. If midline ridging is the only abnormality present, and if the nerve roots are free in the foramen, complete laminectomy of the affected levels with preservation of the facet joints will suffice. If an extrusion of disc material is present, this obviously should be removed, but this is not usually the case in end-stage disc degeneration. The disc space need

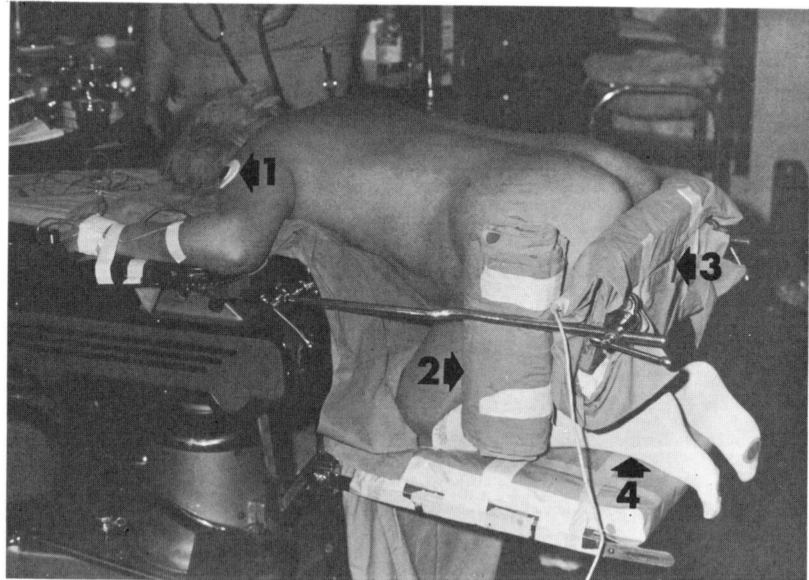

Figure 23–23. Kneeling position used for laminectomy and spinal fusion. Note how, even in this obese patient, the abdomen is completely free, preventing any pressure on the vena cava.

1. ECG monitoring is used because of the difficulty of listening to the heart sounds in this position.
2. Lateral padding is used to stabilize the patient and prevent pressure on the side bars.
3. The patient is stabilized caudally by the use of a seat to prevent extreme flexion at the knees and hips.
4. Elastic stockings or elastic bandages are used to prevent pooling of blood in the calf area.

not be entered in most of these individuals, since little nuclear material will be present.

Although the symptoms may be unilateral, the authors advise a complete bilateral laminectomy to prevent contralateral symptomatology in the future. If foraminal encroachment is present, a thorough foraminotomy is indicated. If a narrow lateral recess is present, this must be unroofed completely. When possible, the lateral portion of the facet joint should be maintained. Often this is not possible, particularly on the symptomatic side. If complete removal of the facets and foraminotomy is undertaken, a fusion should be added.

In certain individuals, even after foraminotomy and unroofing of the lateral recesses, the nerve root will still be tightly tethered between the cephalad pedicle and caudal disc and osteophytes. In these individuals, excision of the pedicle may be necessary. Occasionally a lateral herniation, or osteophytic ridges, will cause a nerve root compression distal to the foramen. These sources of nerve root compression, of course, must be addressed and removed.

It should be reiterated that laminectomy per se does not create sufficient instability to routinely warrant the combined procedure of decompression and spinal fusion. Only demonstrable segmental instability or iatrogenic instability at the same level are indications for spinal fusion in addition to the decompression. A more detailed discussion can be found in Chapter 25.

Indications for Fusion

The questions regarding the ideal surgical procedure and the role of spinal fusion for a degenerated intervertebral disc are as yet unanswered. When reviewing the literature in this field, one is reminded of Josh Billings' cryptic statement, "It ain't what a man don't know that makes him a fool, but what he does know that ain't so." Semmes reviewed 1500 patients in whom only disc excision had been performed and found that 98 per cent considered themselves to have benefited from their operation.[230] Our experience is similar.[87] At the other end of the spectrum, Young and Love[280] reviewed a series of 450 patients who underwent a combined procedure and 558 patients who had disc excision alone, and found that the combined operation relieved both symptoms in 20 per cent more patients than did the operation for removal of the disc alone, and that there were three times as many failures to obtain relief of either back or leg pain when the fusion was not performed. There are innumerable other follow-up studies in the literature that fail to resolve these questions. The answers will not be forthcoming until long-term prospective studies are undertaken in which patients in a definite diagnostic category are treated in a random and variable pattern. Until this is done, the proposed benefits of a considered spinal fusion will rest on less than solid ground.

At our present state of knowledge, spinal fusion for symptoms related to disc herniation and degeneration should be undertaken for the following indications:

1. Acute disc herniations with a protracted significant component of back pain.
2. Chronic disc degeneration with significant back pain and degeneration limited to one or two disc levels.
3. Surgical instability created during decompression.
4. The presence of neural arch defects coincident with disc disease.
5. Symptomatic and radiographically demonstrable segmental instability.

Surgical Technique

Simple Disc Excision

It must be emphasized that the procedure described below is used in people with evidence of acute, single-level soft disc herniation in whom radicular symptoms predominate. This method is designed to minimize the postoperative recovery time, yet effectively treat the source of nerve root compression, which is anticipated to be a frankly herniated or extruded disc.

Anesthesia. This operation may be performed under spinal, epidural, general endotracheal, or local anesthesia. With spinal or epidural anesthesia the patient is able to breathe and cough with minimal disturbance of the physiology. These techniques have proved satisfactory and safe.

Position at Operation. The patient is placed in a kneeling position (Fig. 23–23). The abdomen is free and the intra-abdominal pressure reduced, thereby minimizing epidural venous bleeding. This position has proved to be of benefit, and since its adoption epidural bleeding has virtually been eliminated as a cause of concern during surgery. When operative procedures are performed with the patient in a prone position with pressure on the abdomen, it is not infrequent for the surgeon to visualize distended epidural veins in the operative field. With the use of the abdomen-free kneeling position, however, the epidural veins collapse and offer little problem when encountered. Elastic stockings or leg wraps can be used to decrease venous pooling.

Preparation and Antibiotics. Prophylactic antibiotics are utilized. At this time we prefer intravenous cefazolin sodium, given just before the operation begins. Cefazolin sodium is continued for 24 to 48 hours postoperatively, usually 1 gm intravenously every eight hours. The back is shaved narrowly along the midline and scrubbed with an antiseptic soap solution such as Betadine.

Incision. Because this technique emphasizes a minimum of soft tissue dissection, which enhances early ambulation and recovery, accurate placement of the incision is required. Three techniques are employed to place the incision directly over the affected disc:

1. Notation of the level of the iliac crest on the plain lumbar spine films.
2. Palpation of the last spinous process, which is usually S1. By a combination of these landmarks, the operator ordinarily can satisfactorily locate the precise spinous process of concern, at least for the lower lumbar areas.
3. A preoperative lateral radiograph with skin marker and/or spinal needle.

The incision runs from the centers of the spinous processes of the vertebrae between which the affected disc lies. In an average-sized individual, for a single-level laminotomy/dissection, a 3- to 6-cm incision is usually adequate, if placed correctly, carried down to the fascia. Hemostasis should be obtained with electrocautery at each tissue level. Through this incision the paraspinous muscles are dissected free from the lamina on the appropriate side by subperiosteal stripping with a Cobb or similar-type elevator. A Taylor retractor fits nicely through the incision with its point resting lateral to the facet joints. The Taylor retractor may be either fixed to the drape or held by a roller gauze looped under the surgeon's foot. This retracts the paraspinal muscles. Palpation of the sacrum and the lamina at this point will ascertain the appropriate level. L5 is usually the lowest vertebra to have a definitive lamina or ligamentum flavum, or both. In addition, the operator may grasp the spinous process with a large towel clip. The sacral spinous process does not move, whereas the other lumbar lamina will be somewhat mobile with normal articulations. This maneuver, incidentally, can demonstrate a particularly "loose" lamina suggestive of spinal instability or spondylolisthesis. Localizing radiographs should be taken if any doubt exists. This is particularly important if there are transitional vertebrae or if a proximal lumbar laminectomy is to be performed.

The ligamentum flavum beneath the caudal aspect of the superior lamina is separated (Figs. 23–24, 23–25), and a thumbnail-sized opening is rongeured on the inferior margin of the superior lamina (Fig. 23–26). At this point magnifying loupes of 3.5 power are used, which greatly enhance the surgeon's ability to delineate fine structures. The ligamentum fla-

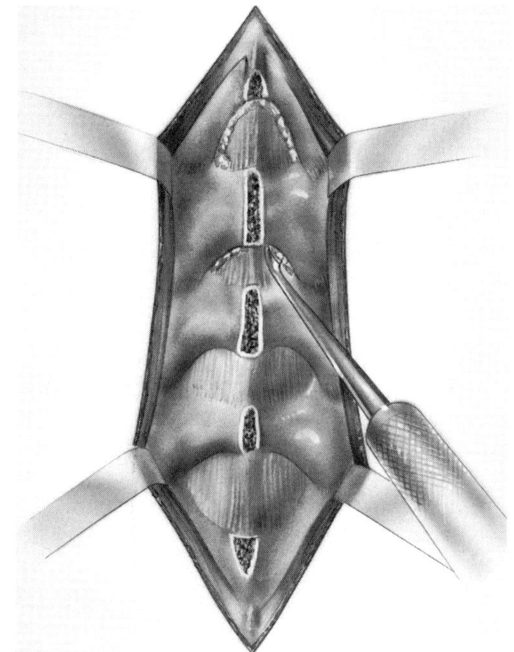

Figure 23–24. Preliminary step for performance of a lumbar decompressive laminectomy. With sharp curets, all soft tissues are removed from the lamina and interlaminar spaces down to the superficial layers of the ligamentum flavum. The curets must be sharp and ventral pressure must be avoided. Curettage should be performed against the bony surfaces.

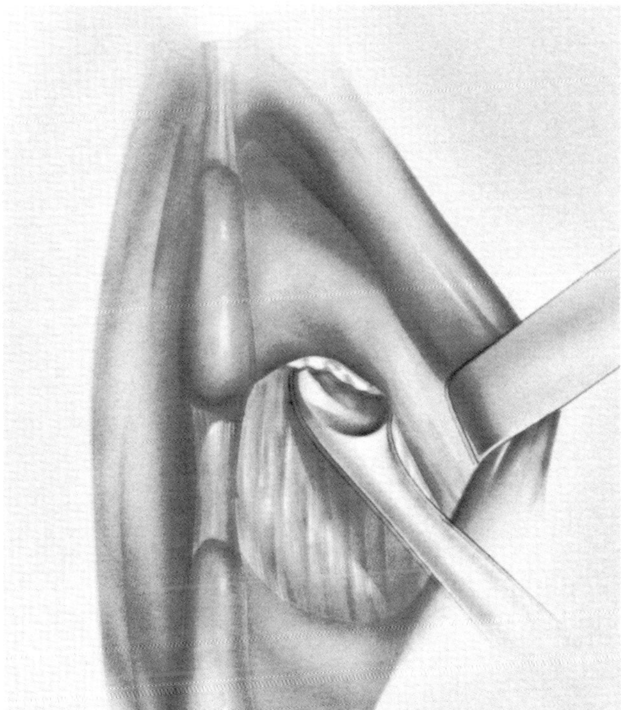

Figure 23–25. The posterior elements of the spine are cleaned of all soft tissue with sharp curets.

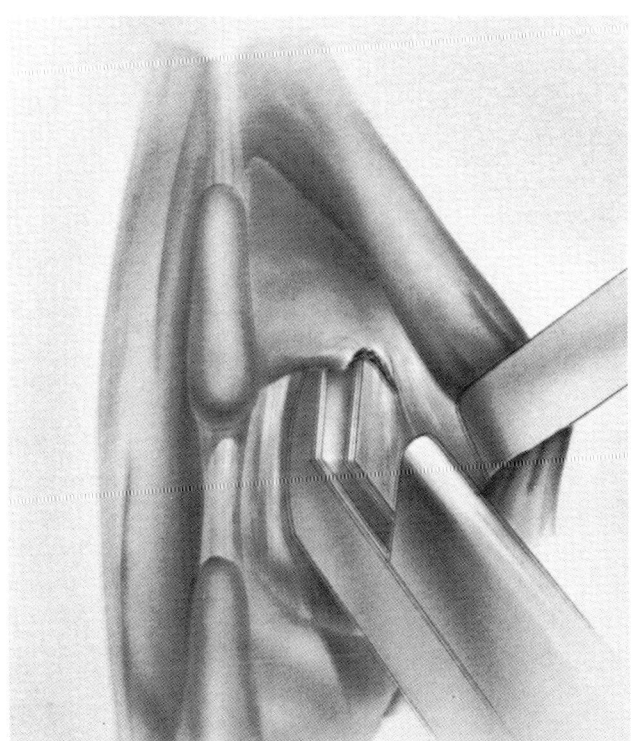

Figure 23–26. The limits of the ligamentum flavum are well defined, as are the bony landmarks.

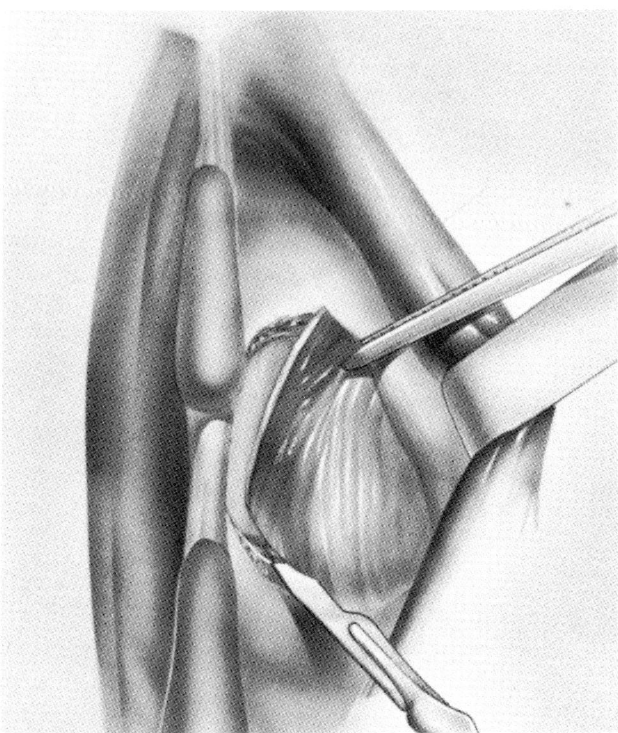

Figure 23–27. The ligamentum flavum is turned down with a fine forceps and excised with a small scalpel. The point of the knife is under direct vision. The dura should be protected by an angled elevator placed between it and the ligamentum flavum, before the knife is used.

Figure 23–28. The extent of bone removal and ligamentum flavum removal before nerve root retraction. The lateral border of the nerve root is well seen before the nerve is retracted. Note the extruded nucleus beneath the nerve root.

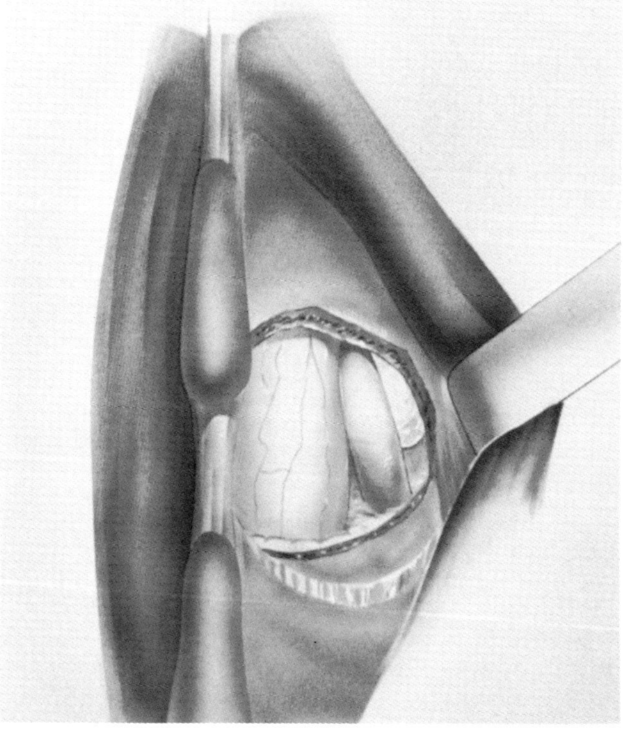

vum is opened with a No. 15 scalpel blade, and a long cottonoid pattie or Frazier dural elevator (protector) is inserted between the ligamentum flavum and the epidural tissue (Fig. 23–27). A long, thin cottonoid pattie is easily accepted in this space, thereby separating the dura from the subsequent dissection of the ligamentum flavum. The remaining ligament can be excised by sharp dissection, or removed piecemeal with a Kerrison rongeur. Epidural fat, if present, is removed gently with forceps. At this point the dura is clearly evident through the laminectomy incision. A separate thin band of ligamentum flavum, which runs along the lateral portion of the spinal canal, may have to be removed separately.

The operator is now prepared to inspect the nerve root (Fig. 23–28). This is the most significant portion of the procedure, because only by palpation can one assume that the appropriate nerve root is under pressure and thereby responsible for the radicular symptoms. The laminotomy should be extended laterally (and superiorly and inferiorly) to expose safely and completely the lateral aspect of the nerve root and to visualize its contact with the offending disc material.

Under loupe or perhaps microscopic magnification, the nerve root is retracted medially with a Penfield 4 elevator. A thin instrument, such as the Penfield dissector, can be used to separate the anterior surface of the nerve root dura from the floor of the spinal canal. When there is a significant disc herniation, these structures are frequently adherent. If frank extrusion is encountered, an effort should be made to remove it fairly early in the dissection in order to avoid significant retraction injury to the nerve root. The extruded fragment should be removed intact, if possible, since portions of a fragmented extrusion may be difficult to find subsequently. If a protruding disc is encountered, 1 × 1 cm cottonoid patties with radiopaque strings can be placed laterally along the root in the epidural space after the nerve root is gently retracted over the dome of the disc. Such patties, above and below the disc herniation, can gently retract the nerve root and thereby reduce traction placed on the root by a metal root retractor. Ultimately, with the nerve root retractor in place, the area of herniated disc should be visible. It may be necessary to further extend the laminectomy laterally to obtain sufficient room. Removal of significant portions of the intervertebral facet joint is not usually necessary in order to expose disc herniations.

An incision into the posterior longitudinal ligament and annulus fibrosus is made with a No. 15 knife blade on a long thin handle. This is often accompanied by a spontaneous extrusion of the nucleus pulposus. Straight and angled intervertebral disc rongeurs are inserted to remove disc material (Fig. 23–29). The surgeon should at all times be aware of the depth to which the rongeur is being inserted into the disc space. Although the jaws of the rongeur are operated by the right hand (for a right-handed surgeon), the left hand holds the shaft of the disc rongeur and prevents it from plunging when vigorous "bites" of disc material are extracted. A sense of bottoming is felt when the jaws of the rongeur are closed. The jaws are then opened and advanced a few millimeters into the disc material before its removal. The jaws of the disc rongeur should be in contact with the cartilaginous plates of the superior or inferior vertebra during the piecemeal removal of disc material. This technique, along with the surgeon's undivided concentration, will prevent plunging of the disc rongeur into the retroperitoneal space. When the central and lateralmost portions of the nucleus pulposus have been removed, the interspace is entered with a right-angled dural separator, and the residual, more fibrotic disc material is separated from the annulus. It is forced into the center of the interspace, and more fragments may be retrieved separately with disc rongeurs. Primary attention should be focused on removing all free or protruding portions of disc material. A complete discectomy is almost impossible from the posterior approach. Aggressive curetting of end plates is not necessary. However, removal of all loose, free fragments is essential to ensure a good result. The right-angled dural elevator is then placed between the nerve root and the site of the former disc herniation in the epidural space. Any residual bulging is flattened by forceful collapse of the elevated area into the interspace.

At this point careful inspection of the epidural space around the nerve root and anterior to the dural sac is made with an appropriate instrument (e.g., a Frazier angled elevator). The nerve root should now be movable with a minimum of force. If there is resistance to movement, or tension, the procedure is not

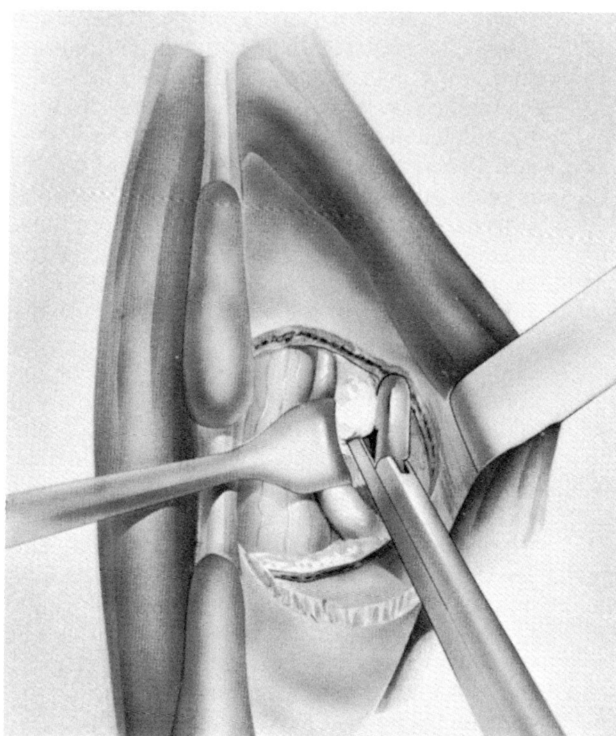

Figure 23–29. Removal of the disc extrusion while the nerve is retracted. The authors recommend retraction of the nerve root with cotton pledgets whenever possible to avoid trauma to the nerve root.

Figure 23–30. Exploration of the intervertebral foramen with a Frazier or malleable probe. The nerve root should be free of both compression and tension.

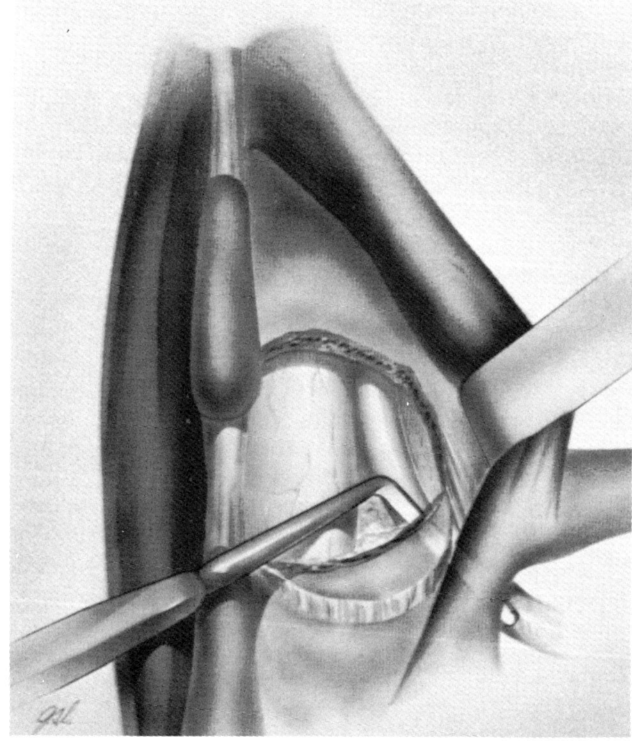

complete. A search must be made for extruded disc fragments, perhaps more remote from the laminotomy area itself (Fig. 23–30). If the nerve root continues to be tense, a "foraminotomy" may be necessary. With a Kerrison rongeur, bone is excised along the course of the exiting nerve root. This may require removal of the medial portion of the articular facet joint. This sacrifice must be made, however, if the nerve root cannot be freed in any other way. Our experience indicates that significant portions of this joint can be excised at one level, unilaterally, without subsequent problems. If persistent tension on the nerve root is due to an underlying spondylotic spur, foraminotomy may be the only technique by which the nerve root can be decompressed. Ultimately the foraminotomy may extend out beyond the confines of the spinal canal to the point at which the nerve root curves around the pedicle. If there is evidence of nerve root tension at this time or location, pedicle removal, or osteophyte impaction, may be required. At this point, the nerve root is usually quite free.

Wound Closure. After the disc material has been removed and the nerve root is free, the entire exposed dura is covered with an autogenous fat graft. This graft is removed with scalpel by dissection from the subcutaneous area, great care being taken not to interfere with the blood supply to the skin. If no fat is available, Gelfoam may be used to cover the dura (see below). The paraspinous muscles and fascia are approximated with heavy absorbable suture. The subcutaneous closure is obtained with absorbable suture in two layers, and skin closure as desired. Drains are placed before closure, deep to the fascia and superficial to it if there is abundant subcutaneous tissue.

Interposition Membrane

Scar formation about the dural sac and nerve roots after surgical intervention constitutes one of the most frequently cited causes of postoperative pain. This scar formation almost always occurs to some extent after any operation. It may act as a constrictive force about the neural elements and tether the nerve roots to the spine. For reasons that are not well explained, this scar formation causes symptomatology in certain patients. It may be present for several months or a year before the symptoms become apparent. Surgical removal of this scar tissue results in its recurrence in a short time. Thus, it was with great interest that surgeons concerned with the spine greeted the research of MacNab[164] on the etiology and prevention of postoperative scar formation in the neural canal. In the experimental animal he showed the relationship of postoperative dural scar to surgically exposed muscle. This tendency toward scar formation could be markedly inhibited by the interposition of a resorbable Gelfoam membrane. Attention to atraumatic technique and complete hemostasis are also of obvious importance.

Subsequently, autogenous fat grafts have been shown to be superior to Gelfoam in the reduction of perineural adhesions. Laboratory studies[94, 128, 155] have indicated that autogenous fat is a more effective deterrent to scar tissue formation than is Gelfoam. Where fat is not available, Gelfoam continues to be used.

Alternatives to Standard Discectomy

Chemonucleolysis Versus Discectomy

The place of chemonucleolysis in relation to discectomy in the treatment of disc herniation remains unsettled. Javid[130] and Ravichandran and Mulholland[218] have reported comparable results comparing the two modalities. Ejeskar and associates'[70] studies have not been able to confirm this. In studies performed by Crawshaw and colleagues[42] and others,[240] patients who had undergone appropriate nonoperative therapy of at least three months' duration and who met strict preoperative criteria were randomly allocated to surgery or chymopapain. An additional 64 patients who did not fulfill all the trial criteria received chymopapain injection. After one year of follow-up the failure rates in the two chymopapain groups were comparable: 52 and 47 per cent, significantly higher than in the surgically treated group, in which the rate was 11 per cent. Eighteen patients from the chymopapain-treated group underwent surgical discectomies; seven of these patients were from the nontrial group, which contained a total of 30 poor results. Six of the seven patients did not improve with surgery. The mean duration between injection and surgery was 4.8 months in the trial group and 6.4 months in the nontrial group.

These studies suggest that there should never be any deviation from strict preoperative selection criteria when recommending invasive treatment of a lumbar disc herniation. Poor results will invariably occur. Furthermore, if chymopapain treatment is selected, the authors suggest that surgery should be considered if a positive clinical response has not occurred by four weeks after the injection. This recommendation, of course, assumes appropriate preoperative findings (positive imaging, positive tension sign, correlative neurologic deficit).

It should be pointed out that at the time of this writing, the use of chymopapain has few strong advocates in North America. Owing to complications, and inappropriate applications of this treatment modality, it draws disfavor as a treatment for disc herniation. It clearly has more successes than a placebo, but the current medical and medicolegal environment makes it difficult to use or recommend.

Our own experience with chemonucleolysis parallels Crawshaw's. In general, we have found that the patients, as a group, improve less rapidly than patients who undergo standard discectomy or microdiscectomy, in terms of their radicular symptoms, and have a significantly increased incidence of persistent low back pain and spasm that may often last as long as six weeks. This is in contradistinction to the dramatic relief of radicular discomfort and transient postoperative pain that the average patient experiences with a technically well performed lumbar discectomy[121] with sufficient bone removal to visualize the lateral border of the nerve root, to check for the presence of concomitant pathosis such as lateral recess stenosis, and to provide sufficient exposure to allow minimal manipulation of the nerve root and strict hemostasis.

To reiterate words of caution, it has been repeatedly documented that for surgery to be effective in the treatment of sciatica, unequivocal evidence of nerve root compression must be found at surgery. To predict this mechanical root compression, one must find firm substantiation, not only in the neurologic evaluation, but also in the roentgenographic data before one proceeds with laminectomy.

In groups of patients in whom there is no radiating dermatomal leg pain, no neurologic deficit, and no positive tension sign and in whom the presumptive diagnosis of spinal stenosis cannot be inferred, surgery should rarely be considered. The person with persistent complaints, and a paucity of findings, should be directed toward a nonsurgical evaluation in an effort to explain this discrepancy.

In our experience, when sympathy for the patient's complaints has outweighed the objective evaluation, surgical endeavors have been fraught with great difficulty and the "explorations" have almost always been unrevealing and unrewarding. In persons who have met firm criteria for lumbar laminectomy the results are overwhelmingly satisfactory, and in our experience 95 per cent of these patients could be expected to show a good or excellent result.[87] The small percentage of patients who do not benefit from a lumbar laminectomy present a difficult challenge. The evaluation of these salvage patients is a thesis in and of itself, and they are submitted to a separate salvage protocol (see Chapter 48).

Percutaneous Discectomy Versus Standard Discectomy

Friedman's[83] percutaneous dissecting technique involves positioning the patient in a lateral decubitus position on the operating table with the painful side down. Under fluoroscopic guidance, a skin incision is made over the disc space to be entered, approximately 10 cm lateral to the midline, and a specially designed speculum is inserted through the psoas muscle to the midpoint of the lateral part of the desired interspace. With special lengthened instruments inserted through the cannula, the annulus is then incised and the disc removed piecemeal with pituitary rongeurs. At the time of Friedman's report, nine patients had undergone the procedure. Seven had clear radiculopathies with appropriate radiographic findings, and they all had excellent relief of symptoms. Two patients presented with intractable low back pain, bilateral posterior thigh pains, and central disc herniations on radiographic examination. One experienced good relief; one did not. Three of the patients had several days of paraspinal spasm after the procedure, and one complained of a lower extremity dysesthetic sensation that persisted for several weeks after the operation. The author presumed that this resulted from damage to the lumbar sympathetic chain. The length of follow-up was six months.

Kambin and Gellman[135] reported a posterolateral technique for percutaneous discectomy using modified Craig needle biopsy instrumentation, followed by evacuation of the disc using aspiration and insertion of specially designed punch forceps. After four to eight months of follow-up, all nine patients in this study were free of radicular symptoms. All were discharged within two to three days of the operation.

Onik and Helms[205] in 1988 introduced the nucleotome, an automated aspiration probe for performing percutaneous discectomies. It consists of a 2-mm blunt probe with a single 6-mm side port. When the probe is positioned in the center of the abnormal disc and suction is applied to the port, disc material can be aspirated. Currently, over 2000 percutaneous discectomies have been performed with this technique. Long-term follow-up evaluation of these patients, however, is lacking, with the exception of a group of fewer than 200 patients. In this selected group, it appears that good results can be achieved in 65 to 75 per cent.

Onik and Helms[205] reported the potential advantages of these procedures, which are similar to those of chemonucleolysis, i.e., no lumbar incision, muscle stripping, or bone removal, and the procedure may take less than 15 minutes. Minimal postoperative pain was encountered by most patients in these studies, the overall hospital stay was shortened, and the epidural space was not violated.

Although injury was not encountered, the potential for injury to the abdominal vasculature and viscera, as well as the sympathetic trunk, lymphatic chains, and lumbar plexus exists. In Friedman's study,[83] all patients underwent preoperative screening to identify aberrant and retroperitoneal structures that might lie in the projected surgical path. This involved performing a transaxial scan at the level of the upper iliac crest four hours after meglumine diatrizoate (Gastrografin) had been administered to the patient orally. One patient was denied percutaneous discectomy because his abdominal CT scan revealed that the ascending colon laid directly in the surgical path.

Because of the height of the iliac crest and the size of the instrumentation used, entry into the L5–S1 interspace is difficult even with surgically designed curved instrumentation. There are many potential disadvantages (including a success rate significantly less than that of standard lumbar laminectomy) associated with these procedures that limit their general use at the present time. It is possible, however, that as a longer follow-up and more experience are accrued by the individuals investigating these techniques, percutaneous discectomy may become a useful alternative to a standard discectomy or microdiscectomy for the herniated disc that is not sequestered or is not too large, and if the patient's preoperative myelogram, CT scan, MRI, and radiographs demonstrate no evidence of anomalous nerve roots, altered intra-abdominal pathology, or anomalies of the osteoarticular structures. At present the results of percutaneous nucleotomy in well-selected patients are comparable with those obtained with chemonucleolysis.

Tension Sign Negative

If the tension sign is negative, particularly in younger patients, and there is no neurologic deficit, we usually recommend an injection of epidural steroids. Dilke and colleagues[63] reported a randomized study of 100 consecutive patients with low back and radicular pain who were treated with 10 ml of normal saline and 80 mg of methylprednisolone acetate injected epidurally. These patients were compared with a control group who received a 1-ml injection of sterile saline in the interspinous ligament area of the lumbar spine. Of the experimental group, 46 per cent reported complete pain relief one week after the injection, compared with 11 per cent of the control group. The study has been criticized, however, for the lack of a true control, and nonblinded assessment of results was not present in the study design. Cuckler and associates[43] reported on a multicenter evaluation of lumbar radicular pain syndromes treated in a prospective, randomized, double-blind fashion with either 7 ml of methylprednisolone acetate and procaine hydrochloride, or 7 ml of physiologic saline solution and procaine hydrochloride. The 73 patients participating in this study had objective roentgenographic confirmation of lumbar root compression consistent with the clinical diagnosis of either acute herniated disc or spinal stenosis. No statistically significant difference was observed between the control and experimental groups for either acute disc herniation or spinal stenosis after an average of 20 months of symptoms. A major criticism of this study, however, is that the results were evaluated very early (24 hours after injection), and there may have been delayed symptom resolution that went undetected. Repeat injections, as recommended by others, may have been useful and were not addressed by the study. Other studies[25, 32] of reasonable design clearly indicate that results are better when the injection is performed sooner rather than later and in patients who have not had previous back surgery. We continue to use epidural steroids and consider them as being possibly effective as a second-level therapeutic intervention. We caution our patients about the negligible but existing complications of this technique, as well as the variable and unpredictable results.

Spinal Stenosis

In the patient who is over 50 years of age and continues to have persistent radicular discomfort despite six weeks of therapy, strong consideration should be given to the possibility of spinal stenosis. Arnoldi and colleagues[9] and others[98, 250] defined lumbar spinal stenosis as a condition involving any type of narrowing of the spinal canal, nerve root canals, or tunnels of the intervertebral foramina. To the purist a lumbar disc herniation is an acquired form of lumbar spinal stenosis. Degenerative changes in the lumbar spine resulting in a global, or more commonly lateral recess, stenotic narrowing of the cross-sectional area of the canal are similar to the herniated nucleus pulposus in that the most common symptoms are low back pain and sciatica. Signs and symptoms of nerve root compression, however, seem to occur later and less acutely than in patients with a disc herniation syndrome. The SLR test is usually negative, and the patient's clinical history and routine lumbosacral spine films usually allow the diagnosis to be inferred. Altered temperature sensation, paresthesias, dysesthesias, and "charley horses" (cramping of the legs) are common subjective symptoms. As many as one third of the patients may report motor weakness, frequently in the L4 or L5 innervated muscles (quadriceps, anterior tibialis, toe extensors). The back pain is usually exacerbated by standing or walking and is less common when the patient is supine or sitting.

The neurogenic claudication syndrome associated with spinal stenosis consists of pain, aching, and cramping, often combined with paresthesias in the lower extremities related to walking or exercise, with weakness or giving way in the lower extremities occurring at the limits of the patient's exercise tolerance. The actual incidence of this clinical syndrome is probably low. The key differential involved in a patient with lower extremity claudicatory disturbance is between a vascular and a neurogenic origin. This assessment can be aided by checking the patient's peripheral pulses; if these are absent or (more significantly) asymmetrically diminished, consultation with a vascular surgeon may be indicated.

If the history is more consistent with neurogenic causes, but the patient has a negative tension sign and no firm neurologic findings, electromyography (EMG) may be considered. If the EMG is positive for radicular dysfunction, imaging (myelo-CT or MRI) is indicated. Occasionally, the EMG will uncover an extraspinal mimicker of true "sciatica" (e.g., peripheral neuropathy, neuromuscular disease). The term sciatica itself is a misnomer since it is commonly used to refer to nerve root entrapment on the basis of lumbar disc disease. True sciatic neuropathy due to entrapment in the sciatic notch or fascial compartments of the thigh is uncommon. Nevertheless, the EMG and nerve conduction study often provide diagnostic clues to the exact anatomic and physiologic causes of the patient's leg pain, sensory loss, or weakness. Table 23–3 illustrates the differential diagnosis of radicular leg pain and segmental sensory disturbances. When the EMG and nerve conduction study demonstrate evidence of an extraspinal cause of the leg symptoms, we routinely advise consultation with a neurologist to expedite the treatment process and aid in the differential diagnosis. EMGs, however, need not be performed routinely, as in most cases the clinical picture and radiographic evaluation reveal the diagnosis. EMGs can be reserved for the unclear case or to rule out nonspinal etiologies for the atypical signs and symptoms.

In a patient with neurologic findings and a strong clinical history, the EMG is usually bypassed. We agree with Wiltse and colleagues' observation[274, 275] that once the patient has severe symptoms from spinal stenosis he or she does not routinely get well with time, as does the younger patient with a herniated disc. It is therefore not our policy to procrastinate in the persistently symptomatic patient whose myelogram, CT scan, or MRI demonstrates nerve root compression consistent with the signs and symptoms.

Epidural steroids, along with other nonoperative measures, can be tried in these patients. Once again, this is tempered by the realization that the algorithm pathways are two-way streets.

Our surgical results in treating patients with degenerative spinal stenosis are significantly better than the 70 per cent figure obtained by other investigators when treating one- or two-level involvement.[114, 227] Our present surgical procedure involves bilateral decompressive lumbar laminectomies of the involved stenotic segments, with foraminotomies as indicated by the symptoms, diagnostic studies, and intraoperative findings. In patients undergoing decompressive laminectomies for spinal stenosis, it is occasionally necessary to perform generous bilateral mesial facetectomies in order to decompress effectively the lateral recess regions of the stenotic segments. When bilateral recess decompressions are performed, a sum total of greater than one facet joint complex is removed, or there is concomitant segmental instability (e.g., degenerative spondylolisthesis with spinal stenosis), strong consideration should be given to performing an intertransverse fusion. We believe that this is justified in order to reduce greatly the chances of the postoperative complication of iatrogenic instability (see Chapter 25).

Low Back Pain Predominant

Further Nonoperative Measures

In patients in whom low back pain is the predominant and persisting symptom despite six weeks of therapy, we advise a technetium diphosphonate bone scan and a more complete medical evaluation. The latter can be directed by an internist, rheumatologist, or neurologist, depending on the patient's particular symptom complex.

We have found the bone scan to be an excellent survey tool, often allowing us to identify early spinal tumors involving bone, and infections not seen on routine roentgenographic examination. It is particularly important to obtain this study in patients with nonmechanical back pain. If the pain is constant, unremitting, and unrelieved by postural changes, it may lead the physician to diagnose an occult neoplasm or metabolic disorder that is not otherwise readily apparent.

As previously mentioned, 3 per cent of apparent cases of back pain presenting to an orthopedic clinic are attributable to extraspinal causes.[253] Our consultants' evaluation of the patient, along with some routine laboratory tests, often expedites the exclusion of such pathologic conditions. In all patients we routinely check the erythrocyte sedimentation rate, which has a reported sensitivity of 59 per cent in detecting occult pathoses, such as infection, tumor, many of the systemic arthritides, and other disorders.

In the older patient, our laboratory investigations routinely include tests for a serum protein or immunoelectrophoresis, alkaline phosphatase, calcium, phosphate, BUN, creatinine, complete blood count and differential, routine urinalysis, and acid phosphatase if the patient is male and over 60 years of age. In the younger patient with decreased lumbar flexion and chest expansion, sacroiliac joint films should be obtained to assess for spondyloarthropathies, such as ankylosing spondylitis.

If any of these diagnostic modalities are positive, the appropriate treatment can be instituted. If patients are not found to have an abnormality on bone scan and have no other medical diseases as a cause for the back pain, they are referred to a low back school. At this time, the inference is that most of these patients are suffering from discogenic pain or a facet joint pain syndrome, and with time, appropriate anatomic-mechanical education, reassurance, and the establishment of an exercise (reconditioning) program under the guidance of the low back school educators, gradual improvement will occur in most individuals.[19, 106]

Measures to Treat or Prevent Chronic Impairment

Back Schools. The concept of a back school is based on the use of a trained therapist as a patient educator. The duration and content of back school programs across the country are highly variable. However, most include discussions of the following: (1) basic spinal anatomy; (2) causative epidemiologic and pain-producing factors; (3) how a patient can reduce the intensity and frequency of low back pain by appropriately modifying activities of daily living; (4) statements on the value of exercise, proper posture, and good body mechanics;

(5) the natural history of low back pain; and (6) perhaps a visit to the patient's work site. Controlled studies[19] have identified that back school education can reduce time off from work after industrial injuries. Hall and Iceton[106] reviewed 6418 participants in the Canadian Back Education Program. Significant subjective improvement occurred in 60 per cent of the participants. This figure rose to 80 per cent when only those patients who experienced back pain for six months or less were considered. Of the participants, 97 per cent rated the program as having significant educational benefit.

Our personal program is now an integral part of our treatment plan and encourages patients to assume greater responsibility for their own health and well-being. The basic program is organized into two sessions. At the initial session the patient is given insight into the epidemiologic, pathologic, and ergonomic factors involved in the common causes of back pain. The second session deals with factors such as nutrition, stress reduction, posture, exercise, and body mechanics. Ample time is allowed for group interaction and practice sessions in body mechanics (see "Body Mechanics"). We advise that any physician involved in treating patients with spinal disorders should participate in or have access to such a program.[126]

Chronic Pain Programs. Nachemson[195] defined the factors that tend to predispose to chronic low back pain. These include alcoholism, psychosocial problems, poor education, very heavy or very sedentary jobs, lack of physical activity, failed back surgery, and increased disability insurance benefits. Epidemiologic studies indicate that recovery from back pain is usually rapid. In fact, 80 per cent of the disability costs are accounted for by only 10 per cent of the back injury patients.[240] In many situations the claim may become a solution to another problem, such as employer or job dissatisfaction, monetary benefits, excessive stress, marital discord, and other, perhaps unidentified factors.

In recent years, management of these patients has led to a proliferation of multidisciplinary pain treatment programs emphasizing work-hardening/work-tolerance conditioning activity, industrial monitoring and treatment protocols, detoxification programs, and psychologic counseling.

The major programs in those centers reporting success include a number of components:[10]

1. Thorough physician assessment to rule out surgically or medically treatable causes of back pain. Patients who have no clearly definable medical or surgical disease are instructed that setting a goal of complete and permanent pain relief may not be realistic, and therefore their treatment will be aimed at providing skills, rehabilitation, and knowledge that in turn will allow them to better cope with their pain and return to a productive, although at times modified, life style.
2. Physical therapy and psychological assessments, again aimed at modifying functional deficits that may be intruding on the patient's ability to function optimally and at times eliminate maladaptive behavior patterns.
3. An occupational assessment that allows the treating group to analyze the patient's present employment and decide on the suitability of his or her return to the previous job. If the work status is not clear, quantitating residual functional capacity after completion of a prescribed treatment program results in recommendations regarding those jobs in which it is hoped that the employee may function with a decreased risk of aggravation of the symptom complex.

The effectiveness of a multidisciplinary approach in dealing with chronic low back pain is well documented in the literature. In Mayer and colleagues' study,[174] patients who had been experiencing low back pain for 30 months were reviewed. The results were compared with those from a retrospective control group that did not participate in the comprehensive program. Their study demonstrated at two years of follow-ups that 80 per cent of the treatment group were actively working compared with 41 per cent of the comparison group. Furthermore, the control group underwent twice as much additional spine surgery and had a five times greater rate of subsequent visits to health care professionals. The repeat injury rate of successfully rehabilitated patients was 4 per cent, which compares favorably with the overall risk of first-time injury in the workplace.

It is our recommendation that early referral to a multidisciplinary, functional restoration type of treatment program should be considered for the patient who is tending toward chronicity and in whom no identifiable source for the pain has been found. In such circumstances, a functional restoration approach that considers both the biologic and the psychosocial elements of chronic disease can be expected to benefit most patients treated.

Psychosocial Evaluation

If the low back school is effective, the patient may return to a normal life pattern. It is critical that before being referred to this type of facility the patient must be thoroughly screened so that there is no question of treating tumors and infections in the classroom. If, however, the low back school has failed, these patients should undergo a thorough psychosocial evaluation in an attempt to explain the failure of the usually effective therapeutic measures for low back pain. The use of a psychosocial evaluation is predicated on the knowledge and belief that the disability is related not only to the patient's pathologic anatomy, but also to the perception of pain and his or her stability in relationship to the sociologic environment.

In addition to the nonorganic physical signs previously mentioned, Waddell and associates[255] supplied a list of symptoms of which the psychologically distressed patient may often complain. These are generally vague and ill localized and lack formal relationships to time, physical activity, and anatomy. The seven symptoms that have the highest degree of reliability in this study were complaints of tailbone pain, whole leg pain, whole leg numbness, the whole leg giving way, no pain-free intervals, intolerance of or inappropriate reaction to treatments, and a history of emergency admission to the hospital for low back pain.

Only the most myopic physician would deny that the patient's psychological profile and ability to function in a specific environment have a part to play in the treatment of low back pain. We all see the patient with a frank herniated disc who is able to continue working and regards this as only a trivial and annoying problem. At the other end of the spectrum is the hysterical patient who takes to the bed immediately upon the slightest twinge of lumbago. If the physician detects a patient with voluminous nonorganic signs and symptoms, further psychological evaluation should be recommended. Southwick and White[236] reviewed the use of psychological tests in the evaluation of low back pain. A pain diagram is also a useful assessment tool: a simple, self-administered test in which the patient pictorially represents the location and character of the pain.[188] Because of its ease of administration, it can be used as a rapid screening test to justify further formal psychological testing.

One frequently used test is the MMPI, a psychologic test composed of 550 items that separate into ten clinical psychological scales and three validity scales.[46] In chronic low back pain sufferers, great importance has been attached to the scores on the three neurotic scales of the MMPI. Abnormally high scores on the hypochondriasis and hysteria scales coupled with a low score on the depressive scale have been termed the "conversion V pattern."[112] The finding of this pattern supplies, at least in part, a functional basis to the patient's chronic low back complaints. We would caution, however, that the specificity of any psychological test is by no means 100 per cent in terms of excluding a true organic disorder.

Pheasant and colleagues[213] performed randomized, blinded, cross-over studies evaluating the effect of antidepressant medication on chronic low back pain patients with known MMPI profiles. They observed a 46 per cent decrease in the use of analgesics while patients were using amitriptyline compared with placebo. The difference was highly significant statistically. Furthermore, the MMPI profile of the compliant patients in this study again demonstrated the conversion V pattern, the interpretation being that these patients tended to focus on physical symptoms as a means of dealing with internal or external stress. The noncompliant patients did not show the conversion V pattern but instead had elevated values on the psychopathic deviance (PD) and schizophrenia (Sc) scales. Sternbach and colleagues[244] labeled this the "litigation profile," the interpretation being that the elevated PD and Sc scale scores point to impulsive and passive-aggressive personality characteristics.

To summarize, at this point in the algorithm the use of psychological testing can be extremely useful, since we know that the test profiles in chronic low back pain patients can be expected to differ significantly from those in healthy persons and are frequently helpful in predicting treatment outcomes.[255] In this regard, the additive effects of multiple variables in the forecasting scheme (such as MMPI scores combined with knowledge of compensation or litigation involvement and formal psychiatric evaluation) will enhance the strength of the examiner's predictions. (See Chapter 51.)

At this point in the algorithm it is not uncommon to uncover drug habituation and psychological causes for magnification and propagation of the pain complaint. Spengler[239] found that by simply instituting a withdrawal program for chronic low back pain patients addicted to narcotics, successful withdrawal from the narcotics will result in a 10 per cent cure rate from pain by itself. If the evaluation is revealing of this type of pathosis, proper measures should be instituted to overcome the disability. We are constantly surprised at the number of ambulatory patients who present with addiction to prescribed narcotics or diazepam (Valium). We believe that the use of these drugs should be kept to an absolute minimum. Oxycodone and similar narcotic analgesics are truly addicting, and diazepam is both habituating and depressing. The complaint of low back pain is a common expression, and to routinely treat these persons with diazepam or other similar drugs is often detrimental to their welfare and may perpetuate maladaptive pain behavior. In patients whose symptoms seem primarily an expression of their depressive reaction, we have found tricyclic antidepressant drugs very useful rather than the previously mentioned agents. The type of psychiatric and psychological treatment indicated depends, in part, on the background of the patient, his or her intelligence and insight, and the means available to afford this type of treatment. Unfortunately, psychiatric therapy is expensive and demanding of a high level of insight and motivation. Psychologists and psychiatric clinics with ancillary personnel such as psychiatric social workers are often a reasonable answer. Programs of behavior modification, such as operant conditioning, have proved useful in certain situations in returning patients to a more productive way of life, but hard data supporting their use are not available at present.

Patients who are unwilling or unable to follow a program outline, continue the use of narcotics, and reject or fail the recommended psychiatric treatment must be considered a failure, and we advocate discontinuing medical therapy. To continue random measures of treatment for these persons without correcting their underlying psychosocial disorder is a waste of time, money, and medical facilities. They should be discharged from therapy with the offer to reevaluate them in the future if they wish to reenter the treatment protocol. If patients are able to rid themselves of narcotics and respond to the psychiatric counseling offered, they can usually return to a normal life pattern without further or regular back treatment. However, Painter and associates[207] found that recidivism is high in this patient group, the most significant factor leading to regression being continued reinforcement for invalidism in the patient's life environment. These reinforcements most often are compensation-litigation issues, a lack of significant support in the family and social environment, and truly functional psychiatric disturbances.

Persistent Pain in Patients Without Psychosocial Abnormality

Instability

In the case of patients with low back pain or sciatica who have arrived at the psychosocial evaluation decision-making point in the algorithm, and in whom no psychosocial abnormality is detected, the lumbar spine roentgenograms should be carefully studied for evidence of instability, or significant degenerative changes in the disc and facet joints. Each region of the vertebral column has an upper limit of what may be considered normal angulation and translational motion. In a normal state a modest amount of angulation occurs but very little translatory movement. With degenerative disc disease the angulatory and translatory motion changes in flexion and extension can be considerable, creating pronounced shearing forces parallel to the plane of the disc, as well as abnormal tensile stresses at the points of ligamentous attachment. MacNab[162] coined the term "segmental instability" to describe this process.

There is a relative dearth of information in the literature as to why certain patients with segmental instability develop back pain and others do not. The evidence is much clearer when one considers the entity of spinal stenosis or radiculopathy from a disc herniation in terms of the effects of compromised space in the spinal and nerve root canals producing restricted motion of the neural elements, along with direct compression effects. This is in contrast with the lack of precision with which we are able to define the anatomic origin of back pain in the setting of roentgenographic instability. The pain experienced in this setting may be related to the soft tissue structures exceeding their viscoelastic limits, thereby stimulating pain-sensitive mesenchymal structures. An acute attack of lumbago, however, may correspond to actual tears of the soft tissue structures, facet arthritis, or herniation of the disc through the outermost fibers of the annulus. Many of these structures receive their afferent nerve supply via the sinuvertebral nerve. Pedersen and associates[210] showed that the individual sinuvertebral nerves are actually connected by an ascending and descending series of interconnected fibers. Therefore, since there is an overlap in the level of the sinuvertebral ramifications, it is possible that lumbago from instability occurring at a single spinal unit may involve more than one recurrent branch of the sinuvertebral nerve. We currently use the roentgenographic criteria developed by White and associates[264] for the diagnosis of clinical instability of the lumbosacral spine (Table 23–5). "Relative" flexion sagittal-plane translation of more than 12 per cent of the anteroposterior diameter of the vertebral body, or a "relative" flexion sagittal-plane rotation (angulation) of greater than 11 degrees, is accepted as significant roentgenographic evidence of instability in the lumbar spine. At the lumbosacral junction the criteria are slightly different: "relative" flexion sagittal-plane translation of more than 25 per cent, "relative" extension sagittal-plane translation of more than 12 per cent, or "relative" flexion sagittal-plane rotation of more than 19 degrees can be accepted as evidence of instability.

Table 23–5. SEGMENTAL INSTABILITY: ROENTGENOGRAPHIC CRITERIA

	Lumbar Spine (L1–L5)	Lumbosacral Spine (L5–S1)
"Relative" flexion sagittal-plane translation	>16%	>25%
"Relative" extension sagittal-plane translation	>12%	>12%
"Relative" flexion sagittal-plane rotation	>11°	>19°

From White, A. A., Panjabi, M. M., Posner, I., et al.: Instruct. Course Lect. *30*:457, 1981.

Spinal Fusion

If these roentgenographic stigmata of instability are present on active flexion-extension lateral views of the lumbosacral spine, or if the patient has a reversal of the normal lordotic position of the motion segment or traction osteophytes at one level, spinal fusion may be indicated. If the decision to proceed with spinal fusion is undertaken, the surgeon and the patient must both be ready to accept a level of effectiveness of approximately 75 per cent. The failure rate for relief of back pain after spinal fusion in these patients is considerably higher than the failure rate after laminectomy using the criteria outlined earlier for the relief of leg pain. If success occurs after a spinal fusion, the patient should be encouraged to return to a normal life pattern. If the spinal fusion has failed, the patient will proceed to the salvage protocol described earlier. It should be emphasized that, for the most part, few patients will find their way toward spinal fusion for the diagnosis of segmental instability. By far the greater number of patients with chronic, persistent, disabling low back pain eventually improve with nonoperative measures, have nondiscogenic causes for low back pain, or have a psychosocial disturbance.

Occasionally, before embarking on the fusion procedure, we obtain further confirmatory evidence to localize precisely the level of origin of the patient's symptoms. Information can be gained by the use of facet injections of local anesthetics with or without steroids, injected under roentgenographic control. Although discography has been discredited as a method of determining back pain disorders,[122] some clinicians still regard it as a valuable technique for determination of pathologic, symptomatic change in a disc space. If the discs above and below the proposed fusion site demonstrate significant degenerative changes and are subjectively painful, this may cause one to reverse a recommendation for fusion in light of the fact that the multilevel arthrodeses have a significantly increased incidence of symptomatic pseudarthroses (and failure).

Additional presumptive evidence for pro-

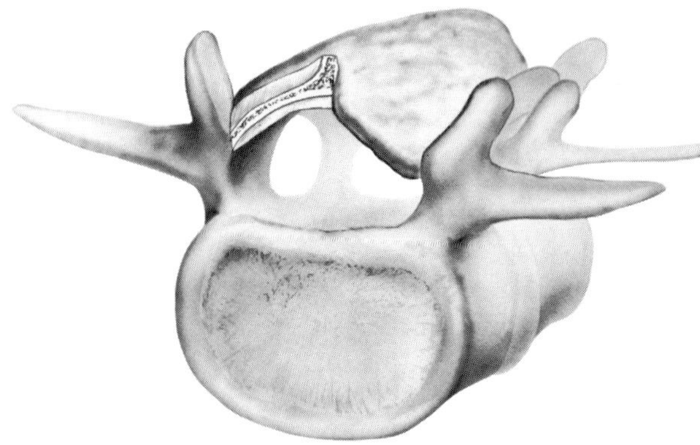

Figure 23–31. Iatrogenic spinal stenosis due to a midline spinal fusion. The decortication of lamina and application of bone graft in the midline create spinal stenosis through two mechanisms. The first of these is thickening of the lamina and the second is overgrowth of the fusion mass at the cranial end of the fusion, dipping into the interspace and compressing the neural elements.

ceeding with a fusion procedure can occasionally be obtained by reinstitution of bracing and observation of the patient for the prompt recurrence of symptoms once the immobilization is removed. Fidler and Plasmans[82] investigated the effects of a canvas corset, Raney and Baycast jackets, and a Baycast spica on the segmental sagittal mobility of the lumbosacral spine. The canvas corset reduced the mean angular movement to two thirds of normal. The Raney and Baycast jackets reduced the mean angular movements in the middle of the lumbar spine to approximately one third of normal. The Baycast spica was most effective of all in immobilization techniques, especially at the L4–L5 interspace. Fidler routinely uses a Baycast spica when considering fusion. The inclusion of the thigh improves control of the pelvis. In our practice we rely on the details obtained from the history, physical examination, and roentgenograms, and do not routinely institute a trial of cast or brace immobilization.

Lateral Spine Fusion

When arthrodesis of the spine is necessary, the authors currently recommend the use of bilateral lateral fusion. Many variations of this technique have been reported in the past.[57, 247, 258, 274] There are several advantages to the use of a lateral fusion. Foremost among these are the certainty of obtaining a solid fusion, the ability to perform the fusion in the absence of the posterior elements, and the prevention of iatrogenic spinal stenosis (Figs. 23–31 and 23–32).

Anesthesia. This operation is performed under spinal or general anesthesia.

Position at Operation. This procedure is performed with the patient in the prone position. If decompressive laminectomy or disc excision is to be performed at the same time, the kneeling position is used to ensure collapse of the epidural veins and to minimize abdominal compression (see Fig. 23–23). If only a spinal fusion is to be performed, the patient can be placed on a flat operating table with

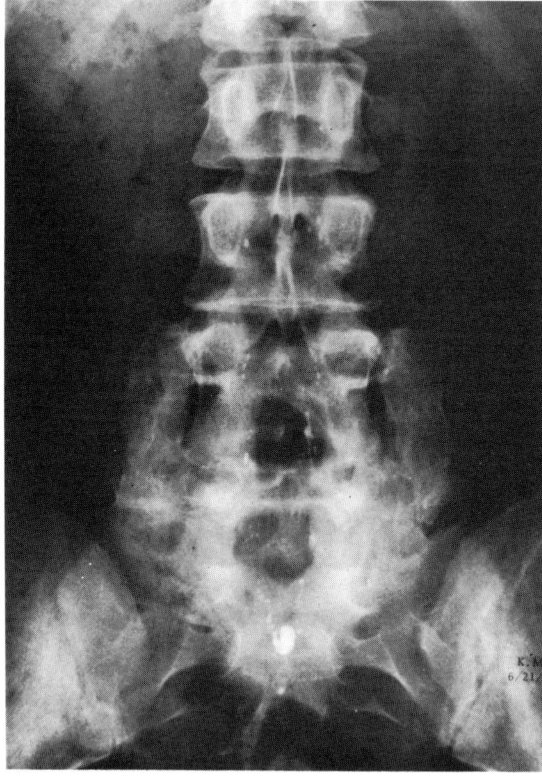

Figure 23–32. Well-formed bilateral lateral spinal fusion from L4 to the sacrum. Note the massive appearance of the bone graft from the transverse process of L4 to the ala of the sacrum. No graft material is placed in the midline.

lateral rolls beneath the chest and abdomen to allow pulmonary excursion. The anterior iliac crest is centered over the kidney rest, permitting flexion of the table, if desired, to reduce the lumbar lordosis. Elastic stockings are placed on the patient to decrease venous pooling.

Antibiotics. The prophylactic use of antibiotics is advised.

Incision. When combined with a laminectomy, a straight incision is made. If a fusion of L4 to the sacrum is to be performed, the incision starts above the third lumbar spinous process and continues in a caudal direction to the sacral spinous process. The vertical incision is carried directly down to the fascia in the midline, without the creation of layers. Absolute hemostasis is obtained at this step. Then, with the electric cutting knife, the fascia is incised from above the third spinous process to the midportion of the sacrum. Subsequently, with a broad, sharp periosteal elevator, the paraspinal muscles are stripped subperiosteally from the spine. This dissection is carried to the facet joints. As this dissection progresses, the wound is packed tightly with sponges to control bleeding. When this is completed, the sponges are removed, and large self-retaining retractors are placed to expose the posterior elements of the spine. At this point the surgeon should orient himself carefully through the sacrum and the lower lumbar vertebrae to be certain the work is being performed at the correct levels.

Nerve root exploration and decompression are undertaken as described previously. Attention is then turned to exposure of the transverse processes. Using either the electric knife or a sharp periosteal elevator, the fascia is incised directly laterally to the facet joints. As this fascia is incised, the periosteal elevator can sweep laterally along the superior articular facets of the lower facets and down onto the transverse process. Paraspinal muscles can then be swept laterally, exposing the entire length of the transverse process. When the process is cleaned of soft tissue and completely exposed on its dorsal aspect, this area should be packed with a sponge to control bleeding. The stripping and exposure should then be continued in a caudal direction. All ligaments and muscles should be dissected well laterally, forming an uninterrupted gutter between the transverse processes and the ala of the sacrum if necessary. After the fifth transverse process is exposed, cleaned, and packed, the approach is continued down to a point distal and lateral to the superior articular facet of the sacrum. Dissection lateral to this element will expose the ala of the sacrum. Many dense ligaments are adherent in this area and must be dissected from the sacrum in order to clearly expose the ala. It is essential to visualize both the transverse processes and the ala clearly in order to obtain an optimal preparation of the fusion bed. The sponges previously used to obtain hemostasis about the transverse processes and the ala of the sacrum are then removed, and a careful decortication of the transverse processes, the lateral portion of the pedicle, and the lateral portion of the articular facets is performed. This is best accomplished with large, sharp curets, although power-driven burrs can be used. Care is required not to fracture the transverse process.

The ala of the sacrum is best decorticated with a narrow, rounded gouge. The lateral portion of the superior articular facet of the sacrum should also be decorticated. A hole is created in the cranial portion of the ala of the sacrum with a large curet, which will ultimately receive a portion of the graft material. This process of exposure and decortication is repeated on both sides of the spine. The wound is again carefully packed, and the midline fascia is closed with a towel clip.

Alternative approaches and a more detailed description of the technique can be found in Chapter 27.

Bone Graft. The posterior iliac crest is exposed by dissecting away the layer of adipose tissue with a large sponge superior to the fascia. The fascia is incised in line with the posterior iliac crest, and the crest is dissected subperiosteally. The gluteal muscles are carefully dissected from the lateral wing of the ilium. Care must be taken to remain beneath the periosteum, or bleeding that is difficult to control may occur. A broad reverse retractor is then inserted to clearly expose the lateral portion of the ilium. With sharp, curved gouges, long strips of cortical and cancellous bone are removed from the ilium until the inner wall of the ilium is exposed. Large amounts of bone are readily obtained from this area. This graft material should be cut into narrow strips and saved in blood-soaked sponges (Fig. 23–33).

Placement of Graft Material and Closure of Wound. The midline wound is reexposed and

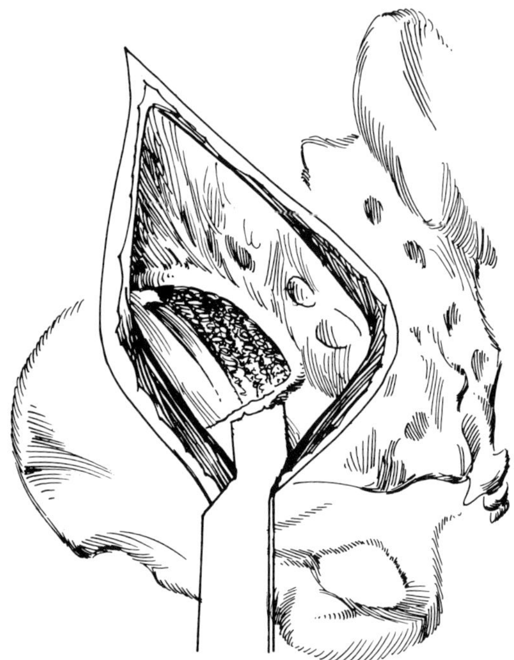

Figure 23–33. Technique of obtaining autogenous graft material from the posterior iliac crest. A large spiked retractor is used to expose the posterior surface of the ilium. Long strips of cortical and cancellous bone are then obtained, using curved gouges. The graft material is saved in blood-soaked sponges and transferred to the previously prepared bed.

the self-retaining retractors are reinserted. All the sponges are removed from the wound, and the wound is checked with careful finger palpation to make sure that none of the recesses harbor a hidden sponge. At this point the preliminary sponge count should be obtained. The graft material is then placed in the trough that has been created from the transverse processes to the ala of the sacrum bilaterally (Fig. 23–34).

The wounds should be frequently irrigated with antibiotic solution, and all devitalized tissue should be debrided. A suction drain is inserted in the midline wound and another at the iliac crest donor site. The fascia is then closed using No. 1 absorbable suture. Subcutaneous closure is obtained with absorbable suture in two layers, over a drain. The skin edges are approximated as desired.

Postoperative Management. The patient is allowed out of bed and walking the day after surgery. If there is difficulty in voiding, the patient may be permitted to stand at the bedside on the night of surgery. This may circumvent the need for catheterization with its attendant risk of infection. An exercise program is started on the second or third postoperative day. Minimal external support in the form of braces or corsets is used for one- or two-level primary fusions. For multilevel fusions or pseudarthrosis repairs, a custom-molded TLSO is recommended. This program of early mobilization has not been shown to lower the rate of successful fusion and has many dramatic advantages. Psychologically, the patient becomes attuned to an optimistic course and early return to productive life. The paraspinal muscles rapidly resume their normal tone, and the resolution of edema and hematoma occurs quickly.

The suction drains are withdrawn at 24 to 48 hours. Antibiotics, as previously noted, are administered for 24 to 48 hours postoperatively.

After discharge the patient is encouraged to gradually increase the level of activity, using pain as a guideline to the appropriate level. Automobile riding is discouraged for the first several weeks, and heavy lifting should be avoided. After four to six weeks the patient may return to light work, at least on a part-time basis. After three months most patients are able to return full time to sedentary and moderately active employment. Heavy physical labor should be restricted for six months, as should vigorous athletics.

The patient is reevaluated at six-week intervals for the first three months and then at three-month intervals for the first year. As recovery progresses the patient is placed on a more vigorous program of exercises and is again instructed in the essential aspects of back hygiene and care. He or she is encouraged to return to a normal way of life as rapidly as possible.

Anterior Interbody Fusion

This type of fusion is often used for patients who have had multiple surgical procedures through the posterior approach to the spine that have failed. Dense posterior scarring, wide resection of the posterior elements of the spine, and a failed lateral spinal fusion are some indications for consideration of this technique. The major disadvantage inherent in this surgical approach is the inability to carefully explore and decompress nerve roots when required.

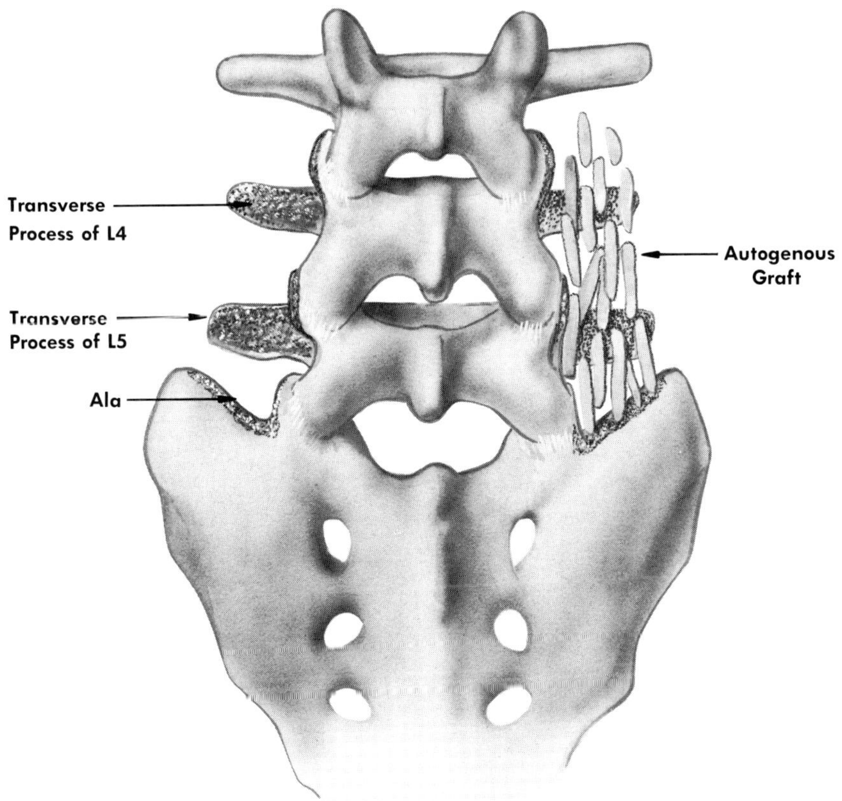

Figure 23–34. Area of the bed of raw cancellous bone for a lateral spine fusion from L4 to the sacrum. The bed is shown on the left and the graft material is in place on the right. In fact a much larger volume of graft material is used. The bed includes the transverse processes, the ala of the sacrum, the lateral portion of the pedicle, and the lateral portion of the superior articular facets.

This operation should be performed by a spinal surgeon and an abdominal surgeon together, unless the former has had extensive experience with the anterior approach.

Anesthesia. A nasogastric tube is used to prevent abdominal distention. Endotracheal anesthesia is preferred, with the patient in the Trendelenburg position.

Approach. A retroperitoneal approach is utilized. A left paramedian incision is made, the anterior rectus sheath opened, and the muscle retracted. The retroperitoneal space is entered, and the peritoneum is dissected bluntly from the undersurface of the posterior rectus sheath.[109] The peritoneum is mobilized, and as the lower lumbar spine is exposed, the ureter is left in its peritoneal bed and reflected to the right. The sacral promontory is identified by palpation. Care should be taken to try not to damage the sympathetic nerves coursing over the sacrum. The major sympathetic chains on either side of the lumbar vertebrae are carefully dissected and retracted in a lateral direction. The L5–S1 interspace is exposed by retracting the left iliac artery and vein to the left and the right iliac artery and vein to the right. To expose the fourth lumbar vertebra, the left artery and vein may need to be displaced to the right side. Spiked, rubber-shod retractors can be driven into the body of the vertebra to maintain exposure.

Anterior Disc Excision and Fusion. The anterior longitudinal ligament and anterior annulus are excised from end plate to end plate with a knife. Exposure can be improved at this time by hyperextension of the operating table and spine. Then, with a sharp osteotome, chisel, curets, and/or rongeurs, the entire disc is excised and subchondral bone is exposed, with bleeding cancellous bony areas burred or curetted. The dimensions of this space are measured and corticocancellous grafts ob-

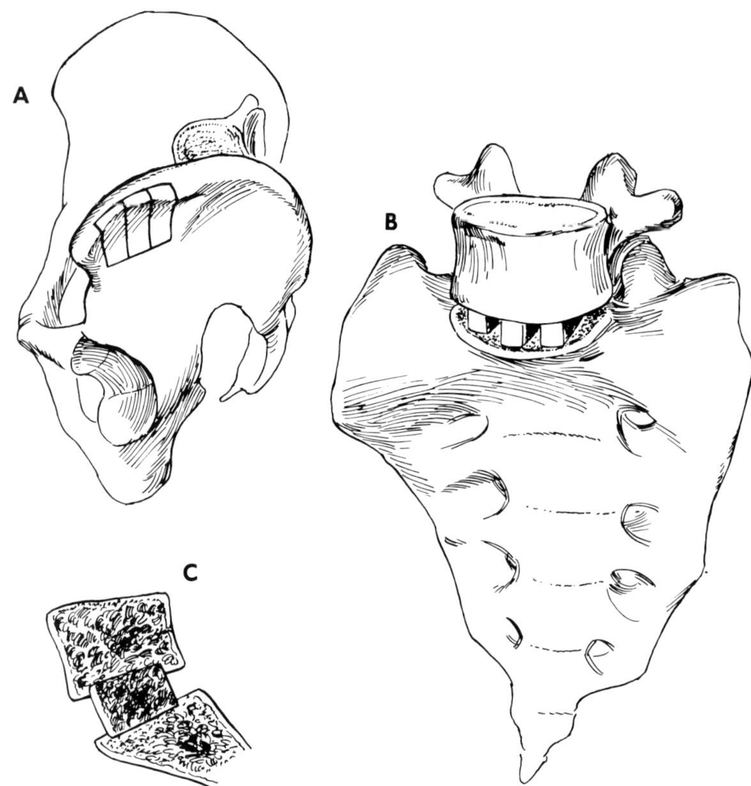

Figure 23–35. Technique of anterior lumbar fusion. After excision of the intervertebral disc, cortical cancellous grafts from the iliac crest are inserted into countersunk panels created in the adjacent vertebral end plates. *A,* Wedges of bone can be taken from anterior iliac crest (bicortical is preferred); or alternatively, fibula or allograft can be employed. *B,* Multiple grafts in place across the disc space. *C,* Sagittal section showing graft seated between the L5 and S1 bodies.

tained from the left iliac crest. Alternatively, for anterior interbody fusions, allograft functions well and heals at a rate similar to autograft. There is significantly less morbidity from use of allograft. The grafts should be slightly larger than the disc space so that firm impaction can be obtained. After insertion of the graft(s) the spine can be brought to a neutral position, locking the grafts in place (Fig. 23–35). The wound is closed in a routine manner after hemostasis is obtained.

Postoperative Management. The nasogastric tube is removed after peristalsis returns. Elastic stockings and early ambulation are utilized to prevent thrombophlebitis. The management in other respects is similar to that after lateral spinal fusion.

Pseudarthrosis

The overall rates of solid fusion in previous series were approximately 90 per cent, with a pseudarthrosis incidence of 8 to 10 per cent. After the advent of the lateral fusion technique, the incidence of pseudarthrosis in two-level fusions has been reported as low as 6 per cent.[55] However, as more modern imaging studies are developed, more attention is paid to patient and radiographic assessment, and longer-term follow-up occurs, it appears that the initial high rates of fusion successes were markedly optimistic. An 80 to 90 per cent fusion rate for one level is more realistic and achievable. As the number of levels increases, the likelihood of obtaining a solid fusion at every level diminishes.

In the hope of learning in detail what the diagnosis of pseudarthrosis portends for a patient, we studied 39 individuals who had this diagnosis. They were compared with a matched group of 39 patients, each having an identical diagnosis and operation in whom the fusion was solid. By comparing these two matched groups, we can determine with some degree of precision the implication of pseudarthrosis for the patient who has undergone a spinal fusion.

In an overall subjective evaluation of the worth of their surgery, 82 per cent of the patients who had developed pseudarthrosis felt

Table 23–6. PERCENTAGE OF PATIENTS WHO CONSIDERED SURGERY WORTHWHILE

Pseudarthrosis	Solid Fusion
82	92

that their surgery was worthwhile, compared with 92 per cent of the group who had solid fusions (Table 23–6). Little difference was found between the pseudarthrosis group and the solid fusion group when they were asked specifically about their overall relief from symptomatology. Fifty-six per cent of patients in the former group and 61 per cent in the latter obtained total relief. It is interesting to note that although there was a slight decrease in the number who obtained total relief in the pseudarthrosis group, three patients who achieved solid fusions obtained no relief, and all patients who developed pseudarthrosis obtained at least partial or temporary relief (Table 23–7).

When back pain alone was considered, of the 92 per cent of patients in the pseudarthrosis group who originally had back pain, 44 per cent still had the symptoms at follow-up evaluation. In the solid fusion group, of the 97 per cent of patients who originally had back pain, 38 per cent had significant back pain at follow-up evaluation (Table 23–8).

Sciatica was eliminated more consistently than back pain at follow-up evaluation. Of the 79 per cent of patients in the pseudarthrosis group who had sciatica, only 25 per cent had their symptoms at follow-up evaluation. In the solid fusion group, of the 85 per cent of patients who originally had sciatica, only 20 per cent had their symptoms at follow-up evaluation (Table 23–9). The subjective factors noted above were submitted to chi-square analysis and in no case was a significant difference noted between the pseudarthrosis and the solid fusion group.

It seems justifiable to draw certain conclusions from the above information. One of two situations must exist: either the pseudarthrosis represents a fibrous stabilization, which is essentially as effective as bony fusion, or the fusion component of these procedures was not essential. The former is not unreasonable, as the amount of motion demonstrated on flexion-extension films of pseudarthrosis is usually minimal and often less than 2 mm. The latter conclusion, however, remains in question.

It would also seem prudent to observe patients with pseudarthrosis for a prolonged period before carefully reoperating in an attempt to achieve union. There seems little rationale for submitting patients to multiple attempts at repair of pseudarthrosis if, as a group, there is little difference in their subjective result when solid fusion is obtained.

The overall picture obtained is that a number of patients who have undergone spinal fusion continue to have back pain and less frequently sciatica, whether or not their fusion has become solid. The success rate, as judged by objective evaluation, is slightly greater in the group that has achieved solid fusion. Pseudarthrosis, of itself, does not appear to be the dreaded complication that is often portrayed. A more precise definition of the role of spinal fusion and evaluation of the essentiality of achieving this fusion will depend on the availability of long-term prospective studies of spinal surgery.

If instability is not present, at this point in the algorithm patients must be considered to have failed treatment, and therapy should be discontinued. There are no further measures that will benefit these persons and they should be offered reevaluation at one year, or referred

Table 23–8. PERCENTAGE OF PATIENTS WITH BACK PAIN AT FOLLOW-UP

	Pseudarthrosis	Solid Fusion
Preoperative	92	97
Postoperative	44	38

Table 23–7. PERCENTAGE OF PATIENTS RECEIVING RELIEF FROM SYMPTOMS

	Pseudarthrosis	Solid Fusion
Total	56	61
Partial	34	26
Temporary	10	5
None	0	8

Table 23–9. PERCENTAGE OF PATIENTS WITH SCIATICA AT FOLLOW-UP

	Pseudarthrosis	Solid Fusion
Preoperative	79	85
Postoperative	25	20

to a pain clinic, to make certain their clinical picture does not change and perhaps to uncover any occult disease process.

Requirements for Successful Spinal Surgery

As one reviews the overwhelming amount of written material pertaining to spinal surgery, certain precepts become clear, and certain requirements evident, if good results are to be obtained:

1. Accurate knowledge of the variable pathology of disc degeneration is essential.
2. Accurate diagnosis of nerve root compression must be made preoperatively.
3. Adherence to the proper criteria for operative intervention maximizes surgical success and decreases unnecessary interventions.
4. The proper surgical procedure should be selected and planned preoperatively.
5. Skillful execution of the surgical procedure by an experienced spinal surgeon should lead to satisfactory results (relief of leg pain) in over 90 per cent of patients.
6. Prompt recognition and treatment of complications is critical.
7. Careful postoperative care and rehabilitation should not be ignored and should be a standard component of all surgical procedures.

If every patient undergoing spine surgery enjoyed the benefit of these principles, the quality of surgical result would improve dramatically, and the gray veil of apprehension, fear, and anxiety that has surrounded spinal surgery for years would be lifted.

References

1. Abdullah, A. F., Ditto, E. W., Byrd, E. B., and Williams, R.: Extreme lateral lumbar disc herniations. J. Neurosurg. *41*:229, 1974.
2. Aitken, A. P., and Bradford, C. H.: End results of ruptured intervertebral discs in industry. Am. J. Surg. *73*:365, 1947.
3. Alcoff, J., Jones, E., Rust, P., et al.: Controlled trial of imipramine for chronic low back pain. J. Fam. Pract. *14*:841, 1982.
4. Amlie, E., Weber, H., and Holme, I.: Treatment of low back pain with piroxicam. Result of a double-blind placebo-controlled trial. Spine *12*:473, 1987.
5. Amundson, G., and Garfin, S. R.: Minimizing blood loss during spine surgery. *In* Garfin, S. R. (ed.): Complications of Spine Surgery. Baltimore, Williams & Wilkins Co., 1989, pp. 29–52.
6. Andersson, G. B., Ortengren, R., and Nachemson, A.: Intradiskal pressure, intra-abdominal pressure and myoelectric back muscle activity related to posture and loading. Clin. Orthop. *129*:156, 1977.
7. Andersson, G. B., Svensson, H. O., and Oden, A.: The intensity of work recovery in low back pain. Spine *8*:880, 1983.
8. Appenzeller, O., Stendefer, J., Appenzeller, J., and Atkinson, R.: Neurology of endurance training. V. Endorphins. Neurology *30*:418, 1980.
9. Arnoldi, C. C., Brodsky, A. E., Cauchoix, J., et al.: Lumbar spinal stenosis and nerve root entrapment syndromes. Definition and classification. Clin. Orthop. *115*:4, 1976.
10. Aronoff, G. M., Evans, W. O., and Enders, P. L.: A review of follow-up studies of multidisciplinary pain units. Pain *16*:1, 1983.
11. Astrand, P. O.: Exercise physiology and its role in disease prevention and in rehabilitation. Arch. Phys. Med. Rehabil. *68*:305, 1987.
12. Balantyne, B. T., Reser, M. D., Lonenz, W., et al.: The effects of inversion traction on spinal column configuration, heart rate, blood pressure and perceived discomfort. J. Orthop. Sports Phys. Ther. *7*:254, 1986.
13. Bartelink, D. L.: The role of abdominal pressure in relieving the pressure on the lumbar intervertebral discs. J. Bone Joint Surg. *39B*:718, 1957.
14. Basford, J. R.: Low energy laser treatment for pain and wounds: hype, hope or hokum? Mayo Clin. Proc. *61*:671, 1986.
15. Bell, G. R., and Rothman, R. H.: The conservative treatment of sciatica. Spine *9*:54, 1984.
16. Bell, G. R., Rothman, R. H., Booth, R. E., et al.: A study of computer-assisted tomography in the diagnosis of herniated lumbar disc and spinal stenosis. Spine *9*:552, 1984.
17. Benn, R. T., and Wood, P. H. N.: Pain in the back. Rheumatol. Rehabil. *14*:121, 1975.
18. Bernini, P. M., and Simeone, F. A.: Reflex sympathetic dystrophy associated with low lumbar disc herniation. Spine *6*:180, 1981.
19. Berquist-Ullman, M.: Acute low back pain in industry. Acta Orthop. Scand. *170*(Suppl.):1977.
20. Biering-Sorenson, F., and Thomson, C.: Medical, social and occupational history as risk factors for low back trouble in a general population. Spine *11*:720, 1986.
21. Bisla, R. S., Marchisello, P. J., Lockshin, M. D., et al.: Auto-immunological basis of disk degeneration. Clin. Orthop. *121*:205, 1976.
22. Bobechko, W. T., and Hirsh, C.: Auto-immune response to nucleus pulposus in the rabbit. J. Bone Joint Surg. *47B*:574, 1965.
23. Boden, S. D., Davis, D. O., and Dina, T., et al.: Incidence of abnormal lumbar spine magnetic resonance imaging scans in asymptomatic patients: a prospective and blinded investigation. Paper presented at 57th Annual Meeting, American Academy of Orthopaedic Surgeons, New Orleans, LA, February 1990.
24. Bogduk, N., and Cherry, D.: Epidural corticosteroid agents for sciatica. Med. J. Aust. *143*:402, 1985.
25. Bogduk, N., and Long, D.: The anatomy of the so-called "articular nerves" and their relationship to facet denervation in the treatment of low-back pain. J. Neurosurg. *51*:172, 1979.

26. Boulos, S.: Herniated intervertebral lumbar disc in the teenager. J. Bone Joint Surg. *55B*:273, 1973.
27. Boumphrey, F. R. S.: Fusion in the Lumbar Spine. Seminars in Neurologic Surgery: Lumbar Disc Disease. New York, Raven Press, 1982.
28. Boumphrey, F., Bell, G., Masaryk, T. J., et al.: Impact of MRI on results of chemonucleolysis. Orthop. Trans. *11*:20, 1987.
29. Bradford, D. S., and Garcia, A.: Lumbar intervertebral disk herniations in children and adolescents. Orthop. Clin. North Am. *2*:583, 1971.
30. Breen, A. C.: Chiropractors in the treatment of back pain. Rheumatol. Rehabil. *16*:46, 1977.
31. Breig, A., and Marions, O.: Biomechanics of the lumbosacral nerve roots. Acta Radiol. *1*:1141, 1963.
32. Brevik, H., Hesla, P. E., Molnar, I., and Lind, B.: Treatment of chronic low back pain and sciatica: Comparison of caudad injections of bupivacaine and methylprednisolone. Adv. Pain Res. Ther. *1*:927, 1976.
33. Brown, M. D., and Tsaltas, T. T.: Studies on the permeability of the intervertebral disc during skeletal maturation. Spine *1*:240, 1976.
34. Bulos, S.: Herniated intervertebral lumbar disc in the teenager. J. Bone Joint Surg. *55B*:273, 1973.
35. Bundschuh, C. V., Modic, M. T., Ross, J. S., et al.: Epidural fibrosis and recurrent disk herniation in the lumbar spine: MR imaging assessment. A. J. R. *150*:923, 1988.
36. Burn, J. M., and Langdon, L.: Duration of action of epidural methylprednisolone. Am. J. Phys. Med. *53*:29, 1974.
37. Burton, C. V.: The gravity lumbar reduction therapy program. J. Musculoskeletal Med. *3*:12, 1986.
38. Cady, L. D., Bischoff, D. P., O'Connell, E. R., et al.: Strength and fitness and subsequent back injuries in firefighters. J. Occup. Med. *21*:269, 1979.
39. Cady, L. D., Thomas, P. C., and Kanwasky, R. J.: Program for increasing health and physical fitness of firefighters. J. Occup. Med. *27*:110, 1985.
40. Caldwell, A. B., and Chase, C.: Diagnosis and treatment of personality factors in chronic low back pain. Clin. Orthop. *129*:141, 1977.
41. Colonna, P. C., and Friedenburg, Z.: The disc syndrome. J. Bone Joint Surg. *31A*:614, 1949.
42. Crawshaw, C., Frazer, A., Merriam, W. F., et al.: A comparison of surgery and chemonucleolysis in the treatment of sciatica: a prospective randomized trial. Spine *9*:195, 1984.
43. Cuckler, J. M., Bernini, P. A., Wiesel, S. W., et al.: A prospective, randomized, double-blind study of the use of epidural steroids in the treatment of lumbar radicular pain. J. Bone Joint Surg. *67A*:63, 1985.
44. Curtis, P.: Spinal manipulation: does it work? State Art Rev. Occup. Med. *3*:31, 1988.
45. Cyriax, J.: Textbook of Orthopaedic Medicine. 7th ed. Vol. 1. London, Baillière Tindall, 1978.
46. Dahlstrom, W. G., Welsh, G. S., and Dahlstrom, L. E.: An MMPI handbook. Vol. 1. Clinical Interpretation. Minneapolis, University of Minnesota Press, 1972.
47. Dan, N. G., and Saccasan, P. A.: Serious complications of lumbar spinal manipulation. Med. J. Aust. 2:672, 1983.
47a. Dandy, W. E.: Loose cartilage from intervertebral disk stimulating tumor of the spinal cord. Arch. Surg. *19*:660, 1929.
48. Danforth, M. S., and Wilson, P. D.: The anatomy of the lumbosacral region in relation to sciatic pain. J. Bone Joint Surg. *7A*:109, 1925.
49. Dapas, F., Hartman, S., and Martinez, L.: Baclofen for the treatment of acute low back syndrome. Spine *10*:345, 1985.
50. Davies, G., and Gould, J.: Trunk testing using a prototype Cybex II isokinetic dynamometer stabilization system. J. Orthop. Sports Phys. Ther. *3*:164, 1982.
51. Davies, J. E., Gibson, R., and Tester, L.: The value of exercises in the treatment of low back pain. Rheumatol. Rehabil. *18*:243, 1979.
52. Dehateur, B. J., Lehmann, J., and Warren, G. G.: Comparison of effectiveness of isokinetic and isotonic exercise in quadriceps strengthening. Arch. Phys. Med. Rehabil. *53*:60, 1982.
53. Delamarter, R. B., Henffle, M., Modic, M., et al.: Postoperative epidural fibrosis versus recurrent lumbar disc herniation: diagnosis by gadolinium-DTPA enhanced MRI. Presented at the 101st Annual Meeting of the American Orthopaedic Association, Hot Springs, VA, June 1988.
54. Deloney, T., Rowlingston, F. C., Carron, H., et al.: Epidural steroid effects on nerves and meninges. Anesth. Anal. *59*:610, 1980.
55. DePalma, A. F., and Rothman, R. H.: The nature of pseudoarthrosis. Clin. Orthop. *59*:113, 1968.
56. DePalma, A., and Rothman, R.: Surgery of the lumbar spine. Clin. Orthop. *63*:162, 1969.
57. DePalma, A. F., and Rothman, R. H.: The Intervertebral Disc. Philadelphia, W. B. Saunders Co., 1970.
58. DeVries, H.: EMG fatigue curve in postural muscles. A possible etiology for idiopathic low back pain. Am. J. Phys. Med. *47*:175, 1968.
59. Deyo, R. A.: Conservative therapy for low back pain: distinguishing useful from useless therapy. J.A.M.A. *250*:1057, 1983.
60. Deyo, R. A., and Diehl, A. K.: Lumbar spine films in primary care: current use and effects of selective ordering criteria. J. Gen. Intern. Med. *1*:20, 1986.
61. Deyo, R. A., Diehl, A. K., and Rosenthal, N.: How many days of bedrest for acute low back pain? A randomized clinical trial. N. Engl. J. Med. *315*:1064, 1986.
62. Deyo, R. A., Loeser, J., and Bigos, S.: Herniated lumbar intervertebral disc. Ann. Intern. Med. *112*:598, 1990.
63. Dilke, T. W. F., Burry, H. C., and Grahame, R.: Extradural corticosteroid injection in the management of lumbar nerve root compression. Br. Med. J. *2*:635, 1973.
64. Dillane, J. B., Fry, J., and Kalton, G.: Acute back syndrome: a study from general practice. Br. Med. J. *2*:82, 1966.
65. Di Maggio, A., and Mooney, V.: Conservative care for low back pain: What works? J. Musculoskel. Med. *4*:27, 1987.
66. DiStefano, V. J., Klein, K. S., Nixon, J. E., et al.: Intra-operative analysis of the effects of position and body habitus on surgery of the low back. Clin. Orthop. *99*:51, 1974.
67. Dolce, J. J., and Baczynski, J. M.: Neuromuscular activity and electromyography in painful backs:

psychological and biochemical models in assessment and treatment. Psychol. Bull. *97*:402, 1985.
68. Dyck, P.: The femoral nerve traction test with lumbar disc protrusions. Surg. Neurol. *6*:163, 1976.
69. Dyck, P., and Doyle, J. B., Jr.: "Bicycle test" of van Gelderen in diagnosis of intermittent cauda equina compression syndrome. J. Neurosurg. *46*:667, 1977.
70. Ejeskar, A., Nachemson, A., Herberts, P., et al.: Surgery versus chemonucleolysis for herniated lumbar discs: a prospective study with random assignment. Clin. Orthop. *174*:236, 1983.
71. Elliott, F. A., and Schutta, H. S.: The differential diagnosis of sciatica. Orthop. Clin. North Am. *2*:477, 1971.
72. Emmett, J., and Love, J.: Vesical dysfunction caused by protruded lumbar disc. J. Urol. *105*:80, 1971.
73. Epstein, B. S., Epstein, J. A., and Jones, M. D.: Lumbar spinal stenosis. Radiol. Clin. North Am. *15*:227, 1977.
74. Evans, J. G.: Neurogenic intermittent claudication. Br. Med. J. *5415*:985, 1964.
75. Evans, W.: Intrasacral epidural injection in the treatment of sciatica. Lancet *2*:1225, 1930.
76. Fairbank, J. C., Park, W. M., McCall, I. W., et al.: Apophyseal injection of local anesthetic as a diagnostic aid in primary low-back pain syndromes. Spine *6*:598, 1981.
77. Farfan, H. F.: Mechanical Disorders of the Low Back. Philadelphia, Lea & Febiger, 1973.
78. Farfan, H. F., Cossette, J. W., Robertson, G. H., et al.: The effect of torsion on the lumbar intervertebral joints: the role of torsion in the production of disc degeneration. J. Bone Joint Surg. *52A*:468, 1970.
79. Farrell, J. P., and Twomey, L. T.: Acute low back pain. Comparison of two conservative treatment approaches. Med. J. Aust. *1*:160, 1982.
80. Fast, A., Shapiro, D., Ducommun, E. J., et al.: Low back pain in pregnancy. Spine *12*:368, 1987.
81. Fidler, M. W., Jowett, R. L., and Troup, J. D. G.: Myosin ATPase activity in multifidus muscle from cases of lumbar spinal derangement. J. Bone Joint Surg. *57B*:220, 1975.
82. Fidler, M. W., and Plasmans, C. M. T.: The effect of four types of support on the segmental mobility of the lumbosacral spine. J. Bone Joint Surg. *65A*:943, 1983.
83. Friedman, W. A.: Percutaneous discectomy: an alternative to chemonucleolysis? Neurosurgery *13*:542, 1983.
84. Friis, M. L., Gulliksen, G. C., Rasmussen, P., and Husby, J.: Pain and spinal root compression. Acta Neurochir. *39*:241, 1977.
85. Frymoyer, J. W., Pope, M. H., Clements, J. H., et al.: Risk factors in low back pain: an epidemiological survey. J. Bone Joint Surg. *65A*:213, 1983.
86. Gallinuro, P., and Cortesegna, M.: Three cases of lumbar disc rupture and one of cauda equina associated with spinal manipulation (chiroprosis) (letter). Lancet *1*:411, 1983.
87. Garfin, S. R., Glover, M., Booth, R. E., et al.: Laminectomy: a review of the Pennsylvania Hospital experience. J. Spinal Dis. *1*:116, 1988.
88. Garvey, T. A., Marka, M., and Weisel, S. W.: A prospective randomized double-blind evaluation of trigger-point injection therapy in low back pain. Spine *14*:962, 1988.
89. Gertzbein, S. D., Tait, J. H., and Devlin, S. R.: The stimulation of lymphocytes by nucleus pulposus in patients with degenerative disk disease of the lumbar spine. Clin. Orthop. *123*:149, 1977.
90. Ghia, J. N., Mao, W., Toomey, T. C., et al.: Acupuncture and chronic pain mechanisms. Pain *2*:285, 1976.
91. Ghormley, R. K.: Low back pain with special reference to the articular facets, with presentation of an operative procedure. J.A.M.A. *101*:1773, 1933.
92. Gibb, D.: Spinal injection: corticosteroids. Med. J. Aust. *2*:302, 1981.
93. Gilbert, J. R., Taylor, D. W., Hildebrand, A., et al.: Clinical trial of common treatments for low back pain in family practice. Br. Med. J. *291*:791, 1985.
94. Gill, G. G., Sakovich, L., and Thompson, E: Pedicle fat grafts for the prevention of scar formation after laminectomy. Spine *4*:176, 1979.
95. Goldner, J. L., Urbaniak, J. R., and McCollum, D. E.: Anterior disc excision and interbody spine fusion for chronic low back pain. Orthop. Clin. North Am. *2*:543, 1971.
96. Goldthwait, J. E.: The lumbosacral articulation: an explanation of many cases of "lumbago," "sciatica," and paraplegia. Boston Med. Surg. J. *164*:365, 1911.
97. Gorshi, D. W., Rao, T. K., Glessor, S. N., et al.: Epidural triamcinolone and adrenal responses to stress. Anesthesiology *55*:A147, 1981.
98. Grabias, S.: Current concepts review: the treatment of spinal stenosis. J. Bone Joint Surg. *62A*:308, 1980.
99. Green, L. N.: Dexamethasone in the management of symptoms due to herniated nucleus pulposus. J. Neurol. Neurosurg. Psychiatry *35*:1211, 1975.
100. Grew, N. D., and Deane, G.: The physical effect of lumbar spinal supports. Prosthet. Orthot. Int. *6*:79, 1982.
101. Gulliver, J.: Acute low back pain in industry. Acta Orthop. Scand. *129*:6, 1970.
102. Hadler, N. M., Curtis, P., Gillings, D. B., et al.: A benefit of spinal manipulation as adjunctive therapy for acute low-back pain: a stratified controlled trial. Spine *12*:703, 1987.
103. Haimovic, I. C., and Beresford, R. H.: Treatment of lumbosacral radicular pain with dexamethasone: a controlled study. Neurology *35*:abstract, 1985.
104. Hakelius, A.: Prognosis in sciatica: a clinical follow-up of surgical and non-surgical treatment. Acta Orthop. Scand. (Suppl.)*129*:1, 1970.
105. Hakelius, A., and Hindmarsh, J.: The significance of neurological signs and myelographic findings in the diagnosis of lumbar root compression. Acta Orthop. Scand. *43*:239, 1972.
106. Hall, H., and Iceton, J. A.: Back school: an overview with specific reference to the Canadian Back Education units. Clin. Orthop. *179*:10, 1983.
107. Hanson, P. G., Griese, M. D., and Corlis, R. I.: Clinical guidelines for exercise training. Postgrad. Med. *67*:120, 1980.
108. Hanvick, L. J.: MMPI profiles in patinets with low back pain. J. Consult. Psychol. *15*:350, 1951.
109. Harmon, P. H., and Abel, M.: Correlation of mul-

tiple objective diagnostic methods in lower lumbar disc disease. Clin. Orthop. *28*:132, 1963.

110. Hazard, R. G., and Buckley, L. M.: Whys and wherefores of treating back pain with NSAID's. J. Musculoskel. Med. *6*:64, 1989.
111. Henderson, R. S.: The treatment of lumbar intervertebral disc protrusion. Br. Med. J. *2*:597, 1952.
112. Hendler, N., Viernstein, M., Gucer, P., and Long, D.: A preoperative screening test for chronic back pain patients. Psychosomatics *20*:801, 1979.
113. Hibbs, R.: An operation for progressive spinal deformities. N.Y. J. Med. *93*:1013, 1911.
114. Hindmarsh, T., Ekholm, S. E., Kido, D. K., et al.: Lumbar myelography with metrizamide and iohexol: a double-blind clinical trial. Acta. Radiol. [Diagn.] (Stockh.) *25*:365, 1984.
115. Hirsch, C.: Efficiency of surgery in low back disorders. J. Bone Joint Surg. *47A*:991, 1965.
116. Hirsch, C., and Nachemson, A.: The reliability of lumbar disk surgery. Clin. Orthop. *29*:189, 1963.
117. Hitselberger, W., and Witten, R.: Abnormal myelograms in asymptomatic patients. J. Neurosurg. *28*:204, 1968.
118. Hochler, F. K., Tobias, J. S., and Buerger, A. A.: Spinal manipulation for low back pain. J.A.M.A. *245*:1835, 1982.
119. Holmes, H. E., and Rothman, R. H.: The Pennsylvania plan: an algorithm for the management of lumbar degenerative disc disease. Spine *4*:156, 1979.
120. Holmes, H. E., and Rothman, R. H.: Technique of lumbar laminectomy. Instr. Course Lect. *28*:193, 1979.
121. Holmes, H. E., and Rothman, R. H.: Technique of lumbar laminectomy. Instr. Course Lect. *28*:200, 1979.
122. Holt, E. P.: The question of lumbar discography. J. Bone Joint Surg. *50A*:720, 1968.
123. Horal, J.: The clinical appearance of low back disorders. Acta Orthop. Scand. (Suppl.) *188*:109, 1969.
124. Hult, L.: The Munkfors investigation. Acta Orthop. Scand. (Suppl.) *16*:5, 1954.
125. Jackson, C. P., and Brown, M. D.: Is there a role for exercise in the treatment of patients with low back pain? Clin. Orthop. *179*:39, 1983.
126. Jackson, C. P., and Klugerman, M.: How to start a back school. J. Orthop. Sports Phys. Ther. *179*:10, 1988.
127. Jackson, R., Montesaro, P., and Jacobs, R.: Facet joint injections in mechanical low-back pain patients: a prospective statistical study. Proceedings of International Society for Study of Lumbar Spine. Orthop. Trans. *10*:509, 1986.
128. Jacobs, R., McClain, O., and Neff, J.: Control of post-laminectomy scar formation: an experimental and clinical evaluation. Spine *5*:223, 1980.
129. Jarrett, R. W., and Richelson, E.: Antidepressants: a clinical update for medical practitioners. Mayo Clin. Proc. *59*:330, 1984.
130. Javid, M. J.: Treatment of herniated lumbar disk syndrome with chymopapain. J.A.M.A. *243*:2043, 1980.
131. Jayson, M. I., Herbert, C. M., and Barks, J. S.: Intervertebral discs: nuclear morphology and bursting pressures. Ann. Rheum. Dis. *32*:308, 1973.
132. Jockheim, K. A.: Lumbaler Bandscheibenverfall. Berlin, Springer-Verlag, 1961.
133. Jones, D. L., and Moore, T.: The types of neuropathic bladder dysfunction associated with prolapsed lumbar intervertebral discs. Br. J. Urol. *45*:39, 1973.
134. Kalenak, A., Medlar, C. E., Fleagle, S. B., et al.: Athletic injuries: heat versus cold. Am. Fam. Physician *12*:131, 1975.
135. Kambin, P., and Gellman, H.: Percutaneous lateral discectomy of the lumbar spine. Clin. Orthop. *174*:127, 1983.
136. Keller, R. H.: Traumatic displacement of the cartilaginous vertebral rim: a sign of intervertebral disc prolapse. Radiology *110*:21, 1974.
137. Kellett, J.: Acute soft tissue injuries: a review of the literature. Med. Sci. Sports Exerc. *18*:489, 1986.
138. Kellgren, J. H.: The anatomical source of back pain. Rheumatol. Rehabil. *16*:3, 1977.
139. Kelsey, J., and White, A. A.: Epidemiology and impact of low-back pain. Spine *5*:133, 1980.
140. Kelsey, J. L.: An epidemiological study of acute herniated lumbar intervertebral discs. Rheumatol. Rehabil. *14*:144, 1975.
141. Kelsey, J. L.: An epidemiological study of the relationship between occupations and acute herniated lumbar intervertebral discs. Int. J. Epidemiol. *4*:197, 1975.
142. Kelsey, J. L.: Demographic characteristics of persons with acute herniated lumbar intervertebral disc. J. Chronic Dis. *28*:37, 1975.
143. Kelsey, J. L., Greenberg, R. A., Handy, R. I., et al.: Pregnancy and the syndrome of herniated lumbar intervertebral disc: an epidemiological study. Yale J. Biol. Med. *48*:361, 1975.
144. Kendall, P. H. G., and Jenkins, J. S.: Exercise for backache: a double-blind controlled trial. Physiotherapy *54*:54, 1968.
145. Klatz, R. M., Goldman, R. M., Pinchuk, B. G., et al.: The effects of gravity inversion procedures on systemic blood pressure, intraocular pressure and central retinal arterial pressure. J. Am. Osteopath. Assoc. *82*:853, 1983.
146. Knutsson, B.: Aspects of the neurogenic electromyographic records of voluntary contraction in cases of nerve root compression. Electromyography *2*:238, 1962.
147. Kopp, P., Alexander, H., Turocy, R., et al.: The use of lumbar extension in the evaluation and treatment of patients with acute herniated nucleus pulposus. Clin. Orthop. *202*:211, 1986.
148. Korenko, P., Boumphrey, F., Bell, G., et al.: McKenzie extension exercises in the treatment of acute disc prolapse: a prospective study. Orthop. Trans. *9*:509, 1985.
149. Kostuik, J. P., Harrington, I., Alexander, D., et al.: Cauda equina syndrome and lumbar disc herniation. J. Bone Joint Surg. *68A*:386, 1986.
150. Kramer, J.: Pressure dependent fluid shifts in the intervertebral disc. Orthop. Clin. North Am. *8*:211, 1977.
151. Kulak, R. F., Belytschko, T. B., Schultz, A. B., and Galante, J.: Nonlinear behavior of the human intervertebral disc under axial load. Orthop. Clin. North Am. *9*:377, 1976.
152. Kulak, R. F., Schultz, A. B., and Belytschko, T. B.: Biomechanical characteristics of vertebral motion

segments and intervertebral discs. Orthop. Clin. North Am. *6*:121, 1975.
153. LaBan, M. M., Perrin, J. C. S., and Latimer, F. R.: Pregnancy and the herniated lumbar disc. Arch. Phys. Med. Rehabil. *64*:319, 1983.
154. Lancourt, J. E.: Traction techniques for low back pain. J. Musculoskel. Med. *3*:44, 1986.
155. Langenskiöld, A., and Kiviluoto, O.: Prevention of epidural scar formation after operation on the lumbar spine by means of free fat transplants. Clin. Orthop. *115*:92, 1976.
156. Larsson, U., Choler, U., Lidstrom, A., et al.: Autotraction for treatment of lumbago-sciatica. Acta Orthop. Scand. *51*:791, 1980.
157. Lassoner, E. M., Alho, A., Karalarju, E. O., and Paavilaimen, T.: Short term prognosis in sciatica. Ann. Chir. Gynaecol. *66*:47, 1977.
158. Lehman, J. S., Warren, C. G., and Scham, S. M.: Therapeutic heat and cold. Clin. Orthop. *99*:207, 1974.
159. Lewis, I. W., Cannon, J. T., and Liebeskind, J. C.: Opioid and non-opioid mechanisms of stress analgesia. Science *208*:623, 1980.
160. Liang, M., and Komaroff, A. L.: Roentgenograms in primary care patients with acute low back pain: a cost-effectiveness analysis. Arch. Intern. Med. *142*:1108, 1982.
161. Lora, J., and Long, D.: So-called facet denervation in the management of intractable back pain. Spine *1*:121, 1976.
162. MacNab, I.: The traction spur: an indicator of segmental instability. J. Bone Joint Surg. *57A*:663, 1971.
163. MacNab, I.: Backache. Baltimore, Williams & Wilkins Co., 1977.
164. MacNab, I.: The laminectomy membrane. J. Bone Joint Surg. *56B*:545, 1974.
165. MacNab, I.: Personal correspondence.
166. Manniche, C., Hesselsøe, G., Bentzen, L., et al.: Clinical trial of intensive muscle training for chronic low back pain. Lancet *2*:1473, 1988.
167. Markolf, K. L., and Morris, J. M.: The structural components of the intervertebral disc. J. Bone Joint Surg. *56A*:675, 1974.
168. Maroudas, A., Nachemson, A., Stockwell, R., and Urban, J.: In vitro studies of the diffusion of glucose into the intervertebral disc. *In* Nachemson, A.: Towards a better understanding of low back pain: a review of the mechanics of the lumbar disc. Rheumatol. Rehabil. *14*:129, 1975.
169. Maruta, T., Swanson, D. W., and Swenson, W. M.: Low back pain patients in a psychiatric population. Mayo Clin. Proc. *51*:57, 1976.
170. Masaryk, T. J., Boumphrey, F., Modic, M. T., et al.: Effects of chemonucleolysis demonstrated by MR imaging. J. Comput. Assist. Tomogr. *10*:917, 1986.
171. Masaryk, T. J., Ross, J. S., Modic, M. T., et al.: High-resolution MR imaging of sequestered lumbar intervertebral disks. A.J.N.R. *9*:351, 1988.
172. Maury, M., Francois, N., and Skoda, A.: About the neurological sequelae of herniated intervertebral disc. Paraplegia, *11*:221, 1973.
173. Mayer, T. G., Gatchel, R. J.: Functional Restoration for Spinal Disorders: The Sports Medicine Approach. Philadelphia, Lea & Febiger, 1988.
174. Mayer, T. G., Gatchel, R. J., Mayer, H., et al.: A prospective two-year study of functional restoration in industrial low back injury. An objective assessment procedure. J.A.M.A. *258*:1763, 1987.
175. Mayer, T. G., Smith, S. S., Kelley, J., and Mooney, V.: Quantification of lumbar function. II. Sagittal plane trunk strength in chronic low-back pain patients. Spine *10*:765, 1985.
176. McCarron, R. F., Wimpee, M. W., and Hudkins, P. G.: The inflammatory effect of nucleus pulposus. Spine *12*:760, 1987.
177. McGill, C. M.: Industrial back problems, a control program. J. Occup. Med. *10*:174, 1968.
178. McKenzie, R. A.: The Lumbar Spine: Mechanical Diagnosis and Therapy. Waikanae, New Zealand, Spinal Publications, 1981.
179. Melzack, R., and Wall, P. D.: Pain mechanism: a new theroy. Science *150*:961, 1965.
180. Mendelson, G., Kidson, M. A., Loh, S. T., et al.: Acupuncture analgesics for chronic low back pain. Clin. Exp. Neurol. *15*:182, 1978.
181. Mendelson, G., Selwood, T. S., Kranz, H., et al.: Acupuncture treatment of chronic back pain: a double-blind placebo-controlled trial. Am. J. Med. *74*:49, 1983.
182. Merrit, J. L., and Hunder, G. G.: Passive range of motion not isometric exercise amplifies urate synovitis. Arch. Phys. Med. Rehabil. *64*:130, 1983.
183. Micheli, L. J., Hall, J. E., and Miller, M. E.: Use of modified Boston brace for back injuries in athletes. Am. J. Sports Med. *8*:351, 1980.
184. Mixter, W. J., and Barr, J. S.: Rupture of the intervertebral disc with involvement of the spinal canal. N. Engl. J. Med. *211*:210, 1934.
185. Modic, M. T., Feiglin, D. H., Piraino, D. W., et al.: Vertebral osteomyelitis: assessment using MRI. Radiology *157*:157, 1985.
186. Modic, M. T., Masaryk, T. J., Boumphrey, F., et al.: Lumbar herniated disc and canal stenosis: prospective evaluation by surface coil MR, CT and myelography. A.J.N.R. *7*:709, 1986.
187. Mooney, V.: Surgery and post-surgical management of the patient with low back pain. Phys. Ther. *59*:1000, 1979.
188. Mooney, V., Cairnes, D., and Robertson, J.: A system for evaluating and treating chronic back disability. West. J. Med. *124*:370, 1976.
189. Mooney, V., and Robertson, J.: The facet syndrome. Clin. Orthop. *115*:149, 1976.
190. Murphy, R. W.: Nerve roots and spinal nerves in degenerative disk disease. Clin. Orthop. *129*:46, 1977.
191. Nachemson, A.: The load on lumbar disks in different positions of the body. Acta Orthop. Scand. *36*:426, 1965.
192. Nachemson, A.: The load on lumbar discs in different positions of the body. Clin. Orthop. *45*:107, 1966.
193. Nachemson, A.: Towards a better understanding of low-back pain: a review of the mechanics of the lumbar disc. Rheumatol. Rehabil. *14*:129, 1975.
194. Nachemson, A.: Work for all. Clin. Orthop. *179*:77, 1983.
195. Nachemson, A.: Advances in low back pain. Clin. Orthop. *200*:266, 1985.
196. Nachemson, A. L.: The lumbar spine: An orthopaedic challenge. Spine *1*:59, 1976.
197. Nachemson, A. L., and Elfstrom, G.: Intravital

dynamic pressure measurements in lumbar discs. A study of common movements, maneuvers and exercises. Scand. J. Rehabil. Med. *7* (Suppl.):5, 1970.

198. Nachemson, A., and Morris, J. M.: In vivo measurements of intradiscal pressure. Discometry, a method for the determination of pressure in the lower lumbar discs. J. Bone Joint Surg. *46A*:1077, 1964.

199. Natchev, E., and Valentino, V.: Low back pain and disc hernia observation during autotraction treatment. Manual Med. *1*:39, 1984.

200. Naylor, A.: Intervertebral disc prolapse and degeneration. The biochemical and biophysical approach. Spine *1*:108, 1976.

201. Naylor, A., Happey, F., Turner, R. I., et al.: Enzymatic and immunological activity in the intervertebral disc. Orthop. Clin. North Am. *6*:51, 1975.

202. Nosse, L. J.: Inverted spinal traction. Arch. Phys. Med. Rehabil. *59*:367, 1978.

203. Ober, R. R.: Back strain and sciatica. J.A.M.A. *104*:1586, 1935.

204. Ohnmeiss, D., Stith, W., Gilbert, P., and Rashbaum, R.: Treatment of acute low back pain. Spine *3*:69, 1989.

205. Onik, G., and Helms, C. (eds.): Automated Percutaneous Lumbar Discectomy. San Francisco, Radiology Research and Education Foundation, 1988.

206. Oudenhoven, R. C.: Gravitational lumbar traction. Arch. Phys. Med. Rehabil. *59*:510, 1978.

207. Painter, J. R., Seres, J. L., and Newman, R. I.: Assessing benefits of the pain center: why some patients regress. Pain *8*:101, 1980.

208. Pamrianpour, M., Nordin, M., Mortiz, U., and Kahanovitz, N.: Correlation between different tests of trunk strength. *In* Buckle, P. (ed.): Proceedings of Musculoskeletal Disorders at Work. University of Surrey, Guildford, England, Taylor & Francis, 1987.

209. Pearce, J., and Moll, J.: Conservative treatment and natural history of acute lumbar disc lesions. J. Neurol. Neurosurg. Psychiatry *30*:13, 1967.

210. Pedersen, H. E., Blunck, C. F., and Gardner, E.: The anatomy of lumbosacral posterior rami and meningeal branches of spinal nerves (sinu-vertebral nerves). J. Bone Joint Surg. *38A*:377, 1956.

211. Perry, J.: The use of external support in the treatment of low back pain. Artif. Limbs *14*:49, 1970.

212. Peyser, E., and Harari, A.: Intradural rupture of lumbar intervertebral disk: report of two cases with review of the literature. Surg. Neurol. *8*:95, 1977.

213. Pheasant, H., Bursk, A., Goldfarb, J., et al.: Amitriptyline and chronic low back pain: a randomized double-blind crossover study. Spine *8*:552, 1983.

214. Quintet, R. J., and Hadler, N. M.: Diagnosis and treatment of backache. Semin. Arthritis Rheum. *8*:261, 1979.

215. Raaf, J.: Some observations regarding 905 patients operated upon for protruded lumbar intervertebral disc. Am. J. Surg. *97*:388, 1959.

216. Ransford, A. O., Cairns, D., and Mooney, V.: The pain drawing as an aid to the psychologic evaluation of patients with low-back pain. Spine *1*:127, 1976.

217. Rashbaum, R. F.: Radiofrequency facet denervation: a treatment alternative in retracting low back pain with or without leg pain. Orthop. Clin. North Am. *14*:569, 1983.

218. Ravichandran, G., and Mulholland, R. C.: Chymopapain chemonucleolysis: a preliminary report. Spine *5*:380, 1980.

219. Resnick, D., and Niwayama, G.: Intervertebral disk herniations: cartilaginous (Schmorl's) nodes. Radiology *126*:57, 1978.

220. Richardson, R. R., Arbit, J., Siqueira, E. B., and Zagar, R.: Transcutaneous electrical neurostimulation in functional pain. Spine *6*:185, 1981.

221. Rippe, J. M., Blair, S. M., Freedson, P. S., et al.: The health benefits of exercise. Part I. Physician Sports Med. *15*:115, 1987.

222. Ross, J. C., and Jackson, R. M.: Vesical dysfunction due to prolapsed disc. Br. Med. J. *3*:752, 1971.

223. Rothman, R. H., and Bernini, R. H.: Algorithm for salvage surgery of the lumbar spine. Clin. Orthop. *154*:14, 1982.

224. Rothman, R. H., and Simeone, F. A.: The Spine. 2nd ed. Philadelphia, W. B. Saunders Co., 1982.

225. Rowe, M. L.: Low back pain in industry: a position paper. J. Occup. Med. *11*:161, 1969.

226. Russin, L. A., and Sheldon, J.: Spinal stenosis: report of series and long-term follow-up. Clin. Orthop. *115*:101, 1976.

227. Saal, J. A., and Saal, J. S.: Non-operative treatment of herniated lumbar intervertebral disc with radiculopathy: an outcome study. Spine *14*:431, 1989.

228. Scavone, J. G., Latshaw, R. F., and Rohrer, F. V.: Use of lumbar spine films: statistical evaluation at a university teaching school. J.A.M.A. *246*:1105, 1981.

229. Scham, S. M., and Taylor, T. K.: Tension signs in lumbar disc prolapse. Clin. Orthop. *75*:195, 1971.

230. Semmes, E.: Ruptures of the Lumbar Intervertebral Disc. Springfield. Charles C Thomas, 1964.

231. Shah, J. S.: Structure, morphology and mechanics of the lumbar spine. *In* Jayson, M. (ed.): The Lumbar Spine and Low Back Pain. London, Pitman Medical, 1980, pp. 359–405.

232. Sharr, M. M., Garfield, J. S., and Jenkins, J. D.: The association of bladder dysfunction with degenerative lumbar spondylosis. Br. J. Urol. *45*:616, 1973.

233. Simmons, J. W.: An algorithmic approach to treatment of low back pain. Orthop. Rev. *2*:86, 1982.

234. Smith-Peterson, M. N.: Arthrodesis of the sacroiliac joint; a new method of approach. J. Orthop. Surg. *3*:400, 1921.

235. Smyth, M. J., and Wright, V. J.: Sciatica and the intervertebral disc. An experimental study. J. Bone Joint Surg. *40A*:1401, 1958.

236. Southwick, S., and White, A. A.: Current concepts review: the use of psychological tests in evaluation of low-back pain. J. Bone Joint Surg. *65A*:560, 1983.

237. Spangfort, E.: Lasègue's sign in patients with lumbar disc herniation. Acta Orthop. Scand. *42*:459, 1971.

238. Spangfort, E. V.: The lumbar disc herniation. A computer-aided analysis of 2,504 operations. Acta Orthop. Scand. (Suppl.) *142*:61, 1972.

239. Spengler, D. M.: Chronic low back pain: the team approach. Clin. Orthop. *179*:71, 1983.

240. Spengler, D. M., Bigos, S. J., Martin, N. A., et al.:

Back injuries in industry: an overview and cost analysis. Spine *11*:241, 1986.
241. Spitzer, W. O., LeBlanc, F. E., Dupuis, M., et al.: Scientific approach to the assessment and management of activity-related spinal disorders: report of the Quebec Task Force on spinal disorders. Spine *12*:S1, 1987.
242. Stambough, J. L., and Booth, R. E.: Complications in spine surgery as a consequence of anatomic variations. *In* Garfin, S. R. (ed.): Complications of Spine Surgery. Baltimore, Williams & Wilkins Co., 1989, pp. 89–110.
243. Steindler, A., and Luck, J. V.: Differential diagnosis of pain low in the back; allocation of the source of pain by procaine hydrochloride method. J.A.M.A. *110*:106, 1938.
244. Sternbach, R. A., Wolf, S. R., Murphy, R. W., and Akeson, W. H.: Traits of pain patients: The low-back "loser." Psychosomatics *14*:226, 1973.
245. Szlachter, B. N., Quagliarello, J., Jeeelewicz, R., et al.: Relaxin in normal and pathogenic pregnancies. Obstet. Gynecol. *59*:167, 1983.
246. Troup, J. D. G., Martin, J. W., and Lloyd, D. C. E. F.: Back pain in industry: a prospective survey. Spine *6*:61, 1981.
247. Truchly, G., and Thompson, W. A.: Posterolateral fusion of the lumbosacral spine. J. Bone Joint Surg. *44A*:505, 1962.
248. Tsairis, P.: Corticosteroid therapy in the management of lumbar radiculopathy. Contemp. Orthop. *17*:53, 1988.
249. Vanharanta, H., Videman, T., and Mooney, V.: McKenzie exercise, backtrack and back school in lumbar syndrome. Orthop. Trans. *10*:533, 1986.
250. Verbiest, H.: Results of surgical treatment of idiopathic developmental stenosis of the lumbar vertebral canal: a review of 27 years' experience. J. Bone Joint Surg. *59B*:181, 1977.
251. Verbiest, H.: Radicular syndrome from developmental narrowing of lumbar vertebral canal. J. Bone Joint Surg. *36B*:230, 1954.
252. Verbiest, H.: Pathomorphologic aspects of developmental lumbar stenosis. Orthop. Clin. North Am. *6*:177, 1975.
253. Waddell, G.: An approach to backache. Br. J. Hosp. Med. *28*:187, 1982.
254. Waddell, G.: A new clinical model for the treatment of low back pain. Spine *12*:632, 1987.
255. Waddell, G., Main, C., Morris, E., et al.: Chronic low-back pain, psychologic distress, and illness behavior. Spine *9*:209, 1984.
256. Waddell, G., McCulloch, J. A., Jummel, E., and Venner, R. M.: Non-organic physical signs in low back pain. Spine *5*:117, 1980.
257. Ward, N. G.: Tricyclic antidepressants for chronic low back pain: mechanisms of action and predictors of response. Spine *11*:661, 1986.
258. Watkins, M. B.: Lumbosacral fusion results with early ambulation. Surg. Gynecol. Obstet. *102*:604, 1956.
259. Weber, H.: Lumbar disc herniation: a prospective study of prognostic factors including a controlled trial. J. Oslo City Hosp. *28*:36, 1978.
260. Weber, H.: Lumbar disc herniation: a controlled, prospective study with ten years of observation. Spine *8*:131, 1983.
261. Weber, H.: Traction therapy in sciatica due to disc prolapse. J. Oslo City Hosp. *23*:167, 1973.
262. Weber, H., Ljunggren, A. E., and Walker, L.: Traction therapy in patients with herniated lumbar intervertebral discs. J. Oslo City Hosp. *34*:61, 1984.
263. Weise, M. D., Garfin, S. R., Gelberman, R. H., et al.: Lower extremity sensibility testing in patients with herniated lumbar intervertebral discs. J. Bone Joint Surg. *67A*:1219, 1985.
264. White, A. A., Panjabi, M. M., Posner, I., et al.: Spinal stability: evaluation and treatment. Instr. Course Lect. *30*:457, 1981.
265. White, A. H.: Injection techniques for the diagnosis and treatment of low back pain. Orthop. Clin. North Am. *14*:553, 1983.
266. Whitman, A.: An anatomic variation of the lumbosacral joint; its diagnosis and treatment. J. Bone Joint Surg. *6*:808, 1924.
267. Wiesel, S. W., Bell, G. R., Feffer, H. L., et al.: A study of computer assisted tomography. Part I. The incidence of positive CAT scans in an asymptomatic group of patients. Spine *9*:549, 1984.
268. Wiesel, S. W., Bernini, P., and Rothman, R. H.: The Aging Lumbar Spine. Philadelphia, W. B. Saunders Co., 1982.
269. Wiesel, S. W., Cuckler, J. M., DeLuca, F., et al.: Acute low back pain: an objective analysis of conservative therapy. Spine *5*:324, 1980.
270. Wiley, A. M., and Trueta, J.: The vascular anatomy of the spine and its relationship to pyogenic vertebral osteomyelitis. J. Bone Joint Surg. *41B*:796, 1959.
271. Williams, P. C.: Lesions of the lumbosacral spine. Part I. J. Bone Joint Surg. *19*:690, 1937.
272. Williams, P. C.: Reduced lumbosacral joint space. J.A.M.A. *99*:1677, 1932.
273. Wilson, C. B., Ehni, G., and Grollimus, J.: Neurogenic intermittent claudication. Clin. Neurosurg. *18*:62, 1971.
274. Wiltse, L. L., Bateman, J. G., Hutchinson, R. H., and Nelson, W. E.: The paraspinal sacrospinalis-splitting approach to the lumbar spine. J. Bone Joint Surg. *50A*:919, 1968.
275. Wiltse, L. L., Kirkaldy-Willis, W. H., and McIvor, G. W. D.: The treatment of spinal stenosis. Clin. Orthop. *115*:83, 1976.
276. Wiltse, L. L., and Rocchio, P. D.: Pre-operative psychological tests as predictors of success of chemonucleolysis treatment of the low back syndrome. J. Bone Joint Surg. *57A*:478, 1975.
277. Wisneski, R. J., and Rothman, R. H.: The Pennsylvania Plan II: an algorithm for the management of lumbar degenerative disc disease. Instr. Course Lect. *34*:17, 1985.
278. Wolkind, S. N.: Psychiatric aspects of low back pain. Psychotherapy *60*:75, 1974.
279. Wood, K. M., Arguelles, J., and Norenberg, M. D.: Degenerative lesions in rat sciatic nerves after local injection of methylprednisolone in sterile aqueous solution. Reg. Anaesth. *5*:13, 1980.
280. Young, H., and Love, J.: End results of removal of protruded lumbar intervertebral discs with and without fusion. Instr. Course Lect. *16*:213, 1959.

CHAPTER

24

ALTERNATIVE FORMS OF DISC EXCISION

John A. McCulloch, M.D.
Joseph C. Maroon, M.D.
Gary Onik, M.D.

CHEMONUCLEOLYSIS

John A. McCulloch, M.D.

In Chapter 22 the authors outlined the clinical syndrome of herniated nucleus pulposus (HNP) causing sciatica and the indications for surgical intervention. They made clear the essential prerequisites for successful surgical intervention (Tables 24–1 and 24–2 summarize those points). There are three procedures available as alternatives to standard laminectomy/discectomy: chemonucleolysis, percutaneous discectomy, and microdiscectomy.

If there is a common thread of failure in these three procedures it is that they fail to live up to the strict definition of indications and prerequisites for successful surgical intervention. They should not be used when a standard laminectomy/discectomy is not desired; they are substitute procedures with specific indications and contraindications.

CHYMOPAPAIN

Since its introduction by Jansen and Balls in 1941, chymopapain has had a chequered course to clinical acceptance.[10] After 1963, when Smith first reported its clinical use in the treatment of lumbar disc herniations, chymopapain was widely used in Canada, Great Britain, France, Germany, and the United States.[27] An American double-blind study in 1975 led to the withdrawal of chymopapain from clinical use in the United States, however.[26] Subsequent double-blind studies by Fraser, Smith Laboratories, and Travenol Laboratories led the United States Food and Drug Administration (FDA) to reconsider its position, and chymopapain was again released for general use in 1982.[3–5, 11, 34]

Surgeons, accustomed to surgically excising space-occupying pathology, were reluctant to embrace the concept of injecting discs with chymopapain, a constituent of meat tenderizer. A report on six deaths and 37 serious neurologic complications in the United States in approximately 80,000 injections done over 18 months (ending time, 1984) served to undermine chymopapain as a clinical tool.[28] One manufacturer's claim that chymopapain was as good as surgery (92 per cent success rate) and unsupported claims of product superiority by competing firms built false hopes in the drug and seriously damaged its credibility as a clinical tool.[29]

In many other countries chymopapain continues to provide acceptable results in the treatment of lumbar disc herniations. Despite the ongoing controversy surrounding chymopapain and despite the fact that its continuing

Table 24–1. CRITERIA FOR DIAGNOSIS OF ACUTE RADICULAR SYNDROME

Symptoms	Signs
Leg pain, including buttock discomfort, dominates over back pain	Marked reduction in SLR ability, bowstring discomfort, crossover pain
Presence of localizing neurologic symptoms (e.g., paresthesia in a dermatomal distribution)	Two of four neurologic signs (wasting, weakness, sensory loss, reflex alteration)

Three or four of these criteria are required for diagnosis. The exception is the young patient (< 25 years) who may have no neurologic symptoms or signs.

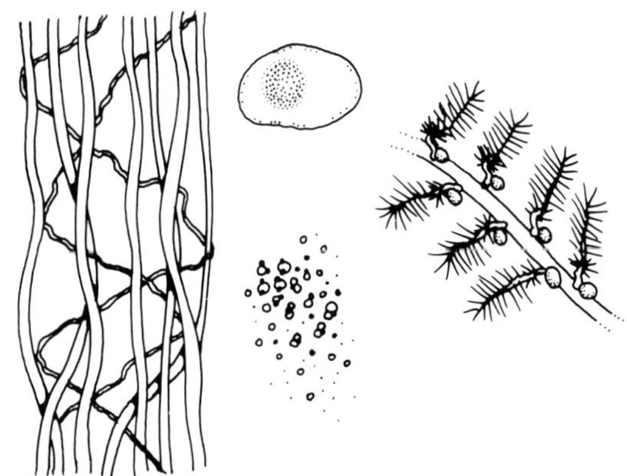

Figure 24–1. The four components of discal connective tissue: *left,* collagen; *middle,* cells and water; *right,* proteoglycan aggregate.

use taxes the physician's credibility, I believe there are continuing limited indications for the use of chymopapain in the treatment of some disc herniations.

Pharmacology

Chymopapain is an extract of latex of the tropical fruit papaya. Of the proteolytic enzymes in papaya, chymopapain is the most specific in its activity on nucleus pulposus and the least antigenic. Despite its being less antigenic than papain, chymopapain is a foreign protein to the human body and capable of precipitating allergic reactions. It is a sulfur-containing enzyme, and therefore reducing agents such as cystine hydrochloride are required to stabilize it. It should be reconstituted immediately before use, and thereafter it maintains effective enzymatic activity for only a few hours, after which the enzyme digests itself and is no longer pharmacologically active.

Mechanism of Action

Connective tissue can be classified into two basic components—cells and noncellular matrix. The cartilage connective tissue of nucleus pulposus contains cartilage cells; the matrix is made up of collagen and proteoglycan water complexes. This noncellular matrix of nucleus pulposus can be thought of as collagen-reinforcing bars laid in a viscoelastic base of proteoglycan and water. It is a pliable structure and, through the various effects of trauma and aging, can be displaced in whole or in part from the disc space cavity into the spinal canal.

Chymopapain's only effect is on the proteoglycan–water aggregates of nuclear tissue (Fig. 24–1). This proteoglycan aggregate imbibes water and cements itself among the collagen fibers to give the nucleus pulposus its viscoelastic structure. Because of the chemical make-up of proteoglycan and its fluid nature,

Table 24–2. INDICATIONS FOR SOME FORM OF SURGICAL INTERVENTION FOR AN HNP

Failure to respond to conservative care
Persisting sciatica
Recurrent sciatica
Increasing neurologic deficit
Bladder and bowel involvement

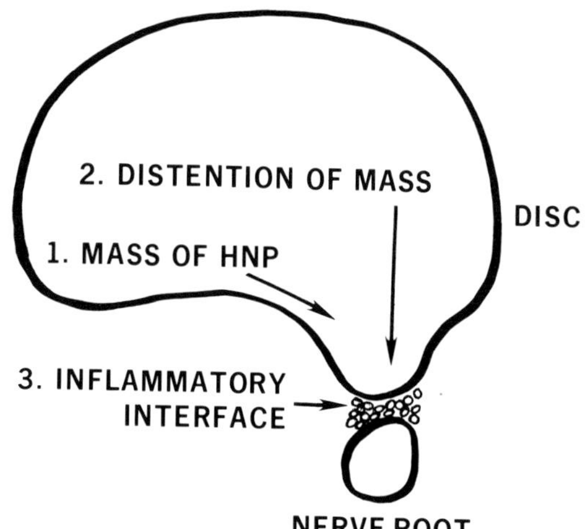

Figure 24–2. The three local factors contributing to sciatic nerve root pressure and irritation.

it has the ability to absorb and release water, thereby absorbing the dissipating forces across the disc space. Proteoglycans are negatively charged.

During displacement of discal nuclear material into the spinal canal, three local components may contribute to the symptom of sciatica (Fig. 24–2). Chymopapain, positively charged, has a direct effect on the negatively charged proteoglycan aggregate by splitting off the glycosaminoglycan side chains, which interferes with the ability of proteoglycan to hold water. This hydrolysis deflates the nuclear bulge and thus reduces pressure on the nerve root. Since collagen is not directly affected, there is still some mass of disc tissue present for weeks or months after chemonucleolysis (Fig. 24–3).[9]

To understand the failure of the action of chymopapain in the extruded/sequestered disc herniation, one must appreciate that in addition to the relatively inaccessible location of the disc fragment to chymopapain, the histologic make-up of this mass of material lying in the spinal canal is almost uniformly collagenous and thus unaffected by the enzyme. At the other end of the spectrum is a disc protrusion, potentially containing a considerable amount of proteoglycan, that responds dramatically to chymopapain. The combination of a displaced fragment and the collagenous nature of that fragment makes chymopapain injection for an extruded/sequestered disc useless.

Toxicology

Except in subarachnoid injection, chymopapain has a wide margin of safety between the effective therapeutic dose and the toxic dose.[36] In animal experiments there is a 100-fold margin of safety between the effective therapeutic dose and the toxic dose. Because

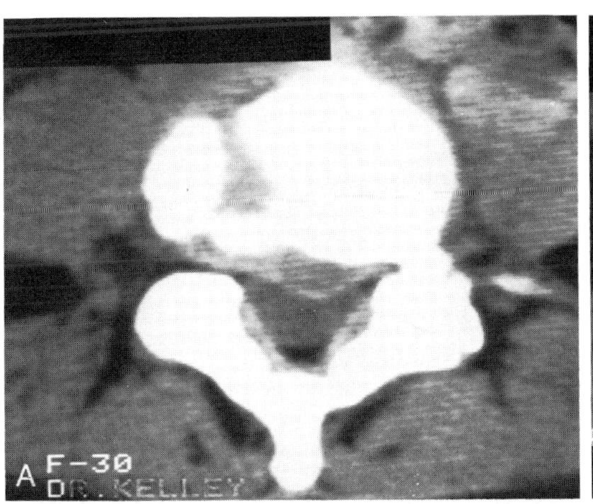

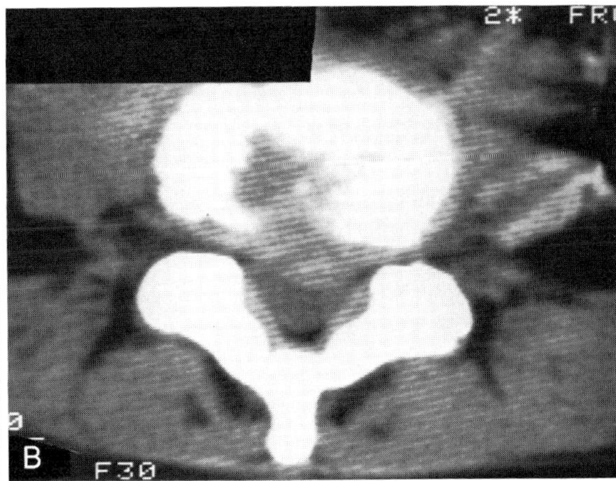

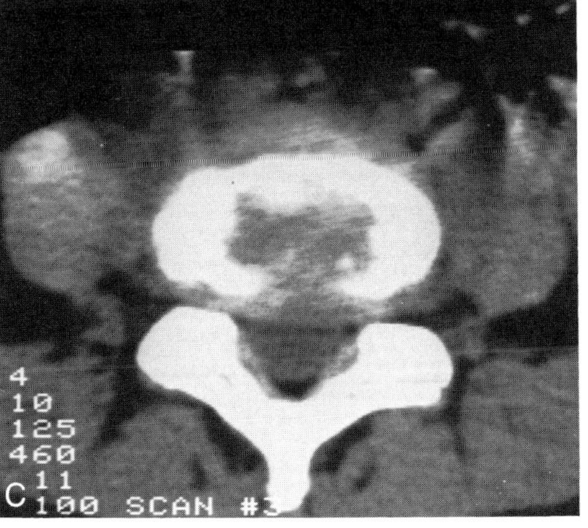

Figure 24–3. *A,* CT scan before chymopapain injection, showing a herniated nucleus pulposus at L4–L5 *(left). B,* CT scan 1 month after the chymopapain injection, showing a persisting defect at L4–L5 *(left)* in spite of relief of symptoms. *C,* CT scan 6 months after the chymopapain injection (and no further treatment), showing the defect to be absent.

chymopapain has no effect on collagenase structures such as bone, ligaments, muscle, nerve, and epidural tissue, it is safe and has virtually no local complications when properly injected. Rydevik and associates reported adverse effects on nerve tissue in rabbit tibial nerves, but this has not been borne out by clinical work.[25, 37]

Chymopapain is dangerous when injected into the subarachnoid space. It dissolves the basement membrane of the pia-arachnoid vessels, resulting in subarachnoid hemorrhage. This hemorrhage can cause a local phenomenon such as arachnoiditis and cauda equina syndrome, or it can spread through the entire cerebrospinal fluid (CSF) space and cause subarachnoid hemorrhage.

In addition, there seems to be a serious, albeit iatrogenic, delayed, possibly hypersensitive effect of chymopapain on the subarachnoid space. This effect has caused transverse myelitis in humans. These topics will be covered in the section on chymopapain complications.

Indications and Contraindications

As with any surgical procedure, it is difficult to obtain good results if one cannot recognize the patients who will respond to treatment. There are clear indications for and contraindications to the use of chymopapain, summarized below.

Indications

There is only one indication for chemonucleolysis with chymopapain—an HNP that causes sciatica (Table 24–1).

Extruded/Sequestered Disc

Within the five criteria listed in Table 24–1, chymopapain is contraindicated in an extruded/sequestered disc, a diagnosis virtually impossible to make on clinical grounds alone. We have reviewed 50 consecutive extruded/sequestered discs (documented at surgery), looking at all aspects of the patient's history and physical examination.[18] Age, sex, type of work, level of disc herniation, side of disc herniation, smoking, onset of symptoms, location of pain, nature of pain, aggravating factors, relieving factors, associated symptoms, progression of symptoms, nerve root tension findings, and neurologic signs offered no clue as to whether or not the disc was an extruded/sequestered fragment. With a few clinical exceptions, the diagnosis of an extruded/sequestered disc is best made on the basis of investigative studies. The following clinical findings suggest an extruded/sequestered fragment, and discolysis is contraindicated:

1. Cauda equina syndrome with bladder and bowel involvement.
2. A large myelographic or computed tomography (CT) defect that is in association with a significant neurologic deficit.
3. Double root involvement, for example, both an L5 and an S1 root lesion.

The following findings on investigation are suggestive of either an extruded/sequestered disc or a chymopapain nonresponsive disc herniation:

1. Large HNP (filling more than 50 per cent of the sagittal diameter on any one magnetic resonance imaging [MRI] or CT scan slice).
2. Pedunculated shape to disc fragment (a disc fragment with a long sagittal dimension and a narrow stalk or coronal dimension).
3. A disc fragment that has migrated away from the disc space.
4. Artifactual changes, such as calcification (osteophyte formation) or air in the fragment.

The following investigative findings suggest that a disc protrusion is present and chymopapain injection may be of benefit:

1. A defect exactly opposite the disc space.
2. A shallow defect with more coronal breadth than sagittal depth (on axial CT or MRI).

Relative Contraindications

Spinal Stenosis

Spinal stenosis affecting the canal or lateral zone never responds to chemonucleolysis. Occasionally these bony defects are complicated by a disc herniation; it is highly unlikely that these combined conditions will be favorably altered by chemonucleolysis. In fact, the postinjection disc space narrowing may aggravate the spinal canal or lateral zone stenosis. This occurrence has led to the false assumption that chymopapain causes spinal stenosis, when in fact stenosis was present but undiagnosed before chemonucleolysis and became a cause of persisting symptoms after injection. The wider use of CT scanning and MRI is eliminating this problem.

Previous Surgery

Patients who have had previous surgery and suffer from recurrent disc herniations at the same level and same side should not have chemonucleolysis. Patients who have had previous surgery and suffer from a disc herniation at a different level or opposite side may benefit from chemonucleolysis.

Strong Contraindications

Degenerative Disc Disease and Facet Joint Disease

Patients with back pain predominantly caused by mechanical instability, either within the disc space or within the facet joint, do not respond to chymopapain injection.

Spinal Instability

Patients with spondylolisthesis do not benefit from the injection of chymopapain at the slip level. In fact, the temporary instability that occurs at a disc space level after the injection of chymopapain could cause an increase in the listhesis.[35] This contraindication applies to both lytic and degenerative spondylolisthesis. A patient with spondylolisthesis may have a symptomatic disc herniation at a level other than the slip level, and that patient would qualify for chymopapain injection, provided he or she fulfills the criteria for diagnosis of a soft disc herniation causing sciatica.

Absolute Contraindications

Sensitivity to Chymopapain

A patient may give a history of an allergy to the ingestion of meat tenderizer or foods containing chymopapain (beer, cheese, and some toothpastes). These patients are at risk for an allergic reaction and should not be considered for chymopapain injection. A positive skin test for chymopapain sensitivity is an obvious contraindication to chymopapain injection.[18] A patient who has had a previous chemonucleoysis may, after a long latent interval, develop another disc herniation at another level. Manufacturers caution against a second chymopapain injection. If that patient has a negative skin test, however, a repeat chemonucleolysis (different level) could be considered.[19]

Disc Herniations at Cord Levels

To date there is no recommendation for chymopapain to be injected into disc herniations at cord levels. The cord level could be either a thoracic or cervical disc. Unfortunately most thoracic discs are calcified, and most cervical radicular syndromes are chronic with an element of bony nerve root entrapment, and a chymopapain injection would be of no benefit. There is ongoing research into the use of chymopapain in the treatment of the infrequent soft cervical disc herniation, and a recommendation for or against injection into soft cervical or thoracic discs cannot be made at this time.

Neurologic Lesion of Unknown Cause

It is unreasonable to risk plant enzyme injection in a patient who has a neurologic problem of obscure cause (e.g., multiple sclerosis).

Pregnant Women

The effect of chymopapain on the fetus has never been documented, and its use in pregnancy is not recommended.

Nonorganic Spinal Pain

Patients with emotional or functional causes of back disability will not benefit from chemonucleolysis.

Patient Age and Duration of Symptoms

Younger patients (below the age of 25) are more likely to have a simple disc protrusion, whereas the more mature patient has a higher incidence of a disc extrusion/sequestration. There is a tendency for the older patient or the patient with many years of symptoms to have associated diagnoses such as spinal stenosis. The adult (average age 40) and the older patient (over 55) often have pathology nonresponsive to chymopapain; thus, the most common use of chemonucleolysis is in the younger patient with a simple disc protrusion.[14]

Aim of Therapy

Most physicians view chemonucleolysis as the last step in conservative treatment before surgical intervention is considered. Since most disc ruptures occur at single levels, chemonucleolysis should be done only at single levels. When selecting patients for chymopapain injection, only those in whom good surgical result are expected should be considered. Chymopapain should not be used as a catch-all for patients rejected for surgery. Almost all patients in whom chymopapain injection fails should have surgical intervention, because most of them will be found to have a sequestered or extruded disc.

PREOPERATIVE CHYMOPAPAIN SENSITIVITY TESTING

The best strategy for coping with chymopapain sensitivity, specifically anaphylaxis, is to identify patients at risk and exclude them from the injection of chymopapain. We have experimented with a sensitive and sufficiently specific skin test, the prick test.[19] Skin testing in 1000 consecutive patients has shown no anaphylactic or other severe immediate hypersensitivity reactions in patients who had a negative skin test.[18] There appears to be a high level of confidence in this approach, enough to recommend the chymopapain skin test to detect chymopapain sensitivity. Tests for chymopapain antibody level (immunoglobulin E), such as ChymoFAST and RAST, are also available but are not considered as reliable as skin testing.

TECHNIQUE OF CHEMONUCLEOLYSIS

Considerable confusion arose when one manufacturer originally recommended the use of general anesthesia, premedication, a needle insertion site 8 cm from the midline, a 45-degree angle to approach the disc space, single-needle technique to get into the L5–S1 disc space, and the use of contrast material for discographic assessment for disc integrity.[30] After the complications that followed the release of chymopapain in the United States, a critical review suggested that a safer protocol was in order, resulting in some changes recommended in the technique of chemonucleolysis.[31] They essentially repeat the recommendations of numerous authors, and include the use of local neuroleptic anesthesia, the selection of a needle insertion site at an adequate distance from the midline (10 cm average), the use of a double-needle technique for at least the L5–S1 disc space, and the avoidance of discography using contrast material.[24, 36]

Whether or not contrast material is used, the basic technical rule is that you must know exactly where the needle tip is before injecting chymopapain. If this requires the use of contrast material and a screening roentgenogram, contrast material must be used. With proper needle insertion technique and two good radiographs at 90 degrees to each other, routine use of contrast material is not necessary to localize needle tip position.

LOCAL VERSUS GENERAL ANESTHESIA

Local anesthesia (augmented with neuroleptic agents) is the anesthetic of choice for the following reasons:

1. It is safer.
2. It is efficient; it shortens operating room (OR) time and the patient's stay in the hospital.
3. The patient avoids the complications of general anesthesia and intubation.
4. It allows for earlier intervention in the event of a complication, such as anaphylaxis.
5. It preserves discometry or discography as a test.

After a negative skin test, it is highly unlikely that a patient will experience a hypersensitivity reaction, and thus the main reason for suggesting general anesthesia is eliminated.

PREMEDICATION—TEST DOSE REGIMEN

I do not premedicate or use a test dose.[30] Rather than assume that all patients are at risk and premedicate, one should attempt to identify reactors with an allergic history and a skin test. Other tests, such as RAST or ChymoFAST, are available.

The reasons for not premedicating are as follows:

1. The incidence of anaphylaxis is low (0.35 per cent), and lower still with skin testing.[8]
2. There is no scientific evidence that premedication lowers the incidence below this figure in our experience.
3. Any treatment considered to be prophylactic should contain the most effective agent; in anaphylaxis this is epinephrine. Obviously it cannot be included in a prophylactic program.
4. Patients who have been premedicated according to recommendations have experienced severe anaphylactic reactions.[28]
5. Patients who have received an intradiscal test dose (not skin test) of chymopapain have experienced severe anaphylactic reactions.[28]
6. Anaphylaxis requires aggressive treatment as follows:
   a. The doses of cortisone and antihistamines required to treat anaphylaxis are much greater than the recommended doses in the premedication regimen.
   b. The addition of epinephrine.
7. The best defense against anaphylaxis is
   a. Identification and exclusion of the hypersensitive patient (skin test).
   b. An alert, well-prepared team of assistants.

OPERATING ROOM OR RADIOLOGY DEPARTMENT

The OR has the greatest concentration of skilled personnel for managing the complications of discolysis. Generally speaking, life-threatening emergencies such as anaphylaxis severely stress a radiology department. If operating room image intensifier capabilities are less than optimal for the performance of chemonucleolysis, however, the radiology department will have to be used.

PRONE OR LATERAL POSITION?

The lateral position is the choice of most users. The prone position is acceptable, provided the puncture site is not too lateral. Theoretically, the bowel has not fallen away from the lateral abdominal gutter in the prone position. In the lateral position, the bowel falls away from the lateral gutter, and a 10-cm insertion site is safe.

Principles of the Lateral Approach

1. Maintain proper position of the patient. If the procedure is being performed with the patient in the lateral position, there is a tendency for the awake patient to roll out of the perfect lateral position. The most common mistake made by the beginner trying to get a needle into a disc space is to miss that the patient has rolled into an oblique position.

2. Select the correct disc. It is important to see the front of the sacrum before selecting the disc space for injection. One can inadvertently put a needle into the L3–L4 disc space, believing it to be at the L4–L5 level. This can be prevented by viewing the front of the sacrum before counting levels. Four or six lumbar vertebrae or other congenital lumbosacral anomalies can confuse the selection of the disc space to be punctured.

3. Select the correct insertion site. It is important to get far enough from the midline. In the average patient 10 cm from the midline, adjacent to the iliac crest, is the correct insertion site. In a larger patient one may have to go further than 10 cm from the midline, and in a smaller patient a needle insertion site closer to the midline should be selected.

4. Approach the disc at the proper angle. The angle of approach to the disc space is

closer to 60 degrees than 45 degrees; however, it is important to remember that the needle must not penetrate the foramen and enter the spinal canal to puncture the subarachnoid space. It is advisable to leave the stylet out of the needle as an additional precaution. Inadvertent puncture of the subarachnoid space is then heralded by the immediate backflow of CSF, signaling the necessity to abort the procedure and reschedule in two to three weeks.

5. Position the needle tip in the center of the disc. The center of the disc space is defined as the middle third of the disc space on lateral roentgenogram and superimposed on the spinous process on anteroposterior (AP) roentgenogram.

6. Discography or discometry. The use of contrast or the water acceptance test will support the fact that the needle tip is within the discal cavity.

7. Dose. The proper amount of active chymopapain to be injected into a clean disc space ranges from 0.75 to 1.0 ml (2000 pKat/cc).

If more than three passes of the needle have occurred without entry to the disc space being achieved, abort the procedure. Similarly, if you penetrate the nerve root (i.e., cause severe leg pain), abort the procedure. I recommend that after puncturing the skin, the stylet should be removed from the needle and the needle advanced toward the disc space with an open lumen. If you inadvertently cross the subarachnoid space on advancing the needle, the immediate backflow of CSF will be ample notification to abort the procedure. Never abandon the lateral approach for the midline transdural approach.

POSTOPERATIVE CARE

The most important thing to recognize about postoperative management of the patient after chemonucleolysis is the tremendous variation in patient response to the procedure and recovery from the chemical disc excision. Approximately 20 per cent of patients have significant back pain (back spasms) immediately after the procedure. This is best managed with an intravenous or intramuscular dose of steroids. This back spasm usually settles a few hours to a few days after the procedure. The pain is severe and is usually more severe than the pain that occurs after surgical intervention.[2] Eighty per cent of the patients do not have excessive back pain, and their symptoms can be controlled by moderate doses of oral analgesics. Most patients benefit from a light canvas corset support, which helps them ambulate in the initial weeks after chymopapain injection.

There are three courses of postinjection leg pain. Often there is dramatic relief of leg pain, but most patients destined for a good result notice a gradual reduction. Leg cramping and paresthetic discomfort in the leg are the last to disappear. Paresthetic discomfort often takes many weeks to go away. A patient may notice a dramatic increase in leg pain immediately after injection. If this happens an unsuspected extruded disc has been made worse by injection. This patient requires swift surgical intervention (within a day or two of the procedure) to remove the extruded or sequestered fragment of disc material.

Patients are usually discharged from the hospital the same day or within one or two days after chymopapain injection.[20] Analgesic or muscle-relaxant medication are usually required for one to two weeks after discharge. Self-employed patients may feel compelled to return to work within the first week after injection, but a patient with light occupational demands should wait two to four weeks before considering a return to work. Patients who have heavier work demands should convalesce for the same amount of time as patients who undergo standard laminectomy/discectomy. The return to leisure activity varies according to its form. The first leisure activity usually available to patients is swimming, which can be started two to four weeks after injection.

It is advisable to see patients one month after the procedure for assessment, including roentgenogram. Patients who have lost most of their leg pain, who have improved in straight leg raising (SLR) ability, and who show disc space narrowing on a plain lateral roentgenogram are destined for an excellent result. Patients with some improvement in leg discomfort and some improvement in SLR may be observed for an additional one to two months before a decision about future treatment intervention is made. Those patients who have unaltered leg pain one month after the procedure usually have persisting SLR reduction and the procedure can be considered a failure. These patients need immediate surgical intervention. As mentioned earlier, most of these patients have an extruded or sequestered disc and benefit from microsurgical intervention.[13] If CT or MRI is used preoperatively, most cases of lateral recess stenosis will have been promptly and correctly diagnosed and not selected for chemonucleolysis. If myelography was the only available method of evaluating patients, however, a number of failures may have lateral recess (zone) stenosis. These patients require appropriate decompression.

RESULTS

The decisive study supporting the efficacy of chemonucleolysis was completed by Fraser.[5,6] Using carefully selected patients he demonstrated a 75 per cent success rate two years after chemonucleolysis compared with placebo (50 per cent) response in saline-injected controls. Other blinded studies have supported Fraser's conclusions.[3,11]

Other publications have reported results varying from poor to 90 to 95 per cent success. I have experienced approximately a 70 per cent good result rate, slightly higher for younger patients, and slightly better at the L5–S1 level in all age groups.[14,20,36]

The most common cause of failure is the sequestered or extruded fragment of disc material that has not been dissolved by chymopapain. Since the nuclear content of the disc space has been dissolved by the chymopapain, little work needs to be done within the disc space itself during surgery. In fact, microsurgery dealing with the spinal canal pathology alone is the treatment of choice in these patients.[13] Chemonucleolysis did not compromise surgical intervention in over 300 personal cases.

It is obvious that the 70 per cent good result rate will be improved on only by correctly identifying patients who have an extruded/sequestered disc and using surgical excision in these cases.

COMPLICATIONS

Anaphylaxis

Anaphylaxis occurs in 0.35 per cent of patients who have not been prescreened. It is manifested by a profound drop in blood pressure and requires vigorous immediate resuscitation to save the patient's life.[8] The cornerstones of treatment for anaphylaxis are appropriate doses of epinephrine, large volumes of intravenous fluids, steroids, and antihistamines.

With the use of skin testing, anaphylaxis is becoming a less frequent problem. I have seen 1000 cases of chymopapain injection preceded by skin testing for chymopapain sensitivity. To date, there has not been an anaphylactic reaction in a patient who has had a negative skin test. This represents data from a combined study in Berlin, Germany, and Akron, Ohio.[20] Thus the management of anaphylaxis has moved into prophylaxis. Any patient with a positive skin test is eliminated from treatment with chymopapain.

Neurologic Complications

Chymopapain, with or without contrast material, injected into the subarachnoid space is almost certain to be disastrous. It is extremely important that the needle tip does not cross the subarachnoid space on insertion into the nuclear cavity or reside in the subarachnoid space at the time of injection. If there is any question about the needle tip position, the procedure should be aborted.

The possibility of a connection between the disc space and the subarachnoid space is the one drawback to not using contrast material at the time of needle placement. It is obvious after injecting contrast material into the disc that when it appears in the subarachnoid space, there is a connection between the disc cavity and the subarachnoid space. The most common cause of this connection is crossing the subarachnoid space on needle insertion. It is my opinion that whenever there is any degree of resistance to injection of test material into the nuclear cavity, it is highly unlikely that there is a connection between the disc space and the subarachnoid space. For this reason, it is possible to use a water acceptance test rather than contrast material at the time of chymopapain injection.

Injection of chymopapain (with or without contrast material) into the subarachnoid space may cause subarachnoid hemorrhage with cerebral complications, a cauda equina syndrome, or a delayed traverse myelitis. Preliminary experimental work suggests that it is not chymopapain alone but the combination of chymopapain and contrast material in the subarachnoid space that causes serious neurologic complications.[29] Other research suggests that chymopapain alone is capable of causing subarachnoid hemorrhage and serious neurologic complications.[37]

Miscellaneous Complications

Two miscellaneous complications of chemonucleolysis require consideration. The first is root damage from penetration of the nerve root at the time of needle insertion. This usually occurs under general anesthesia, and affects the fifth lumbar nerve root, with damage caused by attempting to get the needle into the L5–S1 disc space.[38] Root penetration has led to some permanent causalgic syndromes. Under local neuroleptic anesthesia, this is a rare complication.

A second complication is discitis. This is either low-grade infective discitis or chemical discitis that results in a prolongation of the patient's back pain and a typical roentgenographic picture. Fraser and associates have done the definitive work in this area as well.[6] They have shown that although chymopapain is bactericidal in vitro, it does not appear to prevent a particular type of disc inflammation in vivo. Histologic sections of sheep disc spaces injected with chymopapain and bacteria showed some signs of disc space infection and some cultured out of the bacteria *(Staphylococcus epidermidis)*. They concluded that most cases of discitis, although low grade in severity and often sterile on culture, originate from bacterial contamination of the disc at the time of the procedure.

Other authors have described increased signal intensity on T2-weighted MRI images in the portion of the vertebral bodies adjacent to the disc space injected with chymopapain.[9, 15] Initially this was believed to represent chemical discitis, but when it was also noticed after surgical discectomy and as part of the degenerative process in unoperated and uninjected patients, it was concluded that these changes are nonspecific inflammatory or edematous reactions to disc insult or degeneration.[12] Fulminating septic discitis with systemic manifestations is infrequent. When this does occur, the basic principles of management of any infective discitis apply.

FAILURES

It is possible with any surgical therapy to select a patient with nonphysical disability, to make the wrong diagnosis, or to perform the wrong operation and end up with a poor result. This has happened, and continues to happen, with selection of patients for chymopapain injection. True failures in chymopapain injection should almost always be due to a pathologic condition within the spinal canal, and almost always this is an extruded or sequestered disc.

It should be possible to determine that a patient has failed to respond to chemonucleolysis four to six weeks after injection. Subsequent surgery is not compromised by chemonucleolysis. In fact, there is a discolysis advantage—within a number of weeks after injection of chymopapain into the disc space, the disc space narrowing offers some degree of stability. Furthermore, there is no nuclear material left within the disc space and thus no extensive disc space dissection is needed. Finally, the absence of nuclear material within the disc space and the surgical removal of all nuclear material within the spinal canal should result in an extremely low recurrence rate.[13]

WHAT HAS HAPPENED TO CHEMONUCLEOLYSIS AS A CLINICAL PROCEDURE?

Most surgeons have abandoned the use of chymopapain, and with good reason. The reasons can best be summarized as medical, legal, and political.

1. Medical
    a. Chemonucleolysis does not deliver consistently good results compared with surgery, but chemonucleolysis is the last step in conservative care, and it is unfair to compare the procedure with surgery.
    b. There is more postinjection back pain after chemonucleolysis than after surgical discectomy.
    c. The neurologic complications of cauda equina syndrome, subarachnoid hemorrhage, and transverse myelitis have contributed to the negative image of chemonucleolysis.
    d. The newer diagnostic modalities of CT and MRI have enabled much more ac-

curate diagnosis of the nature and location of the pathology of a disc rupture. This has allowed for a more accurate identification of the patient who will respond to chemonucleolysis, significantly limiting its indications compared with the early days of chemonucleolysis, when diagnoses were supported by oil myelography.

2. Legal
   a. In the United States the legal community has seized on the complications and failures of chemonucleolysis with a fervor that has dampened enthusiasm for the procedure. They have been aided by medical expert witnesses who testify about the negative aspects of chemonucleolysis.
3. Political
   a. The manufacturers of the product have contributed significantly to the demise of chemonucleolysis by building false expectations for outcome, poorly preparing the surgical community for its widespread use, and getting involved in many conflict-of-interest situations such as company officers and stockholders occupying positions of scientific trust without disclosing their conflict.

THE FUTURE OF CHEMONUCLEOLYSIS

Chemonucleolysis with chymopapain is a less invasive, lower-risk, less expensive surgical procedure in patients who have an HNP that causes sciatica. In spite of the recent serious complications and deaths, there is a wide margin of safety between chemonucleolysis and surgical intervention for disc disease (Table 24–3). In the properly selected patient, there is at least a 70 per cent chance of a successful result.

Table 24–3. COMPARISON OF SURGICAL AND CHEMONUCLEOLYSIS COMPLICATIONS

Complications	Surgery (%)	Chemonucleolysis USA (%)	Chemonucleolysis Europe (%)
Mortality	0.3[32]	0.02[23]	0.0[1]
Morbidity			
Serious	0.02[16, 17, 32]	0.05[1]	0.04[1]
Anaphylaxis	0.00	0.5[23]	0.06[1]
Less serious	2.0[16, 32]	0.03[23]	0.8[1]
General	2 to 3	Extremely low	

In my experience chemonucleolysis with chymopapain has been a safe, simple, and effective treatment modality in over 7000 patients. If it is successful, the patient avoids a back incision. The patient is in the hospital for less time, and in some cases a faster return to work is possible. Two studies suggest that the long-term results are excellent and the recurrence rate is extremely low.[14, 33] Finally, failure to respond to chymopapain injection does not compromise future surgical considerations.

References

1. Bouillet, R.: Complications of discal hernia therapy: comparative study regarding surgical therapy and nucleolysis by chymopapain. Acta Orthop. Belg. *49*(Suppl):48, 1983.
2. Brown, M. D., and Tompkins, J. S.: Pain response post-chemonucleolysis or disc excision. Spine *14:*321, 1989.
3. Dabezies, E. J., Langford, K., Morris, J., et al.: Safety and efficacy of chymopapain (discase) in the treatment of sciatica due to a herniated nucleus pulposus: results of a randomized, double-blinded study. Spine *13:*561, 1988.
4. Fraser, R. D.: Chymopapain for the treatment of intervertebral disc herniation: a preliminary resport of a double-blinded study. Spine *7:*608, 1982.
5. Fraser, R. D.: Chymopapain for the treatment of intervertebral disc herniation: the final report of the double-blinded study. Spine *9:*815, 1984.
6. Fraser, R. D., Osti, O. L., and Vernon-Roberts, B.: 1986 Volvo Award in basic science: discitis following chemonucleolysis: an experimental study. Spine *11:*679, 1986.
7. Gentry, L., Turski, P. A., Strother, C. M., et al.: Chymopapain chemonucleolysis: CT changes after treatment. A. J. R. *145:*361, 1985.
8. Hall, B. B., and McCulloch, J. A.: Anaphylactic reactions following the intradiscal injection of chymopapain under local anesthesia. J. Bone Joint Surg. *65A:*1215, 1983.
9. Huckman, M. S., Clark, J. W., McNeill, T. W., et al.: Chemonucleation and changes observed on lumbar MR scan: preliminary report. A. J. N. R. *8:*1, 1987.
10. Jansen, E. F., and Balls, A. K.: Chymopapain: new crystalline proteinase from papaya latex. J. Biol. Chem. *137:*459, 1941.
11. Javid, J. J., Hordby, E. J., Ford, L. T., et al.: Safety and efficacy of chymopapain (chymodiactin) in herniated nucleus pulposus with sciatica. J. A. M. A. *249:*2489, 1983.
12. Katz, M. E., Teitelbaum, S. L., Gilula, L. A., et al.: Radiologic and pathologic patterns of end-plate-based vertebral sclerosis. Invest. Radiol. *23:*447, 1988.
13. Kitaoka, H., and McCulloch, J. A.: Microdiscectomy for failed chemonucleolysis. Neuro-orthopaedics *5:*45, 1988.
14. Lorenz, M., and McCulloch, J. A.: Chemonucleolysis for herniated nucleus pulposus in adolescents. Presented to American Academy of Orthopaedic Sur-

geons, Las Vegas. J. Bone Joint Surg. *67A*:1402–1404, 1985.

15. Masaryk, T. J., Boumphrey, F., Modic, M. T., et al.: Effects of chemonucleolysis demonstrated by MR imaging. J. Comput. Assist. Tomogr. *10:*917, 1986.
16. Mayfield, F. H.: Complications of laminectomy. Clin. Neurosurg. *23*:435, 1976.
17. McLaren, A. C., and Bailey, S. I.: Cauda equina syndrome: a complication of lumbar discectomy. Clin. Orthop. *204:*143, 1986.
18. McCulloch, J. A., and Lambe, D.: Unpublished data.
19. McCulloch, J. A., Dolovich, G., and Canham, W.: Skin testing for chymopapain allergy: a preliminary report. Ann. Allergy *55:*609, 1985.
20. McCulloch, J. A.: Outpatient discolysis with chymopapain. Orthopedics *6:*1624, 1983.
21. McCulloch, J. A., and Brock, M.: Unpublished data.
22. McCulloch, J. A.: Chemonucleolysis for relief of sciatica due to a herniated intervertebral disc. Can. Med. Assoc. J. *124:*880, 1981.
23. Morris, J.: Complications of chemonucleolysis. Presented at Spine Update, San Francisco, 1984.
24. Parkinson, D., and Shields, C.: Treatment of protruded lumbar intervertebral discs with chymopapain. J. Neurosurg. *39:*203, 1973.
25. Rydevik, B., Brånemark, P-I., Norberg, C., et al.: Effects of chymopapain on nerve tissue. Spine *1:*137, 1976.
26. Schwetschenau, P. R., Ramirez, A., Johnston, J., et al.: Double-blind evaluations of intradiscal chymopapain for herniated lumbar discs: early results. J. Neurosurg. *45:*622, 1976.
27. Smith, L.: Enzyme dissolution of nucleus pulposus in humans. J. A. M. A. *187:*137, 1964.
28. Smith Laboratories, Inc., Northbrook, Il. Data from postmarketing surveillance, 1985.
29. Smith Laboratories, Inc., Northbrook, Il. Advertising brochure.
30. Smith Laboratories, Inc., Northbrook, Il. Original product brochure.
31. Smith Laboratories, Inc., Northbrook, Il. Product information letter, July 1984.
32. Spangfort, E. V.: The lumbar disc herniation: a computer-aided analysis of 2,504 operations. Acta Orthop. Scand. *142*(Suppl):1, 1972.
33. Tregonning, G. D., Transfeldt, E. E., McCulloch, J. A., et al.: Chymopapain vs. conventional surgery for lumbar disc herniation: a ten year follow-up. Presented at The Annual Meeting American Academy of Orthopaedic Surgeons. Las Vegas, February 1989.
34. Travenol Laboratories, Inc.: New Drug Application 18-625. Submitted to United States Food and Drug Administration, April 1981.
35. Wakano, K., Kasman, R., Chao, E. Y., et al.: Biochemical analysis of canine intervertebral disc after chymopapain injection: a preliminary report. Spine *8:*59, 1983.
36. Weiner, D. S., and Macnab, I.: The use of chymopapain in degenerative disc disease: a preliminary report. Can. Med. Assoc. J. *102:*1252, 1970.
37. Wiltse, L. L.: Chymopapain chemonucleolysis in lumbar disc disease. J. A. M. A. *233:*1164, 1975.
38. Wiltse, L. L., Widell, E. H., and Hansen, A. Y.: Chymopapain chemonucleolysis in lumbar disc disease. J. A. M. A. *231:*474, 1975.

PERCUTANEOUS AUTOMATED DISCECTOMY

Joseph C. Maroon, M.D.
Gary Onik, M.D.

Approximately 200,000 patients per year undergo surgical removal of lumbar discs in the United States. Surgical results from a laminotomy, laminectomy, or microdiscectomy have a success rate as high as 90 per cent in carefully selected patients. Despite these good results, there is still risk to soft tissues, joints, nerves, and the invariable production of epidural fibrosis. In 1964, Smith suggested that chemonucleolysis with chymopapain introduced percutaneously might be an alternative to open surgical procedures without the attendant risks of surgery.[8] When finally released by the FDA in 1984, over 70,000 papain injections were performed in the United States in the course of a six-month period. Unfortunately, complications such as anaphylaxis, subarachnoid hemorrhage, transverse myelitis, and severe back pain have resulted in marked limitation of this procedure.

Conceptually, however, percutaneous discectomy has continued to be an attractive alternative to many investigators. Hijikata and associates performed the first percutaneous discectomy in 1975 without chemonucleolysis.[3] A cannula approximately 5 mm in diameter was inserted against the lateral annulus, and disc material was removed through long pituitary forceps. Hijikata subsequently used this procedure in over 100 patients with a reported 70 per cent success rate. He experienced one case of discitis and a major vascular injury.[4]

In 1983 Kambin and Gellman reported results using a comparable procedure, again with no complications. A report in 1989 by Kambin on 100 patients revealed a success rate of 85 per cent.[5]

Schreiber and Suezawa modified Hijikata's technique, and through a contralateral percutaneous approach inserted a fiberoptic discoscope to visualize the material actually being removed. They reported a 72 per cent success rate in 109 patients treated over an eight-year period. A 7 per cent incidence of discitis and injury to the lumbar plexis in two patients and a major vessel in another are serious concerns, however.[7]

In 1983 Friedman evaluated a technique previously presented by Jacobson using a straight lateral approach to the disc space and involved the insertion of a 40 French chest tube.[2a] The disc was then extracted with specially designed long instrumentation. He concluded that this procedure was unsafe because of the potential of bowel and nerve injury.

All the above techniques accomplished decompression percutaneously by manually removing disc fragments with long, specially designed grasping forceps. Because of the repeated reentry of the grasping forceps into the discs, the chance for infection is increased. Also, the large size of the instruments resulted in a higher incidence of nerve root injury as well as major vessel damage in at least two instances. Aware of these problems, Onik and associates described an automated percutaneous discectomy technique that used a reciprocating suction cutting device for aspirating, amputating, and then sucking out disc material. The reciprocating guillotine-like knife moved across a single side port enclosed in a blunt-tipped cannula at 180 times per minute. This increased the speed of the procedure and reduced the size of the instrumentation to 2 mm. Since the instrument was placed into the disc space only once, there was a much lower chance for infection. In addition, a curved cannula was designed through which the flexible nucleotome could be placed reliably into the L5–S1 disc space.[6]

Since the introduction of this automated technique, approximately 30,000 of these procedures have been done in the United States with no mortality. The morbidity primarily consists of a 0.2 per cent discitis rate.[1] The purpose of this section is to present the criteria for patient selection, review the technique, and present the results to date in various clinical trials.

PATIENT SELECTION

As with any surgical procedure, success depends on patient selection. Percutaneous automated discectomy (PAD) is effective in treating those patients with small to moderate, well-contained disc herniations that show evidence clinically and radiographically of nerve root compression. The most important clinical symptoms occur in patients who have leg pain greater than back pain and have failed all conservative measures and remain significantly disabled by pain. A history of paresthetic discomfort in a specific dermatomal distribution is significant. Physical findings usually include a positive SLR examination, slight weakness of the extensor hallucis longus or plantor flexors of the foot, mild sensory disturbances, and reflex alterations in a specific dermatome. Posterior leg pain that does not radiate below the knee is viewed with suspicion, particularly if it is not associated with other physical findings. The disruption of other soft tissues, such as facet joints, can cause referred leg pain of this nature, and careful palpation and evaluation of flexion, extension, and rotation of the lumbosacral spine is indicated. If there is marked weakness in any muscle group, bowel or bladder disturbances, or profound sensory loss, this procedure should not be considered. Also, a cross-positive SLR sign is usually a strong indication of a sequestered fragment and contraindicates the use of percutaneous discectomy.

A demonstrated radiographic abnormality on CT, MRI, or intrathecally enhanced CT and myelography must be present and correlate with the patient's physical findings. The ideal candidate is one who has a small to moderate-size focal herniation or bulge that makes an impression on the thecal sac consistent with the patient's symptomatology (Figs. 24–4, 24–5). Patients with degenerative disc disease and diffuse annular bulging extending from the entire circumference of the vertebral body are not candidates for this procedure. Also to be excluded are patients with lateral recess stenosis, calcified disc herniations, or moderate to severe dentral spinal stenosis (Fig. 24–6). Patients with evidence of instability, such as anterolisthesis or retrolisthesis, are also not candidates for the procedure.

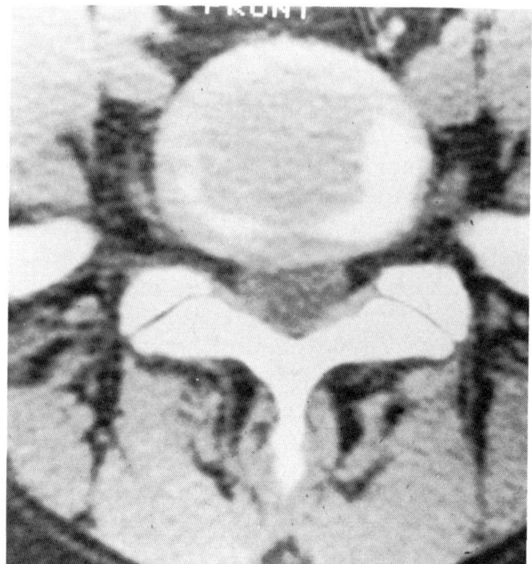

Figure 24–4. CT scan of the L5–S1 level showing a small, well-contained, focal, right-sided HNP. Conservative therapy failed and the patient responded well to a percutaneous discectomy.

A major task in obtaining good results is determining whether the disc is contained by the annulus or posterior longitudinal ligament or whether it has extruded through the posterior longitudinal ligament. The most definitive criterion for a sequestered disc is the demonstration of a fragment superiorly or inferiorly from the disc space by radiographic means (Figs. 24–7, 24–8). In the axial view, because of partial volume averaging, it is possible in contained herniation to see some disc material above or below the disc space; it is important to demonstrate, however, that the epi-center or the largest portion of the herniation is at the disc level, and sagittal MRI can be helpful in this determination. Also, there must be contiguous axial sections on MRI and CT scans from L3 to S1 with no associated gaps to exclude far lateral herniations as well as migrated fragments.

The size of the herniation is also used in determining whether or not it has extruded. Freis and associates have shown that herniations that compromise the thecal sac by 50 per cent or more had a 90 per cent correlation with sequestration.[2] Therefore, any herniation that size should not be considered for percutaneous discectomy. A further radiographic point is that the angle of the herniation of the disc should be obtuse. Acute angulations indicate the extrusions and contraindicate percutaneous discectomy (Fig. 24–9).

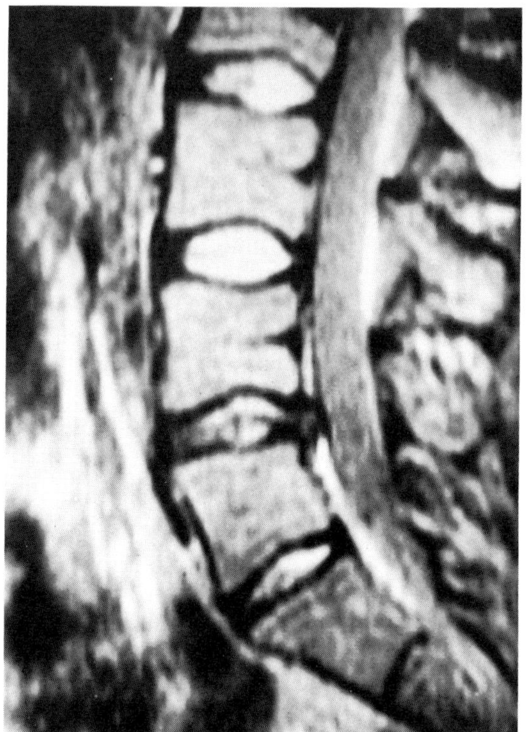

Figure 24–5. Sagittal MRI scan showing a well-contained herniation to the L4–L5 level.

Finally, discography, although controversial, may be helpful in excluding those patients likely to have extruded disc fragments. The most important criterion of discography is

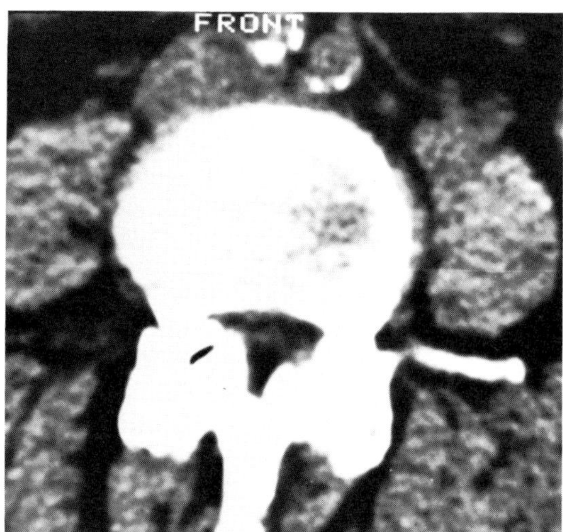

Figure 24–6. CT scan showing severe facet hypertrophy with lateral recessed stenosis as well as central canal stenosis.

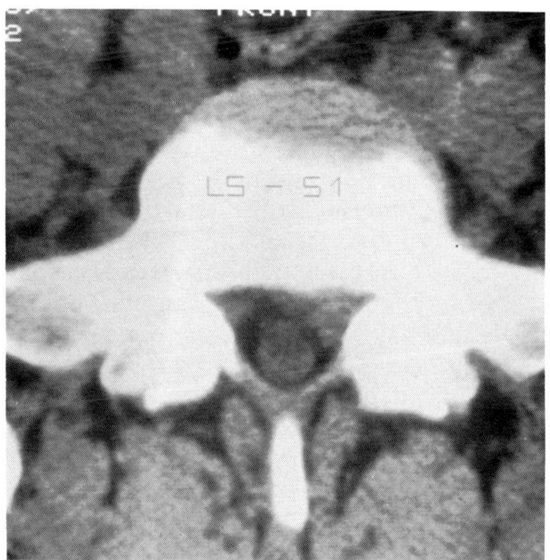

Figure 24–7. CT scan at the L5–S1 level showing a free fragment of disc in the left lateral recess.

whether the herniation fills with contrast medium injected into the center of the disc. If the herniation is well outlined by contrast and is contained by the posterior longitudinal ligament, good results may be anticipated (Fig. 24–10). If there is extravasation of contrast up and down the spinal canal, invariably poor results may be anticipated (Fig. 24–11). It is conceivable that a false-positive diagnosis for

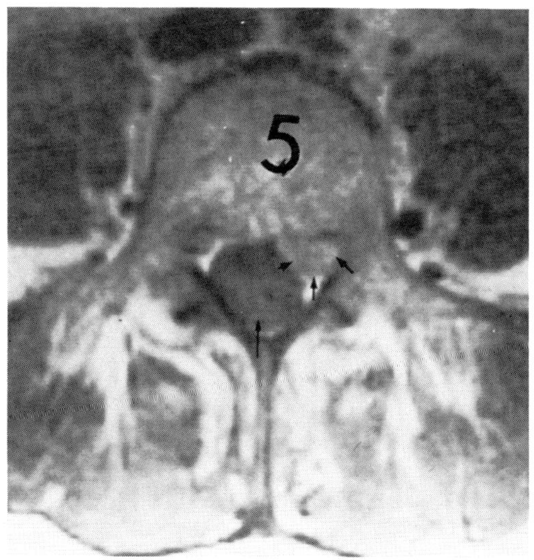

Figure 24–8. Sagittal axial MRI scan showing a free fragment of disc at the L4–L5 level, again in the lateral recess.

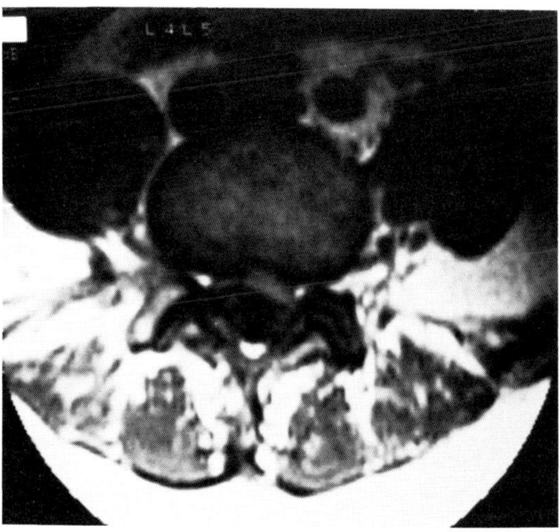

Figure 24–9. Axial MRI scan showing an HNP at the L4–L5 level *(to the left).* Note the sharp angulations of the herniation with disc margin indicated as an extruded fragment.

extrusion can occur if contrast medium flows behind the posterior longitudinal ligament, but if this occurs, we generally do not do the procedure.

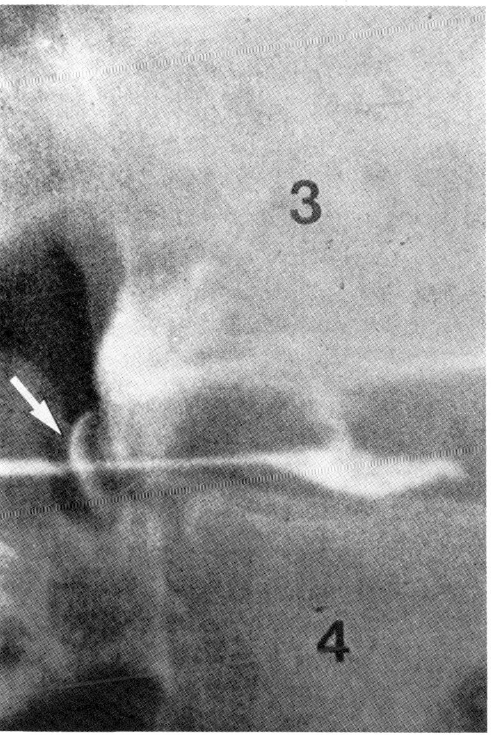

Figure 24–10. Discogram at the L3–L4 level showing contrast material outlining a well-contained herniation *(arrow).* No free flow of contrast is noted here.

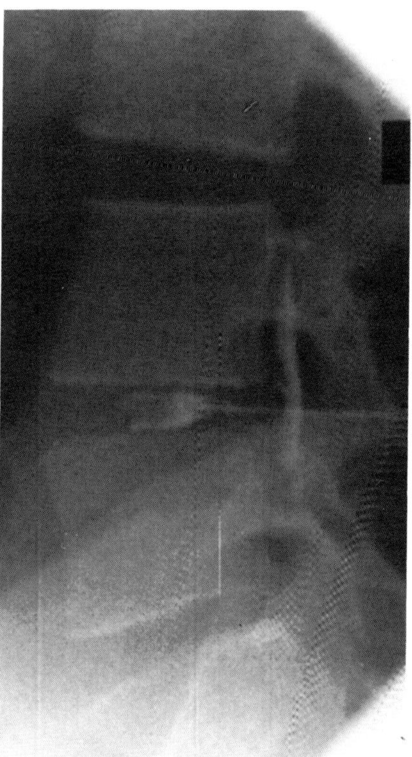

Figure 24–11. Discogram at the L4–L5 level showing free flow of contrast into the epidural space, indicating a complete tear of the annulus posterior longitudinal ligament, which implies a high likelihood of a free fragment.

TECHNIQUE

The safety of PAD relies on guiding the nucleotome into the disc space with precise radiographic control. Since a small but significant number of patients have colon posteriorly behind the psosis, when placed in the prone position, a localizing CT scan is obtained to rule out this possibility. Using this localizing scan, it is also possible to select a tentative entry site using the cursor on the CT scan on the same side as the patient's symptoms.

The procedure is performed in the lateral decubitus position, which minimizes the radiation exposure to the operator and allows flexion and extension of the patient during the procedure. To open the disc space posteriorly and decrease the lumbar lordosis, the patient must be perfectly straight and not rotated. When using the fluoroscope one must count up from the sacrum, viewing with continuous fluoroscopy so that the inadvertent disc space is not punctured by the small fluoroscopic image on some C arms. Since all of the structures to be avoided, such as great vessels and bowels, lie anteriorly, the AP view is inadequate for monitoring. We therefore use the lateral view initially and never insert the tip of the trochar anterior to the line that connects the posterior vertebral bodies (Fig. 24–12). Any trochar placement that strikes the spine anterior to this line will have an anterior trajectory and will be an inadequate placement.

The insertion site is 8 to 14 cm lateral from the midline depending on the patient's body habitus. The procedure is performed under local anesthesia. A 22-gauge spinal needle is used to anesthetize the skin and the deeper tissue. An 18-gauge introduction trochar is then placed into the correct position, abutting the annulus. If radicular pain is experienced with insertion of the trocar, redirection is indicated. When lying against the annulus in the AP view, the trochar should be lateral to a line that joins the medial border of the pedicles. This confirms that it is outside the thecal sac (Fig. 24–13). When in this position, it can

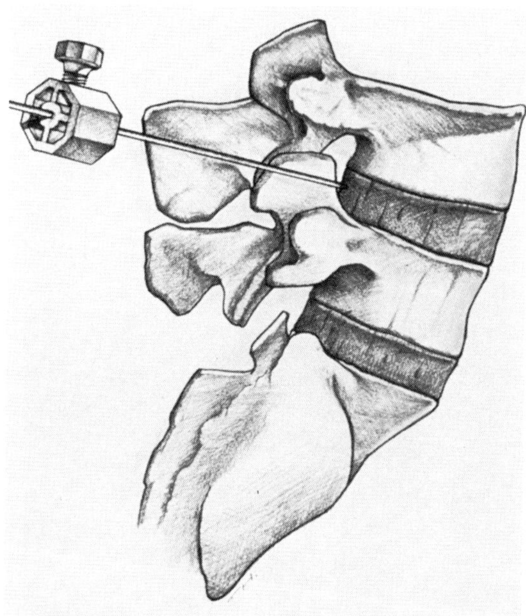

Figure 24–12. Lateral diagram of lumbar spine showing a trocar lying against the annulus at the L4–L5 level. The tip of the trocar is sitting on the imaginary line that connects the posterior vertebral bodies. If the trocar was anterior to the posterior vertebral body line, it would indicate an anterior trajectory and should be replaced.

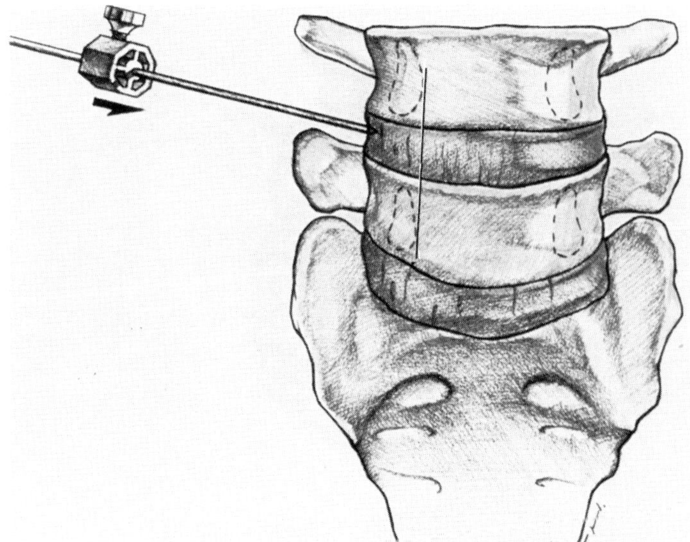

Figure 24–13. In the anteroposterior view, the tip of the trocar is lateral to the line that connects the medial border of the pedicles. Since the thecal sac lies medial to the medial border of the pedicles, this confirms that the tip of the trocar is not traversing the thecal sac on its way to the center of the disc.

be advanced into the center of the disc space (Fig. 24–14). Since we want to be as close as possible to the disc herniation, any placement that has an anterior trajectory is not acceptable and needs to be corrected.

Once the trochar is in the correct position, the tissue dilator and cannula are placed over the trochar down to the annulus (Fig. 24–15) The dilator is then removed and the cannula is pushed the extra few millimeters to rest on the annulus.

At this point, the fluoroscopic beam is brought perpendicular to the cannula. This view ensures that the cannula is absolutely down to the annulus (Fig. 24–16). When this oblique view confirms that the cannula is against the annulus, the trephine is placed over the trochar and through the cannula and the annulus is incised (Fig. 24–17). Only after the incision is made with the trephine can the trochar be removed along with the trephine.

The nucleotome is then placed into the disc through the cannula and confirmed to be within the disc space on both AP and lateral views (Fig. 24–18). At this point the disc is aspirated by activating the foot pedal–controlled suction cutting device. The procedure is monitored by watching the disc material in the aspiration provine. Since the disc is avascular, the aspiration contents should be essentially bloodless. By rotating and elevating and depressing the nucleotome at different depths, access to the disc material is obtained. The procedure is terminated when disc material can no longer be aspirated. This usually takes 20 to 40 minutes.

PERCUTANEOUS DISCECTOMY AT THE L5–S1 LEVEL

Because of the iliac crests and the rather oblique projection that must be made to enter the L5–S1 disc space, a point must be selected that allows medial entry far enough into the disc while still being lateral enough to allow a central to posterior placement. The starting entry point is determined by fluoroscopy. A line drawn tangential to the outside portion of the sacroiliac joint and extending superiorly until it intersects the iliac crest is a reasonable starting point from which to begin the procedure. A line is then drawn to the top of the iliac crest, and the top of the iliac crest is marked fluoroscopically along its length so that when the instruments are placed they are as close to the iliac crest as possible. The insertion is begun where these two lines intersect (Fig. 24–19).

Under lateral fluoroscopy, the needle for anesthesia is placed in its trajectory toward the disc and its angle with the disc is assessed. If the anesthesia needle is in the plane of the disc (Fig. 24–20), the entry point for the pro-

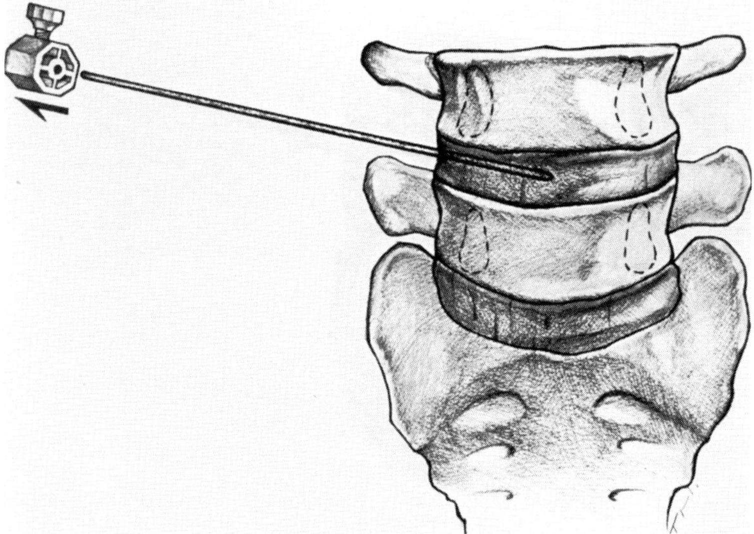

Figure 24–14. The trocar is advanced into the center of the disc in the anteroposterior view and is then confirmed on a lateral view to be the center of the disc also.

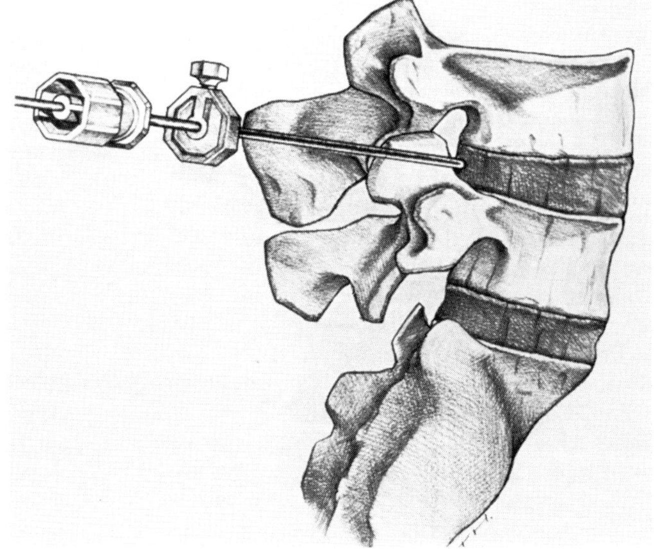

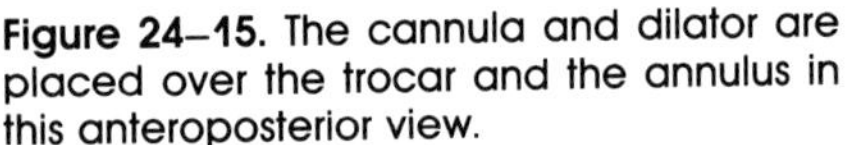

Figure 24–15. The cannula and dilator are placed over the trocar and the annulus in this anteroposterior view.

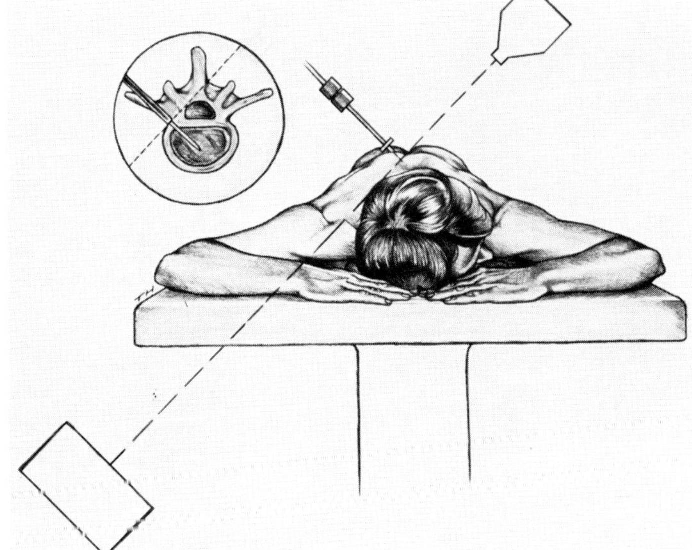

Figure 24–16. An oblique view is obtained that looks at the interface between the cannula and the annulus. In this way, any space between the cannula and the annulus can be identified.

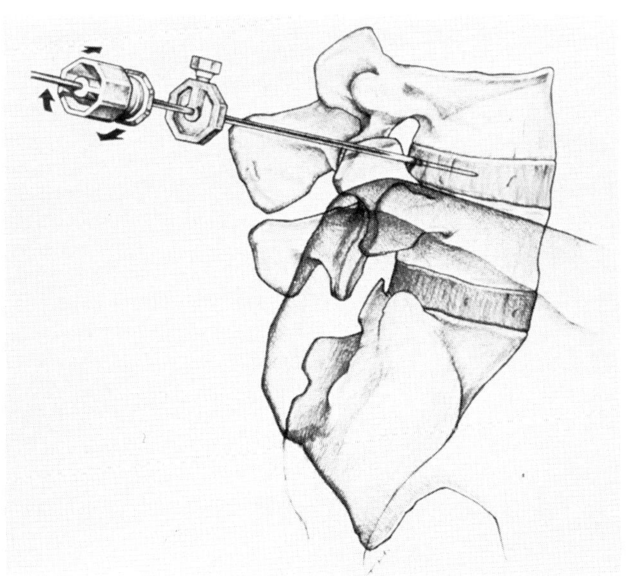

Figure 24–17. Using a circular motion, the trephine is placed over the trocar through the cannula, and the disc is incised.

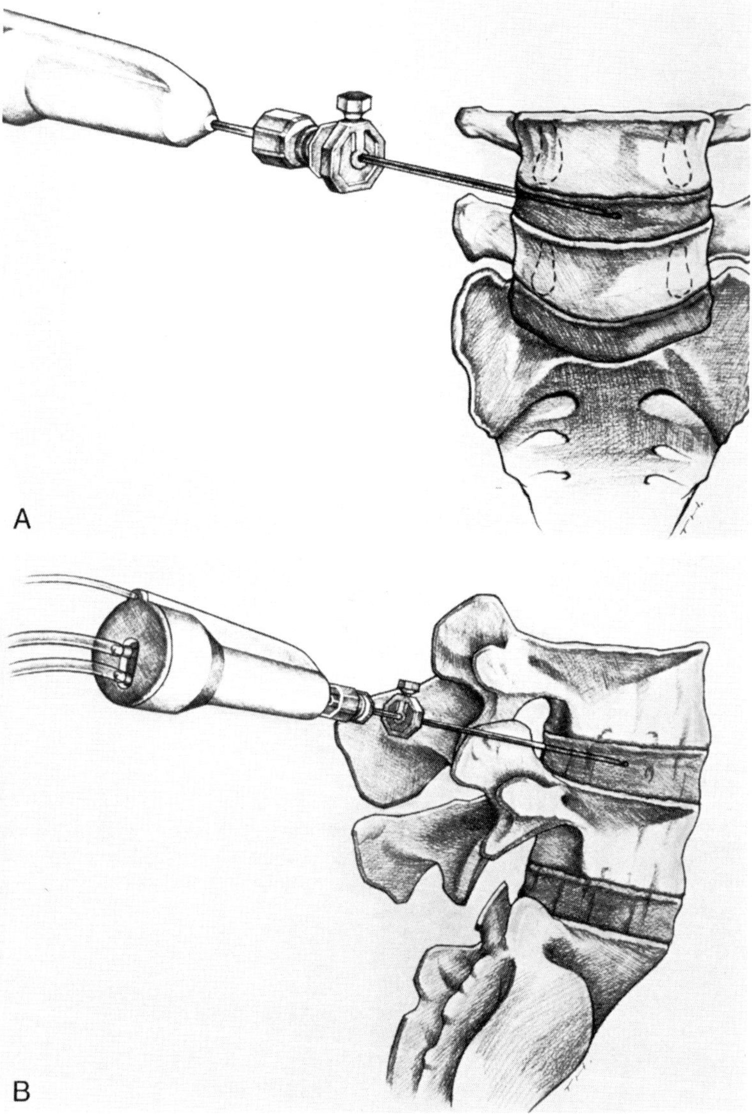

Figure 24–18. *A, B,* The nucleotome is placed within what is confirmed to be the center of the disc in both anteroposterior and lateral views.

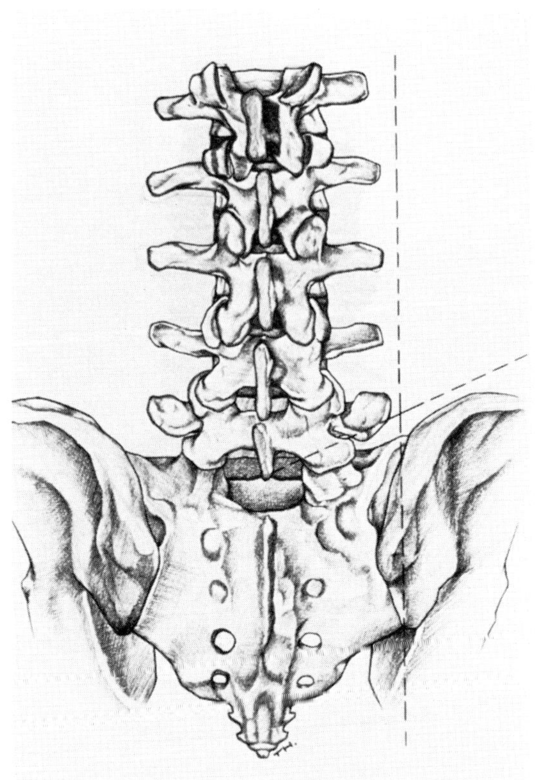

Figure 24–19. A line is drawn along the outside of the sacroiliac joint and across the top of the iliac crest. Where the lines intersect is the initial point for starting the placement at the L5–S1 level.

cedure is empirically moved laterally by approximately 2 cm and the angle of the anesthesia needle to the disc is again noted. If the needle is in the plane of the disc or only slightly angled to the disc (Fig. 24–21), the entry point will again be moved empirically laterally until the angle to the disc has reached its limit in allowing entry into the disc (Fig. 24–22) or to a maximum determined by the planning CT if that limit is not reached. In this way, using a small-gauge spinal needle, the point can be found that is farthest lateral and still allows entry into the disc space. By moving laterally as far as possible, the difficulty of getting to the center of the disc is minimized. If needed, a curved cannula can be used to help bring the instrument back into the plane of the disc (Fig. 24–23).

RESULTS

From 1984 to 1987 a prospective, multi-institutional study was carried out by 18 different investigators to evaluate the safety and efficacy of percutaneous automated discectomy.[6a] To be included in the study, patients had to have leg pain greater than back pain with physical findings and radiography (CT, MRI) that confirmed the presence of an HNP consistent with their symptoms. To be considered successfully treated, the patients had to have moderate to complete pain relief, be on no narcotic medications, return to preinjury functional status, and be satisfied with the procedure. Patients for this study were excluded if they had a history of previous lumbar surgery; previous chymopapain injection; workmen's compensation claim; or any cause of their pain as revealed by CT such as severe degenerative facet disease, lateral recessed stenosis, spinal stenosis, or evidence of a free fragment of disc. Although investigators were encouraged to stay within this study protocol, patients prospectively were treated outside the protocol and recorded as such. Of 506 patients, 11 were lost to follow-up and 327 met the prospective study criteria; 168 were knowingly

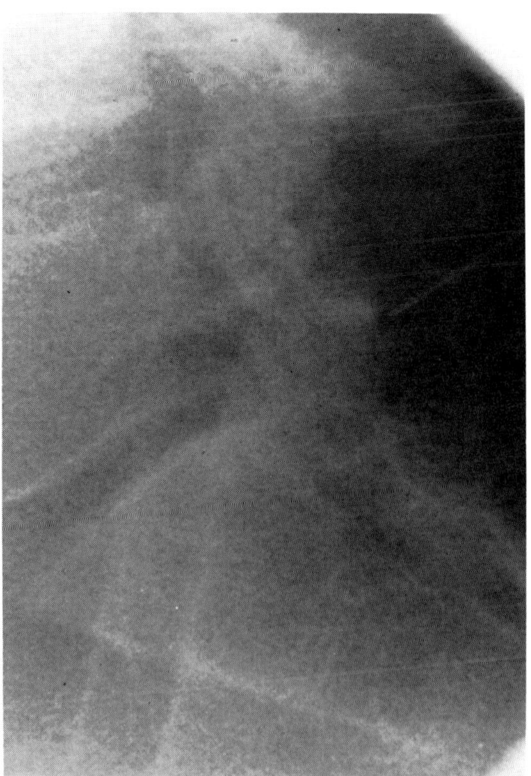

Figure 24–20. In this lateral fluoroscopic view, the anesthesia needle placed in the direction of the disc is in the plane of the disc. The entry point therefore can be moved farther laterally.

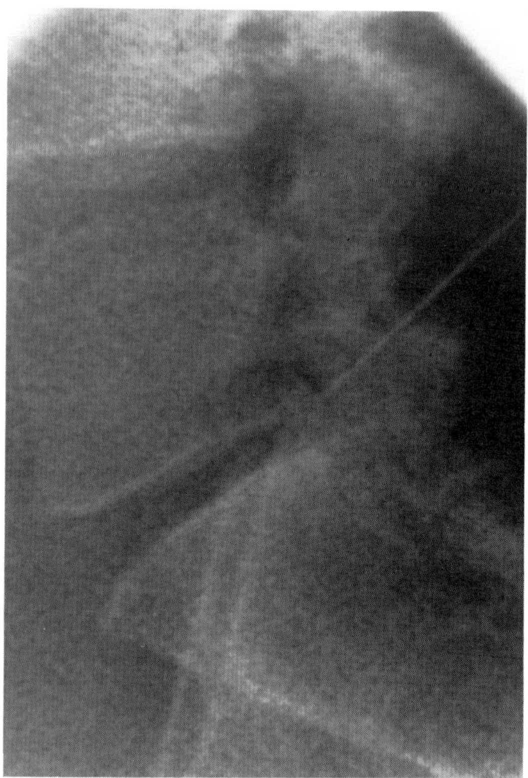

Figure 24–21. In this fluoroscopic view, the entry point has been moved farther laterally. Because of this placement and the upswing of the iliac crest, the needle angulation to the disc has increased. It is clear, however, that the disc with this angulation can still be entered with a needle. The entry is therefore placed farther lateral.

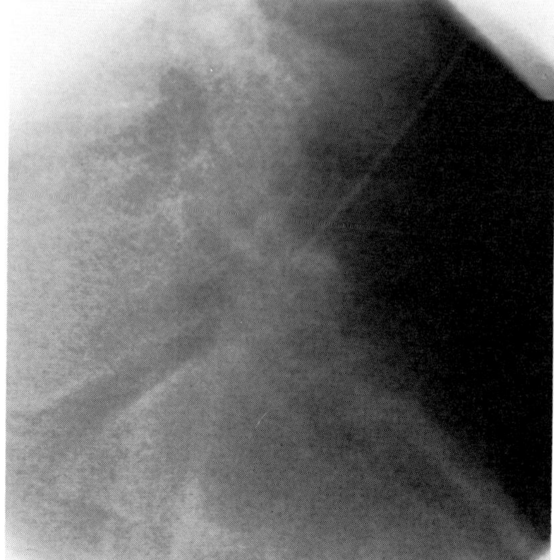

Figure 24–22. In this fluoroscopic view, the entry point has been moved farther laterally and the angle to the disc has increased. It was thought at this point that further angulation of the needle by moving the entry point farther laterally would have included entry of the needle into the disc. This was therefore chosen as the best entry point for entering the L5–S1 level.

treated outside the protocol. The mean patient age was 41 years. The mean duration of preoperative conservative treatment was 11.6 months. Eighty per cent of the procedures were performed at L4–L5 and approximately 20 per cent at L5–S1.

Of the 327 patients with a one-year or greater follow-up within the protocol, the success rate was 75.2 per cent; 24.8 per cent were considered failures. Of patients treated outside the protocol, 49.4 per cent were successful and 50.6 per cent were unsuccessful.

Complications included one case of discitis successfully treated with antibiotics. Another patient had transient paresthesias in the thigh secondary to a psoas hematoma that was not hemodynamically significant. Three patients had transient severe paravertebral spasms, although most experienced only mild discomfort in the area of needle insertion. The mean hospital stay for the procedure was 0.3 days, and most were treated as outpatients.

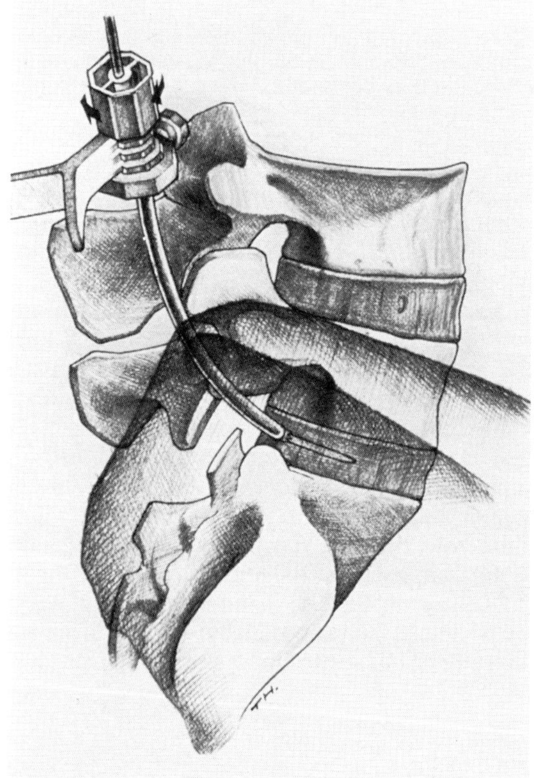

Figure 24–23. The curved cannula here is shown bringing the trephine, in this case, back into the plane of the disc.

These results have been confirmed by a separate multi-institutional study comprising over 600 cases.[1]

The postoperative course after HPD is variable. A patient may obtain immediate, complete relief from sciatica occasionally. Most patients note immediate moderate relief of pain then gradual resolution over six weeks or longer. We have seen an occasional patient who has minimal, if any, relief up to four weeks and then improves progressively. We therefore wait at least six weeks before considering the procedure a failure. Thus far, in our experience, patients who fail to get well have not been made worse by the procedure.

We instituted a postoperative rehabilitation program to correct postural problems with trunk stabilization and strengthening of abdominal and back muscles. Patients with sedentary jobs usually return to work the first week or two after a procedure. All patients who do heavy manual labor go through a work hardening program before returning to work six to 12 weeks after the procedure. We consider this is important since most patients have been off work and have lost muscle tone and strength.

CONCLUSION

PAD appears to be a low-risk procedure effective in 70 to 80 per cent of appropriately selected patients. Advantages include the use of local anesthesia, minimal tissue disruption, performance on an outpatient basis and an earlier return to former activities. Since the spinal canal is not violated, epidural fibrosis and scarring is absent and therefore does not preclude a subsequent open procedure. Subsequent evaluation reveals minimal disc space narrowing; therefore, there should be a negligible biomechanical effect. The problem of differential sequestered versus contained disc remains and is primarily an imaging problem at this point. Discography may be beneficial in helping to evaluate patients with questionable sequestration or tears in the posterior longitudinal ligament. The risks of PAD are significantly lower than those of traditional surgery and therefore this procedure should be considered in properly selected patients.

References

1. Bocchi, L., Ferrata, P., Passarello, F., et al.: La nucleoaspirazione secondo Onik nel trattamento dell'ernia discale lombare analisi multicentrica dei primi risultati su oltre 650 trattamenti. Riv. Neuroradiol. *2*(Suppl. 1):119, 1989.
2. Freis, J., Abodely, D., Vijungo, J., et al.: Computed tomography of herniated and extruded nucleus pulposus. J. Comput. Assist. Tomogr. *6*:874, 1982.

2a. Friedman, W. A.: Percutaneous discectomy: an alternative to chemonucleolysis? Neurosurgery *13*:542–547, 1983.

3. Hijikata, S., Yamagishi, M., Nakayama, T., et al.: Percutaneous discectomy: a new treatment method for lumbar disc herniation. J. Toden. Hosp. *5*:5, 1975.
4. Hijikata, S.: Percutaneous nucleotomy: a new concept technique and 12 years' experience. Clin. Orthop. *238*:9, 1989.
5. Kambin, P., and Schatter, J. L.: Percutaneous lumbar discectomy: review of 100 patients and current practice. Clin. Orthop. *238*:24, 1989.
6. Onik, G., Maroon, J. C., and Davis, G. W.: Automated percutaneous discectomy at the L5–S1 level. Use of a curved cannula. Clin. Orthop. *238*:71–76, 1988.

6a. Onik, G., Mooney, V., Maroon, J. C., et al.: Automated percutaneous discectomy: a prospective multi-institutional study. Neurosurgery *2*:228–233, 1990.

7. Schreiber, A., Suezawa, M. D., and Leu, H.: Does percutaneous nucleotomy with discoscopy replace conventional discectomy? Eight years of experience and results in treatment of herniated lumbar disc. Clin. Orthop. *238*:35, 1989.
8. Smith, L.: Enzyme dissolution of the nucleus pulposus in humans. J.A.M.A. *187*:137–140, 1964.

MICRODISCECTOMY

John A. McCulloch, M.D.

The results of surgery are determined far more by patient selection than by surgical technique. Microsurgery for lumbar spine conditions has to be viewed in this context. The use of the microscope as an aid for disc excision or bony decompression is a technical advancement in spine surgery only. The microscope will not perform the surgery, and it will not assure a good result.

WOUND HEALING

To dismiss microsurgery as irrelevant because wounds heal side to side and not end to end (therefore the length of the incision is not important) is to misunderstand wound healing. Skin heals side to side and the length of the skin incision is not important except for cosmesis, but wounds heal end to end—the longer the paraspinal incision, the greater is the wound hematoma and the more significant is the scar laid down.[16] Laroque and MacNab, in developing their hypothesis for laminectomy membrane, observed that the fibrous response was always more marked when a wide operative exposure was used.[11] Unfortunately this observation was not enlarged on because the thrust of their research was to show the value of a Gelfoam membrane, used to separate the exposed dura and nerve roots from the erector spinae muscles.

Definition

Healing by Primary Intention (First Intention)

Healing by primary intention applies to full-thickness (epidermis and dermis disruption) wounds that meet the following criteria:

1. The wound edges are clean and free of contamination and foreign bodies.
2. They are closely apposed soon after the wound has been made.
3. Adequate blood supply to the wound edges is present.

Primary wound healing occurs with the primary suture of clean skin edges. It meets two closely linked criteria:

1. Dead space is reduced to a minimum.
2. As a secondary phenomenon, granulation tissue is reduced to a minimum.

Healing by Secondary Intention

Healing by secondary intention is healing by granulation tissue. It occurs in two situations: wounds left open, and wounds with dead space.

Although the long skin incision of a paraspinal wound is closed and is expected to heal by primary intention, dead space deep to the skin incision will heal by granulation tissue or secondary intention (Fig. 24–24). Healing by secondary intention involves the two major phenomena of wound healing, that is, inflammation and repair (scar).

The following criteria apply to healing by secondary intention:

1. The larger the dead space, the larger is the clot.
2. The larger the dead space, the greater is

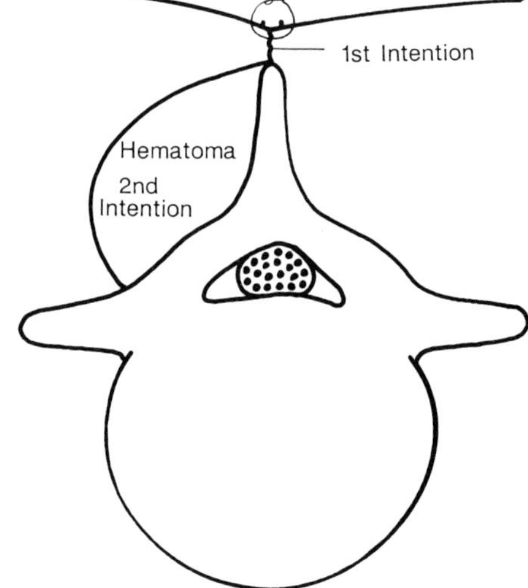

Figure 24–24. Skin is expected to heal by primary intention, but if dead space is left behind by a longer paraspinal incision, it will fill with hematoma and heal by secondary intention (scar). Dead space is reduced when the smallest possible invasion (microsurgery) is used.

the amount of necrotic debris and fibrin that must be removed from the inflammatory reaction.

3. The repair cannot be completed until the inflammatory response has been controlled and the injurious agents and necrotic debris have been removed.

4. The greater the amount of injurious agents, such as suture, and the greater the amount of necrotic debris to be removed, the slower is the repair and the more extensive the repair in the form of scar tissue.

Module of Wound Healing

Figure 24–25 demonstrates the advancing front of wound healing encircling the dead space hematoma that fills a paraspinal incision. There is such an organized mass of cells and events involved in wound healing that the healing wound can be considered a temporary organ.[16] It is turned on through some unknown mechanism that occurs immediately after the skin incision. It is turned off when wound healing is complete, and no one has been able to determine why wound healing ceases when it is no longer needed. It is known that wound healing is affected by general diseases such as malnutrition and is adversely affected by local factors such as the amount of tissue damage made at the time of the incision, the number of sutures inserted, and the presence or absence of other necrotic debris and infection. In the end this healed wound is represented by scar.

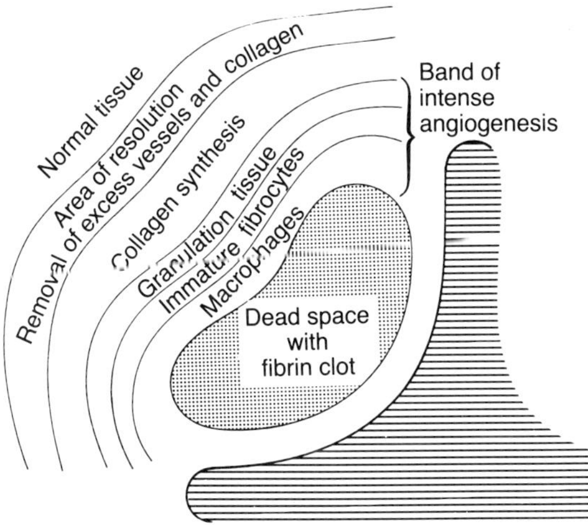

Figure 24–25. The nodule of wound healing—a complicated, multifaceted "organ unto itself."

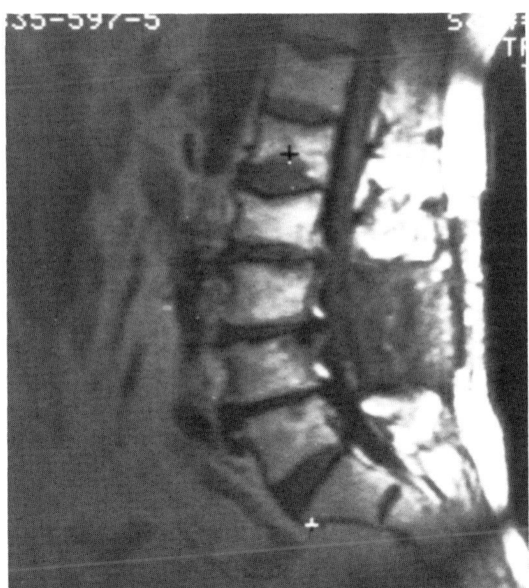

Figure 24–26. Postoperative spinal stenosis on T1-weighted MRI scan, showing extensive scar extending for three segments.

Clinical Relevance

There is only one sure way to stop scarring—not to operate. Obviously some patients require surgical intervention, and the question becomes: what can be done to reduce scarring deep in the wound around the important neurologic structures? The single most important thing is to reduce dead space to a minimum. The volume of dead space can be equated to healing by secondary intention, and healing by secondary intention means scar tissue.

Figure 24–26 shows a postoperative spinal stenosis in which extensive deroofing has been completed and the postoperative scar has formed. Figure 24–27 shows a 1-inch microsurgical incision with little muscle dissection that was closed with virtually no dead space. A laminectomy membrane that was not achieved through the use of Gelfoam or fat resulted.

Another disadvantage of a long paraspinal incision is increased suture material, a foreign body in the wound that slows wound healing. A further disadvantage is the denervation that occurs in paraspinal tissues. This was documented by MacNab and associates in a clinical study of 113 patients who underwent lumbar spine surgery and were examined postoperatively with electromyography.[13] Some measure

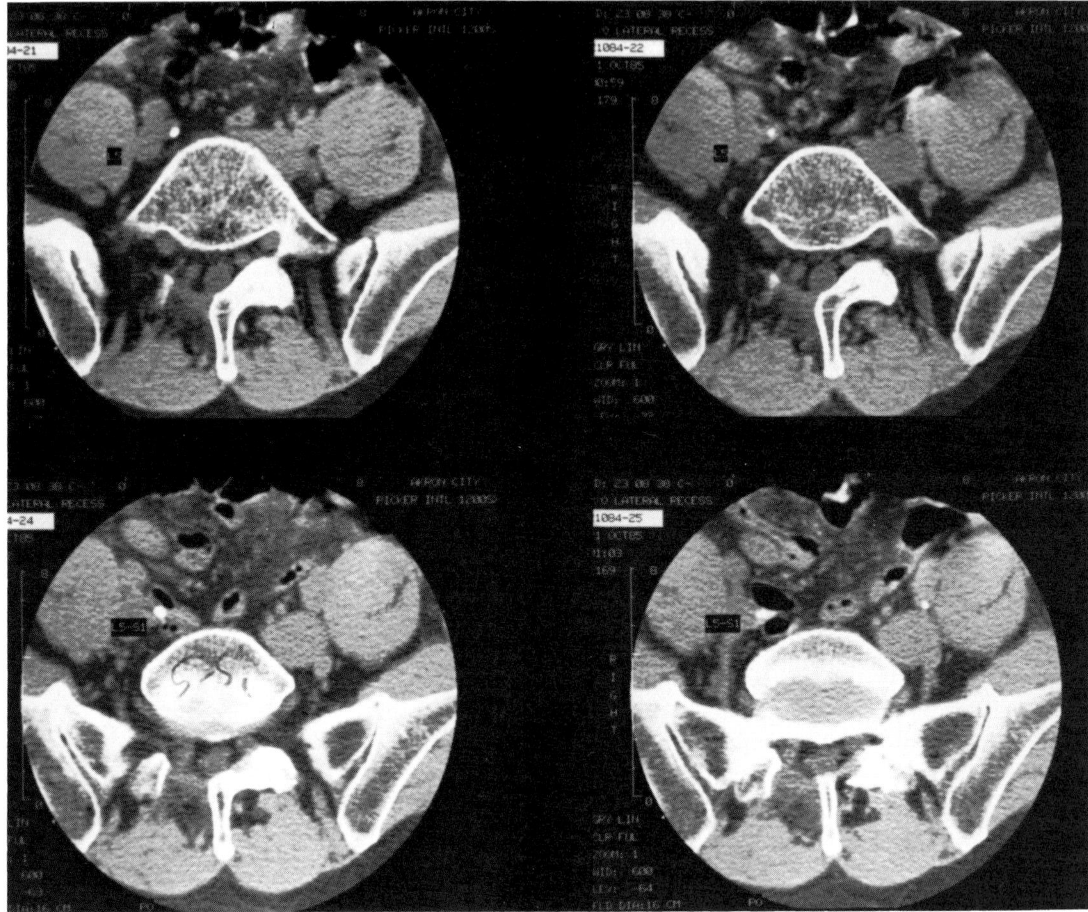

Figure 24–27. Postoperative microdiscectomy on CT. Note the laminectomy membrane and very little scar around the dura and root (right L5–S1).

of denervation of the paravertebral muscles occurred in 96 per cent of the cases. Denervation persisted for many years after surgery, and reinnervation was only partial.

The concept of a microsurgical paraspinal wound was supported further by the study of Kahonovich and associates, which compared a group of patients who had a standard laminectomy to a group of patients who had a microsurgical exposure.[9] The surgical results in the two groups were identical except for postoperative morbidity and length of stay in the hospital. The patients in whom a microsurgical approach was used had a much reduced postoperative morbidity and a much shorter hospital stay.

A final point in support of the smallest possible wound is the observation in repeated spine surgery that the best place to look for normal structures, such as unscarred dura, is behind normal bone or ligamentum flavum. Thus if spine exposure can be accomplished with maintenance of as much normal anatomy as possible, such as bone or ligamentum flavum, the ultimate scar tissue formation around the dura and nerve roots will be reduced. One of the advantages of microsurgery is that it can be accomplished with limited removal of ligamentum flavum and lamina.

EARLY MOBILIZATION

There are many benefits to early mobilization. A patient who can get out of bed the same day as the surgical procedure and be home the next day has an advantage over a patient who has a more painful wound and requires longer bed rest and hospitalization. The general effects of early mobilization include a reduced incidence of pulmonary and vascular complications (such as atelectasis and thrombophlebitis) and an earlier return to the anabolic phase of wound healing.

Local Effects of Early Mobilization

The three basic molecular steps in local wound healing are as follows:[16]

1. Intracellular synthesis of tropocollagen molecules.
2. Extracellular assembly of fibrils and fibers.
3. Formation of ground substance.

A fundamentally important property of the healing wound is its tensile strength, which is directly related to collagen formation and orientation. Salter and associates showed that when healed with continuous passive motion (CPM) healed better both qualitatively and quantitatively when compared with immobilized wounds.[20] These investigators postulated that the tension of CPM enhanced the formation and alignment of collagen.

Little attention has been paid to ground substance formation and stimulation in a mobilized wound. Ground substance is the latticework or template on which the collagen polymerizes; it probably plays an important role in orienting the pattern of the fibrous network. It is possible that early mobilization stimulates early maturation and more vigorous function in ground substance, thereby further enhancing wound healing.

CONCLUSIONS

Before the contributions of Semmelweis and Lister, infection of the surgical wound was expected. The advent of aseptic techniques, the introduction of antibiotics, and the improvements in surgical technique changed all of that. These advances have made modern surgery possible. Before them, avoiding an infection was considered luck; now an infection in a clean wound is rare.

Today's surgeons are at another threshold: we make the incision and we expect a scar. Is there some way we can reduce scar, and when its formation is necessary, is there some way we can control its formation? To a certain extent this has been accomplished with such interposition membranes as fat. It appears that the initial proposal by Larocca and MacNab of using Gelfoam has not stood the test of time.[11, 28] Their observation that the laminectomy should be as restricted as possible, consistent with thorough decompression of the involved nerve, was significant, however. This is the approach that should be taken to paraspinal surgery. In 1913 William Halsted stated, "I believe that the tendency will always be in the direction of exercising greater care and refinement in operating, and that the surgeon will develop increasingly a respect for tissues; a sense which recoils from inflicting, unnecessarily, insult to structures concerned in the process of repair." This historic observation is becoming more important as more surgery is being done through limited exposures. The ability to do spine surgery through limited exposure is brought about by two modern factors. First, there is a much better understanding of syndromes that affect function in the low back. An example is the better distinction between a radicular syndrome resulting from a disc herniation and one resulting from subarticular stenosis. Second, more sophisticated investigative tools, such as CT scanning and MRI allow an accurate clinical diagnosis on which to base a surgical decision. Not only is an accurate clinical diagnosis possible, but an exact definition and localization of the pathology within the spinal canal is also available.

The amount of scar tissue formed around the dura and nerve roots will be directly related to the extent of exposure of the structures. The more limited the exposure of these structures, the less is the scar tissue that will form. This is the essence of microsurgery.

The Role of the Microscope

The basis of any good surgical practice is knowing when and on which patient to operate. Of secondary importance is the technical ability to get the job done without difficulty, thereby avoiding a poor result or a complication. To use the microscope without obeying these principles is to court failure. The microscope is nothing more than an aid that magnifies and illuminates the surgical field so the surgeon can get the job done. It is exceptional for a surgeon to decide to use the microscope in lumbar disc surgery and not have trouble adapting. Most authors who are honest about their results will report that the learning curve leading to the full potential of microscope use was initially associated with increased complications. Perseverance has resulted in a command of the tool and its magnifying and illuminating qualities to enhance the surgeon's skills.

The microscope cannot be used to seek and find pathology. The nature and the location of the pathology has to be pinpointed preoperatively to allow for successful surgical excision through a small incision. The microscope cannot be used to see where you are going; you know where you are going from careful analysis of the patient and the investigation, and you use the microscope to get there.

INDICATIONS FOR MICROSURGERY

A General Statement

A review of the natural history of lumbar disc disease reveals that spinal surgeons play a palliative role in the management of microsurgery. The most outstanding study on the natural history of lumbar disc disease was done by Weber.[21] He randomly divided large groups of patients with unequivocal signs of a disc herniation into surgical and nonsurgical groups. Table 24–4 summarizes his results. Weber showed that although surgery initially increases good results, its advantages disappear after longer follow-up study.

Hakelius also completed a retrospective study of 583 patients with unilateral (L5 or S1) sciatica.[7] His results were similar to Weber's in that the surgically treated patients initially had a better result, but by six months there was no difference between the two groups of patients. He did show that after seven years of follow-up, the conservatively treated group had more low back pain, more sciatic discomfort, more recurrences, and more lost time from work.

Table 24–4. WEBER'S RESULTS

	Nonsurgical Results	Surgical Results
1 year	60% better	92% better
4 years	No statistical difference between the two groups	
10 years	No difference between 4-year and 10-year follow-up	

From Weber, H.: Lumbar disc herniation: a controlled prospective study with 10 years of observation. Spine *8*:131, 1983.

From these and other studies on the natural history of sciatica caused by a disc herniation, one can conclude that sciatica is a transient, self-limiting condition. Satisfactory resolution over time is likely to occur regardless of the method of treatment. If surgical intervention is proposed it is essential to prove that surgery has a high rate of initial success with limited risk to the patient at the lowest possible expense.

Indications for Surgery in HNP

The indications for microsurgical discectomy are no different from those for any discectomy. They include

1. Increasing neurologic deficit.
2. Significant neurologic deficit with significant SLR reduction.
3. Bladder and bowel involvement. The acute massive disc herniation that causes bladder and bowel paralysis is usually a sequestered disc requiring immediate surgical excision for the best prognosis. There is no disc herniation too large to be removed through a microsurgical wound.
4. Failure of conservative treatment. This is the most common reason for surgical intervention in the presence of an HNP. Ideal conservative treatment is treatment that occurs over at least six weeks and not more than three months and results in improvement of symptoms and signs. The amount of complete bed rest should be three to five days. Other conservative measures such as medication (analgesics, anti-inflammatory drugs, and muscle relaxants), modalities (heat and cold), and exercises may be used.[1] The key to measuring the success of conservative treatment is not only relief of pain but also improvement in SLR ability. If a patient goes to bed with appropriate medication for three to five days and there is no improvement in SLR ability, it is likely that the patient will have a protracted conservative course, for which surgical intervention is indicated. It is proposed that surgical intervention in the acute radicular syndrome

Table 24–5. RECURRENT SCIATICA: INDICATIONS FOR SURGERY

First episode of sciatica	90% of patients will get better and stay better
Second episode of sciatica	90% of patients will get better, but 50% of the patients will have a recurrence of symptoms; consider surgery
Third episode of sciatica	90% of patients will get better but almost all will have recurrent episodes of sciatica; propose surgery

This condition is to be distinguished from recurrent HNP (disc herniation recurring after previous surgery).

occur before three months of symptoms to avoid the chronic pathologic changes that can occur within a nerve root. Conservative treatment can also fail in that the patient experiences recurrences of the sciatic syndrome. Table 24–5 outlines the use of recurrences of sciatica as an indication for surgical intervention.

ADVANTAGES OF MICROSURGERY

Greater Visibility

The basic principle of microsurgery is the facilitation of surgical effort by magnification, illumination, and spatially compressed three-dimensional vision (stereopsis) (Fig. 24–28).

The available microscopic magnification is wide ranging and especially precise for viewing the nerve root. There is one basic principle: Before extensive Kerrison use, retraction, or sharp dissection is carried out, the lateral border of the nerve root must be clearly identified. This results in less direct (trauma) and indirect (traction) injury to the root.

The bright coaxial illumination available in the microscope allows for direct vision to great depths and the use of instruments in a shadow-free environment.

Greater Precision

Because of the better visualization of structures, it is possible to limit the extent of the incision by decreasing the extent of soft tissue dissection of fascia and muscle. I assiduously avoid any incision into the supraspinous or interspinous ligaments and dissect muscle off only one interspace. Once one is through the ligamentum flavum, epidural fat can be better preserved to use as an inherent fat graft at the end of the case. It is possible to see epidural veins clearly and, if necessary, to cauterize them with bipolar cautery without damaging the nerve root. In patients with previous surgery the plane between the nerve root and the annulus is blurred by scar tissue. Under the

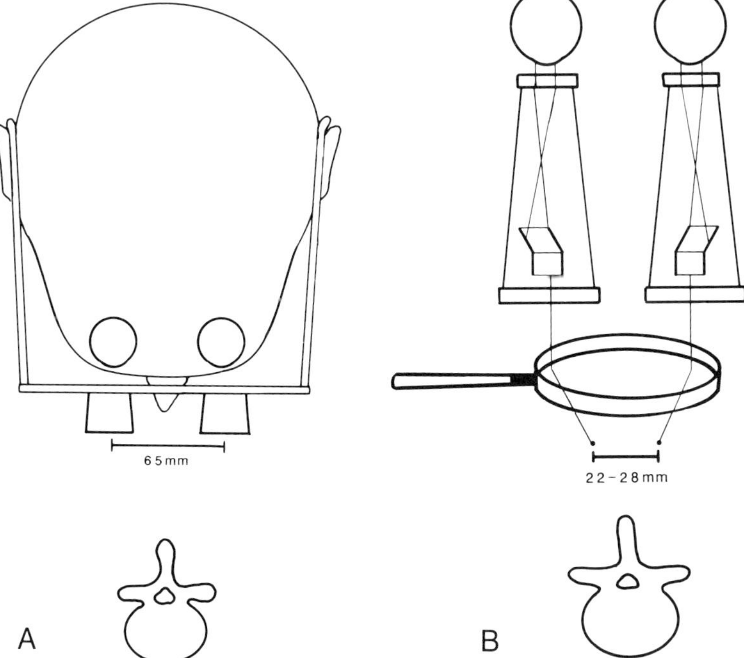

Figure 24–28. *A,* Stereopsis (three-dimensional visualization) with loupes requires an interpupillary distance of approximately 65 mm. *B,* Through the systems of prisms in the construct of the microscope, three-dimensional visualization can be achieved through an interpupillary distance of less than 30 mm, which allows for a smaller incision.

microscope this interval is more easily dissected. With the maneuverability of the microscope head and the depth of the coaxial light, it is possible to look through the subarticular zone into the foramen more readily than without the microscope.

Decreased Morbidity

The smaller wound achievable with microsurgery results in less bleeding and faster patient recovery with earlier hospital discharge.[9] It is likely that a skilled surgeon, fully in charge of the capabilities of the microscope, will complete the disc excision faster than a surgeon using standard laminectomy techniques. This needs to be tested over time by more surgeons. Whether it is important or not is a philosophical question. A smaller scar can be considered more aesthetically pleasing than a larger scar, although no scar at all is preferable. A shorter skin incision theoretically decreases the number of cutaneous nerves cut, and thus decreases the risk of neuroma formation.

Better Results

The most controversial claim of microsurgeons is that their results are better. There is no scientific evidence that this is true; indeed, when the complications of early microsurgical experiences are studied, it seems unlikely that the results could be better than laminectomy/discectomy.

Remember that microsurgery is not seek-and-find surgery. Before the limited incision is made, a carefully thought-out game plan should be in place. This is a hidden benefit of microsurgery—you become more knowledgeable about your patients. There is no room for error and the surgeon does not attempt to "seek-and-find" if pathology is not found. This curtails surgical misadventure and improves results.

The other reasons for better results with microsurgery include a better working relationship with the nerve root, a better view of the pathology, and the ability to look in the subarticular recess and foramen using the coaxial light source. Preserving the interspinous–supraspinous ligament complex theoretically decreases the potential for long-term instability, however, there is no scientific evidence to support these statements—just surgical intuition.

Teaching and Education

There is a general trend to reduce the size of the wound in lumbar disc surgery to reduce postoperative morbidity and achieve an earlier hospital discharge. If this is accomplished with standard operating room lighting or loupes and headlights, the surgical assistant will see even less. It is only when the microscope is used in the limited surgical wound that the surgical assistant achieves equal viewing rights with the operating surgeon. The microscope results in a much better teaching environment in a residency training program. Teaching is further enhanced with the documentation aids of still and motion photography.

DISADVANTAGES OF MICROSURGERY

Knowing the limitations of a technique is the key to avoiding problems and maximizing the potential. Microsurgery has inherent disadvantages that lead to complications if they are not understood and overcome.

Limited Field of Vision

The diameter of the field of vision in microsurgery is less than 50 mm. If that field is not centered over the pathology, fragments of disc and bony encroachment will be missed.

Limited Field of Work

A 1-inch skin incision is the common incision according to microsurgical articles. The incision is usually 1 to 1.5 inches, especially if the patient is large or obese and a deep working wound is anticipated. If a 1.5-inch skin incision is used, and if it is the diameter of the operating field, the area for instrumentation is even less than the potential field of vision (33 mm versus 41 mm). This limited operating field requires special instrumentation (straight and of small diameter), manipulated precisely, to avoid errors and damage to important neurologic structures. Failure to accept this limitation has led to an increased incidence of dural tears and root damage. There are occasions when the surgical exercise will occur near the edge of the microscope field. At this point stop and reposition the microscope so that the working area is centered. Once the limited field of work is acknowledged and instrumentation is adapted, problems will be significantly reduced.

Bleeding

A small amount of bleeding into a limited operative field interferes with visualization and completion of the surgical exercise. The difference between 25 mL of blood loss and 100 mL of blood loss under the microscope is significant. Every effort in preoperative preparation (i.e., stopping anti-inflammatory medication), in patient positioning on the operating room table, and in control of hemorrhage has to be made to avoid this disadvantage.

Infection

Wilson and associates reported an increased rate of disc space infection after microsurgery.[25, 26] This is most likely because of the presence of the microscope directly over the wound. Although the microscope is sterilely draped, there are parts of the microscope that are exposed (eyepieces) that have the potential to contaminate the wound. The limited operating space between the microscope and the wound introduces another element of potential break in proper surgical technique that can result in wound contamination.

THE MICROSCOPE

For years surgeons have used visual assistance to see more of the anatomy that is being dissected. Most spine surgeons use loupes, but these have their disadvantages:

1. Lack of compressed stereotaxis (see Fig. 24–28).
2. Using loupes at a magnification higher than 4× exaggerates head movement and blurs the anatomy.
3. With loupes, it is not possible to change the magnification during the procedure.
4. During long procedures it becomes tedious to use loupes.
5. The surgical assistant also has to use loupes and bumps heads with the surgeon.
6. At best, the lighting system with loupes is paraxial rather than coaxial.

For these reasons, a number of surgeons now use the microscope for better illumination and visualization of the surgical field in lumbar disc disease.

Principles

To assist the surgeon, the microscope must meet the following criteria:

1. It must produce an enlarged image that helps the surgeon to better visualize the anatomy.
2. The enlarged image must be upright and unreversed to eliminate reorientation of the image with the actual surgical field. This is accomplished by the use of prisms built into the microscope.
3. The image must be three-dimensional so that the surgeon can obtain satisfactory depth perception.
4. The working distance between the scope and the focus point must be comfortable enough for the surgeon to work and open enough for the introduction of instruments.
5. The color reproduction of the image must be accurate.

The important points in constructing a microscope for lumbar disc surgery are described below.

The Microscope Head and Optics

The operating microscope is a combination of binocular field glasses and a magnifying glass (Fig. 24–29). Interposed between the binoculars and the magnifying glass is a magnifying chamber that allows for increasing or decreasing image size (Fig. 24–30). The microscope is a series of lenses and prisms that allow for transformation of an image to the retina (Fig. 24–31). Optical deficiencies, such as reflections and glare, have to be factored out of the system to improve image quality. This has resulted in an instrument of complicated design that is impossible to explain here. There are articles that explain the microscope in more detail;

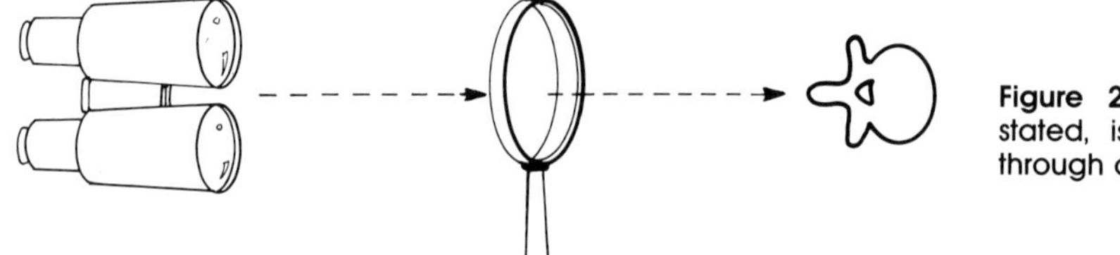

Figure 24–29. The microscope, simply stated, is a pair of binoculars looking through a magnifying glass.

this section will serve as a basic summary of the microscope assembly important for lumbar disc surgery.[10]

Objective Lens (the Magnifying Glass)

Objective lenses with focal length ranging from 150 to 400 mm are available in 25-mm increments. The focal length of an objective lens is a close approximation of the distance between the lens and the point of anatomy that is in focus.

By changing the objective lens, it is possible to change the magnification of the image on the retina, the size of the field of view, the depth of the field of view, and the illumination. By decreasing the focal length of the objective, a smaller visual field is outlined, at a greater magnification, with increased illumination and a smaller depth of field. The reverse, increasing the focal length of the objective, increases the size of the visual field, thereby decreasing the magnification and illumination, and results in a greater depth of field.

A 300-, 350-, or 400-mm lens is generally used in spinal surgery. The surgeon must try the various lenses to choose the most comfortable position for standing at the microscope and operating on the patient. There also must be a comfortable distance between the bottom of the microscope and the depth of the wound in which to manipulate instruments. My preference is a 350-mm lens.

The Binocular Assembly

The binocular assembly consists of two components: the binocular tube and the eyepieces (see Fig. 24–29).

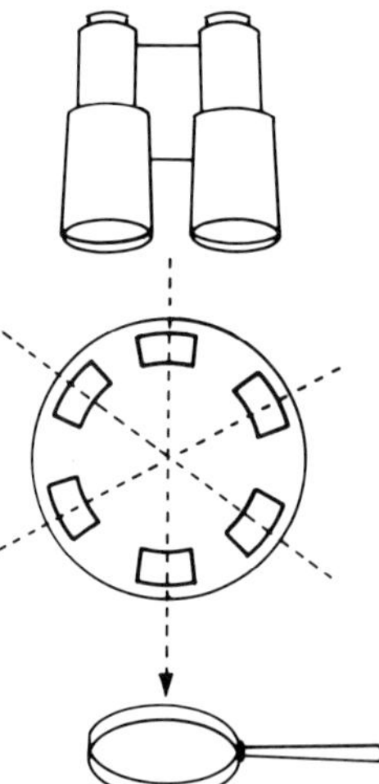

Figure 24–30. A magnifying chamber allows for greater or lesser magnification during the procedure as called for by the surgeon.

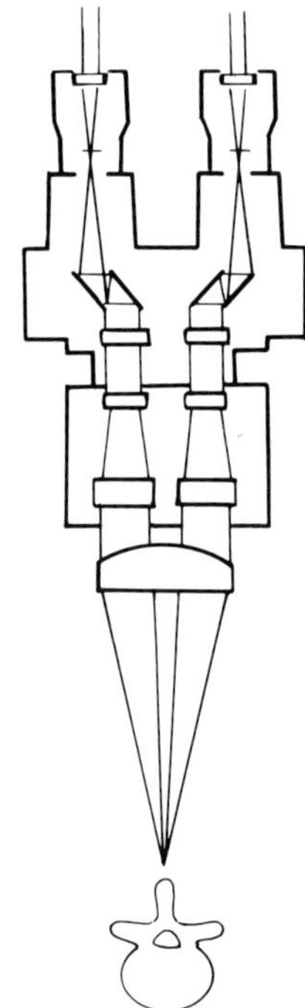

Figure 24–31. The final assembly of the microscope is a complicated series of lenses and prisms that transforms the spinal image onto the retina.

The image formed by the objective lens is magnified by the binocular assembly. The amount of magnification in the objective and in the binocular assembly is represented by the formula

$$\frac{Fb}{Fo}$$

where Fb is the binocular tube length and Fo is the focal length of objective. A popular scope model incorporates a 170-mm binocular tube length. Using a 350-mm objective lens, the magnification factor is represented by the formula

$$\frac{Fb}{Fo} = \frac{170}{350} = 0.486$$

The function of the binocular tubes is to take the image of the objective, which is translated in infinity, and converge it to something that can be viewed by the human eye. With the addition of eyepieces, the optical system in the binocular assembly becomes convergent.

Binocular tubes can be straight or inclined. The most popular model today is the tiltable binocular tube that allows for individual adjustment of the angle of the binocular tube. This is most helpful when the surgeon and surgical assistant are of different heights.

The diameter of the binocular tubes is 20 mm. This along with the binocular tube length and the objective lens determines the diameter of the operating field according to the formula

$$Do = \frac{20 \text{ mm}}{Fb/Fo}$$

$$Do = \frac{20}{170/350} = \frac{20}{0.486} = 41 \text{ mm}$$

Decreasing the objective focal length in turn decreases the diameter of the field.

Eyepieces

Another portion of the magnification equation for the microscope is added by the eyepieces. The convergent system in the binocular tube produces an intermediate-size image, which is magnified by the eyepieces for viewing by the human eye. Eyepieces for the Zeiss microscope are measured at 10×, 12.5×, 16×, and 20×; for the Wild microscope, the eyepieces are 10×, 15×, and 20×. The eyepieces on each of these microscopes are adjustable, with 8 diopters to correct for visual acuity problems. It is possible to wear eyeglasses when using the binocular tube–eyepiece assembly. The rubber cups on the eyepieces need to be folded back in this case. The use of eyeglasses is recommended when correction for astigmatism is necessary. If eyeglasses are required only for myopia or hyperopia, it is possible to operate without eyeglasses, using the diopter adjustments on the eyepieces to achieve focus.

With the addition of the eyepieces, a further calculation of the magnification is represented by the formula

$$\frac{Fb}{Fo} \times Me$$

where Me is the magnification of the eyepieces.

The standard setup for lumbar disc surgery is calculated by the formula

$$\frac{170}{350} \times 12.5 = 6.07$$

Interpupillary Distance

Interpupillary distance varies from surgeon to surgeon. The eyepieces must be adjusted for interpupillary distance so that the two images are fused and stereoscopic or three-dimensional appreciation of the image occurs.

Magnification Chamber

The final piece of the microscope that determines the size of the image structures is the magnification chamber, as depicted in Figure 24–30. A Galilean telescopic system allows for alteration in the magnification setup between the binocular assembly and the objective lens. The actual magnification factor achieved with the chamber can be 0.4×, 0.6×, 1.0×, 1.6×, or 2.5×. The magnification chamber can be a turret drum setup that clicks in at the above-listed magnification factors or a zoom magnifying chamber. The zoom system is a mechanized chamber controlled by a foot pedal or dial on the microscope that gives a continuous magnification range from 0.5 to 2.5, using a single optical system.

Common Optics for Lumbar Disc Surgery

The magnification formula governing any microscope is

$$\text{Mag} = \frac{\text{Binocular tube length}}{\text{Objective focal distance}} \times \text{Eyepieces} \times \text{Mag chamber}$$

$$\text{MT} = \text{Fb/Fo} \times \text{Me} \times \text{Mc}$$

For a Zeiss microscope, the equation would be

$$\text{MT} = \frac{170}{350} \times 12.5 \times 1.0 = 6.07$$

Using the 1.6 magnification setting, the formula would change to

$$\text{MT} = \frac{170}{350} \times 12.5 \times 1.6 = 9.7$$

Illumination Strength

As magnification increases, the amount of illumination decreases, but the change in brightness is not enough to interfere with surgery.

Illumination Systems

An advantage of the illuminating system of the microscope is the coaxial path of the observation and illumination beams (Fig. 24–32). The ideal illumination system provides enough light for the surgeon to see the anatomy clearly. It should also be economical and consistent. In addition, when the source fails (burned-out bulb), it should be easily replaced. A constant problem with all lighting sources in the microscope is the generation of heat; the least amount of heat generation is the most desirable.

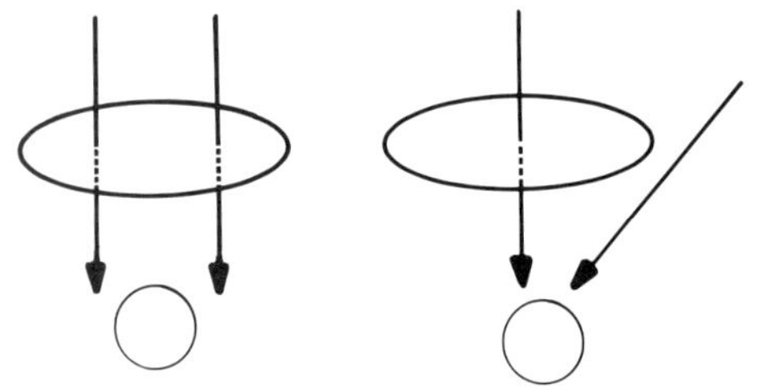

Figure 24–32. *Left,* Coaxial lighting: the light source and the line of vision are parallel. *Right,* Paraxial lighting: the light source comes from a different direction from the line of vision, necessitating a wider incision to get the light into the depths of the wound.

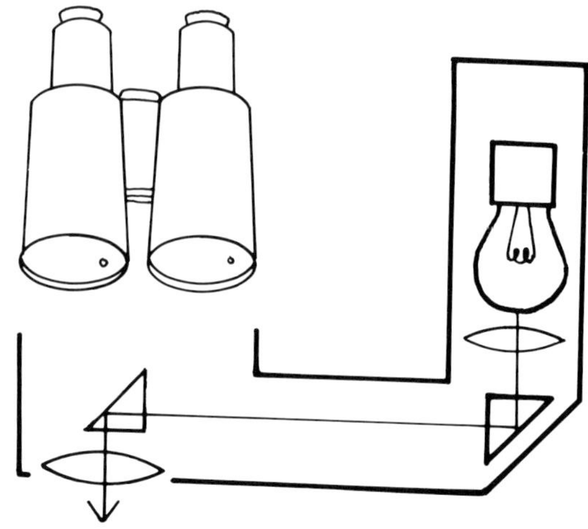

Figure 24–33. A light source close to the microscope has to be reflected into the wound via prisms.

The choices for illuminating the microscope are as follows:

Incandescent (Tungsten Coil) Light. Incandescent light is the oldest and cheapest source of light in the operating microscope. Either 6-volt, 30-watt or 6-volt, 50-watt bulbs have been used, with the higher wattage used when documentation equipment is attached to the microscope. In the early microscopes, the bulb was close to the microscope head and the heat generated was significant.

Halogen (Tungsten Coil) Bulb. The halogen bulb is the most popular choice for illumination today. It is a more sensitive light than the incandescent bulb, with a greater blue spectrum. This results in the surgical site appearing whiter and brighter. The standard halogen bulb used is 12 volts, 100 watts. This produces light with a brightness of 160,000 lux or 14,860 foot-candles.

Light Transfer Systems

Light is transferred through the microscope in one of two ways.

Prisms and Filters. If an incandescent bulb is used close to the microscopic head, its light source is transferred through the objective with a series of prisms and filters, as depicted in Figure 24–33.

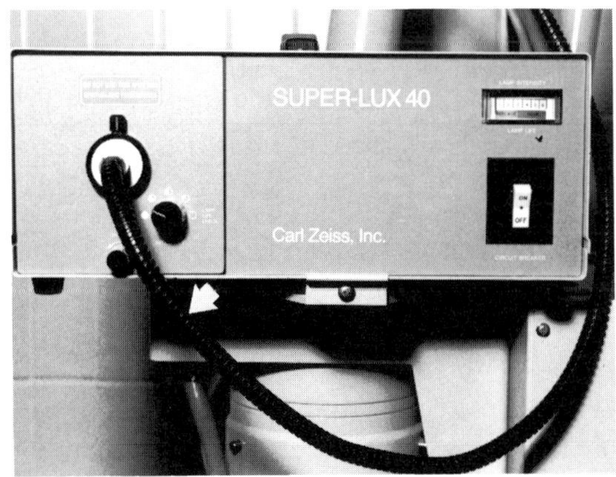

Figure 24–34. A more popular choice that generates less heat within the microscope is a distant light source carried into the microscope via a fiberoptic cable *(arrow)*.

Fiberoptics. A more popular choice is fiberoptics (Fig. 24–34). This allows for placement of the light source at a distance from the microscope head, making it easier to control heat and easier to change bulbs when they burn out during the procedure. The disadvantages of fiberoptic systems is that they are expensive, and with continuing use and bending of the fiberoptic cable, the glass fiberoptic cables break, reducing the light.

My current setup is a Superlux-40 (Zeiss) light source powered by a 12-volt, 100-watt halogen bulb with the light carried to the microscope by a fiberoptic cable (Fig. 24–34).

TECHNIQUE OF MICROSURGERY FOR HERNIATED NUCLEUS PULPOSUS

The most common frame and position are shown in Figure 24–35. The patient is stable in the kneeling position and is not hyperflexed at the hips and knees. The abdomen is free, thereby relieving pressure on the abdominal venous system and in turn decreasing venous backflow through Batson's plexus into the spinal canal. In this position it is easy to obtain an intraoperative lateral roentgenogram of the lumbosacral spine if necessary.

Identification of Level and Side

The level of surgical intervention should be marked before prepping and draping (Fig. 24–36). In most cases, the side of entry is predetermined. A midline disc herniation may be approached from either side but preferably from the most symptomatic side.

Skin Incision and Exposure of Interlaminar Space

The skin incision, 1/2 to 3/4 inch on either side of the marking line, is made beside the

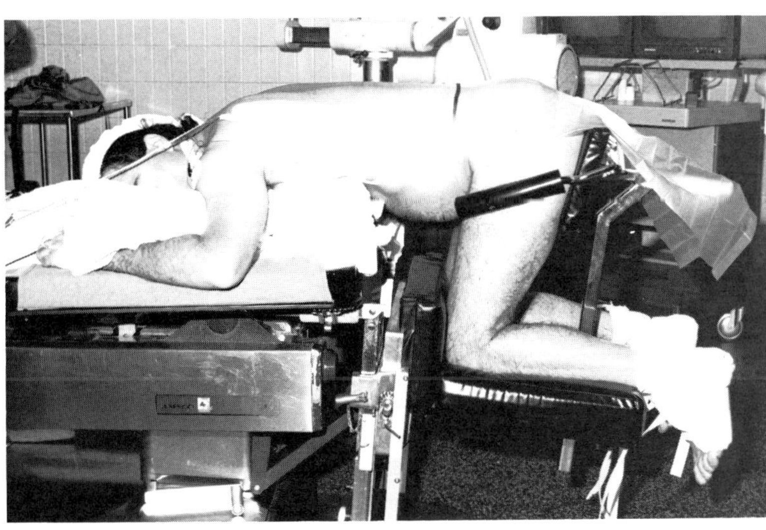

Figure 24–35. The kneeling position.

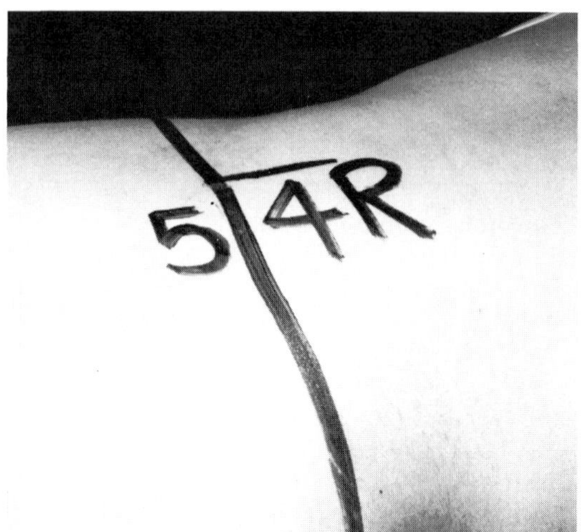

Figure 24–36. The limited surgical incision requires exact preoperative marking.

spinous processes rather than in the midline. Blunt dissection is used to expose the lumbodorsal fascia, which in turn is opened in a curvilinear fashion (Fig. 24–37). The skin opening and fascial incision are designed to do the least amount of damage to the interspinous–supraspinous ligament complex. The subperiosteal muscle dissection and elevation

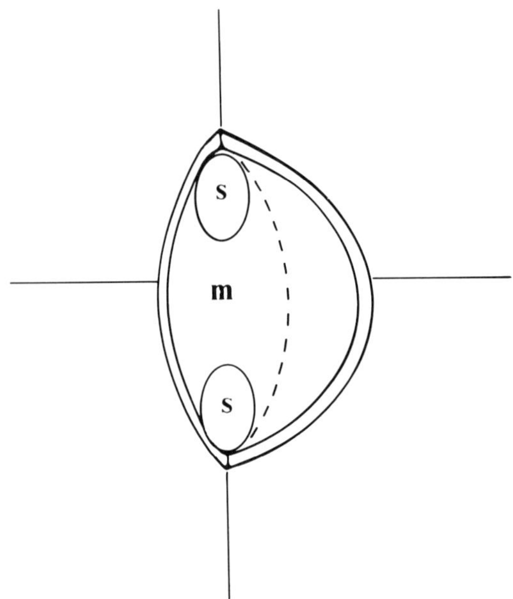

Figure 24–37. The curvilinear incision through lumbodorsal fascia and erector spinae fascia. s, Spinous process; m, midline supraspinous ligament area.

are confined to the interlaminar level being exposed.

Entry to the Spinal Canal

The surgeon should inspect the interlaminar interval and decide which type of entry to the spinal canal to use.

Transligamentous Entry

Crossing the ligamentum flavum to enter the spinal canal is the simplest, most direct route to the pathology. If the interlaminar interval is narrowed by degenerative changes, other routes are necessary.

Partial Hemilaminectomy

Partial hemilaminectomy is a popular neurosurgical approach whereby the inferior portion of the cephalad lamina is removed before the ligamentum flavum. There are many times when a microsurgical disc excision can be accomplished without removing any lamina, which is why most microsurgeons prefer the transligamentous approach.

Through the Safety Net

The base of the superior facet is marked by the inferior pole of the inferior facet and acts as a safety net (Fig. 24–38). In difficult openings, such as in patients who have had previous surgery, this is safe.[22] It is marked by the facet

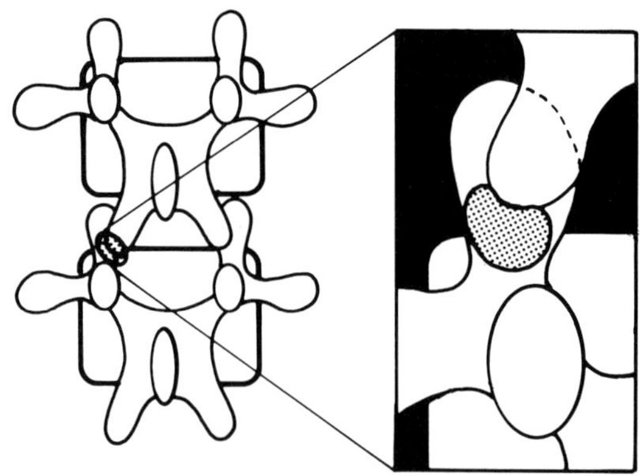

Figure 24–38. The "safety net," so named because the facet fat pad marks the area and the inferior portion of the superior facet protects against damaging the nerve.

fat pad and will lead the microsurgeon out of trouble more often than not. From there exposure can proceed along the inferior border of the cephalad lamina or the superior edge of the caudad lamina.

Across the Pars Interarticularis, Removing the Inferior Facet

This is an aggressive method of entry sometimes used for decompression of a foraminal stenosis or removal of a foraminal disc. This approach raises the problem of instability of the segment.

Extent of Interlaminar Exposure Relative to Pathology

With the knowledge of the location of the pathology in the spinal canal, a plan of cephalad-caudad laminar excision can be followed. For example:

1. A third-storey HNP in the L5 segment requires removal of some of the cephalad and caudad laminar edges during an L4–L5 exposure (Fig. 24–39).
2. A second-storey HNP in the L4 segment requires removal of at least half the cephalad lamina (Fig. 24–40).

The Lateral Edge of the Nerve Root

Once one is in the spinal canal, finding the lateral edge of the nerve root using blunt dissection is the most important step. After the lateral border of the nerve root is defined and the root retracted medially, it is possible to become more aggressive with the Kerrison to achieve the cephalad or caudad laminar excision necessary to deal with the pathology.

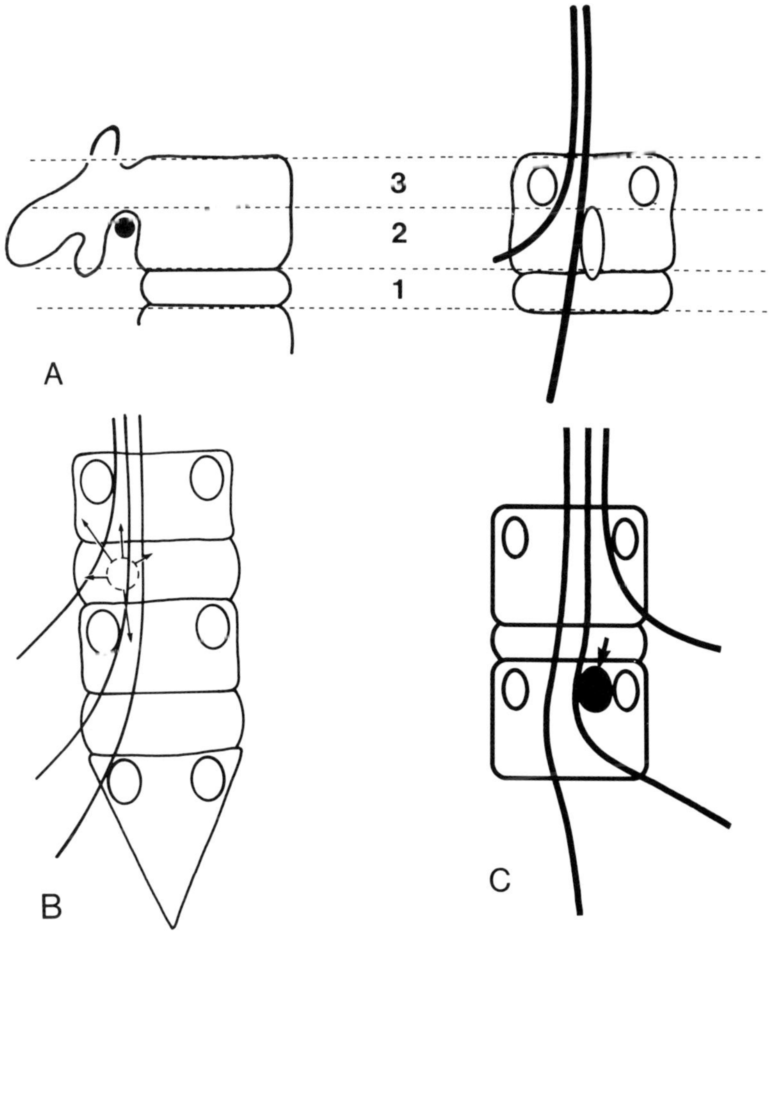

Figure 24–39. *A,* For the purposes of a microsurgical exploration, each lumbar anatomic segment is divided into three levels or stories: first storey, disc level; second storey, foraminal level; third storey, pedicle level. *B,* Disc fragments may migrate down into the third storey of the level below, laterally into the first storey, or up into the second storey of the same segment. *C,* A third-storey (pedicle) HNP from the disc space above *(arrow).*

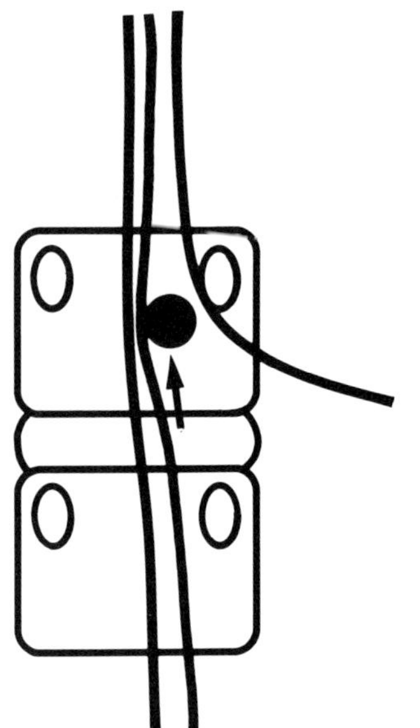

Figure 24–40. A second-storey disc herniation.

If you cannot find the lateral edge of the nerve root, think of the following:

1. An axillary disc displacing the root laterally.
2. Failure to remove an osteophytic lipping of the medial edge of the superior facet.
3. Adhesions.
4. Anomalous roots.

Sharp tools should not be used in the spinal canal until the lateral border of the nerve root has been located.

If you are having trouble finding the lateral edge of the nerve root or are wondering if there is any root lateral to the root you have identified, remember the following basic rule: nerve roots are intimately related to pedicles (Fig. 24–41). If you cannot find a nerve root, find a pedicle and the root will be immediately beside it; if you have a nerve root isolated, check that the medial bony wall of the pedicle is lateral to your probe to prove that no other nerve tissue is lateral to you at that particular point.

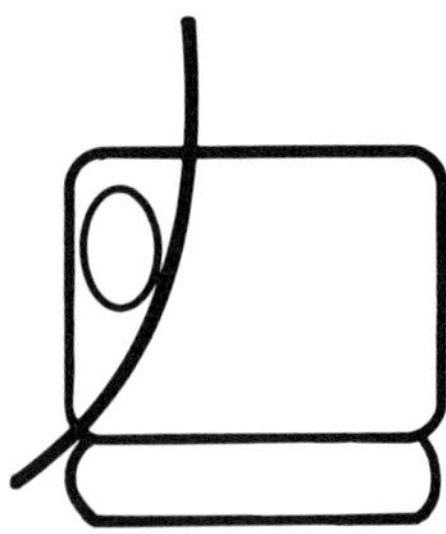

Figure 24–41. Nerve roots are intimately related to pedicles.

Retraction of the Nerve Root

Before retracting the nerve root, be sure that you have its lateral border clearly defined and that no adhesions are present. Microsurgery is a two-handed procedure; one hand holds and manipulates the root, the other hand operates. For this reason, it is best for the surgeon to hold the root retractor, which allows proper positioning and the retraction necessary to complete the operation.

Dealing With Canal Pathology

The object of the surgical exercise is to leave a freely mobile nerve root. This requires removal of the obvious portion of ruptured disc and also includes a search of the canal, along with probing of the foramen, for residual discal or bony pathology.

Removing Intradiscal Tissue

How much disc to remove from within the discal cavity is an unanswered question. Removal of as much disc as possible implies curettage of the interspace, including removal of the end plates. Critics of this approach point out the following drawbacks:

1. It is not possible to remove all intradiscal material in this manner, no matter how long the surgeon works.
2. This aggressive approach increases the risk of damage to visceral structures, anterior to the disc space.
3. The incidence of chronic back pain produced by conditions such as sterile discitis and instability is increased.
4. Although there are some articles in the literature to suggest that this extensive intradiscal debridement decreases the recurrent

HNP rate, there are other articles refuting the position. In the end, the only reasonable prospective controlled study was Spengler's, which suggested that limited disc excision is all that is necessary.[19]

Advantages of Limited Disc Removal

The advantages of limited disc removal are as follows:

1. Less trauma to end plates and less dissection.
2. Less nerve root manipulation.
3. Lower infection rate.
4. Lower complication rate for structures anterior to disc space (vessel perforation).
5. Less disc space settling postoperatively.

RESULTS OF MICROSURGERY FOR LUMBAR DISC DISEASE

Two hundred and fifty-seven patients underwent a lumbar spine microsurgical procedure between September 1983 and December 1986.[4] Surgery was indicated in the presence of acute or chronic radicular symptoms. Patients with an acute radicular syndrome had dominant leg pain and significant reduction in SLR with or without neurologic symptoms and signs. A patient with dominant leg pain and significant SLR reduction was not considered to have an acute radicular syndrome unless a structural lesion was demonstrated on myelography or CT scanning. Patients without this structural lesion on investigation did not undergo microsurgical intervention. Patients with chronic radicular syndromes had a less definitive diagnosis. They all had claudicant leg discomfort in a typical radicular distribution, associated with minor-to-moderate SLR reduction and minimal neurologic symptoms and signs. They also had to have had a structural lesion demonstrated on myelography or CT scanning, with CT scanning being positive more often than myelography. All patients reported in this series failed to respond to standard conservative treatment, which in the acute cases included a minimum of five days bed rest; an ambulatory program consisting of modified activities, corset support, and anti-inflammatory medication lasting a minimum of six weeks; or both. Patients with a chronic radicular syndrome had symptoms for a minimum of three months and failed to respond to an ambulatory conservative treatment program. All patients reported in this series were considered to be significantly disabled from a functional point of view and would have been candidates for a standard laminectomy/discectomy.

Table 24–6. PREVIOUS LUMBAR SPINE PROCEDURES (GROUP I)

Diagnosis	Total	Previous Discolysis	Previous Laminectomy
HPN	185	58 (31.4%)	8 (4.3%)
LZS*	24	7 (29.2%)	2 (8.3%)
HNP and LZS	14	5 (35.7%)	0
	223	70 (31.4%)	10 (4.5%)

*Lateral zone stenosis (subarticular and foraminal).

Methods

The history, physical examination, diagnosis, and intraoperative findings were obtained from the patient's chart. Details of the postoperative course, back-to-work status, and residual leg or back pain were obtained from a follow-up examination and a special questionnaire. Follow-up examination and retrieval of the questionnaire were obtained in 249 patients (97 per cent).

Results

Two groups of patients were studied independently. The first (Group I) consisted of 223 patients who had a microdiscectomy or microdecompression without fusion. The second (Group II) consisted of 26 patients who had a paraspinal fusion, using fresh cancellous autogenous bone, combined with microdecompres-

Table 24–7. COMPENSATION CASES (GROUP I)

Diagnosis	Total Cases	Compensation Cases
HNP	185	41 (22.2%)
LZS*	24	2 (8.3%)
HNP and LZS	14	4 (28.6%)
	223	47

*Lateral zone stenosis.

Table 24–8. LEVEL OF SURGERY (GROUP I)

Level	Number	Frequency
L1–L2	1	0.4%
L3–L4	16	7.2%
L4–L5	106	47.5%
L5–S1	94	42.2%
2 levels	6	2.7%
	223	100.0%

Table 24–10. RESULTS (GROUP I)

Grade I	Excellent	108	48.4%	75.8%
Grade II	Good	61	27.4%	
Grade III	Fair	17	7.6%	24.2%
Grade IV	Poor	37	16.6%	
		223	100%	

sion. These patients are excluded from this discussion.

Group I (223 Patients)

Diagnoses in Group I included herniated nucleus pulposus (185), lateral zone stenosis (24), and a combination of the two (14). There were 154 men and 69 women. The average age was 46 years (15 to 85 years). The average follow-up was 19 months (10 to 28 months). Eighty patients had undergone previous procedures before their microsurgical intervention. Seventy of these had received previous chymopapain treatment; ten had undergone previous laminectomy (Table 24–6).

In Group I there were 47 patients with pending compensation cases (Table 24–7). Table 24–8 shows the distribution of the affected segments. Clinical evaluation was made using a modification of Spangfort's criteria (Table 24–9).

Patients with Grade I or II classification were considered satisfactory. Those with Grade III or IV were considered unsatisfactory. On this functional grading scale, any patient who had limitations in the activity level or had not returned to work was considered a failure. Some patients with an unsatisfactory result were working with continuing symptoms but were not seeking further care. Other patients were relieved of leg pain but were not working, and these were also classified as having an unsatisfactory result.

Table 24–9. FUNCTIONAL GRADE

	Grade	Rating	Description
Satisfactory	I	Excellent	Complete relief of symptoms, back to normal
	II	Good	Mild discomfort, able to participate in all activities; do not require medications or bracing
Unsatisfactory	III	Fair	Better than preoperative status, significant limitations of activities, requiring medications, bracing
	IV	Poor	No better than preoperative status, unable to return to work

Average blood loss was 166 ml. The average postoperative hospitalization lasted 2.3 days. The result of surgery was rated excellent in 108 patients (48.4 per cent), good in 61 patients (27.4 per cent), fair in 17 patients (7.6 per cent), and poor in 37 patients (16.6 per cent) (Table 24–10). Satisfactory and unsatisfactory results were further analyzed by diagnosis and the presence or absence of previous surgery (Tables 24–11 to 24–13).

In patients with pending compensation cases, 31 (66 per cent) obtained a satisfactory result, whereas 16 (34 per cent) obtained an unsatisfactory result. In patients without compensation pending, 138 (79 per cent) obtained a satisfactory result, whereas 38 (21 per cent) had an unsatisfactory result.

A total of 189 patients worked before the operative procedure. Of the 34 patients who were not employed, 21 were retired, 11 were housewives, and two were students. Of the 189, 171 patients (90.5 per cent) returned to their previous work at an average 2.2 months postoperatively, and 18 (9.5 per cent) were unable to return to work because of continuing back or leg symptoms. Thirty-five patients (74.4 per cent) with compensation cases pending returned to work at an average 3.2 months postoperatively, whereas 136 (95.7 per cent)

Table 24–11. RESULTS IN PATIENTS BY DIAGNOSIS (GROUP I)

	HNP	LZS*	HNP and LZS	Total
Satisfactory	146 (78.9%)	12 (50%)	11 (78.6%)	169 (75.8%)
Unsatisfactory	39 (21.1%)	12 (50%)	3 (21.4%)	54 (24.2%)
	185 (100%)	24 (100%)	14 (100%)	223 (100%)

*Lateral zone stenosis (subarticular and foraminal).

Table 24–12. RESULTS IN PATIENTS WITHOUT PREVIOUS SURGERY (GROUP I)

	HNP	LZS*	HNP and LZS	Total
Satisfactory	100 (84%)	8 (53.3%)	8 (88.9%)	116 (81.1%)
Unsatisfactory	19 (16%)	7 (46.7%)	1 (11.1%)	27 (18.9%)

*Lateral zone stenosis (subarticular and foraminal).

without compensation cases pending returned to work at an average 1.6 months postoperatively.

The 10.8 per cent complication rate in Group I patients seems high (Table 24–14). It is important to emphasize that 223 patients in this group represent my first cases of microsurgical intervention. Obviously there was a learning curve, and most of these complications—specifically the dural tear complications—occurred early in the microsurgical experience. The six dural tears were all considered minor punctures, except for one that required suture repair. The other five tears were not repaired, and none of the six tears led to any further complications.

The 3-in-100 incidence of wrong-level explorations was discovered intraoperatively, and the correct level was subsequently exposed. Five of the six cases were one level too high, which is the most common wrong-level error in microsurgery. Wrong-level explorations tend to be one level higher than the level sought, and they occur most commonly in obese and loose-jointed patients in hyperlordosis when on the operating table in the kneeling position. The basic rule to avoid wrong-level explorations is to know before starting exactly what pathology is to be encountered; when that pathology is not encountered on operative exposure, one must be immediately suspicious of wrong-level exploration. If there is any reason for doubt, it is essential to obtain an intraoperative roentgenogram to verify the operative level exposed. I used intraoperative marking infrequently, but I always used it

Table 24–13. RESULTS IN PATIENTS WITH PREVIOUS SURGERY (GROUP I)

	HNP	LZS*	HNP and LZS	Total
Satisfactory	46 (69.7%)	4 (44.4%)	3 (60%)	53 (66.3%)
Unsatisfactory	20 (30.3%)	5 (55.6%)	2 (40%)	27 (33.7%)

*Lateral zone stenosis (subarticular and foraminal).

Table 24—14. COMPLICATIONS (GROUP I)

	Number	%
Dural tear (minor)	6	2.70
Wrong level exploration*	6	2.70
Hemorrhage requiring transfusion	3	1.35
Superficial wound infection	2	0.90
Disc space infection	2	0.90
Increased neurodeficit	2	0.90
Hematoma	1	0.45
Gastritis	1	0.45
Urinary retention	1	0.45

*Recognized during surgery.

whenever the expected pathology was not encountered.

Three patients required blood transfusion for hemorrhage. This is much lower than standard laminectomy/discectomy but is still an unacceptable rate of transfusion for microsurgical intervention for simple disc herniations.[14] These three patients contributed to an average blood loss of 166 ml, which is higher than the values given in previously published reports.[3, 5, 15, 17, 24]

Those patients with minor superficial infections were recorded and easily treated. Of more concern is the almost 1 per cent disc-space infection rate, which is unacceptably high. The probable reason for this is manipulation of the microscope, which has nonsterile exposed eyepieces over the wound. Some of these patients received prophylactic antibiotics and some did not, but the pattern of the use of prophylactic antibiotics did not allow for any conclusions. A review of the literature reveals a range of disc space infection rates. Spangfort's large and comprehensive series reports a rate of 2 per cent.[18] Goald (0 per cent in 477 patients) and Williams (0 per cent in 530 patients) dealt with canal pathology only and did not invade the disc space in the limited fashion used in this series.[5, 24] After reviewing a number of articles, Ebeling and associates concluded that the infection rate is the same for microsurgery and standard laminectomy/discectomy.[3] Using a similar approach, Dauch concluded that the infection rate for standard laminectomy/discectomy (2.8 per cent) was much higher than for microsurgery (0.4 per cent).[2]

Two patients had an increase in neurologic deficits (increased weakness) that was considered minor but definite. Both of these recovered and had no residual problems.

Miscellaneous complications of wound hematoma, gastritis, and urinary retention were also recorded. The low incidence of urinary retention is the result of ambulation of patients on the day of (or the day after) microsurgical intervention. None of the patients with complications, nor any other patient in this report, has had recourse to litigation. Although a complication rate of 10.8 per cent seems unusually high, these were considered minor complications with minimal effect on the hospital stay and no effect on the ultimate result.

In summary, it can be stated that in Group I patients the results of microsurgical intervention for lumbar disc disease, on preliminary evaluation, compare favorably with standard laminectomy/discectomy. The complication rate is also comparable and, with further experience, will probably be reduced.

CONCLUSION

Microsurgical intervention for lumbar disc disease is a controversial subject. To some it is a gimmick. To others it is simply the advancement of surgery to different technical levels that use the combination of magnification and illumination to facilitate and limit operative exposure.[6, 8, 12, 15, 23, 24, 27] This series and other reports leave no doubt about the decreased length of hospitalization after microsurgical intervention, and thus the decreased cost of caring for patients. This decreased cost, along with preliminary results comparable with those of standard laminectomy/discectomy, offers an advantage for microsurgical intervention. A hidden advantage of microsurgical intervention is the necessity for an extremely accurate preoperative diagnosis before the surgical exposure is undertaken. Microsurgery is not seek-and-find surgery, and thus it is imperative that an accurate diagnosis of the level, nature, and extent of pathology be made before a microsurgical procedure is undertaken. Thus, one can refute the accusations of decreased surgical exposure and missed pathology. The increased infection rate in this and other series must be resolved, and probably centers around the presence of a partially nonsterile instrument over the operative field. Wrong-level surgical intervention is a constant problem for microsurgeons.

In spite of these initial setbacks in microsurgical experiences, the procedure has become one of the many options available to the patient with various spine disorders.

References

1. Bell, G. R., and Rothman, R. H.: The conservative treatment of sciatica. Spine *9*:54, 1984.
2. Dauch, W. A.: Infection of the intervertebral space following conventional and microsurgical operation on the herniated lumbar intervertebral disc. Acta Neurochir. (Wien) *82*:43, 1986.
3. Ebeling, U., Reichenberg, W., and Reulen, H. J.: Results of microsurgical lumbar discectomy. Acta Neurochir. (Wien) *81*:45, 1986.
4. Feldman, R., and McCulloch, J. A.: Microsurgery for lumbar root encroachment. Submitted for publication.
5. Goald, H. J.: Microlumbar discectomy: follow-up of 477 patients. J. Microsurg. *2*:95, 1980.
6. Goald, H. J.: A new microsurgical reoperation for failed lumbar disc surgery. J. Microsurg. *7*:63, 1986.
7. Hakelius, A.: Prognosis in sciatica: a clinical follow-up of surgical and non-surgical treatment. Acta Orthop. Scand. *129*(Suppl):1, 1970.
8. Hudgins, W. R.: The role of microdiscectomy. Orthop. Clin. North Am. *14*:589, 1983.
9. Kahanovich, N., Viola, K., and McCulloch, J. A.: Limited surgical discectomy and microdiscectomy: a clinical comparison. Spine *14*:79, 1989.
10. Lang, W. H., and Muchel, F.: Zeiss Microscopes for Microsurgery. Berlin, Springer-Verlag, 1981.
11. Larocca, H., and MacNab, I.: The laminectomy membrane. J. Bone Joint Surg. *56B*:545, 1974.
12. Loew, F.: Different operative possibilities for treatment of lumbar disc herniations. Neurosurg. Rev. *9*:109, 1986.
13. MacNab, I., Cuthbert, H., and Godfrey, C.: The incidence of denervation of the sacro-spinales muscles following spinal surgery. Spine *2*:294, 1977.
14. Mandel, R. J., Brown, M. D., McCullough, N. C., et al.: Hypotensive anesthesia and autotransfusion in spinal surgery. Clin. Orthop. *154*:27, 1981.
15. Merli, C. A., Angiari, P., and Tonell, C.: Three years experience with microsurgical technique in treatment of the protruded lumbar disc. J. Neurosurg. *28*:25, 1984.
16. Peacock, E. E.: Dynamic aspects of collagen biology. Part 1: synthesis and assembly. J. Surg. Res. *7*:433, 1967.
17. Sachde, V. P.: Microsurgical lumbar discectomy: a personal series of 300 patients with at least 1 year follow-up. J. Microsurg. *7*:55, 1986.
18. Spangfort, E. V.: The lumbar disc herniation: a computer aided analysis of 2,504 operations. Acta Orthop. Scand. *142*(Suppl):1, 1972.
19. Spengler, D. M.: Results with limited excision and selective foraminotomy. Spine *6*:604, 1982.
20. Van Royen, B. J., O'Driscoll, S. W., Dhert, W. J. A., and Salter, R. B.: A comparison of the effects of immobilization and continuous passive motion on surgical wound healing in mature rabbits. Plast. Reconstr. Surg. *78*:360, 1986.

21. Weber, H.: Lumbar disc herniation: a controlled prospective study with 10 years of observation. Spine *8:*131, 1983.
22. Weir, B. K. A., and Jacobs, G. A.: Reoperation rate following lumbar discectomy: an analysis of 662 lumbar discectomies. Spine *5:*366, 1980.
23. Williams, R. W.: Microlumbar discectomy: a conservative surgical approach to the virgin herniated lumbar disc. Spine *3:*175, 1978.
24. Williams, R. W.: Microlumbar discectomy: a 12-year statistical review. Spine *11:*851, 1986.
25. Wilson, D. H., and Harbaugh, R.: Microsurgical and standard removal of the protruded lumbar disc: a comparative study. Neurosurgery *8:*422, 1981.
26. Wilson, D. H., and Kenning, J.: Microsurgical lumbar discectomy: preliminary report of 83 consecutive cases. Neurosurgery *4:*137, 1979.
27. Yasargil, M. G.: Microsurgical operation of herniated lumbar disc. Adv. Neurosurg. *4:*81, 1977.
28. Yong-Hing, K., Reilly, J., DeKorompay, V., and Kirkaldy-Willis, W. H.: Prevention of nerve root adhesions after laminectomy. Spine *5:*59, 1980.

CHAPTER

25

SPINAL STENOSIS

Steven R. Garfin, M.D.
Björn L. Rydevik, M.D., Ph.D.
Stephen J. Lipson, M.D.
Harry N. Herkowitz, M.D.
Hani El-Kommos, M.D.
Srdjan Mirkovic, M.D.
Robert E. Booth, Jr., M.D.

PATHOPHYSIOLOGY

Steven R. Garfin, M.D.
Björn L. Rydevik, M.D., Ph.D.
Stephen J. Lipson, M.D.

The symptoms of spinal stenosis are related to a complex series of changes in the spinal column. Most of the alterations observed pathoanatomically and radiographically can be ascribed to the degenerative or aging process. However, in certain individuals these changes lead to symptoms and signs of spinal stenosis. The narrowing of the spinal canal that occurs in spinal stenosis causes mechanical compression of spinal nerve roots. In many individuals this compression is asymptomatic, but in some a variety of clinical symptoms can occur, including weakness, reflex alterations, pain (in characteristic or uncharacteristic patterns), and paresthesias.

Spinal stenosis is a progressive and dynamic process. Because of this, symptoms are not identical from individual to individual, and may vary over time in the same individual. This may relate to such factors as the degree of compression, the location of compression, the amount of inflammation along the nerve root, and disc prominence. Before our more universal awareness of the diagnosis of spinal stenosis, the bizarre or frequently atypical and varying symptoms and inconsistent signs (often with lack of neurologic deficit) commonly led physicians to recommend psychiatric evaluation of these elderly patients. Now, however, the clinical manifestations of spinal stenosis are better understood, and much more precise diagnosis is possible.[15–17, 23, 25, 26, 31, 42, 52, 53, 56, 67, 71, 88, 117, 125, 128, 158, 159, 192, 193]

Unfortunately, the underlying pathophysiologic mechanisms of the signs and symptoms are still incompletely understood. Early descriptions of spinal stenosis focused primarily on factors related to discs, facets, anatomic deformities, facet arthritis, and ligament buckling/hypertrophy. More recently, an appreciation of the involvement of the nerves of the cauda equina has been gaining attention (Fig. 25–1). Although there is much evidence related to peripheral nerve compression, there are very limited data evaluating the spinal nerve root and cauda equina under compression. This chapter focuses on available knowledge in most of the involved areas and tissues, including bone, disc, facets, and neural elements.

The societal and individual aspects of the importance of back and radicular pain date back to early civilization, when witches and demons were thought to be the source of back pain. It was felt at the time that exorcism could play a role in alleviating this pain. Shakespeare, in *Timon of Athens*, noted that sciatica was a crippler and affected the limbs in a most serious way. The medical history of spinal stenosis itself actually began in the 1800s.

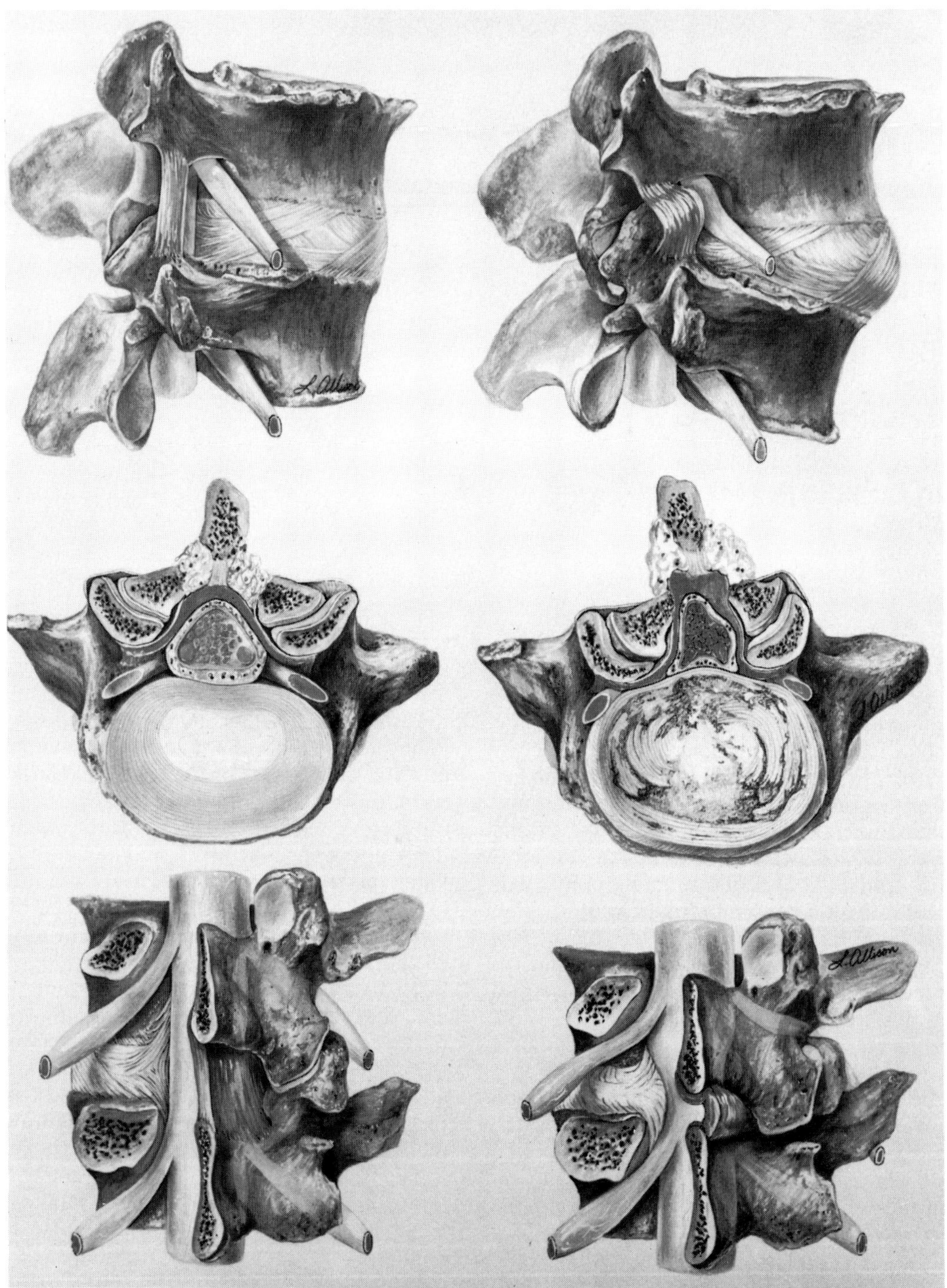

Figure 25–1 *See legend on opposite page*

Portal first raised issues related to some of our modern ideas regarding spinal stenosis when he theorized that back and leg pain could be due to bone impingement on the nerves.[183] Sachs and Fraenkel in 1900 related the sciatic complaints and signs in elderly individuals to pinching of the nerves in the spinal canal.[155a] However, they believed the compression to be due to tumors or infections and recommended that their patients have laminectomies for those disorders. Bailey and Casamajor wrote in 1911 that the spinal nerve symptoms were due to bony stenosis and recommended laminectomy.[9] In 1913 Elsberg became one of the first neurosurgeons to specialize in laminectomies.[49a] Later, Mixter and Barr emphasized the importance of disc pathology in sciatica and altered our concepts of leg pain.[121] In the 1950s and beyond, Verbiest and, separately, Kirkaldy-Willis, contributed immensely to our knowledge of disc disease and spinal stenosis and introduced many of the current clinical and pathoanatomic concepts of the disease.[35, 93–97, 181–184, 186, 188]

DEFINITIONS

Stenosis is a narrowing of a hollow tube or canal. The narrowing in the spinal column can occur in one of a number of places, although usually it is (1) centrally in the spinal column, (2) along the nerve root as it courses anteromedial to the facet joint, or (3) in the intervertebral (subpedicular) foramen. Depending on the amount and location of the stenosis, the symptoms may be restricted to a single isolated root, as in lateral recess stenosis, or may present with a more complex picture involving multilevel, bilateral radicular pains and signs.

Spinal stenosis can be classified into congenital/developmental and acquired types (Fig. 25–2).[5] The congenital/developmental can be subdivided into dwarfism, such as achondroplasia, and idiopathic types. The latter may relate to many normal-size adults seen with these complaints, who have congenitally narrowed canals.[41, 45, 140, 141, 156, 157] Achondroplasts will not be discussed in this chapter.[4, 8, 10, 24, 38, 54, 65, 76, 110, 164, 167, 196]

Acquired stenosis has many etiologies.[5, 42–44, 46, 142] These can be related to defects of the pars interarticularis (isthmic), iatrogenically induced stenosis,[20] post-traumatic stenosis,[79] developmental/degenerative stenosis, and miscellaneous conditions.[69, 82, 91, 190] A subcategory, which combines degenerative changes with congenital/developmental narrowing, probably covers most patients who seek treatment.

Figure 25–1. Artist's compilation of pathologic changes that result in spinal stenosis *(right)* compared with three normal views of the L4–L5 intervertebral joint *(left)*.

The tripod joint complex, composed of the intervertebral disc and two facet joints, must be visualized in order to understand the pathophysiology of stenosis. The articular facets sublux in the axial, sagittal, and front planes, and the disc tends to narrow more in the posterior half than in the anterior half. This leads to a rotation of the superior facet anteriorly toward the posterior lateral corner of the adjacent vertebra. With subluxation of the facet joint, in both an axial and a sagittal plane, joint erosion, recurrent joint effusion, and degenerative changes with osteophyte formation occur. These diarthrodial joints are subject to all the changes that can occur in a peripheral joint. Rotational subluxation affects the inferior facet on one side and the superior facet on the contralateral side, causing them to protrude into the spinal canal. The ligamentum flavum, a passive elastic ligament, shortens with narrowing of the disc and subluxation of the facet joint. As a consequence of this shortening, the elastic ligament thickens. The thickened ligament is passively pushed into the neural space by the osteoarthritic changes, and perhaps subluxation, of the facet joint. These changes are best seen in the transverse view of the intervertebral joint.

The consequences of an anvil effect of the bulging annulus fibrosus, with its marginal osteophytes pushed up against the anterior subluxating superior facet joints, are that it takes up the room lateral or posterior to the nerve roots, which are just anterior and medial to the superior facet. For example, if the intervertebral joint depicted in this illustration is the L4–L5 disc, the L5 nerve roots are displaced by this anvil effect of the superior facet of L5 against the bulging L4 disc. The L5 roots are compressed. There is rotation of the left inferior facet and the right superior facet into the spinal canal. Degenerative changes in the joint and the marginal osteophyte formation are depicted. The ligamentum has thickened and has been passively displaced into the neural space by the subluxed, hypertrophied facet joints. From a posterior view, one can appreciate the natural consequences of central stenosis and the passive constriction of the dura, silhouetted beneath the narrowed interface. The relationship of the L4 nerve root, taking a serpiginous course above the subluxed and rotated superior facet, can also be seen in this diagram. These are all permutations of nerve root entrapment, as a result of disc narrowing and facet joint subluxation. If these changes occur gradually and in the absence of annular tears, pain may not occur until late in the disease process, when ischemia and compression become additive and create symptoms.

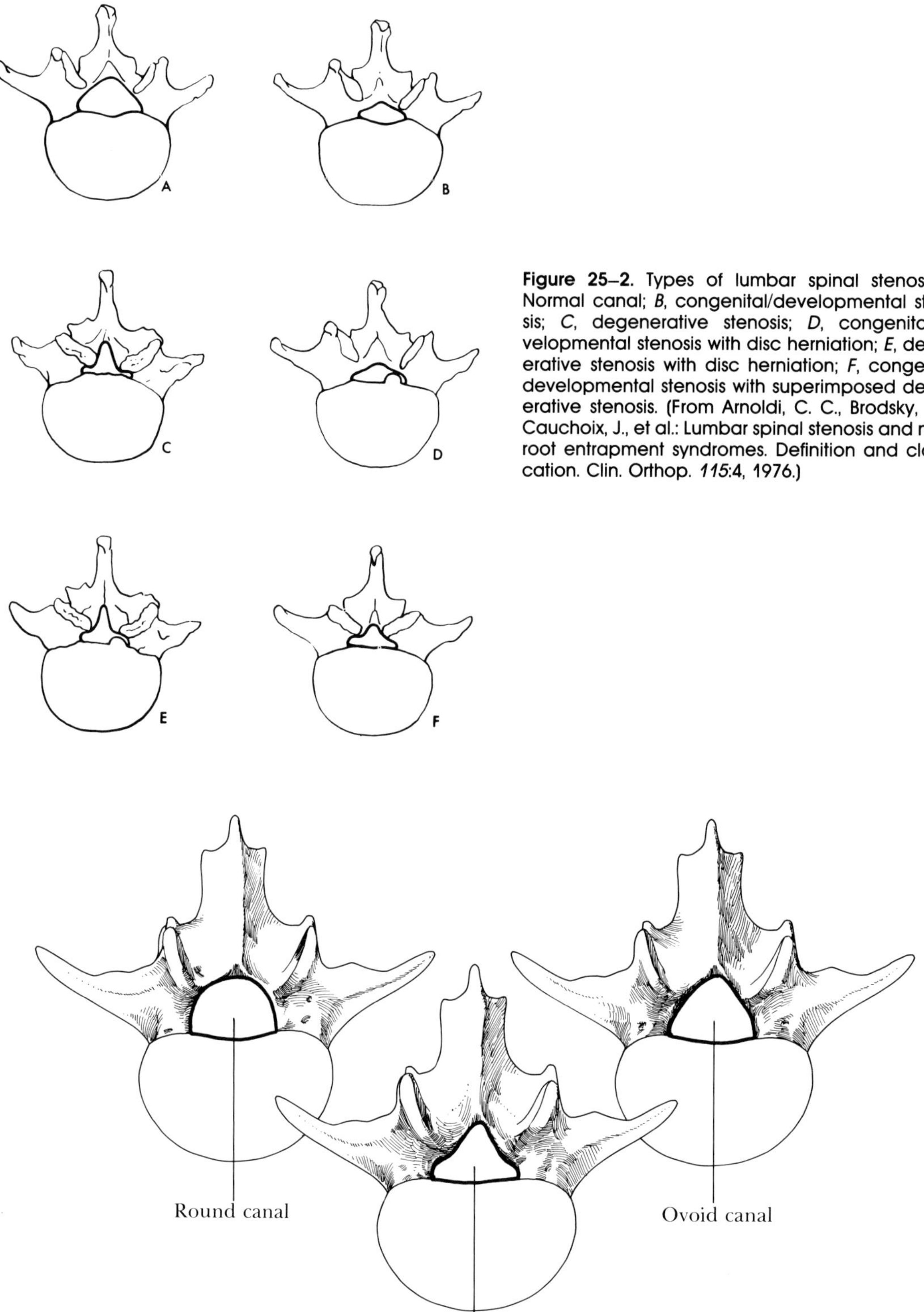

Figure 25–2. Types of lumbar spinal stenosis. *A*, Normal canal; *B*, congenital/developmental stenosis; *C*, degenerative stenosis; *D*, congenital/developmental stenosis with disc herniation; *E*, degenerative stenosis with disc herniation; *F*, congenital/developmental stenosis with superimposed degenerative stenosis. (From Arnoldi, C. C., Brodsky, A. E., Cauchoix, J., et al.: Lumbar spinal stenosis and nerve root entrapment syndromes. Definition and classification. Clin. Orthop. *115*:4, 1976.)

Figure 25–3. The three variations of the spinal canal: round, ovoid, and trefoil. The lateral recesses of the trefoil canal render the lumbar roots particularly vulnerable to compression by extruded disc material. (From DePalma, A. F., and Rothman, R. H.: The Intervertebral Disc. Philadelphia, W. B. Saunders Co., 1970.)

These individuals start with a smaller than normal canal and have superimposed degenerative changes such as bulging discs, facet hypertrophy/arthritis, buckling or hypertrophy of ligaments, and/or spondylolistheses.

PATHOPHYSIOLOGY

Clinical/Experimental

Spinal Column

The spinal canal can have a number of anatomic configurations. The round, or nearly round, canal is the most capacious centrally and laterally (Fig. 25–3).[47, 48, 143, 194] In general a normal lumbar canal has 12 mm or more anteroposterior diameter and a cross-sectional area of at least 77 ± 13 mm^2.[162, 163] Trefoil canals, on the other hand, have an unfavorable configuration, particularly in the lateral recess. Any small lateral bulging discs or facet alterations could lead to compression of the nerve root in the intervertebral canal.[146] However, this anatomic configuration does not absolutely guarantee that a patient will develop symptoms of spinal stenosis.[100]

The main culprit initiating the sequence of events leading to spinal stenosis appears to be disc degeneration.[93–95, 97, 98] Kirkaldy-Willis and Farfan popularized the concept of a three-joint complex.[94, 95, 97] In this depiction the spine motion segment can essentially be visualized as a large tripod, with the disc as one of the joints or legs, and the facets completing the two posterior supports of the three-joint complex (Fig. 25–4). Any alteration in one of these joints, which usually has the disc as the primary dysfunctional unit, can lead to abnormal biomechanical stresses on the others. This results in arthritic/degenerative changes in the facets and further deterioration of the disc itself.

The Disc

Biochemical Changes. In tissue pathology, aging implies an accumulation of changes over time. Degeneration, on the other hand, suggests a deterioration or worsening of the physical properties of a tissue with retrogressive pathologic changes in the cells or tissue, the consequence of which may be destruction or inhibition of function. As the intervertebral disc ages, it undergoes degeneration. Clinicians, however, tend to differentiate aging, as a morphologic anatomic change, from degeneration, which has similar alterations but often is associated with a clinical complaint. Although disc degeneration is often demonstrable radiologically in adults with low back pain,[92] a causal relationship between low back pain and degenerative changes has not been established definitively.[115] Common radiologic degenerative changes in the disc motion segment can be noted in the absence of low back disorders.[86] There is no clear distinction between the normal anatomic changes of degeneration through aging and those that may be considered pathologic.[30, 78] Aging and degeneration are similar pathologic processes, but some physiologic feature, or features, occurring during degeneration cause(s) a clinical complaint.

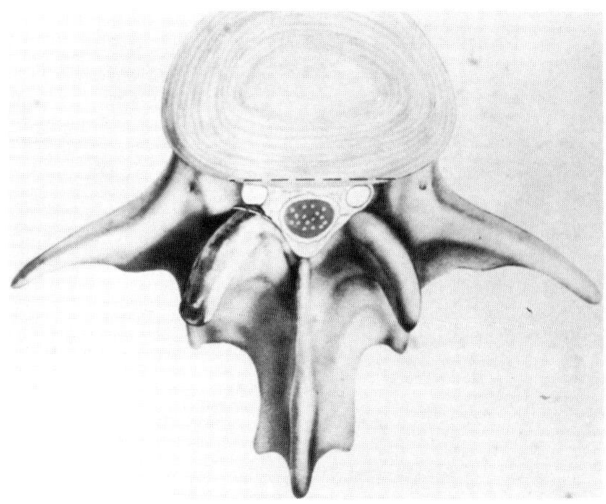

Figure 25–4. A bulging disc that additively narrows the spinal canal in the presence of facet hypotrophy and presumably ligamentous buckling. On the left the fat around the nerve root, as well as the nerve root, is diminished in size because of the disc and facet that narrow the lateral recess.

Pathoanatomic Changes. In most patients, disc degeneration has been shown to be the first stage in the degenerative/aging process ("cascade") of the spine (Fig. 25–5).[97, 98] However, Videman and associates demonstrated that in 20 per cent of degenerative spines, facet arthritis precedes evidence of disc degeneration.[187] In any event, once disc degeneration occurs, it can lead to stenosis through a bulging annulus encroaching on the spinal canal anteriorly, as well as through frank disc herniation, or a slow progressive process with osteophyte formation and other stigmata of spondylosis (see Figs. 25–1 and 25–4).

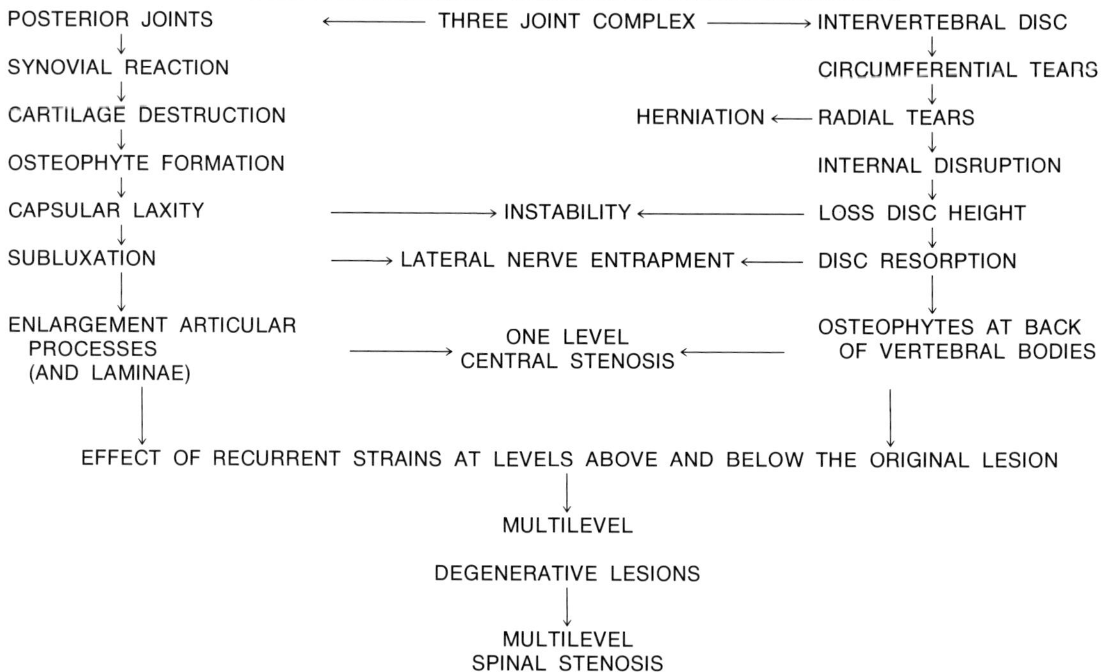

Figure 25–5. Degenerative cascade in the lumbar spine. The interrelationship of multiple factors is depicted. (From Kirkaldy-Willis, W. H., Wedge, I. H., Yong-Hing, K., and Reilly, J.: Pathology and pathogenesis of lumbar spondylosis and stenosis. Spine *3*:319, 1978.)

In youth and in the intact disc, the annular contour is smooth and the nucleus of the disc is gelatinous. The annular material is distinct and has a lamellar structure, which is separate from the nucleus pulposus (Fig. 25–6). As the patient ages, concentric rings in the annulus become more discrete, and there is a less well defined border between the nucleus and the annulus (Fig. 25–7).[30, 66, 78, 180] As shown by Kirkaldy-Willis and colleagues, the first gross stage in the degenerative cascade is circumferential tearing (Fig. 25–8).[97] As the process develops, the circumferential tears coalesce and radial tears become evident (Fig. 25–9). With progression there is further degeneration, coupled with biomechanical and biochemical alterations (proteoglycan and collagen changes and dehydration) that affect the disc and narrow the intervertebral disc space height. As collapse and fissuring occur, there is further bulging posteriorly, particularly along the posterior longitudinal ligament (Fig. 25–10). Finally, marked degeneration and dehydration conclude the degenerative process within the disc itself (Fig. 25–11). These "age-related" changes usually occur first in the lower, more mobile disc segments of L5–S1 and L4–L5, but then proceed cephalically and involve most discs over time.

On the basis of these observations, intervertebral disc degeneration has been graded and classified by Nachemson[124] and Lewin.[103] Nachemson's classification divides disc degeneration into four grades, denoting the range from the young or normal disc to severe degeneration by progressive loss of the nucleus, distinction of the nucleus-annulus border, the appearance of fibrosis and fissuring, and marginal osteophyte formation. In a collected autopsy series,[119] disc degeneration first appeared in the second decade in males and the third in females, with 97 per cent of discs demonstrating degeneration by age 50. L5–S1, L4–L5, and L3–L4 are often the most degenerated discs.

In the fetal and infant nucleus pulposus, notochordal cells are found as clusters of vacuolated cells floating in a basophilic matrix.

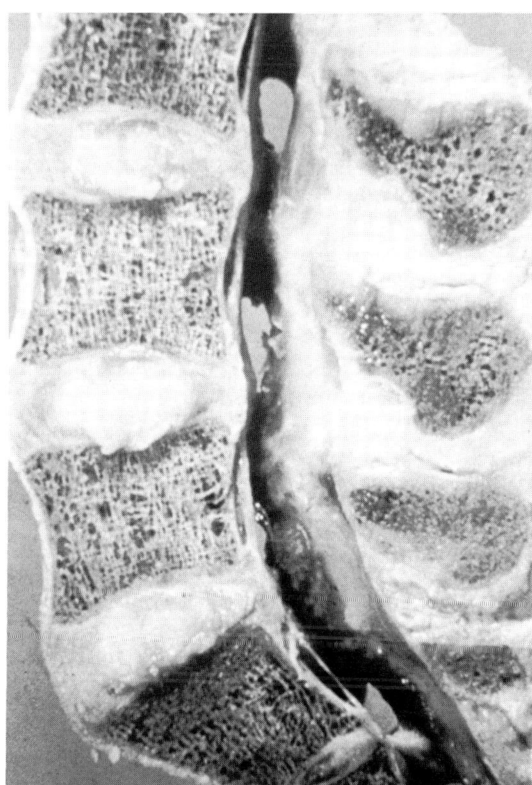

Figure 25–6. Healthy-appearing discs from a young specimen. The gelatinous nucleus bulges and nearly extrudes through the sagittal cut. Discrete annular lamellae can be seen. This is a sagittal section through the midportion of the spinal canal. (From Kirkaldy-Willis, W. H., Wedge, J. H., Yong-Hing, K., and Reilly, J.: Pathology and pathogenesis of lumbar spondylosis and stenosis. Spine *3*:319, 1978.)

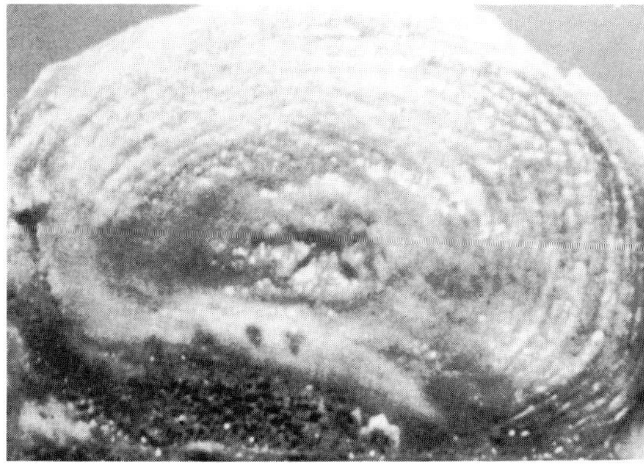

Figure 25–7. A relatively healthy disc. The nucleus can be seen centrally and the annulus is well defined peripherally. (From Kirkaldy-Willis, W. H., Wedge, J. H., Yong-Hing, K., and Reilly, J.: Pathology and pathogenesis of lumbar spondylosis and stenosis. Spine *3*:319, 1978.)

Histochemically the enzymes found in these cells are similar to those in perichordal cells.[195] There is a fine fibrillar structure in the matrix, and both fibroblasts and chondrocytes can be seen along with the notochordal cells. The original peripheral portion of the nucleus is fibrous, blending with the fibers of the annulus fibrosus. This border becomes indistinct after the second decade.[29, 39] Gradual cavitation, apparent desiccation, cellular degeneration, fibroblastic proliferation, and calcium salt deposition follow. The fibroblasts in the nucleus are not orderly as in the annulus, and more chondrocytes appear. With progressive degeneration the annulus fibrosus and nucleus pulposus are indistinct, with fibrocartilage replacing the nuclear area.[29]

The lamellae of the annulus become coarser and hyalinized with age. Fissures become apparent and pigmentation may occur. Nests of

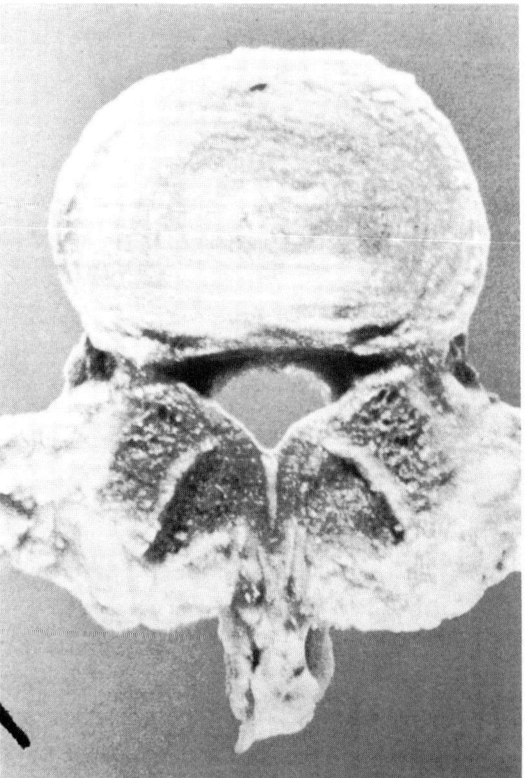

Figure 25–8. With age there is some drying of the annulus and nucleus. Small tears develop in line with the lamellae. These can be seen anteriorly and posterolaterally in this specimen. (From Kirkaldy-Willis, W. H., Wedge, J. H., Yong-Hing, K., and Reilly, J.: Pathology and pathogenesis of lumbar spondylosis and stenosis. Spine *3*:319, 1978.)

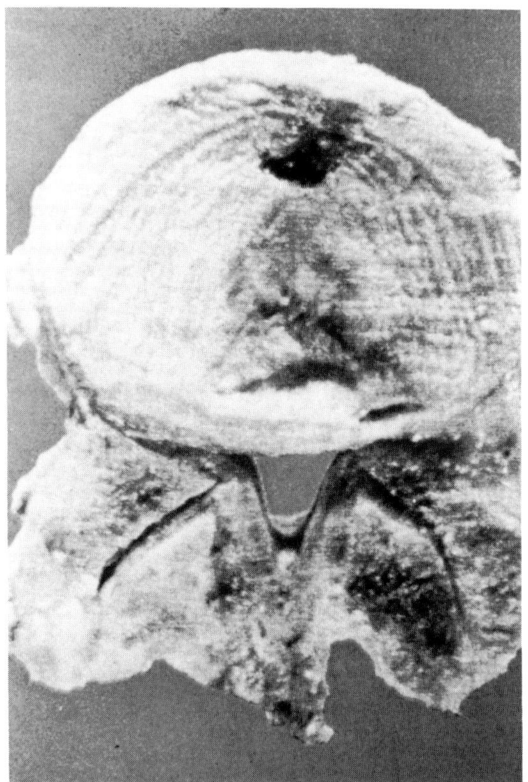

Figure 25–9. As the degenerative process advances, the tears coalesce and become large, radial tears. The annulus and nucleus become less distinct and dehydration proceeds. In addition, as seen in the lower portion of the illustration, the facet joints develop arthritic changes and occupy a broader area of the spinal canal. (From Kirkaldy-Willis, W. H., Wedge, J. H., Yong-Hing, K., and Reilly, J.: Pathology and pathogenesis of lumbar spondylosis and stenosis. Spine *3*:319, 1978.)

chondrocytes can be noted by the fourth decade, and progression of fibrocartilaginous change is frequently observed. Vascular invasion occurs. Progression of disc degeneration is associated with further conversion to more disorganized fibrocartilage. In the annulus fibrosus, with age, the pericellular area loses a periodic acid–Schiff (PAS) positive component, enhanced Alcian blue staining occurs, and the matrix becomes more granular.[180] While the lamellae become disordered, more random PAS-reactive fibrous material appears, implying an alteration in the collagen-proteoglycan relationship. These changes, which lead to alteration in the mechanical properties of the annulus fibrosus, may be considered "regressive."[180]

With nucleus pulposus degeneration, PAS positivity increases and corresponds to age pigment, while Alcian blue proteoglycan staining decreases.[144] These changes are concomitant with fibrocartilaginous metaplasia of the annulus, where chondrocytes and chondrons appear, starting in the inner lamellae; Alcian blue territorial matrix appears as the once orderly annulus fibrosus becomes more random.

The fine structure of human intervertebral discs, shown by electron microscopy, has been extensively reviewed.[21] Cell activity, collagen, proteoglycan, and noncollagenous proteins can

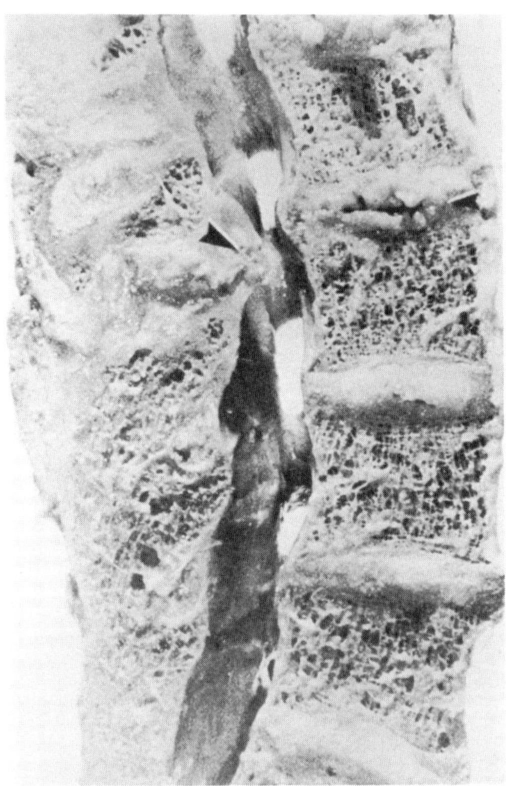

Figure 25–10. In this specimen there is a posterior fusion that begins distal to the arrowhead. The first motion segment is, therefore, at the level of the arrowhead where the posterior fusion ends. Across from the fusion the discs are well maintained and bulge through this sagittal cut. However, at the first motion segment (at the arrowhead), marked disc degeneration can be seen with narrowing and fissuring. The end plate also is more osteoporotic centrally than the bone below. This is similar to what frequently happens at L5–S1. It demonstrates the importance of motion and mechanical stresses to the degenerative process. (From permission Kirkaldy-Willis, W. H., Wedge, J. H., Yong-Hing, K., and Reilly, J.: Pathology and pathogenesis of lumbar spondylosis and stenosis. Spine *3*:319, 1978.)

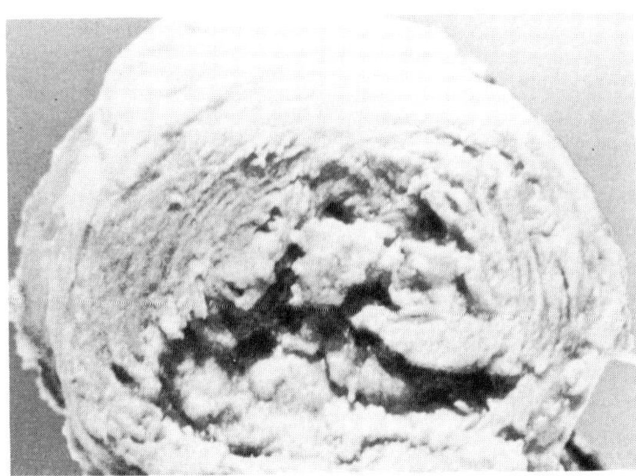

Figure 25–11. The termination of this process is significant degenerative change with marked dehydration, fissuring, and erosions. The dried nucleus is indistinguishable from the annulus. (From Kirkaldy-Willis, W. H., Wedge, J. H., Yong-Hing, K., and Reilly, J.: Pathology and pathogenesis of lumbar spondylosis and stenosis. Spine *3*:319, 1978.)

be localized and "observed" microscopically. The collagen fibrils of the lamellae of the annulus fibrosus provide tensile strength and are architecturally organized in layers, with an angle of 40 to 70 degrees between layers. Occasional granules are found adherent to the fibril surface. The fibrils are tightly packed and increase in diameter and variability with age. Near the nucleus-annulus border, fibrils are less dense and less organized. In the nucleus pulposus they form a loose network, with more varied diameters. Proteoglycan and noncollagenous proteins coat the collagen fibrils of the nucleus pulposus. With age, fibrillar diameter increases and the fibrils of the nucleus become more dense.

Proteoglycans provide resistance to compression in the discs, as in other cartilaginous tissues. Proteoglycans form small granules in the extracellular matrix, often in association with collagen fibrils. Electron microscopy, using a monolayer technique,[22] demonstrates that infant proteoglycans form aggregates with hyaluronic acid, but to a lesser degree and smaller than those in articular cartilage. It is thought that regional differences in these chemical structures and aggregate formation allow variation in the hydrodynamic and, therefore, mechanical properties of the tissue.

Histologic studies at the light and electron microscopic level demonstrate that the biochemical constituents of the intervertebral disc display an architectural array that reflects their gross structure and, therefore, properties. Alteration in the constituents with regard to content, structure, and array can be expected to parallel degenerative change. What is not known is which factor, or factors, provoke(s) these degenerative alterations.

Biochemistry of Structural Components

The major structural components of intervertebral discs are collagen, proteoglycans, and water, together making up 90 to 95 per cent of the volume of normal discs. The collagen network provides the intervertebral connection, while its lamellar structure permits motion. Proteoglycans maintain hydration of the disc tissues and, through their osmotic properties, imbibe water, swell the disc, and provide tissue turgor. Through high concentrations, with their hydrodynamic and electrostatic properties, proteoglycans regulate fluid loss.

Water. The intervertebral disc normally is highly hydrated. The nucleus pulposus consists of about 85 per cent water and the annulus fibrosus 78 per cent. In both tissues water content falls to about 70 per cent with degeneration.[62, 73, 84, 127, 147] Proteoglycan content and hydration decrease with age, especially in the nucleus pulposus.[111, 120] An investigation of water content with respect to proteoglycan content, age, spinal level, and degeneration[179] demonstrates that proteoglycan content and hydration fall with age and vary with spinal level. The relationship of swelling pressure and hydration, however, is dependent on the intervertebral disc proteoglycan:collagen ratio, rather than age or degeneration.

Collagen. The intervertebral disc contains Types I and II collagen.[59] Overall the human annulus is about 60 per cent Type II and 40 per cent Type I. There is an interchanging radial distribution of collagen types in the annulus. The nucleus contains exclusively Type II collagen.[61, 81] Type II fibrils from the nucleus exhibit greater intermolecular spacing than Type I when examined by x-ray diffraction.[74] It is a feature associated with increased water content, implying that highly hydrated Type II fibrils may better deform and absorb compressive forces.

In both young and old human discs, the collagen content is higher in the outer portions of the annulus than in the inner annulus and nucleus.[2, 19] In younger spines total collagen content varies little, but in older spines the collagen content of the annulus increases caudally along the spine, as well as peripherally in the annulus. Total collagen content undergoes alteration with age and topographically increases by a small amount.[19] This change also occurs in the nucleus. There is, however, a change in the proportion of Type I to Type II, Type I increasing in content with age.[19] This pattern is noted in both animals (pigs) and humans.[58]

Irreducible cross linking in the collagen accumulates with age, and in the disc reducible cross links are absent by age 25.[81] In a study of intervertebral discs above degenerated discs, reducible cross links have been found along with the appearance of Type I collagen.[81] This finding indicates new synthesis of collagen. Reducible cross links have been found with topographic variation in discs, and although the content is lower with age, new synthesis can be found if discs are sampled regionally.[19] Hydroxypyridinium (HP) is the major irreducible cross link in adult collagen and increases with age.[123] Intervertebral discs and articular cartilage are the tissues most rich in HP.[59] Type II collagen contains more HP than Type I.[59] A study of HP in human herniated disc tissue has shown a decrease in HP content relative to that in the normal annulus, indicating new synthesis of collagen.[105]

Immunofluorescent studies of human disc material have shown no qualitative difference in collagen types in surgical and postmortem tissue. However, Type III collagen, associated with fibril formation in reticular networks, has been found in pericellular areas along with proteoglycans.[170] No change has been observed in patients with only posterior annular tears.[147] Similar studies in discs at levels of spondylolisthesis showed a reduction in Types I and III. Type III collagen therefore appears to arise regionally during disc degeneration.

In summary, current information in collagen biochemistry indicates that disc degeneration is accompanied by alterations in the array of collagen subtypes, with Type I replacing Type II, the appearance of Type III, and an overall accumulation of irreducible cross links, but a regional appearance of newly synthesized collagen. The regional changes imply that new synthesis reflects areas of tensile, as opposed to compressive, loads and may be a cellular response to these mechanical loads.[19]

Proteoglycans. Proteoglycans of intervertebral discs are homologous to those from articular cartilage.[169] They contain a core protein and glycosaminoglycans of chondroitin sulfate (CS) and keratan sulfate (KS) attached to the core, and are able to aggregate with hyaluronic acid, stabilized by link protein. They have shorter KS and CS chains than articular cartilage proteoglycans and a shorter core protein. Proteoglycans from the annulus have a higher proportion of aggregating proteoglycans than those from the nucleus. The smaller size of proteoglycans from discs is an intrinsic property.[168]

The nucleus pulposus is richer in proteoglycans than the annulus.[2, 84, 118, 175] With age and degeneration, total proteoglycan content decreases,[75, 84, 120, 126, 179] the ratio of KS to CS increases,[3, 73, 75, 112, 113] extractability increases, and aggregation decreases,[3] although the hyaluronic acid content of the disc is in excess of that needed for maximal aggregation.[77] A study of the proteoglycan content in discs, graded by the Lewin method,[103] demonstrated a decreasing proteoglycan content with increasing grades of disc degeneration.[137] Regional studies of the disc show that water and proteoglycan content are lost with degeneration, especially in the nucleus, and that the proteoglycans lose the ability to aggregate, in association with a decrease in the size of the core protein.[111] It has been suggested that degradation occurs in the hyaluronic acid–binding region, and that proteoglycan synthesis is slower in degenerative discs. A study of surgical and postmortem tissues showed that, except in the youngest patients, proteoglycans were of similar size in all patients and a wide range of aggregating proteoglycans were present.[170] No correlations could be made with clinical diagnosis.

Link proteins are the glycoproteins that stabilize the noncovalent bonding of aggregating proteoglycan to hyaluronate. All cartilage link proteins appear to be derived from the same protein core, but differ in core length and degree of glycosylation. During age and degeneration there is an increase in nonaggregating proteoglycans and an increase in smaller and fragmented link proteins.[37, 138] Changes in disc proteoglycan components are due to proteolysis. Intervertebral discs elaborate neutral collagenolytic, gelatinolytic, and elastinolytic enzymes,[165] and serine proteinases.[116] Three link proteins have been isolated in discs, the largest occurring in young ones.[138] In adults, discs contain much less link protein than in articular cartilage, and the three proteins are greater in abundance in the annulus fibrosus than in the nucleus pulposus. With age the smallest link proteins accumulate along with fragmentation products. Activation of proteolytic activity in the disc may play a role in degenerative changes.

Biochemical Changes in Animal Models

Animal modeling has allowed some insight into biochemical changes in the disc. A rabbit model of surgically induced ventral herniation has been studied in which progressive fibrocartilaginous metaplasia occurs, with the proliferation of tissue altering the disc architecture.[106, 107] Morphologically, an end-stage degenerative disc is reached. Water content is acutely lost and regained by the fourth day after injury, parallel to the initial loss and apparent rapid synthesis of proteoglycans. Progressive water and proteoglycan content loss then follows. The aggregating population of proteoglycans reaccumulate at about three weeks after injury, but then diminish by six to seven weeks. The size of the monomeric proteoglycans does not change with degeneration, but newly synthesized proteoglycan monomers are always larger than the average population. This model postulates an acute response of inner annulus fibrosus cells to the surgical injury and raises the possibility of a repair attempt by the tissue.

Proteoglycans have been studied in fused canine spines.[27, 28] In chondrodystrophic dogs, discs in the fused and parafusion areas were studied.[27] The proteoglycans isolated had decreased ability to aggregate and a slightly smaller hydrodynamic size at six months, though they were larger 12 months after fusion. Chondroitin sulfate increased proportionately. These studies concluded that a new proteoglycan population is synthesized, of a type seen in younger, less mature tissues. A similar study was done in nonchondrodystrophic dogs.[28] In this series proteoglycans increased in content, extractability, and size. The ability to aggregate was increased. There was no change in the CS:KS ratio. The difference in behavior of these two breeds, under the same experimental fusion conditions, was hypothesized to be due to differences in the matrices and cells that are genetically determined.

Disc degeneration has been morphologically defined and represents a tissue change that includes a loss of tissue and chemical components. In summary, histologic and fine structure studies indicate a progressive remodeling of the tissues. A loss of the normal array of matrix components is seen. Biochemical studies indicate that disc degeneration is not just progressive fibrosis of the disc, but a structural process on a regional basis with the replacement of Type II collagen with Type I and the appearance of Type III collagen. Qualitative changes occur in the proteoglycan component. Animal studies indicate that disc cells are responsive to mechanical alteration but may be governed by constitutional factors. Disc degeneration should be viewed not necessarily as simply a deteriorative, destructive process, but rather as a remodeling process. An understanding of cell regulation and expression may allow further insight into this process. Better delineation of these microscopic level alterations may provide an understanding of the mechanical factors involved (primarily or secondarily) and the radiographic findings observed.

As the disc degenerates, abnormal biomechanical stresses occur across the motion segment. These abnormal stresses lead to the radiographic picture of a collapsed disc space with end-plate sclerosis (Fig. 25–12). In the extreme this can present a picture similar to infection, but the sclerosis is confined to the motion segment and areas adjacent to the disc space (Fig. 25–13). The "instability" and reactive changes are associated with large osteophytes. This is the "end-stage" clinical (radiographic) picture of the process detailed chemically above. This advanced stage has been called benign idiopathic vertebral sclerosis.

Facets

As the disc space narrows, there is of necessity a concomitant "settling" or "erosion" of the facet joints (Fig. 25–14).[72, 197] Because of this mechanical abnormality, increased stresses are placed upon the facet joints.[7, 102, 108] This leads to less space, or cross-sectional area, in the neuroforamen and causes some degree of compromise of the spinal nerve root as it exits the canal.[122] Also, in the early stages of degen-

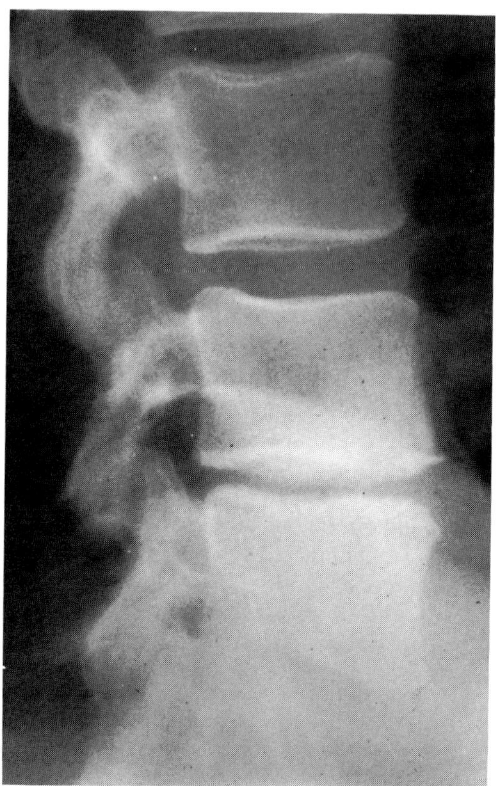

Figure 25–12. An example of a single-level degenerative disc. Small traction spurs can be seen anteriorly, beginning approximately 2 mm from the end plate. There is slight retrolisthesis of L4 on L5. Sclerosis starting at the end plate and extending into the body can be seen. In some cases this benign vertebral sclerosis becomes so extensive that it can be confused with tumor or infection, and occasionally a biopsy is required.

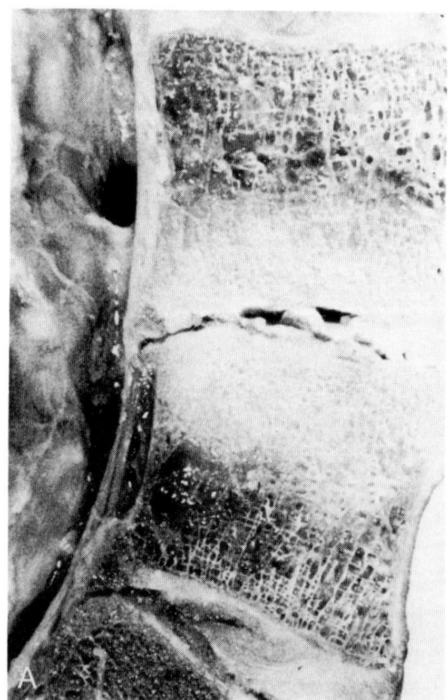

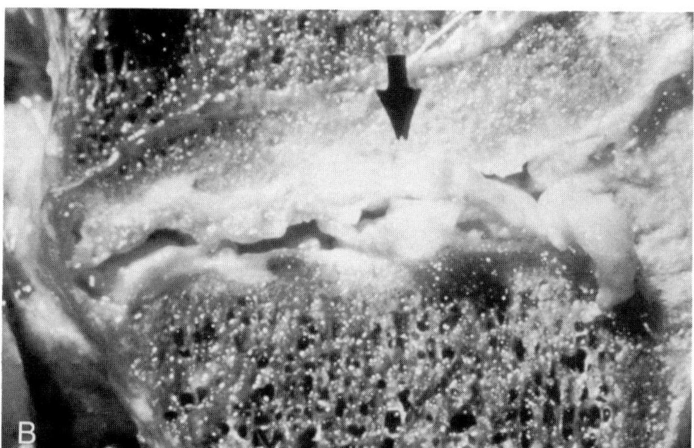

Figure 25–13. Cadaveric specimen through a motion segment that has significant degenerative changes. *A*, The disc is nearly absent. There is retrolisthesis of the more cephalad vertebra on the caudal one. Small osteophytes can be seen posteriorly. Significant sclerosis is demonstrated at the end plate and extends proximally and distally. *B*, Close-up view of a cadaveric specimen with significant disc degeneration *(arrow)*. The end plate margin is difficult to discern. There is fissuring and dehydration of the disc itself. No clear discrete nucleus or annulus can be seen. (From Kirkaldy-Willis, W. H., Wedge, J. H., Yong-Hing, K., and Reilly, J.: Pathology and pathogenesis of lumbar spondylosis and stenosis. Spine *3*:319, 1978.)

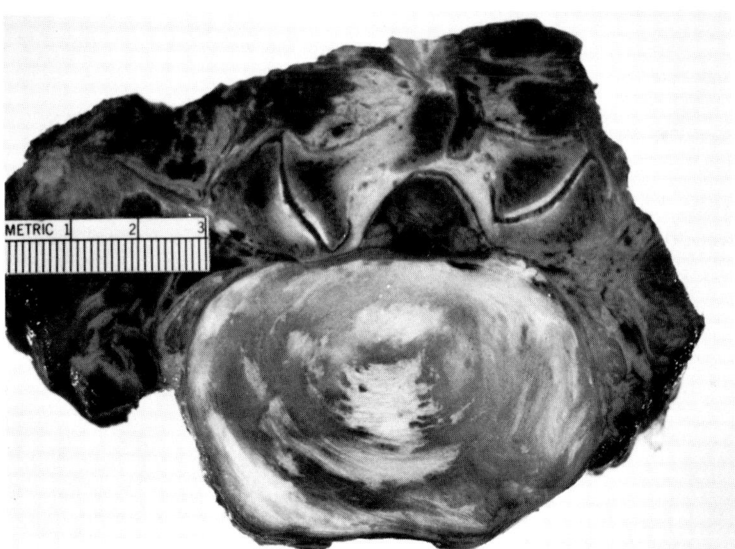

Figure 25–14. Transverse section of L4–L5 intervertebral joint demonstrating severe disc degeneration associated with asymmetric, degenerative facet joints. Note the compromise of the lateral recess, affecting the L5 nerve root.

eration, there frequently is a subtle retrolisthesis of the superior vertebral body on the subjacent one, coupled with overriding facets and bulging disc spaces (Fig. 25–15). This causes entrapment of the nerve root between the pedicle superiorly, the bulging disc inferiorly, the vertebral body osteophytes anteriorly, and the hypertrophied degenerative facets posteriorly (Fig. 25–16). In addition, if there are osteophytes that develop along the facet joints, these may impale the nerve root as the degenerative process, and hence stenosis, increases (Fig. 25–17).[99]

The symptoms of spinal stenosis frequently involve the lower lumbar nerve roots. This can be explained on a pathoanatomic, as well as a structural-anatomic, basis. Most degenerative discs are seen at the L4–L5 and L5–S1 levels. These levels involve the L4, L5, and S1 roots and provide a physiologic explanation why most symptoms occur along these nerve roots. Separately, the pedicles in the lower lumbar spine[174] are larger and have a more transversely oriented caudal border than the more superior lumbar pedicles, which are concave inferiorly (Figs 25–18 and 25–19). Initially, the disc heights in the lower lumbar spine are higher and the neuroforamen is "large." With age-related changes and disc narrowing, however, there is less room in the neuroforamen for the spinal nerve roots, particularly as the pedicles encompass a relatively larger area and do not have a concave surface, as seen in the upper segments, to "bridge" the exiting nerve root (Fig. 25–20).

The neuroforamen is bounded by the facet

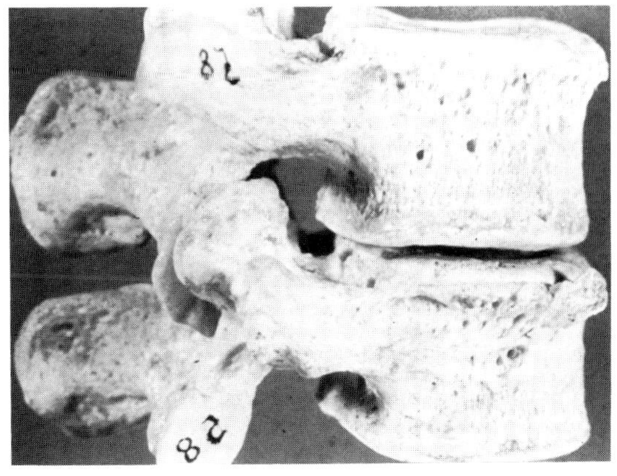

Figure 25–15. This cadaver specimen shows an example of retrolisthesis, facet subluxation, and disc space narrowing. An important observation is the protrusion into the neuroforamen from bone and facets, which can be seen in this specimen. (From Kirkaldy-Willis, W. H., Wedge, J. H., Yong-Hing, K., and Reilly, J.: Pathology and pathogenesis of lumbar spondylosis and stenosis. Spine *3*:319, 1978.)

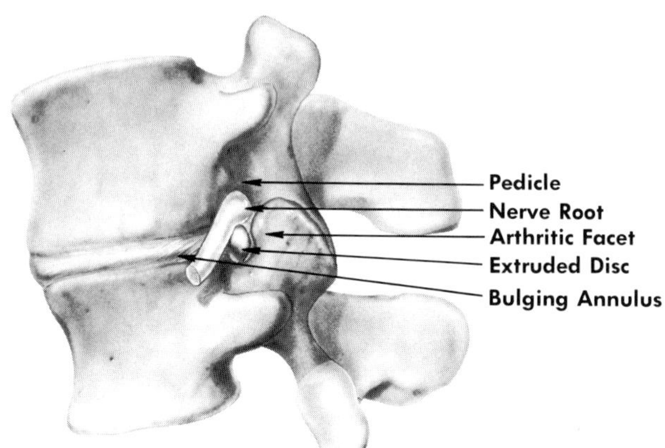

Figure 25–16. Foraminal encroachment secondary to chronic disc degeneration. The nerve root exiting the foramen will be compressed by the arthritic facet joint posteriorly, the relative descent of the pedicle superiorly, and the posterior bulge of the annulus or disc extrusion anteriorly. The surgeon must be satisfied that the nerve root is entirely free throughout the entire course of the foramen when the nerve root is decompressed.

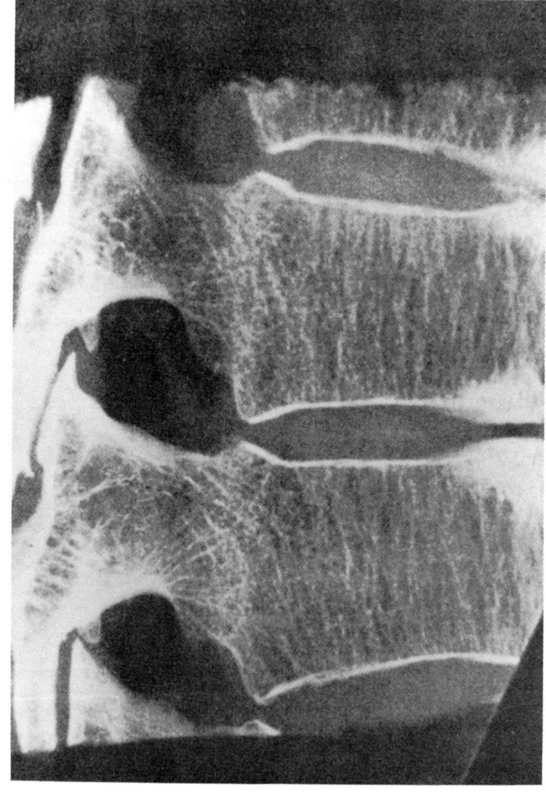

Figure 25–17. Small osteophytes can be seen coming from the inferior facet surfaces in this radiograph. The osteophyte enters the neuroforamen superiorly, where the nerve root also lies. This could lead to symptoms of spinal stenosis, but most likely would require a larger osteocartilaginous prominence. (From Sutro, C. J.: Lumbar facets—spinal stenosis and intermittent claudication: a mini review. Bull. Hosp. Joint Dis. *40*:13, 1979.)

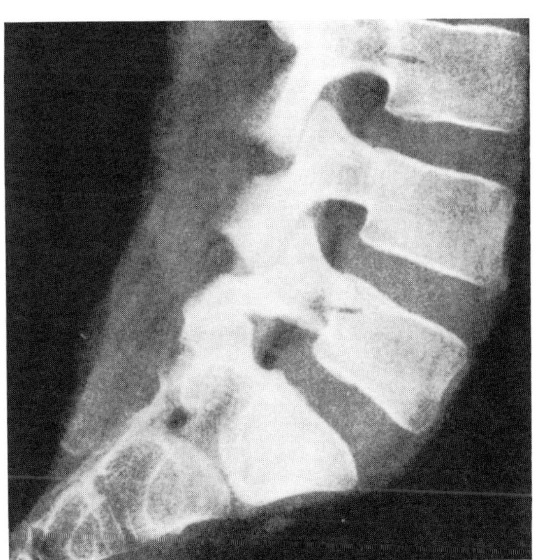

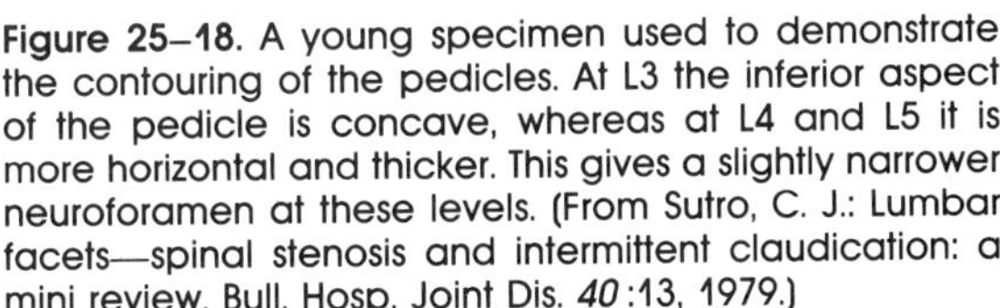

Figure 25–18. A young specimen used to demonstrate the contouring of the pedicles. At L3 the inferior aspect of the pedicle is concave, whereas at L4 and L5 it is more horizontal and thicker. This gives a slightly narrower neuroforamen at these levels. (From Sutro, C. J.: Lumbar facets—spinal stenosis and intermittent claudication: a mini review. Bull. Hosp. Joint Dis. *40*:13, 1979.)

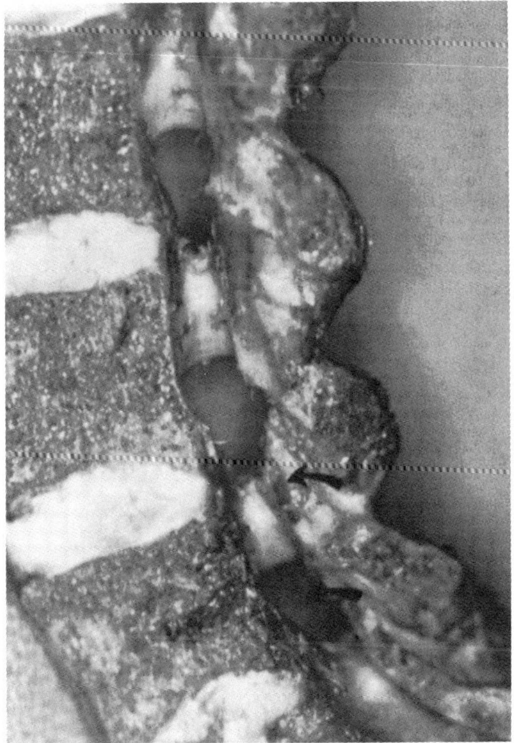

Figure 25–19. Fairly normal-appearing lumbar spine. The upper two discs appear relatively normal and healthy with a visible nucleus and discrete annulus. The lower disc has degenerative changes and erosions into the lower body (sacrum). A loss of the regular nuclear-annular outline is seen in the discs above. The upper arrow points to the L5 pedicle and the lower one to the L5–S1 neuroforamen. Note the transverse nature of the pedicle of L5 compared with the more concave inferior margin of L4 and particularly L3. (From Lancourt, J. E., Glenn, W. V., and Wiltse, L. L.: Multiplanar computerized tomography in the normal spine and in the diagnosis of spinal stenosis. Spine *4*:379–390, 1979.)

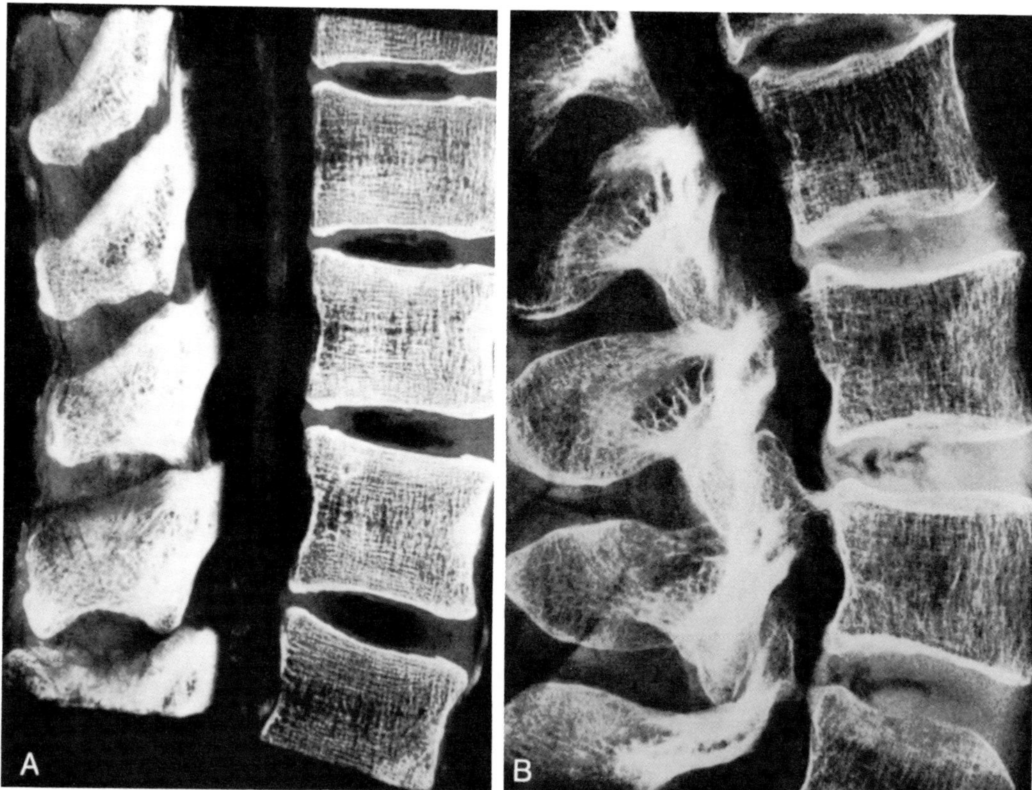

Figure 25–20. Sagittal cuts through a cadaveric spine. *A*, Sagittal cut through the central portion of the spinal canal. Note the slight decrease in size from cephalad to caudal. *B*, Same specimen, although the cut is slightly off center. Again the narrowing of the neuroforamen distally, compared with more proximally, can be seen. This may be one reason why more symptoms are related to the L5 root in spinal stenosis than to more proximal roots. This is an anatomic explanation, but there also is a higher incidence of disc degeneration at L4–L5 and L5–S1 that contribute significantly to the pathophysiology of the symptoms. (From Sutro, C. J.: Lumbar facets—spinal stenosis and intermittent claudication: a mini review. Bull. Hosp. Joint Dis. *40*:13, 1979.)

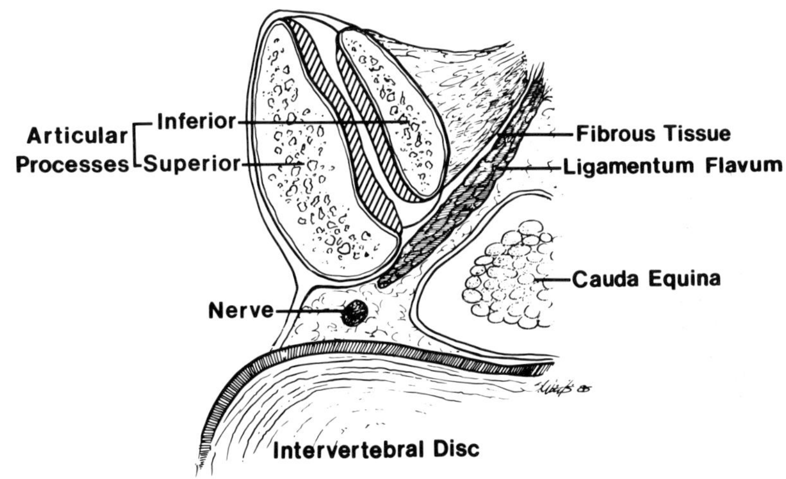

Figure 25–21. Artist's conception of a lateral recess. The inferior and superior facets are labeled. The anterior margin of the superior articular process lies just posterior to the nerve root. The nerve root is bound anteriorly by the intervertebral disc and posterior aspect of the vertebral bodies, superiorly by the pedicle, and posteriorly and medially by the facet joint.

joints posteriorly, the pedicles superiorly and inferiorly, and the vertebral body and disc anteriorly (Fig. 25–21) A change in any of these structures, or concomitant degenerative processes, leads to compromise of the space available for the spinal nerve root (Fig. 25–22).

The arthritic processes in the facet follow the course observed in most other joints.[49–51, 102, 104, 176] Initially, in a well-preserved facet joint, the cartilage is intact and has a well-contoured, gliding surface (Fig. 25–23). The joints are covered with synovium and a capsule. The central portion of the facet is cancellous, although there is impaction centrally, most likely related to mechanical stresses. Isolated radiographs of normal facet joints show evidence of some sclerosis, particularly in the concavity of the superior facets. With further aging the porosity of the bone in the facet increases (Fig. 25–24). Concurrently, there is a loss of joint space (Fig. 25–25). There is also a decrease in subchondral sclerosis, suggesting an alteration in the stress distributions across the facet joints. Osteophytes begin developing at this stage. With aging and degeneration the cartilage surface begins to erode further (Fig. 25–26). As the cartilage fails, the bone loses its mass and its normal function. The joint surfaces become markedly irregular and override (Fig. 25–27). Arthritic changes can occur unilaterally but more frequently are bilateral.

Segmental Instability

Instability across the motion segment (vertebral body–disc–vertebral body) can occur as

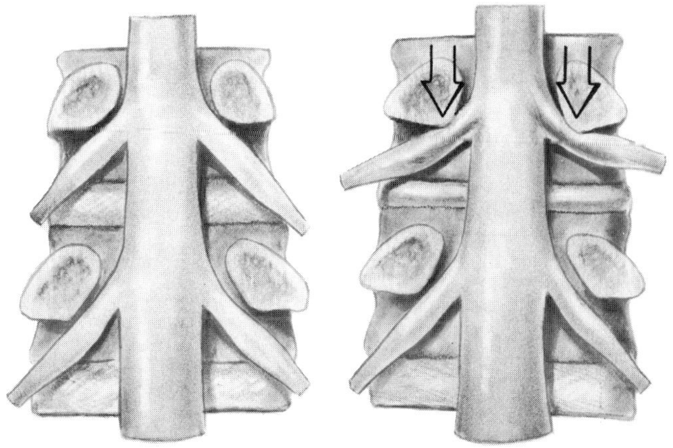

Figure 25–22. The relative caudal migration of the pedicles during disc degeneration, which may trap the nerve roots between the pedicle above and the bulging disc and osteophytes below. During exploration of a nerve root it must be ascertained that the root is free not only of compression, but also of tension. If the root is tethered about the pedicle, trimming of the offending pedicle may be necessary.

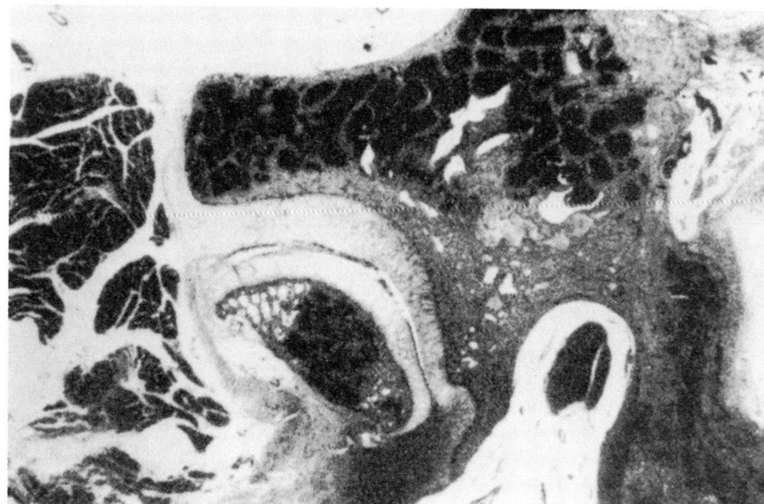

Figure 25–23. Histologic example of a facet joint. The cartilage is seen centrally with joint space visible. Bone is seen centrally and laterally.

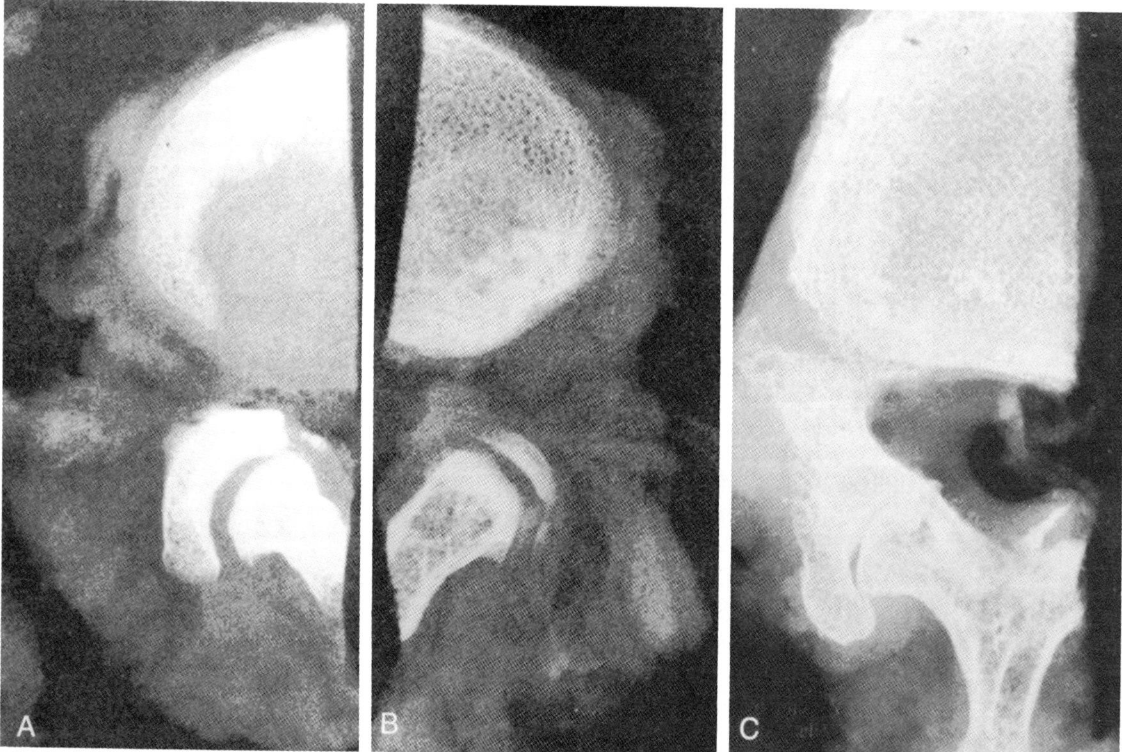

Figure 25–24. Series of radiographs through facet with varying degrees of degenerative change. Increasing porosity in the bone can be seen. *A*, Facet joint is seen in the central lower portion of the picture; the disc is above. This cadaveric tomogram shows a relatively congruous facet. Although separated because of an artifact of preparation, the joint space is maintained. There are no osteophytes and the bone density appears grossly normal. *B*, An example of slightly more advanced degenerative joint disease. In this case the joint surfaces are not completely opposed and are dyscongruous. There is sclerosis of the subchondral bone but osteoporosis of the facet itself. There is thinning of the component of the facet joint on the right. *C*, A more advanced case of an osteoarthritic facet joint, which is dyscongruous. Osteophytes and overlapping of the joint can be seen. Osteoporosis is seen in the spinous process, lamina, and facet. Medially, there appears to be almost no cartilage. (From Sutro, C. J.: Lumbar facets—spinal stenosis and intermittent claudication: a mini review. Bull. Hosp. Joint Dis. *40*:13, 1979.)

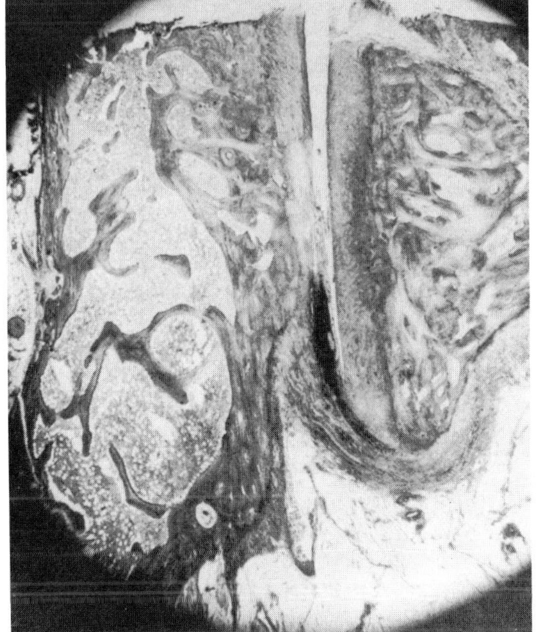

Figure 25–25. Longitudinal section through a facet joint. Centrally and inferiorly there is separation of the cartilage from the underlying bone. There is some mild associated osteoporosis on the right but normal bone configuration on the left.

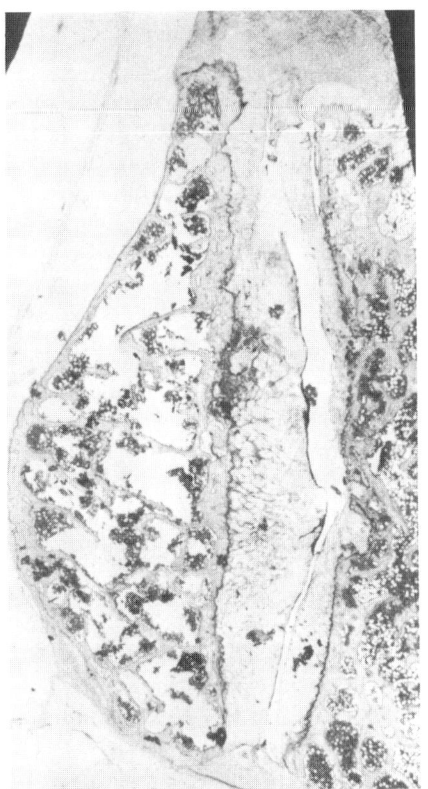

Figure 25–26. A slide of a facet joint with evidence of mild arthritis. Centrally, and to the top of the illustration, the cartilage is nearly absent. Lucencies (osteoporosis) of the bone can be seen. Some fissuring of the cartilage can be noted on the superior aspect of this slide. (From Sutro, C. J.: Lumbar facets—spinal stenosis and intermittent claudication: a mini review. Bull. Hosp. Joint Dis. *40*:13, 1979.)

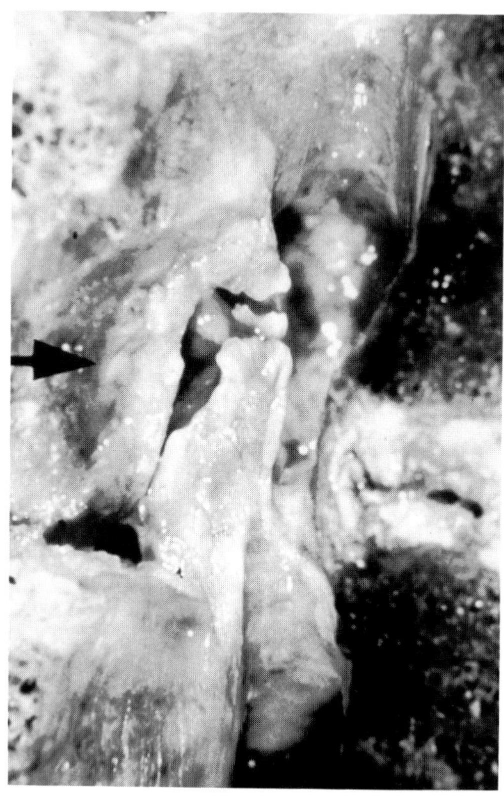

Figure 25–27. Facet joint is shown at the arrow. This should be a smooth contiguous surface, but in this case the cartilage is eroded and a large gap can be seen between the joint surfaces. The pedicle is in the superior central aspect of the illustration, and the disc is the irregular white structure to the right. (From Kirkaldy-Willis, W. H., Wedge, J. H., Yong-Hing, K., and Reilly, J.: Pathology and pathogenesis of lumbar spondylosis and stenosis. Spine *3*:319, 1978.)

the degenerative/aging process progresses.[64, 68, 70, 172] Although it cannot perhaps be grossly detected radiographically, this instability can be related to translational or rotational abnormalities. Normally, because of the "tripod" configuration of the spine with normal disc, facet joints, ligaments, and joint capsules, the spinal motion segment, and particularly the neuroforamen, can smoothly and symmetrically accommodate rotational motions, as well as flexion and extension, without significant alteration in the space available. However, as the discs degenerate anteriorly, the ligaments buckle and/or hypertrophy,[177] and the changes associated with facet arthritis progress, the central canal, as well as the neuroforamen, is less accommodating in rotation (Fig. 25–28). As the body rotates, because of the altered anatomy and mechanics, narrowing occurs and can lead to altered torsional stresses.[97, 178] This can produce irritation/inflammation (and perhaps pain) of the spinal nerve roots and cauda equina.

Separately, subluxations (anterior or posterior) can occur.[55, 57, 63, 89, 129, 148] If the disc collapse exceeds the facet arthritic changes, there may be some retrolisthesis of the superior vertebral body on the subadjacent one, with posterior overriding of the facet joints (Fig. 25–29). However, if the anterior and posterior column degeneration occurs relatively concurrently, the facet joint begins to erode, hypertrophic changes develop, and a gradual realignment and redistribution of forces across the facet joint can occur. This may allow anterior subluxation of the vertebra above on the vertebra below. This most commonly occurs at the L4–L5 level, presumably because of the restraining effects of the iliolumbar ligaments on the L5 vertebral body and transverse processes, allowing relatively more motion at L4–L5, and therefore subluxation.[101]

The changes described above for spinal stenosis are also a function of aging. With degeneration there is a progressive loss of disc space height, which, in addition to the degenerative changes, leads to a gradual increase of lordosis. Breig noted that as the spine aligns into progressively more extension, the ligamentum flavum, and the nerves within the cauda equina, become broader and wider.[18] This, coupled with the posterior bulging of the discs and the smaller space available to take up relatively wider neural tissue elements, leads to a relative

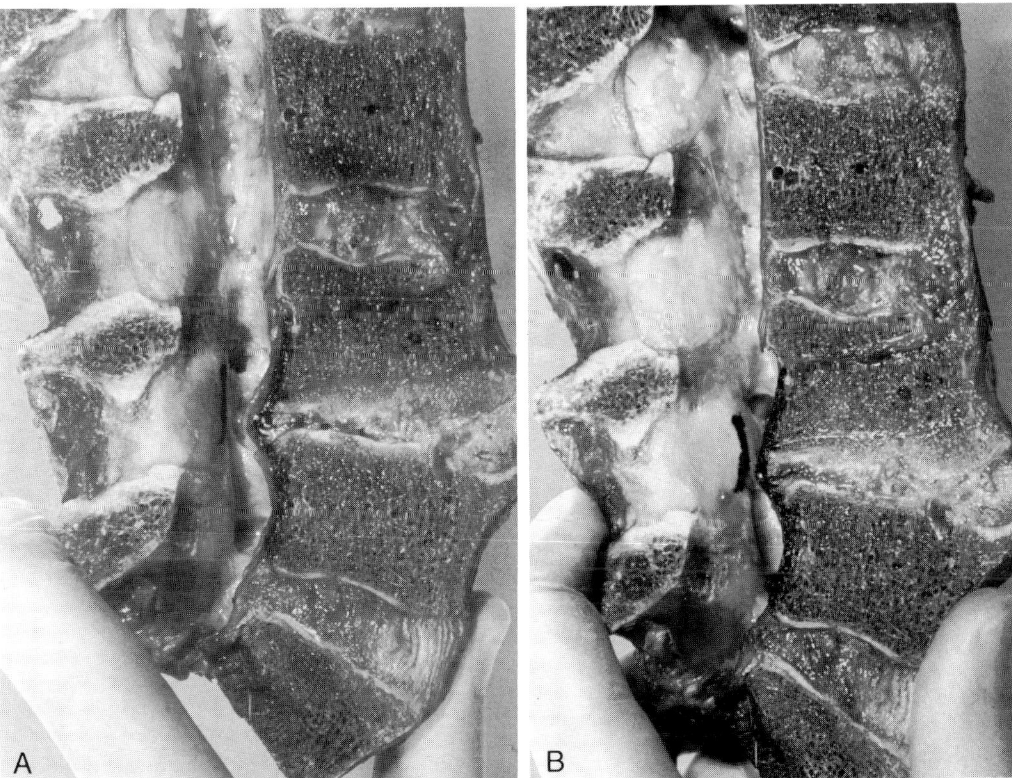

Figure 25–28. The effect of rotation on canal-neuroforamen size. *A*, This specimen, cut sagittally, has a clockwise force applied to it. The space between the posterior aspect of the markedly degenerative bulging intervertebral disc and the posterior ligaments and facets are shown between the black lines. *B*, Same specimen as in *A*, except now a counterclockwise force is applied. There is significantly less space between the lines. In this space lie the nerve roots as they exit to the neuroforamen. This mild rotational change narrows the available space, as shown in this specimen, and can contribute to stenosis and its symptoms. (From Kirkaldy-Willis, W. H., Wedge, J. H., Yong-Hing, K., and Reilly, J.: Pathology and pathogenesis of lumbar spondylosis and stenosis. Spine 3:319, 1978.)

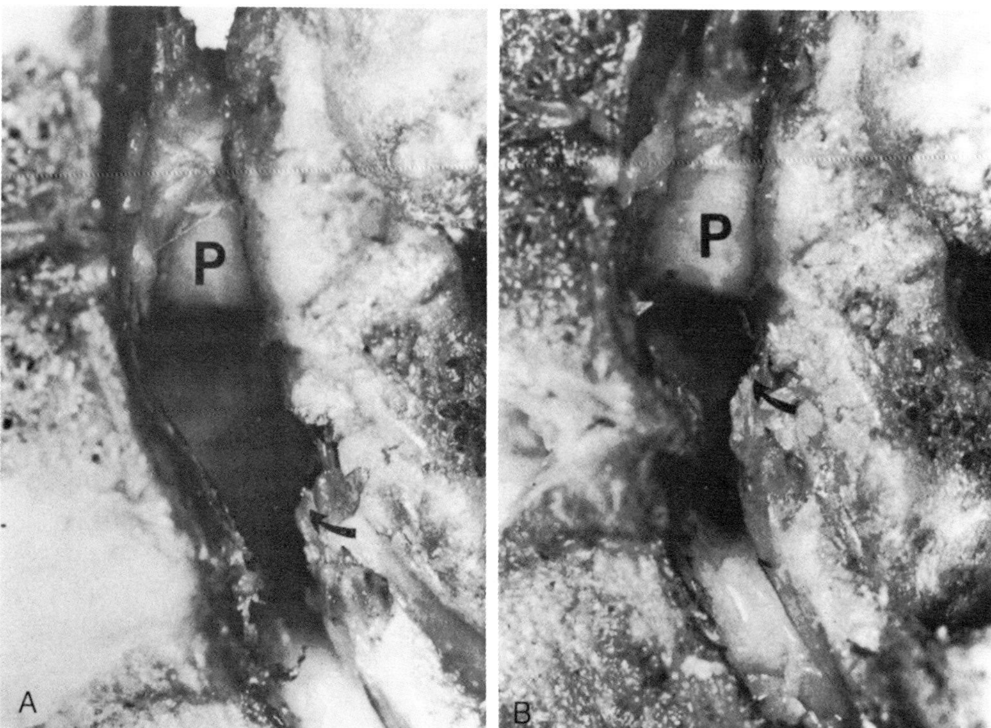

Figure 25–29. The effect on the neuroforamen of disc space collapse. *A*, The L4–L5 facet joints have been debrided of capsular tissue. The pedicle (P) is of L4. The arrow is at the superior margin of L5, which also has a small osteophyte. *B*, Same specimen as in *A*, except the L4–L5 disc has been surgically removed. The specimen is then compressed. This simulates a degenerative disc. In this example the arrow is now significantly closer to the inferior margin of the pedicle, and the posterior longitudinal ligament and posterior annulus bulge laterally and posteriorly into the neuroforamen. The space available for the neurovascular bundle as it exits through the L4–L5 neuroforamen is markedly stenotic, comparing *A* and *B*. (From Lancourt, J. E., Glenn, W. V., and Wiltse, L. L.: Multiplanar computerized tomography in the normal spine and in the diagnosis of spinal stenosis. Spine *4*:379–390, 1979.)

increase in the spinal stenosis—perhaps greater than what is actually measured anatomically. Degenerative changes in the facet joints, degenerative spondylolisthesis, and osteophyte formation contribute markedly to this stenotic pattern, both dynamically and statically (Figs. 25–30 to 25–34).[114]

Pathophysiology of Pain in Spinal Stenosis: Experimental Studies

If spinal stenosis is a normal function of aging, why do some people have pain? A number of theoretical reasons have been proposed to explain symptoms and signs associated, in some individuals, with spinal stenosis. One explanation is that the pain is due to mechanical instability and concomitant nerve root compression. However, as described above, the changes observed in patients with spinal stenosis are related to aging and can be found in a large number of asymptomatic individuals (Fig. 25–35). It is unlikely that pure mechanical instability (rotational or translational), or isolated nerve root compression, can by themselves explain the pain felt by these patients (Fig. 25–36). These factors do not independently explain why the symptoms of spinal stenosis tend to be intermittent, or why only a limited number of individuals in the population develop them.

However, there are some elegant studies evaluating the effect of compression on the cauda equina. Using cadaver spines and circumferential clamps to narrow the cauda equina (Fig. 25–37), Schönström and colleagues evaluated the pressure changes within the cauda equina related to degree of restriction (Fig. 25–38).[161–163] These authors found

Text continued on page 817

Figure 25–30. Radiograph illustrates a traction osteophyte at the L3–L4 level. Note that the osteophyte is horizontally oriented and 2 mm away from the disc space. Note the marked narrowing of the disc space and the vacuum phenomena at L3–L4.

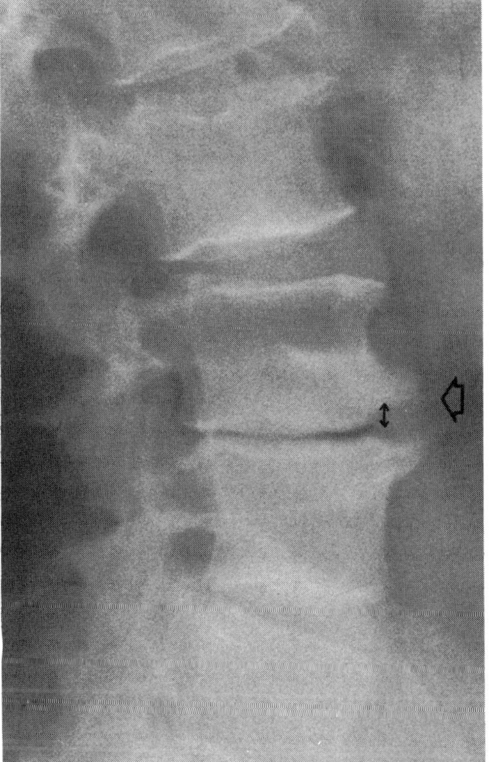

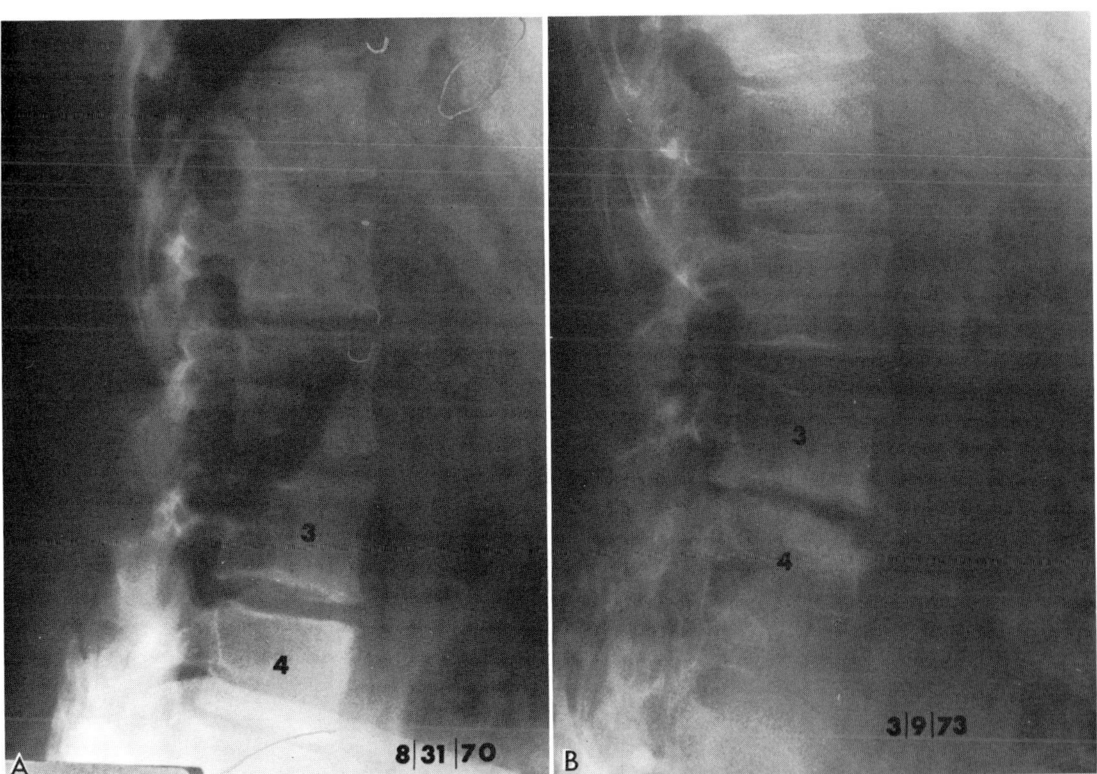

Figure 25–31. Radiographs illustrate the development of disc degeneration at the L3–L4 disc space over a period of three years. Note the loss of height of the space, osteophyte formation, and sclerosis of the end plates. In this instance the radiographic appearance was suggestive of infection, and biopsy was performed but revealed only evidence of chronic disc degeneration. At times the sclerosis can be so marked as to simulate a neoplasm of the vertebral body. *A*, Presenting lateral radiograph. *B*, Three years later, same patient.

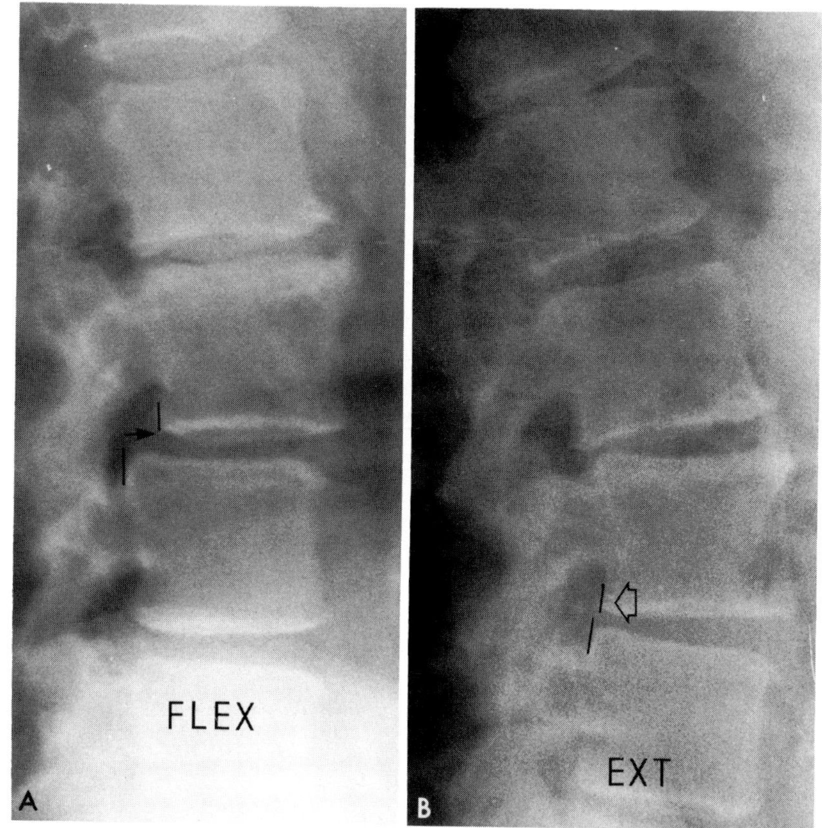

Figure 25–32. Radiographs illustrating segmental instability due to disc degeneration on flexion and extension views. *A*, Note that in flexion there is a 3.5-mm anterior migration of the cranial vertebra. *B*, In extension there is almost complete realignment of the vertebral body. This was productive of both back pain and sciatica.

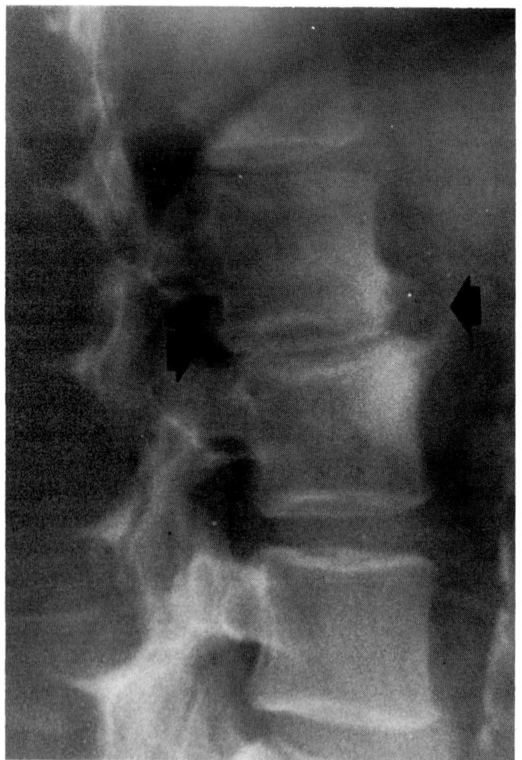

Figure 25–33. Radiograph illustrating marked disc degeneration at the L3–L4 level. There is associated loss of height of the disc space, sclerosis of the adjacent vertebral body, osteophyte formation, and a 2-mm retrospondylolisthesis.

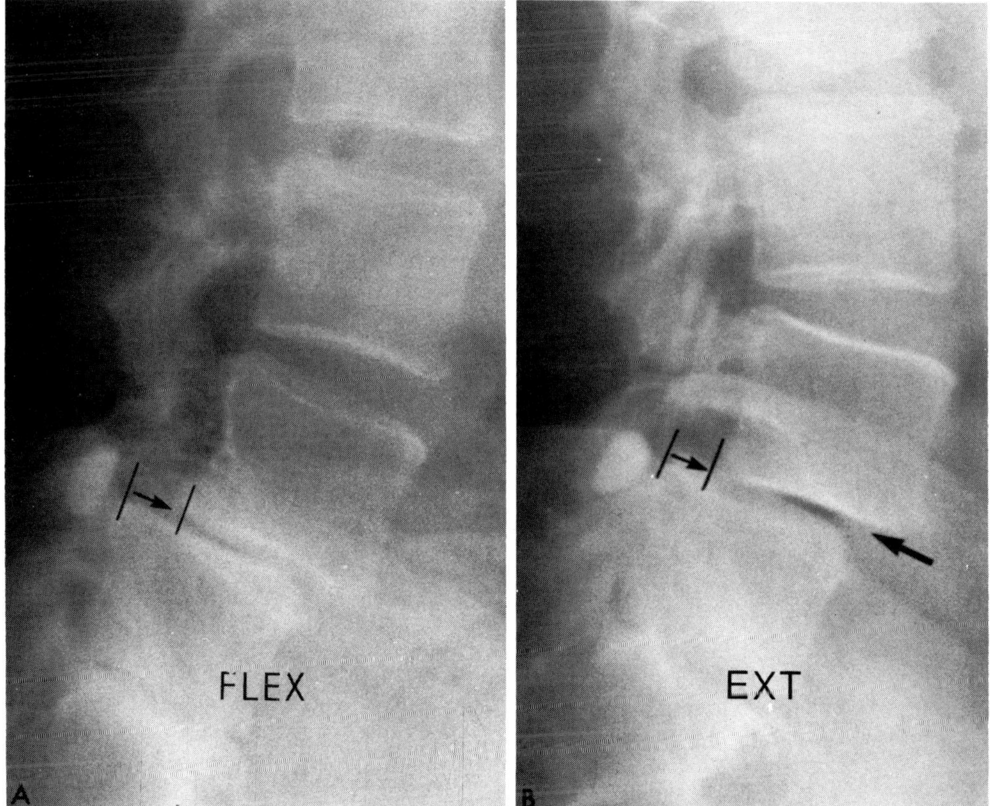

Figure 25–34. Radiographs illustrating segmental instability at L4–L5 secondary to disc degeneration. This is also termed "degenerative spondylolisthesis." *A*, Note that in flexion there is a 5-mm anterior migration of L4 relative to L5. *B*, In extension there is only partial reduction of this subluxation together with production of a vacuum phenomenon at the affected area.

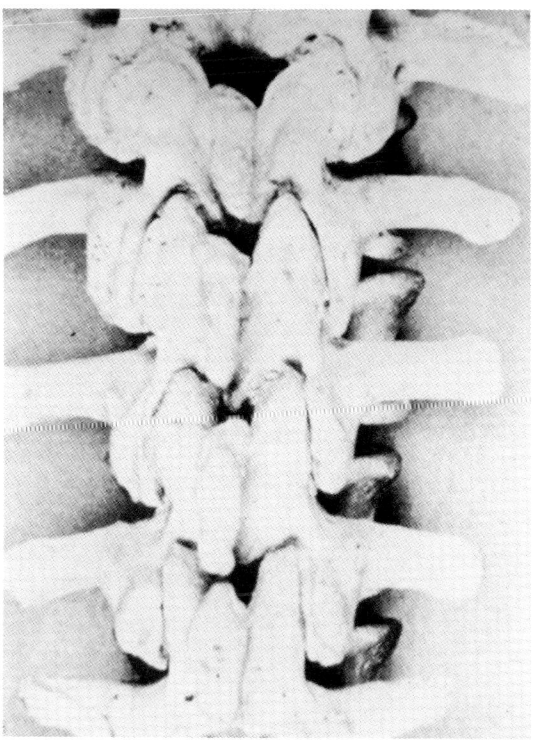

Figure 25–35. Cadaveric specimen showing changes characteristic of spinal stenosis. The posterior elements are thickened. In the midportion there are narrow interlaminar spaces. The spinous processes nearly abut. There is facet hypertrophy, which is particularly visible in the more sagittally oriented lower facet joints. There is a suggestion of rotation through the midportion of this specimen. The spinous processes are bulbous posteriorly and irregular inferiorly.

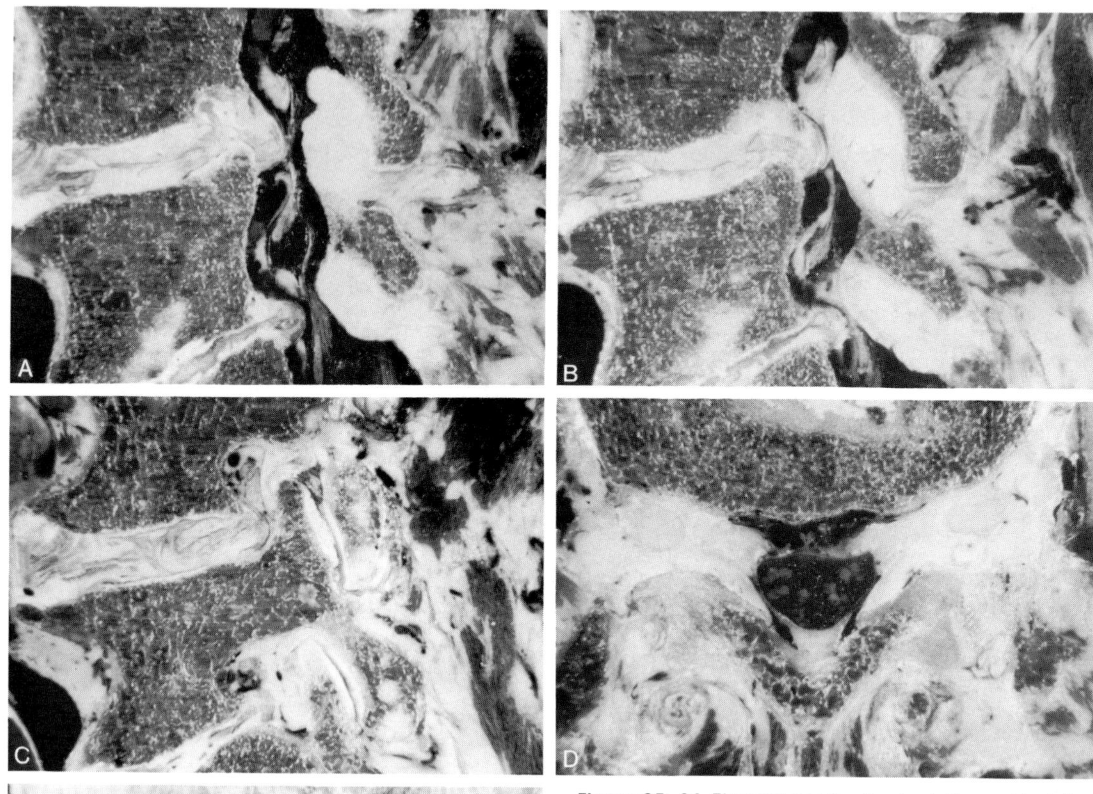

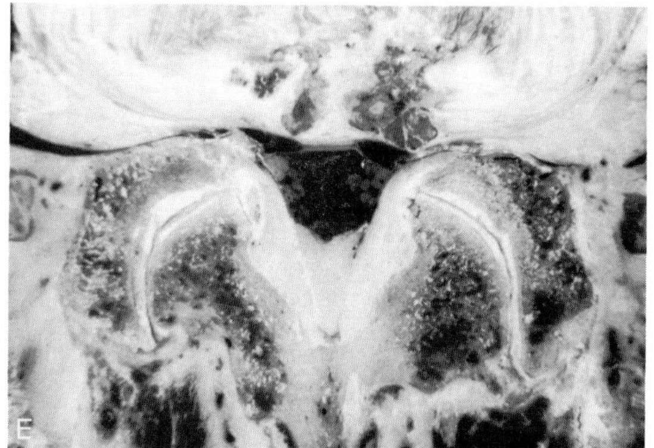

Figure 25–36. Elegant anatomic depictions of bulging discs and degenerative (aging) changes. *A*, This picture is taken slightly off center in the sagittal plane and is extending toward the neuroforamen. The irregular contour of both of the discs shown in this specimen can be seen. The inferior one is markedly narrowed with erosion of the end plates. *B*, A slightly more lateral section than in *A*. The disc, seen centrally, is now more prominent. The section is beginning to enter the neuroforamen. Facet capsule and ligament can be seen. Centrally, there is almost no space for the neural elements. *C*, A cut directly through the neuroforamen. Both the inferior and superior facets can be seen, as can the prominent disc. The spinal nerve and surrounding vessels can be seen in the superior portion of the neuroforamen. In this particular specimen, because of the facets and the prominent disc, the space available for the spinal nerve is limited. *D*, Cross section through a relatively normal lumbar spinal canal. The cauda equina is well seen centrally (in black). Epidural veins are seen between the cauda equina and the body. The nerve roots are well visualized in the lateral foramen. There is no evident compromise of the cauda equina or the nerve roots. The body is on the top portion of this picture. *E*, A patient who could have symptoms of spinal stenosis. The facet joints are irregular and arthritic. The cartilage of the joints is narrowed, as is the joint space. There is sclerosis of the bone of the facet joint anteriorly, but osteoporosis posteriorly (suggesting alterations in weight bearing). This cut through the disc (top of illustration) shows vascular intrusion into the posterior aspect of the bulging disc. There is no discrete annulus. The disc bulges centrally and laterally. The lateral recess is markedly narrowed because of the combination of a degenerative disc and facet and perhaps some vascular engorgement. (From Rauschning, W.: Normal and pathologic anatomy of the lumbar root canals. Spine *12*:1008–1019, 1987.)

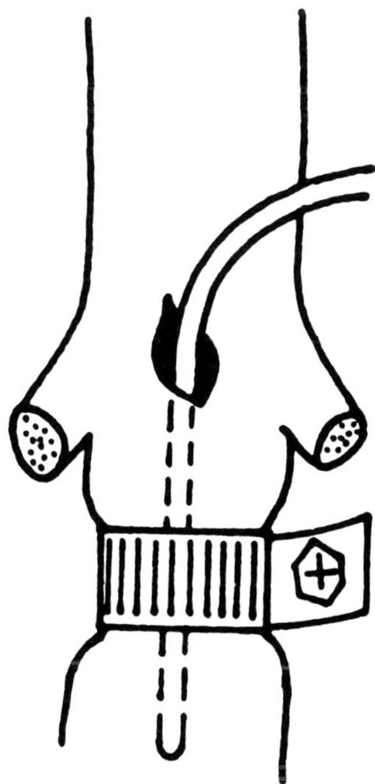

Figure 25–37. The system used by Schönström to measure intrathecal pressure after application of a circumferential band. The percentage narrowing was determined and depicted as shown in Figure 25–38. The catheter measured intrathecal pressure at and distal to the circumferential band. (From Schönström, N., Lindahl, S., Willen, J., et al.: Dynamic changes in the dimensions of the lumbar spinal canal. An experimental study in vitro. J. Orthop. Res. 7:115–121, 1988.)

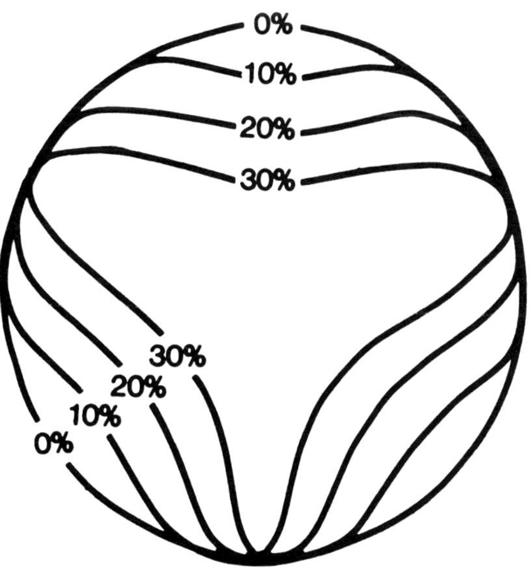

Figure 25–38. Narrowing of the spinal canal (spinal stenosis) as depicted by Schönström. This demonstrates canal volume diminution as a percentage of original volume. (From Schönström, N., Lindahl, S., Willen, J., et al.: Dynamic changes in the dimensions of the lumbar spinal canal. An experimental study in vitro. J. Orthop. Res. 7:115–121, 1988.)

that the minimal cross-sectional area necessary to accommodate the neural elements of the cauda equina, including the dural sac, was 77 $\pm$ 13 mm^2 at L3. The first signs of a pressure increase along the nerve roots during progressive gradual constriction occurred when the cross-sectional area decreased below that figure (Fig. 25–39). This value (77 $\pm$ 13 mm^2) is approximately 45 per cent of the normal cross-sectional area of the dural sac at this level (L3).[160] To create a pressure of 50 mm Hg among the nerve roots of the cauda equina, the cross-sectional area had to be further narrowed to an area of 63 $\pm$ 13 mm^2 (37 per cent of the normal, noncompressed dural sac area). To develop a pressure of 100 mm Hg, the neural tissues had to be narrowed to 33 per cent of their normal size. These data suggest that constriction of the cauda equina in the midlumbar spine requires narrowing to approximately 50 per cent or more of normal, before significant pressure, and therefore perhaps symptoms, develop. The 50 mm Hg value noted above is significant, in that Rydevik and associates have demonstrated that pressures above 50 mm Hg lead to capillary restriction (Fig. 25–40) and electrophysiologic alteration in spinal nerve roots.[130, 132, 133, 139, 155]

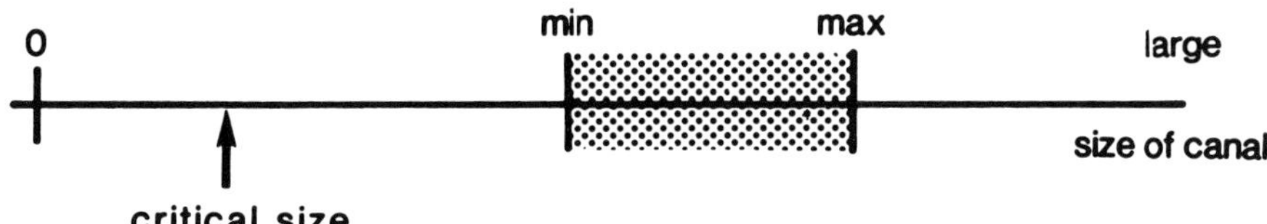

Figure 25–39. The concept of a critical canal size diminution necessary for symptoms to develop in spinal stenosis was proposed by Schönström. There is a minimal and maximal size of the canal based on extension and flexion, respectively, of the spine. In the example shown here the minimal size of the canal, even with extension and disc bulging, does not decrease the area/volume to the critical point (size). Presumably no symptoms would develop. If the size of the canal were smaller and the minimum extended below the critical size, symptoms would occur.

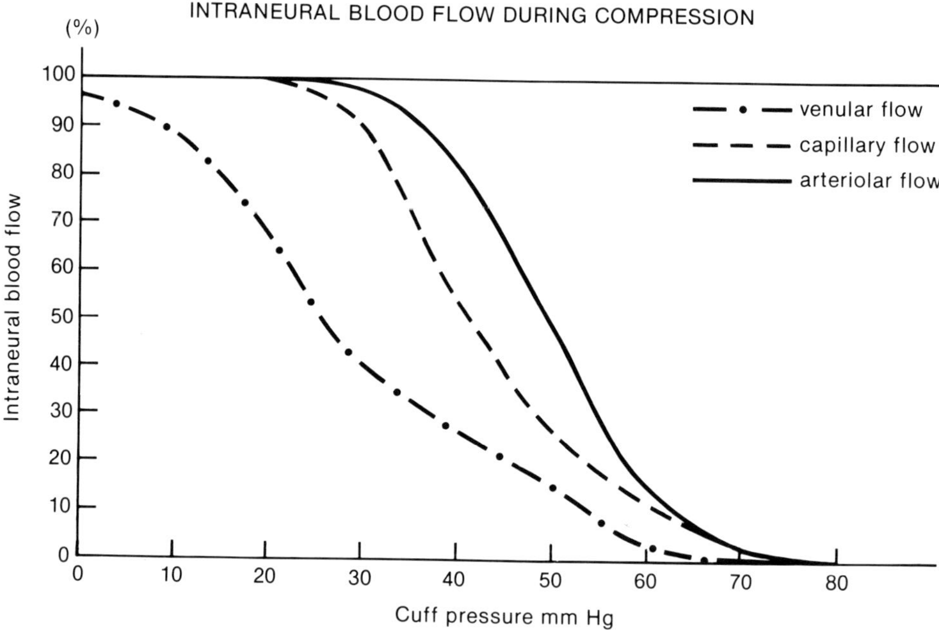

Figure 25–40. Intraneural blood flow during compression. This graph, with data based on intravital microscopy, demonstrates the change in intraneural blood flow during extrinsic compression. The ordinate is the percentage of intraneural blood flow. As shown, venular flow drops off rapidly between 20 and 30 mm Hg pressure, while arteriolar flow falls dramatically at approximately 50 mm Hg. In the animal model used, the mean arterial blood pressure was approximately 80 mm Hg. (From Rydevik, B., Lundborg, G., and Bagge, U.: Effects of graded compression on intraneural blood flow. An in vivo study on rabbit tibial nerve. J. Hand Surg. *6*:3–12, 1981.)

Because there are considerable variations in the size of the human lumbar spinal canal, and these are affected by changes in axial loading, flexion-extension, degenerative discs, and so forth, it is clear that symptoms may not be the same in every individual.[18, 41, 85, 90, 191] Also, they may not occur with the same degree of "degenerative change," depending on other factors. The absolute cross-sectional area available for the nerve root, which also interrelates with the size of the nerves and the induced pressure, may vary from individual to individual, and perhaps suggests why the signs and symptoms are so variable within an individual, as well as throughout the population.

Mechanical compression of the nerve roots in the lumbar spine can create a number of intraneural tissue reactions which may lead to pain or neurologic alterations.[33, 80, 109, 149, 150, 173] Rydevik and colleagues[33, 80, 109, 149, 150, 173] showed in an animal model that compression of the nerve roots, even with low pressure (5 to 10 mm Hg), leads to venous congestion of the intraneural microcirculation (Fig. 25–40).[133] With 130 mm Hg compression (in a porcine model), complete ischemia of the compressed nerve root segments occurs. This pressure correlates with the systolic pressure of the animal. In addition, solute transport (H_3-labeled methylglucose) reduces approximately 45 per cent across a nerve root segment that is compressed at 10 mm Hg.[130] Intraneural edema (demonstrated with fluorescence microscopy) was noted after 50 mm Hg compression for only two minutes.[131] In a related series of experiments, porcine cauda equina compression at 100 mm Hg for two hours led to significant electrophysiologic impairments in both afferent and efferent conduction (Fig. 25–41). Interestingly, in these studies, motor nerves recovered faster and to a more complete degree than the sensory nerve roots after pressure release. This may have implications in explaining continued subjective complaints of pain and discordant neurologic findings in patients with documented spinal nerve root compression.

In an unrelated animal study, Delamarter and associates evaluated the effect of constriction bands across the cauda equina on neurologic deficits.[34] They did not assess intra- or interneural pressure related to the compression

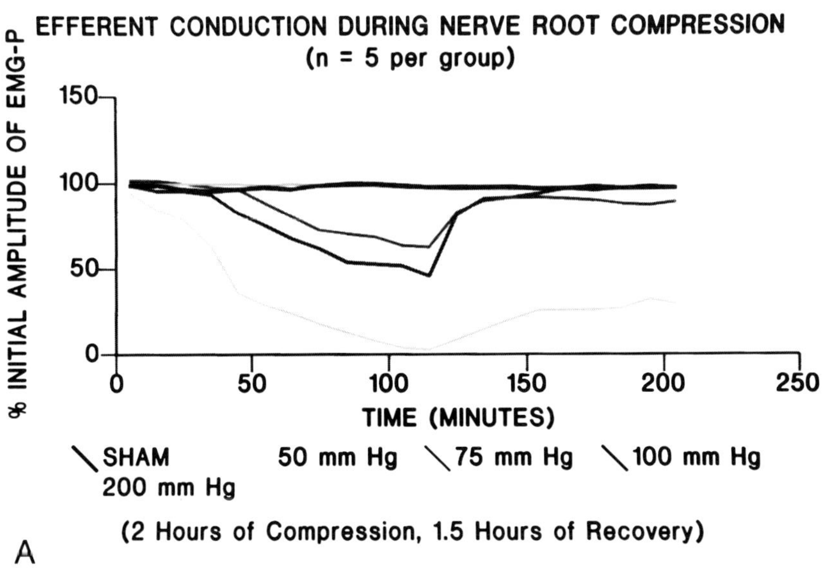

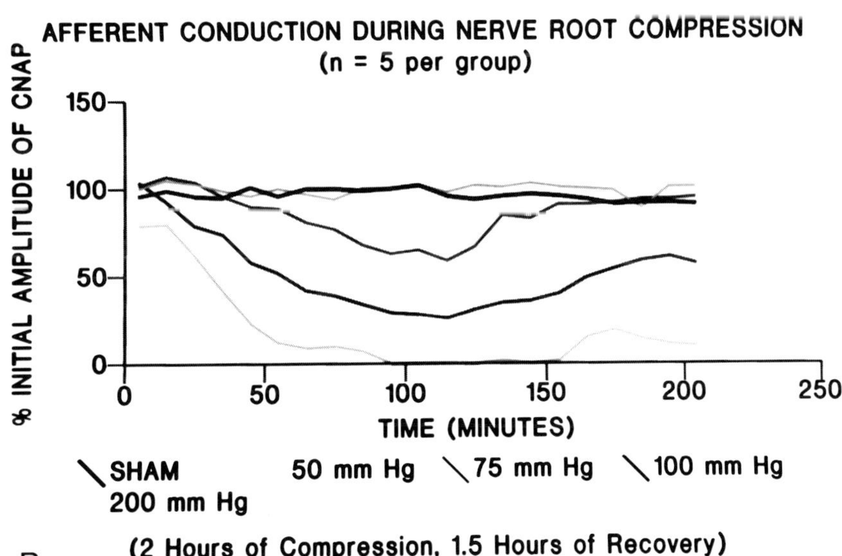

Figure 25–41. The effect of compression pressure on porcine cauda equina electrophysiologic function. *A, Efferent* conduction during experimental nerve root compression in a pig model of cauda equina compression. As shown in this graph, with two hours of compression at 200 mm Hg *(lower line)*, there is rapid loss of conduction with almost no improvement during the recovery period. (Compression is released after 120 minutes.) At 75 and 100 mm Hg, there is a gradual diminution of efferent conduction, but this returns rapidly toward normal with the cessation of compression. *B, Afferent* conduction during experimental nerve root compression in a pig model of cauda equina compression. As shown in this example, with two hours of compression at 200 mm Hg *(lower line)*, there is rapid loss of conduction with almost no improvement during the recovery period. (Compression is released after 120 minutes.) At 100 mm Hg, there is a relatively rapid drop-off of afferent conduction, with limited recovery. At 75 mm Hg there is nearly complete recovery after two hours of compression. At 50 mm Hg external compression does not affect the electrophysiologic function.

(unlike Schönström and associates). They found that with 25 per cent circumferential narrowing in the group of animals studied there were no neurologic deficits; however, with 50 per cent or more restriction of the cross-sectional area, motor and sensory deficits were observed. This is consistent with Schönström's findings using absolute values of cross-sectional area, as described previously.

As gleaned from the above studies, mechanical compression of the cauda equina nerve roots could lead to acute and possibly long-term impairment of neurologic function, cauda equina blood supply, and transport of nutrients to the nerve fibers.[152, 154] Similarly, waste product clearance from the nerve root tissue may be decreased because of this mechanical compression. These changes may be enhanced by chronic inflammatory changes in and around the nerve tissues. Prolonged mechanical compression, combined with metabolic alterations, may lead to demyelinization. It has been observed that demyelinated roots are frequently pain sensitive.[189]

These studies all suggest that mechanical compression may have a significant role in the symptoms and signs of spinal stenosis, help explain the discrepancy seen between individuals, and suggest why plain radiographs or CT or MRI scans do not adequately explain the entire pattern, although they do accurately describe the anatomy and the gross pathologic changes.

Some authors have described the source of the pain in spinal stenosis and degenerative disc disease as related to the nerves to the spinal column, including the sinuvertebral nerve or the posterior ramus (Fig. 25–42).[40, 87, 166, 171] This may be particularly true when mechanical instability leads to irritation/inflammation of these nerves. However, they are extremely small, are present in all humans, are difficult to study or isolate, and are therefore impossible at this point to implicate as the source of pain with any degree of assuredness.

Venous hypertension and venous stasis have also been proposed as mechanisms in creating pain in spinal stenosis. Arnoldi and associates demonstrated increased venous pressures within the vertebral body in patients with spinal stenosis.[5] However, if this is the explanation, it is unclear why the symptoms should be intermittent. Symptoms of spinal stenosis are frequently relieved by flexion and increased by extension, yet patients are still in the upright position (whether flexed or extended), so the veins should not rapidly decompress just by postural changes. This suggests that stasis is not the sole factor. There is also a generous anastomosis of veins in and around the spine. This is a valveless system, and it again suggests that stasis is not the major culprit in the pathoetiology of spinal stenosis. If the symptoms are related to venous congestion or hypertension, the relief of pain with decreased activity should be slow. How-

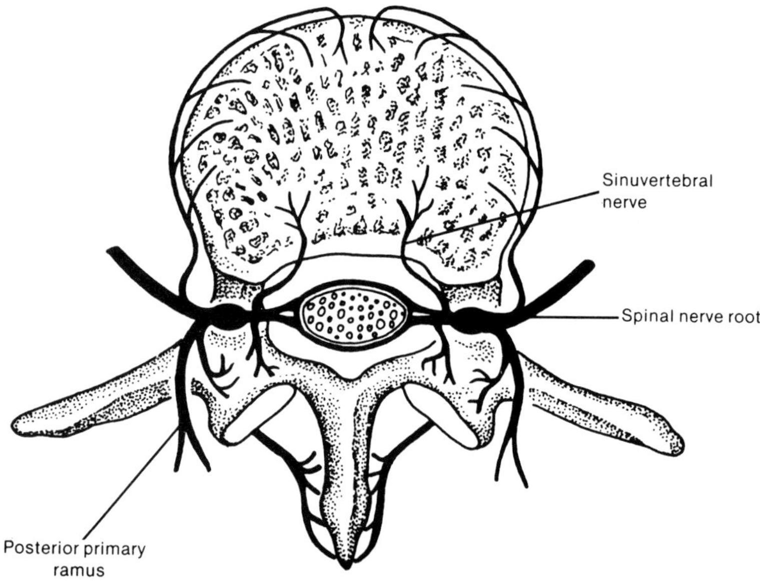

Figure 25–42. Diagrammatic demonstration of the sinuvertebral nerve and the posterior primary ramus. These structures innervate the posterior column, the posterior longitudinal ligament, the annulus, and the facet joints, as well as the dura. They can contribute to the symptoms of low back pain, as well as some of the referred leg symptoms, seen in degenerative disc disease and spinal stenosis.

ever, patients with spinal stenosis frequently obtain relatively rapid relief of pain with merely a change in posture. In addition, if the symptoms are related to venous hypertension in the bone, a narrow laminectomy may often be sufficient to "decompress the veins." However, unless the nerve roots are adequately decompressed, symptoms often persist. Again, this suggests that the venous system is not the primary component in the symptoms and signs of spinal stenosis.

More reasonable explanations relate to the arterial and nutritional support systems of the cauda equina.[6, 32, 36, 134, 188] Parke and associates showed that the cauda equina nerve roots are supplied with blood from arteries that come from the spinal artery centrally, as well as radicular or segmental arteries laterally.[135, 136] It has been shown that these arteries dilate with exercise, and that with stimulation of the nerve, oxygen use increases in that nerve.[11, 12] With narrowing of the canal (by bone and soft tissue components) and subsequent ischemia, there would be diminished oxygen supply, occurring particularly during exercise, when the needs are greatest, and when the vessels do not have room to dilate. Also, at the area where the central and radicular systems approach each other, there is an area of relative hypovascularity along the spinal nerve roots and cauda equina.

Studies of the vascularity of the human cauda equina and peripheral nerves show decreased microvessels per cross-sectional area in the former.[136, 188] This is distinct from the dorsal root ganglion, where there is a very rich and extensive microvascular network.[6] These vessels along the dorsal root ganglion are also more permeable than intraneural blood vessels at other levels.[6, 134] This vascular supply, coupled with the permeability of the microvessels in the dorsal root ganglion, suggests an increased metabolic demand. In addition, this area where the sensory nerve cell bodies are situated is the locale of synthesis of several essential substances.[6] Therefore, any compromise in the blood supply and flow may lead to alterations in solute transport or manufacture and be a focus for pain. Separately, nutritional transport has been shown to occur through the cerebrospinal fluid (CSF).[151, 153] Such factors as chronic compression, inflammation, fibrosis, ischemia, and diminution in protein synthesis and metabolism may slow the diffusion process, limit transport, and lead to a relative toxic and deprived state, which can further contribute to the symptoms and signs of spinal stenosis.

In summation, the pathoanatomy and pathoetiology of the symptoms and signs of spinal stenosis have not been fully elucidated. However, important basic facts are known. The degenerative processes seen in the spine, related to chemical and mechanical alterations, lead to clinical and mechanical changes that can affect and inflame the neural elements in the lumbar spine. This, coupled with compression (static and dynamic), vascular occlusion, ischemia, and metabolic-nutritional effects, may lead to pain and neurologic dysfunction.

References

1. Adam, M., and Deyl, Z.: Degenerated annulus fibrosus of the intervertebral disc contains collagen type III. Ann. Rheum. Dis. *43*:258–263, 1984.
2. Adams, P., Eyre, D. R., and Muir, H.: Biochemical aspects of development and ageing of human lumbar intervertebral discs. Rheumatol. Rehab. *16*:22–29, 1977.
3. Adams, P., and Muir, H.: Qualitative changes with age of proteoglycans of human lumbar disc. Ann. Rheum. Dis. *35*:289–295, 1976.
4. Alexander, E.: Significance of the small lumbar spinal canal: cauda equina compression syndromes due to spondylosis. Part 5. Achondroplasia. J. Neurosurg. *31*:513–519, 1969.
5. Arnoldi, C. C., Brodsky, A. E., Cauchoix, J., et al.: Lumbar spinal stenosis and nerve root entrapment syndromes. Definition and classification. Clin. Orthop. *115*:4–5, 1976.
6. Arvidson, B.: Distribution of intravenously injected protein tracers in peripheral ganglia of adult mice. Exp. Neurol. *63*:388–410, 1979.
7. Badgley, C. E.: The articular facets in relationship to low back pain and sciatic radiation. J. Bone Joint Surg. *23A*:481–496, 1941.
8. Bailey, J. A.: Orthopaedic aspects of achondroplasia. J. Bone Joint Surg. *52A*:1295–1301, 1970.
9. Bailey, P., and Casamajor, L.: Osteoarthritis of the spine as a cause of compression of the spinal cord and its roots. J. Nerv. Ment. Dis. *38*:588–609, 1911.
10. Bergstrom, K., Laurent, U., and Lundberg, P. O.: Neurological symptoms in achondroplasia. Acta Neurol. Scand. *47*:59–70, 1971.
11. Blau, J. N., and Logue, V.: Intermittent claudication of the cauda equina. An unusual syndrome resulting from central protrusion of a lumbar intervertebral disc. Lancet *1*:1082–1086, 1961.
12. Blau, J. N., and Rushworth, G.: Observations on the blood vessels of the spinal cord and their responses to motor activity. Brain *81*:354–363, 1958.
13. Bogduk, N., and Engel, R.: The menisci of the lumbar zygoapophyseal joints—a review of their anatomy and clinical significance. Spine *9*:454–460, 1984.

14. Bogduk, N., Tynan, W., and Wilson, A. S.: The nerve supply to the human lumbar intervertebral disc. J. Anat. *132*:39, 1981.
15. Bowen, V., et al.: Lumbar spinal stenosis. Childs Brain *4*:257, 1978.
16. Brailsford, J. F.: Chondro-osteo-dystrophy. Am. J. Surg. *7*:404–410, 1929.
17. Brailsford, J. F.: Chondro-osteo-dystrophy. J. Bone Joint Surg. *34B*:53–63, 1952.
18. Breig, A.: Adverse Mechanical Tension in the Central Nervous System. New York, John Wiley & Sons, 1978.
19. Brickley-Parsons, D., and Glimcher, M. J.: Is the chemistry of collagen in intervertebral discs an expression of Wolff's law? A study of the human lumbar spine. Spine *9*:148–163, 1984.
20. Brodsky, A. E.: Post-laminectomy and post-fusion stenosis of the lumbar spine. Clin. Orthop. *115*:130, 1976.
21. Buckwalter, J. A.: The fine structure of human intervertebral disc. *In* White, A. A., III, and Gordon, S. L. (eds.): Symposium on Idiopathic Low Back Pain. St. Louis, C. V. Mosby Co., 1982, pp. 108–143.
22. Buckwalter, J. A., Pedrini-Mille, A., Pedrini, V., and Tudisco, C.: Proteoglycans of human infant intervertebral disc. Electron microscopic and biochemical studies. J. Bone Joint Surg. *67A*:284–294, 1985.
23. Burton, C. V.: On the diagnosis and surgical treatment of lumbar subarticular and "far out" lateral spinal stenosis. *In* Watkins, R. G., and Collis, J. S., (eds.): Lumbar Discectomy and Laminectomy. Rockville, MD, Aspen Publishers, 1987, pp. 195–202.
24. Caffey, J.: Achondroplasia of pelvis and lumbosacral spine. Some roentgenographic features. A. J. R. *80*:449–457, 1958.
25. Ciric, I., et al.: The lateral recess syndrome. J. Neurosurg. *53*:433–443, 1980.
26. Clark, K.: Significance of the small lumbar canal: cauda equina compression syndromes due to spondylosis. Part 2. Clinical and surgical significance. J. Neurosurg. *31*:495–498, 1969.
27. Cole, T. - C., Burkhardt, D., Ghosh, P., and Taylor, T.: Effects of spinal fusion on the proteoglycans of the canine intervertebral disc. J. Orthop. Res. *3*:277–291, 1985.
28. Cole, T. - C., Ghosh, P., Hannan, N. J., et al.: The response of canine intervertebral disc to immobilization produced by spinal arthrodesis is dependent on constitutional factors. J. Orthop. Res. *5*:337–347, 1987.
29. Coventry, M. B., Ghormley, R. K., and Kernohan, J. W.: The intervertebral disc: its microscopic anatomy and pathology. Part II. Changes in the intervertebral disc concomitant with age. J. Bone Joint Surg. *27A*:233–247, 1945.
30. Coventry, M. B., Ghormley, R. K., and Kernohan, J. W.: The intervertebral disc: its microscopic anatomy and pathology. Part III. Pathologic changes in the intervertebral disc. J. Bone Joint Surg. *27A*:460–474, 1945.
31. Crock, H. V.: Isolated lumbar disk resorption as a cause of nerve root canal stenosis. Clin. Orthop. *115*:109, 1976.
32. Crock, H. V., and Yoshizawa, H.: The Blood Supply of the Vertebral Column and Spinal Cord in Man. New York, Springer-Verlag, 1977.
33. Dahlin, L. B., Rydevik, B., McLean, W. G., et al.: Changes in fast axonal transport during experimental nerve compression at low pressures. Exp. Neurol. *84*:29–36, 1984.
34. Delamarter, R. B., Bohlman, H. H., Dodge, L. D., and Miro, C.: Experimental lumbar spinal stenosis: analysis of the cortical evoked potentials, microvasculature, and histopathology. J. Bone Joint Surg. *72A*:110–120, 1190.
35. Dupuis, P. R., Yong-Hing, K., Cassidy, J. D., and Kirkaldy-Willis, W. H.: Radiologic diagnosis of degenerative lumbar spinal instability. Spine *10*:262, 1985.
36. Dommisse, G.: Morphological aspects of the lumbar spine and lumbosacral region. Orthop. Clin. North Am. *6*:163–175, 1975.
37. Donohue, P. J., Jahnke, M. R., Blaha, J. D., and Caterson, B.: Characterization of link protein(s) from human intervertebral-disc tissues. Biochem. J. *251*:739–747, 1988.
38. Duvoisin, R. C., and Yahr, M. D.: Compressive spinal cord and root syndromes in achondroplastic dwarfs. Neurology *12*:202–207, 1962.
39. Eckert, C., and Decker, A.: Pathological studies of intervertebral discs. J. Bone Joint Surg. *29A*:447–454, 1947.
40. Edgar, M. A., and Ghadially, J. A.: Innervation of the lumbar spine. Clin. Orthop. *11*:35, 1976.
41. Edward, W. C., and LaRocca, S. H.: The development of segmental sagittal diameter in combined cervical and lumbar spondylosis. Spine *10*:42–49, 1985.
42. Ehni, G.: Effects of certain degenerative diseases of the spine, especially spondylosis and disk protrusion, on the neural contents, particularly in the lumbar region. Mayo Clin. Proc. *50*:327, 1975.
43. Ehni, G.: Significance of the small lumbar spinal canal: cauda equina compression syndromes due to spondylosis. Part 1. Introduction. J. Neurosurg. *31*:490–494, 1969.
44. Ehni, G.: Significance of the small lumbar spinal canal: cauda equina compression syndromes due to spondylosis. Part 4. Acute compression artificially induced during operation. J. Neurosurg. *31*:507–512, 1969.
45. Eisenstein, S.: Measurements of the lumbar spinal canal in two racial groups. Clin. Orthop. *115*:42, 1976.
46. Eisenstein, S.: The morphometry and pathologic anatomy of the lumbar spine in South African Negroes and Caucasoids with specific reference to spinal stenosis. J. Bone Joint Surg. *59B*:173–180, 1977.
47. Eisenstein, S. M.: The trefoil configuration of the lumbar vertebral canal. J. Bone Joint Surg. *62B*:73–77, 1980.
48. Eisenstein, S.: Lumbar vertebral canal morphometry for computerized tomography in spinal stenosis. Spine *8*:187–191, 1983.
49. Eisenstein, S. M., and Parry, C. R.: The lumbar facet arthrosis syndrome—clinical presentation and articular surface changes. J. Bone Joint Surg. *69B*:3–7, 1987.
49a. Elsberg, C. A.: Experiences in spinal surgery. Observations upon 60 laminectomies for spinal disease. Surg. Gynecol. Obstet. *16*:117–132, 1913.

50. Engel, R., and Bogduk, N.: The menisci of the lumbar zygoapophyseal joints. J. Anat. *135*:795–809, 1982.
51. Epstein, J. A., Epstein, B. S., Lavine, L. S., et al.: Lumbar nerve root compression of the intervertebral foramina caused by arthritis of the posterior facets. J. Neurosurg. *39*:362, 1973.
52. Epstein, J. A., Epstein, B. S., and Lavine, L.: Nerve root compression associated with narrowing of the lumbar spinal canal. J. Neurol. Neurosurg. Psychiatry *25*:165, 1962.
53. Epstein, J. A., Epstein, B. S., and Lavine, L.: Nerve root compression due to stenosis of the lumbar canal. J. Neurol. Neurosurg. Psychiatry *29*:315, 1966.
54. Epstein, J. A., and Malis, L. I.: Compression of spinal cord and cauda equina in achondroplastic dwarfs. Neurology *5*:875–881, 1955.
55. Epstein, J. A., et al.: Degenerative spondylolisthesis. J. Neurosurg. *44*:139, 1976.
56. Epstein, J. A., Epstein, B. S., Rosenthal, R. C., and Lavine, S. L.: Sciatica caused by nerve root entrapment in the lateral recess: the superior facet syndrome. J. Neurosurg. *36*:584–589, 1972.
57. Epstein, N. E., Epstein, J. A., Carras, R., and Lavine, L. S.: Degenerative spondylolisthesis with an intact neural arch: a review of 60 cases with an analysis of clinical findings and the development of surgical management. Neurosurgery *13*:555–561, 1983.
58. Eyre, D. R.: Biochemistry of the intervertebral disc. Int. Rev. Connective Tissue Res. *8*:227–291, 1979.
59. Eyre, D. R., Koob, T. J., and Van Ness, K. P.: Quantitation of hydroxypyridinium cross links in collagen by high-performance liquid chromatography. Anal. Biochem. *137*:380–388, 1984.
60. Eyre, D. R., and Muir, H.: Collagen polymorphism: two molecular species in pig intervertebral disc. FEBS Lett. *42*:192–196, 1974.
61. Eyre, D. R., and Muir, H.: Types I and II collagens in intervertebral disc. Interchanging radial distributions in annulus fibrosus. Biochem. J. *157*:267–270, 1976.
62. Eyring, E. J.: The biochemistry and physiology of intervertebral disk. Clin. Orthop. *67*:16–28, 1969.
63. Farfan, H. F.: The pathological anatomy of degenerative spondylolisthesis in a cadaver study. Spine *5*:412, 1980.
64. Farfan, H. F., and Gracovetsky, S.: The nature of instability. Spine *9*:714, 1989.
65. Freund, E.: Spastic paraplegia in achondroplasia. Arch. Surg. *27*:859–867, 1933.
66. Friberg, S., and Hirsch, C.: Anatomical and clinical studies on lumbar disc degeneration. Acta Orthop. Scand. *19*:222–242, 1949.
67. Friedman, E.: Narrowing of the spinal canal due to thickening of the laminae, a cause of low back pain and sciatica. Clin. Orthop. *21*:190–197, 1961.
68. Frymoyer, J. W., and Selby, D. K.: Segmental instability, rationale for treatment. Spine *10*:280, 1985.
69. Gelman, M. I.: Cauda equina compression in acromegaly. Radiology *112*:357–360, 1974.
70. Gertzbein, S. D., et al.: Centrode patterns in segmental instability in degenerative disc disease. Spine *10*:257, 1985.
71. Gill, G. G., and White, H. L.: Mechanisms of nerve root compression and irritation in backache. Clin. Orthop. *5*:66, 1955.
72. Gotfried, Y., Bradford, D. S., and Oegema, T. R.: Facet joint changes after chemonucleolysis induced disc and space narrowing. Spine *11*:944–954, 1986.
73. Gower, W. E., and Pedrini, V.: Age related variations in protein-polysaccharides from human nucleus pulposus, annulus fibrosus and costal cartilage. J. Bone Joint Surg. *51A*:1154–1162, 1969.
74. Grynpas, M. D., Eyre, D. R., and Kirschner, D. A.: Collagen type II differs from type I in native molecular packing. Biochim. Biophys. Acta *626*:346–355, 1980.
75. Hallen, A.: Hexosamine and ester sulphate content of the human nucleus pulposus in different ages. Acta Chim. Scand. *12*:1869–1862, 1958.
76. Hancock, D. O. and Philliphs, D. G.: Spinal compression in achondroplasia. Paraplegia *3*:23–33, 1965.
77. Hardingham, T. E., and Adams, P.: A method for the determination of hyaluronate in the presence of other glycosaminoglycans and its application to human intervertebral discs. Biochem. J. *159*:143–147, 1976.
78. Harris, R. I., and MacNab, I.: Structural changes in the lumbar intervertebral discs. Their relationship to low back pain and sciatica. J. Bone Joint Surg. *36B*:304–322, 1954.
79. Hasue, M., et al.: Post-traumatic spinal stenosis of the lumbar spine. Spine *5*:259–263, 1980.
80. Hasue, M., Kikuchi, S., Sakuyama, Y., and Ito, T.: Anatomic study of the interrelation between lumbosacral nerve roots and their surrounding tissues. Spine *8*:50–58, 1983.
81. Herbert, C. M., Lindberg, K. A., Jayson, M. I. V., and Bailey, A. J.: Changes in the collagen of human intervertebral discs during ageing and degenerative disc disease. J. Mol. Med. *1*:79–81, 1975.
82. Herzberg, L., and Bayliss, E.: Spinal-cord syndrome due to noncompressive Paget's disease of bone: a spinal artery steal phenomenon reversible with calcitonin. Lancet *2*:13, 1980.
83. Hirsch, C., Ingelmark, V. E., and Miller, N.: The anatomic basis for low back pain: studies on the presence of sensory endings in ligamentous capsular and intervertebral disc structures in the human lumbar spine. Acta Orthop. Scand. *33*:1–17, 1963.
84. Hirsch, C., Paulson, S., Sylven, B., and Snellman, O.: Biophysical and physiological investigations on cartilage and other mesenchymal tissues. Acta Orthop. Scand. *22*:175–181, 1952.
85. Huizinga, J., Heiden, J. A., and van der Vinken, P. J. J. G.: The human vertebral canal: a biometric study. Proc. R. Neth. Acad. Sci. *C55*:22–33, 1952.
86. Hult, L.: Cervical, dorsal and lumbar spine syndromes. Acta Orthop. Scand. (Suppl. 17):65–73, 1954.
87. Inman, V. T., and Saunders, J. B.: Referred pain from skeletal structures. J. Nerv. Ment. Dis. *99*:660–667, 1944.
88. Joffe, R., Appleby, A., and Arjona, V.: Intermittent ischemia of the cauda equina due to stenosis of the lumbar canal. J. Neurol. Neurosurg. Psychiatry *29*:315, 1966.
89. Johnson, K. E., Willner, S., and Johnsson, K.:

Postoperative instability after decompression for lumbar spinal stenosis. Spine *11*:107–110, 1986.
90. Kadziolka, R., Asztely, M., Hanai, K., et al.: Ultrasonic measurement of the lumbar spinal canal. J. Bone Joint Surg. *63B*:504–507, 1981.
91. Karpman, R. J., et al.: Lumbar spinal stenosis in a patient with diffuse idiopathic skeletal hypertrophy syndrome. Spine *7*:598–603, 1982.
92. Kellgren, J. H., and Lawrence, J. S.: Osteoarthrosis and disc degeneration in an urban population. Ann. Rheum. Dis. *17*:388–397, 1958.
93. Kirkaldy-Willis, W. H.: The relationship of structural pathology to the nerve root. Spine *9*:49, 1984.
94. Kirkaldy-Willis, W. H., and Farfan, H. F.: Instability of the lumbar spine. Clin. Orthop. *165*:110, 1982.
95. Kirkaldy-Willis, W. H., and Paine, K. W.: Lumbar spinal stenosis. Clin. Orthop. *99*:30, 1974.
96. Kirkaldy-Willis, W. H., et al.: Lumbar spinal nerve entrapment. Clin. Orthop. *169*:171–178, 1982.
97. Kirkaldy-Willis, W. H., Wedge, J. H., Young-Hing, K., and Reilly, J.: Pathology and pathogenesis of lumbar spondylosis and stenosis. Spine *3*:319, 1978.
98. Knuttsen, S.: The instability associated with disc degeneration in the lumbar spine. Acta Radiol. *25*:593, 1944.
99. Lancourt, J. E., Glenn, W. V., and Wiltse, L. L.: Multiplanar computerized tomography in the normal spine and in the diagnosis of spinal stenosis. Spine *4*:379–390, 1979.
100. Larsen, J. L., and Smith, D.: Vertebral body size in lumbar spinal canal stenosis. Acta. Radiol. (Diagn.) *21*:785–788, 1980.
101. Leong, J. C. Y., Luk, K. D. K., Chow, D. H. K., and Woo, C. W.: The biomechanical functions of the iliolumbar ligament in maintaining stability of the lumbosacral junction. Spine *12*:669–674, 1987.
102. Lewin, T.: Osteoarthritis in lumbar synovial joints. A morphologic study. Acta Orthop. Scand. (Suppl.) *73*:1–112, 1964.
103. Lewin, T.: Osteoarthritis in lumbar synovial joints. A morphologic study. Acta Orthop. Scand. (Suppl.) *73*:31, 1964.
104. Lewinnek, G. E., and Warfield, C. A.: Facet joint degeneration as a cause of low back pain. Clin. Orthop. *213*:216–222, 1986.
105. Lipson, S. J.: Metaplastic proliferative fibrocartilage as an alternative concept to herniated intervertebral disc. Spine *13*:1055–1060, 1988.
106. Lipson, S. J., and Muir, H.: Experimental intervertebral disc degeneration. Morphologic and proteoglycan changes over time. Arthritis Rheum. *24*:12–21, 1981.
107. Lipson, S. J., and Muir, H.: Proteoglycans in experimental disc degeneration. Spine *6*:194–210, 1981.
108. Lorenz, M., Patawardhan, A., and VanDerby, R.: Load-bearing characteristics of lumbar facets in normal and surgically altered spinal segments. Spine *8*:122–130, 1983.
109. Lundborg, G.: Nerve Injury and Repair. Edinburgh, Churchill Livingstone, 1988.
110. Lutter, L. D., and Langer, I. O.: Neurological symptoms in achondroplastic dwarfs. Surgical treatment. J. Bone Joint Surg. *59A*:87–92, 1977.
111. Lyons, G., Eisenstein, S. M., and Sweet, M. B. E.: Biochemical changes in intervertebral disc degeneration. Biochim. Biophys. Acta *673*:443–453, 1981.
112. Lyons, H., Jones, E., Quinn, F. E., and Sprunt, D. H.: Protein-polysaccharide complexes of normal and herniated intervertebral discs. Proc. Soc. Exp. Biol. *115*:610–614, 1964.
113. Lyons, H., Jones, E., Quinn, F. E., and Sprunt, D. H.: Changes in the protein-polysaccharide fractions of nucleus pulposus from human intervertebral disc with age and disc herniation. J. Lab. Clin. Med. *68*:930–939, 1966.
114. MacNab, I.: The traction spur: an indication of segmental instability. J. Bone Joint Surg. *53A*:663, 1971.
115. Magora, A., and Schwartz, A.: Relation between the low back pain syndrome and x-ray findings. 1. Degenerative osteoarthritis. Scand. J. Rehabil. Med. *8*:115–125, 1976.
116. Malinsky, J.: Histochemical demonstration of carbohydrates in human intervertebral discs during postnatal development. Acta Histochem. *5*:120–128, 1958.
117. McIvor, G. W. D., and Kirkaldy-Willis, W. H.: Pathologic and myelographic changes in the major types of spinal stenosis. Clin. Orthop. *115*:72–76, 1976.
118. Melrose, J., Ghosh, P., and Taylor, T. K. F.: Neutral proteinases of the human intervertebral disc. Biochim. Biophys. Acta *923*:483–495, 1987.
119. Miller, J. A. A., Schmatz, C., and Schultz, A. B.: Lumbar disc degeneration: correlation with age, sex, and spine level in 600 autopsy specimens. Spine *13*:173–178, 1988.
120. Mitchell, P. E. G., Hendry, N., and Billewicz, W. T.: The chemical background of intervertebral disc prolapse. J. Bone Joint Surg. *43B*:141–151, 1961.
121. Mixter, W. J., and Barr, J. S.: Rupture of the intervertebral disc with involvement of the spinal canal. N. Engl. J. Med. *211*:210, 1934.
122. Mooney, V., and Robertson, S.: The facet syndrome. Clin. Orthop. *115*:149–156, 1976.
123. Moriguchi, T., and Fujimoto, D.: Age related changes of the collagen cross-link, pyridinoline. J. Biochem. (Tokyo) *84*:933–935, 1978.
124. Nachemson, A.: Lumbar intradiscal pressure. Acta Orthop. Scand. (Suppl. 43):43–44, 1960.
125. Naylor, A.: Factors in the development of the spinal stenosis syndrome. J. Bone Joint Surg. *61B*:306, 1979.
126. Naylor, A.: The biophysical and biochemical aspects of intervertebral disc herniations and degeneration. Ann. R. Coll. Surg. Engl. *31*:91–114, 1962.
127. Naylor, A., and Horton, W. G.: The hydrophilic properties of the nucleus pulposus of the intervertebral disc. Rheumatism *11*:32–35, 1955.
128. Nelson, M. A.: Lumbar spinal stenosis. J. Bone Joint Surg. *55B*:506, 1973.
129. Newman, P. H.: Stenosis of the lumbar spine in spondylolisthesis. Clin. Orthop. *115*:116, 1976.
130. Olmarker, K., Rydevik, B., Hansson, T., and Holm, S.: Compression-induced changes of the nutritional supply to the porcine cauda equina. J. Spinal Dis. *3*:25–29, 1990.
131. Olmarker, K., Rydevik, B., and Holm, S.: Edema formation in spinal nerve roots induced by experimental, graded compression. An experimental study on the pig cauda equina with special reference to differences in effects between rapid and slow onset of compression. Spine *14*:569–573, 1989.

132. Olmarker, B., Rydevik, B., Holm, S., et al.: Graded compression of the porcine cauda equina modifies nerve root nutrition, blood flow and impulse conduction. Transactions of the Orthopaedic Research Society, 33rd Annual Meeting, San Francisco, January 1987.
133. Olmarker, K., Rydevik, B., Holm, S., and Bagge, U.: Effects of experimental, graded compression on blood flow in nerve roots. A vital microscopic study on the porcine cauda equina. J. Orthop. Res. *7*:817–823, 1989.
134. Olsson, Y.: The involvement of vasa nervorum in the diseases of peripheral nerves. *In* Vinken, P. J., and Bruyn, G. W. (eds.): Handbook of Clinical Neurology. Vol. 12. Vascular Diseases of the Nervous System. Part II. New York, American Elsevier, 1972, pp. 644–664.
135. Parke, W. W., Gammell, K., and Rothman, R. H.: Arterial vascularization of the cauda equina. J. Bone Joint Surg. *63A*:53–62, 1981.
136. Parke, W. W., and Watanabe, R.: The intrinsic vasculature of the lumbosacral spinal nerve roots. Spine *10*:508–515, 1985.
137. Pearce, R. H., Grimmer, B. J., and Adams, M. E.: Degeneration and the chemical composition of the human lumbar intervertebral disc. J. Orthop. Res. *5*:198–205, 1987.
138. Pearce, R. H., Mathieson, J. M., Mort, J. S., and Roughley, P. J.: The effect of age on the abundance and fragmentation of link protein of the human intervertebral disc. J. Orthop. Res. *7*:861–867, 1989.
139. Pedowitz, R. A., Garfin, S. R., Massie, J. B., et al.: Effects of magnitude and duration of compression on spinal nerve root conduction. Spine 1991 (in press).
140. Porter, R. W., et al.: Measurements of the spinal canal by diagnostic ultrasound. J. Bone Joint Surg. *60B*:481–484, 1978.
141. Porter, R. W., and Hibbert, C.: Relationship between the spinal canal and other skeletal measurements in a Romano-British population. Ann. R. Coll. Surg. Engl. *63*:437, 1981.
142. Porter, R. W., Wicks, M., and Hibbert, C.: The size of the lumbar spinal canal in the symptomatology of disc lesion. J. Bone Joint Surg. *60B*:485–487, 1978.
143. Postacchini, F., Ripani, M., and Carpano, S.: Morphometry of the lumbar vertebrae. An anatomic study in two Caucasoid ethnic groups. Clin. Orthop. *172*:296–303, 1983.
144. Pritzker, K. P. H.: Aging and degeneration in the lumbar intervertebral disc. Orthop. Clin. North Am. *8*:65–77, 1977.
145. Puschel, J.: Der Wassergehalt normaler und degenerierter Zwischenwirbelscheiben. Beitr. Pathol. Anat. *84*:123–130, 1930.
146. Rauschning, W.: Normal and pathologic anatomy of the lumbar root canals. Spine *12*:1008–1019, 1987.
147. Roberts, S., Beard, H. K., and O'Brien, J. P.: Biochemical changes of intervertebral discs in patients with spondylolisthesis or with tears of the posterior annulus fibrosus. Ann. Rheum. Dis. *41*:78–85, 1982.
148. Rosenberg, N. J.: Degenerative spondylolisthesis. J. Bone Joint Surg. *57A*:467, 1975.
149. Rydevik, B., Brown, M., and Lundborg, G.: Pathoanatomy and pathophysiology of nerve root compression. Spine *9*:7–15, 1984.
150. Rydevik, B., and Garfin, S.: Spinal nerve root compression. *In* Szabo, R. M. (ed.): Nerve Compression Syndromes—Diagnosis and Treatment. Thorofare, NJ, Slack, 1989, pp. 247–262.
151. Rydevik, B., Holm, S., Brown, M. D., and Lundborg, G.: Diffusion from the cerebrospinal fluid as a nutritional pathway for spinal nerve roots. Acta Physiol. Scand. *138*:247–248, 1990.
152. Rydevik, B., Lundborg, G., and Bagge, U.: Effects of graded compression on intraneural blood flow. An in vivo study on rabbit tibial nerve. J. Hand Surg. *6*:3–12, 1981.
153. Rydevik, B., and Lundborg, G.: Permeability of intraneural microvessels and perineurium following acute, graded experimental nerve compression. Scand. J. Plast. Reconstr. Surg. *11*:179–187, 1977.
154. Rydevik, B., and Nordborg, G.: Changes in nerve function and nerve fibre structure induced by acute, graded compression. J. Neurol. Neurosurg. Psychiatry *43*:1070–1082, 1981.
155. Rydevik, B. L., Pedowitz, R. A., Hargens, A. R., et al.: Effects of acute, graded compression on spinal nerve root function and structure. An experimental study of the pig cauda equina. Spine *16*:487–493, 1991.
155a. Sachs, B., and Fraenkel, J.: Progressive ankylotic rigidity of the spine (spondylose rhizomelique). J. Nerve. Ment. Dis. *27*:1–15, 1900.
156. Sarpyener, M. A.: Congenital stricture of the spinal canal. J. Bone Joint Surg. *27*:70–79, 1945.
157. Sarpyener, M. A.: Spina bifida aperta and congenital stricture of the spinal canal. J. Bone Joint Surg. *29*:817–821, 1947.
158. Schatzker, J., and Pennal, G. P.: Spinal stenosis, a cause of cauda equina compression. J. Bone Joint Surg. *50B*:606, 1968.
159. Schlesinger, P. T.: Incarceration of the first sacral nerve in a lateral bony recess of the spinal canal. J. Bone Joint Surg. *37A*:115–124, 1955.
160. Schönström, N., Bolender, N., and Spengler, D.: The pathomorphology of spinal stenosis as seen on CT scans of the lumbar spine. Spine *10*:806–811, 1985.
161. Schönström, N., Bolender, N. F., Spengler, D. M., et al.: Pressure changes within the cauda equina following constriction of the dural sac. Spine *9*:604–607, 1984.
162. Schönström, N., and Hansson, T.: Pressure changes following constriction of the cauda equina. An experimental study in situ. Spine *13*:385–388, 1988.
163. Schönström, N., Lindahl, S., Willen, J., et al.: Dynamic changes in the dimensions of the lumbar spinal canal. An experimental study in vitro. J. Orthop. Res. *7*:115–121, 1988.
164. Schreiber, F., and Rosenthal, H.: Paraplegia from ruptured discs in achondroplastic dwarfs. J. Neurosurg. *9*:648–651, 1952.
165. Sedowofia, K. A., Tomlinson, I. W., Weiss, J. B., et al.: Collagenolytic enzyme systems in human intervertebral disc. Their control, mechanism, and their possible role in the initiation of biomechanical failure. Spine 7:213–222, 1982.
166. Sinclair, D. C., Feindel, W. H., Weddell, G., and Falcon, M. A.: The intervertebral ligament as a source of segmental pain. J. Bone Joint Surg. *30B*:515, 1948.

167. Spillane, J. D.: Three cases of achondroplasia with neurological complications. J. Neurol. Neurosurg. Psychiatry *15*:246–252, 1952.
168. Stevens, R. L., Dondi, P. G., and Muir, H.: Proteoglycans of intervertebral disc. Absence of degradation during isolation of proteoglycans from the intervertebral disc. Biochem. J. *179*:573–578, 1979.
169. Stevens, R. L., Ewins, R. J. F., Revell, P. A., and Muir, H.: Proteoglycans of the intervertebral disc. Biochem. J. *179*:561–572, 1979.
170. Stevens, R. L., Ryvar, R., Robertson, W. R., et al.: Biological changes in the annulus fibrosus in patients with low-back pain. Spine *7*:223–233, 1982.
171. Stillwell, D. L.: Nerve supply of vertebral column. Anat. Rec. *125*:139–142, 1956.
172. Stokes, I. A. F., and Frymoyer, J. W.: Segmental motion and instability. Spine *12*:688, 1987.
173. Sunderland, S.: Nerves and Nerve Injuries. 2nd ed. Edinburgh, Churchill Livingstone, 1978.
174. Sutro, C. J.: Lumbar facets—spinal stenosis and intermittent claudication: a mini review. Bull. Hosp. Joint Dis. *40*:13, 1979.
175. Sylven, B.: On the biology of the nucleus pulposus. Acta Orthop. Scand. *20*:275–279, 1951.
176. Taylor, J. R., and Twomey, L. T.: Age changes in lumbar zygoapophyseal joints—observations on structure and function. Spine *11*:739–745, 1986.
177. Towne, E. B., and Reichert, F. L.: Compression of the lumbosacral roots of the spinal cord by thickened ligamenta flava. Ann. Surg. *94*:327–336, 1931.
178. Troup, J. D. G.: Biomechanics of the lumbar spinal canal. Clin. Biomech. *1*:31–43, 1986.
179. Urban, J. P. G., and McMullin, J. F.: Swelling pressure of the lumbar intervertebral discs: influence of age, spinal level, composition, and degeneration. Spine *13*:179–187, 1988.
180. Van Den Hoof, A.: Histological age changes in the anulus fibrosus of the human intervertebral disk. Gerontologia *9*:136–149, 1964.
181. Verbiest, H.: A radicular syndrome from developmental narrowing of the lumbar vertebral canal. J. Bone Joint Surg. *36B*:230–237, 1954.
182. Verbiest, H.: Further experiences on pathologic influence of a developmental narrowing of the lumbar vertebral canal. J. Bone Joint Surg. *38B*:576–583, 1956.
183. Verbiest, H.: Pathomorphologic aspects of developmental lumbar stenosis. Orthop. Clin. North Am. *6*:177–196, 1975.
184. Verbiest, H.: Neurogenic intermittent claudication in cases with absolute and relative stenosis of the lumbar vertebral canal (ASLC and RSLC), in cases with narrow lumbar intervertebral foramina, and in cases with both entities. Clin. Neurosurg. *20*:204–214, 1973.
185. Verbiest, H.: Neurogenic intermittent claudication. Lesions of the spinal cord and cauda equina, stenosis of the vertebral canal, narrowing of intervertebral foramina and entrapment of peripheral nerves. *In* Vinken, P. J., and Bruyn, G. W. (eds.): Handbook of Clinical Neurology. Vol. 20. Part II. New York, North Holland/American Elsevier, 1976, pp. 611–807.
186. Verbiest, H.: Fallacies of the present definition, nomenclature and classification of the stenoses of the lumbar vertebral canal. Spine *1*:217–225, 1976.
187. Videman, T., Malmivaara, A., and Mooney, V.: The value of axial view in assessing diskograms. An experimental study with cadavers. Spine *12*:299–304, 1987.
188. Watanabe, R., and Parke, W. W.: Vascular and neural pathology of lumbosacral spinal stenosis. J. Neurosurg. *64*:64–70, 1986.
189. Weinstein, J. N., La Motte, R., Rydevik, B., et al.: Nerve. *In* Frymoyer, J. W., and Gordon, S. L. (eds.): New Perspectives on Low Back Pain. Park Ridge, IL, American Academy of Orthopaedic Surgeons, 1989, pp. 35–130.
190. Weisz, G.: Lumbar spinal canal stenosis in Paget's disease. Spine *8*:192–198, 1983.
191. Weisz, G. W., and Lee, P.: Spinal canal stenosis: concept of spinal reserve capacity: radiologic measurements and clinical applications. Clin. Orthop. *179*:134–140, 1983.
192. Wilson, C. B.: Significant of the small lumbar spinal canal: cauda equina compression syndromes due to spondylosis. Part 3. Intermittent claudication. J. Neurosurg. *31*:499, 1969.
193. Wilson, C. B., Ehni, G., and Grollmus, J.: Neurogenic intermittent claudication. Clin. Neurosurg. *18*:62, 1970.
194. Winston, K., Rumbargh, C., and Colucci, V.: The vertebral canal in lumbar disc disease. Spine *9*:414, 1984.
195. Wolfe, H. J., Putchar, G. J., and Vickery, A. L.: Role of the notochord in human intervertebral disk. I. Fetus and infant. Clin. Orthop. *39*:205–212, 1965.
196. Yamada, H., Nakamura, S., Tajami, M., and Kageyama, N.: Neurological manifestations of pediatric achondroplasia. J. Neurosurg. *54*:49–57, 1981.
197. Yang, K. H., and King, A. I.: Mechanism of facet load transmission as a hypothesis for low back pain. Spine *9*:557–565, 1984.

CLINICAL EVALUATION AND DIFFERENTIAL DIAGNOSIS

Harry N. Herkowitz, M.D.
Hani El-Kommos, M.D.

Since its initial description by Verbiest in 1954,[27] spinal stenosis has become a well-recognized clinical entity. Its symptoms and signs have been confused with those of vascular claudication, and in fact peripheral vascular disease remains the primary clinical disorder in the differential diagnosis.[12] The purpose of this section is to outline the natural history and clinical evaluation of a patient with suspected spinal stenosis. In addition, the differentiating factors in lumbar disc herniations, peripheral vascular disease, and peripheral neuropathy will be highlighted.

NATURAL HISTORY

It is essential to know the natural history of any disorder so that rational decisions can be made on the type and timing of treatment.

Johnsson and colleagues studied three groups of patients with myelographically proved spinal stenosis.[14] Group I (conservative treatment) consisted of 19 patients. Group II contained 30 surgical patients without a complete myelographic extradural block, and Group III 30 surgical patients with total myelographic occlusion of the dural sac. The mean duration of follow-up was 29, 41, and 43 months, respectively. Of patients not operated on there was improvement in eleven (58 per cent), no change in seven (37 per cent), and worsening of symptoms in one. Of patients operated on without a complete myelographic block there was improvement in 19 (63 per cent) and no change in 11 (36 per cent). No patient deteriorated as a result of the surgery. Of the 14 patients with complete block operated on, nine (64 per cent) improved, four (29 per cent) were unchanged, and one was more debilitated than before the surgery.

Diminished walking capacity, a common indication for surgery, was evaluated in the three groups. In the nonoperated patients there was improvement in eight (42 per cent), no change in six (32 per cent), and worsening in five (26 per cent). In the operated group without a complete block, 15 (50 per cent) improved, eight (27 per cent) were unchanged, and seven (23 per cent) were worse. In the operated group with complete myelographic blockage, 11 (79 per cent) were improved and three (32 per cent) had reduced walking capacity.

The authors also compared the postoperative results with the duration of symptoms in the different groups. Although better results were noted in patients with a shorter duration of symptoms (mean of 28 ± 22 months, improved; mean of 38 ± 42 months, not improved), this was not statistically significant.

Thus, it appears from this study that a significant number of patients with spinal stenosis do not demonstrate a progressive deterioration over time.

HISTORY

The age of onset of symptoms is related in part to the type of spinal stenosis. Patients with congenital or developmental stenosis often note symptoms beginning in their early 30s. Whether the patient is of normal stature with a congenitally narrow canal or an achondroplastic dwarf, symptom onset coincides with the development of osteoarthritis in a spinal canal with no reserve space.[15, 20, 23]

Degenerative spinal stenosis is the most common form of spinal stenosis and the type on which this discussion centers. Its onset is in the middle to late 50s or early 60s. Several early series report significantly more males than females, but with the increased recognition of this disorder the ratio appears to favor females over males (3:1 to 5:1).[10, 11, 26] For patients with degenerative spondylolisthesis, females are also affected significantly more often than males, which may be related to hormonal factors leading to ligamentous laxity of the motion segment along with facet joint degeneration.[4, 9]

Although low back pain is commonly associated with spinal stenosis, this symptom usually is not the reason for referral to the orthopedic surgeon. The quality of back pain is that of osteoarthritis, i.e., ache and stiffness, often worse in inclement weather.[1] In addition, the back pain usually is of insidious onset rather than an acute "jolt." Patients rarely have a "sciatic list" or significant back spasm, as seen with a herniated disc. The back pain is mechanical in that activity aggravates it while rest relieves the discomfort. Radiation of pain to the coccyx or buttocks is typical.[13] A clue that the low back pain is associated with spinal stenosis is noted in its early stages with progressive buttock discomfort, tightness, or burning brought about by walking or standing. The patient also may complain of walking bent over because the buttock or low back pain is lessened by this maneuver. Complaints of limited spine movement are common but much fewer than in patients with a lumbar disc herniation. Most patients complain of limitations in extension of the spine such as in reaching up to get something out of a cabinet rather than in forward bending.[22, 29] Often the extension leads to "jolts of lightning" down the buttocks or legs. Patients with degenerative spondylolisthesis tend to have quantitatively and qualitatively more back pain than those with stenosis secondary to lumbar osteoarthritis alone.[2]

Referral to the orthopedic surgeon is prompted by complaints of pain in the leg(s). These can be grouped into two types. Type I is described as typical sciatica. This usually involves one extremity with aching or sharp pain following a specific dermatomal distribution. Reflex changes or motor weakness may occur. The fifth lumbar nerve root is the one most commonly involved, producing weakness in the extensor hallucis longus or tibialis anterior.

Neurogenic claudication or pseudoclaudication is the more common form of leg pain associated with spinal stenosis (Type II). Complaints of pain, numbness, tingling, weakness, cramping, or burning in one lower extremity, or more commonly both, are the typical words used to describe the symptoms.[8, 16] Classically the pain begins in the low back or buttocks and radiates into the legs without following a specific dermatomal distribution. The symptoms may stop at the knee, but as activity increases or the condition progresses, they radiate to the foot.[21] Typically, walking or standing precipitates symptoms, whereas sitting and leaning forward or lying down alleviates the discomfort.[17] A sudden worsening of symptoms or progression of neurologic findings may indicate disc herniation associated with the spinal stenosis.

Claudication due to vascular disease may be confused with that related to spinal stenosis.[6] Patients with peripheral vascular disease usually complain of cramping or tightness in the calves, with symptoms beginning distally and progressing proximally, which is the opposite of the situation in spinal stenosis. In addition, patients with vascular claudication obtain relief by standing, while those with neuroclaudication note persistent pain with standing and improvement by sitting forward.[7] The claudication of vascular disease usually occurs with a constant distance, while patients with spinal stenosis usually note a variable distance before symptoms occur (Table 25–1).

Peripheral neuropathy is another condition that may be confused with neuroclaudication. In an elderly population, diabetes is often present in patients with suspected spinal stenosis. Burning or hypersensitivity beginning in the feet and progressing proximally is typical.[25] Usually the pain is worse at night and has no relation to activity. Patients may also complain of being unable to feel their feet owing to posterior column involvement. In severe cases, weakness may occur in one lower extremity or both. A "stocking glove" distribution of discomfort below the knees unrelated to activity is the hallmark of neuropathy. This can be confirmed by prolonged nerve conduction velocities.

Table 25–1. COMPARISON OF VASCULAR WITH NEUROGENIC CLAUDICATION

Evaluation	Vascular	Neurogenic
Claudication distance	Fixed	Variable
Relief of pain	Standing	Sitting—flexed
Walk uphill	Pain	No pain
Bicycle ride	Pain	No pain
Type of pain	Cramp, tightness	Numbness, ache, sharp
Pulses	Absent	Present
Bruit	Present	Absent
Skin	Loss of hair Shiny	Normal
Atrophy	Rarely	Occasional
Weakness	Rarely	Occasional
Back pain	Uncommon	Common
Limitations of spine movement	Uncommon	Common

Urinary dysfunction is uncommon in patients with stenosis, occurring in 3 to 4 per cent of cases.[19] Because of the advanced age of individuals it is not uncommon to have bladder abnormalities unrelated to stenosis. Bladder complaints related to the spinal stenosis are usually those of incontinence.

PHYSICAL EXAMINATION

Palpation of the lower back usually does not produce severe tenderness. Patients usually complain of discomfort "deep down" within the muscles. Occasionally, point tenderness may be elicited over the sacroiliac joint(s) and in the sciatic notch area. In performing range of motion maneuvers patients often can forward flex without difficulty, but extension is significantly limited. Brieg showed in cadaver studies that when the spine moves from flexion to extension, the following occurs: (1) the spinal canal is shortened by 2.2 mm, (2) nervous tissue shortens and becomes broader, (3) the ligamentum flavum shortens and broadens, (4) posterior protrusion of the disc occurs, and (5) there is interference with the microcirculation of the nerve roots and cauda equina.[3] All these factors may contribute to the precipitation of buttock and leg pain when extension of the spine is attempted.

The straight leg raising (SLR) test is usually negative in spinal stenosis. It is more likely to be positive in cases with an associated disc herniation.

Strength testing more often than not reveals minimal or no loss of function.[17] Because L4–L5 is the level most commonly involved, the usual neurologic findings are mild extensor hallucis longus or tibialis anterior weakness. At the time of examination the neurologic evaluation may be normal.[18] In view of the pathogenesis and pathophysiology of spinal stenosis, exercise may induce the muscular weakness or a loss of a reflex. In the office setting patients are asked to walk the hallway or climb stairs, and then are reexamined when the history is suggestive of stenosis without there being objective clinical findings.[24] Atrophy may be seen in the thighs or calves in patients with long-standing neural compression. Patients with lateral recess stenosis tend to have weakness or atrophy more often than those with central stenosis only.[5] The fifth lumbar nerve root is also the most common spinal level involved in lateral recess stenosis.

Reflex testing is often unreliable, since loss of a reflex is common in the elderly population. Sensory deficits also are uncommon, but when present are seen most often in the L5 or S1 dermatome. Diffuse sensory loss is more indicative of peripheral neuropathy.

Since spinal stenosis may present with a paucity of physical findings, the clinician may be confused initially as to the cause of the patient's complaints. Confirmation of the diagnosis requires imaging studies, which will be discussed in the next section.

References

1. Blau, J. N., and Logue, V.: Intermittent claudication of the cauda equina. Lancet *1*:1081–1086, 1961.
2. Bolestra, M., and Bohlman, H.: Degenerative spondylolisthesis. Instr. Course Lect. 10:157–169, 1989.
3. Brieg, A.: Biomechanics of the Central Nervous System. Stockholm, Almquist & Wiksell, 1960.
4. Cauchoix, J., Benoist, M., and Chassaing, V.: Degenerative spondylolisthesis. Clin. Orthop. *115*:122–129, 1976.
5. Ciric, I., Mikhael, M., Tarkington, J., and Vick, N.: The lateral recess syndrome. J. Neurosurg. *53*:433–443, 1980.
6. Dodge, L., Bohlman, H., and Rhodes, R.: Concurrent lumbar spinal stenosis and peripheral vascular disease. Clin. Orthop. *230*:141–148, 1988.
7. Dyke, P., and Doyle, J.: "Bicycle test" of Van Gelderen in diagnosis of intermittent cauda equina compression. J. Neurosurg. *46*:667–670, 1977.
8. Evans, J.: Neurogenic intermittent claudication. Br. Med. J. *2*:985–987, 1964.
9. Fitzgerald, J. A. W., and Newman, P. H.: Degenerative spondylolisthesis. J. Bone Joint Surg. *58B*:184, 1976.
10. Grabias, S.: Current concepts review. The treatment of spinal stenosis. J. Bone Joint Surg. *62A*:308–313, 1980.
11. Hall, S., Bartleson, J., Onfrio, B., et al.: Lumbar spinal stenosis. Clinical features, diagnostic procedures and results of surgical treatment in 68 patients. Ann. Intern. Med. *103*:271–275, 1985.
12. Hawkes, C., and Roberts, G.: Neurogenic and vascular claudication. J. Neurol. Sci. *38*:337–345, 1978.
13. Joffe, R., Appleby, A., and Arjona, V.: Intermittent ischemia of the cauda equina due to stenosis of the lumbar canal. J. Neurol. Neurosurg. Psychiatry *29*:315–318, 1966.
14. Johnsson, K., Uden, A., and Rosen, I.: The effect of decompression on the natural course of spinal stenosis. Unpublished.
15. Jones, R., and Thomson, J.: The narrow lumbar canal. J. Bone Joint Surg. *50B*:595–605, 1968.
16. Kirkaldy-Willis, W. H., Paine, K. W. E., Cauchoix, J., and McIvor, G.: Lumbar spinal stenosis. Clin. Orthop. *99*:30–50, 1974.
17. Lipson, S.: Clinical diagnosis of spinal stenosis. Semin. Spine Surg. *1*:143–144, 1989.

18. McNab, I.: Spondylolisthesis with an intact neural arch—the so-called pseudospondylolisthesis. J. Bone Joint Surg. *32B*:325, 1950.
19. Nelson, M. A.: Lumbar spinal stenosis. J. Bone Joint Surg. *55B*:506–512, 1973.
20. Newman, P. H.: Stenosis of the lumbar spine in spondylolisthesis. Clin. Orthop. *115*:116–121, 1976.
21. Paine, K.: Results of decompression for lumbar spinal stenosis. Clin. Orthop. *115*:96–100, 1976.
22. Rosenberg, N. J.: Degenerative spondylolisthesis. J. Bone Joint Surg. *57A*:467–474, 1975.
23. Schatzker, J., and Pennal, G.: Spinal stenosis, a cause of cauda equina compression. J. Bone Joint Surg. *50B*:606–618, 1968.
24. Spengler, D. M.: Current concepts review—degenerative stenosis of the lumbar spine. J. Bone Joint Surg. *69A*:305, 1987.
25. Thomas, P. K.: Clinical features and differential diagnosis. *In* Dyck, P. J., Thomas, P. K., Lambert, E. H. and Bunge, R. (eds.): Peripheral Neuropathy. 2nd ed. Philadelphia, W. B. Saunders Co., 1984, pp. 1169–1190.
26. Tile, M., McNeil, S. R., Zarins, R. Z., et al.: Spinal stenosis: results of treatment. Clin. Orthop. *115*:104–108, 1976.
27. Verbiest, H.: A radicular syndrome from developmental narrowing of the lumbar vertebral canal. J. Bone Joint Surg. *36B*:230–237, 1954.
28. Wilson, C.: Significance of the small lumbar spinal canal: cauda equina compression syndromes due to spondylosis. J. Neurosurg. *31*:499–506, 1969.
29. Wiltse, L. L., Kirkaldy-Willis, W. H., and McIvor, G. W. D.: The treatment of spinal stenosis. Clin. Orthop. *115*:83–91, 1976.

RADIOLOGIC AND ELECTRODIAGNOSTIC EVALUATION

Harry N. Herkowitz, M.D.

The confirmation of a clinical diagnosis of spinal stenosis is made by radiographic studies that include plain x-ray, computed tomography (CT), myelography, and magnetic resonance imaging (MRI). In addition, electrodiagnostic studies of the lower extremities consisting of electromyography (EMG), nerve conduction velocity, and somatosensory evoked potentials are often useful as an adjunct to the imaging studies in establishing the diagnosis.

ANATOMY

Before discussing the radiology of spinal stenosis, it is important to define several anatomic areas of the vertebral segment. The spinal canal is the area formed anteriorly by the back of the vertebral body, disc, and posterior longitudinal ligament. The posterior border consists of the lamina, pars interarticularis, and facet joints (Fig. 25–43). Its shape may be circular, oval, or trefoil (Fig. 25–44).[21] Normally, 15 per cent of the lumbar spinal canals are trefoil in shape, predisposing these individuals to lateral recess stenosis.[96]

The second anatomic region is the lateral recess or nerve root canal. It is bordered laterally by the pedicle, posteriorly by the superior articular facet, and anteriorly by the posterolateral surface of the vertebral body and adjacent disc (Fig. 25–45).[16] The narrowest portion of the lateral recess is at the superior border of the corresponding pedicle, because the horizontal portion of the superior articular facet lies at the superior border of the pedicle.[64]

The final anatomic area to define is the intervertebral foramen, which is shaped like an inverted teardrop. Its superior border is formed by the posterior wall of the vertebral body above; the inferior border by the posterior wall of the vertebrae below; and the posterior border by the pars interarticularis, the ligamentum flavum, and the apex of the superior articular facet of the inferior vertebrae.[28]

The clinical syndrome of spinal stenosis may involve only the central canal (central canal stenosis) or the nerve root canal or foramen (lateral recess spinal stenosis).[34, 35, 38, 40, 43, 55, 59, 83, 84, 89, 98, 125] In addition, both may occur at the same level or independently at different levels in the same patient.[3, 7, 10, 12, 13, 103–105, 107, 114, 115, 118]

Lee and associates classified the nerve root canal into three zones to clarify the anatomy and to describe the pathologic structures responsible for nerve root compression within the three zones (Fig. 25–46).[70] The entrance zone is the superior most portion of the nerve

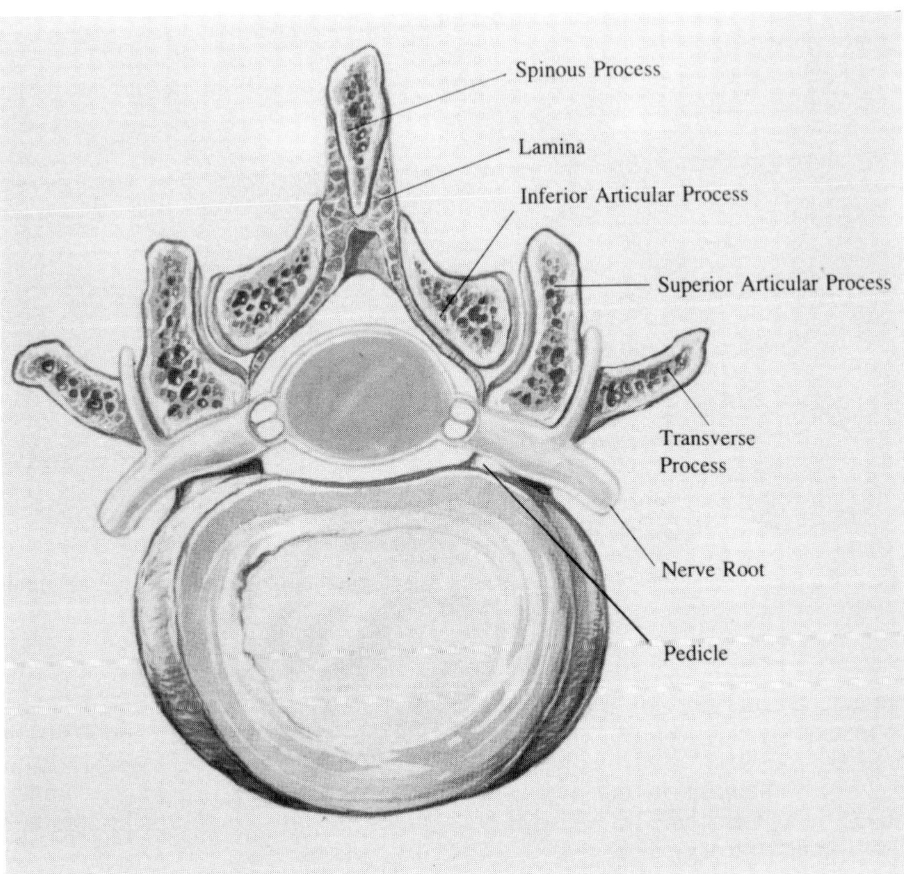

Figure 25–43. Anterior, posterior, medial, and lateral borders of spinal canal. Anterior: back of the vertebral body; posterior: lamina; medial and lateral: facet joints and pedicles.

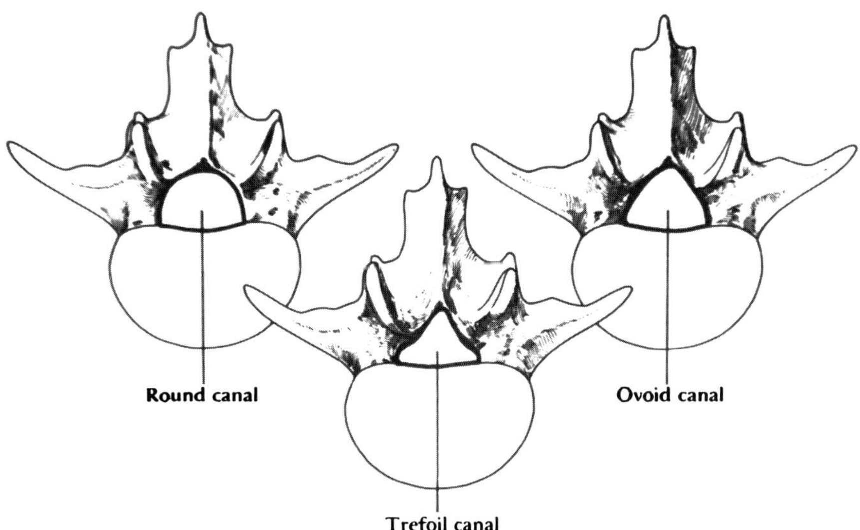

Figure 25–44. Various configurations of the spinal canal.

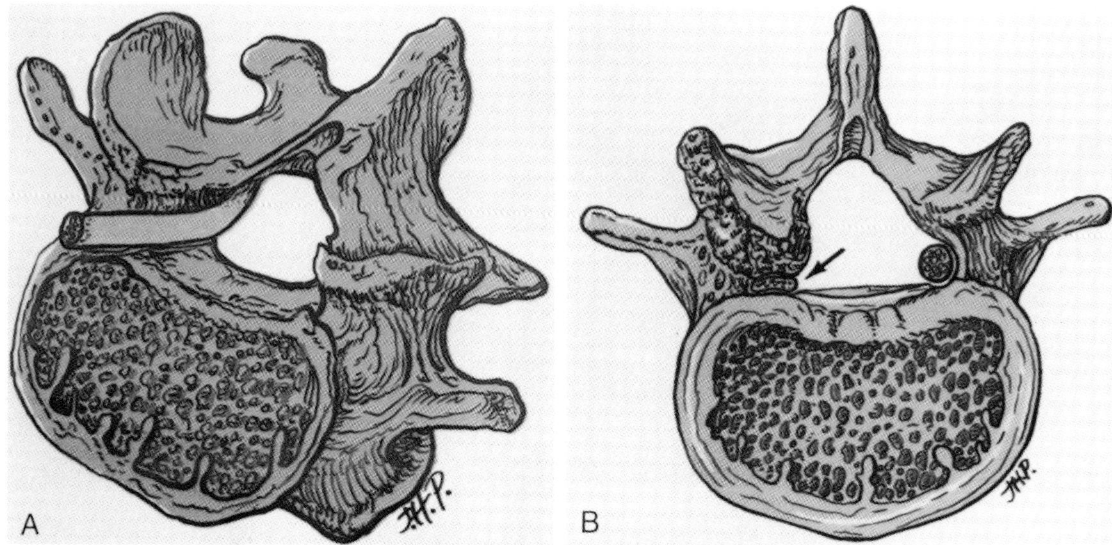

Figure 25–45. *A,* The nerve root canal with its boundaries. *B,* Entrapment of the nerve root by the superior articular facet on the right.

canal containing the nerve root, with the anterior wall formed by the posterior surface of the disc and the posterior wall by the facet joint (Fig. 25–47). Stenosis in this region is usually caused by hypertrophic osteophytes of the superior articular facet (Fig. 25–48).

The middle zone boundaries are (1) anterior border: posterior vertebral body; (2) posterior border: pars interarticularis; and (3) medial border: open. The contents of this zone are the dorsal root ganglion and ventral root (Fig. 25–49). Middle zone stenosis is most commonly caused by osteophytes under the pars interarticularis, or fibrocartilage build-up under a spondylotic defect (Fig. 25–50).

The exit zone is formed by the intervertebral foramen whose borders are, posteriorly, the lateral aspect of the facet joint below the facet

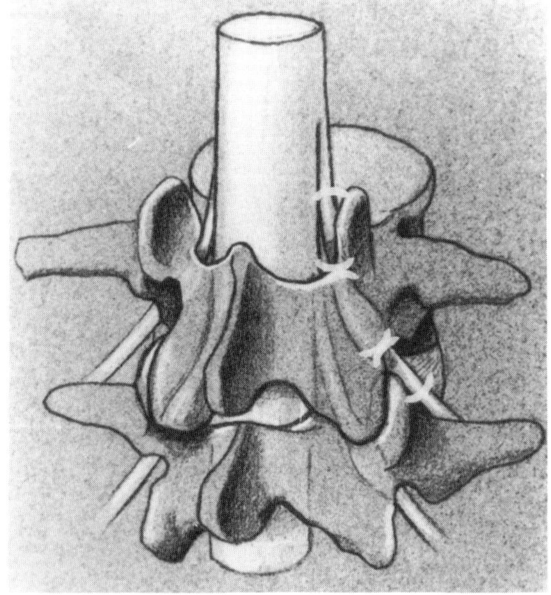

Figure 25–46. Three zones of the lateral spinal canal of the lumbar spine. The entrance zone is the upper circle, the middle zone is represented by the middle circle, and the exit zone is the end circle.

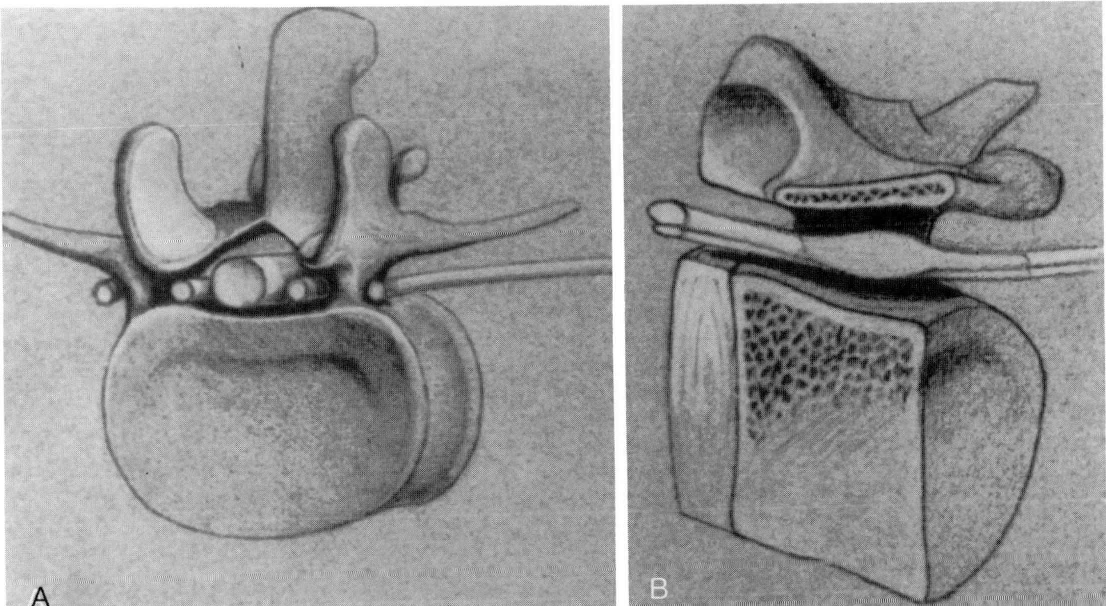

Figure 25–47. *A,* Axial and *B,* parasagittal views of the entrance zone of the lateral recess. The axial view shows the disc or vertebral end plate, superior margin of the lamina, and facet joint. The nerve root is shown end on *(A)* and longitudinally on sagittal section *(B).*

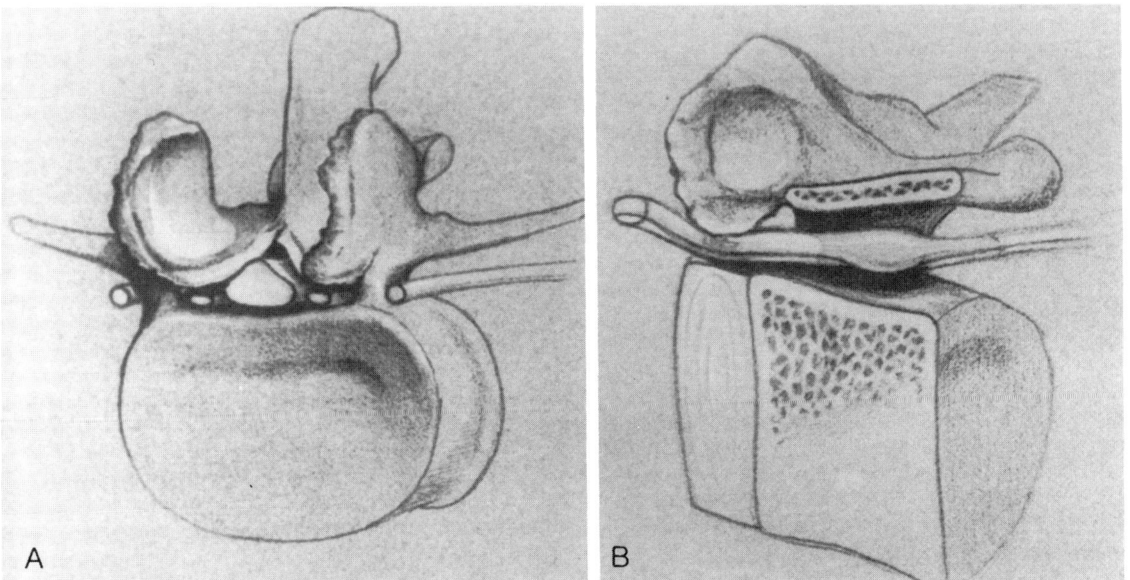

Figure 25–48. Nerve root entrapped by hypertrophic facet and thickened ligamentum flavum demonstrated on axial *(A)* and parasagittal *(B)* views.

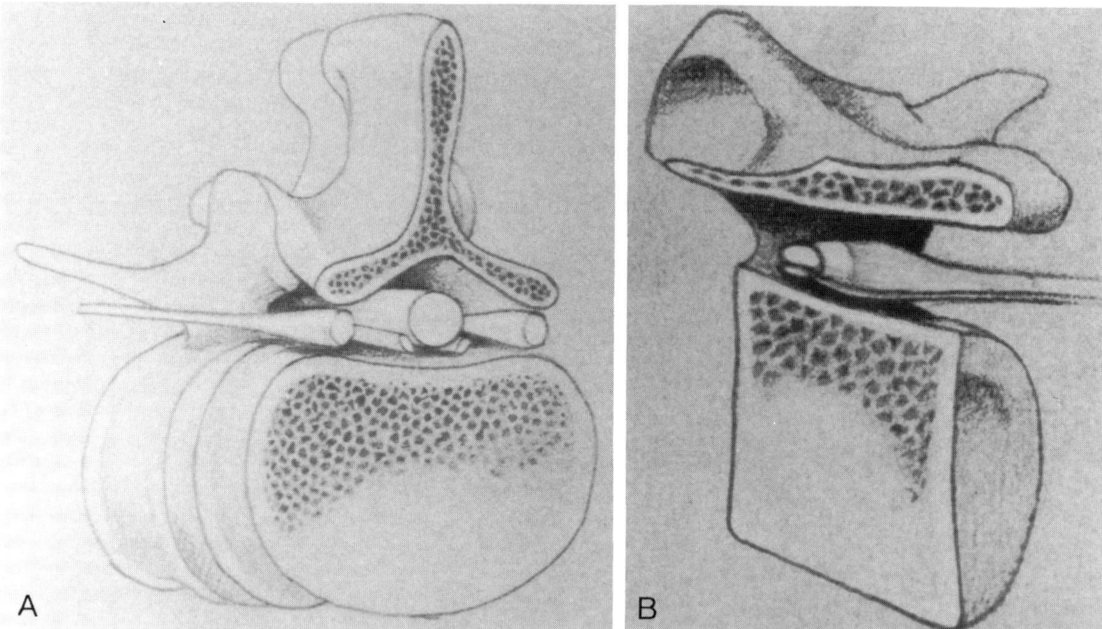

Figure 25–49. Midzone region on axial *(A)* and parasagittal *(B)* views. *A* shows cut surfaces of the spinous process, pars interarticularis, and vertebral body. The ventral nerve root and dorsal root ganglion are also showing at the cut surface.

of the entrance zone, and anteriorly, the disc that is one segment below the disc of the entrance zone. The neural contents of this zone consist of the peripheral nerve (Fig. 25–51). Exit zone stenosis is caused by hypertrophic facets with subluxation (Fig. 25–52). This descriptive anatomy lends itself to a better understanding of the nerve root canal and the pathologic conditions causing compression of the nerve within the three zones. It also facilitates a better understanding of the diagnostic studies necessary to detect neural compression and the surgical techniques required to alleviate the compression.

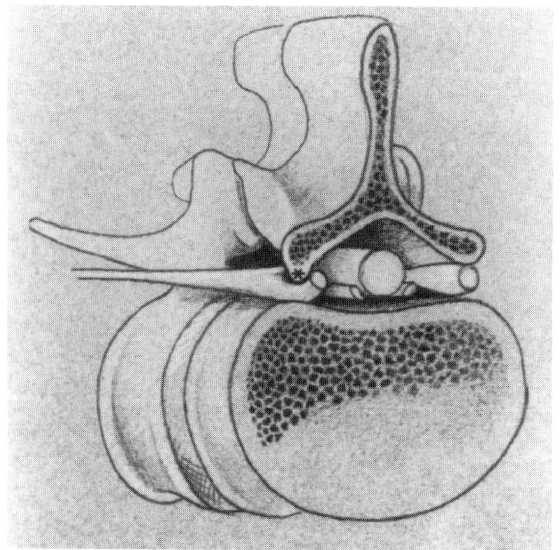

Figure 25–50. Axial view of midzone stenosis. The localized bony hypertrophy or ridge (*) under the lamina where the ligamentum flavum attaches may cause entrapment of the dorsal root ganglion.

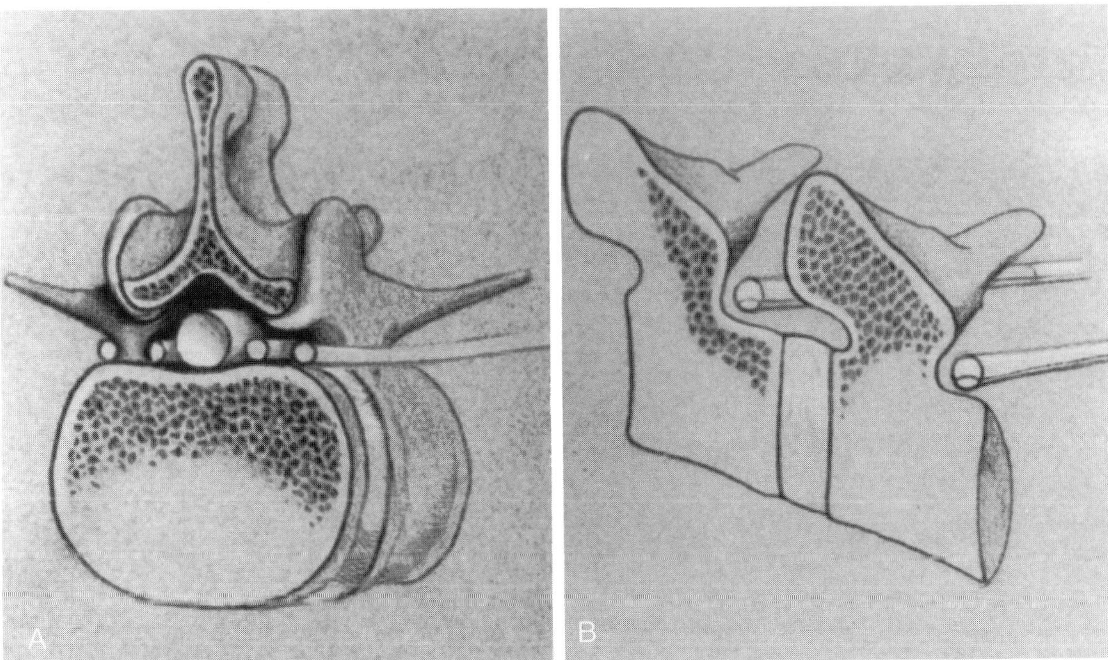

Figure 25–51. *A,* Axial and *B,* parasagittal views of the exit zone. The cut surface shows the spinous process, lamina, and inferior facet posteriorly and the vertebral body or inferior end plate anteriorly. An exiting nerve is shown along with a nerve root medially.

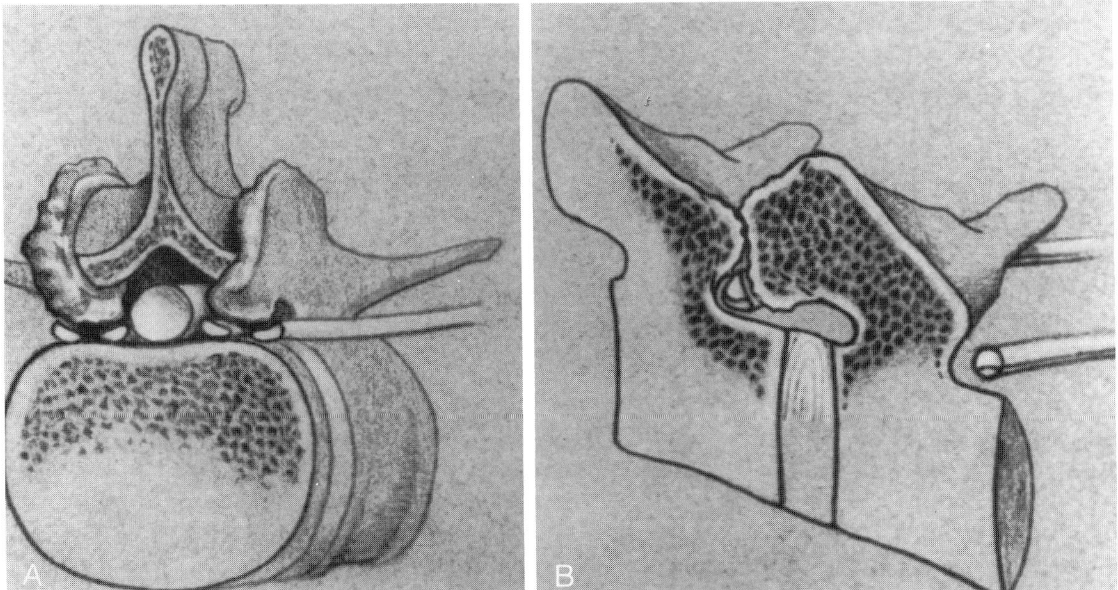

Figure 25–52. *A,* Axial and *B,* parasagittal views of exit zone stenosis. Hypertrophic arthritis of the superior articular facet can entrap the spinal nerve at its exit from the spinal column.

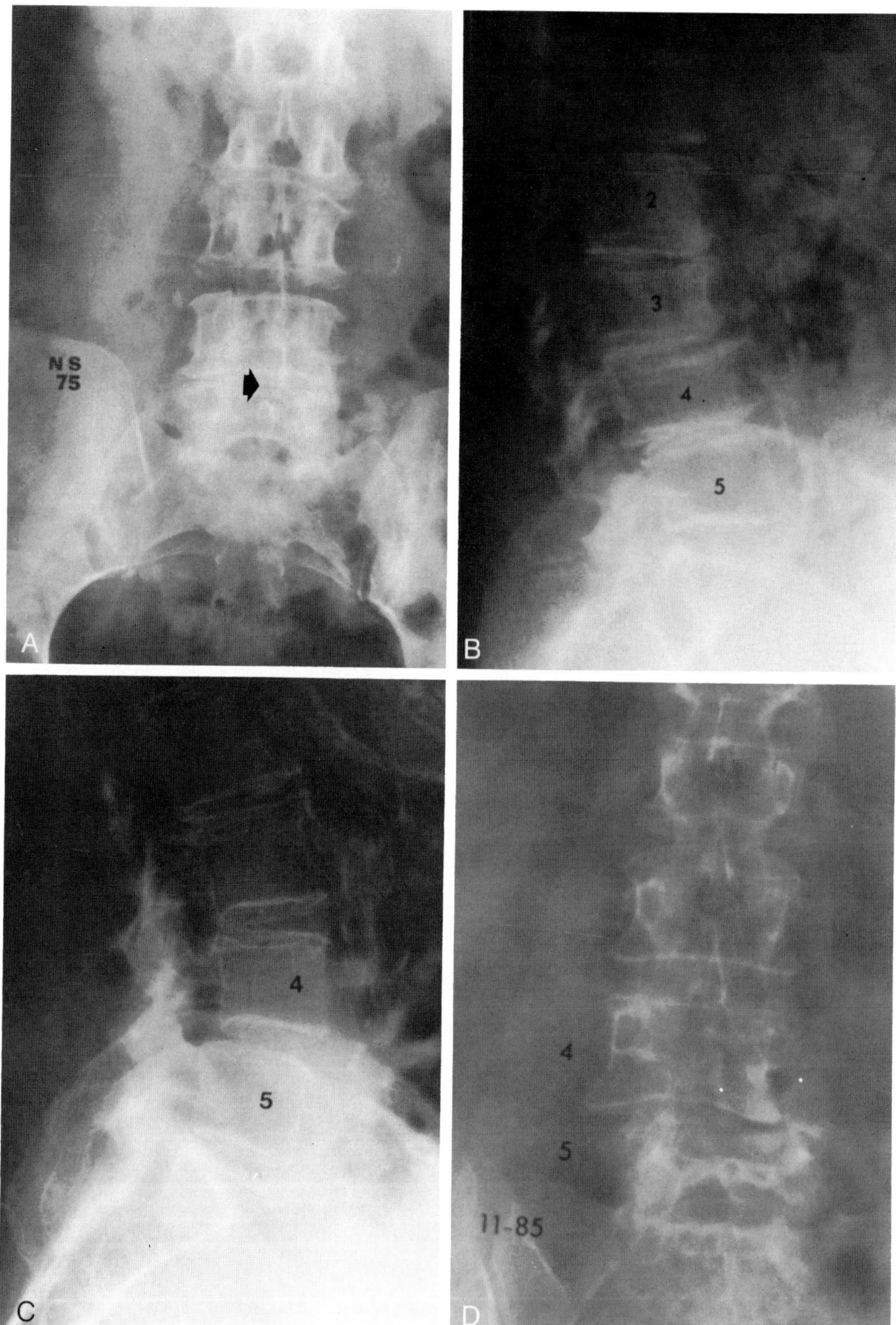

Figure 25–53. *A*, Anteroposterior radiograph demonstrating multiple-level spondylosis with facet arthritis and spinous process settling at L4–L5 *(arrow)*. *B*, Lateral view of multiple-level disc degeneration, spondylosis, and loss of lumbar lordosis. *C*, Lateral view of degenerative spondylolisthesis at L4–L5. *D*, Anteroposterior view of lateral spondylolisthesis at L4–L5.

RADIOLOGY

Plain X-ray

Plain x-ray evaluation includes anteroposterior, lateral, right and left oblique, standing, and flexion-extension lateral views. The plain film abnormalities include disc space narrowing due to degeneration of the disc, inferior or superior facet osteoarthritis, spondylosis, degenerative scoliosis, spondylolisthesis, spinous process settling ("kissing spines"), and finally narrowing of the interpedicular distance in cases of congenital spinal stenosis. These abnormalities may be present singly or in combination (Fig. 25–53).[19, 57, 63, 110, 120]

Standing films are helpful in patients presenting with scoliosis or spondylolisthesis. Lowe and colleagues demonstrated an increase in the amount of displacement in 26 per cent of 50 patients with spondylolisthesis.[71] Flexion-extension x-rays in the lateral position may be performed in the standing or lying position to demonstrate motion occurring at a potentially unstable segment. This motion may be horizontal or angular (Figs. 25–54 and 25–55). Bending x-rays may also be performed in the anteroposterior projection (left and right bending) to determine the flexibility of a scoliotic curve.

It is important to remember that "abnormalities" present on a plain x-ray film should not necessarily be construed as responsible for the patient's complaints.[128] Frymower and associates showed that there is no statistical difference between symptomatic and asymptomatic individuals when their plain films are compared.[37]

The dimensions of the spinal canal have previously been measured on x-ray and by actual anatomic specimen, both in vitro and in vivo.[58, 90, 91] Verbiest was the first to apply numbers to the diameter of the canal, using a special caliper intraoperatively. He divided the measurements of the midsagittal canal into three groups: (1) pure absolute stenosis that measured 10 mm or less, (2) pure relative stenosis measuring between 10 and 12 mm, and (3) mixed stenosis that was a combined form of absolute and relative stenosis.[113]

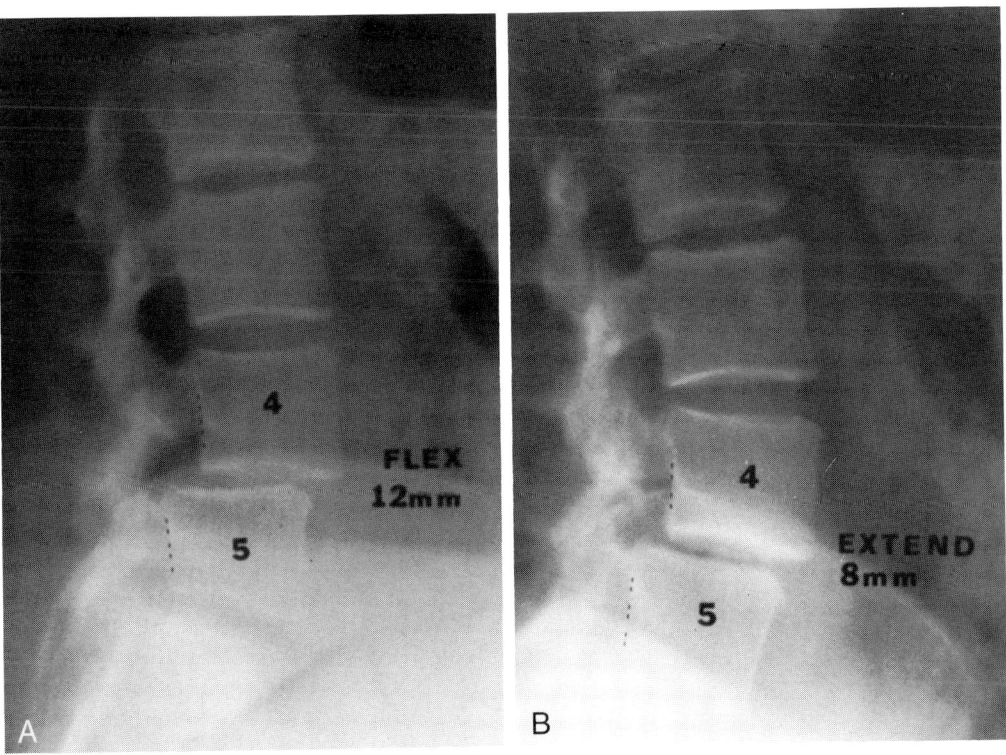

Figure 25–54. Standing lateral radiographs demonstrating excessive translational motion in flexion *(A)* and extension *(B)*.

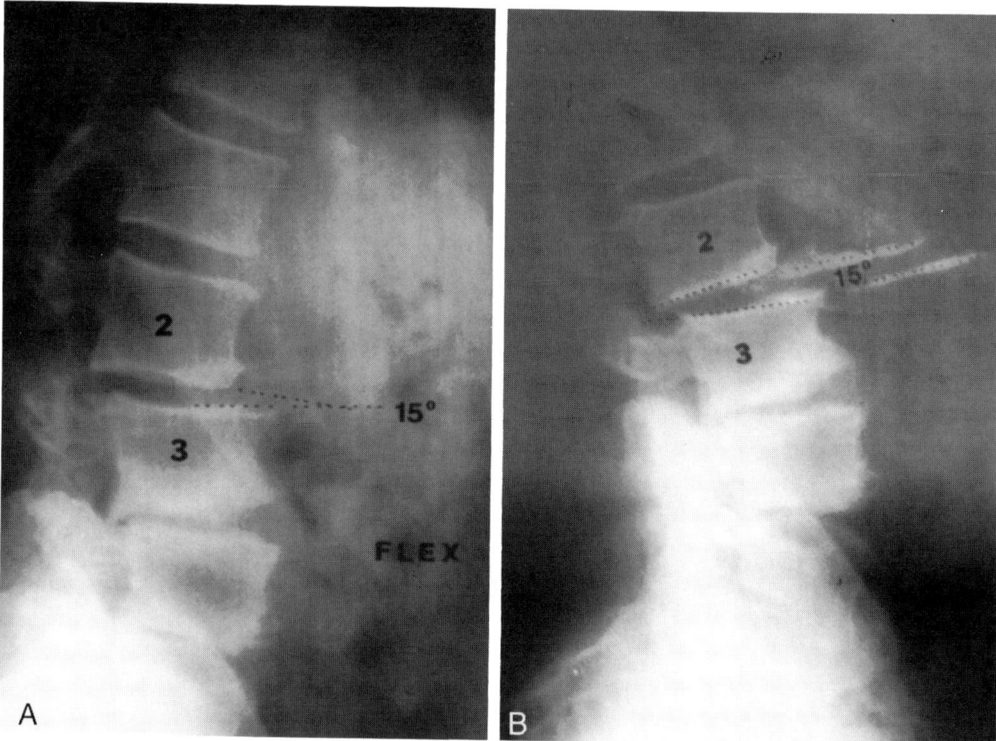

Figure 25–55. Lateral radiographs demonstrating excessive angular motion in flexion *(A)* and extension *(B)* at L2–L3.

Eisenstein described both the radiologic and actual bony measurements of over 1000 lumbar vertebrae in 433 adult black and white skeletons. He found that the overall limit of the midsagittal diameter was 15 mm and the transverse diameter 20 mm on radiographs. The skeletal (actual) dimensions were 18 mm as the lower limit of normal for the interpedicular (transverse) distance and 13 mm for the midsagittal distance. The greatest narrowing was found at L2–L4.[27–29]

Winston and colleagues reviewed the dimensions of the spinal canal in 29 patients undergoing decompressive lumbar laminectomy compared with a matched control group of 30 individuals.[127] Although they found that the sagittal canal diameter in the operated group was significantly smaller than that in the control group, they concluded that a small canal by itself does not establish the diagnosis in symptomatic patients and does not have any predictive value in asymptomatic patients.

In the normal skeleton, the interpedicular distance gradually widens in the lumbar canal from L1 to L5 (Fig. 25–56).[124] In degenerative spinal stenosis the interpedicular distance is not affected, but in developmental spinal stenosis, such as exhibited by achondroplastic dwarfs, the interpedicular distance narrows as one proceeds distally down the lumbar canal.[17, 25, 26] This is due to the short, thick pedicles and small laminae in the achondroplast (Fig. 25–57).[1, 117]

The shape of the canal may have a significant effect on the production of symptoms in spinal stenosis. A round spinal canal with an anteroposterior dimension of 10 mm may not produce symptoms, whereas a trefoil canal with a dimension of 15 mm may show significant symptoms. This is because flattening of the lateral recesses is more likely to occur in the trefoil canal than in the round or oval canal (see Fig. 25–44).[33, 96]

The lateral recess measurements have been well delineated by CT scanning using the bone window setting. Absolute stenosis occurs with narrowing of 3 mm or less and relative stenosis with narrowing of 3 to 5 mm.[16]

Kirkaldy-Willis and colleagues emphasized two important points regarding the interpre-

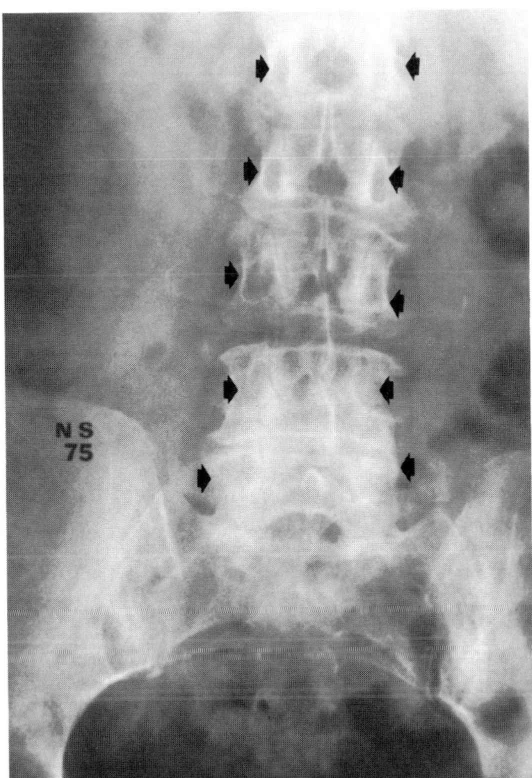

Figure 25–56. Anteroposterior radiograph demonstrating widening of the pedicles distally in the lumbar spine *(arrows).*

tation of lateral recess abnormalities.[62–65] First, the lumbar nerve at the affected joint passes laterally below the pedicle of the upper vertebrae. This is where the measurement must be taken. Narrowing below is not significant because the nerve root is not present there. Second, superior articular facet osteophytes entrap the root exiting one joint below; e.g., hypertrophy of the first sacral superior articular facet entraps the first sacral nerve root exiting below.

Until recently the concept of spinal stenosis has been based only on the bony measurement of the canal. Weisz and Lee outlined the concept of spinal reserve capacity in describing central spinal stenosis that takes into account both the bony and the soft tissue contents (dural sac, ligamentum flavum, and surrounding fat) within the spinal canal. The capacity is measured by the difference between the sagittal diameter of the canal (C1) and the sagittal diameter of the dural sac and the surrounding soft tissue (C2).[121]

Bolender and associates reviewed the value of CT and myelography in the diagnosis of central lumbar stenosis.[9] They concluded that the dimensions of the bony canal as seen on CT provided an accurate diagnosis in only 20 per cent of cases. Measuring the effect of soft tissue compression on the dimensions of the dural sac by computing the cross-sectional area of the dural sac on the CT scan (100 mm, absolute stenosis; 100 to 130 mm, relative stenosis; above 130 mm, normal) or measuring the anteroposterior diameter of the dural sac on myelography (stenosis less than 13 mm) increased the diagnostic accuracy to 83 per cent.

Degenerative spondylolisthesis is a common radiographic finding in spinal stenosis (Fig. 25–58). It occurs four times more often in females than in males, three times more often in blacks than in whites, and six to nine times more often at the L4–L5 interspace. It rarely occurs before the fifth decade and forward displacement does not exceed 30 per cent.[95] The patho-

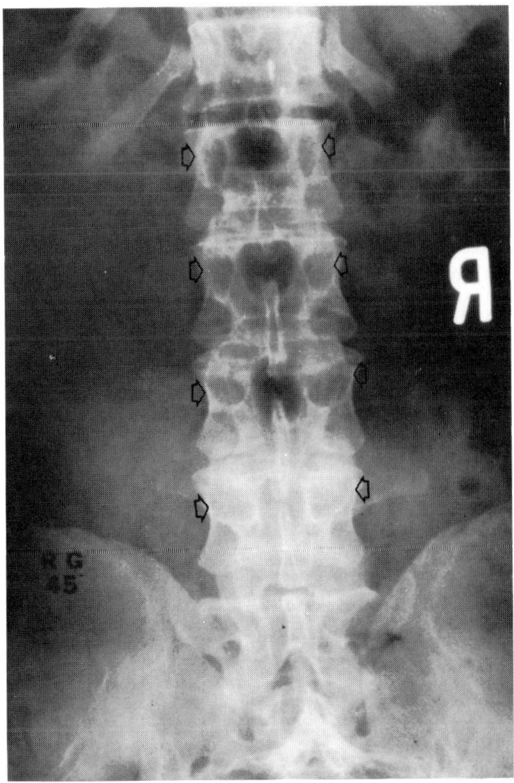

Figure 25–57. Anteroposterior radiograph of an achondroplastic dwarf demonstrating the gradual narrowing of the pedicles distally in the lumbar spine *(arrows).*

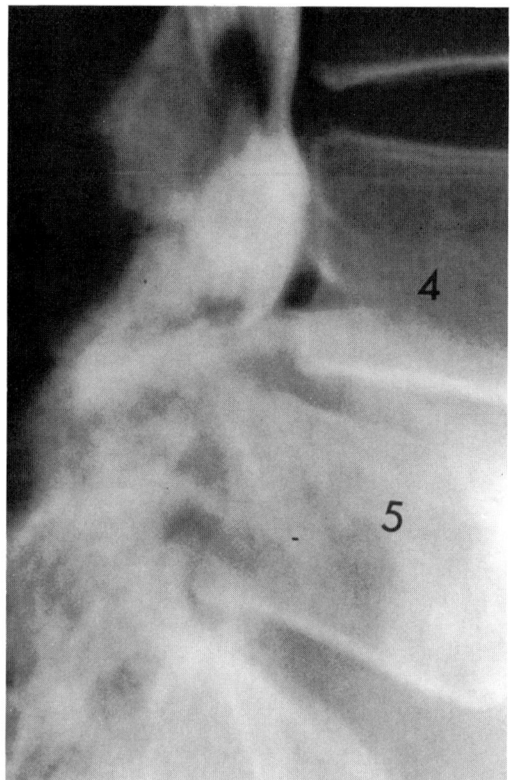

Figure 25–58. Lateral myelogram of a patient with spinal stenosis secondary to degenerative spondylolisthesis at L4–L5 demonstrating complete block.

genesis is related to osteoarthritis of the facet joints.[73] Most patients have a reduction in the lumbar lordosis, thus increasing the lumbosacral angle and causing increased stress at the L4–L5 facet joints. In addition, the configuration of the lumbosacral facet joints and the stabilizing effect of the iliolumbar ligament predispose the L4–L5 level to slippage.[15] The most common symptoms are back pain and neurogenic claudication or radiculopathy. The amount of slippage does not correlate with the symptoms.

Surgery is required in approximately 10 per cent of patients with symptomatic degenerative spondylolisthesis.[32, 60, 67, 74, 87, 97, 116, 126]

Instability

Perhaps the most controversial area in radiographic diagnosis is the definition of instability. In the broadest sense, instability is defined as the loss of ability of the spine under physiologic loads to maintain relationships between vertebrae in such a way that there is neither initial damage nor subsequent irritation to the spinal cord or nerve roots, and also no development of incapacitating deformity or pain due to structural changes.[122]

Table 25–2. Checklist for the Diagnosis of Clinical Instability in the Lumbar (L1–L5) Spine

Element	Point Value*
Cauda equina damage	3
Relative flexion sagittal plane translation >8% or extension sagittal plane translation >9%	2
Relative flexion sagittal plane rotation <−9°	2
Anterior elements destroyed	2
Posterior elements destroyed	2
Dangerous loading anticipated	1

*Total of 5 or more = clinically unstable.

From Posner, I., White, A. A., III, Edwards, W. T., and Hayes, W. C.: A biomechanical analysis of the clinical stability of the lumbar and lumbosacral spine. Spine 7:386, 1982.

Using cadaveric lumbar spines, Posner and colleagues developed a checklist for instability of the lumbar and lumbosacral spine (Tables 25–2 and 25–3). This assigns points to horizontal and angular displacement, nerve damage, and destruction of the anterior or posterior elements. A score greater than 5 indicates clinical instability.[92] Although this scale provides an excellent guideline for the diagnosis of instability, it does not correlate symptoms with instability. The first article to relate clinical symptoms to the amount of motion was by Friberg.[36] Instead of flexion-extension x-rays, traction-compression films are used. The patient hangs from a trapeze for the traction film and stands with a weighted knapsack for the compression film. The upper vertebrae

Table 25–3. Extreme Test Values to Define Clinical Thresholds of Stability

	Flexion		
	Lumbar (L1–L5)	*Lumbosacral (L5–S1)*	Extension (L1–S1)
Z^C (maximum)	2.3 mm	1.6 mm	2.8 mm
Z^C% (maximum)	8%	6%	9%
Θc (minimum)	−9°	1°	*

*No test value is given for Θ with extension forces since there was no significant difference between intact and maximal displacements when the FSUs were physiologically loaded with preload and extension forces.

From Posner, I., White, A. A., III, Edwards, W. T., and Hayes, W. C.: A biomechanical analysis of the clinical stability of the lumbar and lumbosacral spine. Spine 7:386, 1982.

move posteriorly during traction and anteriorly during compression. Friberg determined that symptoms are not necessarily related to the amount of forward or backward motion, but rather to the total amount of forward and backward motion combined (Fig. 25–59).

Myelography

Myelography has been the "gold standard" study for the confirmatory diagnosis of spinal stenosis.[6] In evaluating a diagnostic tool for accuracy, both the sensitivity and specificity of the test must be evaluated. Sensitivity is defined as the ability of a test to detect a disease when it is present; specificity refers to the ability of a test to remain normal when no disease is present. The corollary of each, respectively, is represented as false negativity and false positivity. Bell and associates, reporting on 122 surgically confirmed cases of lumbar disc herniation and spinal stenosis, compared the accuracy of myelography to that of CT. Myelography was found to be more accurate than CT for the diagnosis of lumbar disc herniation: 83 versus 72 per cent, respectively.[6] For the diagnosis of spinal stenosis, myelography was also found to be more accurate than CT: 93 versus 89 per cent, respectively.

The myelographic dye in clinical use today is a second-generation water-soluble agent. The two available agents are iohexol (Omnipaque) and iopamidol (Isovue). The advantages of these are a significant reduction in the side effects of headache, nausea, and seizure activity compared with the first-generation myelographic dye. A review of 300 patients who had undergone myelography with iohexol revealed headache in 11 per cent of patients and nausea in 6 per cent. No seizures or mental aberrations were noted.[129] This represents a three- to fivefold reduction in side effects com-

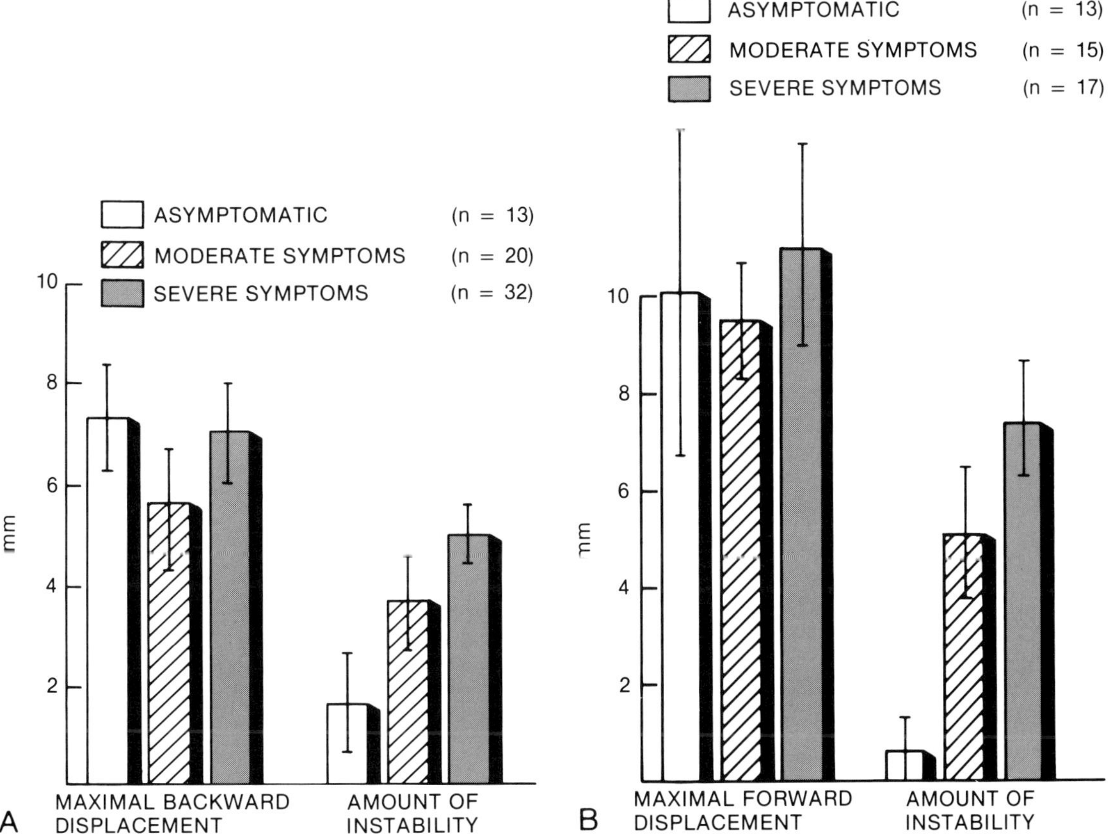

Figure 25–59. Schematics demonstrating no significant difference in low back symptoms with maximal forward *(A)* and backward *(B)* displacement. Symptoms are related to the total amount of forward and backward motion.

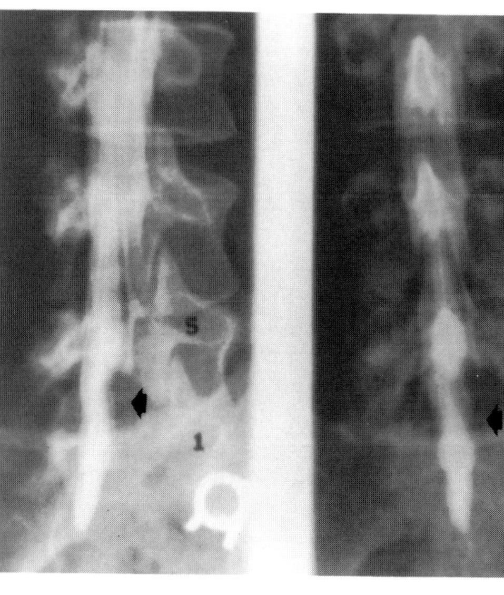

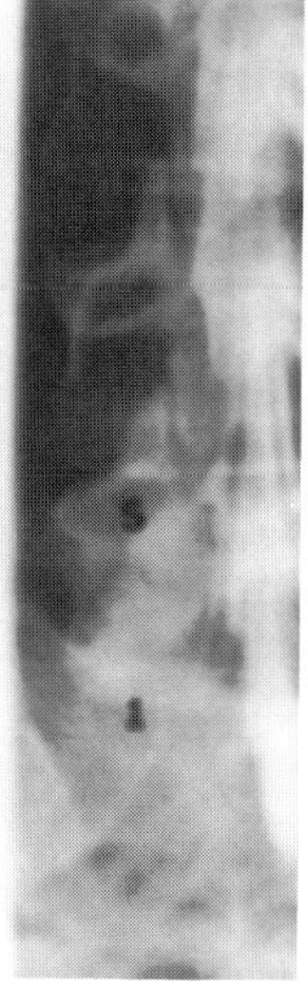

Figure 25–60. Unilateral extradural myelographic defect at L5–S1 on the right due to a herniated lumbar disc *(arrows).*

pared with the first-generation agent.[14, 51] Thanks to the reduction in side effects, myelography has become an outpatient procedure.

There are several differences between the myelographic appearance of a lumbar disc herniation and that of spinal stenosis.[4, 20, 24, 30, 31, 45, 78, 88] First, the plain x-rays of a disc herniation are usually normal, owing to the younger age group in which lumbar disc herniations commonly occur. Second, the myelographic picture of a disc herniation is usually an unilateral extradural defect at L4–L5 or L5–S1 (Fig. 25–60). In contrast, the myelographic appearance of spinal stenosis is usually described as an "hourglass" constriction at one or multiple levels (Figs. 25–61 to 25–63).[75, 84–86, 99, 108, 109, 111]

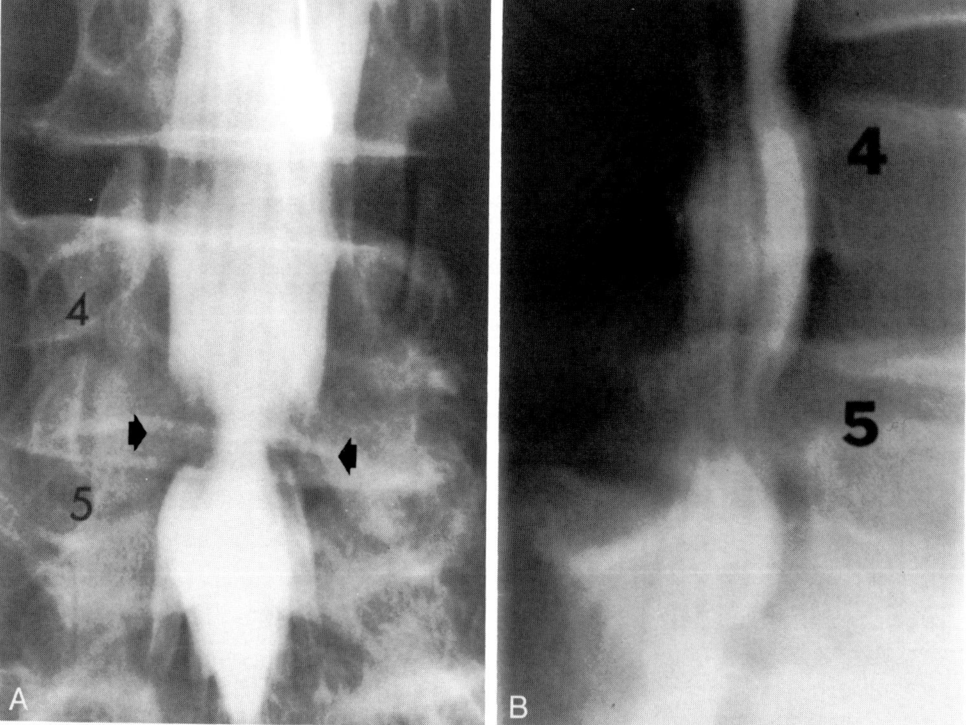

Figure 25–61. Anteroposterior *(A)* and lateral *(B)* myelograms demonstrating the "hourglass" constriction typical of spinal stenosis *(arrows).*

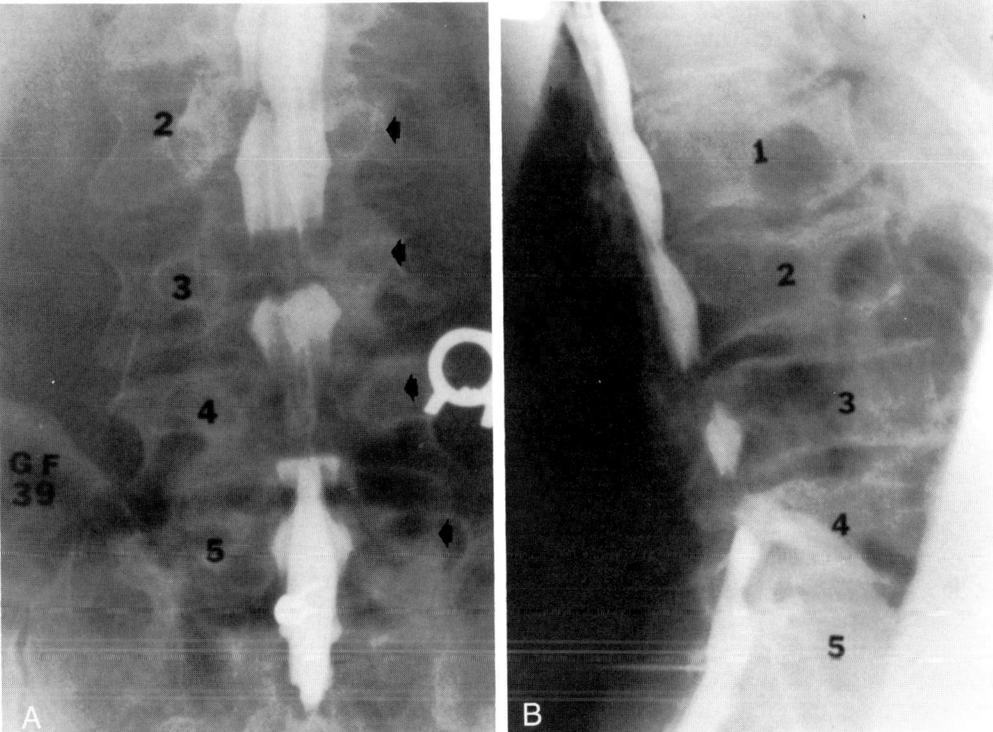

Figure 25–62. Anteroposterior *(A)* and lateral *(B)* myelograms showing multiple-level spinal stenosis in an achondroplastic dwarf.

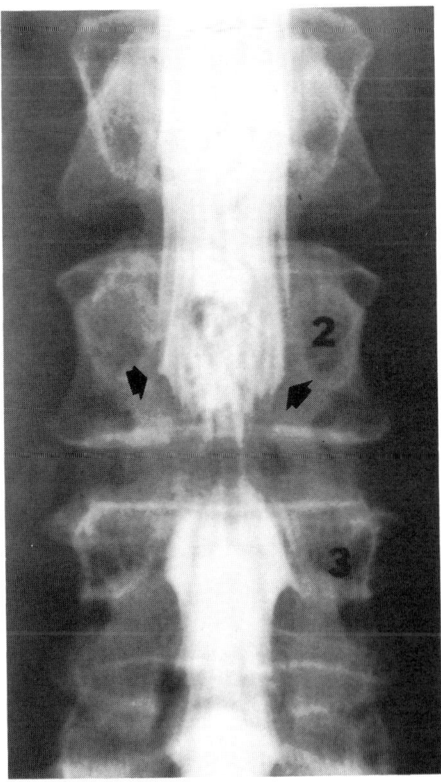

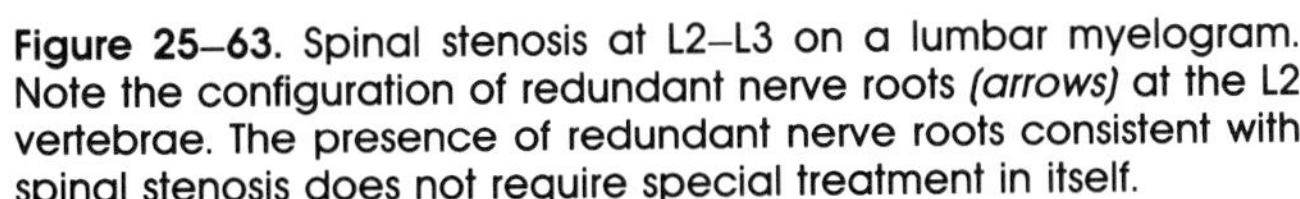

Figure 25–63. Spinal stenosis at L2–L3 on a lumbar myelogram. Note the configuration of redundant nerve roots *(arrows)* at the L2 vertebrae. The presence of redundant nerve roots consistent with spinal stenosis does not require special treatment in itself.

It is important to remember that defects present on the myelogram must be correlated with the clinical evaluation. Hitselberger and Witten reported a group of patients undergoing myelography for evaluation of an acoustic neuroma who had no history of a lumbar disc herniation or spinal stenosis. A significant lumbar myelographic defect was noted in 24 per cent of the patients.[50]

The advantages of myelography are first, that it visualizes the entire lumbar spine to the conus medullaris; second, that there is extensive clinical experience; and third, that patients are positioned in extension for the test, which accentuates the stenotic levels. In addition, hyperextension may be performed during the study in patients with a clinical picture consistent with spinal stenosis but whose myelographic results are equivocal in the standard position.[103]

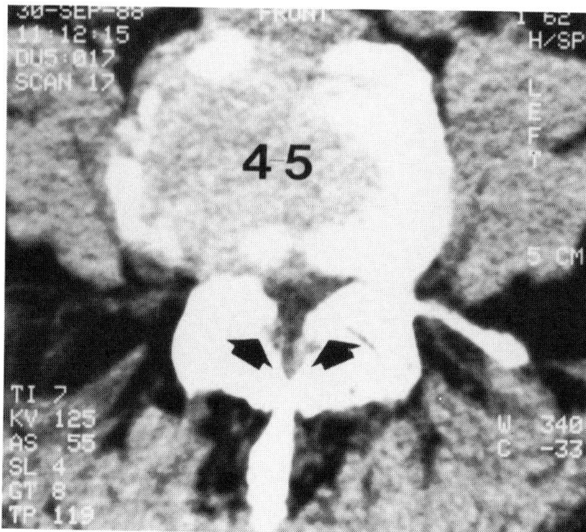

Figure 25–64. Severe spinal stenosis on CT. The dural sac *(arrows)* is compressed by the hypertrophic facet joints and thickened ligamentum flavum.

The disadvantages of myelography are first, that it is an invasive study. Second, side effects of headache, nausea, or seizure activity may occur. These can be minimized by eliminating patients as candidates for myelography who have a history of seizures, phenothiazine intake, or alcoholism. In addition, patients with inconsistent subjective complaints and a normal examination with a normal myelogram have a threefold increased incidence of complications compared with a group with a positive myelogram consistent with the clinical examination.[46] Third, patients with known iodine allergy may not be able to undergo myelography. Tallroth reported 26 patients with iodine allergy who had received myelography.[106] After the patients were pretreated with atropine, valium, and steroids, no allergic reactions occurred. At the present time, patients with a previous allergy to iodine are referred for MRI. In individuals unable to tolerate MRI, a one-week steroid preparation is given before myelography unless a previous anaphylactic reaction to iodine has occurred. Fourth, CT provides a more direct and accurate evaluation of the lateral recesses than does myelography.[77]

Computed Tomography

CT has several advantages over myelography for the evaluation of spinal stenosis.[54, 93, 94] First, it provides an accurate representation of the size and shape of the spinal canal (Fig. 25–64).[68] Second, it directly visualizes the lateral recesses and neuroforamen, whereas myelography indirectly identifies the nerve root canal (Figs. 25–65 and 25–66).[69, 112] Third, it is useful in identifying pathologic levels below a complete block. In a series of 32 patients with a complete lumbar myelographic block, CT demonstrated a herniated lumbar disc or spinal stenosis at 30 of 50 nonvisualized levels (60 per cent) (Fig. 25–67).[47] Finally, it is a noninvasive outpatient procedure.

The disadvantages of CT are first, that routine scanning is performed from L3 to S1, and therefore the conus medullaris or stenotic seg-

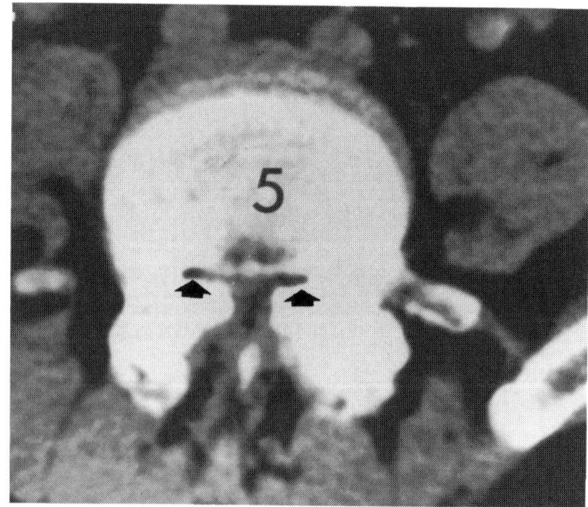

Figure 25–65. CT scan demonstrating severe narrowing of the lateral recess on the left and right at L5 *(arrows)*.

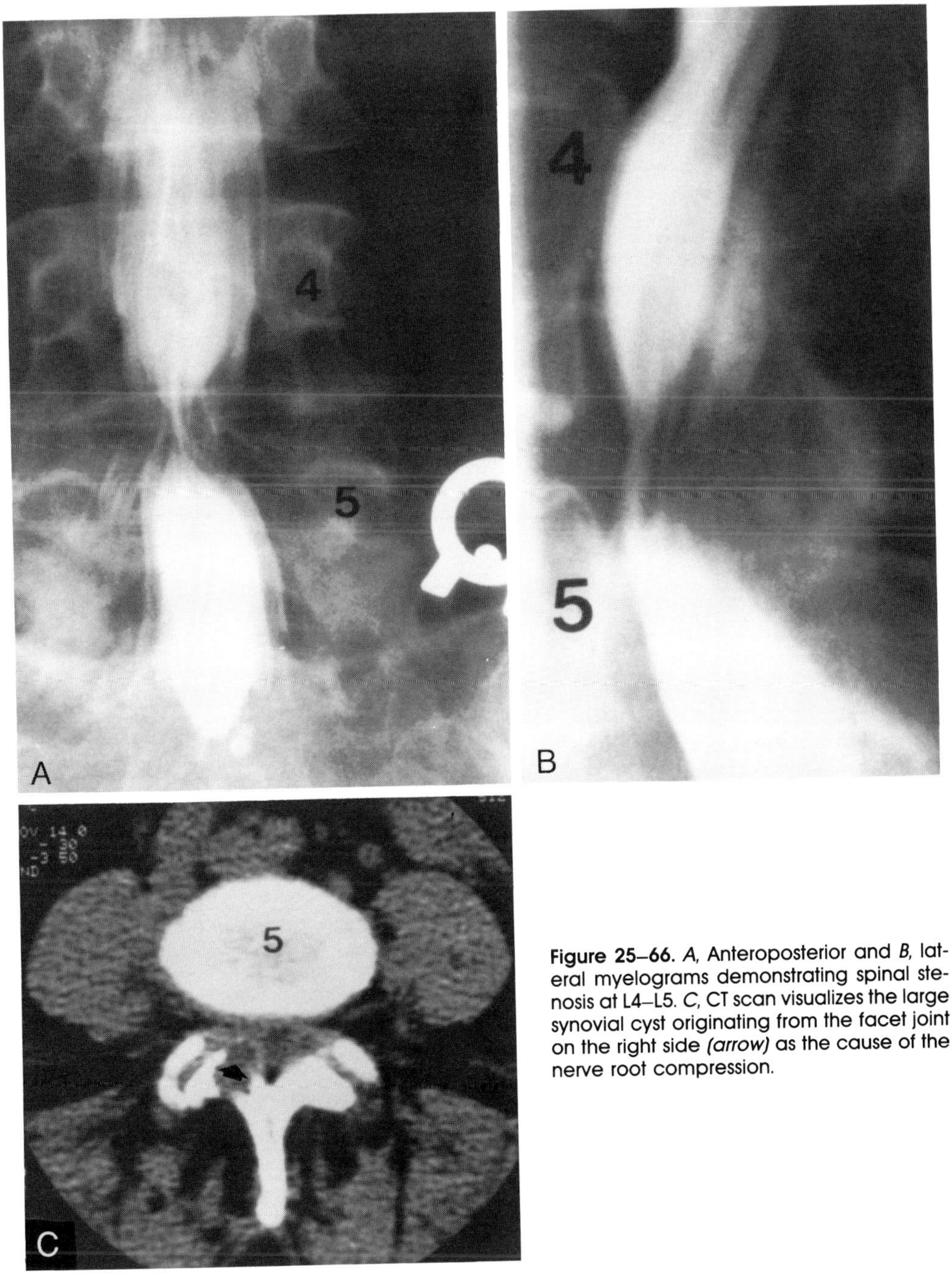

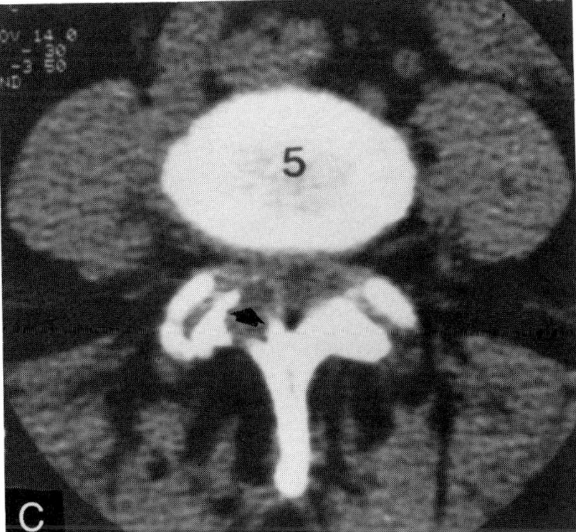

Figure 25–66. *A*, Anteroposterior and *B*, lateral myelograms demonstrating spinal stenosis at L4–L5. *C*, CT scan visualizes the large synovial cyst originating from the facet joint on the right side *(arrow)* as the cause of the nerve root compression.

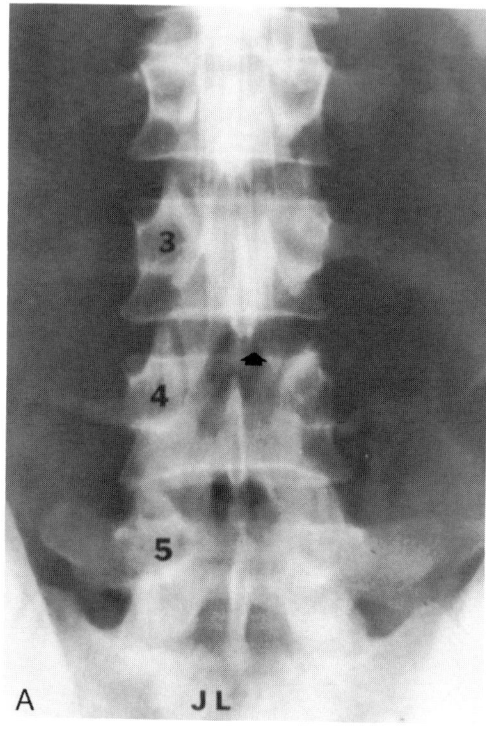

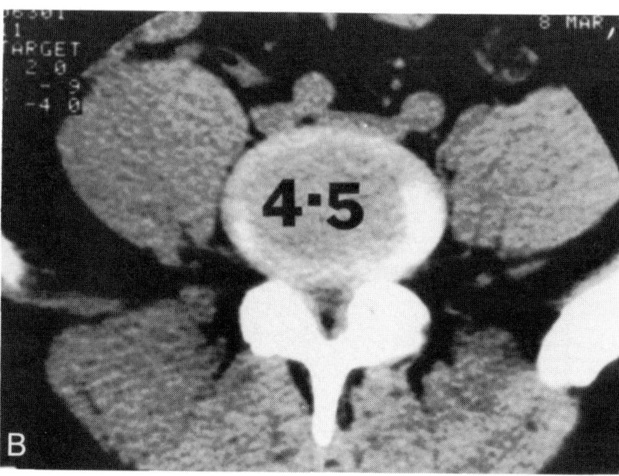

Figure 25–67. *A,* Anteroposterior myelogram demonstrating a complete block at L3–L4 due to congenital spinal stenosis. *B,* CT scan showing severe central canal stenosis below the myelographically blocked level at L3–L4.

ments above the third lumbar vertebrae are not visualized on the routine scan. Second, to accommodate for lumbar lordosis, the gantry may be tilted up to 15 degrees, but this may not allow parallel scanning of the L5–S1 segment if lordosis exceeds that amount.[101] Along with the thickness of the CT slice, a nonparallel image may distort the final picture produced owing to the partial volume effect. That is, a computer average of all the tissues present in that CT slice occurs; thus, thicker sections that contain a larger amount of bone will cause the less dense tissues (e.g., dura, ligamentum, flavum, or epidural fat) to appear denser than they actually are. This may lead to a false-positive image of a narrow central canal, lateral recess, or herniated disc (Fig. 25–68).[102] When a doubt remains, reformatting in a sagittal or coronal plane may be helpful.[11] Third, the results of the scan are open to interpretation. A study from Boston University asked five neuroradiologists to interpret ten CT scans and report on the presence of central canal or lateral recess spinal stenosis.[5] The results showed a strong correlation among the radiologists for central canal measurements, but a significant *negative* correlation for lateral recess measurements. This report emphasized the wide variability among neuroradiologists in their interpretation of the CT scan, and points out to the clinician the importance of evaluating all diagnostic studies in relation to the clinical examination.

The accuracy of CT as compared with mye-

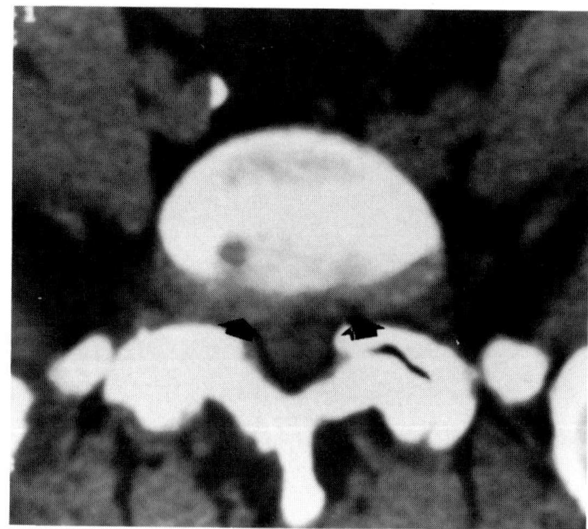

Figure 25–68. False-positive CT scan at L5–S1 suggesting a disc protrusion *(arrow)* owing to the image not being taken parallel to the disc space.

lography was described by Bell and associates in 122 patients in whom the diagnosis was surgically confirmed.[122] Myelography was found to be more accurate than CT for herniated lumbar disc (83 versus 72 per cent, respectively) and for spinal stenosis (93 versus 89 per cent, respectively). However, these results were not statistically significant. CT provides a direct view of the nerve root canal and the causes of compression within the spinal canal. Wiesel and colleagues reported the incidence of *positive* CT scans in an *asymptomatic* group of individuals.[123] For all age groups, the incidence of false-positive scans was 35.4 per cent. For individuals under 40 years of age, an abnormal scan was noted in 19.5 per cent, with the diagnosis of herniated disc in all cases. For individuals over 40 the incidence was 50 per cent, the diagnosis of facet degeneration, herniated disc, or spinal stenosis being the most common. This study also emphasized the importance of correlating the diagnostic studies with the clinical evaluation.

Does performance of a CT scan immediately after myelography increase the diagnostic accuracy of either one by itself? In a review of 80 surgical patients with the diagnosis of a herniated disc or spinal stenosis who were undergoing myelography followed CT, the accuracy of CT alone was 82 per cent, myelography alone 77 per cent, and the two combined 91 per cent.[119] For patients with spinal stenosis, CT was correct in 83 per cent, myelography in 76 per cent, and the combined studies in 91 per cent. However, the results were not statistically significant. Myelography and CT complement each other in the surgical evaluation of spinal stenosis. The normal sequence of events is to obtain the CT scan early in the surgical evaluation, while the myelogram is obtained before the confirmed surgical date. For spinal stenosis there appear to be no documented advantages in combining the studies.

Magnetic Resonance Imaging

MRI is the newest diagnostic tool for evaluation of the spine. With MRI, anatomic images are created by radiowaves absorbed and remitted from protons rotating about their axis in a magnetic field. The intensity and distribution of the signal are reflections of various tissue characteristics, which include the density of the resonating protons, the states of motion of the proton, and the chemical parameters, which are known as T1 and T2 relaxation times. T1 describes the interaction that occurs between the nucleus of the proton and its environment, and depends on the surrounding tissue chemistry. T2 depends on the interaction among the surrounding nuclei. The differences between T1 and T2 in normal and abnormal tissues are what produces an anatomic image.[44]

The amount of T1 and T2 present is governed by varying the pulse sequence technique that controls how long the signal is allowed to grow or decay. By means of changes in the T1 and T2 relaxation times, specific anatomic structures can be enhanced.[80]

Magnetic resonance is a sensitive indicator of changes in tissue water content. For spine evaluation, both T1- and T2-weighted images are obtained.[81, 82] T1 images provide excellent resolution among the soft tissue structures (Fig. 25–69). T2 images increase the signal intensity of the normal nucleus pulposus and CSF because of their high water content, and the result is the MRI myelogram (the image of the dural sac appears similar to that seen with conventional myelography) (Fig. 25–70).[76]

The films generated by MRI are routinely presented in sagittal, transverse, and coronal planes, while those from CT usually provide transverse images unless reformatting is requested. The advantages of MRI are that it is a noninvasive study that does not rely on radiation to produce its images. Its disadvantages are that a significant number of patients (15 per cent) will be unable to tolerate the procedure owing to claustrophobia, implanted metallic objects, or obesity. Also, the quality of MRI scans varies considerably from institution to institution. It is essential that the surgeon review the films personally to ensure that the quality is sufficient for a surgical evaluation.

What is the accuracy of MRI in comparison with myelography or CT? Before the use of surface body coils, which improve resolution and allow thinner cuts to be made, two studies reported the value of MRI in the diagnosis of spinal stenosis. In a review of 17 patients, Edelman found MRI to be comparable with CT in diagnostic accuracy.[23] The advantage

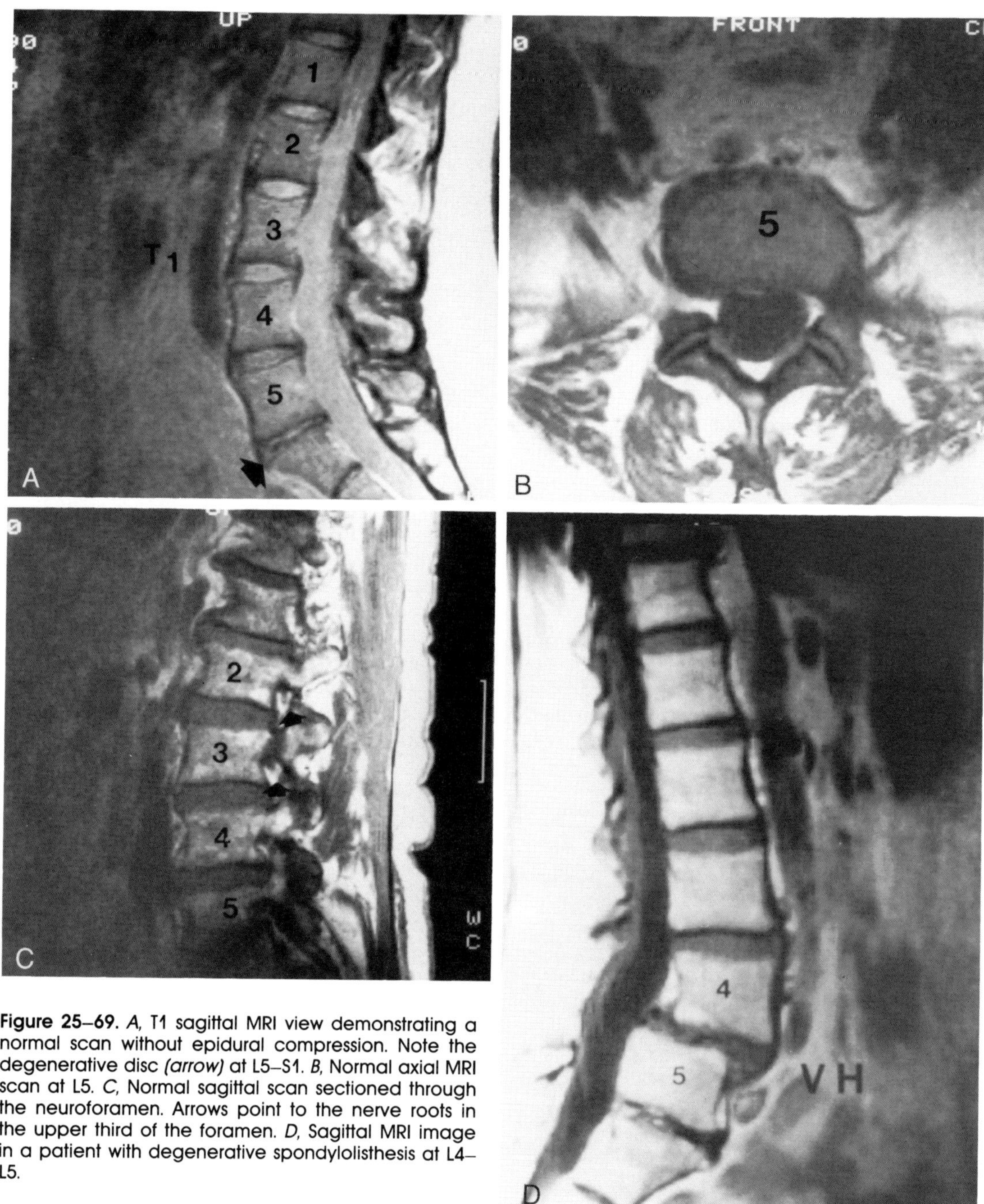

Figure 25–69. *A,* T1 sagittal MRI view demonstrating a normal scan without epidural compression. Note the degenerative disc *(arrow)* at L5–S1. *B,* Normal axial MRI scan at L5. *C,* Normal sagittal scan sectioned through the neuroforamen. Arrows point to the nerve roots in the upper third of the foramen. *D,* Sagittal MRI image in a patient with degenerative spondylolisthesis at L4–L5.

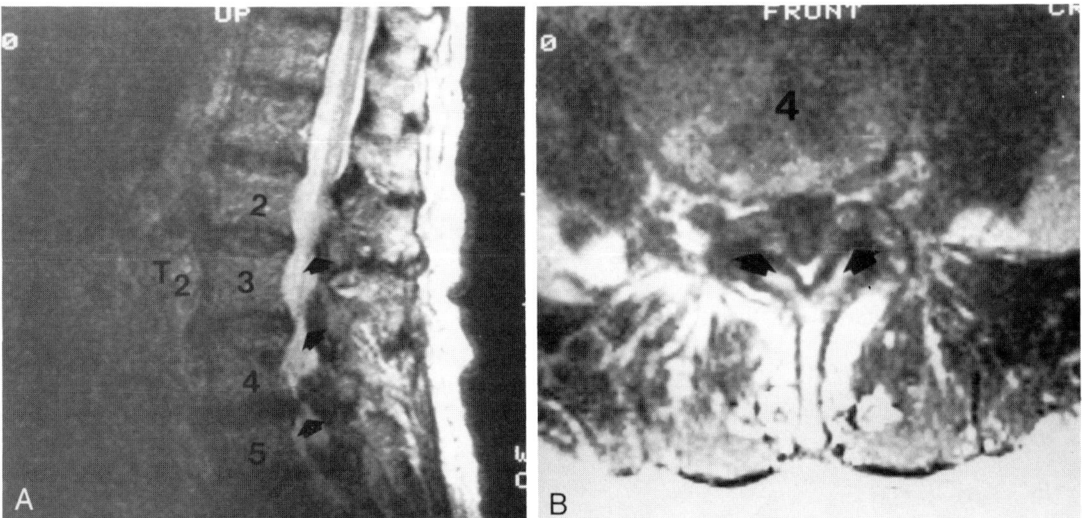

Figure 25–70. *A*, T2 sagittal MRI view showing the "myelogram effect" with multiple-level spinal stenosis *(arrows)*. *B*, Axial MR image through L4 demonstrates the facet joint hypertrophy *(arrows)* with compression on the dural sac.

over myelography was MRI's noninvasiveness; MRI's advantage over CT was its ability to obtain parallel images at the lumbosacral junction. Cranshaw and associates reported 21 patients who showed clinical evidence of lateral recess spinal stenosis.[18] MRI demonstrated reduction of epidural fat in the lateral recesses in eight patients, which was thought to be consistent with lateral recess spinal stenosis. However, there was no surgical confirmation in this series.

The accuracy of MRI using surface coils for the diagnosis of lumbar disc herniation and spinal stenosis was reported by Modic and associates.[79] The series consisted of 48 surgical patients operated on at 62 lumbar levels. Agreement between MRI and CT was noted in 86.8 per cent of levels; for MRI and myelography there was 82.6 per cent agreement. The surgical correlation was 82.6 per cent between MRI and surgical findings for both type and location of disease, while for CT and surgical findings it was 83 per cent, and for myelography and surgery, 71.8 per cent. When MRI and CT were combined, 92.5 per cent agreement was noted; myelography and CT combined demonstrated 89.4 per cent agreement. For spinal stenosis the T1 images were useful in evaluating the size and contour of the neural canal foramen and conus medullaris. The T2-weighted images gave an accurate assessment of the extradural–CSF interface and canal dimensions. The results of this study supported MRI as being equivalent to CT and myelography for spinal stenosis and lumbar disc herniation.

A comparison of MRI with contrast-enhanced CT in 41 patients with the diagnosis of spinal stenosis or lumbar disc degeneration demonstrated agreement between these modalities at 96.6 per cent of the levels studied.[100] The conclusions of this study pointed to comparable accuracy between contrast CT and MRI for the diagnosis of spinal stenosis. MRI was found to be more sensitive than contrast CT for the diagnosis of disc degeneration.

It appears that the sensitivity of MRI is comparable with or surpasses that of myelography or CT in the diagnostic evaluation of lumbar spinal stenosis. The specificity, i.e., the ability of a test to remain normal when no disease is present, has been reported by Bowden and colleagues.[8] They described 67 asymptomatic volunteers ranging in age from 20 to 80 years who had undergone a lumbar MRI scan. Three neuroradiologists independently interpreted the scans. The results were reported for three age brackets: 20 to 39, 40 to 59, and 60 to 80.

For the 20 to 39 age group, herniated disc was reported in 22 per cent and spinal stenosis in 1 per cent. For the 40 to 59 age group, herniated disc was reported in 22 per cent and spinal stenosis in none. In the 60 to 80 age group, herniated disc was reported in 36 per cent and spinal stenosis in 21 per cent. Overall,

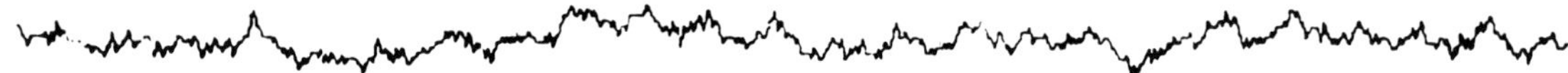

Figure 25–71. Normal electromyelogram of the lower extremity at rest.

30 per cent of the MRI scans were abnormal, with the diagnosis of herniated disc in 25 per cent and spinal stenosis in 5 per cent. This study points out the importance of correlating the clinical examination with the diagnostic studies. This is especially true in the older age population in whom the incidence of false-positive results is so high.

Discography

Discography has two components: the pattern identified by injection of contrast medium into the disc space, and the reaction of the patient to the injection of saline into the disc space (saline acceptance test). In patients with spinal stenosis, the pattern noted on discography is of little benefit in evaluating the individual because disc degeneration is common in the older age group and surgery is done for nerve compression, not disc degeneration. The value of the saline acceptance test likewise is of no benefit in the surgical evaluation of spinal stenosis, for two reasons. First, surgery is indicated for nerve root compression, not disc degeneration. Second, Holt, in a study of asymptomatic volunteers, demonstrated a 38 per cent positive pain response in normal discs, indicating low specificity and a high false-positive rate.[52] In a study of the value of discography in patients with lower back problems, Grubb and colleagues concluded that discography has no role in the evaluation of spinal stenosis.[41]

ELECTRODIAGNOSIS

Electromyography (EMG)

Electromyography evaluates the physiology of the nerve roots, which is useful in diagnosis of motor unit disorders. A motor unit consists of one anterior horn cell, its axon, and the muscle fibers it innervates. Therefore, EMG evaluates lower motor neuron dysfunction only. It does not evaluate sensory disturbance or upper motor neuron abnormalities.

EMG is performed by inserting an electrode into the desired muscle and recording its electrical activity at rest and with stimulation. Duration, amplitude, and the numbers of phases of the voluntary motor unit are then recorded to arrive at a diagnosis (Fig. 25–71). Radiculopathy may express itself as prolonged, shortened, or absent insertional potentials; ongoing spontaneous activity at rest (fibrillation potentials, fasciculations, or positive sharp waves); abnormal potentials (polyphasia, giant

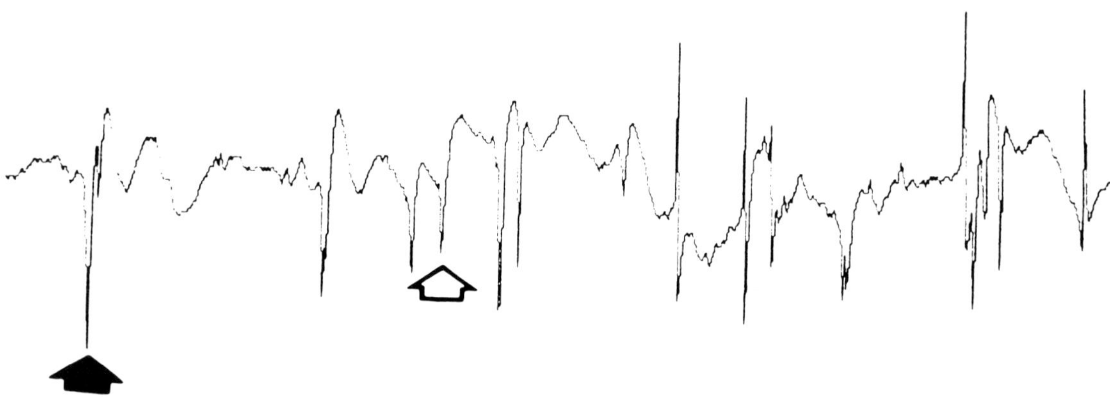

Figure 25–72. Fibrillations *(black arrow)* and positive waves *(white arrow)* recorded from an involved muscle in lumbar radiculopathy at rest.

motor units, increased duration, doublets); and abnormal recruitment and diminished interference patterns (Fig. 25–72).[42]

In lumbar radiculopathy due to a disc herniation, the classic EMG will reveal single root unilateral findings in the paraspinals and affected extremity, while in spinal stenosis it often reveals bilateral multiradicular findings whether or not the patient's symptoms are bilateral.[33] Jacobson, in his review of the use of EMG in spinal stenosis, found 41 of 53 patients (77 per cent) with a bilaterally positive EMG result; 28 of the 41 (68 per cent) had bilateral symptoms. Of patients with a herniated lumbar disc, only 8 of 42 had multiradicular or bilateral EMG findings.[53]

Johnsson and associates performed EMG on 64 patients with myelographically proved spinal stenosis.[56] Of 16 patients with a complete myelographic block, 87.5 per cent demonstrated bilateral EMG changes. Of those without a complete block, 81 per cent exhibited bilateral changes, while of 24 patients with a normal myelogram, only 29 per cent displayed bilateral changes. Multisegmental EMG changes were noted in 94 per cent of patients with a complete block, 75 per cent of those with an incomplete block, and 21 per cent of those with a normal myelogram. This is the first published series to correlate the degree of myelographic block with the EMG findings. This study also demonstrated that the EMG findings are not predictive of surgical outcome.

Although EMG is a useful diagnostic test, it has several limitations. First, it requires a minimum of 10 days before the abnormalities register. Second, false-negative results may occur, since the involved muscle groups may be multiply innervated, with the uninvolved roots supplying sufficient strength. Finally, it must be remembered that the EMG is a measure of the motor nerve end, and therefore sensory dysfunction is not evaluated by this modality.[42] This is especially important in spinal stenosis because this condition often presents only as a sensory disturbance producing claudicatory leg pains on a neuroischemic basis. Thus, it is not uncommon to have normal EMG findings in a case of classic spinal stenosis.

Nerve Conduction Studies

While EMG measures the nerve effect on muscle, the nerve conduction velocity test measures the speed at which the nerve impulse travels. This test is most helpful in differentiating peripheral neuropathy from radiculopathy.[49] Slowed nerve conduction velocity and EMG findings of low-amplitude action potentials and diffuse fibrillation potentials are common in neuropathy (Fig. 25–73). Radiculopathy usually exhibits more focal distal fibrillation potentials with localized unilateral or bilateral paraspinal muscle denervation and normal nerve conduction velocities.

Somatosensory Evoked Potentials (SSEPs)

In the broadest sense, evoked potentials are defined as electrical responses of the nervous system to sensory stimulation. Their greatest use has been for intraoperative monitoring in scoliosis and major spinal reconstructive surgery.

The spinal evoked potential is transmitted through the dorsal columns and is mediated

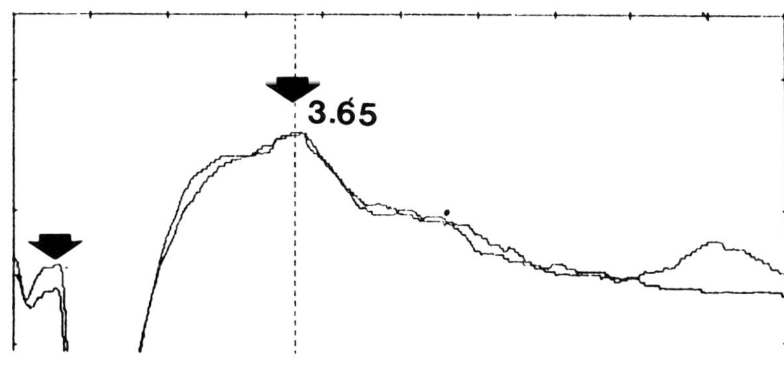

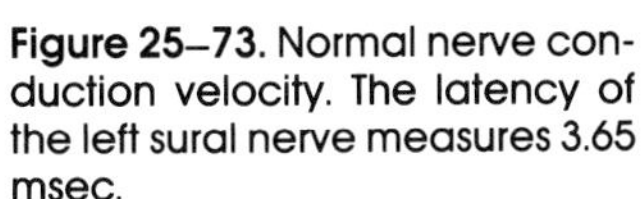

Figure 25–73. Normal nerve conduction velocity. The latency of the left sural nerve measures 3.65 msec.

by large myelinated fibers that are sensitive to both mechanical compression and ischemia.[39] Diseases affecting peripheral nerves, nerve roots, the spinal cord, or brain lesions will affect the evoked response. Lesions of the peripheral nerve prolong the latency response, while root and cord lesions cause changes in the waveform.

For testing SSEPs, the technique involves stimulation of a peripheral nerve (e.g., the posterior tibial) with the signal being picked up by scalp electrodes in preset locations on the sensory cortex and recorded by microprocessor.[48] Evoked potentials seem particularly suited to the neuroclaudication of spinal stenosis because the SSEP measures the sensory component of the nerve, unlike EMG, which measures only the motor side (Fig. 25–74).

Keim and associates reported 20 patients with spinal stenosis: the posterior tibial nerve (L5–S1) was abnormal in 95 per cent, the peroneal (L5) in 90 per cent, the sural (S1) in 60 per cent, and the saphenous (L4) in 12 per cent. In addition, the SSEP response revealed bilateral involvement in patients with unilateral pain and also multiple root involvement,

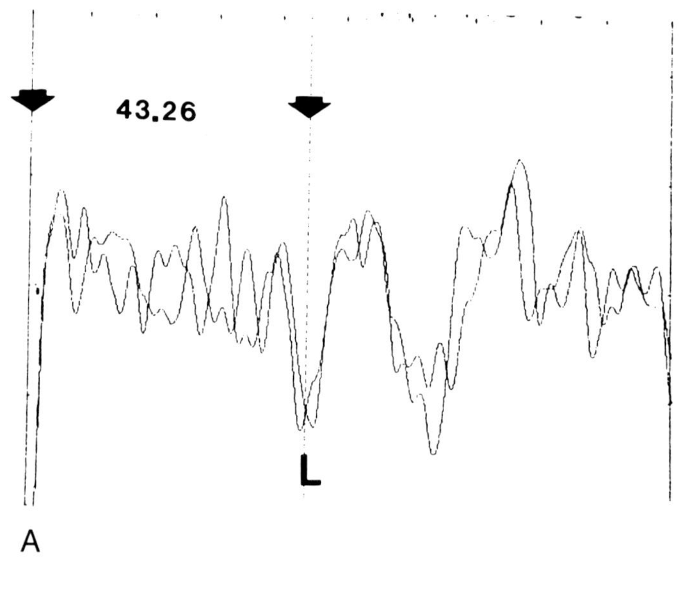

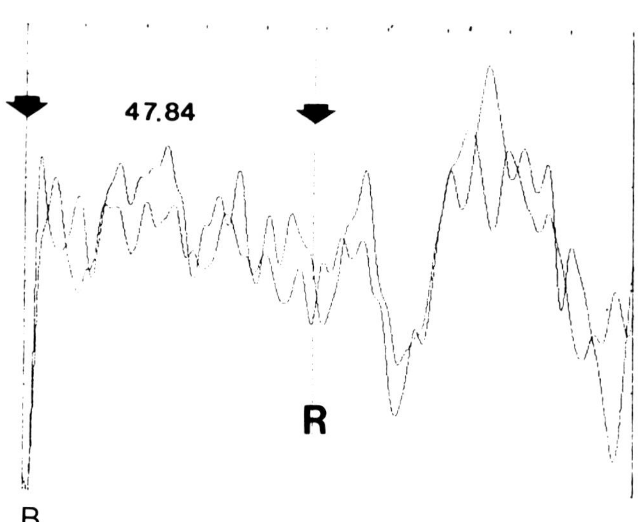

Figure 25–74. *A, B,* Somatosensory evoked potentials in an individual with right lower extremity radiculopathy due to spinal stenosis. The waveform is elicited by stimulating the peroneal nerve at the ankle and recording the stimulus from the sensory cortex on the scalp. The latency is prolonged over 4 msec in the right lower extremity. (More than 2.5 msec difference is significant.)

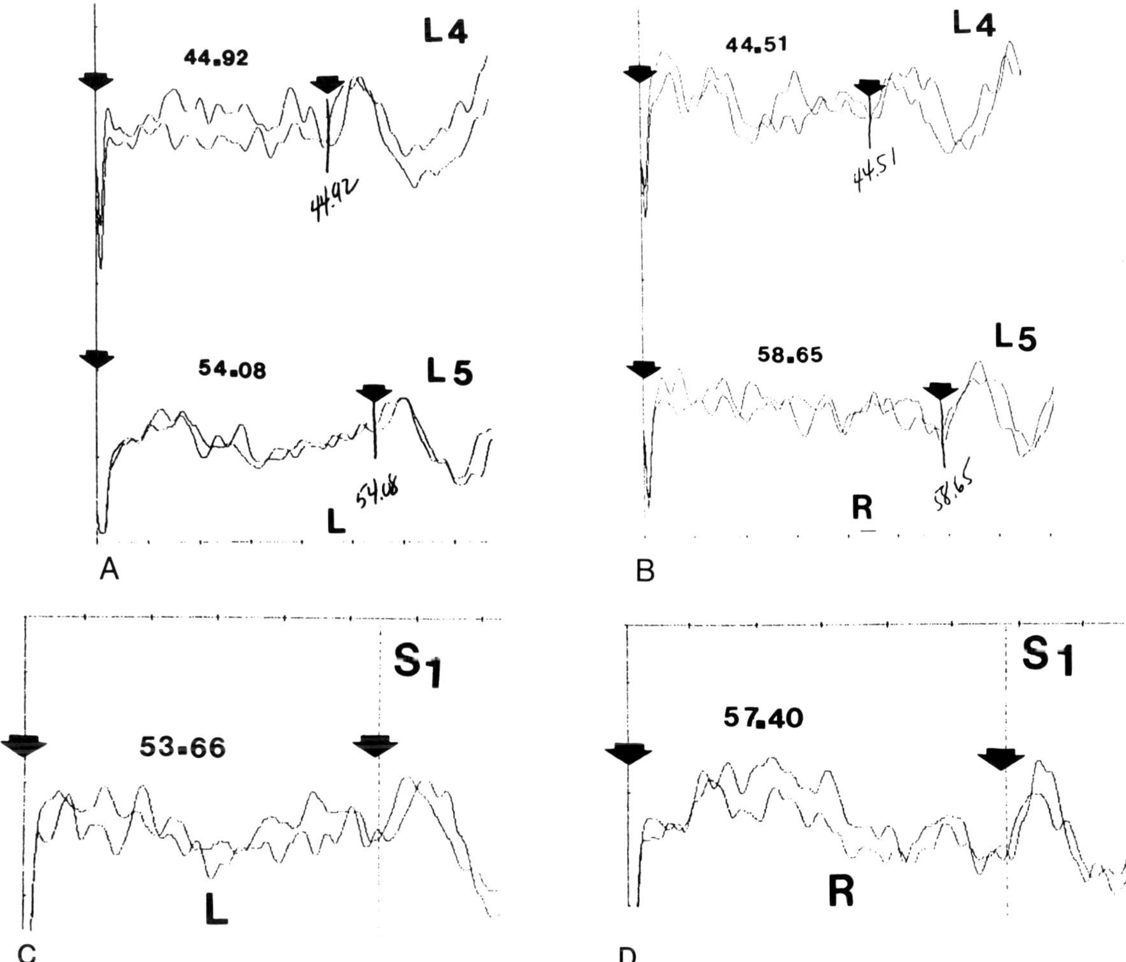

Figure 25–75. *A* to *D*, Dermatomal somatosensory evoked potentials are recorded by stimulating a specific dermatome and recording over the sensory cortex on the scalp. This is an example of stimulation of the L4, L5, and S1 dermatome in a patient with proved spinal stenosis. The latency is prolonged for the right L5 and S1 dermatome. A 5-msec delay indicates significant slowing.

which is more indicative of spinal stenosis than of a disc herniation.[61]

Dvonch and colleagues reported their results in the use of dermatomal somatosensory evoked potentials (DSSEPs) for disc herniation and spinal stenosis.[22] Instead of stimulating a peripheral nerve, electrodes stimulate the dermatomal distribution of the L5 nerve (first web space) and the S1 nerve (fifth metatarsal) and are relayed to electrodes on the sensory cortex (Fig. 25–75). The results of DSSEP were compared with those of myelography in 70 patients. The accuracy was 86 per cent, sensitivity (ability of the test to detect disease when it is present) 89 per cent, and specificity (ability of the test to remain normal when no disease is present) 81 per cent. In 33 of those patients an EMG was performed. The accuracy was 71 per cent, the sensitivity 76 per cent, and the specificity 68 per cent. A second group of 38 surgically treated patients were evaluated: 35 of these (87.5 per cent) had positive evoked potentials correlating to the involved nerve root.

Machida and colleagues reported the use of DSSEP for lumbar disc herniation. Although they confirmed six false-negative results in 40 patients, they recommended this as a valuable diagnostic tool.[72]

On the other side is the study of Aminoff and colleagues involving 19 patients with L5 or S1 radiculopathy evaluated by DSSEP.

They found that it localized the lesions correctly in five patients, localized the lesion to the uninvolved leg in one, and was normal in 12.[2]

The use of stress SSEPs has been described by Kondo and associates.[66] Thirty-seven patients with degenerative spinal stenosis were subjected to SSEP testing before and after walking stress. In 21 of the 37 the amplitude was reduced after walking. The authors concluded that this test is useful as a diagnostic tool and is helpful in differentiating neurogenic from vascular claudication.

Of the available studies (myelography, CT, and MRI), the clinician may be confused as to which to order and when. For the consulting surgeon, most patients have already received a course of conservative management along with a CT scan before the referral. For the preoperative evaluation the patient will have received a myelogram or MRI scan. Therefore, the vast majority of patients will have undergone two studies before surgery, a CT scan along with a myelogram or MRI. The rationale for this is twofold. First, CT provides the best images for evaluation of the lateral recesses. Second, myelogram or MRI provides imaging of the conus medullaris and upper lumbar levels (L1–L2, L2–L3), which the CT scan may not include.

References

1. Alexander, E: Significance of the small lumbar spinal canal: cauda equina compression syndromes due to spondylosis. Part 5. Achondroplasia. J. Neurosurg. *31*:513–519, 1969.
2. Aminoff, M. J., et al.: Dermatomal somatosensory evoked potentials in unilateral lumbosacral radiculopathy. Ann. Neurol. *17*:171–176, 1985.
3. Arnoldi, C. C., et al.: Lumbar spinal stenosis and nerve root entrapment syndromes. Definition and classification. Clin. Orthop. *115*:4, 1976.
4. Asztely, M., et al.: A comparison of sonography and myelography in clinically suspected spinal stenosis. Spine *18*:885–890, 1983.
5. Beers, G. J., et al.: Interobserver discrepancies in distance measurements from lumbar spine CT scans. A.J.N.R. *5*:787–790, 1984.
6. Bell, G. R., et al.: A study of computer assisted tomography: comparison of metrizamide myelography and computed tomography in the diagnosis of herniated lumbar disc and spinal stenosis. Spine *9*:552–556, 1984.
7. Blau, J. N., and Logue, V.: Intermittent claudication of the cauda equina. Lancet *1*:1081, 1961.
8. Bowden, S., Davis, D., Dina, T., et al.: Abnormal MRI scans of the lumbar spine in asymptomatic subjects. J. Bone Joint Surg. *72A*:403–409, 1990.
9. Bolender, N. F., Schönström, N., and Spengler, D. M.: Role of computed tomography and myelography in central spinal stenosis. J. Bone Joint Surg. *67A*:240–246, 1985.
10. Bowen, V., et al.: Lumbar and spinal stenosis. Childs Brain *4*:257, 1978.
11. Braun, I., et al.: Pitfalls in the computed tomographic evaluation of the lumbar spine in disc disease. Neuroradiology *26*:15–20, 1984.
12. Brodsky, A. E.: Post-laminectomy and post-fusion stenosis of the lumbar spine. Clin. Orthop. *115*:130 1976.
13. Brodsky, A. E.: Post-laminectomy and post-fusion stenosis of the lumbar spine. Clin. Orthop. *115*:130, 1976.
14. Burrows, E. H.: Myelography with iohexol (Omnipaque): review of 300 cases. A.J.N.R. *6*:349–351, 1985.
15. Cauchoix, J., et al.: Degenerative spondylolisthesis. Clin. Orthop. *115*:122–129, 1976.
16. Ciric, I., et al.: The lateral recess syndrome. J. Neurosurg. *53*:433–443, 1980.
17. Clark, K.: Significance of the small lumbar canal: cauda equina compression syndromes due to spondylosis. Part 2. Clinical and surgical significance. J. Neurosurg. *31*:495, 1969.
18. Cranshaw, C., et al.: The use of nuclear magnetic resonance in the diagnosis of lateral canal entrapment. J. Bone Joint Surg. *66B*:711–715, 1984.
19. Crock, H. V.: Isolated lumbar disc resorption as a cause of nerve root canal stenosis. Clin. Orthop. *115*:109, 1976.
20. DeVilliers, P. D., and Booysen, E. L.: Fibrous spinal stenosis. A report on 850 myelograms with a water-soluble contrast medium. Clin. Orthop. *115*:140, 1976.
21. Dommisse, G.: Morphological aspects of the lumbar spine and lumbosacral region. Orthop. Clin. North Am. *6*:163–175, 1975.
22. Dvonch, V., Scoff, T., Bunch, W. H., et al.: Dermatomal somatosensory evoked potentials: their use in lumbar radiculopathy. Spine *9*:291–293, 1984.
23. Edelman, R. R.: High resolution surface coil imaging of lumbar disc disease. A.J.N.R. *6*:479–485, 1985.
24. Ehni, G.: Effects of certain degenerative diseases of the spine, especially spondylosis and disk protrusion, on the neural contents, particularly in the lumbar region. Mayo Clin. Proc. *50*:327, 1975.
25. Ehni, G.: Significance of the small lumbar spinal canal: cauda equina compression syndromes due to spondylosis. Part 1. Introduction. J. Neurosurg. *31*:490, 1969.
26. Ehni, G.: Significance of the small lumbar spinal canal: cauda equina compression syndromes due to spondylosis. Part 4. Acute compression artificially induced during operation. J. Neurosurg. *31*:507, 1969.
27. Eisenstein, S.: Measurements of the lumbar spinal canal in two racial groups. Clin. Orthop. *115*:42, 1976.
28. Eisenstein, S.: Lumbar vertebral canal morphometry for computerized tomography in spinal stenosis. Spine *8*:187–191, 1983.
29. Eisenstein, S.: The morphometry and pathologic anatomy of the lumbar spine in South African Negroes and Caucasoids with specific reference to

spinal stenosis. J. Bone Joint Surg. *59B*:173–180, 1977.

30. Epstein, J. A., Epstein, B. S., and Levine, L.: Nerve root compression associated with narrowing of the lumbar canal. J. Neurol. Neurosurg. Psychiatry *29*:315, 1966.
31. Epstein, J. A., Epstein, B. S., and Levine, L.: Nerve root compression due to stenosis of the lumbar canal. J. Neurol. Neurosurg. Psychiatry *29*:315, 1966.
32. Epstein, J. A., et al.: Degenerative spondylolisthesis. J. Neurosurg. *44*:139, 1976.
33. Epstein, J. A., et al.: Sciatica caused by nerve root entrapment in the lateral recess. J. Neurosurg. *36*:584–589, 1972.
34. Epstein, N., et al.: Coexisting cervical and lumbar spinal stenosis. Neurosurgery *15*:489–497, 1984.
35. Farfan, H.: Symposium on the lumbar spine. Orthop. Clin. North Am. *6*:163–196, 1979.
36. Friberg, O.: Lumbar instability: a dynamic approach by traction compression radiograph. Spine *12*:119–129, 1987.
37. Frymower, J. W., et al.: Spine radiography in patients with low back pain. J. Bone Joint Surg. *66A*:1048–1055, 1984.
38. Gill, G. G., and White, H. L.: Mechanisms of nerve root compression and irritation in backache. Clin. Orthop. *5*:66, 1955.
39. Gonzales, E., Hajdu, M., Bruno, R., et al.: Lumbar spine stenosis. Analysis of pre- and post-operative somatosensory evoked potentials. Arch. Phys. Med. Rehab. *66*:11–15, 1985.
40. Gooding, et al.: Intraoperative sonography during lumbar laminectomy. A.J.N.R. *5*:751–753, 1984.
41. Grubb, S. A., Lipscomb, H. J., and Guilford, W. B.: The relative value of lumbar roentgenograms, metrizamide myelography and discography in the assessment of patients with chronic low back syndrome. Spine *12*:282–286, 1987.
42. Haldeman, S.: The electrodiagnostic evaluation of nerve root function. Spine *9*:42–48, 1984.
43. Hasue, M., et al.: Post-traumatic spinal stenosis of the lumbar spine. Spine *5*:259–263, 1980.
44. Helms, C., et al.: Magnetic resonance imaging. Orthopedics *7*:1429–1435, 1984.
45. Herkowitz, H. N., et al.: Metrizamide myelography and epidural venography: their role in the diagnosis of lumbar disc herniation and spinal stenosis. Spine *7*:55–64, 1982.
46. Herkowitz, H. N., et al.: The indications for metrizamide myelography. J. Bone Joint Surg. *65A*:1144–1150, 1983.
47. Herkowitz, H. N., Garfin, S. R., Bell, G., et al.: The use of computerized tomography in evaluating non-visualized vertebral levels caudad to a complete block on a lumbar myelogram. J. Bone Joint Surg. *69A*:218–224, 1987.
48. Herron, L., Trippi, A., and Gonyeau, M.: Intraoperative use of dermatomal somatosensory evoked potentials in lumbar stenosis surgery. Spine *12*:379–383, 1987.
49. Hirsch, L. F.: Diabetic polyradiculopathy simulating lumbar disc disease. J. Neurosurg. *60*:183–186, 1984.
50. Hitselberger, W., and Witten, R.: Abnormal myelograms in asymptomatic patients. J. Neurosurg. *28*:204–206, 1968.
51. Holder, J. C., et al.: Iohexol lumbar myelography: clinical study. A.J.N.R. *5*:399–402, 1984.
52. Holt, E. P.: The question of lumbar discography. J. Bone Joint Surg. *50A*:720–726, 1968.
53. Jacobson, R.: Lumbar stenosis: an electromyographic evaluation. Clin. Orthop. *115*:68–72, 1976.
54. Jacobson, R. E., Gargano, F. P., and Rosomoff, H. L.: Transverse axial tomography of the spine. J. Neurosurg. *42*:406, 1975.
55. Joffe, R., Appleby, A., and Arjona, V.: Intermittent ischemia of the cauda equina due to stenosis of the lumbar canal. J. Neurol. Neurosurg. Psychiatry *29*:315–318, 1966.
56. Johnsson, K. E., Rosen, I., and Uden, A.: Neurophysiologic investigation of patients with spinal stenosis. Spine *12*:483–487, 1987.
57. Jones, R. A. C., et al.: The narrow lumbar canal: a clinical and radiological review. J. Bone Joint Surg. *50B*:595–605, 1968.
58. Kadziolka, R., Asztely, M., Hanai, K., et al.: Ultrasonic measurement of the lumbar spinal canal. J. Bone Joint Surg. *63B*:504–507, 1981.
59. Karpman, R. J., et al.: Lumbar spinal stenosis in a patient with diffuse idiopathic skeletal hypertrophy syndrome. Spine *7*:598–603, 1982.
60. Kawai, S., et al.: Enlargement of the lumbar vertebral canal in lumbar canal stenosis. Spine *6*:381–387, 1981.
61. Keim, H. A., et al.: Somatosensory evoked potentials as an aid in the diagnosis and intraoperative management of spinal stenosis. Spine *10*:338–344, 1985.
62. Kirkaldy-Willis, W. H.: The relationship of structural pathology to the nerve root. Spine *9*:49, 1984.
63. Kirkaldy-Willis, W. H., and Paine, K. W.: Lumbar spinal stenosis. Clin. Orthop. *99*:30, 1974.
64. Kirkaldy-Willis, W. H., et al.: Lumbar spinal nerve entrapment. Clin. Orthop. *169*:171–178, 1982.
65. Kirkaldy-Willis, W. H., et al.: Lumbar spondylosis and stenosis: correlation of pathologic anatomy with high resolution CT scanning. *In* Post, M. J. D. (ed.): Computed Tomography of the Spine. Baltimore, Williams & Wilkins Co., 1984, 546–569.
66. Kondo, M., Matsuda, H., Kureya, S., and Shimazu, A.: Electrophysiological studies of intermittent claudication in lumbar stenosis. Spine *14*:862–866, 1989.
67. Kornberg, M., et al.: The treatment of a herniated lumbar disc in a young adult with developmental spinal stenosis. Spine *9*:541–545, 1984.
68. Lancourt, J. E., et al.: Multiplanar computerized tomography in the normal spine and in the diagnosis of spinal stenosis. A gross anatomic–computerized tomographic correlation. Spine *4*:379, 1979.
69. Lee, B., et al.: Computed tomography of the spine and spinal cord. Radiology *128*:95–102, 1978.
70. Lee, C. W., Rauschning, W., and Glenn, W.: Lateral lumbar spine canal stenosis. Spine *13*:313–320, 1988.
71. Lowe, R., Hayes, T., Kaye, J., et al.: Standing roentgenograms in spondylolisthesis. Clin. Orthop. *117*:80–84, 1976.
72. Machida, M., Asai, T., Sato, K., et al.: New approach for diagnosis in herniated lumbosacral disc. Spine *11*:380–384, 1986.

73. MacNab, I.: Spondylolisthesis with an intact neural arch—the so-called pseudospondylolisthesis. J. Bone Joint Surg. *32B*:325, 1950.
74. MacNab, I.: Negative disc exploration. J. Bone Joint Surg. *53A*:891, 1971.
75. McIvor, G. W. D., and Kirkaldy-Willis, W. H.: Pathologic and myelographic changes in major types of spinal stenosis. Clin. Orthop. *115*:72–76, 1976.
76. Maravicla, K. R., et al.: Magnetic resonance imaging of the lumbar spine with CT correlation. A.J.N.R. *6*:237–245, 1985.
77. Mikhael, M., et al.: Neuroradiological evaluation of the lateral recess syndrome. Radiology *140*:97–107, 1981.
78. Mixter, W. J., and Barr, J. S.: Rupture of the intervertebral disc with involvement of the spinal canal. N. Engl. J. Med. *211*:210, 1934.
79. Modic, M. T., Masaryk, T., Boumphrey, F., et al.: Lumbar herniated disc disease and canal stenosis: prospective evaluation by surface coil MR, CT and myelography. A.J.R. *147*:757–765, 1986.
80. Modic, M., et al.: Nuclear magnetic resonance imaging of the spine. Radiology *148*:757–762, 1983.
81. Modic, M., Hardy, R. W., Jr., Weinstein, M. A., et al.: NMR of the spine: clinical potential and limitation. Neurosurgery *15*:583–592, 1984.
82. Modic, M., et al.: Magnetic resonance imaging of intervertebral disc disease. Radiology *152*:103–111, 1984.
83. Naylor, A.: Factors in the development of the spinal stenosis syndrome. J. Bone Joint Surg. *61B*:306, 1979.
84. Nelson, M. A.: Lumbar spinal stenosis. J. Bone Joint Surg. *55B*:506, 1973.
85. Newman, P. H.: Stenosis of the lumbar spine in spondylolisthesis. Clin. Orthop. *115*:116, 1976.
86. Paine, K. W. E.: Clinical features of lumbar spinal stenosis. Clin. Orthop. *115*:77–85, 1976.
87. Paine, K. W. E.: Results of decompression for lumbar spinal stenosis. Clin. Orthop. *115*:83–91, 1976.
88. Paine, K. W. E., and Haung, F.: Lumbar disc syndrome. J. Neurosurg. *37*:75–82, 1972.
89. Pennal, G. F., and Schatzker, J.: Stenosis of the lumbar spinal canal. Clin. Neurosurg. *18*:86, 1971.
90. Porter, R. W., et al.: Measurements of spinal canal by diagnostic ultrasound. J. Bone Joint Surg. *60B*:481–484, 1978.
91. Porter, R. W.: The spinal canal in symptomatic lumbar disc lesions. J. Bone Joint Surg. *60B*:485–487, 1978.
92. Posner, I., White, A., Edwards, W., and Hayes, W.: A biomechanical analysis of the clinical stability of the lumbar and lumbosacral spine. Spine *7*:374–389, 1982.
93. Post, M. J. D.: Computed Tomography of the Spine. Baltimore, Williams & Wilkins Co., 1984.
94. Raskin, S.: Degenerative changes of the lumbar spine—assessment by computed tomography. Orthopedics *4*:186–195, 1981.
95. Rosenberg, N. J.: Degenerative spondylolisthesis. J. Bone Joint Surg. *57A*:467, 1975.
96. Rothman, R. H., and Simeone, F. A.: Lumbar disc disease. *In* Rothman, R. H., and Simeone, F. A. (eds.): The Spine. 2nd ed. Philadelphia, W. B. Saunders Co., 1982, pp. 508–585.
97. Russin, L. A., and Sheldon, J.: Spinal stenosis: report of series and long-term follow-up. Clin. Orthop. *115*:101, 1976.
98. Rydevik, B., et al.: Pathoanatomy and pathophysiology of nerve root compression. Spine *9*:7, 1984.
99. Schatzker, J., and Pennal, G. P.: Spinal stenosis. A cause of cauda equina compression. J. Bone Joint Surg. *50B*:606, 1968.
100. Schnebel, B., Kingston, S., Watkins, R., and Dillin, W.: Comparison of MRI to contrast CT in the diagnosis of spinal stenosis. Spine *14*:332–337, 1989.
101. Shapiro, R.: Computed tomographic anatomy of the lumbosacral spine. *In* Post, M. J. D. (ed.): Computed Tomography of the Spine. Baltimore, Williams & Wilkins Co., 1984, pp. 78–93.
102. Sheldon, J., and Leborgne, J. M.: Computed tomography of central lumbar stenosis. *In* Post, M. J. D. (ed.): Computed Tomography of the Spine. Baltimore, Williams & Wilkins Co., 1984, pp. 570–590.
103. Sortland, O., et al.: Functional myelography with metrizamide in the diagnosis of lumbar spinal stenosis. Acta Radiol. (Suppl.) *355*:42–54, 1977.
104. Spengler, D.: Degenerative stenosis of the lumbar spine. Current concepts review. J. Bone Joint Surg. *69A*:305–308, 1987.
105. Sutro, C. J.: Lumbar facets—spinal stenosis and intermittent claudication: a mini review. Bull. Hosp. Joint Dis. *40*:13, 1979.
106. Tallroth, R.: Metrizamide myelography in patients with iodine allergy or previous adverse reactions to iodinated contrast media. Spine *12*:574–576, 1987.
107. Tarvin, G., and Prata, R. G.: Lumbosacral stenosis in dogs. J. Am. Vet. Med. Assoc. *177*:154, 1980.
108. Teng, P., and Papatheodorou, C.: Myelographic findings in spondylosis of the lumbar spine. Br. J. Radiol. *36*:122, 1963.
109. Tile, M., et al.: Spinal stenosis: results of treatment. Clin. Orthop. *115*:104–108, 1976.
110. Tsukamoto, Y., Onitsuka, H., and Lee, K.: Radiologic aspects of diffuse idiopathic skeletal hyperostosis in the spine. A.J.R. *129*:913–918, 1977.
111. Uden, A., et al.: Myelography in the elderly and the diagnosis of spinal stenosis. Spine *10*:171–174, 1985.
112. Ullrich, C. G., et al.: Quantitative effect of the lumbar spine canal by computed tomography. Radiology *134*:137–143, 1980.
113. Verbiest, H.: A radicular syndrome from developmental narrowing of the lumbar vertebral canal. J. Bone Joint Surg. *36B*:230–237, 1954.
114. Verbiest, H.: Further experiences of pathologic influence on a developmental narrowing of the lumbar vertebral canal. J. Bone Joint Surg. *38B*:576–583, 1956.
115. Verbiest, H.: Pathomotphologic aspects of development of lumbar scoliosis. Orthop. Clin. North Am. *6*:177–196, 1966.
116. Verbiest, H.: Results of surgical treatment of idiopathic developmental stenosis of the lumbar vertebral canal. J. Bone Joint Surg. *59B*:181–188, 1977.
117. Verbiest, H.: The significance and principles of CAT in idiopathic developmental stenosis of the bony lumbar vertebral canal. Spine *4*:369–377, 1979.

118. Verbiest, H.: Neurogenic intermittent claudication in cases with absolute and relative stenosis of the lumbar vertebral canal (ASLC and RSLC), in cases with narrow lumbar inter-vertebral foramina, and in cases with both entities. Clin. Neurosurg. *16*:204, 1972.
119. Voelker, J. L., Mealey, J., Eskridge, J., and Gilmore, R.: Metrizamide enhanced computed tomography as an adjunct to metrizamide myelography in the evaluation of lumbar disc herniation and spondylosis. Neurosurgery *20*:379–384, 1987.
120. Weisz, G.: Lumbar spinal canal stenosis in Paget's disease. Spine *8*:192–198, 1983.
121. Weisz, G. W., and Lee, P.: Spinal canal stenosis: concept of spinal reserve capacity: radiologic measurements and clinical applications. Clin. Orthop. *179*:134–140, 1983.
122. White, A., and Panjabi, M.: Clinical Biomechanics of the Spine. Philadelphia, J. B. Lippincott Co., 1978.
123. Wiesel, S. W., et al.: A study of computer assisted tomography: the incidence of positive CAT scans in an asymptomatic group of patients. Spine *9*:549–551, 1984.
124. Wilson, C. B.: Significance of the small lumbar spinal canal: cauda equina compression syndromes due to spondylosis. Part 3. Intermittent claudication. J. Neurosurg. *31*:499, 1969.
125. Wilson, C. B., Ehni, G., and Grollmus, J.: Neurogenic intermittent claudication. J. Neurosurg. *31*:499, 1969.
126. Wiltse, L. L., et al.: The treatment of spinal stenosis. Clin. Orthop. *115*:83–91, 1976.
127. Winston, K., Rumbargh, C., and Colucci, V.: The vertebral canal in lumbar disc disease. Spine *9*:414, 1984.
128. Witt, I., Vestegaard, A., and Rosenklit, A.: A comparative analysis of x-ray findings of a lumbar spine in patients with and without lumbar pain. Spine *9*:398–400, 1984.
129. Witwer, G., et al.: Iopamidol and metrizamide for myelography: prospective double-blind clinical trial. A.J.N.R. *5*:403–407, 1984.

NONOPERATIVE AND OPERATIVE TREATMENT

Steven R. Garfin, M.D.
Harry N. Herkowitz, M.D.
Srdjan Mirkovic, M.D.
Robert E. Booth, Jr., M.D.

NONOPERATIVE CARE

The nonoperative management of spinal stenosis uses, for the most part, modalities similar to those necessary to treat pain from lumbar disc degeneration and disease. The cyclic course of the process, which is frequently seen in the early stages, lends itself to some success in nonoperative management of symptoms. However, since the stenosis generally persists, and if it does not slowly progress, many of these patients (unlike younger patients with a herniated disc) may ultimately need surgical decompression. It must be kept in mind that this is an older population, many of whom have significant medical risk factors that may contraindicate surgical intervention.

In most of these patients, leg pain increases with activity and decreases somewhat with rest. However, this age group often cannot afford inactivity. Heart and lung rehabilitation frequently mandates ambulation and activity, which is often restricted by pain. Therefore, attempts to diminish discomfort in a nonoperative fashion often meet with a degree of success, and therefore satisfaction, on the patient's part. Limited activity does not mean bed rest, which in older individuals may be detrimental, but rather restriction of activities such as reduced lifting, twisting, and repeated forward bending. It should be emphasized to patients that their symptoms generally will not lead to paralysis or loss of bowel or bladder function, and that if they can tolerate the pain, they can participate in nearly all activities that are enjoyable or necessary to them.

Physical therapy, particularly in the form of deep heat, ultrasonography, and massage, may alleviate some of the low back symptoms associated with degenerating discs and spinal stenosis. Often, however, this provides only temporary relief, and individuals on limited income cannot afford it on a regular basis. Nevertheless, for acute flare-ups, physical therapeutic "passive" modalities may have some utility. Traction, on the other hand, has little effect on the neurogenic claudication component of stenosis and should not be routinely employed. Gravity traction, which has been shown to be effective in the short term for low back pain, has not proved useful in this older age group with symptoms of spinal stenosis.

In our opinion one of the main benefits of physical therapy is to help the patient initiate an exercise program. This program should consist of aerobic exercise (e.g., stationary bicycle, treadmill, swimming, water exercise, brisk walking) that is tolerated by the cardiopulmonary system but is aerobic in nature, improving conditioning and fitness and helping to release endogenous endorphins to ease pain.

Anti-inflammatory medication, particularly on a short-term basis, may reduce the symptoms of low back and leg pain. Most of these, however, must be used cautiously in older individuals because of the associated risks of harm to the renal and hepatic systems and of sodium retention, and therefore hypertension. As with other forms of arthritis, anti-inflammatory agents may provide some relief and should be considered to help decrease pain and increase the patient's tolerance of activity. Frequent monitoring of renal function, liver function, and blood pressure should be performed when these medications are used on a regular basis. Muscle relaxants tend to sedate older patients and are not usually recommended for symptoms of spinal stenosis. The pain in these patients is related to nerve compromise and not muscle spasm per se.

A lumbosacral corset may be a useful adjunct in individuals with a significant component of low back pain and degenerative joint disease. The corset provides some abdominal support and serves to remind the patient to restrict lumbar motion. Studies have shown a diminution in abdominal tone when a corset is worn for over six weeks. It should therefore be emphasized that the corset is most useful when, for example, the individual is in a car or is up and about for a prolonged period. It should not be worn during sleep or during regular household activities. Isometric abdominal and aerobic exercises should also be encouraged.

A course of epidural steroid injections may also be considered. In this age group, subject to progressive degeneration, symptomatic relief may be temporary. However, the injections may diminish the pain and allow an increased level of function.

A transcutaneous neuroelectric stimulator (TENS) may also have a role to play. This is reserved for older individuals who cannot tolerate surgery or for whom the risk of a surgical procedure may be so great (as in a patient with marked scoliosis, osteoporosis, and advanced age) that an operation would be unwise or the anticipated results less than satisfactory. In these instances a TENS unit has provided some degree of relief. There may not be strong scientific evidence that it is useful on a routine basis, but it does provide some degree of comfort in selected individuals.

One final medication category to consider is antidepressants. At low dosages these drugs have an effect on neurogenic-type pain that is probably related to alterations in cell membrane characteristics or metabolism. Also in low dosages, taken at nighttime, they have a sedative effect. Often, older individuals with increasing pain and decreasing social support mechanisms (family, friends, finance) are depressed, with sleepless nights and decreased activity. The antidepressants (such as amitriptyline, 25 to 50 mg at night) appear to supply some pain relief, may offer a minor degree of antidepressant activity, and help produce sounder sleep. In many patients this is beneficial, at least in allowing increased daytime activity. Which of the components of the anti-depressants' effect provides improvement is unclear, but they may be worth considering in individuals strongly opposed to surgery or medically incapable of tolerating it.

In patients with established symptoms of neurogenic claudication, physical therapy and other nonoperative measures are useful to diminish pain in the short term, but rarely provide long-term relief. In our experience, patients continue to function with a steadily reduced activity level, often becoming more and more sedentary. This may occur so gradually that they do not realize how much their life style has been altered. For individuals with significant daily activity restrictions due to neurogenic claudication, associated with positive imaging studies, surgery often provides the most effective and long-lasting relief. However, the nonoperative approach may provide some relief and allow older patients to prepare for an operation. Although most individuals would actively choose surgery, older patients are often more frightened and more resistant to this than others and need more time to be medically and mentally prepared.

OPERATIVE TREATMENT

Surgery for spinal stenosis is one of the more extensive and technically demanding, yet common, procedures performed on the spine. Surgical success hinges on an in-depth understanding of the pathophysiology involved and a thorough knowledge of spinal anatomy. Insight into spinal instability is also required. A simple and disciplined approach, despite the wide spectrum of surgical pathology and diversity of surgical skills involved, should yield almost the same excellent results as disc surgery, although symptoms may last longer and the patients may be significantly older.[7, 8, 17, 33, 46, 54, 55]

An unsuccessful decompressive laminectomy leads to a "failed back" with decreasing rates of good results and increasing disability with each subsequent salvage attempt. This can have particularly disastrous consequences in older patients with their associated complicated medical histories and perhaps already limited function.

Evaluation of the surgical records of patients who have had unsuccessful spinal surgery reveals four problems that often beset the surgical treatment of this disorder.[4] These are highlighted in the following discussion and include (1) techniques of hemostasis; (2) surgical orientation; (3) delineation of what constitutes an adequate decompression of cauda equina, as well as of the individual spinal nerve roots; and (4) indications for the appropriate use of spinal stabilization, including instrumentation.

Techniques of Spinal Stenosis Surgery

Positioning

The kneeling position with the chest and knees supporting the body, and the abdomen hanging free, is currently favored by most spine surgeons (Fig. 25–76). With the abdomen hanging uncompressed, intra-abdominal pressure is reduced and the epidural veins are not compromised. This reduces hemorrhage and facilitates visualization of the neural elements, as well as the surgical pathology. It also significantly decreases the risk for postoperative epidural hematoma development. A number of surgical positioning frames are available that support the patient in this position. The potential for deep venous thrombosis and subsequent pulmonary embolism in this flexed position can be reduced through the use of elastic stockings (to decrease venous pooling) and pulsed, alternating air stockings. These should be worn intra- and postoperatively.

The kneeling position also gives the surgeon the option of placing the lumbar spine in flexion or hyperextension. The hyperextended position increases the difficulty of performing a laminectomy and decompressing the neural elements and the facet joints because of "shingling" of the posterior elements. However, unlike the flexed position, it most closely duplicates the anatomic configuration and therefore the associated stenosis of a standing individual. Thus, with the spine in the hyperextended posture, a more accurate assessment of the stenosis can be made and a more appropriate surgical decompression undertaken. In addition, complete decompression in the extended position assures the adequacy of the decompression in almost any other position the patient may assume once ambulatory and independent.

Determination of the appropriate level for the spinal incision begins with examination of the anteroposterior radiograph, placed as if the examiner were viewing the patient's back; i.e., the patient's right side on the radiograph is placed to the right side on the view box and corresponds to the examiner's right side. One should search for spinal anomalies such as transitional vertebrae, asymmetric transverse processes, and other structural irregularities that may help identify specific levels during dissection. The anteroposterior film is particularly important in ruling out spina bifida, as this may avoid the potentially disastrous consequences of plunging a sharp instrument through the defect into the cauda equina. The information gained from the films can then be used to guide the palpation of the lumbar spine, which in the kneeling position is relatively subcutaneous in most individuals. An assessment of the distance between and the size of the spinous processes, as well as the presence of a step-off, may indicate the location of the lumbosacral junction, while detection of the iliac crest level, discounting the supplemental thickness of skin, fat, and muscle, can often help determine the correct interspaces.

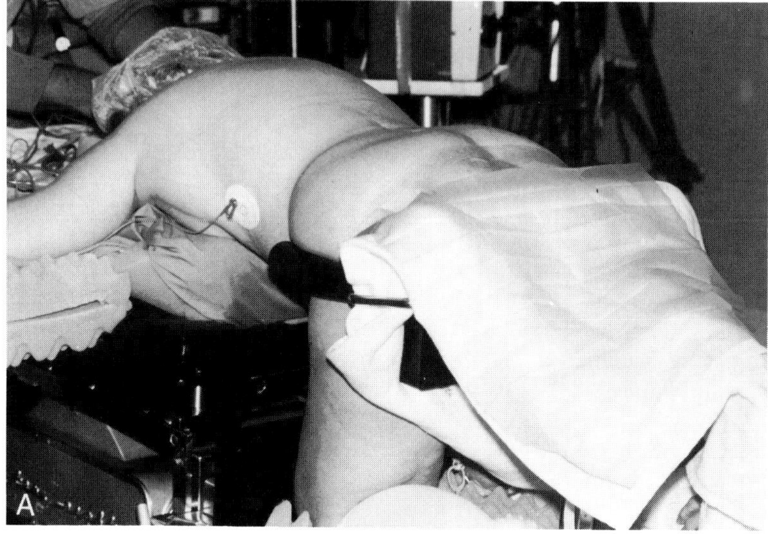

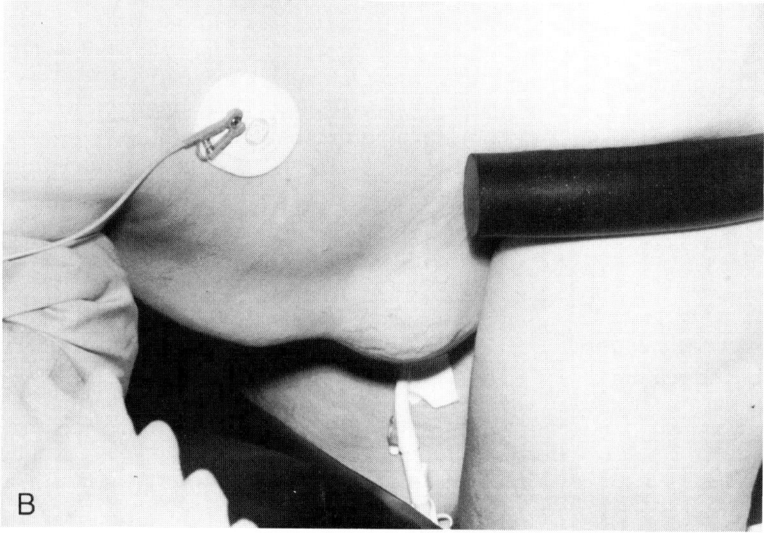

Figure 25–76. Kneeling position used for laminectomy and spinal fusion. *A*, Lateral padding is used to stabilize the patient, who is held caudally by the use of a seat to prevent extreme flexion at the knees and hips. Elastic stockings or elastic bandages are used to prevent pooling of blood in the calf area. *B*, Note how, even in this obese patient, the abdomen is completely free, preventing any pressure on the vena cava.

Spinal Incision

Before the initial incision is made, the paravertebral muscles can be infiltrated with a 1:500,000 epinephrine in saline solution. The incision is made in the midline directly over the spinous processes. The dissection is carried down through the dermis and the subcutaneous fat to the whitish lumbodorsal fascia, a very thick structure easily determined by its consistency and color. The lumbodorsal fascia envelops the erector spinae muscles, coalescing with the psoas fascia anteriorly and the periosteum of the laminae and the spinous processes medially (Fig. 25–77). It is useful to preserve this envelope by performing a subperiosteal dissection to the bony elements of the spine. This avoids violating the intramuscular vessels and thus causing unnecessary hemorrhage, which is often difficult to control. A further clue to the site of the lumbosacral junction can be obtained by appreciating the decussation of the fascial fibers of the lumbodorsal fascia at the L5–S1 interspace. Self-retaining retractors are placed at each end of the wound, while skin and fascial vessels are coagulated with electrocautery. It is imperative that all blood vessels be coagulated as they are encountered, at each step of the dissection.

The subperiosteal dissection is begun by scoring the spinous processes with electrocautery. We prefer to retract the soft tissues bilaterally with Hibbs retractors as we carefully begin dissection of the spinous processes' pos-

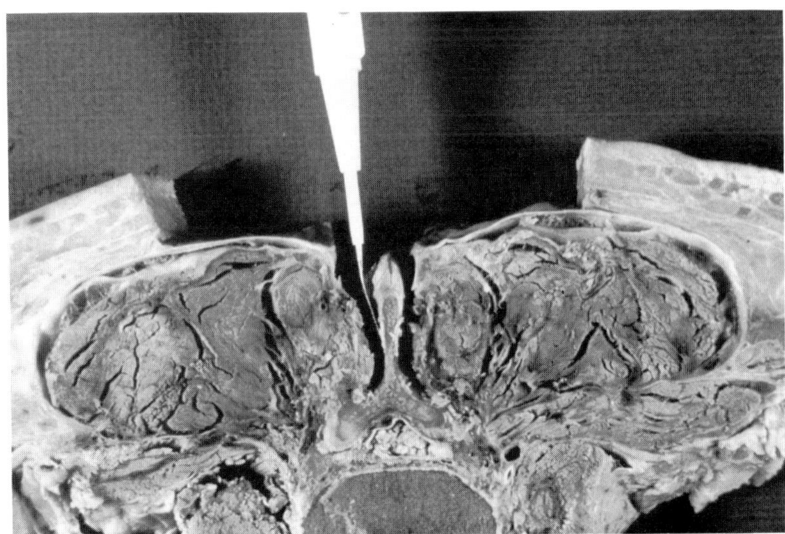

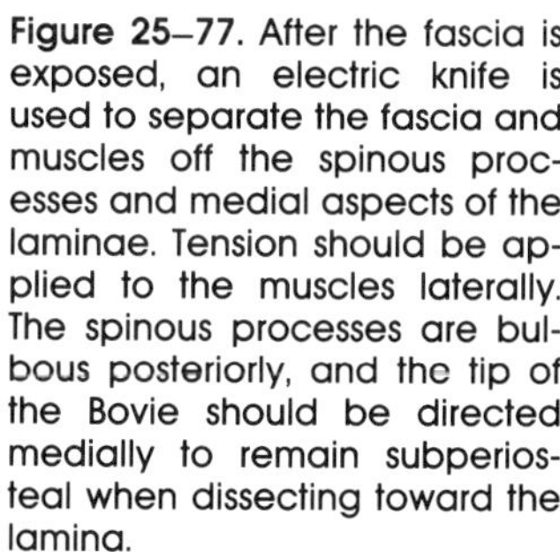

Figure 25–77. After the fascia is exposed, an electric knife is used to separate the fascia and muscles off the spinous processes and medial aspects of the laminae. Tension should be applied to the muscles laterally. The spinous processes are bulbous posteriorly, and the tip of the Bovie should be directed medially to remain subperiosteal when dissecting toward the lamina.

terior enlargements (Fig. 25–77). These bulbous posterior tips are part of the pathophysiology of spinal degeneration and should be recognized in order to avoid plunging directly anteriorly into the paraspinal envelope of fascia and muscle. One should note that paraspinal muscles attach obliquely from caudal-lateral to cephalad-medial. Therefore, a cleaner dissection can be achieved by proceeding in this direction (caudal to cephalad) and keeping the dissecting instruments close to the bone.

Once the paravertebral muscles have been separated from the spinous processes with electrocautery, lateral exposure of the laminae to the facet joints is carried out using periosteal elevators (Cobb elevators) in a scraping fashion (Fig. 25–78). This can be facilitated by pushing a sponge ahead of the elevator, which at the same time achieves hemostasis through a tamponade effect. Even the most effective subperiosteal dissection leaves some short muscle fibers attached to the laminae and ligamentum flavum. These can be excised, or removed, with a large curet or rongeurs, preferably moving from the lateral area of the facet joint to the midline of the spinous process in order not to traumatize the perifacetal arteries, or the paraspinal muscles laterally.

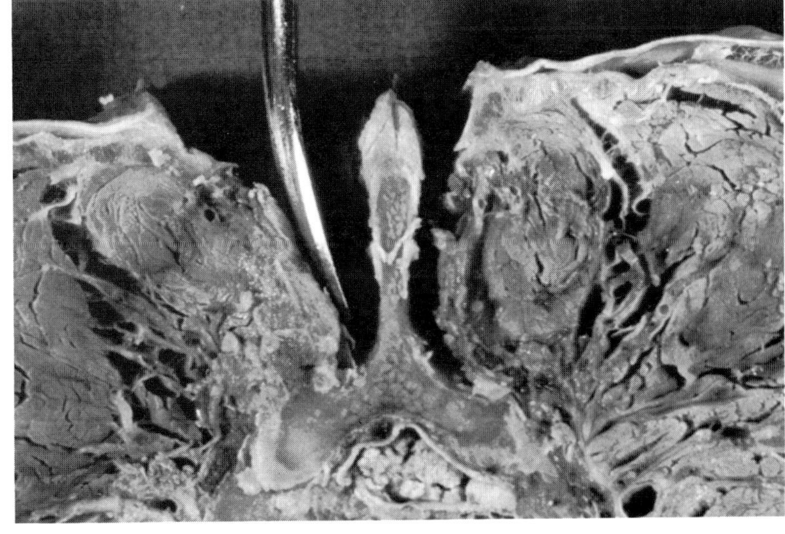

Figure 25–78. A subperiosteal elevator is used to complete the subperiosteal dissection over the laminae and out to the facets.

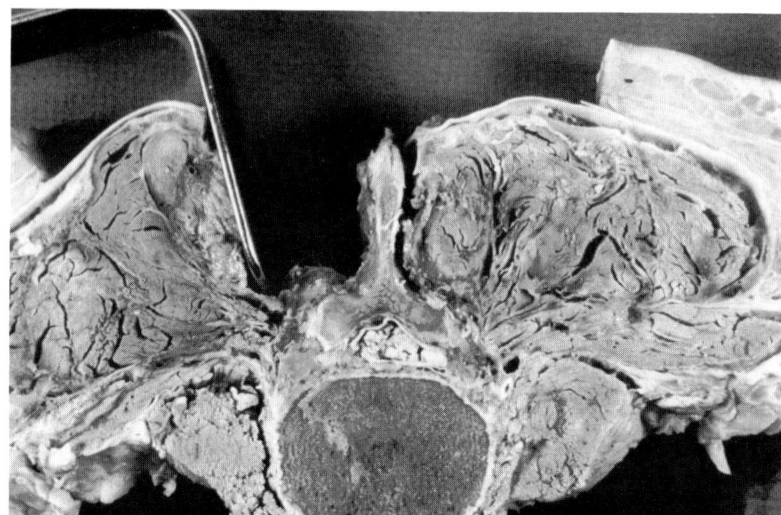

Figure 25–79. At this point self-retaining retractors can be applied. Further soft tissue debridement of the spinous processes, laminae, and interlaminar spaces should be performed.

At this time self-retaining instruments are placed to retract the paraspinal muscles (Fig. 25–79). If a fusion is planned, further dissection to the tips of the transverse processes is required and may be performed at this time (Fig. 25–80). Many types of self-retaining and hand-held retractors have been devised. We prefer to use the Taylor retractor for a one-level unilateral approach because of its safety, simplicity, and ease of transfer. Taylor retractors are held with the help of a gauze connected to the surgeon's foot and wrapped around the retractor handle. These retractors use the facet joints as the point of leverage and are slid down the spinous processes and out obliquely along the lamina over the edge of the facet joint. In most cases, however, multilevel decompression is needed, for which we commonly use the Crank Retractor (Codman). This modular retractor, with blades of varying depths and widths, allows for adaptation to the individual morphologic structures and provides increased visualization of the surgical field. Additional retraction in the caudal and cephalad corners is facilitated with cerebellar retractors. If spinal fusion is not planned, the tips of the blades are carefully placed over the facet joints to ensure preservation of the facet capsules, as well as their innervation and muscular attachments.

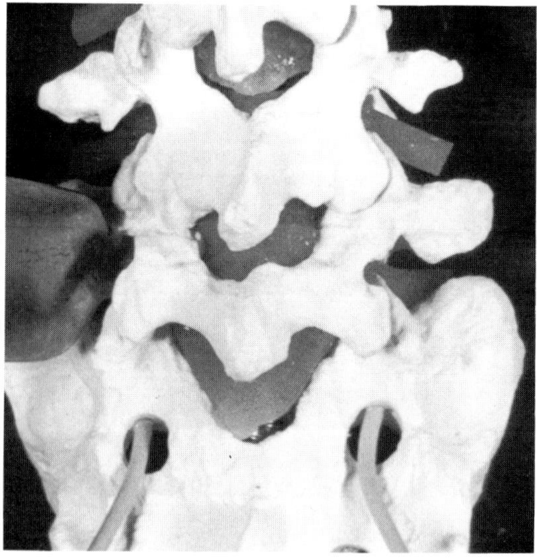

Figure 25–80. At the completion of the dissection, the laminae, the facets, and if necessary the transverse processes of the appropriate segments to be fused should be exposed. Hemostasis should be performed at each tissue level to maximize visualization in the depth of the wound.

If a fusion is planned, paravertebral muscles are elevated laterally with the aide of Hibbs or Cobb elevators, separating muscular attachments from bone and facets with electrocautery. This dissection is carried over the facet joints, sacrificing the capsules, and extending laterally to the tip of the transverse processes (Fig. 25–80). Bleeding within the soft tissue between the transverse processes is carefully coagulated using bayonet forceps and cautery. These exposed lateral gutters should then be packed off to create hemostasis while the decompressive laminectomy is undertaken.

Some additional bleeding may be encountered from the small facetal arteries that course

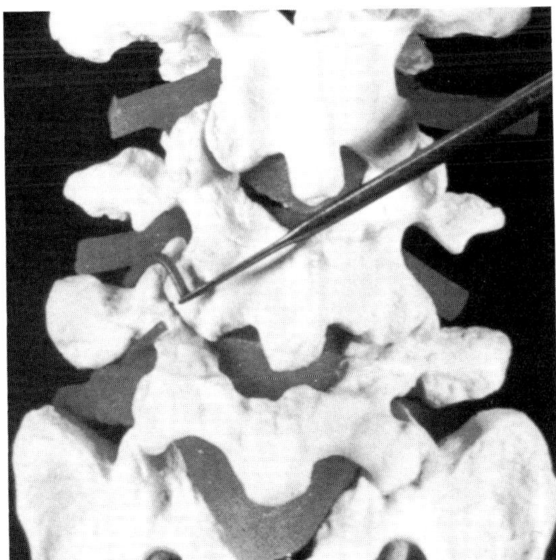

Figure 25–81. If the transverse processes are to be exposed, and particularly if pedicle screws are added, the small perifacetal vessels should be coagulated. These vessels course posteriorly toward the facet joints, cephalad and caudal to the transverse process. If stripping is performed rapidly in this area without attention to these vessels, brisk bleeding can be encountered, associated with significant blood loss. If the arteries are transected near the transverse processes, they may retract and be difficult to locate and coagulate.

around the medial aspect of each facet joint (Fig. 25–81). These vessels provide the primary source of intraoperative bleeding outside the spinal canal. Awareness of their location means that they often can be addressed before being transected.

Identification of Correct Level

Identification of the sacrum remains the most accurate anatomic technique for identifying the appropriate level during spinal surgery. However, if any questions exist as to location or level, intraoperative radiographs should be obtained. In fact, many surgeons routinely obtain intraoperative lateral radiographs before beginning the laminectomies. Identification of the sacrum is facilitated by palpating the termination of the interlaminar spaces, listening to the hollow sound of the sacrum when it is tapped by a dissecting instrument, and palpating the alar prominence laterally. Another useful technique is to grasp the spinous processes with towel clips to demonstrate the presence or absence of motion at the lowest level. Particular care in counting levels should be taken in the presence of transitional vertebrae, if these are demonstrated on the preoperative films. A sacralized transitional lumbar vertebra may at times lead to surgery at an incorrect level. This can be avoided by using the above techniques and by noting the presence of a narrowed lamina and fused facet joints and the location of the sacral foramina relative to the last mobile spinous process. Again, if there is any doubt about the correct level, a lateral intraoperative radiograph with a metallic instrument to mark the levels in question should be obtained. Lateral films with the patient in the kneeling position are easy to obtain and are relatively clear. It is far more prudent to spend additional time confirming the level of surgery than to decompress levels without surgical pathology. In our experience, surgery at the incorrect level generally tends to be too high, rather than too low. Exploration for the correct level should proceed proximally, once the sacrum has been identified and the orientation confirmed.

Surgical Anatomy

With the correct levels identified and the spine exposed with a clean, dry bed, and before opening the spinal canal itself, the surgical anatomy and the planned dissection should be reviewed. The surgeon should particularly note the correct location of the pedicles and the pars interarticularis. These usually are present, even after the remainder of the posterior spinal elements have been removed, and are therefore the key to the subsequent anatomic dissection, particularly in a repeat operation. It is easy to become disoriented once the usual posterior bony landmarks have been removed and the spinal canal is completely open. Pedicles are especially useful in locating and numbering nerve roots as they course around them, thus facilitating assessment of the two areas most commonly at risk for spinal stenosis, the lateral recess and the foramen. The pedicles are beneath the inferior corner of the facet joint, above the mamillary process, at the level of a line bisecting the two transverse processes of a vertebral body (Figs. 25–82 and 25–83).

Decompression

At this time we prefer to remove the spinous processes with a large bone biter such as a

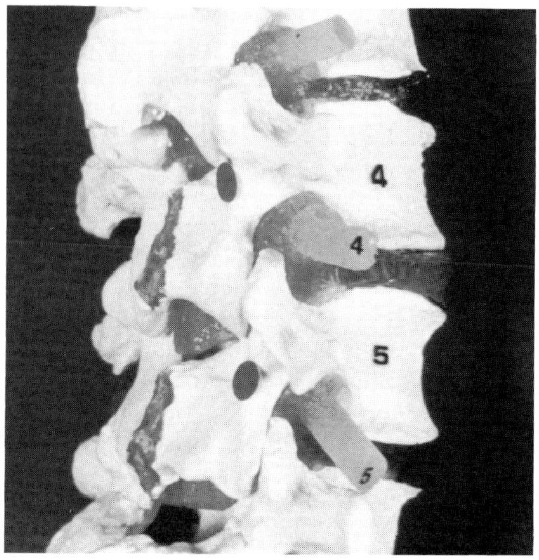

Figure 25–82. If the pedicles are to be entered *(small circles)* the pars interarticularis and mamillary processes should be well exposed. There is usually a bleeding vessel adjacent to the pars interarticularis that requires electrocoagulation.

Horsley rongeur (Fig. 25–84). Bleeding within the exposed venous sinuses of the soft cancellous bone can be controlled with the aid of bone wax.

Before bone is removed, the ligamentum

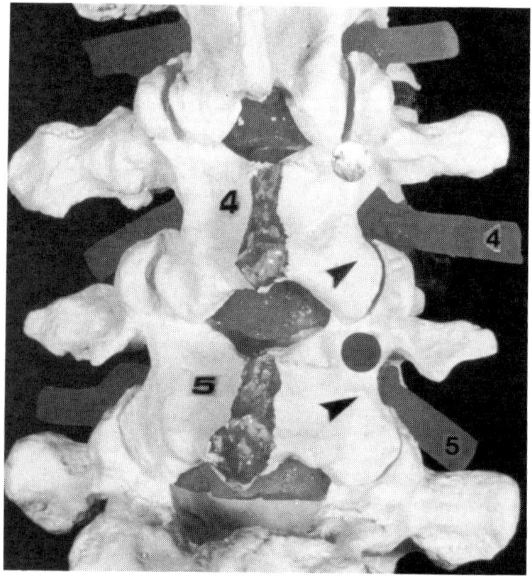

Figure 25–83. In this model the spinous processes have been removed, the facet joints exposed and cleaned, and the transverse processes identified. The center of the pedicle is under the circle at L5 (shown on the right). At L4 the pedicle has been entered.

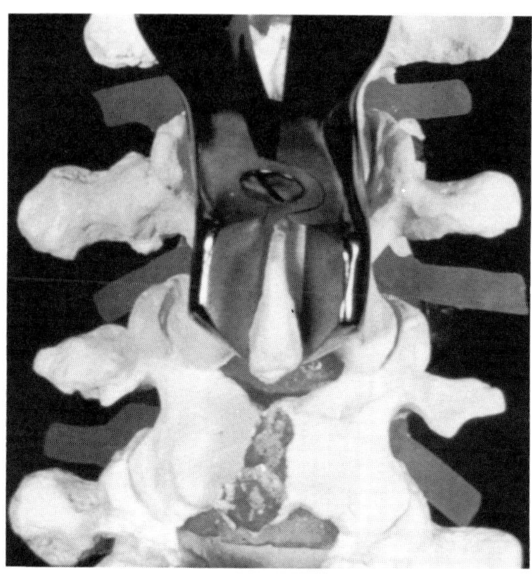

Figure 25–84. A bone cutter can be used to remove the spinous processes and intervening ligaments. Bone wax should be applied over the cancellous bone, as necessary.

flavum should be cleaned of soft tissue and exposed. A small, straight, long-handled curet is then used to gently dissect the insertion of the ligamentum flavum from the undersurface of the lamina of the vertebra above (Fig. 25–85). This need be done only to initiate the laminectomies at the most caudal level to be included. Curets are effective at this task, as they are easy to control; they also are relatively safe since they present a round bowl to the delicate neural elements beneath. This step, and all subsequent steps, are undertaken by beginning in the midline and proceeding laterally toward the facets and foramina. We prefer to proceed in this fashion because the midline of even the most narrow spinal canal is often the last area to develop significant stenosis, and consequently the safest area to begin a dissection.

To expedite the laminectomy, we prefer to thin the posterior aspect of the lamina of all involved segments with a rongeur, or a large cutting burr if the bone is extremely hard or thick. Throughout the procedure bleeding from cancellous bone should be controlled with bone wax (Fig. 25–83). This aids visualization more than reducing major blood loss.

With the inferior anterior surface of the laminar edge exposed, a Kerrison punch can be used to perform the midline laminectomy (Fig. 25–86), which is then extended to the

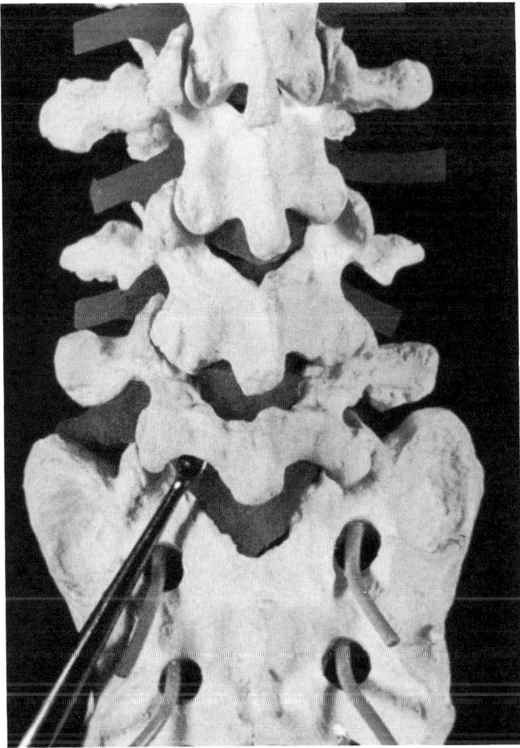

Figure 25–85. Before the laminectomy is begun a small curet can be placed under the inferior edge of the caudal lamina and used to separate the underlying ligamentum flavum from its insertion onto the lamina.

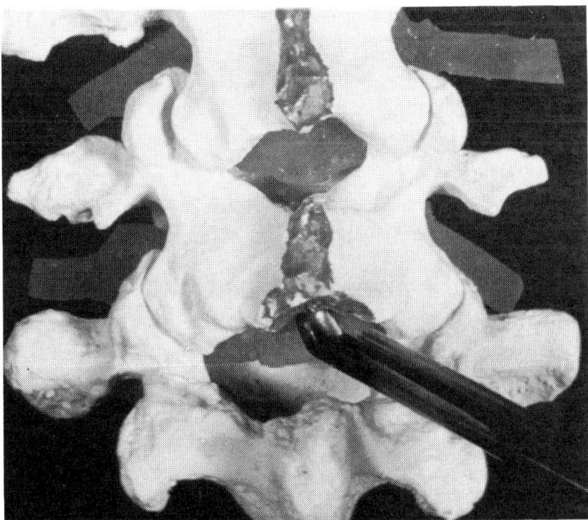

Figure 25–86. After separating the ligamentum flavum, a rongeur or Kerrison punch can be used to perform the midline laminectomy. The central laminectomy should be completed before proceeding laterally.

lateral edges of the dural sac (Fig. 25–87). The rounded edge of the Kerrison punch usually (but not always) protects the neural elements, particularly if dorsal pressure is exerted against the undersurface of the lamina. In patients with spinal stenosis the dura may be quite thin, and the epidural fat often may be absent, and the space available for instruments may be extremely narrow and treacherous. In inflammatory spondylopathies the dura may be adherent to the undersurface of the lamina, and even greater care must be taken in the dissection. We prefer to use a flat dental pick to dissect any adhesions of the dura to the bone itself, although a small, straight curet or a No. 4 Penfield dissector can be used. Generally, as we proceed cephalad with the laminar dissection, we employ a Penfield to palpate and ensure that the path ahead is free of any adhesions. When using the Kerrison, its shoe should be slid gently under the lamina parallel to it; it should not be forced and should not be rocked from side to side in removing pieces of bone. This helps protect the dura from abrasion or laceration by edges of the bony fragments. An awareness of the existing planes during lumbar laminectomy (lamina, ligamentum flavum, epidural fat, epidural veins, scar, and dura) leads to quicker and safer surgery, as well as early control of bleeding.

The final result of this part of the procedure is a central trough extending proximally and distally over the appropriate levels, and laterally to the medial edge of the facet joints (Fig. 25–87). The dura should be readily visible, and any residual bleeding from the epidural

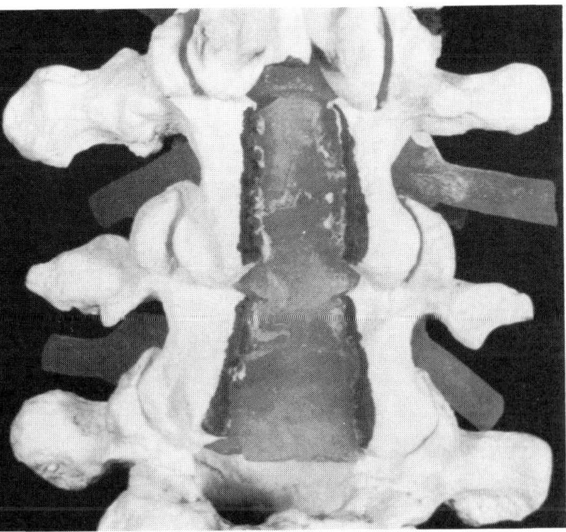

Figure 25–87. At this point the lateral edge of the thecal sac should be visible. No remaining central stenosis should be present.

vessels should be controlled by bipolar electrocautery, Surgicel, thrombin-impregnated Gelfoam, Avitene, and/or cottonoids. Once the decompressive laminectomy is completed centrally, the surgical field should be completely dry before proceeding to the examination of the spinal nerve roots. In young patients with central spinal stenosis due to a congenitally narrow spinal canal secondary to short pedicles, a central decompressive laminectomy alone may be adequate to alleviate neurologic symptoms.

In the vast majority of patients, however, the pathophysiology involves the lateral recess(es) and/or foraminal nerve root compression created by hypertrophic, arthritic superior facet joints, and prominent discs, in which case lateral recess decompressions and foraminotomies are necessary. An appreciation of the foraminal stenosis can be gained by placing an angled Frazier dural elevator from medial to lateral along the path of the nerve root(s) in question, out of the foramina (Fig. 25–88).

Foraminotomy is the most difficult part of the procedure, because nerve roots are often obliterated within the hypertrophied mass of the facets above, as well as surrounded by large epidural veins. To facilitate further decompression we prefer to unroof the lateral recess (Fig. 25–89) and the foramina by performing a less than 50 per cent medial facetectomy using straight osteotomes or Kerrison punches (Fig. 25–90). This should be undertaken carefully, avoiding the temptation to remove large fragments at one time. The dura, as well as the nerve root, must be visualized

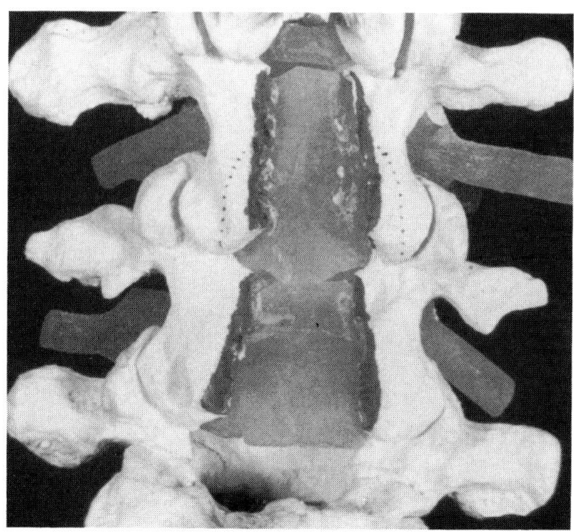

Figure 25–89. Widening of the laminectomy should be performed to decompress the nerve roots. If a total of one facet remains intact, there theoretically is enough structural support for a fusion to be unnecessary. However, concern over performing a fusion should not be the limiting factor, and the decompression should be performed as necessary to free the nerve. Use of a small spinal osteotome, or a Kerrison directed under the pars interarticularis and facet, may preserve stability and help avoid the need for a fusion.

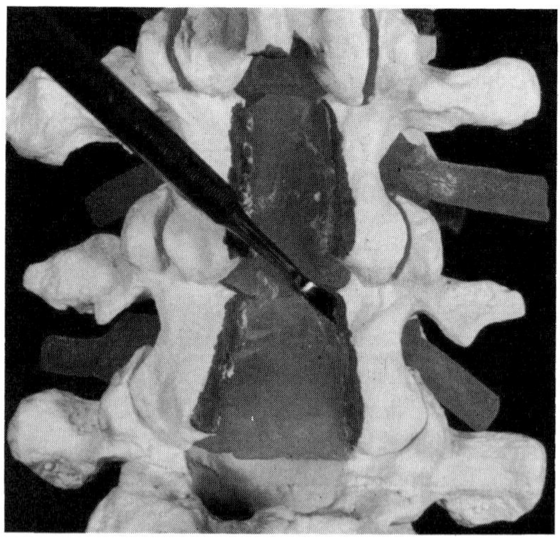

Figure 25–88. An angled Frazier elevator should be placed out along the nerve roots. If there is any obstruction to easy passage of this instrument, a widening of the laminectomy and a foraminotomy should be performed.

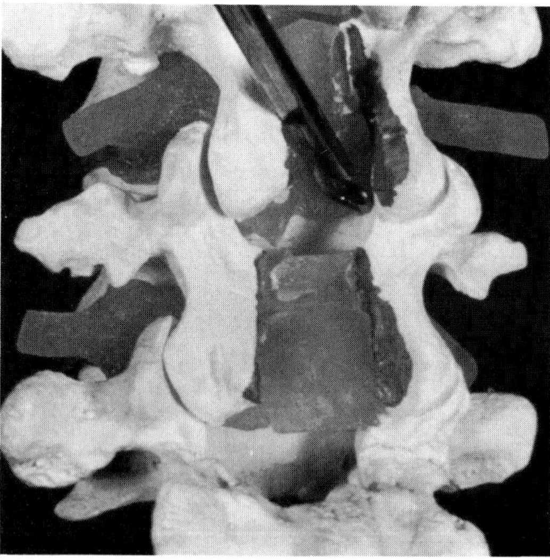

Figure 25–90. After the central laminectomy is completed, a Kerrison can be used to widen the laminectomy to the dural edge. In this model the Kerrison is angled from posteromedial to anterolateral to parallel the nerve roots. This minimizes the risk of transection of a nerve root with the instrument.

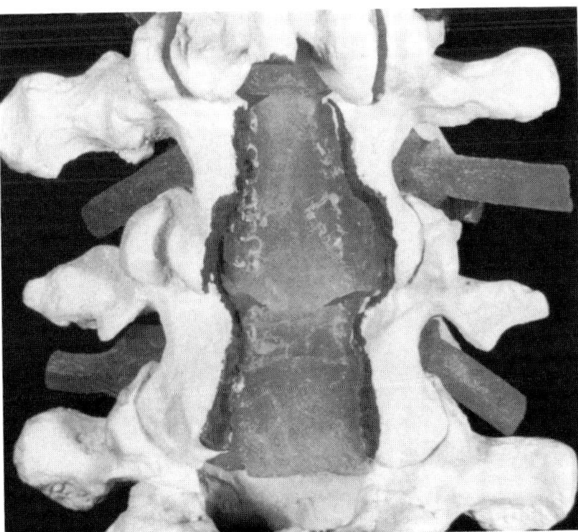

Figure 25–91. A completed laminectomy. The pars interarticularis has not been violated and a total of one facet (combining left and right at L4–L5) remains, so a fusion is not necessary.

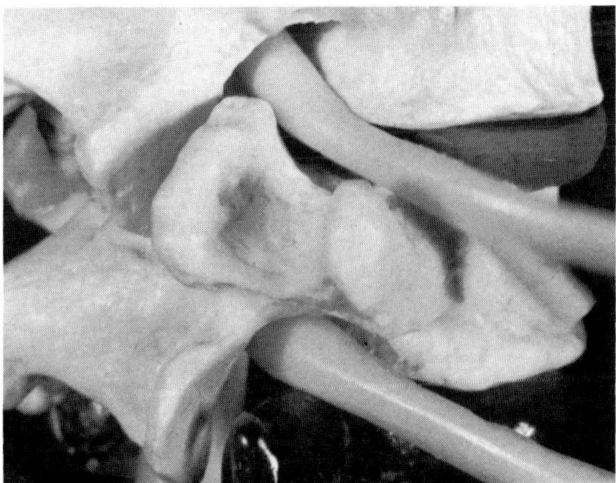

Figure 25–92. Occasionally the root is trapped between the posterior inferior edge of the vertebral body and bulging disc anteriorly and inferiorly, and the facet posteriorly.

and protected at all times by a Penfield elevator or cotton patties placed over the dura. At times a hypertrophied facet may be thinned down with a cutting burr. The more delicate, and directed, foraminotomy is performed with Kerrison rongeurs by undercutting the facets (Fig. 25–90), removing the encroachment of the lateral recess without, it is hoped, destabilizing the facet joint and therefore the spinal motion segment at that particular level. Troublesome bleeding is often encountered at this stage, and one must be patient in achieving hemostasis with bipolar electrocautery, as well as other hemostatic agents. Complete release of the lateral recess without jeopardizing spinal stability should be accomplished, if possible. However, in narrow canals with significant degenerative changes, facet stability is frequently compromised or lost (Fig. 25–91).

Neural Decompression

Crucial in the treatment of spinal stenosis[2, 3, 6] is successful handling of the intra- and extraforaminal sources of nerve compression. Although the anatomic variance causing foraminal and extraforaminal stenosis may be wide, four common problems should be considered when a nerve root, decompressed to the extent of the lateral recess, fails to move easily with direct palpation. The first involves entrapment of the spinal nerve root between the superior facet of one vertebra and the inferior posterolateral aspect of the vertebral body above (Fig. 25–92). To resolve this, the surgeon needs to undercut the superior facet further, or at times excise the facet joint itself. A related problem is when the nerve root is caught between the superior facet of one vertebra and the inferior aspect of the pedicle of the vertebra above (Fig. 25–93). Here again the nerve can be freed by excising the tip of the superior facet, or less preferably the entire facet joint, or burring or curetting away the caudal edge of the pedicle (Fig. 25–94).

The most common of lateral syndromes is seen when the nerve root is entrapped between the bulging (often calcified) degenerated disc anteriorly, the pedicle superiorly, and the facet

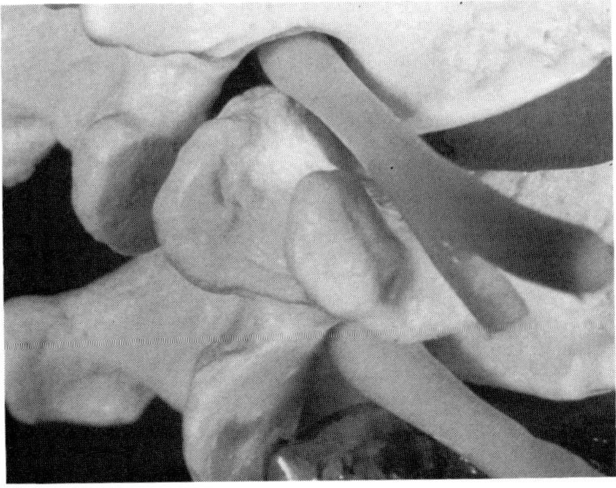

Figure 25–93. Viewing the nerve roots from lateral to the foramen demonstrates the possible compromise from the superior facet of the caudal lamina. This can trap the nerve root between osteophytes posteriorly, the pedicle superiorly, and vertebral body/osteophyte and disc anteriorly and inferiorly.

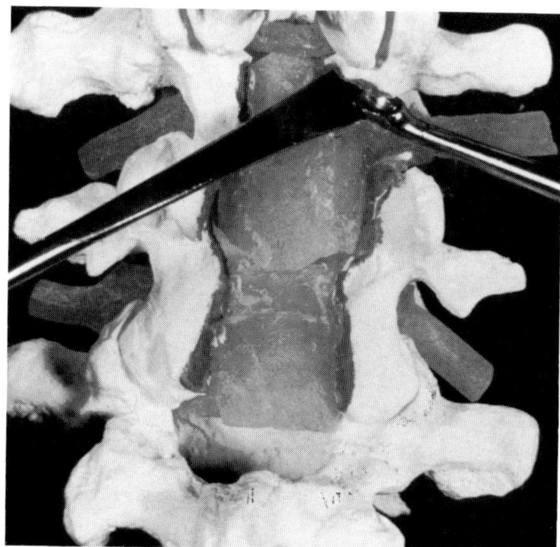

Figure 25–94. Occasionally, more often in spinal stenosis, a discectomy, particularly if there is an osteophytic ridge, cannot be performed or is not helpful. In this case the root should be retracted medially and protected, and a curet or small burr used to remove the inferomedial aspect of the pedicle and decompress the root.

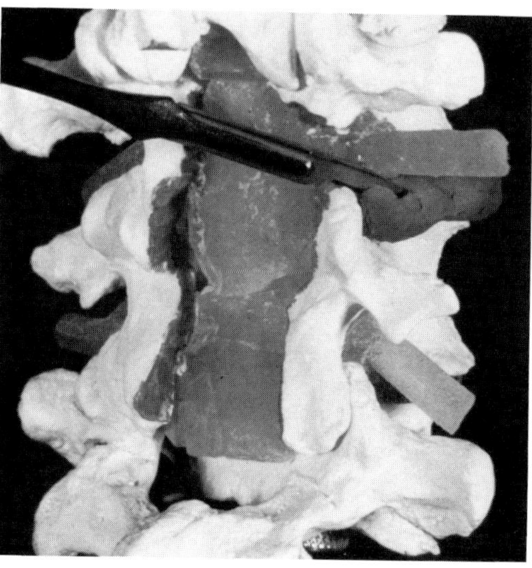

Figure 25–96. To completely free the nerve (see Fig. 25–95) requires a wide foraminotomy. When approached from the central aspect, through the laminectomy defect, it is not uncommon for the facets and pars to be removed. The root can then be retracted proximally and a knife used to excise the disc, as shown in this example.

of the adjacent vertebra posteriorly (Fig. 25–95). This hard and soft tissue problem, at times difficult to appreciate, is usually a consequence of severe disc degeneration that has led to collapse of the intervertebral disc, overriding of the facet joints, and diminution of the foraminal space. Two techniques can be used to resolve this problem. One is to excise the lateral annulus with a No. 15 blade (Fig. 25–96) or a straight pituitary rongeur (Fig. 25–97). A blade is preferable because it minimizes the scarring, which may cause the symptoms to recur. However, it is often difficult to remove hard, calcified, degenerative disc material. These techniques are complex and may

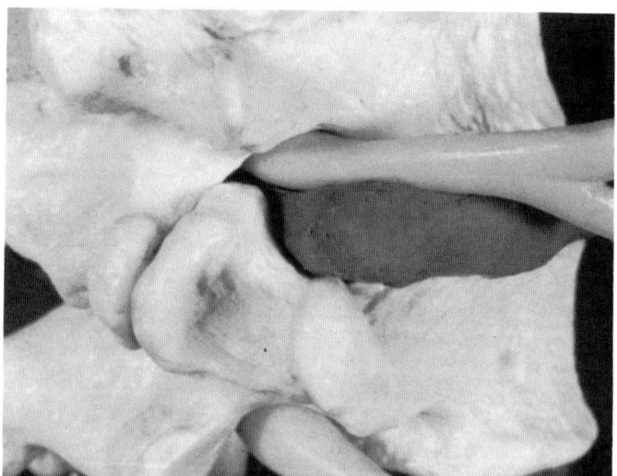

Figure 25–95. Occasionally the nerve is trapped laterally from a large herniated, or protruding, disc. This leads to entrapment of the root between the pedicle above, the disc below, and the facet posteriorly.

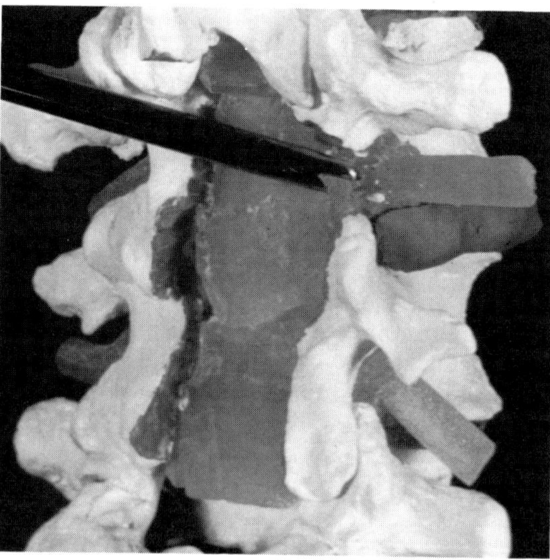

Figure 25–97. A pituitary rongeur can be used to remove disc fragments if they are soft, widen the lateral recess, and decompress the nerve root.

lead to subsequent fibrosis and recurrence of pain, so we often use a second approach, which involves taking down the inferomedial aspect of the vertebral pedicle with a curet or burr (see Fig. 25–94). All these delicate techniques entail a thorough visualization of the neural elements and adequate protection during the procedure itself. Hemostasis once again plays an important role.

The fourth pattern of lateral stenosis is related to degenerative spondylolisthesis. This is most commonly seen at the L4–L5 level. In this case the L5 root is caught between the L4–L5 disc, the superior posterior edge of the vertebral body of L5, and the advancing inferior face of L4 that has "eroded" into the L5 superior facet (Fig. 25–98). Again, appropriate treatment may entail freeing the entrapped nerve root at the expense of the facet joint.

Foraminotomies are often painstakingly difficult, the nerve root being entangled in fibrous, inflammatory tissues and epidural veins. However, despite the potential for instability, root decompression must be completed even if bilateral foraminotomies have to be performed at each level.

Accuracy of Decompression

This is an area in which the surgeon unfortunately must rely heavily on experience, judgment, and the "feel" of the decompressed nerve root. The best general guideline is to "think nerve." CT and MRI scans are only guidelines to the site of the pathology. Surgeons must rely on their tactile and visual senses at the time of surgery to ensure that the central canal, the lateral recesses, the foramina, and all nerve roots are free of compression. This must be done while bearing in mind the occasionally delicate balance between complete neural freedom and spinal stability/instability. No surgical dissection should be terminated until each nerve root at jeopardy is no longer mechanically compromised. A disciplined systematic approach, addressing each entity causing stenosis and paying careful attention to hemostasis, will usually lead to a successful clinical result. At this point a fusion should be performed if indicated (Fig. 25–99).

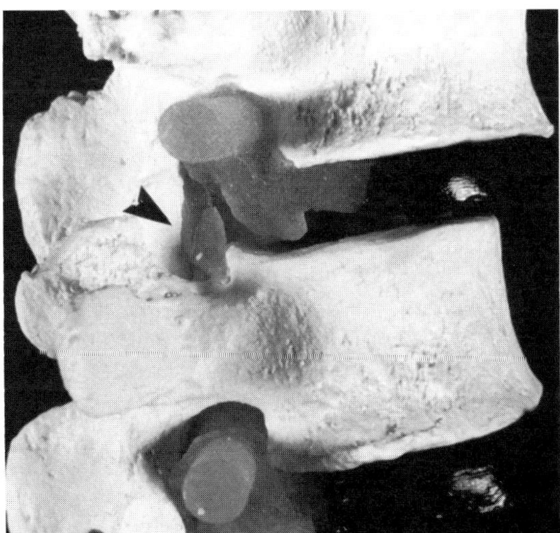

Figure 25–98. Anterolisthesis of the cephalic vertebra. The nerve root *(arrowhead)* is "dragged" anteriorly and trapped by the facets posteriorly and disc and body anteriorly.

Fusion: Indications

Usually the indications for decompression of the lumbar spine to treat the symptoms and signs of spinal stenosis are relatively straightforward. The most common decisions are how long and how wide the laminectomy and root exploration should be. Increasingly, however, concerns relating to the risk of decompression include issues of stability and whether fusion and/or instrumentation without anatomic realignment should be performed. These issues, unfortunately, remain unsolved and difficult to define. In the late 1970s, while Tile and associates coined the phrase "think nerve" as related to the surgical decompression for spinal stenosis, they brought to light the importance of the mechanical compression of the nerve and the need to completely free it posteriorly, superiorly, inferiorly, and laterally to relieve the symptoms of spinal stenosis.[56] However, more extreme decompression may compromise the stability provided by the facet joints, leading to increased incidences of postoperative instability and spondylolisthesis. This created its own problems and additional failed back surgery syndromes.

The literature contains a number of articles regarding fusion after lumbar laminectomy for spinal stenosis, particularly in association with decompressive surgery in patients with preexisting degenerative spondylolisthesis.[3, 7–10, 14, 15, 18, 23–26, 30, 32, 36, 43, 60] Few of these articles, however, are prospective double-blinded studies, the majority being retrospective or chart re-

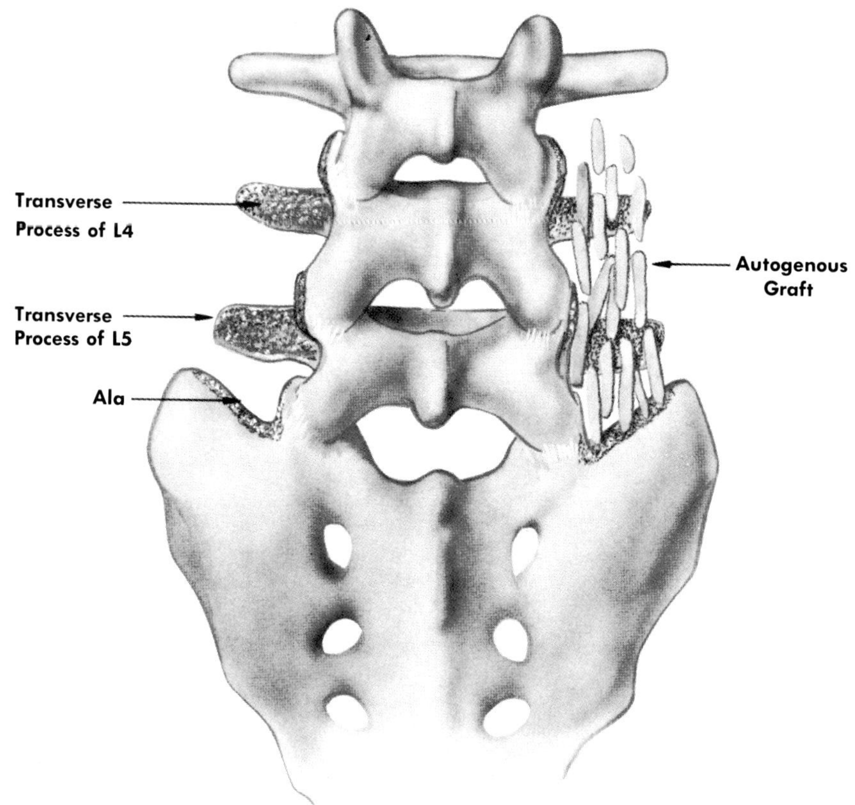

Figure 25–99. On the left is shown the area of decorticated raw cancellous bone for a lateral spine fusion from L4 to the sacrum. The bed is shown on the left and the graft material is in place on the right. In fact a much larger volume of graft material is used. The fusion area includes the transverse processes, the ala of the sacrum, the lateral portion of the pedicle, and the lateral portion of the superior articular facets.

views. Nonetheless, sufficient information is presently available in the literature on which patient selection for a spinal fusion can be based.

We will try to define the indications for fusion after spinal stenosis decompression, and determine which factors, if any, can help predict which patients will benefit from a spine fusion performed at the time of lumbar laminectomy for spinal stenosis.

Rosenberg in 1975 presented one of the first reports in the literature directed toward lumbar decompression in patients with degenerative spondylolisthesis.[49] He described a 10 per cent incidence of postoperative slips in 29 patients who had extensive decompression. There was no correlation between slippage and surgical outcome.

A number of papers have been contributed by Wiltse and associates.[38, 60–62] Writing with Lombardi and colleagues, they compared wide decompression, midline decompression with attempt to preserve a portion of the facet joints, and decompression and fusion in 47 patients (including 40 women) undergoing surgery for degenerative spondylolisthesis.[38] The mean age was 65 years. Forty of these patients had degenerative spondylolisthesis at L4–L5, five at L3–L4, and one at L5–S1. One had multiple-level spondylolisthesis. The spondylolisthesis patient who had decompression with only partial medial facetectomy had an 80 per cent chance of an excellent or good result. If a more radical decompression was performed, for the most part removing complete facet joints, but not including fusion, excellent and good rates dropped to 33 per cent. If, after a wide decompression, a fusion was added, the excellent to good rate was 90 per cent. In this series the best results were in the latter group of patients: those undergoing decompression and fusion. These authors noted two important factors that contributed to the development of the postoperative slip: (1) a preoperative disc height greater than 6 mm and (2) the extent of facet decompression. They also noted that a postoperative slip of more than 50 per cent of the vertebral body width was often associated with pain and a poor result. They concluded that in most cases of degenerative spondylolisthesis when fusion was not included, most patients postoperatively developed a progression of the slip.

White and Wiltse reviewed 182 cases of extensive laminectomies, of which 120 were for lumbar disc herniation and 15 were in patients who had degenerative spondylolisthesis.[60] Of the 182 cases, 13 (7 per cent) developed a slip postoperatively. Ten of these 13 (60 per cent) were decompressions associated with degenerative spondylolisthesis. Because of these results, the authors recommended fusion when decompression for degenerative spondylolisthesis is performed. On the basis of the results of this review, and of other work by the senior author, White and Wiltse developed criteria for spinal fusion in conjunction with decompression for spinal stenosis. These were: (1) a patient who is 60 years of age or less, with a degenerative spondylolisthesis, particularly when a total facetectomy is performed; (2) a patient 55 years of age or less, with degenerative spondylolisthesis; and (3) a patient under 50 with isthmus spondylolisthesis. These recommendations appear relatively straightforward, but because of physiologic differences in individuals, variations in anatomy, and varying surgical techniques and requirements, it is difficult to base decisions solely on age; many other factors intervene and must be considered.

Feffer and associates in 1985 reported 19 patients undergoing surgery for degenerative spondylolisthesis.[14] Eleven of these underwent decompression only, while eight had decompression and bilateral fusions. In the group of patients with fusions, the authors reported 100 per cent success in relieving pain. Of those without a fusion, the results in eight of 11 (72 per cent) were described as good to excellent. Four of these latter patients were noted to have a postoperative slip, but this was not correlated to the results in the report. Brown and Lockwood described postoperative slipping in two of 17 patients (12 per cent) who underwent decompression for symptoms of spinal stenosis with degenerative spondylolisthesis.[7] The mean age of their patients was 63.5 years. The authors concluded that postoperative slip correlated with a poor result. Because of this, although the patient numbers were small, they recommended fusion along with decompression when spondylolisthesis exists, regardless of age. Lee reported 27 patients who underwent surgical decompression for spinal stenosis.[36] Of these, five had decompression only and 22 had decompression and fusion. He observed that 3.7 per cent of the patients slipped postoperatively. Of patients who had presurgical degenerative spondylolisthesis, all had an increase in the amount of slip postoperatively. Herron and Trippi described their large series of patients with decompression for spinal stenosis.[26] They observed an 84 per cent improvement rate in low back pain and 92 per cent improvement in leg pain. However, in this group of patients who had undergone decompression without fusion, only 17 per cent had *complete* relief of back pain and 54 per cent noted *complete* leg pain relief. Dall and Rowe compared six patients undergoing laminectomy and complete facetectomy with 11 who underwent laminectomy and foraminotomy with preservation of a portion of the facets.[10] No fusion was performed in these patients. In addition, discectomy was performed in two of those undergoing radical decompression and in six with decompression with partial facetectomies. The authors observed slipping of up to 3 mm postoperatively in both groups, with a 53 per cent overall improvement rate. Bolesta and Bohlman compared results in 24 patients with decompression only against those in 18 patients who underwent decompression and fusion for degenerative spondylolisthesis.[3] Overall, the satisfactory results were 50 per cent in the decompression group and 100 per cent in those patients who underwent decompression and fusion. Two of the 24 in the decompression group noted no pain, while 13 of 18 in the fusion group reported no pain. Leg pain was present in three of 24 when only decompression was performed and two of 18 when a fusion was added. A progressive slip was observed in 17 of the patients who had decompression without fusion and 10 when fusion was added to the decompression. Patients who were fused had less back and leg pain, less postoperative slippage, and significantly better results than the group with decompression only. The authors recommended posterolateral fusion following decompression for spinal stenosis associated with degenerative spondylolisthesis.

Unfortunately, most of the studies reviewed above were retrospective or associated with chart review. The first prospective study in the English language literature was reported by Johnsson and colleagues, who evaluated 45 patients who had undergone decompression for spinal stenosis.[29] The mean age in this series was 64 years, with a mean follow-up of 46 months. Sixty-five per cent (13 of 18) of the patients with degenerative spondylolisthesis slipped postoperatively, compared with 20 per cent (five of 25) of patients who had spinal stenosis without associated degenerative spondylolisthesis. However, in the 13 patients with degenerative spondylolisthesis who had increased slippage postoperatively, seven were classified as a good result, while five patients with the postoperative slip following laminectomy for stenosis, but no preoperative slippage, were all classified as poor results. The authors thought the reason might be that the nerve roots had already adapted to some degree of deformity/tension when a preoperative spondylolisthesis existed. Because of this increase of slippage in patients undergoing lumbar laminectomy for spinal stenosis, Johnsson and colleagues recommended fusion if the structural integrity of the facets was disturbed. A follow-up study by Johnsson and colleagues on 61 patients who had undergone decompression for spinal stenosis (31 patients) or spinal stenosis associated with degenerative spondylolisthesis (30 patients) noted vertebral slipping in eight patients who had good results and in 18 who had poor results.[30] In this group of patients, 40 were male and 21 female. The mean age was 65 years. No patient had an associated fusion with the laminectomy. The authors identified what they considered to be significant factors leading to *increased slippage:* (1) a female patient, (2) a difference in flexion-extension radiographs, (3) patients who underwent complete facetectomy at surgery, and (4) patients with preexisting degenerative spondylolisthesis. The significant factors leading to a *poor surgical result* in this study were (1) a female patient, (2) a significant difference in flexion-extension radiographs, and (3) a postoperative slip. If the presurgical factors exist, fusion at the time of surgery might be considered. However, these data are not included in this important and useful paper. In this regard, Hopp and Tsou suggested the following criteria for fusion in patients undergoing decompression for spinal stenosis: (1) slippage greater than 2 mm, or a lumbar scoliosis of 10 degrees or more; (2) disc space narrowing of 25 per cent; (3) a decompression that included the L4–L5 level; and (4) any patient who undergoes a radical decompression.[28]

Herkowitz and Kurz, in a prospective study, reported 50 patients undergoing surgery for spinal stenosis symptoms, 25 of whom had only decompression and 25 of whom had decompression and fusion.[25] In this series degenerative spondylolisthesis was observed at a single segment, with a clinical picture of spinal stenosis confirmed by CT and myelogram or CT and MRI. Thirty-six of the patients were female and 14 male. Patients undergoing fusion averaged 63.5 years and those without fusion 65 years of age. Forty-one patients had surgery at L4–L5 and nine at L3–L4. The mean follow-up was three years. The authors reported excellent to good results in 24 patients who had fusion included with the decompression and only 11 patients without fusion. In patients who had fusion, the preoperative degenerative spondylolisthesis averaged 4.8 mm and postoperative 5.3 mm. In patients who did not have fusion, preoperative degenerative spondylolisthesis averaged 5.3 mm and increased postoperatively to 7.9 mm, a statistically significant alteration. There was also a statistically significant difference in the millimeters of slippage that occurred on flexion-extension films, comparing the fusion with the nonfusion group and in the angular motion seen between the two groups. In both instances the nonfusion group had an increase in motion and the fusion group had diminution in these motions postoperatively. In patients who underwent fusion, 36 per cent had pseudarthrosis. Interestingly, these were all rated excellent or good.

The incidence of postoperative slip after decompression for spinal stenosis ranges from 2 to 20 per cent in published series.[20, 23, 24, 28–30, 36, 43, 52, 53, 55] Patients with preexisting degenerative spondylolisthesis have a higher percentage of postoperative slippage. The factors that may influence this increase in slippage in patients with spinal stenosis and degenerative spondylolisthesis include (1) the extent of the decompression, (2) the amount of slippage present preoperatively, (3) the sex of the individual, (4) the severity of spondylosis of the anterior column, (5) the number of levels decompressed, (6) abnormal frontal or lateral plane alignment, and (7) penetration of the disc space at the time of decompression. From this discussion and a review of the literature, certain trends appear that can be used as predictors for postoperative instability. These are as follows: (1) the larger the preoperative slip, the greater is the risk of postoperative slip; (2) postoperative slip does not necessarily correlate with the development of symptoms, particularly when degenerative spondylolisthesis existed preoperatively; (3) decompression across a disc space of normal height has an increased likelihood to lead to postoperative slip; (4) excision of over 50 per cent of both facets at the same level increases the risk of slip; (5) increasing the number of levels of decompression increases the risk of slip; (6) penetration of the disc space at a decompressed level increases the risk of slip; and (7) females are at higher risk than males for development of a postoperative slip.

In the above paragraph we have specifically used the word "trend" since only two of the articles listed are prospective. Hard, reproducible data are lacking. However, these trends do suggest certain indications for fusion after decompression lumbar surgery. In surgery for spinal stenosis without degenerative spondylolisthesis, fusion should be considered when there has been (1) disruption of each facet joint at the same level or a total disruption of one facet joint at the involved segment and/or (2) previous decompression at the same level. For patients undergoing decompression with coexisting degenerative spondylolisthesis, fusion should be considered when there is (1) a documented preoperative progressive slip, (2) minimal anterior column degenerative changes and osteopytes at the level(s) of decompression, (3) a high lumbosacral angle, (4) sacralization of L5 with an L4–L5 spondylolisthesis, (5) disruption of 50 per cent of each facet joint or one total facet joint at the surgical level(s) at the time of surgery, (6) previous decompression at the same level, or (7) laminectomy associated with penetration of the disc space at the time of decompression.

When surgery is performed for symptoms of spinal stenosis with associated degenerative scoliosis, fusion should be considered if (1) a large flexible curve exists (greater than 35 degrees), (2) the decompression occurs within the apex of the curve, (3) there is a lateral spondylolisthesis or multiplane instability, (4) decompression is performed along the entire length of the curve when there is minimal anterior column degeneration, and (5) curve progression has been documented before surgery.

The next question to consider is the role of instrumentation after decompression. The goals of internal fixation are to stabilize the spine, reduce deformity, and improve the fusion rate. Unfortunately, even though the literature on decompression and spinal stenosis is limited, that on instrumentation associated with decompressive surgery for lumbar laminectomy is almost nonexistent. Kaneda and associates reported an 85 per cent success rate after fusion with instrumentation for degenerative spondylolisthesis.[32] In this series a solid fusion was obtained in 96 per cent of cases. However, instrumentation failure was noted in 11 per cent (six patients). In addition the percentage slip, slip angle, and lumbar lordosis were unchanged by the fixed instrumentation system. The article does not cover long-term follow-up. The success rate reported was comparable to with that described for in situ fusions. Another series reported by Chang and McAfee, using a different instrumentation system, gave similar results.[9] However, the percentage of solid fusion was not discussed. Newer, more modular systems allowing multiplane reductions are available. Their use is increasing and the short-term results appear to show greater success and diminish patients' need for analgesic medication. The authors recommend instrumentation, reduction/realignment, and fusion after decompressive laminectomy in the following situations: (1) previous lumbar decompression with progressive spondylolisthesis, (2) symptomatic pseudarthrosis where compression may be useful, (3) scoliosis with a flexible curve and/or documented preoperative curve progression, (4) previous lumbar decompression with progressive scoliosis, and (5) multiplane instability.

References

1. Boccanera, L., and Laus, M.: Cauda equina syndrome following lumbar spinal stenosis surgery. Spine *12*:712–715, 1987.
2. Bohlman, H. H., and Cook, S. S.: One-stage decompression and interbody fusion for lumbosacral spondyloptosis through a posterior approach. J. Bone Joint Surg. *64A*:415, 1982.

3. Bolesta, M., and Bohlman, H.: Degenerative spondylolisthesis: the role of arthrodesis. Presented at A.A.O.S. Annual Meeting, Las Vegas, February 1989.
4. Booth, R. E.: Spinal stenosis. Instr. Course Lect. *35*:420–435, 1986.
5. Boxall, D., Bradford, D. S., Winter, R. B., and Moe, J. H.: Management of severe spondylolisthesis in children and adolescents. J. Bone Joint Surg. *61A*:479, 1979.
6. Bradford, D. S., and Gotfried, Y.: Staged salvage reconstruction of grade IV and V spondylolisthesis. J. Bone Joint Surg. *69A*:191, 1987.
7. Brown, M., and Lockwood, S.: Degenerative spondylolisthesis. Instr. Course Lect. *28*:162–169, 1983.
8. Cauchoix, J., Benoist, M., and Chassaing, V.: Degenerative spondylolisthesis. Clin. Orthop. *115*:122, 1976.
9. Chang, K. W., and McAfee, P. C.: Degenerative spondylolisthesis and degenerative scoliosis treated with a combination segmental rod-plate and transpedicular screw instrumentation system: a preliminary report. J. Spinal Dis. *1*:247, 1989.
10. Dall, B., and Rowe, D.: Degenerative spondylolisthesis: its surgical management. Spine *10*:668–672, 1985.
11. DeWald, R. L., Fault, M. M., Taddonio, R. F., and Neuwirth, M. G.: Severe lumbosacral spondylolisthesis in adolescents and children. Reduction and staged circumferential fusion. J. Bone Joint Surg. *63A*:619, 1981.
12. Epstein, J. A., Epstein, B. S., and Lavine, L.: Nerve root compression associated with narrowing of the lumbar spinal canal. J. Neurol. Neurosurg. Psychiatry *25*:165, 1962.
13. Epstein, J. A., Epstein, B. S., Lavine, L. S., et al.: Degenerative lumbar spondylolisthesis with an intact neural arch (pseudospondylolisthesis). J. Neurosurg. *44*:139, 1976.
14. Feffer, H., Wiesel, S., Cuckler, J., and Rothman, R. H.: Degenerative spondylolisthesis: to fuse or not to fuse. Spine *10*:287–289, 1985.
15. Fitzgerald, J. A. W., and Newman, P. H.: Degenerative spondylolisthesis. J. Bone Joint Surg. *58B*:184, 1976.
16. Freebody, D., Bendall, R., and Taylor, R. D.: Anterior transperitoneal lumbar fusion. J. Bone Joint Surg. *53B*:617, 1971.
17. Garfin, S., Glover, M., Booth, R., et al.: Laminectomy: a review of the Pennsylvania Hospital experience. J. Spinal Dis. *1*:116–133, 1988.
18. Hanley, E. N.: Decompression and distraction—derotation arthrodesis for degenerative spondylolisthesis. Spine *11*:269, 1986.
19. Hanraets, P.: The Degenerative Back and Its Differential Diagnosis. New York, Elsevier, 1959.
20. Hazlett, J. W., and Kinnarel, P.: Lumbar apophyseal process excision and spinal instability. Spine *7*:171, 1982.
21. Harris, R. I.: Modern Trends in Diseases of the Vertebral Column. New York, Appleton, 1967.
22. Helfet, A. J., and Gruebal, L. D. M.: Segmental intervertebral instability and its treatment. *In* Helfet, A. J., and Lee, D. M. G. (eds.): Disorders of the Lumbar Spine. Toronto, J. B. Lippincott Co., 1978, pp. 69–111.
23. Herkowitz, H. N.: The role of fusion in decompressive surgery of the lumbar spine. Presented to the Spine Study Group, 6th Symposium, Palm Springs, CA, November 1988.
24. Herkowitz, H. N., and Garfin, S. R.: Decompressive surgery for spinal stenosis. Semin. Spine Surg. *1*:163–167, 1989.
25. Herkowitz, H. N., and Kurz, L. T.: Degenerative spondylolisthesis. Prospective study comparing decompression versus decompression and intertransverse process fusion. Presented to the International Society for the Study of the Lumbar Spine, Boston, May 1990.
26. Herron, L., and Trippi, A.: L4–L5 degenerative spondylolisthesis. Spine *14*:534–538, 1989.
27. Hodgson, A. R., and Wong, S. K.: A description of a technique and evaluation of results in anterior spinal fusion for deranged intervertebral disc and spondylolisthesis. Clin. Orthop. *56*:133, 1968.
28. Hopp, E., and Tsou, P.: Post-decompression lumbar instability. Clin. Orthop. *227*:143–151, 1988.
29. Johnsson, K. E., Willner, S., and Johnsson, K.: Postoperative instability after decompression for lumbar spinal stenosis. Spine *11*:107, 1986.
30. Johnsson, K. E., Johnell, I., Udena, A., and Willner, S.: Pre-operative and post-operative instability in lumbar spine stenosis. Spine *14*:591–593, 1989.
31. Jones, A. M., McAfee, P. C., Robinson, R. A., et al.: Failed arthrodesis of the spine for severe spondylolisthesis. J. Bone Joint Surg. *70A*:25, 1988.
32. Kaneda, K., Kazamma, H., Satoh, S., and Fujiga, M.: Follow-up study of medial facetectomies and posterolateral fusion with instrumentation in unstable degenerative spondylolisthesis. Clin. Orthop. *703*:159, 1986.
33. Kirkaldy-Willis, W. H., Pain, K. W. E., Cauchoix, J., and McIvor, G.: Lumbar spinal stenosis. Clin. Orthop. *99*:30, 1974.
34. Kirkaldy-Willis, W. H., Wedge, I. H., Yong-Hing, K., and Reilly, J.: Pathology and pathogenesis of lumbar spondylosis and stenosis. Spine *3*:320, 1978.
35. Laurent, L. E., and Osterman, K.: Operative treatment of spondylolisthesis in young patients. Clin. Orthop. *117*:85, 1976.
36. Lee, C. K.: Lumbar spinal instability (olisthesis) after extensive posterior spinal decompression. Spine *8*:429, 1983.
37. Lee, C. K., Hansen, H. T., and Weiss, A. B.: Developmental lumbar spinal stenosis. Spine *3*:246, 1978.
38. Lombardi, J. S., Wiltse, L., Reynolds, J., et al.: Treatment of degenerative spondylolisthesis. Spine *10*:821–827, 1985.
39. McNab, I.: Spondylolisthesis with an intact neural arch—the so-called pseudospondylolisthesis. J. Bone Joint Surg. *32B*:325, 1950.
40. McNab, I., and Dall, D.: The blood supply of the lumbar spine and its application to the technique of intertransverse lumbar fusion. J. Bone Joint Surg. *53B*:628, 1971.
41. Nachemson, A.: The role of spine fusion. Spine *6*:306–307, 1981.
42. Nachemson, A.: Lumbar spine instability. Spine *10*:290–291, 1985.
43. Nasca, R.: Surgical management of lumbar spinal stenosis. Spine *12*:809–816, 1987.
44. Newman, P. H.: Surgical treatment for spondylolisthesis in the adult. Clin. Orthop. *117*:106–111, 1976.

45. Newman, P. H.: Stenosis of the lumbar spine in spondylolisthesis. Clin. Orthop. *115*:116–121, 1976.
46. Paine, K.: Results of decompression for lumbar spinal stenosis. Clin. Orthop. *115*:96–100, 1976.
47. Posner, I., White, A., Edward, W., and Hayes, W.: Biomechanical analysis of the clinical stability of the lumbar and lumbosacral spine. Spine *7*:374–390, 1982.
48. Reynolds, J. B., and Wiltse, L. L.: Surgical treatment of degenerative spondylolisthesis. Spine *4*:148, 1979.
49. Rosenberg, N. J.: Degenerative spondylolisthesis. J. Bone Joint Surg. *57A*:467–474, 1975.
50. Runbold, C.: Treatment of spondylolisthesis by posterolateral fusion, resection of the pars interarticularis and prompt immobilization of the patient. J. Bone Joint Surg. *48A*:1282, 1966.
51. Sacks, S.: Anterior interbody fusion of the lumbar spine. J. Bone Joint Surg. *47B*:211, 1965.
52. Shenkein, H. A., and Hush, C. J.: Spondylolisthesis after multiple bilateral laminectomies and facetectomies for lumbar spondylolisthesis. J. Neurosurg. *50*:45, 1979.
53. Sienkiewicz, P. J., and Flatley, T. J.: Postoperative spondylolisthesis. Clin. Orthop. *221*:172, 1987.
54. Spengler, D. M.: Current concepts review: degenerative stenosis of the lumbar spine. J. Bone Joint Surg. *69A*:305, 1987.
55. Stauffer, R. N., and Coventry, M. B.: Anterior interbody spine fusion. Analysis of the Mayo Clinic series. J. Bone Joint Surg. *54A*:756, 1972.
56. Tile, M., McNeil, S. R., Zarins, R. Z., et al.: Spinal stenosis: results of treatment. Clin. Orthop. *115*:104, 1976.
57. Turner, R. H., and Bianco, A. J.: Spondylolysis and spondylolisthesis in children and teenagers. J. Bone Joint Surg. *53A*:1298, 1971.
58. Verbiest, H.: Results of surgical treatment of idiopathic developmental stenosis of the lumbar vertebral canal. J. Bone Joint Surg. *59B*:181, 1977.
59. White, A. A., Panjabi, M. M., Posner, I., et al.: Spinal stability: evaluation and treatment. Instr. Course Lect. *30*:457, 1981.
60. White, A. H., and Wiltse, L. L.: Postoperative spondylolisthesis. *In* Weinstein, P. R., Ehni, G., and Wilson, C. B. (eds.): Lumbar Spondylosis: Diagnosis, Management, and Surgical Treatment. Chicago: Year Book Medical Publishers, 1977, pp. 184–194.
61. Wiltse, L. L., Kirkaldy-Willis, W. H., and McIvor, G. W. D.: The treatment of spinal stenosis. Clin. Orthop. *115*:83, 1976.
62. Wiltse, L. L., and Winter, R. B.: Terminology and measurement of spondylolisthesis. J. Bone Joint Surg. *65A*:768, 1983.

SECTION 4

DEFORMITY

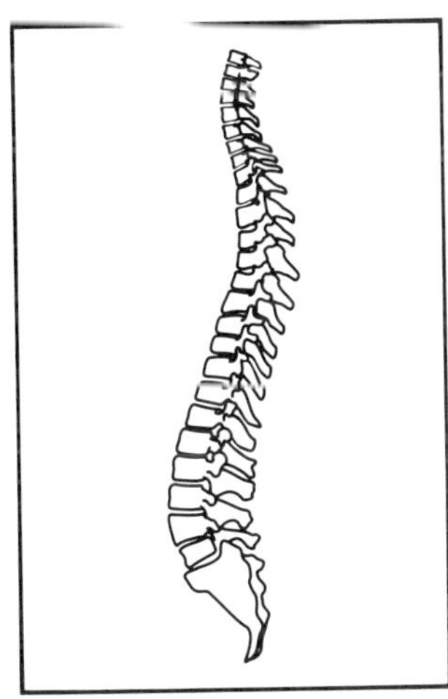

CHAPTER

26

ADULT SCOLIOSIS

John P. Kostuik, M.D.

Adult scoliosis has been defined as scoliosis occurring after skeletal maturity. Some definitions have included all deformities that occur after the age of 20.

Adult scoliosis has two basic forms: that which has its onset before skeletal maturity; and the form that arises early in adult life secondary to either osteoporosis, osteomalacia, or iatrogenic causes such as multiple-level decompressions for spinal stenosis, and from degenerative changes.

This chapter discusses deformities that occur in adult life as a result of onset before skeletal maturity. The principles discussed apply to all scoliosis patients regardless of cause, however.

Until the late 1960s it was believed that surgical treatment of scoliotic deformities in the adult, with the exception of thoracic curves in people in their third decade, could not be treated surgically. Many authors have shown that curves in the adult may progress and that frequently these same curves were painful.[4, 8, 11, 12, 26, 35, 50–53, 56–61, 63, 64, 68, 69] The advent of Harrington instrumentation in the late 1950s, the subsequent improvements in instrumentation by Dwyer, Zielke, and Cotrel and Dubousset, and advances in preoperative assessment and postoperative care have led to marked improvement in the ability to deal with the complex problems of scoliosis in the adult.[9, 10, 15, 20, 21, 40, 41, 69, 70]

Today there is greater recognition not only by family physicians, but also by paramedical personnel, that the adult scoliosis patient who requires surgery can safely undergo surgical intervention.

CURRENT PROBLEM

In 1981 Kostuik and Bentivoglio found that 3.9 per cent of adults had curves that involved the thoracolumbar and lumbar spine.[32] They believed that these curves were structural in nature and had started in adolescence and progressed in adult life; these were not curves secondary to osteoporosis or to local degenerative changes.

In 1968 Vanderpool and associates stated that 6 per cent of adults over the age of 50 showed radiographic evidence of scoliosis, but they believed that most were due to compression fractures, osteoporosis, and osteomalacia.[65]

In the early 1950s Dewar discovered an incidence of structural thoracic scoliosis of 4 per cent after reviewing 10,000 consecutive chest radiographs done for routine hospital admission (unpublished data).

Since many of these curves are mild to moderate in adolescence and do not become apparent until the fourth, fifth, and sixth decades of life, there is no doubt that there will continue to be patients, especially in industrialized countries, in whom surgical intervention will be warranted.

Work by Weinstein and Ponseti has shown etiologic factors responsible for continued progression in adult life.[67] Thoracic curves between 50 and 75 degrees at skeletal maturity increased an average of 30 degrees over the follow-up period. Thoracolumbar curves 50 to 75 degrees at skeletal maturity increased 22.3 degrees over 40 years. Lumbar spine curves in which the fifth lumbar vertebra was not well seated and apical rotation was greater than 33 per cent progressed the most.

In my experience the curve with the worst prognosis in adult life occurs in the young adult or adolescent who has an imbalanced lumbar curve or thoracolumbar curve in which the fifth lumbar vertebra is not parallel with the sacrum and the curve emanates from the lumbosacral junction (Fig. 26–1). This curve presents the greatest technologic difficulties for correction in later adult life and I believe is best treated at an early age if possible.

Other curves with a poor prognosis include those whose apices fall at the L2–L3 or L3–L4 area with significant Grade 3 rotation; are imbalanced; and have a secondary, sharp and angular compensatory curve at the L4–L5 or L5–S1 area. In the young adult or adolescent these curves can be treated and rebalanced by dealing with the compensatory curve at one or two levels rather than dealing with the entire more proximal curve over five to seven levels.

With the increasing age of the patient population it is not uncommon for the spinal surgeon to see an increasing deformity associated with pain, loss of lumbar lordosis, imbalance, osteoporosis, and spinal stenosis. Today with the better understanding of spinal mechanics, improved instrumentation, improved postoperative care, and the better understanding of screw fixation in bone, it is possible to treat these people with little morbidity (Fig. 26–2).

In a review of adult patients with curves in the lumbar and thoracolumbar spine Kostuik and Bentivoglio found an incidence of back pain in 60 per cent of patients.[32] This was similar in incidence to an unselected consecutive series of 100 patients with the same age range without scoliosis. These figures are also comparable with local population studies in the industrialized world in which the incidence of back pain is between 60 and 70 per cent in

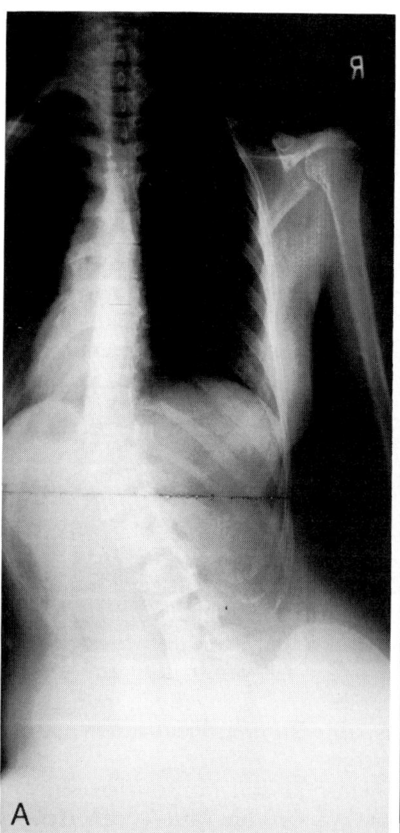

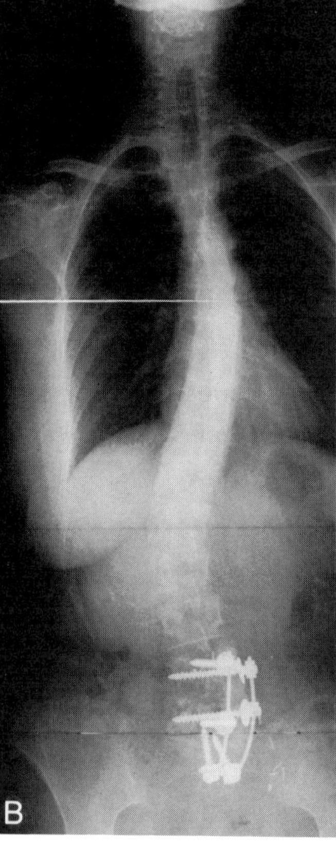

Figure 26–1. *A,* Female age 26 with painful scoliosis. Note the marked imbalance to the left. Pain was reproduced on discography at both L4–L5 and L5–S1 discs. *B,* Rebalanced with relief of pain secondary to lateral closing wedges. Note the double Zielke rods to control rotational forces.

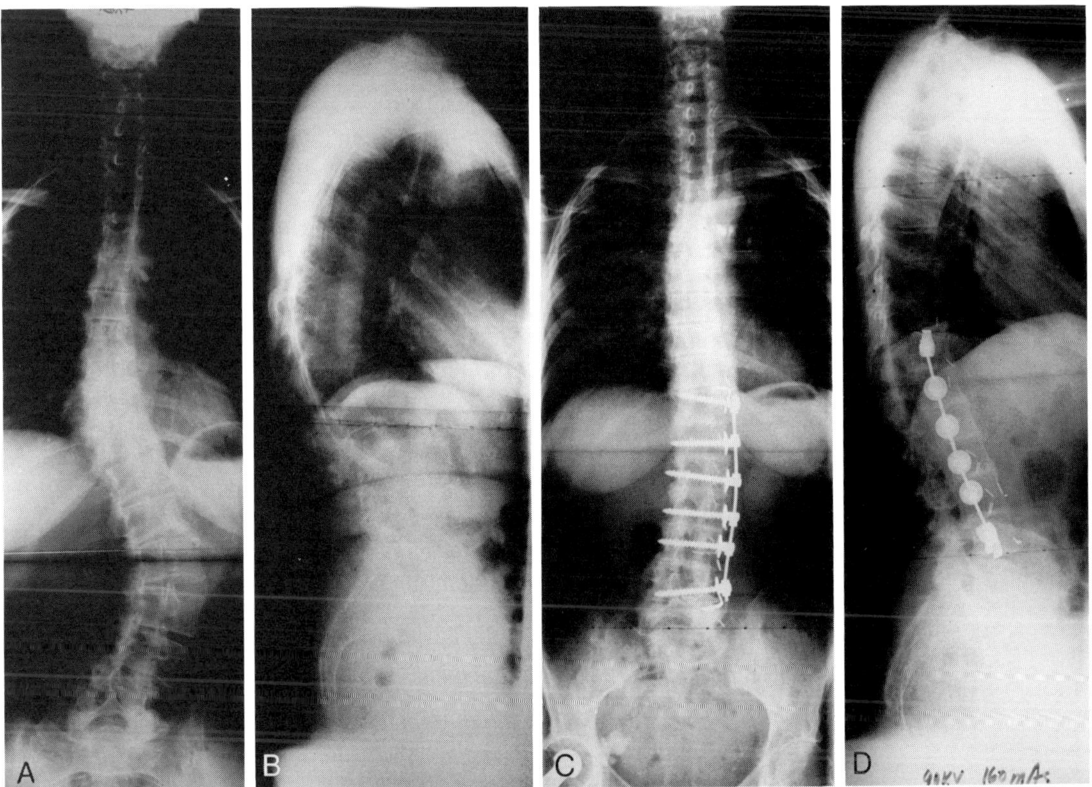

Figure 26–2. *A*, Female age 65 with a documented, progressive, painful curve of 44 degrees. L4–L5 and L5–S1 discs were not painful on discography; L4–L5 and L5–S1 facet blocks did not relieve pain. *B*, Preoperative lateral view, 66 degrees. *C*, Postoperative Zielke instrumentation, 2 degrees. Six-year follow-up, no pain. Note the previous total hip. *D*, Lordosis has been fully preserved.

the general adult population. These authors also noted that in curves greater than 45 degrees the incidence of pain increased markedly. The pain reached its maximum between the ages of 40 and 60 years, similar to the spondylogenic or discogenic pain patterns in the general population. Nachemson found a similar incidence of pain among patients with scoliosis.[44, 45] In contrast to Kostuik and Bentivoglio, however, Nachemson noted the pain always seemed to be mild and rarely required treatment. The degree of deformity is not as paramount in adults as in adolescents. The patient's symptoms should be treated. Most patients should be given a course of nonoperative or conservative treatment first. The exception is the patient with significant progression, evidenced either radiologically or by loss of height, who is imbalanced and has a good deal of rotation radiologically with significant disabling pain (Fig. 26–3). In my experience thoracic curves in the adult with scoliosis are rarely painful.

Other problems confronting the orthopedic surgeon dealing with adult scoliosis are those related to iatrogenic flat-back secondary to distraction fusions with Harrington instrumentation and extending to the distal lumbar spine, usually L5 or S1.[14, 17, 22, 37, 39] This problem may occur as a result of the degenerative changes and loss of disc height below a fusion mass ending at L2–L5, and may occur above a fusion, for instance, from L4 to the sacrum in a woman secondary to osteopenia and loss of disc height. The other problem is a result of precocious degenerative changes that occur below a fusion done in adolescence or young adult life.

Cochran and associates, in a long-term anatomic and functional review of patients with adolescent idiopathic scoliosis treated by Harrington rod fusion, showed a proportionally increased incidence of degenerative changes the more distal the fusion performed in adolescence.[6] There was an approximately 20 per cent incidence of degenerative changes with pain below fusions ending at L2, approximately 40 per cent at L3, 60 per cent at L4, and 80 per cent at L5. Edgar and Mehta found an increased incidence of degenerative changes associated with pain at levels below a posterior fusion that extended to L3 or L4.[16]

When pain is correlated with age, the pattern seems to follow a bell curve, with most patients with pain in the sixth, seventh, and eighth decades of life. Pain appeared to reach its maximum between the ages of 40 and 60 years, which corresponds to the maximal incidence of pain from a spondylogenic or discogenic cause in the nonscoliotic population. When occupation and pain are correlated there appears to be a distinct preference for lighter work by scoliosis patients, although only 21 per cent of patients in the review done by Kostuik and Bentivoglio were aware they had a scoliosis.[32] Rogala and associates also suggested a preference for lighter work by scoliosis patients.[54] The type of occupation was not a predisposing factor to pain in this review, although those with jobs that involved heavier work seemed to be less able to cope and missed more time from work or were more likely to be incapacitated. Patients with curves greater than 45 degrees had a greater degree of incapacitating pain than patients with curves less than 45 degrees and the difference was statistically significant. The increasing incapacity due to pain with greater curves and the increasing severity of pain with increasing age suggest that curves 45 degrees or greater at the end of growth tend to become more clinically significant with increasing age. For both lumbar curves and thoracolumbar curves pain was more noticeable the more severe the curve. All patients with radiographic changes of degenerative processes at the apex of curves also demonstrated similar changes at the lumbosacral junction. Facet sclerosis correlated with a history of pain in 64 per cent of patients.

PATIENT EVALUATION

As with most spinal problems, history is the prime means of evaluation of the patient with

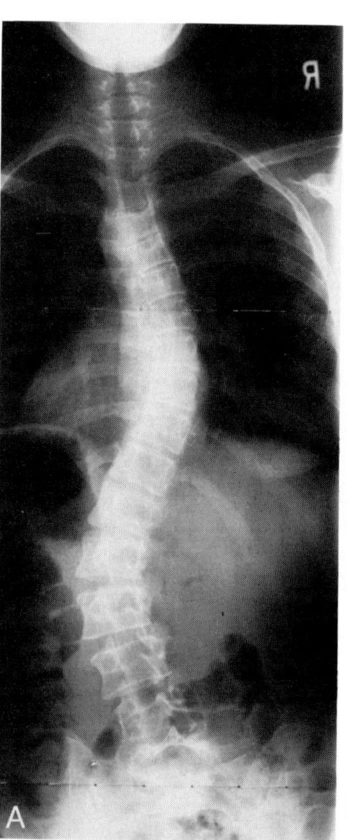

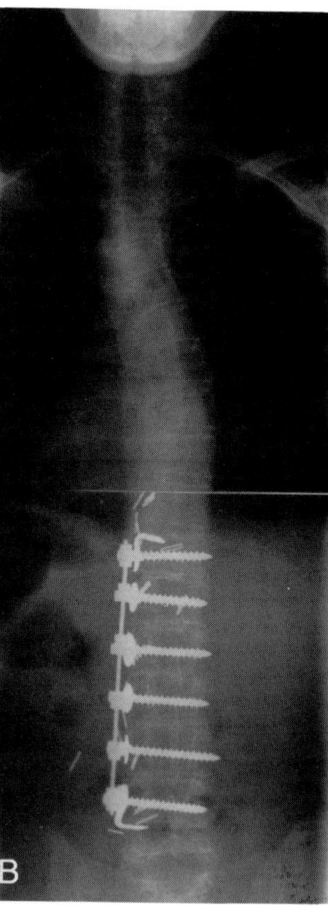

Figure 26–3. *A*, Female age 24 with a lumbar curve of 60 degrees and a thoracic curve of 52 degrees. Note the obliquity of L5. *B*, Postoperative lumbar curve of 15 degrees, and the thoracic curve reduced to 40 degrees. L5 is more parallel to the horizontal plane (i.e., floor) when standing.

scoliosis. A relevant family history of deformity may give some indication of prognosis. For example, a close relative who has a progressive severe deformity and is older than the patient may give some insight as to the patient's future. The date of onset of the deformity should be considered but in itself is not usually important.

A history of curve progression can be determined using information obtained from the patient or the relatives. For example, a change in the way clothes fit, increasing rib hump, a loss of height, or a loss of waistline are relevant. Progression is best documented by serial roentgenograms but these are often not available, particularly in the case of thoracolumbar or lumbar curves where the deformity may not be noticed until adult life. The psychologic aspects of the patient's deformity should be considered. Many adults are reluctant to discuss their deformity unless asked directly. Many of them have learned to live with their deformity and it does not present a problem. Conversely, there are a number of patients in whom deformity continues to play a significant psychologic role. This has occurred in 10 per cent of cases in my series.

A pain questionnaire is important to help determine the location of pain. Pain may be apical or below the apex. Often the patient may indicate the source of pain. It is important to know the duration of pain and how it affects activities of daily living, social function, occupation, and home and sexual life. It is important to know what aggravates and what alleviates the pain. If the pain is radicular in nature and suggestive of root irritation, it is important to get a history of this as well. Radicular pain may be related to nerve root compression at the apex of the curve, and in the thoracic or thoracolumbar curve area it may be costal in nature. In a thoracolumbar curve, radicular pain may also arise from the compensatory curve.[25] If the curve is in the lumbar area, pain may be referred into the lower extremities. True sciatica goes below the knee; pain above the knee may be referred pain, but can be of nerve root origin as well.

It is important to obtain a history of bowel and bladder function. An associated spinal stenosis may occur, presenting initially with bladder incontinence, particularly in women. Incontinence in the elderly woman is often due to spinal stenosis, and should not be assumed to be the aftereffect of childbearing. The history frequently reveals a recent, rather than a chronic, onset of bladder incontinence.

Respiratory malfunction may be the presenting symptom in scoliosis but it usually occurs in paralytic or severe congenital curves only. The patient may describe such respiratory problems as shortness of breath while climbing stairs or performing other activities, or simply tiredness. A good history of respiratory function is important. My review of 200 consecutive adults with idiopathic scoliosis revealed no cases of severe dysfunction, even in curves of 100 degrees or more. Ventilation was often decreased to as little as 25 per cent of predicted normal value, but this rarely was of functional significance. Arterial blood gases were generally normal. Severe problems in perfusion or ventilation in the presence of a scoliosis indicates a congenital scoliosis unless otherwise ruled out. There appears to be a correlation between curve size and pulmonary insufficiency above 60 degrees, but I have seen no pulmonary deaths associated with idiopathic scoliosis in over 20 years of experience. All deaths were in patients with congenital or paralytic curves. The only exception to this rule is the patient who has a marked thoracic lordosis.

Current theories as to the cause of thoracic curves suggest an anterior tether of the thoracic spine resulting in lordosis and scoliosis. In patients with a marked thoracic lordosis, pulmonary function may be severely affected. Pulmonary function tests are done routinely for thoracic curves greater than 60 degrees or in cases of paralytic or congenital scoliosis.

Physical examination focuses on the spinal deformity. A complete examination is necessary, however, including a full neurologic examination as well as a cardiopulmonary evaluation. The three-dimensional nature of the curve should be assessed. A kyphotic or lordotic element should be looked for in the presence of scoliosis and its effect on pulmonary function assessed.

The degree of decompensation, the flexibility, and the size of the rib hump should be measured, as well as the patient's height. Signs of subtle neurologic dysfunction should be looked for, particularly in left thoracic idiopathic curves, which are often associated with syringomyelia. Mild clawing of the toes may indicate a tethered cord. Muscle fatigue in the legs after exercise suggests the presence of spinal stenosis associated with scoliosis.

ROENTGENOGRAPHY

After the clinical determination of scoliosis or kyphosis, initial radiographic analysis should include standing posteroanterior and lateral thoracolumbosacral roentgenograms on a three-foot cassette. These indicate the degree of the deformity, local pathology, and decompensation. In the presence of pain, localized roentgenograms should be taken to look for findings such as enlarged facets, congenital anomalies, disc narrowing, and other specific findings.

Bending roentgenograms indicate flexibility of the curve, if present, but do not provide any formula as to the degree of correction that might be expected by surgical intervention. In mobile thoracolumbar curves treated by anterior Zielke instrumentation, the amount of correction obtained was twice that obtained on bending roentgenograms.

Traction films are occasionally of value in attempting to show whether distraction will overcome decompensation. A supine posteroanterior film may also help.

Hyperextension views of the kyphotic area are of value only if the kyphosis is flexible. Lateral flexion views are used for evaluation of excessive lordosis.

Since scoliosis is a rotational deformity, Stagnara views, particularly in cases of kyphoscoliosis, often best demonstrate the deformity. They are essentially oblique views. Special studies to consider obtaining preoperatively, or during the assessment if concerns of neurologic dysfunction or congenital anomalies exist, include bone scans, myelography, discography, computed tomography (CT), and magnetic resonance imaging (MRI). Bone scans are rarely necessary, but are sometimes of value in the young adult with a minor curve, or a patient with persistent, unexplained pain, to rule out pathology such as a tumor as a cause of the scoliosis. Myelography, or MRI, is indicated in patients with neuropathology and congenital curves. In any patient undergoing surgical correction for painful deformity, preoperative myelography is of value to rule out cauda equina or cord compression before corrective surgery.

CT has not proved of great value in assessing the contents of the dural canal in scoliosis, and in my experience it is best combined with myelography using nonionic dyes. The scan is done three to four hours after the myelogram. In low back problems of a degenerative nature, myelography or CT scans often have a 30 per cent false-positive value. The combination of myelography and CT scanning has proved accurate in more than 90 per cent of cases, however. The role of MRI appears to be promising, but it is still unproved in the study of spinal deformity.

Discography and the use of facet blocks are discussed under Pain Assessment.

NONOPERATIVE CARE

Nonoperative care is used primarily in those patients in whom operative indications are not present, or in whom other factors preclude operative intervention. Among those factors that may preclude surgical intervention are serious cardiac or respiratory disease, or psychologic reasons.

The mainstays of nonoperative treatment are drugs (anti-inflammatories and/or non-narcotic analgesics), physical therapy modalities, and orthotic devices, as well as a general understanding of the patient's condition and prognosis (education).

Excluding cosmetic deformity, significant progression, or neurologic problems, the major indication for operative intervention is pain. Before operative intervention, and in the absence of neurologic problems, nonoperative treatment should be attempted.

The use of nonsteroidal anti-inflammatory medications may be of value. Enteric coated aspirin is often as valuable as more expensive nonsteroidal anti-inflammatory drugs and can be used for long-term treatment. Medications such as muscle relaxants or analgesics with high doses of narcotics such as codeine (30 mg or greater), or some of the synthetic narcotic drugs such as Percodan should be avoided except in very acute phases of severe pain.

Physical therapy, particularly exercises, are rarely successful in controlling pain in adult scoliosis patients. In the adult, motion usually aggravates pain. Flexibility and stretching exercises may be useful for a period of time. Exercises must be tailored to those motions that do not cause pain. Low-impact aerobics, cycling exercises, and swimming are of value.

No physical therapy modality or exercise will prevent the progression of a curve, but they may maintain flexibility to some degree and render subsequent surgical treatment easier.

In the elderly patient with scoliosis who is over 50 years of age, the use of an orthosis, particularly in women, may be useful in decreasing pain and increasing function. Orthoses should be rigid and formed to the patient's deformity. They should be worn while the patient is ambulatory and may help the patient for months or years. In my experience, however, most patients who have worn an orthosis that helped subsequently needed operative intervention. If an orthosis is provided an attempt should be made to involve the patient in an exercise program of a general conditioning nature to maintain mobility of the deformity and general muscle tone.

Other nonoperative treatments that must be considered are diet, providing the patient with a general understanding of the cause of scoliosis, and a prognosis for the individual deformity. A normal regular diet is advised.

Since osteoporosis plays a major role in the progression of deformity in postmenopausal women, it is important that these individuals exercise. Twenty minutes of general low-impact aerobics four times a week before menopause will help diminish the risks and complications of postmenopausal osteoporosis in most women. In postmenopausal women the use of exercise combined with hormonal therapy and calcium under the supervision of a physician may help control the symptoms and signs of osteoporosis after menopause.

SURGICAL INDICATIONS

The general indications for surgery are pain, progression of deformity, neurologic disability, cosmesis, structural imbalance in paralytic or neuromuscular disease, curve progression associated with pain below previous fusions for spinal deformity, and iatrogenic flat-back (kyphosis).

In my estimation the younger adult below the age of 35 without pain but with obvious documented increasing curvature, whose lumbar or thoracolumbar curve measures approximately 45 degrees, and who is unbalanced is best treated surgically, since often disease in these patients continues to progress and they develop a painful lower back.

This is particularly true in women with a significant lumbar or thoracolumbar curve who, because of degenerative changes, may later go from primarily having scoliosis with retention of lumbar lordosis to having kyphoscoliosis that becomes rigid and may require two-stage surgery. The younger adult can be readily treated anteriorly with good correction of deformity using Zielke instrumentation with minimal morbidity (Fig. 26–3). The unanswered question is what happens to the levels below the fusion. Edgar and Menta, and Cochran and associates pointed out that the problem related to posterior instrumentation extending to the L3, L4, or L5 level is an increased incidence of degenerative changes below the fusion associated with pain.[6, 16] My advice to these patients, as for all patients, particularly younger patients, is that they exercise after surgery to maintain a satisfactory level of physical fitness. They must practice good back hygiene and do low back exercises daily. The same endeavors are attempted in elderly patients, but because of their age and a previous sedentary life style this is often not as practical as it is in the younger adult.

The unbalanced younger patient whose major curve measures 40 degrees or more and extends to L3 or L4, but who has a compensatory curve at L4–L5 or L5–S1, may have the primary curve significantly reduced by being rebalanced through the lower curve. This should be done only if the lower curve is painful. These patients run the risk of progression of the upper curve at a later date and it should be explained that they may require extension of their fusion more proximally later. To date, however, the technique has worked satisfactorily in a small group of patients (six), and although the follow-up is short, the average degree of correction of the major curve has been more than 40 per cent (see Fig. 26–1). Pain patterns must be proved preoperatively by discography and facet blocks.

Progression is best documented by a careful history taken from both the patient and the relatives with particular attention paid to their current height and their height at the completion of growth. A loss of height indicates progression of the spinal deformity. Radiologic documentation is ideal but rarely available in these more mature adults. Weinstein and Ponseti showed that curves in the thoracolumbar spine and lumbar spine may progress, particularly if the fifth lumbar vertebra is not well seated (oblique) and apical rotation is greater than 33 per cent.[67] In my estimation imbalance seems to play a major role in progression of the curve, together with a significant degree of rotation.

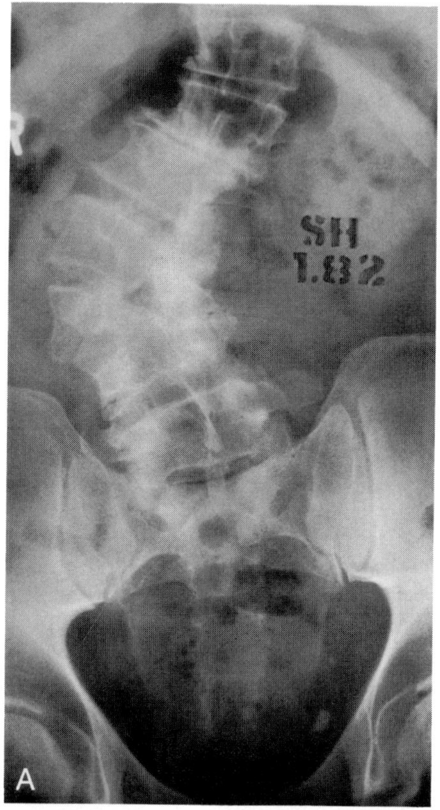

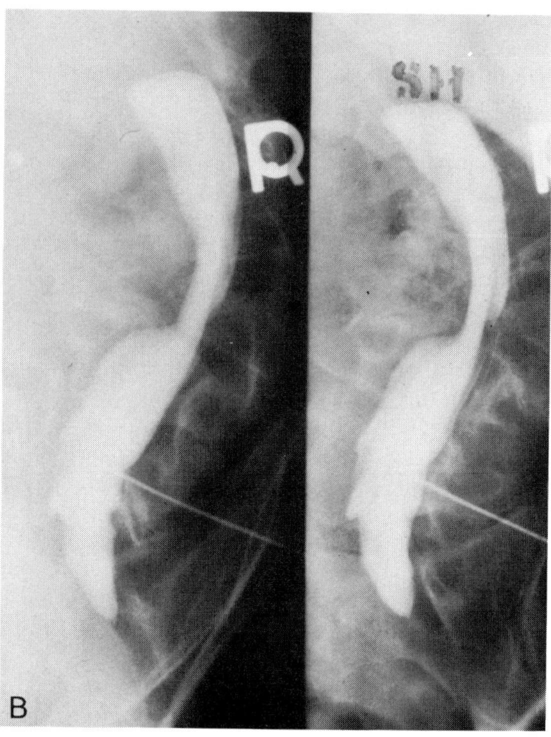

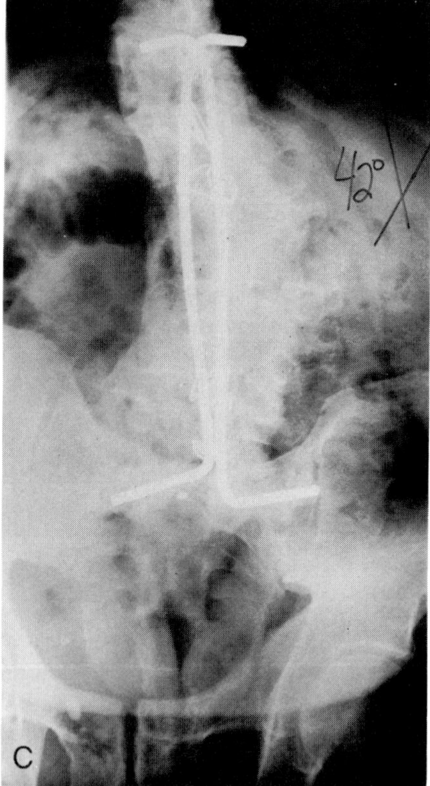

Figure 26–4. *A*, Male age 56 with a curve of 68 degrees and marked symptoms and mild signs of spinal stenosis. *B*, Preoperative myelogram indicates severe compromise of the canal at the apex of the curve. *C*, Postoperative anteroposterior curve of 42 degrees. Five years later the patient was pain free and working.

In our series of more than 1000 adults with scoliosis treated surgically, neurologic deficit was rarely an indication for surgical intervention. With an increasingly aging population, however, greater numbers of patients have an associated spinal stenosis (Fig. 26–4). Surgical decompression by laminectomy is rarely indicated, and in my review in 1979 only five of 227 patients treated surgically for painful scoliosis required associated decompression.

Jackson and associates showed that patients with radicular symptoms that arise from the compensatory curve may show marked improvement in their leg pain postoperatively after correction of the major curve by an anterior procedure.[25] In my experience this has not been particularly successful.

All patients who complain of significant pain preoperatively should undergo preoperative myelography to rule out other causes of pain such as intradural or extradural tumors. Adults with significant lumbar and thoracolumbar curves above 45 degrees should have preoperative myelography, particularly if they have radiating pain, since their problem may also be spinal stenosis.

The problem of cosmesis in the lumbar and thoracolumbar spine in adults is rare except in the young adult who is imbalanced. Many adults with scoliosis (10 per cent) have thoracic curves that are not painful but require surgical correction for cosmetic reasons. After a thorough explanation of the complexities of the surgery and the associated risks, if the patient has a strong psychologic desire for improvement of the deformity even if it is believed that the scoliosis is unlikely to lead to pain later in life or to significant progression, surgical intervention can be considered.

The advent of Cotrel-Dubousset (C-D) instrumentation, as well as other segmental instrumentation devices, allows excellent cosmetic correction to be obtained relatively safely in the adult, especially if the patient is hypokyphotic in the thoracic spine. The use of thoracoplasty (partial rib excision) may also enhance the postoperative cosmetic appearance.

A functional analysis of 100 patients followed for more than ten years postoperatively found that body image and cosmesis played a much greater role in the adult patient's decision to have surgery than was previously suspected.[38]

POSTOPERATIVE CARE

Postoperative care of the adult is much easier today. Recumbency is often not necessary; patients usually become ambulatory by the third or fourth postoperative day. Patients with thoracolumbar curves are usually fitted with either a modular Boston overlap type of brace or molded plastic orthoses postoperatively. Thoracic curves frequently require limited external support or none.

Pain Assessment

Early attempts in the late 1960s and 1970s to treat painful lumbar and thoracolumbar curves with Harrington instrumentation and fusion of the curve without preoperative pain assessment by discography and facet blocks resulted in a significant number of patients complaining of pain postoperatively.[35] The results of pain relief averaged from 65 to 70 per cent. Subsequent evaluation of pain using discography and facet blocks has improved patient results to between 80 and 90 per cent with good pain relief.[31]

Careful assessment of the patient using a careful history is most important. The patients may localize their pain in the low back, or at the apex of their curvature, or both. Frequently, however, the symptoms may be vague. MacNab showed that a hypertonic saline injection into the supraspinous ligament at the thoracolumbar junction can produce pain at the lumbosacral junction.[42]

I performed a prospective study using discography to help differentiate sources of pain.[31] The correct use of discography is limited to an assessment of the lower levels of the lumbar spine, namely L3–L4, L4–L5, and the lumbosacral junction. Rarely are discograms performed at the apex of the curve.

Discography can be used to assess whether or not these levels are degenerative or painful. Facet blocks are similarly used. Discography is usually done from a posterolateral approach, although occasionally, because of deformity, it may be necessary to transgress the dura. Facet blocks are performed using bupivacaine hydrochloride (Marcaine) with infiltration of the posterior ramus. It is recognized that levels other than the L5–S1 articulation have multiple innervation, and if the L4–L5 level is to be assessed the L3–L4 level must be infiltrated as well. It is my practice to use discography in painful lumbar and thoracolumbar curves at the lower levels of the lumbar spine, and facet blocks at the lowest level, L5–S1, which has a single innervation, or at L4–L5.

If facet blocks relieve pain and discography reproduces pain at the lumbosacral junction, it is my feeling that the fusion should be extended to the sacrum. Previous results before discography, when the fusion was not extended to the sacrum, resulted in many patients continuing to complain of pain despite correction of the deformity, when either a posterior or anterior approach was used.[35] Extension of the fusion to the sacrum with preservation of lumbar lordosis and the ability to obtain a solid arthrodesis has resulted in good results in 90 per cent of such cases.

Conversely, if discograms do not reproduce the patient's pain and facet blocks at the lumbosacral junction do not relieve pain, it is assumed that the pain arises in the curve itself. If L5–S1 is not a part of the curve, the curve alone is corrected and the lumbosacral junction is not fused.

It is important to have a thorough mechanical understanding of the patient's pain that is not clouded by significant psychologic difficulties or factors.

SURGICAL TECHNIQUES

Harrington posterior instrumentation is rarely indicated for treatment of scoliotic deformity in adults, especially in the lumbar and thoracolumbar spine. The reason is, even with the use of sacroalar hooks, broad sleeves, or contouring of rods, or the use of square-ended rods with distraction, inevitable loss of lumbar lordosis occurs. Most lumbar and thoracolumbar curves are handled by anterior instrumentation using the Zielke technique.

Zielke instrumentation is not useful if there is a true kyphosis, however (see Fig. 26–10). This can be evaluated by oblique Stagnara views only. If there is a significant kyphosis, Zielke instrumentation may increase it. In kyphoscoliosis in the lumbar spine, which is a common problem in patients over the age of 50, to restore balance and relieve pain it is necessary to restore lumbar lordosis. This can be achieved only in cases where kyphosis is present using a two-stage procedure. An anterior approach is done initially with multiple-level discotomies and fusions, followed two weeks later by posterior segmental (e.g., C-D) instrumentation (Figs. 26–5 and 26–6). If the kyphoscoliosis is mobile, however, this may be achieved by single-stage posterior segmental instrumentation. C-D instrumentation, for example, derotates the spine, restores lordosis, and increases spinal rigidity in comparison with other forms of spinal fixation.[9, 10, 13]

With the advent of Luque instrumentation in 1976, the use of segmental fixation posteriorly has gained great popularity.[10, 41] I do not believe that in lumbar or thoracolumbar curves Harrington instrumentation with segmental wiring suffices. The use of double-L or rectangular rods may be indicated (see Fig. 26–10). Initially, fixation to the pelvis with Luque rods contoured using the Galveston technique showed great promise.[1] However, many of these patients develop pain related to the sacroiliac joint in the presence of a solid fusion of the lumbar spine. With the advent of C-D instrumentation, sublaminar wiring has been abandoned, except in cases of tumor and in some cases of paralytic, or neuromuscular, scoliosis.[7, 19, 23, 24, 27, 36, 48, 55, 62, 66]

Zielke Instrumentation

The prime indication for Zielke instrumentation is a thoracolumbar or lumbar curve that does not require extension of the fusion to the sacrum, is mobile on bending roentgenograms, and has preserved lordosis. If these painful cases are accurately assessed preoperatively with discography and facet blocks, correction of the deformity often can be obtained by Zielke instrumentation inserted anteriorly. In the mature adult the entire curve should be incorporated in the instrumentation. In younger patients levels comparable with those in adolescents suffice.

For fixation, the screw should be angled toward the contralateral junction of the pedicle with the vertebral body. This necessitates careful cleaning of the disc space, including the end plates, back to the posterior longitudinal ligament so that an accurate line can be obtained for insertion of the screws. To ensure that the opposite cortex is penetrated, a depth gauge is used to measure to the line in the interspace that the screw follows. After this, 2 mm can be added to the depth of the screw,

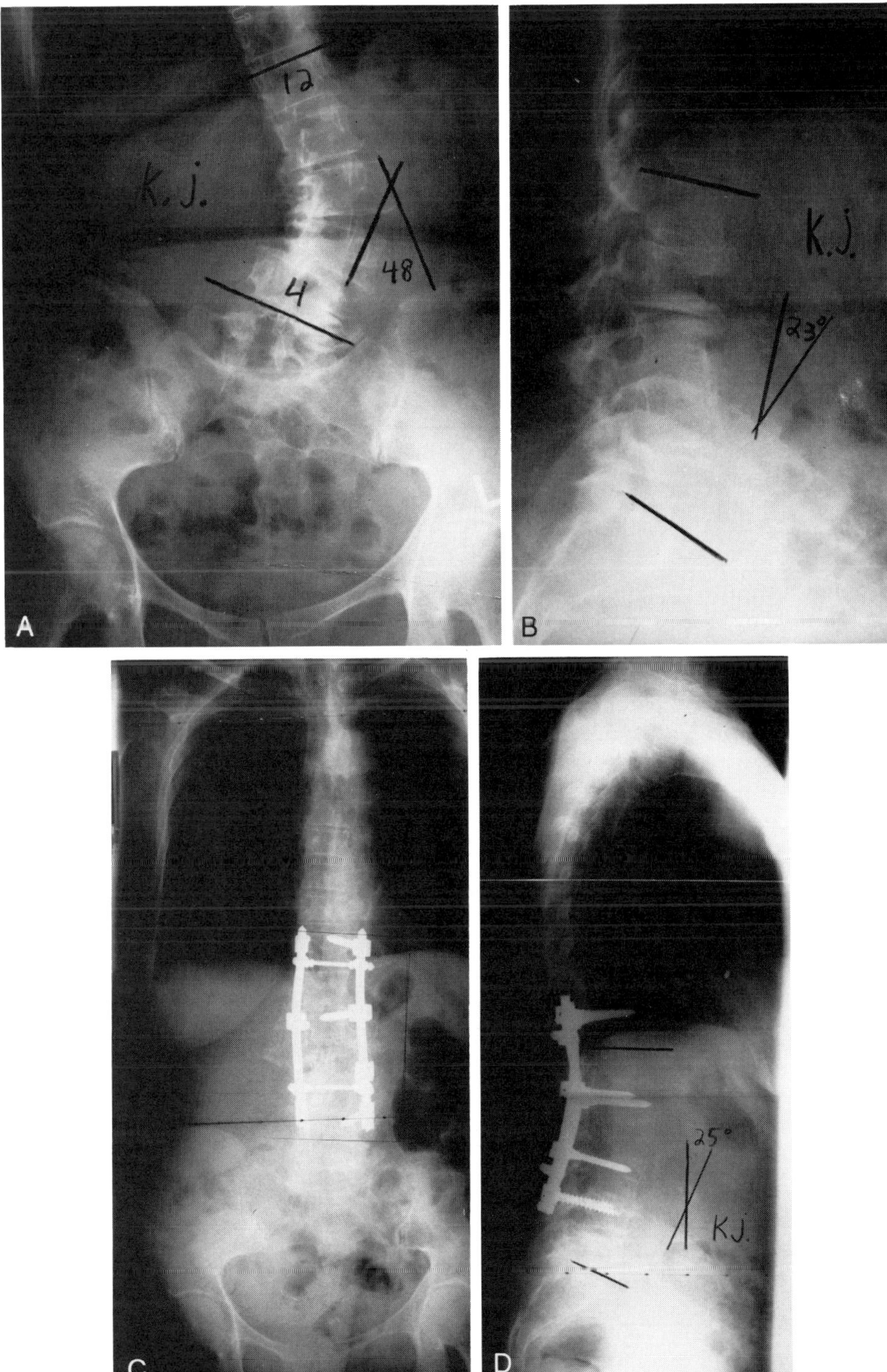

Figure 26–5. *A*, Female age 58 with a progressive painful curve. Stage 1: Multiple anterior discotomies with insertion of morselized bone graft. Stage 2: Cotrel-Dubousset (C-D) instrumentation and fusion. *B*, Preoperative lateral view. Note the significant loss of lordosis (−23 degrees L1–S1). *C*, Postoperative anteroposterior view. *D*, Postoperative lateral view. Note the significant return of lumbar lordosis due to derotation and anterior release (increase of 48 degrees).

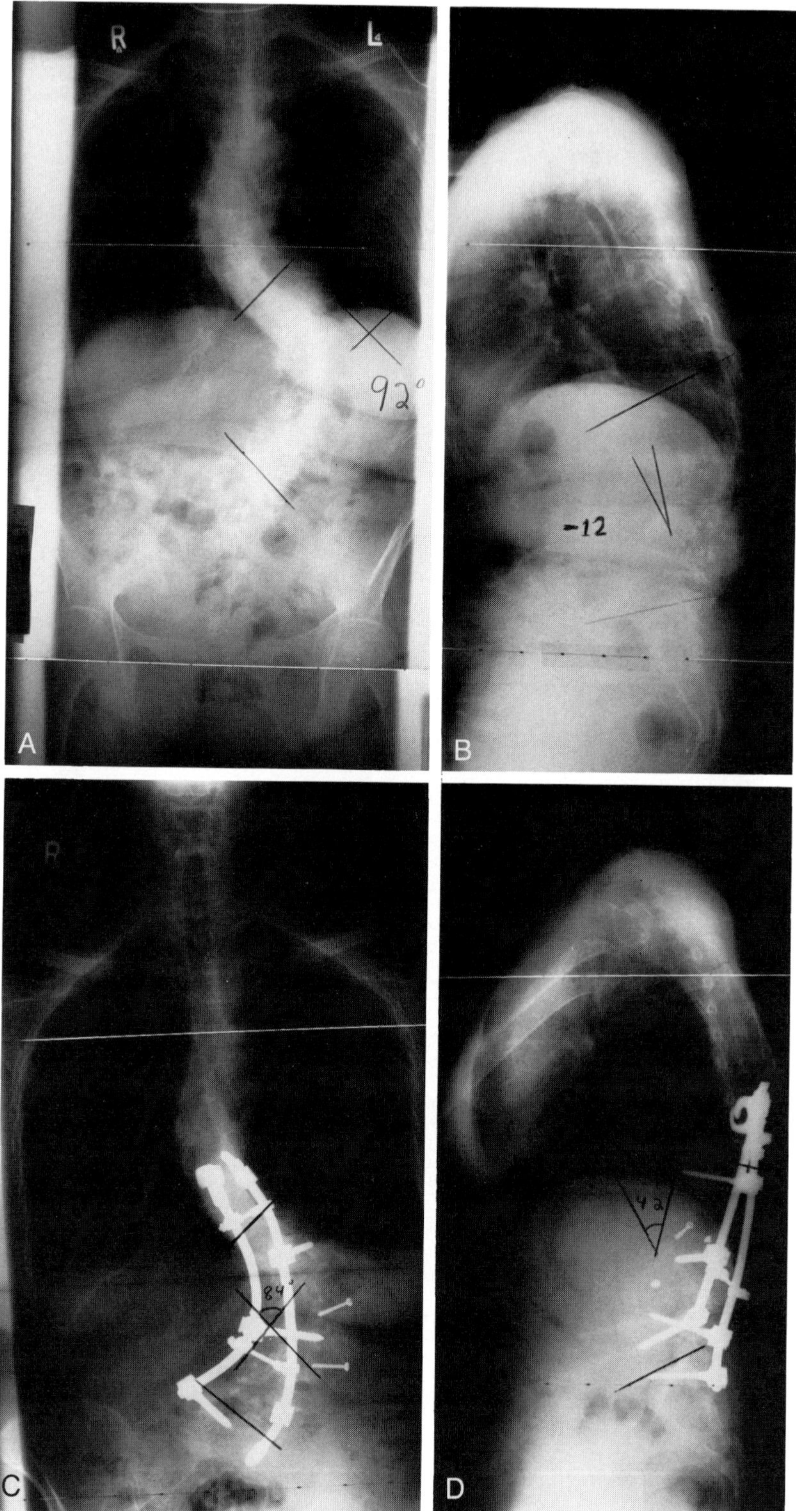

Figure 26–6. *A*, Female age 63 with progressive kyphoscoliosis and a curve of 92 degrees. Stage 1: Multiple anterior discotomies, morselization of L2–L3. Stage 2: C-D instrumentation and fusion. *B*, Preoperative lateral view (−12 degrees of lordosis). *C*, Postoperative anteroposterior view. Minimal correction. *D*, Postoperative lateral view. Marked restoration of lordosis to 42 degrees (gain 54 degrees).

although frequently if there is lipping of the vertebral body, particularly in cases associated with marked degeneration, this is not necessary. From a technical viewpoint, the major problem in many adults has to do with osteoporosis. This can be overcome with the injection of methylmethacrylate into predrilled screw holes in the vertebral bodies. Cooling the methylmethacrylate or using low-viscosity methylmethacrylate allows increased working time for injection of methylmethacrylate into enlarged screw holes. The use of a curette inside the screw hole enlarges the space within the vertebral body for retention of the cement to enhance fixation of the screws (Fig. 26–7).

The most significant difficulty encountered technically has been pull-out of the most proximal screw. I do not believe that an extra level should be incorporated across a nonfused space to prevent this problem (Fig. 26–8). In postmenopausal women I routinely add cement to the upper level at the time of screw insertion.

There have been no difficulties with fusions extending from L5 proximally. However, it is important that the iliolumbar veins at the L5 level be ligated to allow mobilization of the common iliac system.

Extension with Zielke instrumentation to the sacrum is used only in those cases where fusion to the sacrum is done based on preoperative assessment, as indicated previously, and combined with a posterior fusion. Extension of Zielke instrumentation above T9 or T10 is rarely of value since the disc spaces are so narrow that little correction can be obtained. The use of the derotator is almost routine to reproduce lordosis, or reduce kyphosis, of the thoracolumbar spine. This has been a marked advantage over the previously used Dwyer instrumentation, which I no longer use, and which tended frequently to produce a kyphosis despite accurate screw placement.

Autogenous bone graft has been used; this may consist of the excised rib cut into small fragments. The use of bits of block graft or placement of minced graft more anteriorly in the disc space helps to maintain or increase lordosis with the use of Zielke instrumentation. I do not use iliac crest bone, although

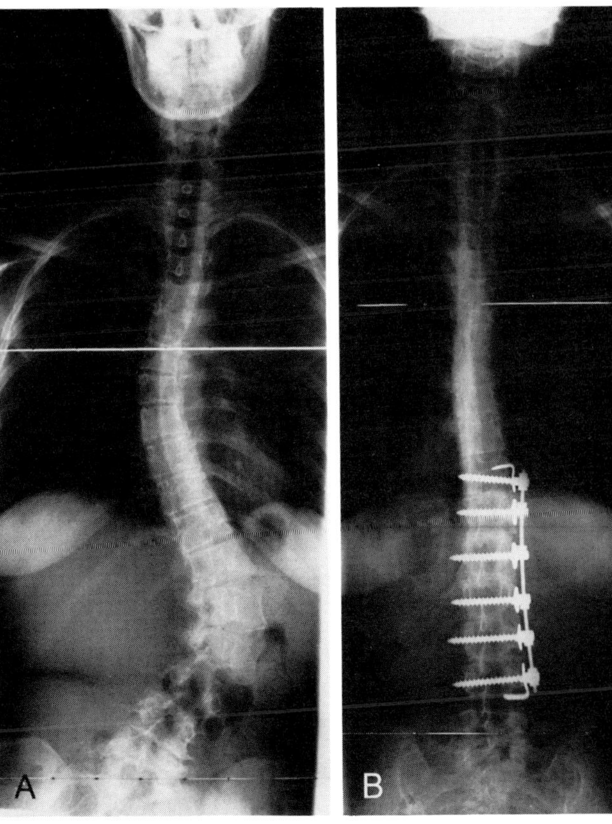

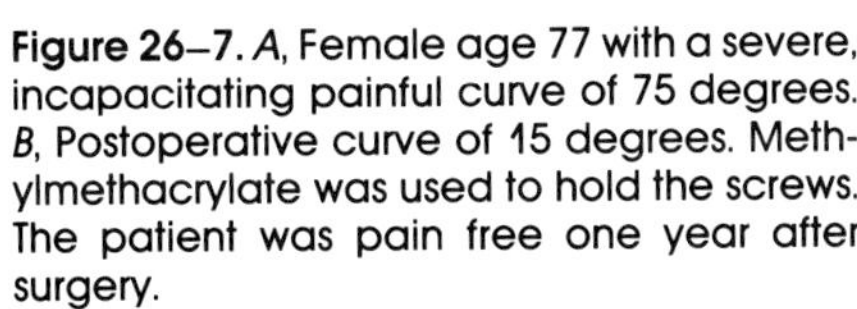

Figure 26–7. *A*, Female age 77 with a severe, incapacitating painful curve of 75 degrees. *B*, Postoperative curve of 15 degrees. Methylmethacrylate was used to hold the screws. The patient was pain free one year after surgery.

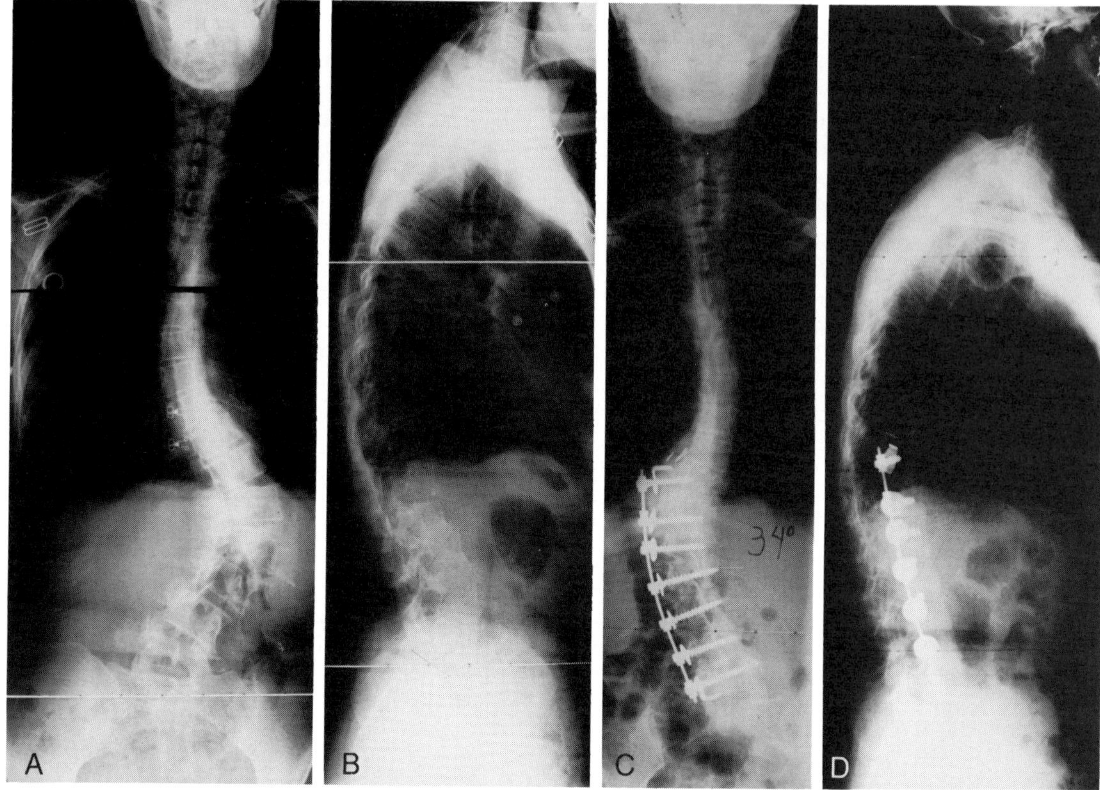

Figure 26–8. *A*, Female age 52 with a curve of 68 degrees that was painful, progressive, and rigid. *B*, Preoperative lordosis of 50 degrees at L1–S1. *C*, Postoperative curve of 34 degrees. Note the proximal hook pull-out. *D*, Postoperative lateral 38 degrees, across L1–S1, with a good long-term result.

this is a reasonable option. Some surgeons increasingly have found success with frozen allograft anteriorly. With the use of hypotensive anesthesia and cell savers, average blood loss has been 1750 ml. Transfusions using bank blood have been kept to a minimum. Hypotensive anesthesia is not routinely used in people over the age of 50.

Zielke instrumentation can be used safely in patients over the age of 70, although it is usually necessary to incorporate methylmethacrylate with the screws (see Fig. 26–7).

Correction using Zielke instrumentation is markedly improved over Dwyer instrumentation and posterior segmental instrumentation.[15, 20, 28, 33, 43, 51, 69, 70] A long-term review of the first 57 patients treated by Zielke instrumentation revealed the average correction was 70 per cent versus 45 per cent with Dwyer instrumentation, with no pseudarthrosis.[33]

The use of a derotational device improved correction of the curve in both the sagittal and anteroposterior planes with improved rotation by approximately one grade using the Nash-Moe method of classification for rotation.[46] Intraoperative complications included five fractured vertebral bodies. This problem was overcome by the use of methylmethacrylate. Postoperative complications included three lateral femoral cutaneous nerve entrapments, one of which required surgical decompression. Two post-thoracotomy syndromes were encountered that settled down with time. There were ten cases of atelectasis and pleural effusions that did not require major treatment. One case of proximal staple pull-out at two levels occurred that required subsequent posterior surgery. Nuts backed out of the screw head in ten cases without any curve deterioration or rod displacement. Rod disengagement from the screw head was noted in six cases without loss of correction over the immediate postoperative roentgenogram. Six patients had partial staple disengagement including the case noted. At an average follow-up of two years, mean loss of correction was less than 1 degree.

In double idiopathic curves the average correction was 62 per cent. At 24 months the mean loss was 3.4 degrees (4 per cent). The noninstrumented proximal thoracic curve improved 38 per cent after correction of the distal lumbar curve without deterioration at follow-up.

All surgical results revealed an improvement of 50 per cent correction over that anticipated from preoperative lateral bending anteroposterior radiographs.

An analysis of Zielke instrumentation, designed for anterior derotation, used posteriorly as pedicle fixation for degenerative disease in cases of scoliosis revealed a high incidence of rod breakage. As a result of this review, it is my policy not to use Zielke instrumentation posteriorly. It has been replaced by the use of C-D instrumentation.

Zielke instrumentation has also been used in the distal convex side of fractional lumbosacral curves for six patients with imbalance and pain (see Fig. 26–1). This has resulted in slightly greater than 40 per cent correction of the proximal major curve. This was done only in patients in whom the distal fractional curve was a source of pain, the patients were imbalanced, and balance was not restored on bending roentgenograms of the major curve. The follow-up period has been only four years in these patients and they may require further treatment of their major curve at a later date. I believe this technique should be reserved for those fractional curves in the lower lumbar and lumbosacral spine where this is the source of the pain, as shown on discography and facet blocks, and the patient is imbalanced.

Cotrel-Dubousset Instrumentation

The universal instrumentation system of Cotrel and Dubousset is now available.[9, 10, 13] The C-D instrumentation system attempts to combine the rigidity of segmental fixation with the concept of curve derotation to obtain correction. This report details my initial experience with the use of C-D instrumentation in the treatment of adult idiopathic scoliosis.

Between August 1985 and June 1988, 49 patients who had developed their deformity secondary to idiopathic scoliosis were treated surgically. There were 43 women and 6 men. An additional 45 patients underwent C-D instrumentation for other causes, but are not reviewed here.

The average age of the patients was 43 years with a range from 21 to 75 years. There were 19 patients older than 50 years at the time of surgery.

The curve distribution was 16 primary thoracic, 15 primary lumbar, 14 double major, and 4 thoracolumbar. Twelve patients had previous spinal fusions.

For the entire series, the patients that were instrumented had an average curve of 60 degrees preoperatively in the frontal plane, with a range of 13 to 115 degrees. Preoperatively the primary thoracic curves averaged 58 degrees, the primary lumbar curves averaged 48 degrees, the thoracolumbar curves averaged 55 degrees, and in the double-major curves, the thoracic curve averaged 76 degrees and the lumbar curve 66 degrees.

The surgical indications were disabling back pain or disabling back pain and neurologic symptoms in 44 patients. In five patients the indication for surgery was progression of the curve.

The technical details regarding the use of C-D instrumentation are extensively described elsewhere.[9, 10] In general, for previously unoperated thoracic curves, the selection of fusion levels as advocated by King and associates and the hook and rod placement as described by Cotrel and Dubousset were used.[9, 10, 29]

In patients with a severe, rigid thoracic curve greater than 90 degrees or in the previously fused patient, either an anterior or posterior release was performed as appropriate before C-D instrumentation. In the interval between the two stages, halo-dependent traction was used to improve curve flexibility and correction. This was done in four patients.

The treatment of thoracolumbar and lumbar curves often involved staged surgery. This was to reduce the high rate of complications associated with single-stage posterior surgery, including pseudarthrosis, poor curve correction, residual truncal imbalance, and loss of or failure to improve lumbar lordosis (see Figs. 26–5 and 26–6). A flexible thoracolumbar or lumbar curve with reasonable preservation of lumbar lordosis in which the fusion need not be extended to the sacrum may be treated with either a single-stage anterior Zielke procedure or single-stage posterior C-D instrumentation.

For rigid lumbar kyphoscoliosis, an initial anterior lumbar release with morselized bone grafting of the interspaces, followed by second-stage C-D instrumentation to derotate the curve and restore lumbar lordosis, was performed (see Figs. 26–5 and 26–6).

In rigid lumbar kyphoscoliosis, if the fusion had to be extended to the sacrum because of painful disc degeneration, an anterior release extending the length of the curve, including the L4–L5 interspaces. Wedge-shaped bone blocks were then inserted at the lower lumbar levels for fusion and to improve lumbosacral lordosis. This was supplemented by anterior internal fixation at these two levels (Fig. 26–9). The remaining levels were grafted anteriorly with morselized bone. Second-stage C-D instrumentation extending posteriorly to the sacrum was subsequently performed seven to ten days later. In four patients fusions extended to the sacrum.

Nineteen patients had staged or associated surgery including two anterior thoracic releases, two posterior thoracic releases, ten anterior thoracolumbar or lumbar releases, four nerve root decompressions, and one thoracoplasty.

Braces or casts were not routinely used except in elderly osteoporotic patients in whom fixation of the instrumentation was believed to be at risk. In these patients a custom-molded polypropylene thoracolumbar orthosis was provided. This was necessary in 14 patients.

Length of follow-up averaged 28 months, with a range of 15 to 49 months.

In the entire series, the average preoperative scoliosis was 60 degrees with a range of 13 to 115 degrees. At final follow-up the curves were reduced to an average of 35 degrees, or 42 per cent correction. In the subset of previously unoperated patients, curve correction averaged 50 per cent. In those patients with an associated anterior release, curve correction averaged 63 per cent. Correction in those patients fused previously averaged 35 per cent.

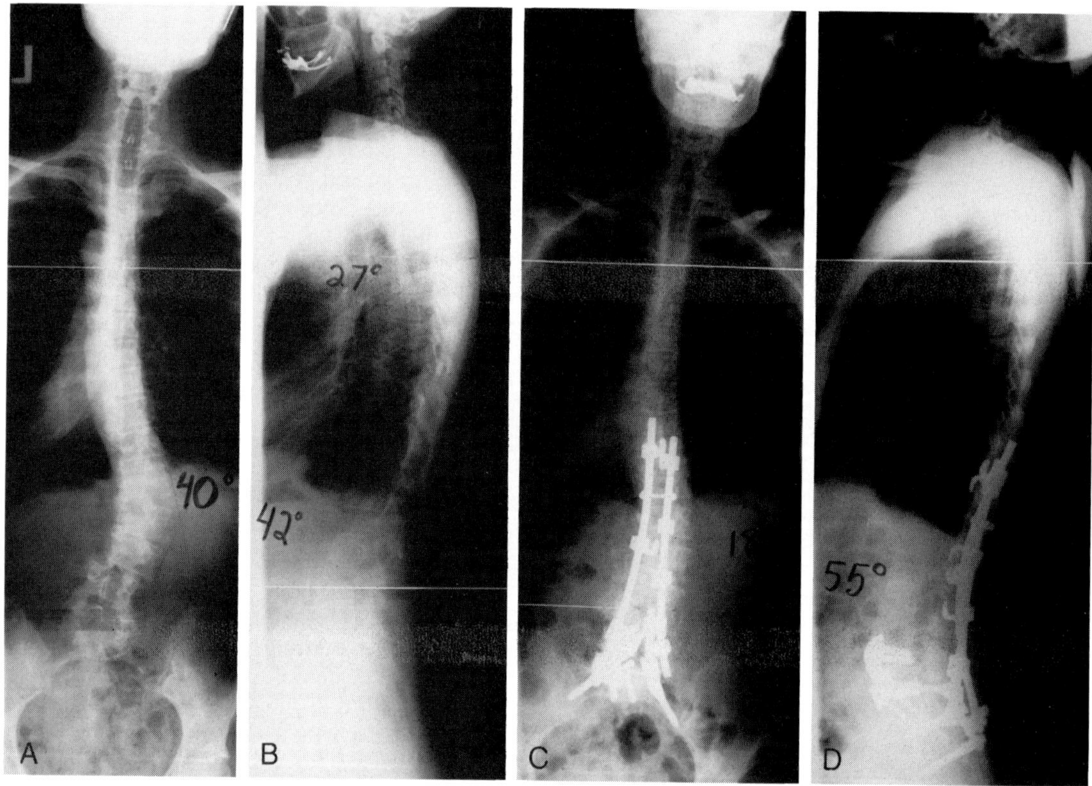

Figure 26–9. *A,* Female age 53 with progressive painful scoliosis of 40 degrees. *B,* The curve was flexible. Preoperative discography revealed painful degenerative L4–L5 and L5–S1 discs. *C, D,* In order to achieve solid fusion, two-stage surgery was performed. The first stage consisted of anterior L4–L5, L5–S1 discectomies, interbody iliac crest grafts, and internal fixation with an "I" beam Yuan plate at L4–S1 and two AO 6.5-mm screws at L5–S1. The second stage C-D instrumentation and fusion derotated the spine and increased the lordosis. The pain was relieved.

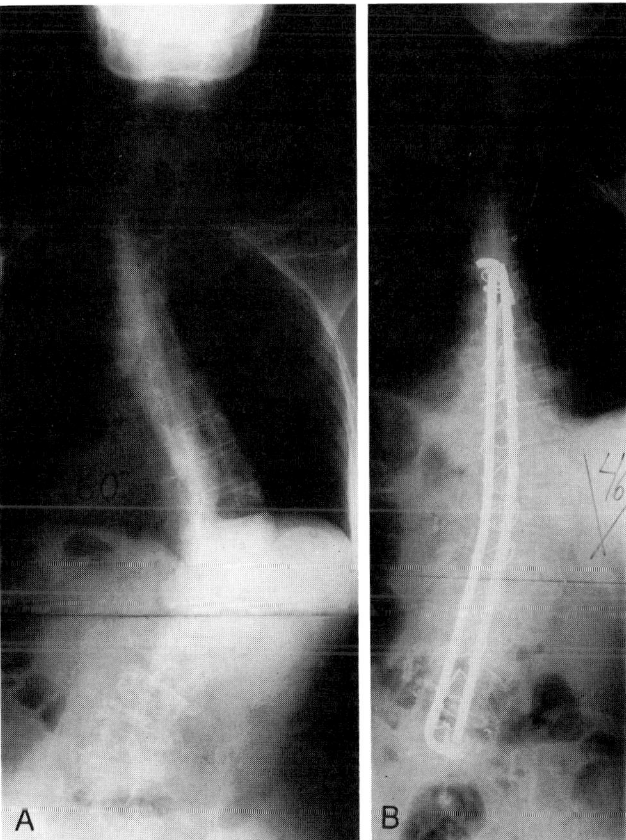

Figure 26–10. *A, B,* Luque instrumentation in a female age 58 with progressive and painful thoracolumbar kyphoscoliosis. The kyphosis precluded the use of Zielke instrumentation. Today, C-D instrumention with derotation would be used.

Percentage correction by curve type revealed significantly greater correction in the primary lumbar and thoracolumbar curves. This was due to the influence of an associated anterior release performed more often in this group. In thoracic curves, correction at final follow-up averaged 45 per cent. In lumbar curves, correction averaged 58 per cent. In thoracolumbar curves, correction averaged 60 per cent. In double-major curves, average correction of both the lumbar and thoracic component averaged 41 per cent.

Loss of correction for the entire series was negligible. There was a significant loss of correction (i.e., greater than 5 degrees) in seven patients. This averaged 13 degrees with a range of 6 to 28 degrees or 49 per cent (range 19 to 93 per cent) of initial correction.

Changes in the sagittal plane curves were a function of their preoperative size. In the relatively kyphotic lumbar spine (less than 20 degrees) lordosis improved an average of 133 per cent, from a preoperative average of 15 degrees to 35 degrees after operation (see Figs. 26–5 and 26–6). In the 20- to 50-degree range (average 38 degrees) lordosis improved only 32 per cent (average 47 degrees). In the relatively hyperlordotic lumbar spine (greater than 50 degrees; average 66) the postoperative lumbar lordosis declined an average of 11 per cent to 59 degrees.

In the hypokyphotic thoracic spine (less than 20 degrees; average 11 degrees) the thoracic kyphosis improved an average of 173 per cent to 30 degrees. In the 20- to 60-degree range the change was insignificant. In the excessively kyphotic spine (average 73 degrees) the thoracic kyphosis decreased an average of 11 degrees.

Apical vertebral rotation, as determined by the method of Nash and Moe, improved an average of one-half a grade, from 2.5 before operation to 2.0 after operation.[46] Preoperatively 30 patients were imbalanced; postoperatively 36 were balanced. Significant imbalance postoperatively (greater than 2 cm) remained in five patients.

Fourteen patients, usually the more elderly

and osteoporotic, wore orthoses postoperatively, usually for four to six months. Blood loss averaged 1400 ml.

Significant or disabling pain present in 44 patients before surgery was eliminated in 30, was significantly improved in six, and was the same or worse in eight patients.

Twenty-eight complications occurred in 20 patients. There were two pneumothoraces, one case of pancreatitis, three urinary tract infections, one dural tear closed primarily, and one superficial wound infection that responded to dressing changes. One patient, age 66, developed a hemothorax after a thoracoabdominal approach for an anterior release that required repeat thoracotomy for control of the bleeding. This patient developed chronic post-thoracotomy incisional pain.

Eight patients complained about prominent rods; five of them have undergone partial removal because of persistent irritation. Neurologic complications were transient and consisted of neuropraxias. Two patients developed complications after anterior approaches. The first was a fourth lumbar nerve root neuropraxia with associated quadriceps weakness that resolved. The second was persistent pain in the distribution of the genitofemoral nerve that resolved after its resection. The only injury directly attributable to the C-D instrumentation procedure was a fourth nerve root neuropraxia that resolved.

The most frequent complication readily attributable to the instrumentation system was that of hook pull-out due to bone failure, that is, lamina fractures. This occurred in five patients. Fortunately, a pattern was apparent, and a reasonable solution seems possible. Four of the five failures occurred in the lumbar region at the distal fixation site. These occurred in patients over 50 years of age who had undergone a preliminary anterior lumbar release before C-D instrumentation. These four failures occurred among ten anterior lumbar releases performed. It would seem prudent in the elderly patient in whom a preliminary anterior release has been performed to supplement the distal lumbar fixation with pedicle screws when possible, instead of relying on laminar hooks. In ten similar subsequent cases in which lumbar pedicle screw fixation was used instrumentation failure has not occurred.

The last fixation failure occurred in the thoracic region in a previously multiply operated patient who had also undergone a first-stage anterior thoracic release. Four of the five instrumentation failures were reinstrumented in the immediate perioperative period. Two of these had a good final result.

One of the five patients with an instrumentation failure had a delayed revision ten months later. She had fused, but had loss of lumbar lordosis and the development of a flat-back syndrome. This was corrected with a lumbar extension osteotomy and she now has a good result.

Thus, three of the five instrumentation failures were ultimately salvageable. The remaining two patients have both fused with loss of lumbar lordosis. Both have pain and fatigue with ambulation.

One patient required extension of her fusion to the sacrum 18 months after C-D instrumentation. At age 16 she had undergone Harrington instrumentation, but developed multiple pseudarthroses in the lumbar region with progressively debilitating pain. Her pain was attributed to the pseudarthroses, however discography at L5–S1 was not performed before the C-D instrumentation. Because of persistent pain after instrumentation, discography was performed and demonstrated a painful lumbosacral disc. She improved after extension of the fusion to the sacrum.

The pseudarthrosis rate appears low. One patient had an obvious pseudarthrosis at L4–L5 despite a circumferential fusion attempt at that level. She has persistent pain but refused further surgery. A 54-year-old woman was found to have three pseudarthroses in the lumbar region after instrumentation of a double major curve. Tomograms were not helpful in confirming the pseudarthroses, but she had persistent pain and lost some correction, prompting exploration and pseudarthrosis repair.

Another patient had a pseudarthrosis in the thoracic region with persistent pain and loss of correction. A bone scan demonstrated uptake in the midthoracic region. Surgical exploration revealed two pseudoarthroses that were corrected and refused.

C-D instrumentation seems to have its greatest benefit in the maintenance or improvement of sagittal plane curves in both the thoracic and lumbar region. In the initial enthusiasm for frontal plane curve correction with Harrington instrumentation the sagittal plane curves were often ignored (Fig. 26–10).

The results from this series indicate that C-D instrumentation causes salubrious changes in lumbar lordosis and thoracic kyphosis. The degree of change is a function of the preoperative size of the curve.

Improvement in lumbar lordosis using C-D instrumentation is in marked distinction from the other instrumentation systems described above. This success was influenced by the use of a staged anterior release in many cases. C-D instrumentation allows the surgeon to take the most advantage of the benefits available from staged anterior surgery.

There were several complications in the series, but it must be realized that several of these patients had complex deformities and 12 patients had undergone previous fusions. Also, 19 patients had staged surgery in the course of their treatment with C-D instrumentation.

All neurologic injuries were neuropraxias and all resolved. Two of these occurred in multiply operated patients and only one could be attributed to the C-D instrumentation procedure. The wound infection rate was low despite multiple procedures that were often long and complex.

A 16 per cent incidence of rod irritation occurred and is somewhat high. C-D instrumentation is bulky compared with Harrington instrumentation. Instrument removal is commonly performed after other orthopedic procedures, however, such as fracture fixation. Thus, instrument removal after scoliosis surgery may be a reasonable trade-off if the initial fixation is enhanced by a somewhat bulkier segmental system such as C-D instrumentation.

Loss of fixation occurred in five patients and resulted from lamina fractures, not from hook dislodgment, which usually occurred with the Harrington system. These occurred in elderly patients who had undergone a staged anterior release. This might be preventable by supplementing the lumbar fixation with pedicle screws instead of relying on laminar hooks in older patients in whom an anterior release has been performed.

Ultimate satisfaction with the procedure must be judged in terms of pain relief because this was the primary indication for surgery in 85 per cent of the patients. Preoperative pain was relieved in 30 patients and in six it was reduced so that they required only occasional non-narcotic analgesics.

Eight patients continued to complain of pain postoperatively that was the same as or worse than before surgery. Three of these patients appeared to have pseudarthroses. One patient appeared to have developed symptoms of spinal stenosis after fusion of her thoracic scoliosis. Ultimately, 86 per cent of the patients had improvement in their preoperative pain.

C-D instrumentation is a complex system, but it is this complexity that provides the surgeon with the versatility necessary to tackle difficult surgical problems. Certainly there is a learning curve involved, but with experience operative time approaches that of other scoliosis reduction systems.

COSMESIS

A review of the first 1000 patients with scoliosis I treated revealed that approximately 10 per cent were treated essentially for cosmetic reasons. These were primarily thoracic curves with a range from 45 to 75 degrees. The age range was from 20 to 42 years. Ninety per cent of the patients were women.

The correction of thoracic deformities for cosmetic reasons in the adult should be given serious consideration. After careful assessment of the reasons for the desire for surgery and a careful explanation of the procedure and its postoperative course and complications, such surgery can be performed on adults, provided that the surgeon is experienced and there is full back-up of institutional facilities and care.

The past few years have seen a return to excision of the rib hump. This is particularly valuable in rigid curves in the thoracic spine and especially in the sagittal plane when there is a hypokyphosis. In more mobile curves the advent of C-D instrumentation to derotate the spine helps to decrease the rib hump. An associated rib excision can be done at the same time.

A review of 20 patients who underwent rib excision consisting of five to six ribs on the convexity with rigid deformities of 90 degrees or greater revealed no untoward morbidity. There were no changes in preoperative and postoperative ventilation studies. Rib hump excision in the presence of a severe rigid thoracic scoliosis can markedly improve the cosmetic result.

In mobile curves the use of C-D instrumentation is preferred. Because of its enhanced stability C-D instrumentation can be used in rigid curves as well. Postoperative orthoses are often not necessary.

At the time of rib excision, bone may be cut into small fragments to be used as graft. The ribs are excised subperiosteally through an incision created at right angles to the longitudinal spinal excision. Two myocutaneous flaps are created to expose the ribs.

SEVERE RIGID SCOLIOTIC DEFORMITIES

I have reported on 85 patients with deformities of 90 degrees or greater, whose curves on bending roentgenograms failed to change.[31]

Fifteen of these patients were primarily kyphotic, 42 had idiopathic curves, and 28 had congenital curves. Most were thoracic and thoracolumbar curves. Thirty-two patients had fusions either as a result of congenital failures (28) or spontaneously (4). Thirty-three patients had been untreated, but were rigid on bending roentgenograms, and were found at the time of surgery to have no spontaneous fusion. Twenty patients had had previous fusions and had progression of their deformity and pain. All patients underwent posterior releases, including osteotomies of previous fusions for congenitally fused spines when necessary. Posterior osteotomies were done at multiple levels, usually four. These were associated with rib releases over three to four levels on the concavity, transverse process osteotomies, and rib resections of five to six ribs on the convexity. Forty patients also had anterior osteotomies. The age range of the patients was from 20 to 55; curve magnitude was from 75 to 180 degrees.

Second-stage surgery was performed two weeks later. At the time of primary release surgery, traction was applied in the initial form of halofemoral traction in 32 patients, and halopelvic distraction later. The latter form of traction continues to be used in severe curves. It has been replaced to some degree by halo-dependent traction either in the circoelectric bed at 30 degrees of dependency or associated with halo wheelchair traction. The second-stage procedure done two weeks later consisted of posterior instrumentation originally with Harrington instrumentation, superseded by sublaminar wiring techniques, and more recently C-D instrumentation.

The degree of correction averaged 40 per cent with halopelvic and 32 per cent with halofemoral distraction. Subsequent Harrington instrumentation added a further 8 per cent to correction. Overall correction in the rigid group of curves was 40 per cent. This was comparable with a series previously reported on mobile curves. Idiopathic curves were corrected an average of 48 per cent, congenital curves 33 per cent.[31]

As previously indicated, the use of sublaminar wiring described by Luque has been abandoned in the treatment of scoliosis with the exception of some cases of paralytic scoliosis.[40, 41] This follows its use in over 200 cases of adult spinal deformity. The reason for changing instrumentation systems is that with the advent of C-D instrumentation and pedicle fixation, more rigid fixation and true means of deformity correction, particularly derotation, are possible. In mobile curves in which it is believed that anterior surgery may not be justified—for example, in cases of significant arteriosclerosis with anterior calcification of the aorta, or cases of marked anterior osteopenia where the curve is still mobile—C-D instrumentation can derotate the spine and restore lordosis.

In cases of significant rigid kyphoscoliosis C-D instrumentation has proved invaluable for restoring lordosis and relieving pain when performed after anterior supplemented discectomies with minced bone graft in the interbody spaces. The instrumentation is carried out two weeks after anterior surgery and can be used in the presence of extensive laminectomies for spinal stenosis (see Figs. 26–5 and 26–6). To date my experience has proved exciting and offers a means of dealing with rigid, painful kyphoscoliosis, particularly in the elderly, with excellent results and decreased risks of neurologic and vascular complications related to instrumentation.

STRUCTURAL DISABILITIES

Patients who have a paralytic scoliosis may find sitting at a desk or wheelchair difficult because of marked pelvic obliquity and/or associated kyphosis with a collapsing spine or hyperlordosis (Fig. 26–11). The latter is encountered particularly in patients who had peritoneal shunts in childhood. Patients with paralytic scoliosis are treated best by using a combined anterior and posterior approach that eliminates the need for heavy postoperative

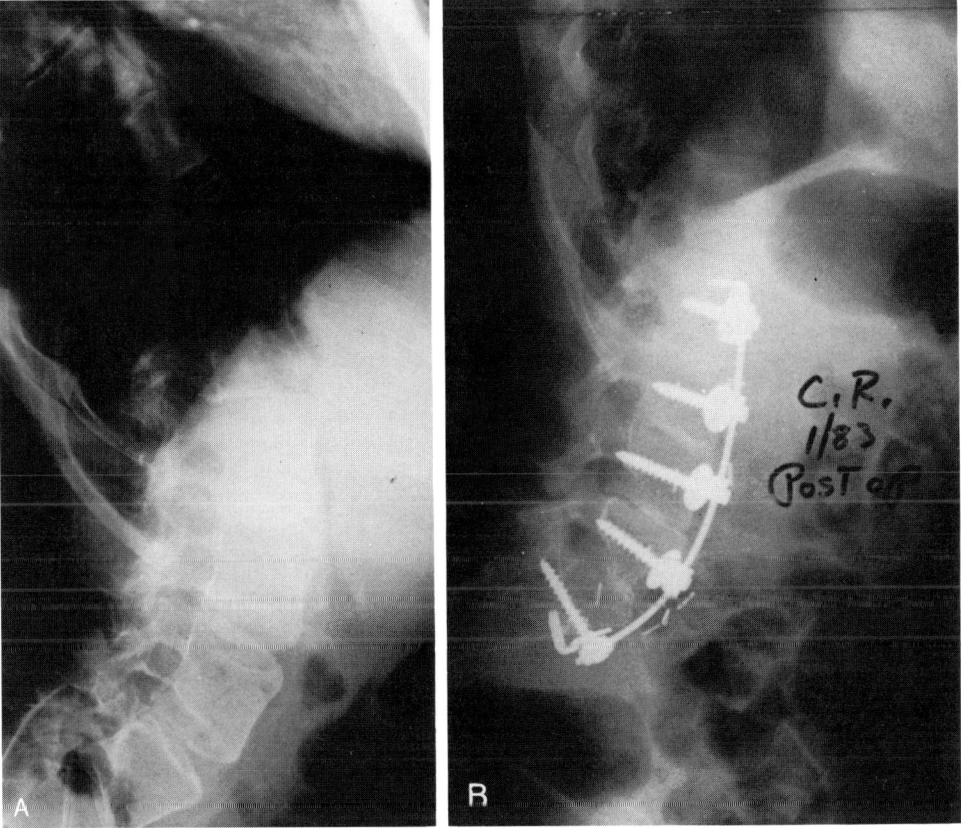

Figure 26–11. *A*, Marked paralytic hyperlordosis. *B*, The lordosis has been reduced to 60 degrees at L1–S1 by anterior Zielke instrumentation. Note the anteroposterior orientation of the screws.

immobilization and allows for early ambulation in a wheelchair.

Certain paralytic curves of a collapsing nature in which respiratory function is decreasing can be significantly helped by correction of the deformity. This results in improved diaphragmatic breathing. A preoperative trial of halo-dependent traction may show an improvement in respiratory function and point out the advantages of surgical correction of the deformity to improve respiratory function by lifting the diaphragm out of the abdomen.

The use of C-D instrumentation has not proved to be sufficient in the treatment of paralytic deformities that extend into the distal lumbar spine and I advocate an anterior and posterior approach. In children the use of Luque instrumentation to the pelvis using L rods, or the Galveston technique, or other modifications has proved of value. In adults, however, this is insufficient and a two-stage anterior and posterior procedure is necessary.

SPINAL DEFORMITIES OVER THE AGE OF FIFTY

The adult over 50 represents a complex problem. The deformity is often rigid and may be associated with significant imbalance and loss of normal lordosis of the lumbar spine. The bone is frequently osteopenic and there may be associated neurologic problems related to spinal stenosis. The major complaint at presentation is pain. My early experience was that major spinal deformities in patients over the age of 50 could be corrected in terms of deformity only at great risks to the neurologic structures, since most of these curves are rigid. As a result, in the early literature most such deformities were stabilized with Harrington instrumentation with little attempt at correction. This often resulted in continuing kyphosis.

With the addition of improved techniques of

anterior fixation such as Zielke instrumentation, and posterior fixation techniques such as C-D instrumentation, correction can now be safely achieved.[9, 70] In the presence of a thoracolumbar or lumbar deformity with good preservation of lordosis, anterior Zielke instrumentation can be safely used. The use of methylmethacrylate has greatly enhanced the holding power of screws in the vertebral bodies. Methylmethacrylate should not routinely be used posteriorly in the pedicles, with the exception of the first sacral pedicle, as the cement may exude from the osteopenic pedicle in elderly adults and result in canal compromise. In the presence of rigid kyphoscoliosis or where there is minimal lumbar lordosis, a two-stage procedure is preferable. The first stage consists of multiple disc excisions and interbody graft using small bone fragments, followed ten days later by posterior derotation using C-D instrumentation to correct the curve and restore lumbar lordosis. This has proved of great value over the last few years.

I performed a long-term review of 80 patients over the age of 50. Fifty patients had idiopathic curves and the remainder had a congenital curve, a paralytic curve, or a pure kyphotic deformity. Twelve of the idiopathic curves were thoracic, nine thoracolumbar, and 17 lumbar. There were 12 double curves. All patients had back pain. Eight patients had progressive pulmonary dysfunction, usually related to an increasing kyphosis. Fifty-seven per cent had documented evidence of progression of greater than 10 degrees three years preoperatively. Sixteen patients had associated nerve root pain. These 80 patients underwent 100 procedures. Twenty patients had a second-stage procedure, either anterior or posterior, for increased stabilization. Twelve patients had concurrent anterior and posterior procedures performed largely for correction of flat-back syndrome through a single-stage combined posterior and anterior osteotomy with anterior and posterior fixation. Although 20 patients underwent a second-stage procedure for stabilization, most had rigid kyphoscoliosis. Fourteen also had a second-stage anterior procedure since fusion was carried to the sacrum posteriorly and, to ensure a solid fusion, anterior fixation and fusion was carried out as described under fusions to the sacrum. A review of all cases showed excellent to good results in 69 per cent, 56.5 per cent of which were good and 12.5 per cent were excellent. Fair and poor results occurred in 6 and 25 per cent, respectively. No pain was noted in 27 patients postoperatively (34 per cent), and radicular pain was relieved in all patients.

In the presence of spinal stenosis or other causes of nerve root pain in scoliosis, performing a posterior decompression alone, particularly if more than one side at one level is decompressed, often leads to increased deformity, instability, pain, and further surgery. An associated stabilization procedure should almost always be performed. I have encountered many patients who have undergone posterior decompression for spinal stenosis in the presence of scoliosis who presented within months to years with significant collapsing, progressive, painful scoliosis (Fig. 26–17). These patients have marked difficulty in obtaining a subsequent stable fused spine because of lack of bone stock as a result of the decompression and subsequent scarring.

In this group of 80 patients over the age of 50, curve correction was 22 per cent with Harrington instrumentation and 22 per cent with sublaminar wired Harrington rods. Twenty-one per cent correction was achieved with Harrington rods combined with L rods and 33 per cent with double-L rods. Curve correction with Dwyer instrumentation was 42 per cent and 67 per cent with Zielke instrumentation (see Figs. 26–2 to 26–7). This compares favorably with the 70 per cent of all adults over the age of 20 corrected by Zielke instrumentation reported previously.[33] The average correction obtained with C-D instrumentation was 50 per cent (see Figs. 26–5 and 26–6). Thirteen of the patients treated with Harrington instrumentation alone developed flat-back syndrome. Pure posterior distraction in the lumbar spine at any age should be avoided. Kyphotic deformities are best treated by anterior instrumentation. Instrumentation failure in this group of elderly adults occurred in 11 cases. Harrington rod fractures occurred in six cases, dislodgment of the rod in one case, L-rod migration in two cases, anterior screw breakage in one case, and posterior Zielke rod breakage in one case.

Intraoperative bone fracture of either lamina or vertebral bodies occurred in seven cases and was salvaged with the use of methylmethacrylate, associated with internal fixation devices. Thirteen patients developed iatrogenic flat-back deformities secondary to Harrington distraction. Four of these patients subsequently underwent restoration of lordosis by single-stage anterior and posterior osteotomies. One patient became paraparetic as a result of surgery, but partially improved. Pseudarthrosis occurred in 21 per cent of patients, primarily in the Harrington instrumentation series. There were no pseudarthroses with the use of Zielke instrumentation or C-D instrumentation. Twenty-five per cent of pseudarthroses occurred in fusions carried to L5 and 24 per cent occurred when carried to the sacrum. All pseudarthroses to the sacrum occurred before the development of two-stage surgery for fusions to the sacrum, as described elsewhere in this chapter. Nine patients developed kyphosis secondary to osteopenic fractures proximal to their instrumentation. Because of improved diagnostic capabilities, improved postoperative care, and the advent of improved fixation such as posterior pedicle fixation, particularly of the C-D type, and anterior Zielke instrumentation, morbidity has been significantly lowered in the past five years. The infection rate was 1 per cent. Pulmonary complications including atelectasis, pneumonia, and/or adult respiratory distress syndrome occurred in 24 per cent of patients.

The importance of restoration of lordosis cannot be overemphasized, particularly in cases of kyphoscoliosis. The use of multiple-level releases anteriorly followed by posterior derotation with C-D instrumentation and, if necessary, posterior osteotomy through the pars interarticularis to increase lordosis markedly improve the quality of life of these older patients.

FUSIONS TO THE SACRUM

A 1978 review by the Morbidity Committee of the Scoliosis Research Society noted that 4 per cent of all scoliosis fusions resulted in a clinically significant loss of lumbar lordosis (unpublished data). This included all forms of posterior instrumentation in all areas of the spine. In a review of fusions to the sacrum, loss of lumbar lordosis was noted in approximately 50 per cent of adult cases and was clinically significant, requiring revision surgery in half of these patients.[34] Balderston and associates experienced similar results.[2] It was not recognized until the late 1970s that distraction of the thoracolumbar and lumbar spine might result in loss of lordosis even with contouring of the Harrington rod together with the use of square-ended Moe rods and sacral-alar hooks[5] as described by Casey and associates. The advent of Luque L rods across the sacroiliac joint and the refinement of this with the Galveston technique resulted in improved maintenance of lordosis and enhanced the rate of fusion for posterior instrumentation to the sacrum.[41] The initial incidence of pseudarthrosis to the sacrum using Harrington rods either with a sacral bar or alar hooks was 40 per cent.[34] A review of Luque instrumentation to the sacrum revealed that the incidence of pseudarthrosis decreased to 15 per cent.[36] The incidence of flat-back deformity in fusions to the sacrum occurred in only 20 per cent of patients and was significant in only one-fifth of these. This occurred despite marked contouring of the rods into lordosis, and primarily only in patients who were kyphoscoliotic. C-D instrumentation has not had this problem because of the possibility of obtaining increased lordosis with segmental fixation. Fusion to the sacrum in idiopathic scoliosis is indicated only if the last motion segment is a source of the pain, or if this motion segment is included in the curve (abnormal L5–S1 take-off).

Since 1981, when fusion to the sacrum was indicated, a two-stage procedure has been performed.[30] If the patient is scoliotic with reasonable lordosis, initially anterior instrumentation using Zielke instrumentation is done. The use of Zielke instrumentation anterior to the sacrum, although technically demanding, has not resulted in any problems related to the common iliac vessels, either artery or vein. Careful technique avoiding any impingement of screw heads against the vessels has resulted in no vascular complications. The rod can safely pass beneath the common iliac vessels, since the rods are small and close to the vertebral body. Occasionally two rods at the distal two to three levels are necessary to help control rotation at the lumbosacral junction. A second-stage posterior fusion using segmental wiring was initially done, but this has been replaced by the use of pedicle fixation (C-D or plate instrumentation).

If the patient has rigid kyphoscoliosis and requires fusion to the sacrum, the first stage is also anterior, consisting of multiple anterior discotomies. The interbody spaces are filled with bone chips, except for the L4–L5 and the L5–S1 interspaces. At those levels interbody bicortical or tricortical grafts are used to maximally fill the disc spaces and increase lordosis. Internal fixation is performed to enhance stability over these two levels. This is followed either at two weeks or preferably at the same sitting by posterior instrumentation that derotates the lumbar spine and restores lordosis.

If the kyphoscoliosis is mobile, the scoliosis is corrected and lordosis restored by first-stage posterior C-D instrumentation and fusion followed by a second-stage anterior L4–S5 fusion with solid interbody grafts and instrumentation. When instrumentation from L4 to the sacrum is indicated, a rigid contoured I plate designed by Yuan or two 6.5-mm AO cancellous screws have replaced Zielke instrumentation (see Fig. 26–9).

I have not encountered any late vascular problems in over 450 cases of anterior instrumentation in both the thoracic and lumbar spine.

During anterior instrumentation, particularly through a left retroperitoneal approach, ligation of the segmental vessels allows the aorta and common iliac vessels to fall away from the vertebral bodies and provides room for placement of the internal fixation devices. Since most lumbar and thoracolumbar curves are left-sided, this approach is most commonly used.

Bicortical grafts from the iliac crest in younger patients, or tricortical grafts in more osteoporotic patients, are used to maintain disc height at L4–L5 and L5–S1 and to increase lordosis anteriorly. Internal fixation is used to enhance fixation since iliac crest bone is unable to support loads much heavier than body weight in the erect position without the use of internal fixation. With the use of combined anterior and posterior approaches the incidence of pseudarthrosis has been reduced to 5 per cent in the last 30 cases.

EXTENSIONS OF FUSIONS IN THE LUMBAR SPINE

Reports by Edgar and Mehta and Cochran and associates, and a review of my statistics show that patients who have had previous fusions to L2, L3, L4, or L5 are at increased risk to develop degenerative changes below their fusion (Fig. 26–12).[6, 16] These patients require extension of their fusion if nonoperative means fail to control pain and the problem becomes progressive, often associated with some degree of spinal stenosis at the level immediately below the fusion. If after investi-

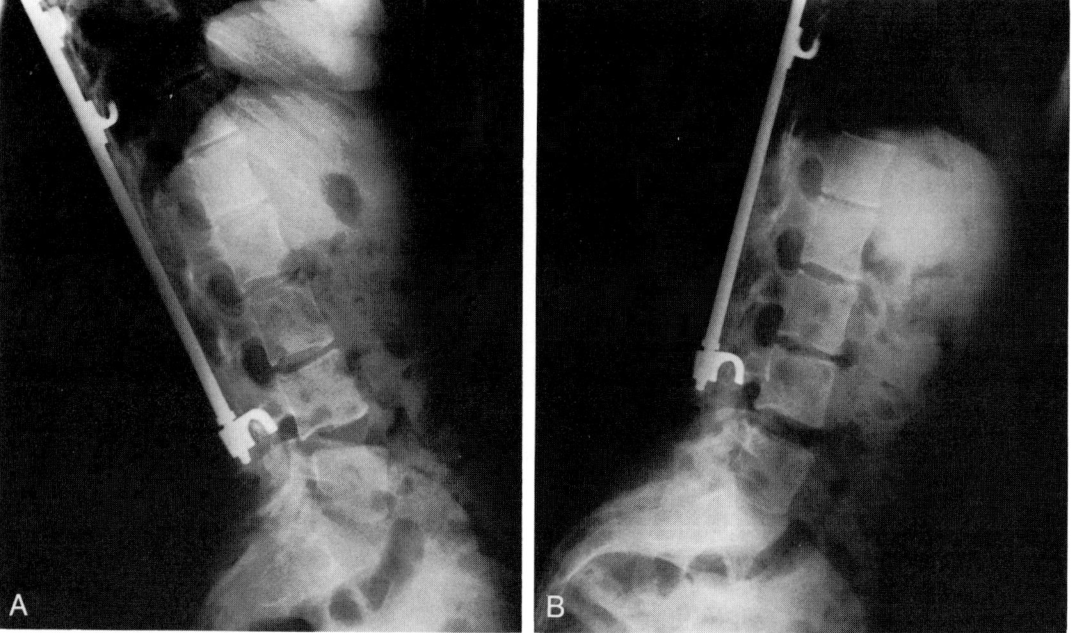

Figure 26–12. *A, B,* Flexion-extension views demonstrate marked instability at the L4–L5 disc space. The patient had undergone Harrington instrumentation 12 years before.

gative studies, including myelography, CT, discograpy, and facet blocks, a fusion does not require extension to the sacrum, posterior instrumentation or anterior instrumentation alone frequently suffices. If extension of the fusion to the sacrum is required, however, a combined approach is necessary.[3] Extension of a fusion to the sacrum is usually done as a single-stage procedure using posterior pedicle fixation and anterior instrumentation. To improve lordosis some of the posterior lamina at L4–L5, L3–L4, or L5–S1 can be removed and compression applied through the pedicles. Anterior interbody grafts are done after opening the disc space as widely as possible. Anterior instrumentation using Zielke rods or a plate helps to enhance the fusion rate (Fig. 26–13). The best results have been obtained with removal of posterior bone to increase lordosis, rather than fusing the spine in situ with instrumentation posteriorly and then anteriorly with an interbody graft and instrumentation. A review of 24 cases of extension fusion to the sacrum revealed that of six fused posteriorly with Harrington rods only, five failed because of development of pseudarthrosis and flat-back (unpublished data). Nine patients fused in situ anteriorly with interbody grafts to maintain lordosis and supplemented either at the same stage or at a second-stage with posterior instrumentation and fusion resulted in three failures with pseudarthrosis and flat-back. Ten fused at a single stage with associated removal of bone posteriorly through the pars interarticularis to increase lordosis and an increased opening of interbody space anteriorly did well, however, with only one pseudarthrosis. Review (unpublished) of a further 32 cases similarly performed reveals the same results as those ten obtained at a single stage earlier.

RESTORATION OF IATROGENIC LUMBAR LORDOSIS

As noted previously, fusions to the sacrum with posterior instrumentation, particularly Harrington instrumentation, have resulted in a 50 per cent loss of lumbar lordosis. Many of these patients require restoration surgery.[14, 17, 34, 39] Although adolescents recover well, it is not unusual for an adolescent who has had fusion to the sacrum to complain of fatigue symptoms and pain in the lower back when he or she reaches the third, fourth, or fifth decade of life. Care must be taken to ascertain that pain does not arise from the sacroiliac joint. Loss of lumbar lordosis results in an increasingly forward flexed posture as the day progresses and the patients walk with their knees and hips flexed. This is an unsightly deformity (Fig. 26–14). Despite a solid fusion, these patients complain of increasing pain and fatigue. This problem was not recognized until the late 1970s. I presented a review of 54 cases in which a combined anterior and posterior osteotomy was used for restoration of lordosis.[37] A combined approach offers better results than a posterior osteotomy of an old fusion mass. Greater correction can be obtained and is not necessary to immobilize the patients in a hip spica postoperatively. Moreover, the use of posterior osteotomy alone has resulted in late recurrence of deformity in at least two cases. A report by Lagrone and associates also indicated that the best results can be obtained with anterior and posterior procedures.[39] A combined anteroposterior approach, together with internal fixation and the use of a lumbar orthosis postoperatively, allows for early ambulation.

Causal factors that result in loss of lumbar lordosis are, in descending order of frequency, distraction instrumentation of the lumbar spine that ends caudally at the L5 or S1 vertebral level; a thoracolumbar junction kyphosis greater than 15 degrees, especially if associated with a kyphotic thoracic spine; and degenerative changes above and/or below a previous fusion caused by loss of disc height that occurs more commonly below a previous fusion ending at L3, L4, or L5.

If loss of lumbar lordosis is also associated with a pseudarthrosis, repair of the pseudarthrosis alone will not relieve the symptoms.

If the patient is imbalanced in the anteroposterior plane, a quadrilateral wedge osteotomy done anteriorly and posteriorly can restore balance in the frontal plane and restore lumbar lordosis in the sagittal plane. If the fusion is solid the osteotomy is usually carried out at the L3–L4 level; otherwise it may be carried out through the posterior pseudarthrosis that is enlarged. The nerve roots at the level of the posterior osteotomy must be clearly identified, and an osteotomy analogous to that described by Smith-Peterson is used. The use of Dwyer screws in the lateral fusion mass posteriorly and the use of cables to close the osteotomy site are preferable. Eight screws

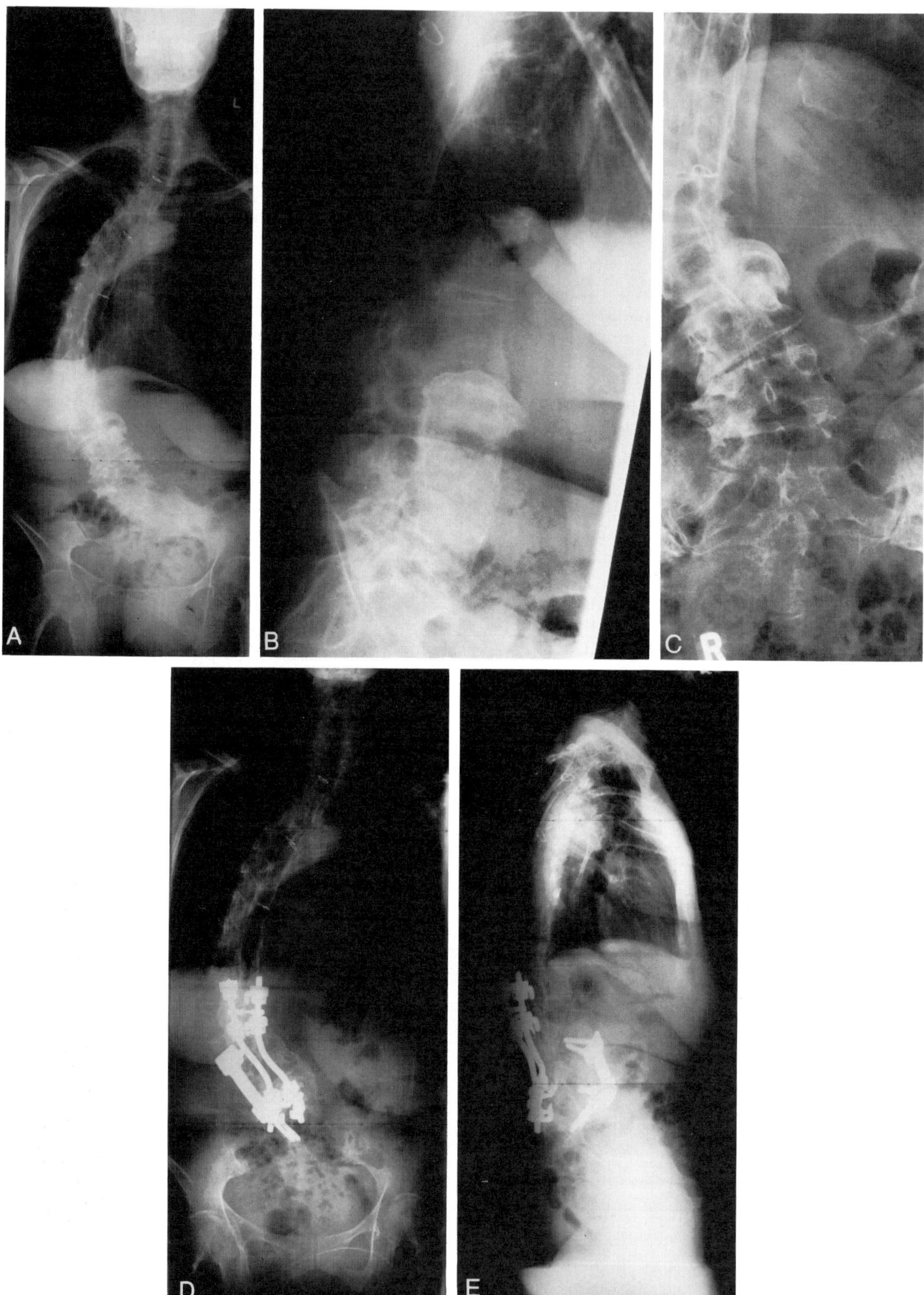

Figure 26–13. *A, B,* Female age 56 who had undergone a posterior fusion 25 years previously. *C,* Anteroposterior view demonstrates marked degenerative changes at L4–L5, L5–S1 with a flat back. *D, E,* Postoperative anteroposterior and lateral views showing extension of fusion to S1. Note the restoration of lordosis. Preoperative discography reproduced pain at L4–L5 and L5–S1. Relief was obtained temporarily by means of facet blocks.

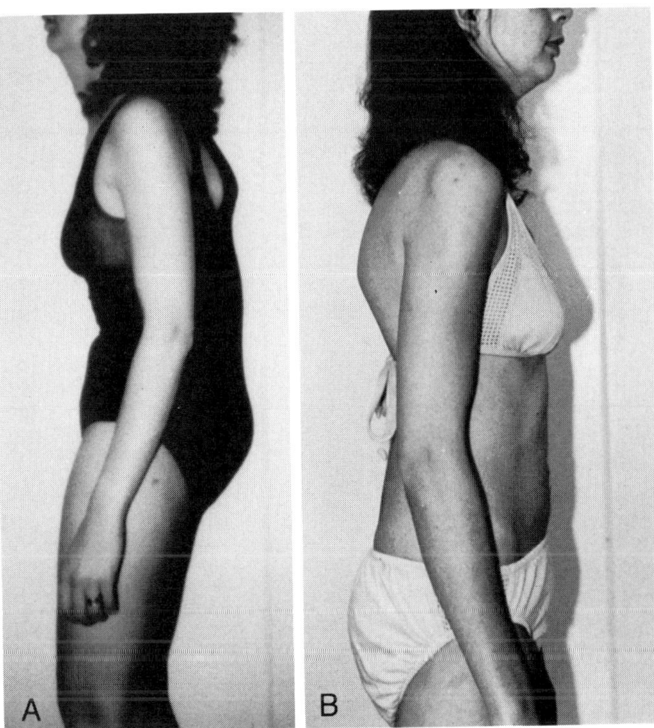

Figure 26–14. *A*, Female age 24 with previous lumbar fusion. Note the marked kyphosis (flat back) secondary to distraction. *B*, Postoperative view. Note the restoration of lordosis.

are used in all, consisting of four screws proximal and four screws distal to the osteotomy site (Fig. 26–15*A*). They are used at either side of the midline. This is simpler to use than other forms of fixation. A midline contoured AO plate is used to help control rotation, with at least two screws proximal and distal to the osteotomy site. Simultaneous with the posterior approach, an anterior approach is carried out, preferably at the L3–L4 level or at the apex of the frontal curve, and corresponding to the posterior osteotomy. An opening wedge osteotomy is done through the disc or if there has been previous anterior fusion through the anterior fusion mass. The opening of the osteotomy anteriorly is carried out simultaneously with Kostuik-Harrington instrumentation while the posterior osteotomy is closed with Dwyer instrumentation. A tricortical or bicortical iliac crest graft is used anteriorly (Figs. 26–15*B* and 26–16). A review of 54 patients treated using this method revealed excellent results, with pain relief in 48 (90 per cent).[37] Union did not occur in three patients because of anterior graft collapse. One of these patients requested reoperation. Neurologic complications occurred in two patients; one had permanent weakness of the dorsal extensors and plantar flexors of her feet and inconsistent bladder control. The minimal follow-up was four years. Average preosteotomy lordosis L1–S1 was 21.5 degrees and was restored to 49 degrees, which was equal to lordosis before initial posterior scoliosis surgery. This is an average of 29 degrees of correction with a range of 24 to 63 degrees.

Prevention of this complication is paramount. This has been described previously under Fusions to the Sacrum.

DEGENERATIVE ADULT SCOLIOSIS

Considerable controversy has existed over the definition of adult scoliosis and the differentiation between adolescent-onset scoliosis and the subsequent development of scoliosis from a preexisting straight spine in the frontal plane.

Vanderpool and associates, in a study performed in Edinburgh, where the incidence of osteoporosis and osteomalacia is known to be high, found an incidence of scoliosis in approximately 6 per cent of an adult group.[65] Many of these patients had evidence of osteo-

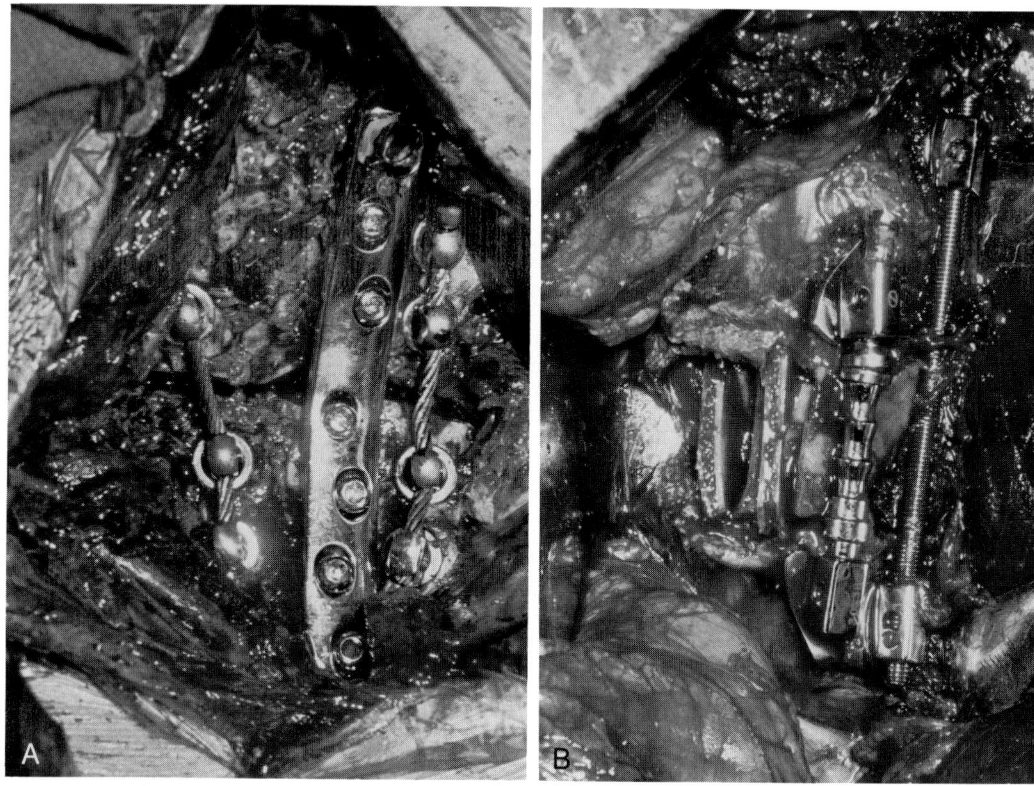

Figure 26–15. *A*, Posterior osteotomy has been closed by the application of Dwyer screws in the lateral fusion mass. An AO plate has been added in the midline to help control rotation. *B*, Simultaneous with posterior closure, the anterior osteotomy site is opened with Kostuik-Harrington instrumentation. Iliac crest grafts are added and a second Kostuik-Harrington compression rod is added to enhance stability.

porosis and osteomalacia, and a significant percentage of onset of these curves was believed to result from these disease states.

Kostuik and Bentivoglio, in a review of 5000 intravenous myelograms, found a 3.9 per cent incidence of thoracolumbar and lumbar curves.[32] These were all of adolescent onset.

The difficulty in differentiating between the two groups lies in the fact that lumbar and thoracolumbar curves in the frontal plane are frequently not noted until the onset of back pain, or until progression occurs as a result of degenerative changes in a preexisting adolescent curve in the late decades of life.

Grubb and associates compared two groups: those with onset in adolescent life and those with later onset where the deformity was believed to occur as a result of degenerative changes.[18] They found significant differences in densitometry measurements between the idiopathic and adult degenerative curves when measurements were made for age-matched controls.

Pain patterns in both groups occurred predominantly in the lower back, buttock, and leg, but the adult degenerative patients had a much higher incidence of stenotic symptoms, with up to 90 per cent aggravated by activity compared with 31 per cent in the idiopathic group. Activities that provoked stenosis-like symptoms were those involving extension of the lumbar spine. The curve magnitude was significantly greater in the idiopathic group, ranging from 34 to 78 degrees with a mean of 52 degrees, while curves in the degenerative group ranged from 15 to 53 degrees with a mean of 28 degrees. Although the curvature in the idiopathic group was significantly greater, the mean degree per segment was 9 degrees in both groups. All patients in the idiopathic scoliotic group in Grubb's series were women, with a mean age of 42 years, whereas in the degenerative groups the men and women were equal and the mean age was 60 years.

Radiologic studies showed that the idio-

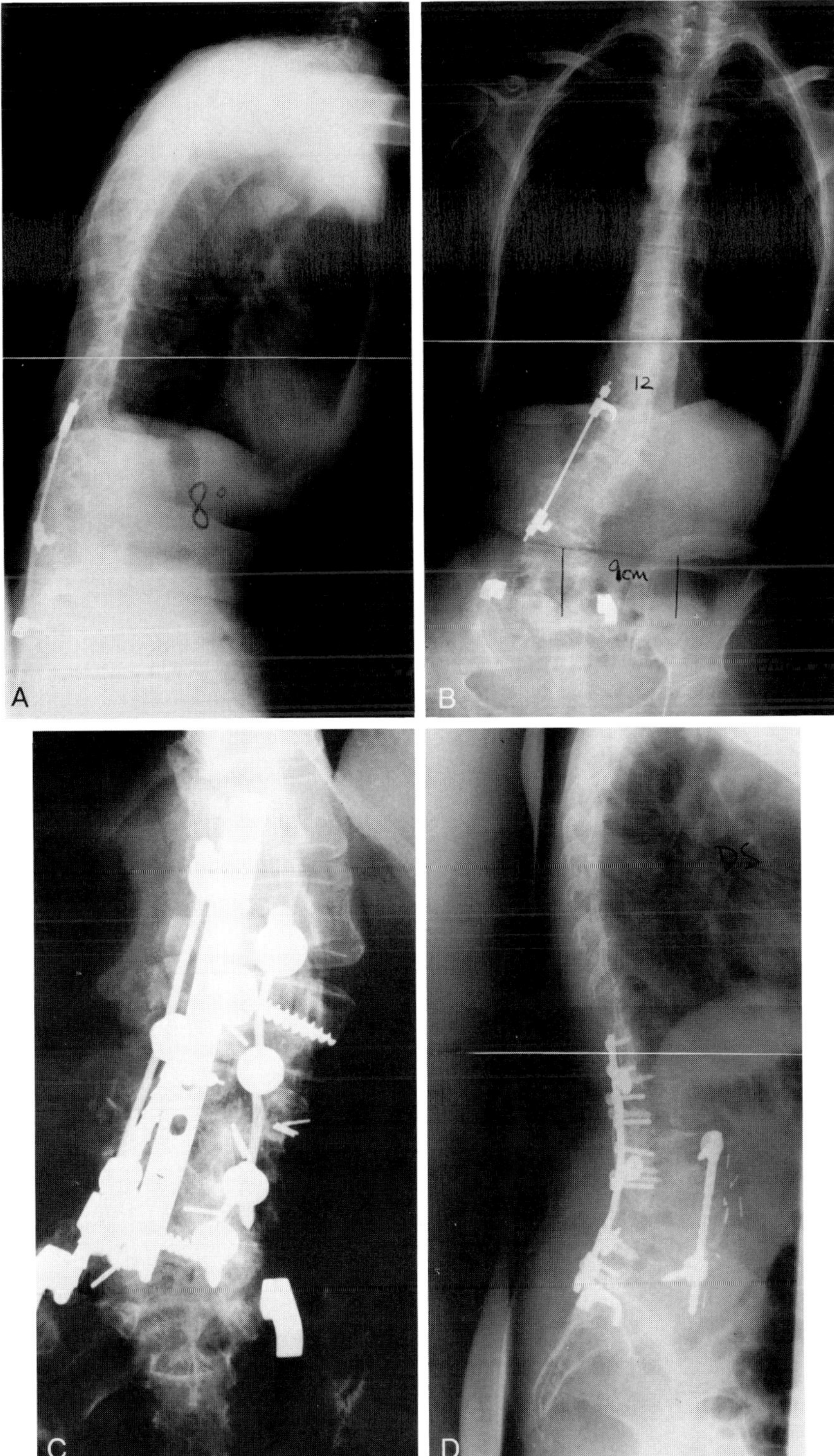

Figure 26–16. *A,* Female age 45. Note the loss of lordosis and marked flat back secondary to distraction and fusion of the lumbar spine. *B,* Anteroposterior view shows imbalance 9 cm to the right. The Harrington distraction rod has been removed. *C, D,* Lordosis and balance have been restored by a single-stage anterior and posterior osteotomy.

pathic group had myelographic defects primarily in the compensatory lumbosacral curve, whereas in the degenerative-onset group, the myelographic defects were seen most frequently within the curve. Using discography, Grubb and associates noted that in the adult-onset group there were grossly degenerative discs throughout the lumbar spine.[18] Pain was frequently not reproduced on distention of the disc. An explanation for this is that in markedly degenerative discs it is impossible to distend the disc quickly enough to reproduce pain. Thus, it is my belief that their study is not valid. In idiopathic patients with mechanical back pain, discography revealed abnormal painful discs with reproduction of symptoms frequently within the curve, as noted previously.[31] Grubb and associates noted that in the untreated group pain was often commonly reproduced on discography at the lower end of the curve in the lumbar spine or in the compensatory lumbosacral curve.[18] Grubb and associates also concluded that the assumption that a structural problem alone is always the direct cause of pain cannot be made.[18] The pain may arise below the curve in a compensatory part of the lumbosacral curve. The structural problem may contribute to development of pain, producing pathology within and below the curve.

The cause of adult progression of an adolescent curve is usually related to degenerative change. In the lumbar and thoracolumbar spine lordosis is initially well preserved, and with progressive degeneration of discs in the fifth and sixth decades of life the patient may change from being lordotic in the lumbar spine to developing kyphosis. The management of such curves is discussed elsewhere in this chapter.

Since a majority of patients with adult-onset deformities developed spinal stenosis, in this group, as in the idiopathic adolescent-onset group, decompression alone should be avoided unless it can be limited to one nerve root with preservation of the facet joints. Any more than this should be accompanied by fusion in situ or by correcting the deformity (Fig. 26–17).

Nash and associates analyzed fusion done in the lumbar spine to see whether the criteria

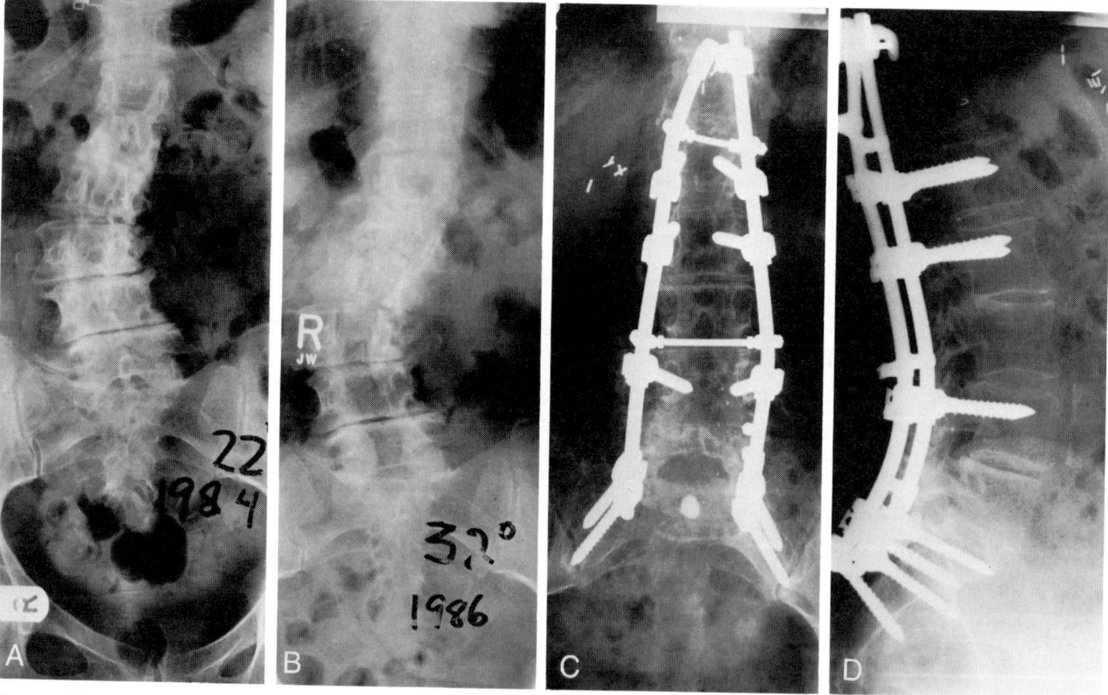

Figure 26–17. *A, B,* Female age 68. Prelaminectomy scoliosis measured 22 degrees. After decompression the deformity increased to 32 degrees together with totally disabling back pain, and subsequently to 50 degrees. There was also a marked loss of lumbar lordosis after decompression. *C, D,* Two-stage surgery restored lordosis and relieved pain. The first stage consisted of multiple anterior discectomies and bone graft. In the second stage, C-D instrumentation and fusion corrected the deformity and restored lordosis.

used for adolescents was valid in adults.[47] Criteria selected were the stable zone, central sacral line, neutrally rotated vertebrae, degenerative arthritis, displaced wedging, rotatory subluxation, vertebral body wedging, lumbosacral take-off, and hemisacralization. They concluded that multiple pathoanatomic factors need to be considered when selecting lumbar vertebrae for fusion in adult scoliosis patients. They believed that the stable zone, although helpful in younger patients for correction in the upper lumbar vertebrae, was not valid in older patients. Degenerative and deforming factors play a role in older patients who have increased disease in the lower lumbar spine, and necessitate fusions to lower levels, as has been pointed out in previous studies.[31] This substantiates the value of doing facet blocks and discography at these lower levels to determine all painful levels.

Nash and associates concluded that patients undergoing fusion into the lumbar area appeared to have a significant improvement in their pain and were satisfied with the surgery in 89 per cent of cases when the selection criteria were applied.[47] They believed that the central sacral line determination was not helpful in the selection of the lumbar fusion vertebrae in adult scoliosis patients.

Unfortunately, the criteria listed above were rarely useful. Indeed, one factor was useful in only 16 of 53 cases; two factors were useful in 20 of 53 cases; three factors were useful in 11 of 53 cases; four factors were useful in three of 53 cases; and five factors were useful in two of 53 cases in Nash's series. As has been previously noted, degenerative changes including rotatory subluxation, disc narrowing, and disc space wedging must be included in the fusion level. In fusion to L2, most patients had two or fewer of the criteria for selection. Most of the patients fused to L3 had two or more criteria. This is also true in patients fused to L5 and to S1. The stable zone is believed to be a factor in most cases fused to L2, L3, and L4. Displaced wedging was a factor in only 53 per cent of cases fused between L2 and L5 and rotatory subluxation was a factor in only slightly more than 50 per cent of cases fused to L4 or L5. This was also true for oblique take-off in patients fused to L5 or S1, and hemisacralization affected only 25 per cent of patients fused to S1. The most important conclusion of this review is that degenerative changes must be included in the fusion and are best evaluated using discography and facet blocks.

References

1. Allen, B. L., Jr., and Ferguson, R. L.: The Galveston technique for L rod instrumentation of the scoliotic spine. Spine *7*:276–284, 1982.
2. Balderston, R. A., Winter, R. B., Moe, J. H., et al.: Fusion to the sacrum for nonparalytic scoliosis in the adult. Spine *11*:824–829, 1986.
3. Byrd, J. A., III, Scoles, P. V., Winter, R. B., et al.: Adult idiopathic scoliosis treated by anterior and posterior spinal fusion. J. Bone Joint Surg. *69A*:843–850, 1987.
4. Bradford, D. S.: Adult scoliosis: current concepts of treatment. Clin. Orthop. *229*:70–87, 1988.
5. Casey, M. P., Asher, M. A., Jacobs, R. R., and Orrick, J. M.: The effect of Harrington rod contouring on lumbar lordosis. Spine *12*:750–753, 1987.
6. Cochran, T., Irstam, L., and Nachemson, A.: Long-term anatomic and functional changes in patients with adolescent idiopathic scoliosis treated by Harrington rod fusion. Spine *8*:576–584, 1983.
7. Coe, J. D., Becker, P. S., McAfee, P. C., and Burr, K. R.: Neuropathology with spinal instrumentation. J. Orthop. Res. 7:359–370, 1989.
8. Collis, D. K., and Ponseti, I. V.: Long-term follow-up of patients with idiopathic scoliosis not treated surgically. J. Bone Joint Surg. *51A*:425–445, 1969.
9. Cotrel, Y.: New Instrumentation for Surgery of the Spine. London, Freud Publishing House, 1986.
10. Cotrel, Y., Dubousset, J., and Guillaumat, M.: New universal instrumentation in spinal surgery. Clin. Orthop. *227*:10–23, 1988.
11. Cummine, J. L., Lonstein, J. E., Moe, J. H., et al.: Reconstructive surgery in the adult for failed scoliosis fusion. J. Bone Joint Surg. *61A*:1151–1161, 1979.
12. Dawson, E. G., Caron, A., and Moe, J. H.: Surgical management of scoliosis in the adult. J. Bone Joint Surg. *61A*:1151–1161, 1973.
13. Denis, F.: Cotrel-Dubousset instrumentation in the treatment of idiopathic scoliosis. Orthop. Clin. North Am. *19*:291–311, 1988.
14. Doherty, J.H.: Complications of fusion in lumbar scoliosis. J. Bone Joint Surg. *55A*:438, 1973.
15. Dwyer, A. F.: Experience of anterior correction of scoliosis. Clin. Orthop. *93*:191–206, 1973.
16. Edgar, M. A., and Mehta, M. H.: A long-term review of adults with fused and unfused idiopathic scoliosis. Orthop. Trans. *6*:462–463, 1982.
17. Grobler, L. J., Moe, J. H., Winter, R. B., et al.: Loss of lumbar lordosis following surgical correction of thoracolumbar deformities. Orthop. Trans. *2*:239, 1978.
18. Grubb, S. A., Lipscomb, H. S., and Conrad, R. W.: Diagnostic findings in painful adult scoliosis. S. R. S. Meeting, Amsterdam, Sept. 1989.
19. Haher, J. E., Devlin, V., Freeman, B., and Rondon, B.: Long-term effects of sublaminar wires on the neural canal. Orthop. Trans. *11*:106, 1987.
20. Hall, J. D.: Dwyer instrumentation in anterior fusion of the spine. J. Bone Joint Surg. *63A*:1188, 1981.

21. Harrington, P. R., and Dickson, J. H.: An eleven-year clinical investigation of Harrington instrumentation: a preliminary report on 578 cases. Clin. Orthop. *93*:113–130, 1973.
22. Hasday, C. A., Passoff, T. L., and Perry, J.: Gait abnormalities arising from iatrogenic loss of lumbar lordosis secondary to Harrington instrumentation in lumbar fractures. Spine *8*:501–511, 1983.
23. Herndon, W. Q., Sullivan, J. A., Yngve, D. A., et al.: Segmental spinal instrumentation with sublaminar wires. J. Bone Joint Surg. *69A*:851–859, 1987.
24. Herring, J. A., and Wenger, D. R.: Segmental spinal instrumentation: a preliminary report of 40 consecutive cases. Spine *7*:285–298, 1982.
25. Jackson, R. P., Simmons, E. H., and Stripinus, D.: Incidence and severity of back pain in adult idiopathic scoliosis. Spine *8*:749–756, 1983.
26. Johnson, J. R., and Holt, R. T.: Combined use of anterior and posterior surgery for adult scoliosis. Orthop. Clin. North Am. *19*:361–370, 1988.
27. Johnston, C. E., II, Happel, L. T., Jr., Norris, R., et al.: Delayed paraplegia complicating sublaminar segmental spinal instrumentation. J. Bone Joint Surg. *68A*:556–563, 1986.
28. Kaneda, K., Fujiya, N., and Satoh, S.: Results with Zielke instrumentation for idiopathic thoracolumbar and lumbar scoliosis. Clin. Orthop. *205*:195–203, 1986.
29. King, H. A., Moe, J. H., Bradford, D. S., and Winter, R. B.: The selection of fusion levels in thoracic idiopathic scoliosis. J. Bone Joint Surg. *65A*:1302–1313, 1983.
30. Kostuik, J. P.: Treatment of scoliosis in the adult thoracolumbar spine with special reference of fusion to the sacrum. Orthop. Clin. North Am. *19*:371–381, 1988.
31. Kostuik, J. P.: Decision-making in adult scoliosis. Spine *4*:521–525, 1979.
32. Kostuik, J. P., and Bentivoglio, J.: The incidence of low back pain in adult scoliosis. Spine *6*:268–273, 1981.
33. Kostuik, J. P., Carl, A., and Ferron, S.: Anterior Zielke instrumentation for adult spinal deformity. J. Bone Joint Surg. *71A*:898–912, 1989.
34. Kostuik, J. P., and Hall, B. B.: Spinal fusions to the sacrum in adults with scoliosis. Spine *8*:489–500, 1983.
35. Kostuik, J. P., Israel, J., and Hall, J. E.: Scoliosis surgery in adults. Clin. Orthop. *93*:225–234, 1973.
36. Kostuik, J. P., Maurais, G. R., and Richardson, W. J.: Primary fusion to the sacrum using Luque instrumentation. Spine. Submitted for publication.
37. Kostuik, J. P., Maurais, G. R., Richardson, W. J., and Okajima, Y.: Combined single stage anterior posterior osteotomy for correction of iatrogenic lumbar kyphosis. Spine *13*:257–266, 1988.
38. Kostuik, J. P., Worden Hawker, R., and Salo, P.: Long-term functional outcome following surgery for adult scoliosis. Presented at the A. O. A., Boston, June 1990.
39. Lagrone, M. O., Bradford, D. S., Moe, J. H., et al.: Treatment of symptomatic flatback after spinal fusion. J. Bone Joint Surg. *70A*:569–580, 1988.
40. Luque, E. R.: The anatomic basis and development of segmental spinal instrumentation. Spine *7*:256–259, 1982.
41. Luque, E. R.: Segmental spinal instrumentation for correction of scoliosis, Clin. Orthop. *163*:192–198, 1982.
42. Macnab, I.: Backache. Baltimore, Williams & Wilkins, 1977.
43. Moe, J. H., Purcell, G. A., and Bradford, D. S.: Zielke instrumentation (VDS) for the correction of spinal curvature: analysis of results in 66 patients. Clin. Orthop. *180*:133–153, 1983.
44. Nachemson, A.: A long-term follow-up study of non-treated scoliosis. Acta Orthop. Scand. *39*:489 500, 1983.
45. Nachemson, A.: A long-term follow-up study of non-treated scoliosis. J. Bone Joint Surg. *50A*:203, 1969.
46. Nash, C. L., Jr., and Moe, J. H.: A study of vertebral rotation. J. Bone Joint Surg. *51A*:223–228, 1969.
47. Nash, C. L., Goldstein, J. M., and Wilham, M. R.: Selection of lumbar fusion levels in adult idiopathic scoliosis patients. S. R. S. Meeting, Amsterdam, Sept. 1989.
48. Nicastro, J. F., Hartjen, C. A., Traina, J., and Lancaster, J. M.: Intraspinal pathways taken by sublaminar wires during removal: an experimental study. J. Bone Joint Surg. *68A*:1206–1209, 1986.
49. Nilsonne, U., and Lundgren, D. D.: Long-term prognosis in idiopathic scoliosis. Acta Orthop. Scand. *39*:455–465, 1968.
50. Nuber, G. W., and Schafer, M. F.: Surgical management of adult scoliosis. Clin. Orthop. *208*:228–237, 1986.
51. Ogiela, D. M., and Chan, D. P. K.: Ventral derotation spondylodesis: a review of 22 cases. Spine *11*:18–22, 1986.
52. Ponder, R. C., Dickson, J. H., Harrington, P. R., and Erwin, W. D.: Results of Harrington instrumentation and fusion in the adult idiopathic scoliosis patient. J. Bone Joint Surg. *57A*:797–801, 1975.
53. Ponseti, I. V.: The pathogenesis of adult scoliosis. *In* Zorab, P. A. (ed.): Proceedings of Second Symposium on Scoliosis. Cansation, Edinburgh, E. & S. Livingstone, 1968.
54. Rogala, E. J., Drummond, D. S., and Gurr, J.: Scoliosis: incidence and natural history. A prospective epidemiological study. J. Bone Joint Surg. *60A*:173–176, 1978.
55. Schrader, W. C., Betham, D., and Scherbin, V.: The chronic local effects of sublaminar wires: an animal model. Orthop. Trans. *11*:106, 1987.
56. Sponseller, P. D., Cohen, M. S., Nachemson, A. L., et al.: Results of surgical treatment of adults with idiopathic scoliosis. J. Bone Joint Surg. *69A*:667–675, 1987.
57. Stagnara, P.: Scoliosis in adults: surgical treatment of severe forms. Excerpta Med. Found. Int. Cong. 192:1969.
58. Stagnara, P., Jouvinoux, P., Peloux, J., et al.: Cyphoscoliosis essentielles de l'adulte: formes severe de plus de 100. Redressment partial et arthrodese. Presented at the XI Sicot Congress, Mexico City, 1969.
59. Stagnara, P.: Utilization of Harrington's Device in the Treatment of Adult Kyphoscoliosis Above 100 Degrees. *In* Fourth International Symposium, 1971. Stuttgart, George Thieme Verlag, 1973.
60. Stagnara, P., Fleury, D., Faucher, R., et al.: Scoliosis majeures de l'adultes superieures a 100–183 cas traites chirurgicalement. Rev. Chir. Orthop. *61*:101–122, 1975.

61. Swank, S., Lonstein, J. E., Moe, J. H., et al.: Surgical treatment of adult scoliosis: a review of two hundred and twenty-two cases. J. Bone Joint Surg. *63A*:268–287, 1981.
62. Thompson, G. H., Wilber, R. G., Shaffer, J. W., et al.: Segmental spinal instrumentation in idiopathic scoliosis: a preliminary report. Spine *10*:623–630, 1985.
63. van Dam, B. E.: Nonoperative treatment of adult scoliosis. Orthop. Clin. North Am. *19*:347–351, 1988.
64. van Dam, B. E., Bradford, D. S., Lonstein, J. E., et al.: Adult idiopathic scoliosis treated by posterior spinal fusion and Harrington instrumentation. Spine *12*:32–36, 1987.
65. Vanderpool, D. W., James, J. I. P., and Wynne-Davies, R.: Scoliosis in the elderly. J. Bone Joint Surg. *51A*:446–455, 1969.
66. Wilber, R. G., Thompson, G. H., Shaffer, J. W., et al.: Postoperative neurologic deficits in segmental spinal instrumentation: a study using spinal cord monitoring. J. Bone Joint Surg. *66A*:1178–1187, 1984.
67. Weinstein, S. L., and Ponseti, I. V.: Curve progression in idiopathic scoliosis. J. Bone Joint Surg. *65A*:447–455, 1983.
68. Winter, R. B., Lonstein, J. E., and Denis, F.: Pain patterns in adult scoliosis. Orthop. Clin. North Am. *19*:339–345, 1988.
69. Winter, R. B.: Combined Dwyer and Harrington instrumentation and fusion in the treatment of selected patients with painful adult idiopathic scoliosis. Spine *3*:135–141, 1978.
70. Zielke, K., Stunkat, R., and Beaujean, F.: Ventrale derotations–spondylodese. Arch. Orthop. Unfallchir. *85*:257–263, 1976.

CHAPTER

27

SPONDYLOLISTHESIS

Glenn Amundson, M.D.
Charles C. Edwards, M.D.
Steven R. Garfin, M.D.

The body's center of gravity lies anterior to the lumbosacral joint. As a result, the lumbar spine tends to slip forward and rotate anteriorly into flexion about the sacral dome. In the normal spine, the inferior facets of L5 buttress against the superior facets of S1 to block slippage and rotation. The pars defect or elongation that characterizes spondylolisthesis functionally cleaves the inferior facets from L5, allowing the lumbar spine to slip forward. This causes anterior shear forces in the lumbosacral disc with progressive disc degeneration. As anterior column height is lost, the lumbar spine begins to tilt into flexion (kyphosis). Depending on the patient's age when this process begins, the architecture of L5 and the sacrum, the degree of sacral lordosis, and the amount of ligamentous laxity, the deformity progresses in some patients and remains stable in others.

HISTORY AND CLASSIFICATION

Spondylolisthesis was first recognized in 1782 by the Belgian obstetrician Herbiniaux.[56a] In 1854 Kilian used the term "spondylolisthesis" to describe the gradual displacement of the fifth lumbar vertebra on the first sacral segment caused by the superimposed body weight.[66] The terms "spondylolisthesis" and "spondylolysis" derive from the Greek roots *spondylo*, meaning spine; *listhesis*, to slip or slide down a slippery path; and *lysis*, to dissolve.

Neugebauer (1888) first classified two distinct types of spondylolisthesis: one caused by a defect in the pars interarticularis, and a second less common type with an intact but narrowed and elongated pars.[82] Newman, in his 1963 review of 319 cases, described five distinct groups using a classification method that remains widely accepted.[83] Recently a postsurgical category has been added. The groups are:

1. ***Congenital (dysplastic) spondylolisthesis.*** Congenital anomalies of the lumbosacral junction, including dysplasia of the fifth lumbar and sacral arches and facets, compromise the buttress mechanism to allow gradual forward displacement of the fifth lumbar vertebra. Three subtypes include dysplastic facets with axial orientation, dysplastic facets with sagittal orientation, and other congenital anomalies of the lumbosacral junction.
2. ***Isthmic (spondylolytic) spondylolisthesis.*** A defect in the pars interarticularis allows forward slipping of the fifth lumbar vertebral body. This is the most common form. Three

subtypes include lytic fatigue fracture of the pars, elongated but intact pars interarticularis, and acute fracture.

3. ***Degenerative spondylolisthesis.*** With long-standing segmental instability and degeneration of the disc and facets, forward displacement occurs.

4. ***Traumatic spondylolisthesis.*** Acute fracture around the L5–S1 facet disrupts the facet buttress to allow anterior displacement. The slipping is often a secondary phenomenon; it may occur weeks after initial injury, distinguishing it from an acute fracture dislocation.

5. ***Pathologic spondylolisthesis.*** Destruction or attenuation of the pars, pedicle, or facets allows secondary slipping.

a. *Subtype A.* Generalized. Widespread, generalized bony changes allow the slip to occur, as in osteoporosis, arthrogryposis, and syphilitic disease.

b. *Subtype B.* Localized. Due to localized bone destruction such as tumor or infection.

6. ***Postsurgical spondylolisthesis*** (spondylolisthesis acquisita). Iatrogenic disruption of ligamentous, discal, or bony structures can allow displacement.

This chapter discusses all types of spondylolisthesis, but focuses on categories 1 and 2, the most common causes of juvenile and adolescent low back pain and sciatica.[70]

Congenital (Dysplastic) Spondylolisthesis

Incidence

In dysplastic spondylolisthesis, the only true congenital spondylolisthesis, displacement occurs early and is often severe. There is a 2:1 female-to-male ratio.[85, 141] Symptoms usually appear during the adolescent growth spurt; however, Taillard[123] quotes a report of a dysplastic slip in a 3.5-month-old infant. Dysplastic slips account for about 14 to 21 per cent of spondylolisthesis cases.[13, 85]

Cause

Congenital deficiencies of the upper sacrum or the arch of L5 prevent the development of a proper "hooking" mechanism. Without an effective facet buttress, the superior vertebra slips forward on the inferior one.[141] The pars may remain intact but usually is poorly developed, elongated, or occasionally even lysed. When the arch remains intact, slipping of greater than 35 per cent may produce cauda equina pressure secondary to spinal stenosis, or root compression secondary to the inferior articular process of L5 compressing the S1 root.

Subtype A. The dysplastic articular processes have a transverse (horizontal) orientation (Fig. 27–1). Spina bifida frequently accompanies the deformity and contributes to the instability resulting in the slippage. Severe hamstring spasm is common. The olisthesis often appears earlier than in other types and may be severe. Fusion is usually required.

Subtype B. Dysplastic facets have an asymmetric sagittal malorientation (Fig. 27–2). The posterior arch is usually intact, minimizing the chance of a high-degree slip occurring. Leg pain, altered gait, and back and hamstring spasm are the most common presenting complaints. The cauda equina distal to the L5 nerve roots can be compressed by the intact arch of L5. If decompression or reduction does not accompany fusion, recovery from altered gait and hamstring spasm is usually prolonged.

Subtype C. Other congenital anomalies at the lumbosacral junction allow spondylolisthesis. Congenital kyphosis due to failure of vertebral body formation and angulatory deformities of the sacrum, as described by Armstrong and Chen, are representative examples.[5, 145]

Isthmic Spondylolisthesis

Incidence

In isthmic spondylolisthesis, the most common spondylolytic disorder, 50 per cent of cases present with only spondylolysis and do not slip.[142] The sex ratio is reversed from the congenital type, that is, there is a 2:1 male-to-female ratio.[42, 127, 137, 138] A pars defect at birth has been sought by gross and histologic sectioning of the pars in hundreds of stillborn infants, but never found.[24, 83, 123, 127, 137–139] Isolated cases have been reported at ages ranging from 6 weeks to 10 months, however.[123, 127, 139] More often this type of spondylolysis occurs only after walking begins. It is rarely seen before 5 years of age, and most commonly occurs at age 7 to 8 years.[83, 137–139] Wiltse found

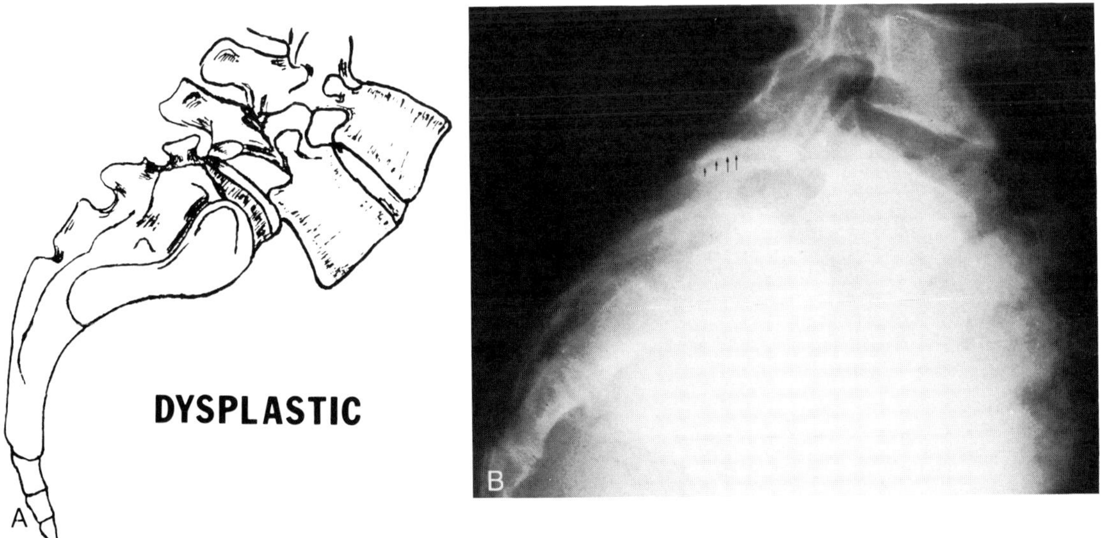

Figure 27–1. Type I congenital (dysplastic) spondylolisthesis. *A*, Insufficiency of the lumbosacral facets, allowing forward subluxation of the fifth lumbar vertebra on the sacrum. *B*, Roentgenogram of a 13-year-old female with Grade I spondylolisthesis. She has dysplastic articular processes *(arrows)* at the level of the olisthesis, which are axially oriented (Type IA). The pars is elongated; this subtype is frequently associated with spina bifida.

a 5 per cent incidence of spondylolysis in children 5 to 7 years of age, with an increase to 6 to 7 per cent by age 18. Most of the increase occurred between 11 and 15 years of age, corresponding to the adolescent growth spurt.[42, 70, 139] Participation in vigorous exercise such as gymnastics, weight lifting, and football can cause new cases to appear into early adulthood.

The incidence among adults in the United States is reported to be from 5 to 7 per cent and varies according to race.[24, 42, 68, 123, 127, 139, 146] Rowe and Roche reported an incidence of 6.4 per cent in white American men, 2.8 per cent in black men, 2.3 per cent in white women, and 1.1 per cent in black women.[102] Although pars defects are only half as frequent in girls as in boys, high-grade slips are four times more likely in women. Stewart found a 50 per cent incidence in Eskimos, with an increased incidence until age 34 years.[122] This remarkably high incidence is believed to be due to both genetic and environmental factors.

Cause

The isthmic defect appears to result from a combination of a hereditary dysplasia of the pars interarticularis and stresses imposed on the lower lumbar spine by an upright bipedal posture and extension loading (repeat microfractures) (Fig. 27–3).[33, 79, 138] The isthmic defect is commonly associated with hypoplastic maloriented facets and spina bifida occulta. Family members of patients with spondylolysis or spondylolisthesis have a reported incidence of 28 to 69 per cent, establishing a strong genetic factor.[6, 123, 127, 137, 138, 146] Female gymnasts have an incidence of spondylolysis four times that of age-matched nongymnasts.[140]

Therefore, the susceptible individual is born with a weak but intact pars interarticularis that after weight bearing and stress, either fractures acutely or gradually attenuates (fatigue fractures) (Fig. 27–4). Bosworth reported four histopathologic patterns resulting in the defect: thin, tenuous, fibrous bands bridging the defect; thick, heavy fibrous columns in the same location; a bony bridge across the portion of the arch, and a false joint.

Mechanical stresses play an important role in producing spondylolysis; erect posture produces a constant downward and forward thrust on the lower lumbar vertebrae, concentrating forces on the pars interarticularis.[33, 83] Spondylolisthesis has never been reported in quadrupeds, nor has it been observed in chronic bedridden patients (humans).

Subtype A. Wiltse states that except for

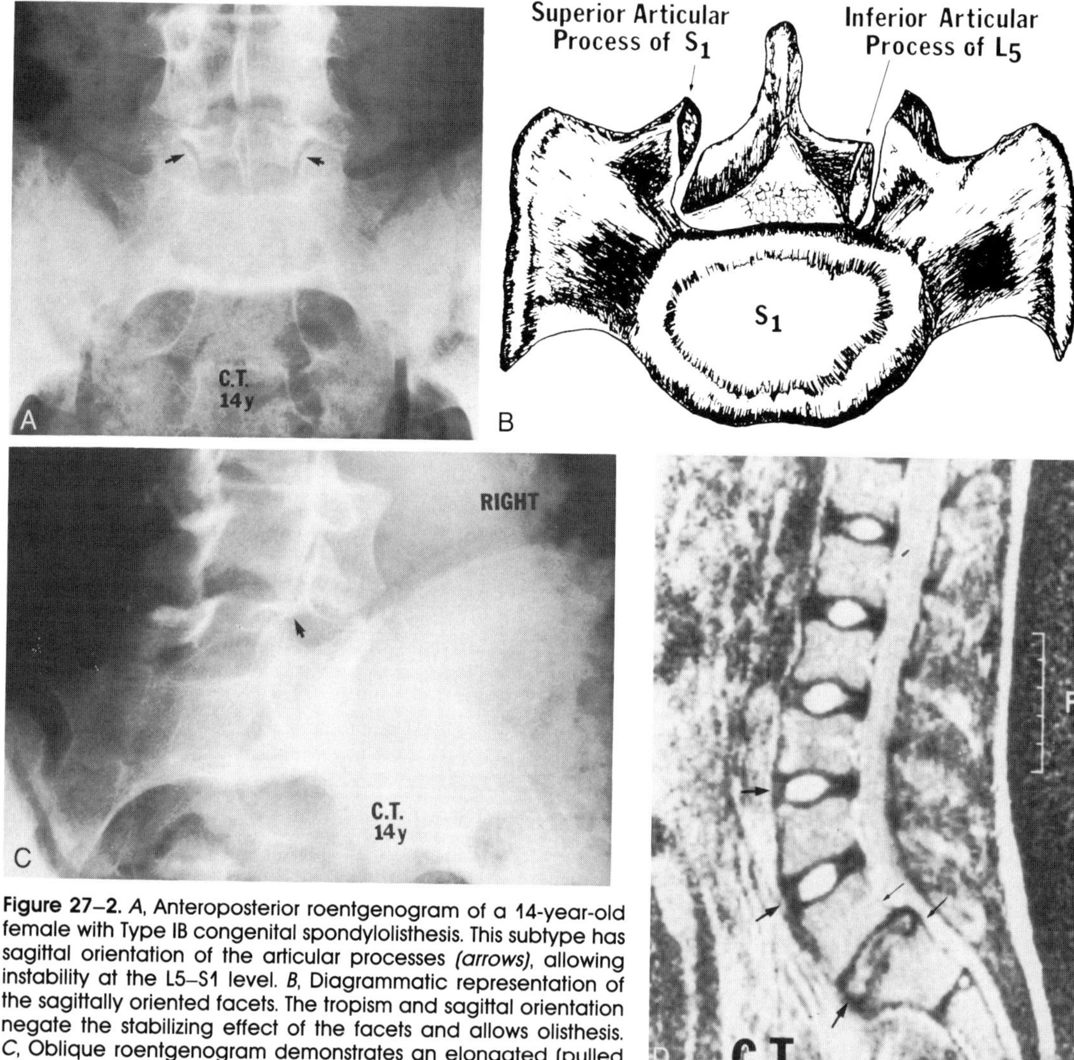

Figure 27–2. *A*, Anteroposterior roentgenogram of a 14-year-old female with Type IB congenital spondylolisthesis. This subtype has sagittal orientation of the articular processes *(arrows)*, allowing instability at the L5–S1 level. *B*, Diagrammatic representation of the sagittally oriented facets. The tropism and sagittal orientation negate the stabilizing effect of the facets and allows olisthesis. *C*, Oblique roentgenogram demonstrates an elongated (pulled taffy) dysplastic pars interarticularis *(arrow)*. *D*, Sagittal plane magnetic resonance imaging (MRI) view of the same patient demonstrates the olisthesis *(thin arrows)* and commonly associated degenerative disc signal (*thick arrows* at L5–C1, compared with upper two arrows), despite the youth of the patient.

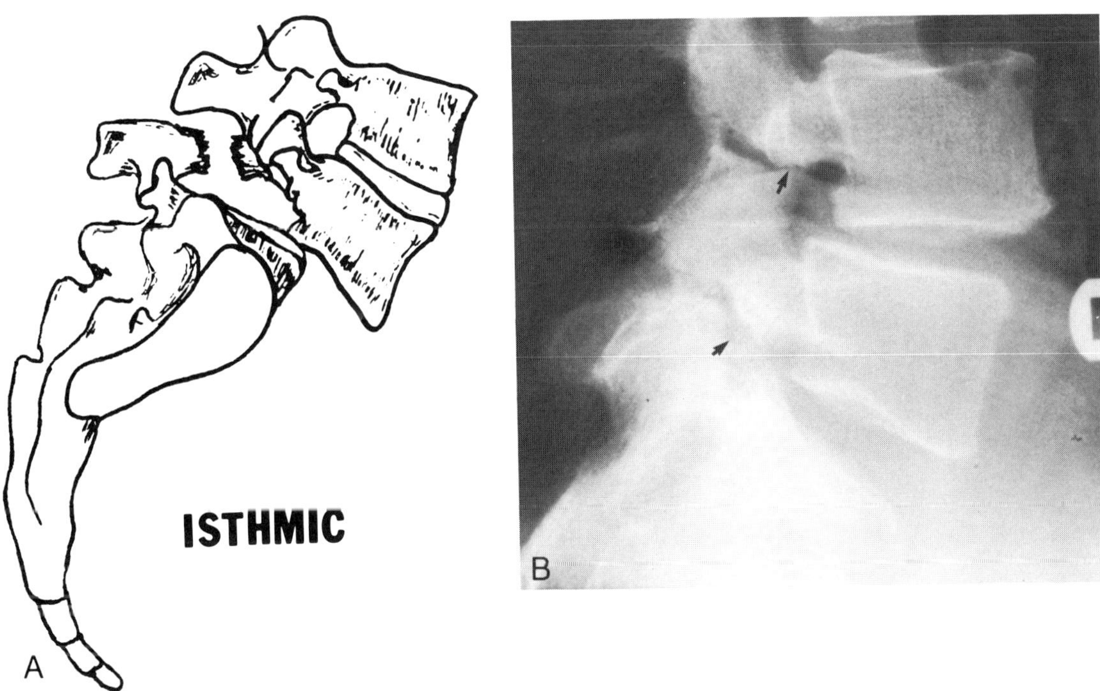

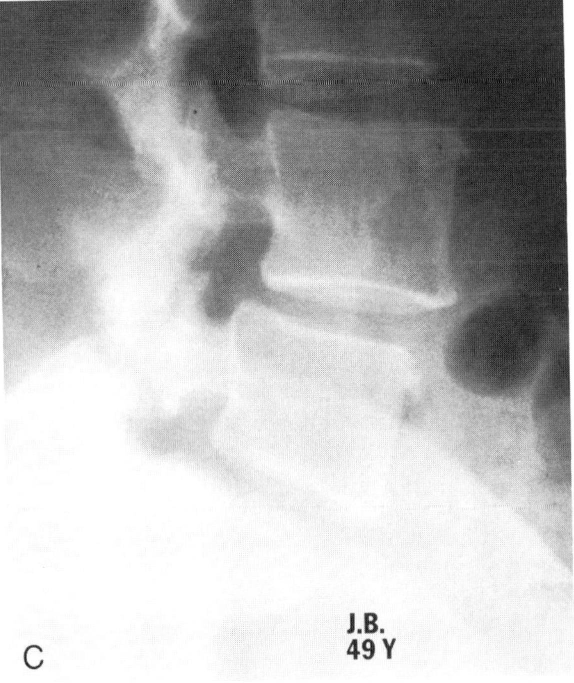

Figure 27–3. *A*, Type II isthmic spondylolisthesis (the most common form). The pars interarticularis defect allows forward slipping of the fifth lumbar vertebral body. The facet joints remain intact. *B*, Roentgenogram of a 38-year-old male who presented with low back pain and sciatica, demonstrating lytic L4 and L5 pars defects, allowing two-level olisthesis. *C*, Roentgenogram of a 49-year-old-female demonstrating L5 isthmic spondylolisthesis and degenerative L4–L5 spondylolisthesis. Degenerative spondylolisthesis is due to long-standing intersegmental instability and degeneration of the disc and facets that allows forward displacement.

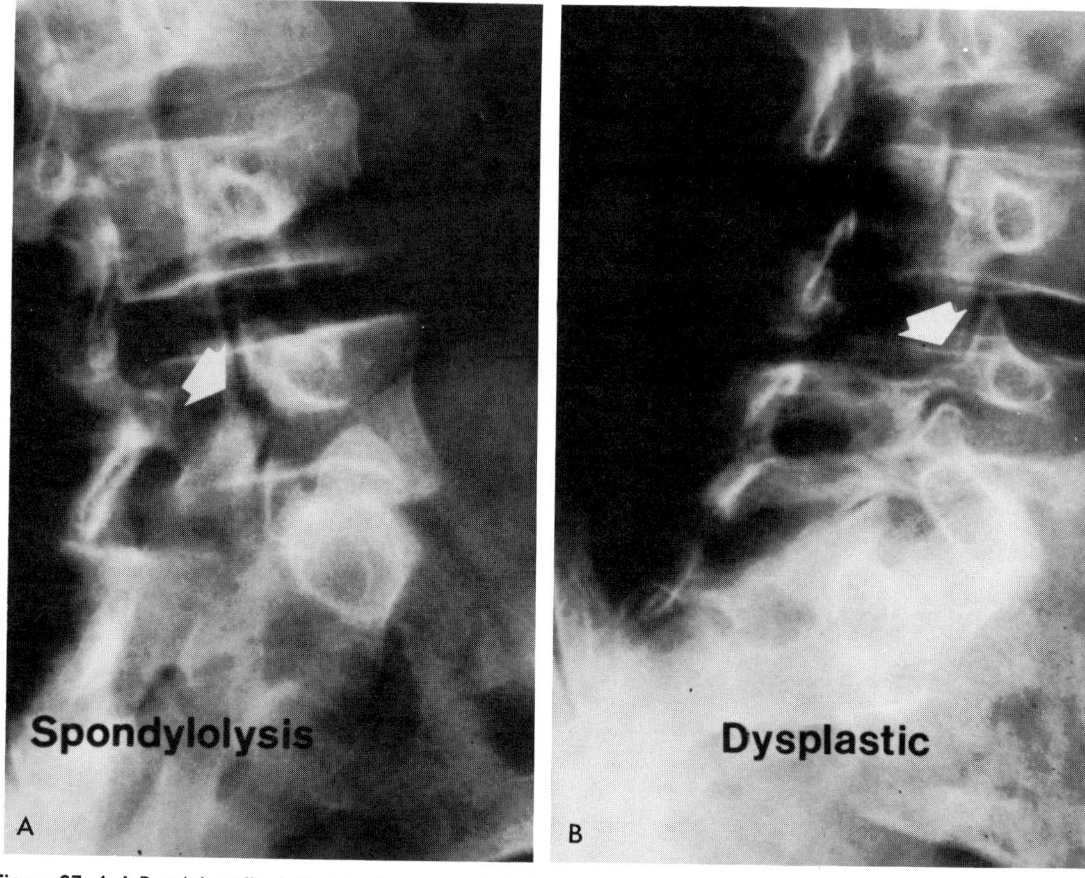

Figure 27–4. *A*, Pars interarticularis defect, spondylolysis *(arrow)* as seen on oblique roentgenographic view, typically found with the isthmic type of spondylolisthesis (Type II). *B*, Similar oblique view of a patient with spondylolisthesis demonstrating elongation and attenuation of the pars interarticularis, perhaps a prespondylolytic lesion.

occasional acute fractures of the pars interarticularis, isthmic spondylolysis or spondylolisthesis begins as a fatigue fracture.[142] This differs from other fatigue fractures in long bones because it develops at an earlier age. Callus is rarely seen and the defect persists, probably because of constant motion and a poor mechanical environment for healing.

Subtype B. Subtype B of isthmic spondylolisthesis, represented by elongation of the pars without separation, is believed to be caused by repeated microfractures that heal in an elongated position (Fig. 27–5).

Subtype C. This type results from an acute pars fracture after severe trauma, and slippage is rare. There is no hereditary factor. In contrast to subtype A, this pars fracture usually heals if immobilized.

Additional etiologic theories for isthmic spondylolisthesis, proposed but subsequently disproved, include the following:

1. The defect is caused by a separate ossification center. This was disproved by consistent findings in stillborn infants and cadavers that ossification occurs at the vertebral body and lateral masses, not at the pars.[67, 137]
2. The defect results from a birth fracture. This was disproved by Rowe and Roche, who found that extreme force was required to produce the fracture experimentally.[102]
3. The defect results from an acute fracture in the postnatal period. This is unlikely since fractures in infancy always heal.
4. Ligamentous laxity and weakness of supporting structures of the back predispose to spondylolysis. Several factors negate this proposal. Many children with a pars defect show no evidence of ligamentous laxity. Women have a lower spondylolytic incidence than men, but in general have greater ligamentous laxity; also, polio victims do not have an increased incidence of spondylolisthesis.[67]

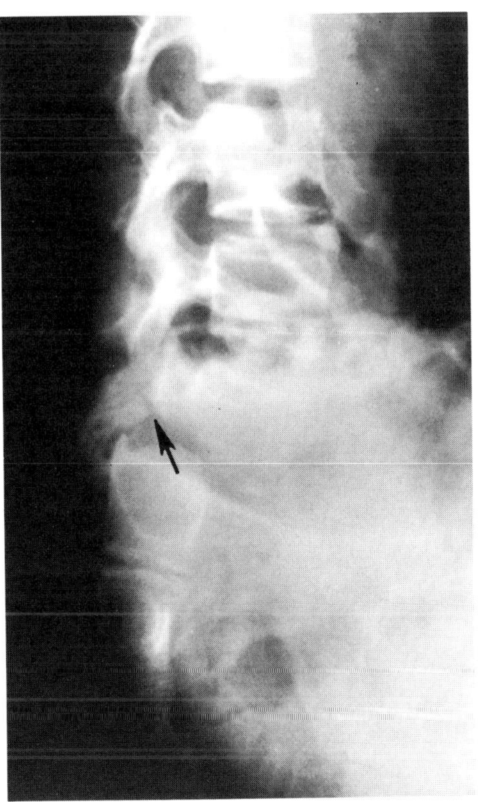

Figure 27–5. Spondylolisthesis due to subluxation of the facets. The pars interarticularis has become attenuated like pulled taffy, and a defect has appeared in the center *(arrow)*. The break in the neural arch may permit further subluxation.

In summary, the following are established observations and factors for type II (isthmic) spondylolysis and spondylolisthesis. Humans are not born with the pars defect. The defect has only rarely been reported below the age of 5 years. It appears most commonly at 6 years of age and seldom occurs after age 8; however, late development has been observed. There is a genetic predisposition. The incidence varies by race. There is a definite familial component. Congenital weakness or dysplasia of the pars interarticularis combined with upright posture and extension loads predispose to the defect and appear to prevent normal healing. Repeated exaggerated spinal motion, such as lumbar hyperextension in gymnastics, increases the incidence of spondylolysis.

Natural History

An excellent prospective study of 500 randomly selected first-grade students was performed by Fredrickson and colleagues.[42, 140] At age 6 they found a 4.4 per cent incidence of spondylolysis and a 2.6 per cent incidence of spondylolisthesis; at adulthood the incidence was 5.4 per cent and 4.0 per cent, respectively. Healing of the pars defect occurred in only one patient who had a unilateral defect. In all patients, the development of the pars defect and slip occurred concomitantly. Slipping was noted to occur during both decades under study, with the largest change during the early teen years.

The likelihood of slip progression is low. It most often occurs in the child or adolescent with more than 50 per cent slip (Fig. 27–6).[117] Women are at greater risk for progressing to higher grade slips once initial slip has occurred.[13, 14, 27, 89, 112] After skeletal maturity, slip progression is usually minimal.[42, 79, 140]

Degenerative Spondylolisthesis

Incidence

Degenerative spondylolisthesis is five times more frequent in women than in men and usually occurs after age 40. Degenerative spondylolisthesis occurs three times more often in black women than in white.[101] The L4–L5 interspace is six to ten times more frequently involved than adjacent levels (see Fig. 27–3*C*). A transitional vertebra with sacralization of L5 is four times more frequent in people with degenerative spondylolisthesis than in the general population.

Etiology

The degenerative lesion is due to long-standing intersegmental instability.[145] Degeneration of the disc coupled with severe degenerative changes of the facet joints allows vertebral slippage. The degenerative changes in the facets often include a more horizontal orientation and tropism. Subsequent anterior and lateral olisthesis and rotatory subluxation can then become manifest. The slip seldom exceeds 33 per cent if no surgery is performed.

Two pain patterns are possible. A claudicant type is characterized by an activity-related aching, and fatigue-like pain in the back, buttocks, thighs, or calves depending on the level of the stenosis. The symptoms of spinal claudication

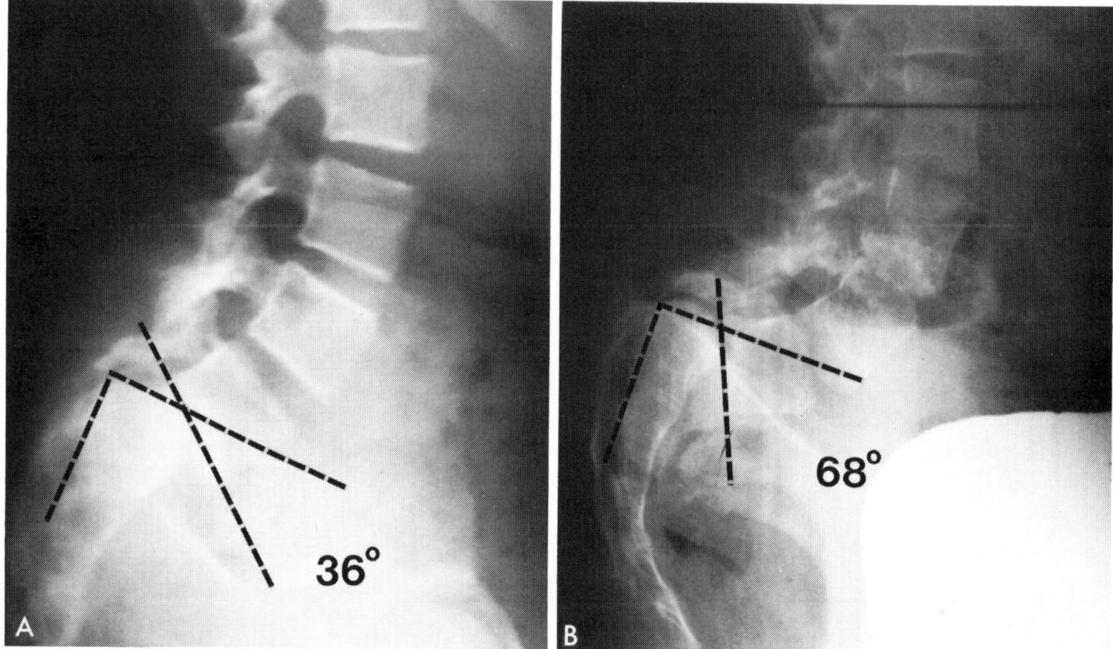

Figure 27–6. Dysplastic (congenital) spondylolisthesis. *A*, Lateral roentgenogram at age 10 with Grade III tangential slip and significant angle of tilt (36 degrees) of L5 on the sacrum. *B*, Same patient at age 13 untreated. Note moderate progression of the tangential slip and marked increase in the angle of tilt (68 degrees), with increase in the lumbar lordosis and sagittal inclination of the sacrum. The patient now has perineal anesthesia and a neurogenic bladder.

are usually relieved by sitting or recumbency, in contrast to vascular claudication, which is usually relieved by standing in place. The other common pattern is that of typical sciatica. The primary site of neural compression in L4–L5 degenerative spondylolisthesis is narrowing in the lateral recess with nerve root compression between the hypertrophied and subluxed facet joints and the posterior superior aspect of the L5 vertebral body.[101] Sciatic tension signs are often absent regardless of presentation.

Pain is usually of slow onset, progressive, rarely severe, and usually is present for several months or years. Most patients describe previous episodes of similar pain. Long periods of remission are common.[10] A more detailed discussion of this entity and its treatment can be found in Chapter 25.

SYMPTOMS

Pain is the most common symptom of spondylolysis and spondylolisthesis. It typically begins with the adolescent growth spurt.[13, 24, 27, 70, 84, 85, 89] Although spondylolisthesis is the most common cause of low back pain and sciatica in children and adolescents, most adolescents with spondylolysis are asymptomatic.[70] Fredrickson and associates found that none of the children in their series complained of pain during the time the defect developed.[42] Wiltse and Jackson found that although most slips progress between ages 10 and 15 years, few were symptomatic.[140] LaFond, in a review of 415 patients, found that only 9 per cent were troubled enough to seek medical attention during childhood or adolescence.[68] Therefore, when evaluating a symptomatic adolescent with radiographic evidence of spondylolysis, other possible causes (e.g., infection, tumor, osteoid osteoma, disc herniation) for pain should be explored before attributing the symptoms to spondylolisthesis.[68]

In a long-term follow-up study of spondylolysis and spondylolisthesis, Saraste found that in the L5 spondylolysis group, the mean age at onset of symptoms was 19 years, and radiographic diagnosis was made at 23 years.[105] Corresponding figures for an L4 spondylolysis group were 20 and 30 years, respectively. Although 91 per cent of patients in the series experienced some form of back pain, and 55 per cent complained of sciatica, disabling pain was reported by only 13 per cent. In contradistinction, symptomatic children with L5 spondylolisthesis or adults with Grade 2+ L4 or L5 degenerative spondylolisthesis are both likely to have recurrent problems. Saraste reported that patients with greater than Grade I spondylolisthesis of L4 or L5 had a 40 per cent incidence of sciatica, and that 90 per cent of these patients required treatment.[105] Children and adolescents with one episode of back pain related to spondylolisthesis of any degree are likely to have recurrent painful episodes.[55, 127]

The most common pain pattern associated with low-grade spondylolisthesis is a dull, aching pain in the back, buttocks, and posterior thigh. It probably originates from several sources. The pars nonunion may be a source of pain.[148] Additionally, the unstable vertebral body segment may cause ligamentous stretch and also incite local muscle spasm.

Saraste's study of spondylolysis and spondylolisthesis suggests that disc degeneration may contribute to symptoms, since a strong correlation occurred between disc degeneration and low back symptoms in patients with spondylolysis.[105] Bosworth and associates noted evidence of disc degeneration at the level of the slip in 67 per cent of their population.[12]

In the second, less common pattern the child has pain radiating into the lower extremities with little or no back pain. This pattern, more typical of dysplastic spondylolisthesis, suggests nerve root irritation and usually involves the fifth lumbar or first sacral root (congenital spondylolisthesis) with pain radiating into the posterior thigh. Adolescents rarely experience pain below the knee. Occasionally they complain only of an ache in the greater trochanteric area, sometimes causing the examining physician to focus too specifically on the hip as the cause of the pain.

Some children have neurologic signs and symptoms including paresthesias, weakness, and incontinence of bowel and bladder. The first two are more common with isthmic spondylolisthesis from L5 root compression, and the latter, particularly cauda equina syndrome, usually occurs with the congenital types.

Forward slips up to 10 per cent appear not to increase the likelihood of future back problems, even with heavy work. With higher grade slips, however, the literature suggests an increased chance of low back symptoms over what would be expected in a population without pars defects.[145] Saraste has observed that adaptive changes, such as wedging of the body of L5, also increase the frequency of symptoms.[104]

Symptoms in adults are often different from those described for children and adolescents. Back pain in adults associated with spondylolisthesis is usually heralded by back pain in the late teens or early 20s. The cause of back pain presenting after age 30 or 35 in a patient with spondylolisthesis may not be due to the pars defect or slippage. Those anatomic changes have most likely been present since childhood, and therefore the symptoms noted in middle age usually have another cause (degenerative disc, strain/sprain, etc.). When there is no history of back pain before age 30, and particularly 40, another reason for the pain should be sought despite the radiographs. Leg pain, especially an L5 radicular pattern, with or without neurologic findings or tension signs, however, may be related to the pars defect and fibrocartilaginous bar, even with a middle-age presentation. The leg pain is often posterolateral, down the leg, or in the hip, increases with activity, and decreases with rest. It often is not associated with a neurologic deficit and has an insidious (although possibly acute) onset.

PHYSICAL FINDINGS

All grades of symptomatic spondylolisthesis can give rise to local signs and hamstring tightness. Deep palpation of the spinous process above the slip (typically L4) may reproduce local, and sometimes radicular, pain. With grade 2 (25 to 50 per cent) or greater slips, a step-off immediately above the slip level (i.e., L4 or L5) can be appreciated.[24, 27, 66] Spasm and eventual foreshortening occurs in the paraspinous muscles and hamstrings. This gives rise to limited forward flexion of the trunk and decreased straight leg raising.[127] Originally, hamstring tightness was believed to represent traction on the cauda equina; however, hamstring tightness occurs with all grades of spondylolisthesis and is seldom accompanied by neurologic signs.[56, 84, 92] It may be that hamstring spasm and tightness represent either an attempt by the body to control an unstable L5–S1 level, or an attempt to rotate the pelvis into a more vertical position to help reestablish the patient's center of gravity.[8, 13, 24, 27, 56, 84, 92, 127, 138] Interestingly, patients requiring surgical fusion of an unstable L5–S1 segment do not resolve their hamstring tightness for 6 to 8 months after surgery, corresponding to the mean 7.5 months required for radiographic consolidation of the fusion mass (Figs. 27–7 and 27–8).[140]

Patients with a significant slip (approximately 50 per cent or greater) have additional physical findings secondary to lumbosacral kyphosis and trunk shortening. When the slip progresses in childhood, the posterior portion of the fifth lumbar vertebra comes to rest on the anterior portion of S1. Concentration of axial loads over such a small area erodes or leads to remodeling of the posteroinferior corner of L5 and the anterosuperior corner of the sacrum. The result is a trapezoidal or wedge-shaped L5 body and a rounded sacral dome. Once this geometry occurs, the rate of anterior lumbar tilt accelerates and the lumbar spine proceeds to rotate about the sacral dome into lumbosacral kyphosis. This throws the upper body's center of gravity anterior to the hip joints resulting in sagittal decompensation (Figs. 27–7 to 27–9).

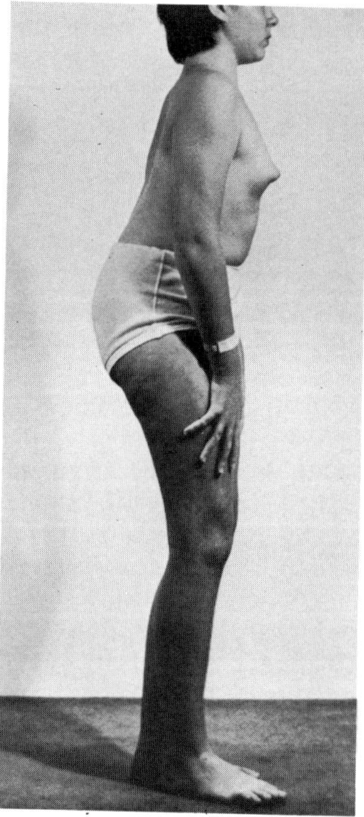

Figure 27–7. Teenager with severe hamstring tightness and the typical posture: flexion of the hips and knees, the pelvis tilted backward, and flattening of the normal lumbar lordosis.

To stand erect the patient must compensate for every degree of lumbosacral kyphosis. This is accomplished in several ways: the hamstrings and iliopsoas muscles contract to rotate the pelvis into a more vertical position and the patient arches the thoracolumbar spine into maximal lordosis. If these measures are not sufficient, the patient must flex the hips and knees to restore an erect posture and sagittal balance (Fig. 27–7). The kyphotic deformity between the low lumbar spine and pelvis makes the wings of the ilia appear widened with the buttocks "flattened," thus producing the typical flat, square buttocks or "sweetheart pelvis" (Fig. 27–10). The forward slip of the lumbar spine and compensatory thoracolumbar hyperlordosis are reflected clinically by an anteriorly protruding inferior rib cage (Figs. 27–11 and 27–31).

The advanced spondylolisthesis deformity is always associated with foreshortening of the trunk.[24, 27, 138] This is from the slippage of L5 from the top of the sacrum into the pelvis, combined with the accordion effect of lumbosacral kyphosis and compensatory thoracolumbar lordosis. Loss of trunk height is responsible for such clinical signs as waist line absence and flank creases (see Fig. 27–11). It is also most likely responsible for the 12 to 40 per cent reduced abdominal and erector spinae muscle strength found in patients with spondylolisthesis since these muscles become shorter than their optimal length on the Blix curve.[52, 77] In very high-grade spondylolisthesis and spondyloptosis, the rib cage often abuts the iliac crest, adding another source of discomfort. Substantial loss of trunk height is responsible for a disproportionate body; this combined with the absence of a waist and redundant belly and flank tissues is cosmetically offensive to the young person afflicted with high-grade spondylolisthesis.

Gait abnormalities are common. The spondylolisthetic gait is characterized by a waddle with limited hip flexion, shortened stride length, and a wide base of support. This gait results from hamstring tightness, vertical tilting of the pelvis (lumbosacral kyphosis), compensatory lumbar hyperlordosis, and the flexion deformity of the hips and knees.[8, 24, 84, 127]

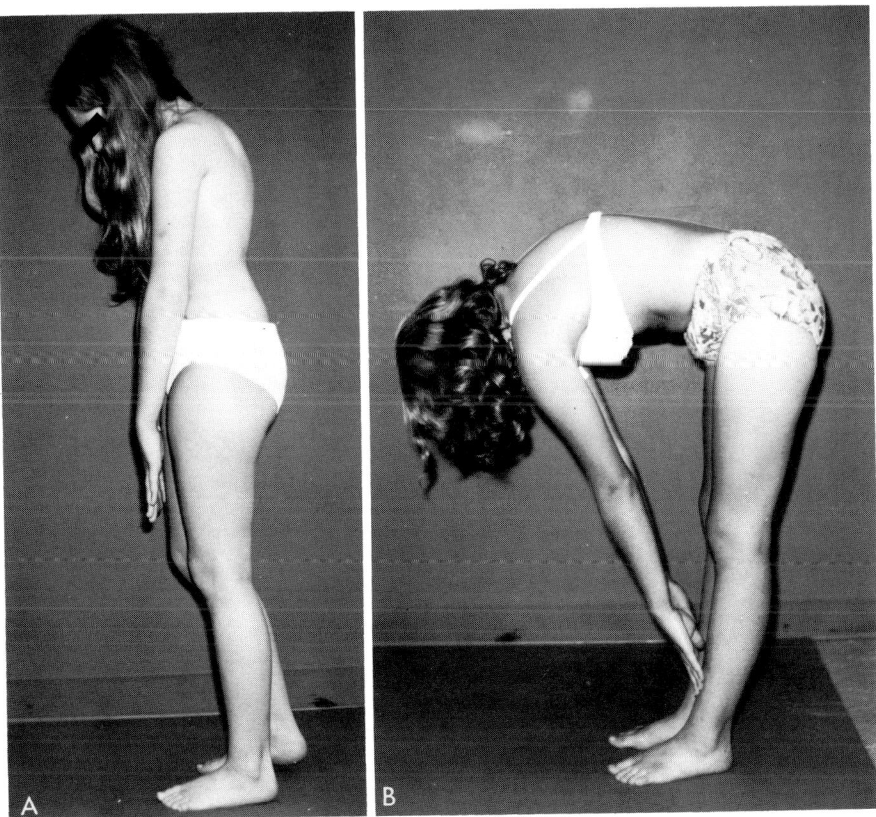

Figure 27–8. *A*, Preoperative appearance of a 12-year-old female with severe hamstring tightness and symptomatic Grade III spondylolisthesis. The patient is attempting to touch her toes, demonstrating marked restriction of forward bending. *B*, Eighteen months after surgery there is complete resolution of hamstring tightness. The patient is now capable of full flexion of the hips with the knees in extension.

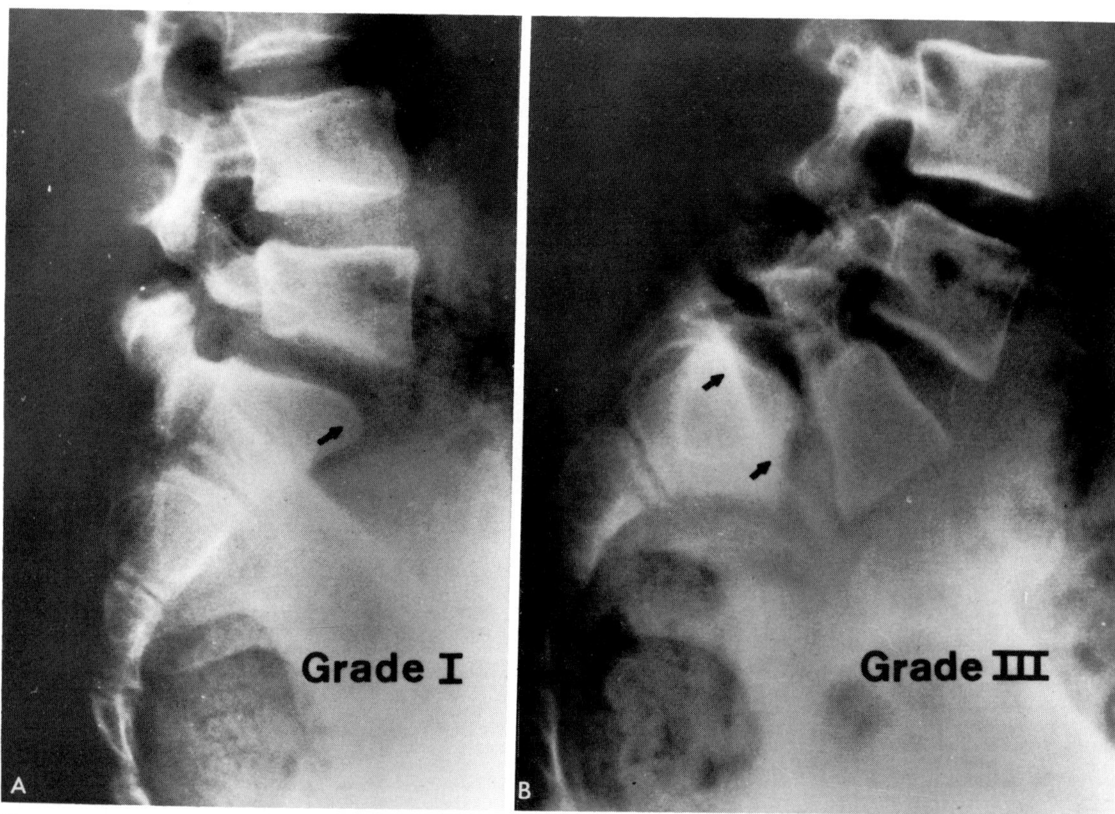

Figure 27–9. Instability of the body of L5 on the sacrum. *A*, A 10-year-old male with Grade I spondylolisthesis, demonstrating mild anterior erosion of the sacrum *(arrow)*. *B*, A 13-year-old male with Grade III spondylolisthesis, demonstrating mild anterior erosion of the sacrum *(arrows)*.

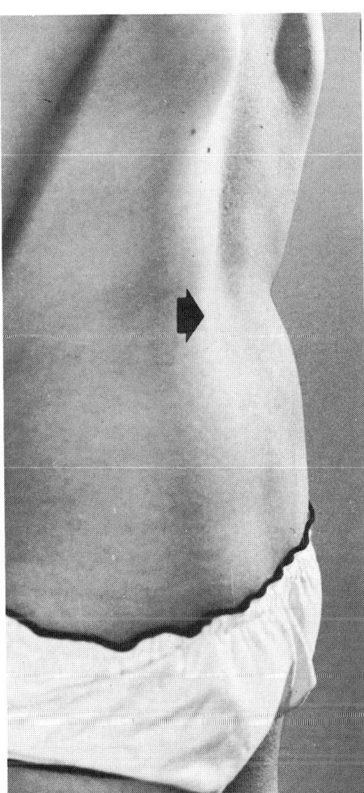

Figure 27–10. Flattening of the buttocks and flaring of the ilia, typical clinical findings in the latter stages of spondylolisthesis. The palpable step-off *(arrow)* is the prominent fifth lumbar spinous process, due to the sliding forward of the fourth with the spondylolisthesis.

The physical manifestations of spondylolisthesis correlate with the degree of slip and primarily with the amount of lumbosacral kyphosis. Wiltse found that some patients demonstrate the typical findings with only a 25 per cent slip. With a 33 per cent slip most patients have the physical examination characteristics associated with spondylolisthesis. With more than a 50 per cent slip, almost all patients demonstrate the classic physical manifestations.[138, 140]

Radicular pain and varying degrees of nerve root dysfunction are present in roughly half of spondylolisthesis patients requiring surgery for pain.[28, 46, 87] Most often there is compression of the fifth lumbar roots as they approach the L5 foramina. Typically they are trapped under the fibrocartilage filling the pars defect, or its adjacent osteophyte, in cases with isthmic spondylolisthesis, or compressed by hypertrophic facets in degenerative spondylolisthesis. Anterior translation of L5 on the sacrum stretches the sacral roots over the posterosuperior corner of the sacral endplate. Urologic examination, including a cystometrogram, may detect and document altered bladder function from sacral root involvement.

ASSOCIATED CONDITIONS

Spina bifida occulta commonly accompanies isthmic defects, with a reported incidence of 24 to 70 per cent.[24, 42, 70, 127] Spina bifida occulta also occurs in approximately 40 per cent of patients with dysplastic spondylolisthesis. In contrast, Brailsford's 1929 population studies reported the normal incidence of spina bifida occulta in adults without spondylolisthesis as 6 per cent.[19a] Some postulate that an incomplete posterior arch (spina bifida occulta) allows added stresses to concentrate on the pars, predisposing to fracture.

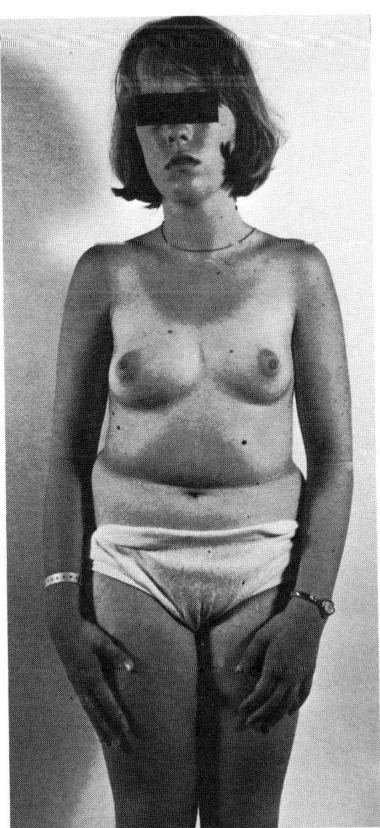

Figure 27–11. Grade III spondylolisthesis. Forward thrust of the lower abdomen forming a transverse abdominal crease at the umbilicus, typically found in Grades III and IV.

Scoliosis occurs in 5 to 7 per cent of all patients with spondylolysis and spondylolisthesis (Fig. 27–12).[11, 24, 27, 77, 99] It is found in approximately 30 per cent of patients requiring surgery for spondylolisthesis (range 23 to 48 per cent).[12, 40, 59, 70, 77, 92] Typically, if the scoliosis is related to the spondylolisthesis, the curve is a long C-shaped curve beginning at the L4–L5 level (Figs. 27–12 and 27–13). The scoliosis may be due to spasm and often corrects with fixation and fusion of the spondylolisthesis.[40, 77] In Bradford's series, 11 of 21 mild curves resolved with treatment of the slip.[14] Larger curves may be torsional with a structural component.[40] The structural variety tends to have asymmetric slippage at the lumbosacral joint, which acts as the apex of the curve, with rotational scoliosis extending proximally to the upper lumbar vertebrae. When torsional-structural scoliosis is clinically significant, we recommend instrumented correction of both deformities.

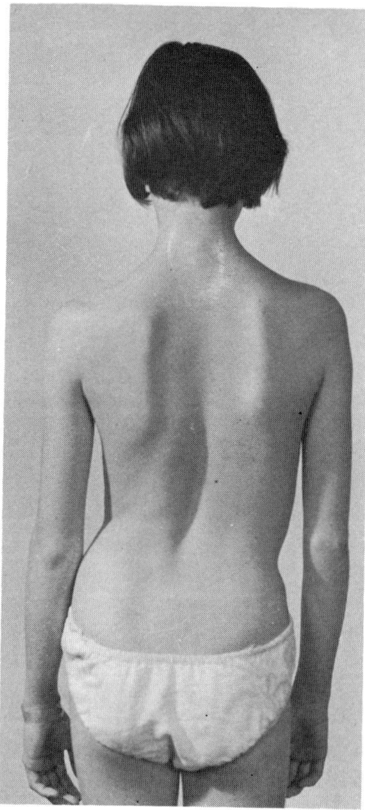

Figure 27–12. Typical "lumbar sag" associated with spondylolisthesis and found in most symptomatic patients. It is probably caused by reflex spasm and splinting from lumbar irritation. This is generally not a structural curve, as it usually resolves with reclining or remission of symptoms.

Although disc degeneration is always associated with spondylolisthesis, posterior disc protrusion at the level of the slip is rare (less than 5 per cent incidence) (Fig. 27–14).[13, 27, 105, 127] Associated lumbarization and sacralization is reported in 7 to 9 per cent of the patients with spondylolysis.

RADIOGRAPHIC STUDIES

Diagnostic Radiographs and Bone Scans

Initial films for backache usually include anteroposterior (AP) and lateral lumbosacral spine radiographs. If spondylolysis is suspected and not seen on these studies, oblique views can be obtained (see Fig. 27–4). In classic cases of a defect in the pars interarticularis, a break in the "Scottie dog's neck" can be observed. To adequately document slipping (spondylolisthesis), and particularly to monitor the possibility of a progressive slip, standing lateral radiographs are required (Fig. 27–15*A,B*).[13, 79] Boxall and associates found significant changes in both the percentage and angle of slip with changes in position (Fig. 27–16).[13] On standing, 40 per cent of their patients demonstrated a percentage slip increase averaging 17 per cent. The slip angle increased an average of 5 degrees with standing in 85 per cent of their patients.[13] Thus, both standing and supine lateral views are recommended.

The AP radiograph adds little in minor cases. In severe slips, however, the L5 vertebra is viewed "end-on" through the sacrum, the so-called reverse Napoleon hat sign (le chapeau) (Figs. 27–17 and 27–18). The hat is actually upside-down and not reversed. A standing AP view is needed to evaluate associated scoliosis.

After the initial films have confirmed the diagnosis, follow-up radiography can be confined to standing lateral views of L5–S1. These films are taken at intervals of six to 12 months during the adolescent growth spurt, a period during which slips are most likely to progress.

Twenty per cent of patients with spondylolysis have unilateral defects that can be difficult to detect. Spondylolysis should be suspected if there is asymmetry of the neural arch and unilateral wedging of the vertebral body.[10]

Text continued on page 932

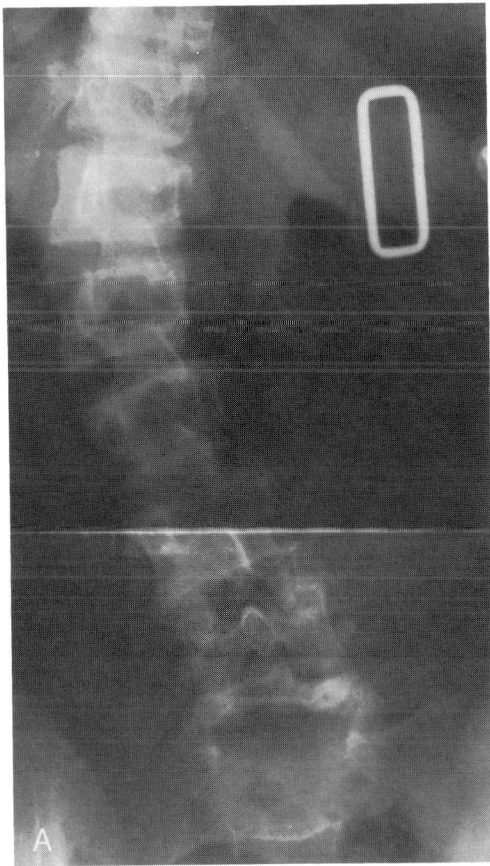

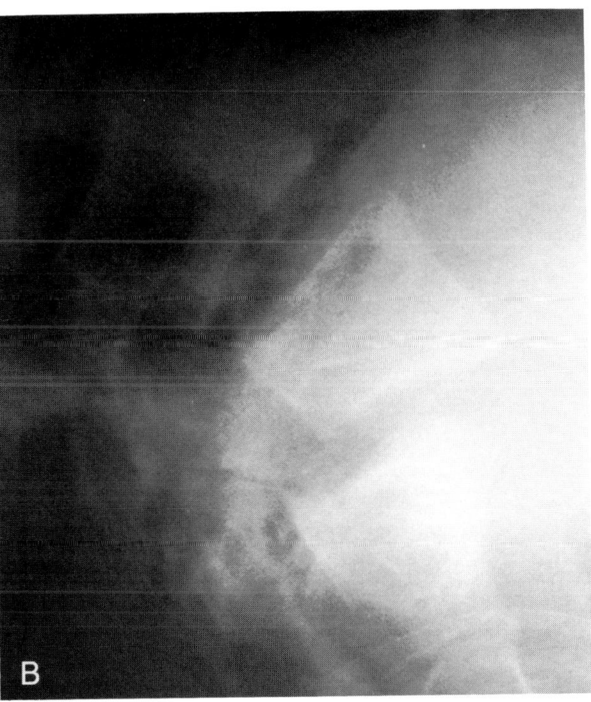

Figure 27–13. Anteroposterior radiographs demonstrating scoliosis. *A*, Large C-shaped curve with take-off at the L4–L5 level. *B*, Lateral radiograph showing the spondylolisthesis of L5 on S1. This patient was treated with fusion of L5 to the sacrum and postoperative bracing. The scoliosis itself was not treated but corrected after the fusion solidified.

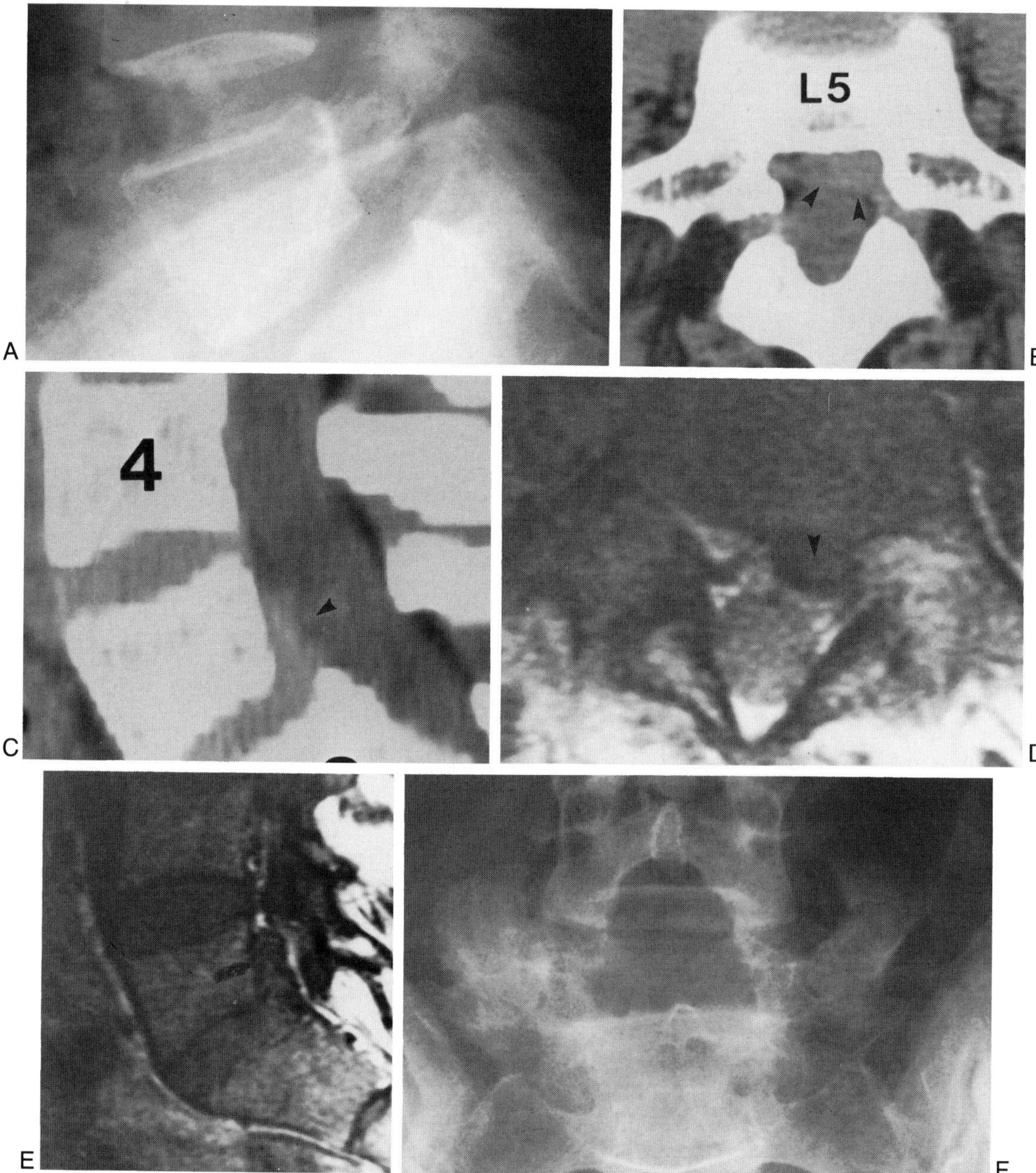

Figure 27–14. A 35-year-old female with an intermittent history of low back pain since adolescence developed gradual onset of posterolateral leg pain. The radiculopathy was primarily in the L5 nerve root distribution. Before the increasing leg pain developed, the patient was an active triathlete. *A*, Lateral radiograph demonstrating Grade I spondylolisthesis. *B*, CT scan shows a disc herniation *(arrowhead)* posterior to the L5 body. The pars defect can be seen on this soft tissue window. *C*, Lateral reconstruction from CT scan shows a large disc herniation from the L5–S1 disc space that has protruded proximally. The L4–L5 disc does not appear to be prominent on this scan. *D*, MR scan shows a large disc protruding behind the L5 body *(arrow)*. *E*, Sagittal MR scan shows a large disc herniation from the L5–S1 disc extruded in the cephalic direction almost to the L4–L5 space. *F*, The patient was treated with an L5 laminectomy, an L5–S1 discectomy, L5 nerve root foraminotomies, and bilateral-lateral fusion of L5 to the sacrum. She healed uneventfully and returned to athletic activities.

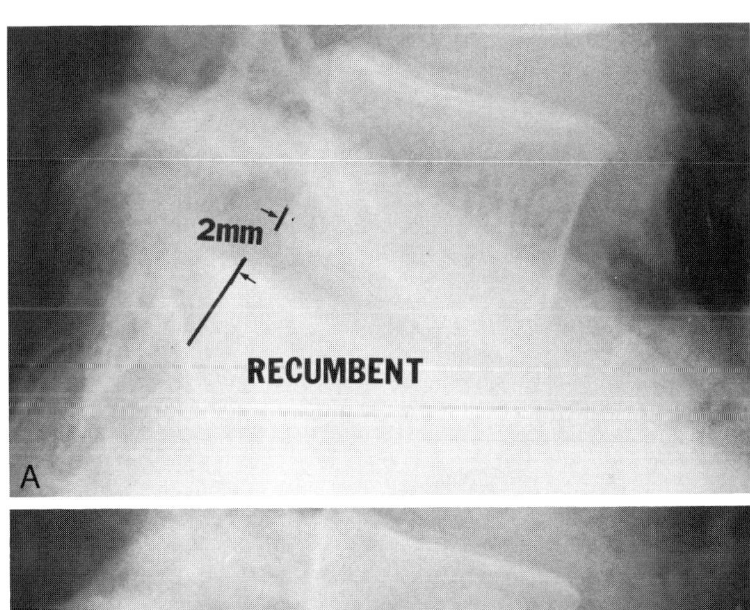

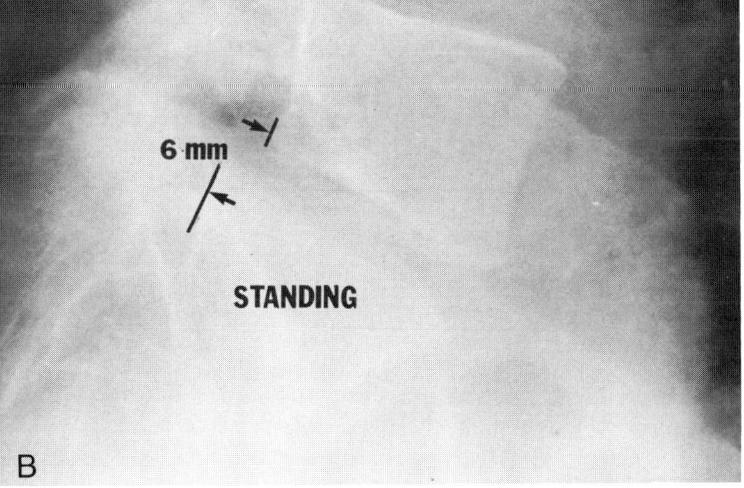

Figure 27–15. *A*, Lateral roentgenogram of a Type II spondylolisthesis, with the patient in the recumbent position: 2-mm olisthesis. *B*, Lateral roentgenogram of the same patient in the standing position: 6-mm olisthesis. Boxall and colleagues clearly demonstrated the importance of standing radiographs, noting significant changes in the percentage and angle of slip with changes in body position.[13]

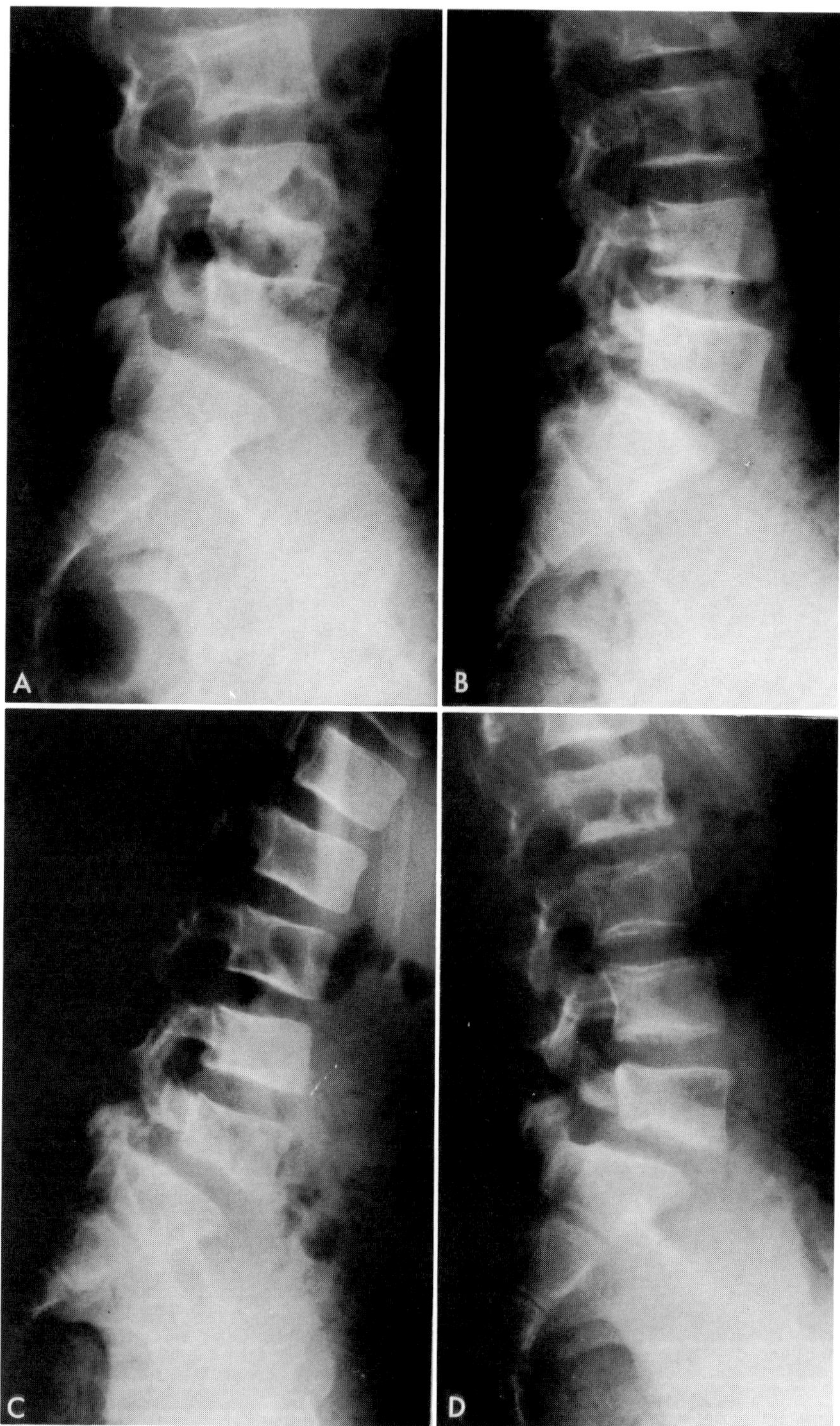

Figure 27–16. A 9-year-old discovered to have spondylolisthesis. *A*, Lateral roentgenogram. *B*, Extension view at the same age demonstrating that the gap can be closed and the fifth lumbar body reduced by positioning. *C*, Flexion. *D*, Extension. Note the widening of the defect and progression of the spondylolisthesis. The patient is no longer able to reduce the gap or subluxation of the body with extension. (Roentgenograms provided courtesy of James A. Averett, Jr., M.D., Atlanta, Georgia.)

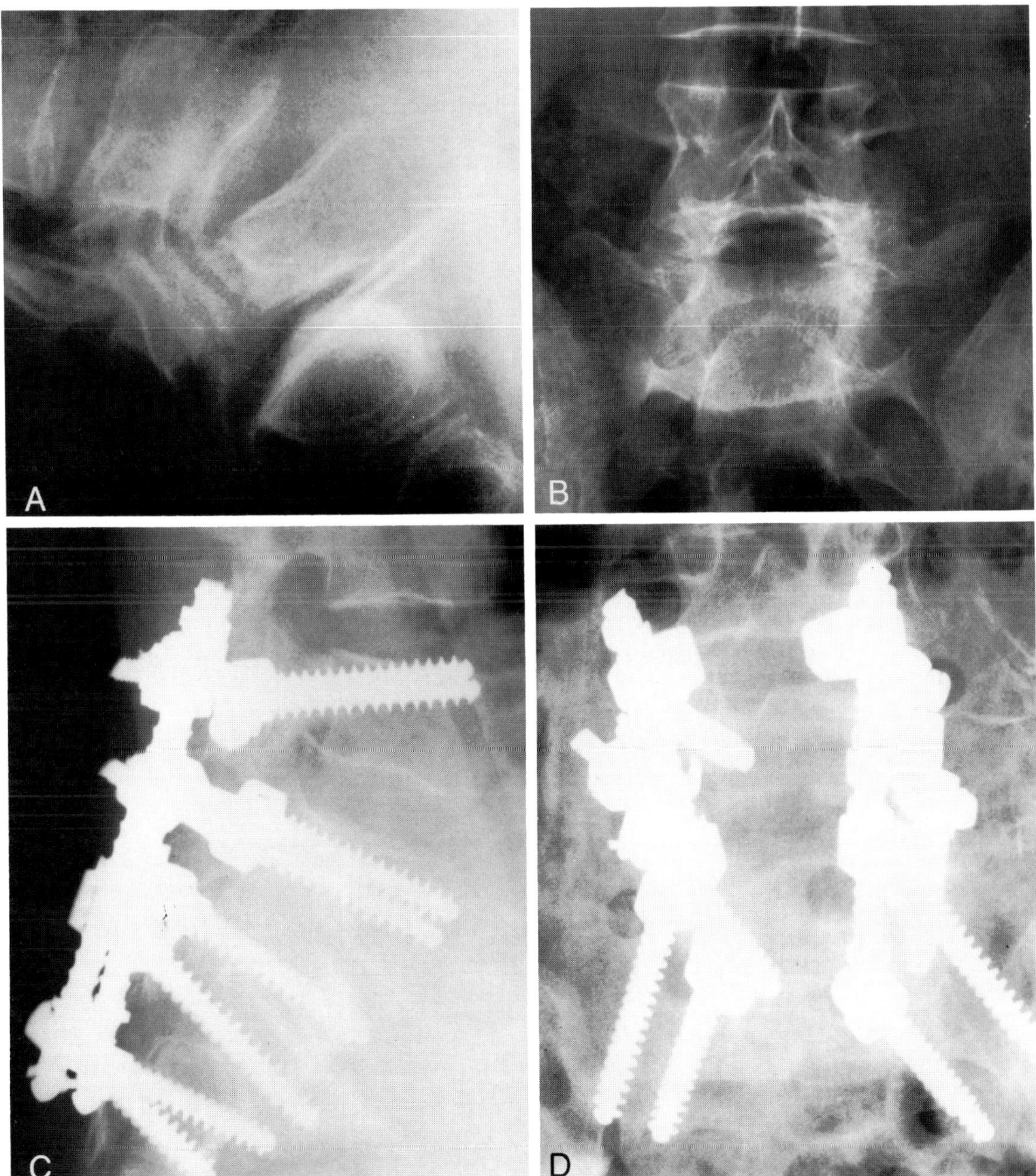

Figure 27–17. Patient with documented progressive spondylolisthesis and neurologic deficit, treated with posterior instrumented reduction and fusion. *A*, Spondylolisthesis L5 on S1. Note the rounding of the sacral dome, angulation of L5 on the sacrum, and vertical orientation of the sacrum. *B*, Anteroposterior radiograph demonstrating essentially a view through the L5 end plate: "Napoleon's hat." *C*, Instrumented reduction of spondylolisthesis. *D*, Although it is difficult to see between the Edwards rods, "Napoleon's hat" is no longer visible.

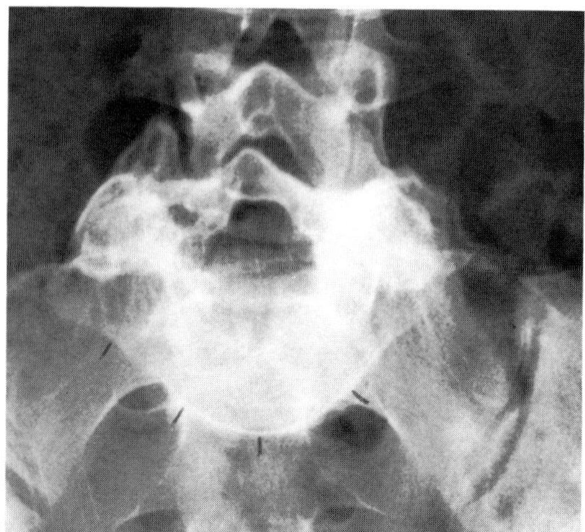

Figure 27–18. Postoperative anteroposterior radiograph demonstrating the standard "Napoleon's hat." Bilateral solid fusion can be noted.

Often the oblique views are hard to interpret and are negative early. Technetium pyrophosphate bone scanning may be used in acutely symptomatic patients to determine whether an acute injury or repair process has occurred. This may be helpful in distinguishing between an acute fracture and preexisting spondylolysis in the victim of multiple trauma.[72] In an acute injury the bone scan may be positive, although radiographic evidence of the pars defect has not yet developed.

A bone scan can also be used to determine whether a spondylolytic lesion is acute enough to merit immobilization with a cast. A positive bone scan and negative radiograph suggests a recent injury that may benefit from immobilization. A negative bone scan with positive radiographs implies an old lesion that will not heal. Additionally, this correlation of clinical, radiographic, and bone scan data is beneficial in clarifying medicolegal aspects of spondylolysis.

Radiographic Measurements

Many measurements have been proposed to evaluate severity, associated changes, and probability of progression in spondylolisthesis. In 1932 Meyerding divided the anteroposterior diameter of the superior surface of the first sacral vertebra into quarters and assigned a grade of I, II, III, or IV to slips of one, two, three, or four quarters (Fig. 27–19).[144] Taillard's method, which describes the degree of slip as a percentage of the anteroposterior diameter of either the top of the first sacral or fifth lumbar vertebra, is used by the authors (Fig. 27–20).[13, 123]

The angular relationship between the fifth lumbar and first sacral vertebrae describes lumbosacral kyphosis (see Fig. 27–19). It is re-

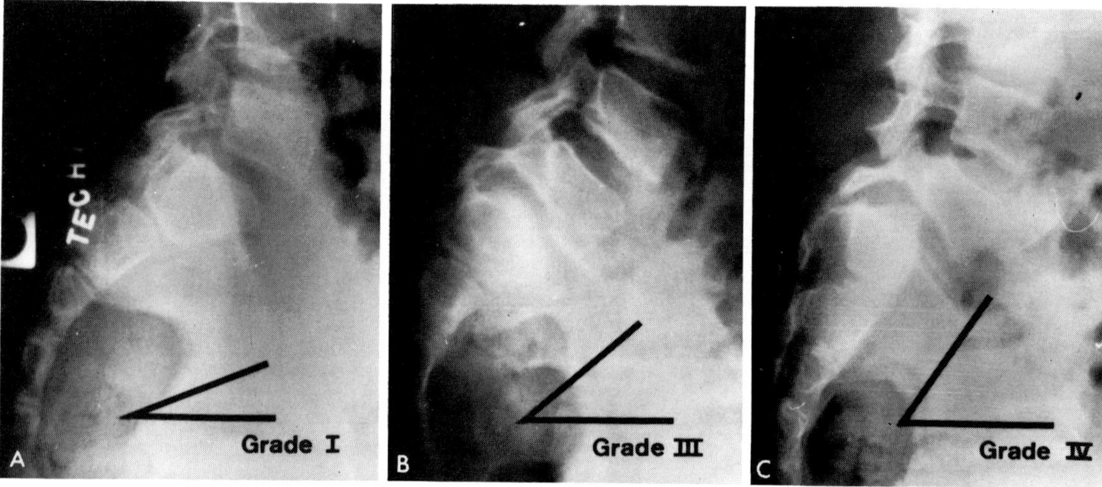

Figure 27–19. Three patients with different degrees of spondylolisthesis, *A*, *B*, and *C* (Grades I, III, and IV). As the slip advances, the sacrum and pelvis become more vertical, in part owing to the backward pull of the tight hamstrings. The lumbar spine moves forward with increasing lordosis, giving rise to the typical clinical appearance. Often it is easier to understand the clinical problem if one considers the lumbar spine to be stable and observes the degree of motion of the pelvis.

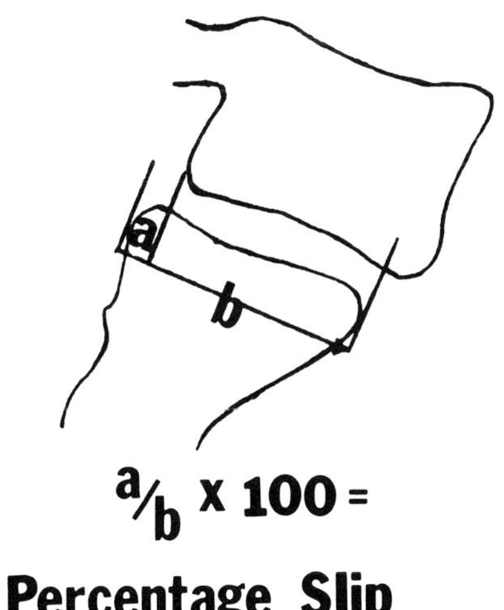

Figure 27–20. A method of quantitating the severity of slip and reporting it as a percentage.

ferred to variably as sagittal roll, sagittal rotation, angle of kyphosis, or slip angle. The term slip angle is most commonly accepted.[13, 27, 144] A reproducible method for measuring the slip angle (kyphosis) in spondylolisthesis involves measuring the angle between the perpendicular of a line drawn along the posterior cortex of the S1 and S2 bodies and a line drawn along the superior endplate of L5 (Fig. 27–21).[117] These two surfaces provide a more reproducible measurement than basing the L5 measurement on the inferior end plate since the lower end plate can be severely distorted.

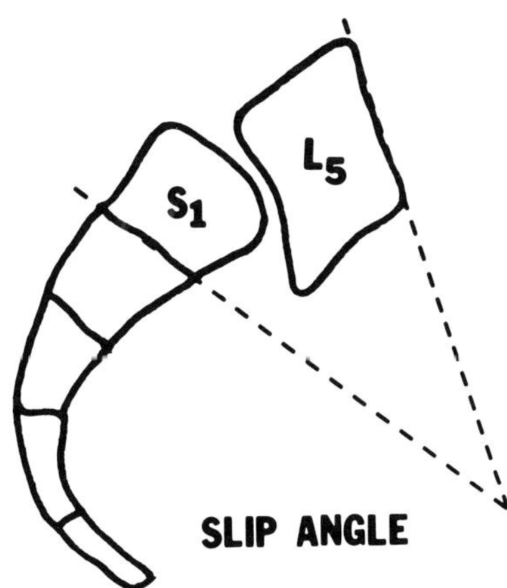

Figure 27–21. A reproducible method of measuring the angular relationship between L5 and S1. An increased slip angle is associated with greater instability and the potential for progressive slip.

The slip angle is the most sensitive indicator of potential instability.[13, 56, 117] It can be used to prognosticate slip progression in spondylolisthetic patients both before and after fusion (Fig. 27–22). A high slip angle indicates potentially greater instability, greater risk of progression, and a poorer biomechanical environment for healing.[13, 56, 117]

Neuroradiographic Studies

Myelography has traditionally been used in the evaluation of spondylolisthesis patients who have no improvement after bed rest, pain or symptoms out of proportion to the severity of the lesion, suspicion of a coexistent lesion, severe slip, and predominant neurologic signs or sciatica.[13, 15, 26, 56, 85, 127] Conversely, in Boxall and associates' review, myelography never showed a lesion of the nerve root or a herniated disc, and the block was always due to the tenting of the dura over the body at the level of slip of the first sacral vertebra. It is also difficult to evaluate the root sleeve at the level of slip.[13, 28] We have rarely obtained

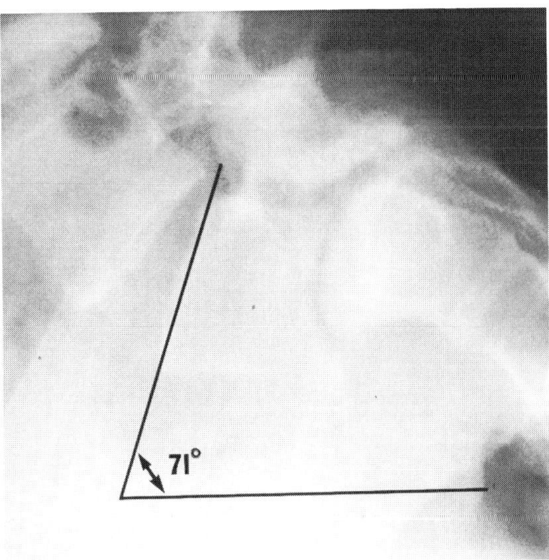

Figure 27–22. Sacrohorizontal angle. When a solid fusion has been obtained from L5 to S1, the top of L5 becomes the new sacrohorizontal angle. Wiltse and Rothman[145] suggested 55 degrees as the break-off point for one-level fusions. Beyond 55 degrees they recommended a two-level fusion from L4 to S1. This lateral roentgenogram also demonstrates anterior erosion of the sacrum, adaptive changes that contribute to instability.

information at the spondylolisthetic level from this invasive study; however, myelograms or other imaging studies may be indicated in the preoperative evaluation to ensure there is no other coexistent lesion that may be mimicking the symptoms of spondylolisthesis or producing the symptoms and signs (Figs. 27–14 and 27–23).

If there is a question as to the source of symptoms or site of root compression, computed tomographic (CT) examination better defines the pathology (see Figs. 27–14 and 27–23). McAfee found that CT demonstrated specific sites for neural encroachment in 13 of 15 patients.[76] Nonmechanical events explained the neurologic compromise in two patients. CT is also helpful in assessing pedicle size when young patients are scheduled for surgical reconstruction.

Magnetic resonance imaging (MRI) may be

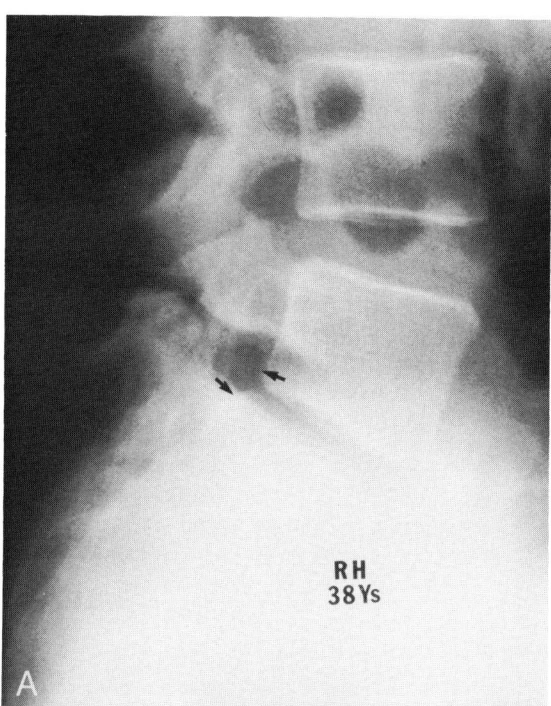

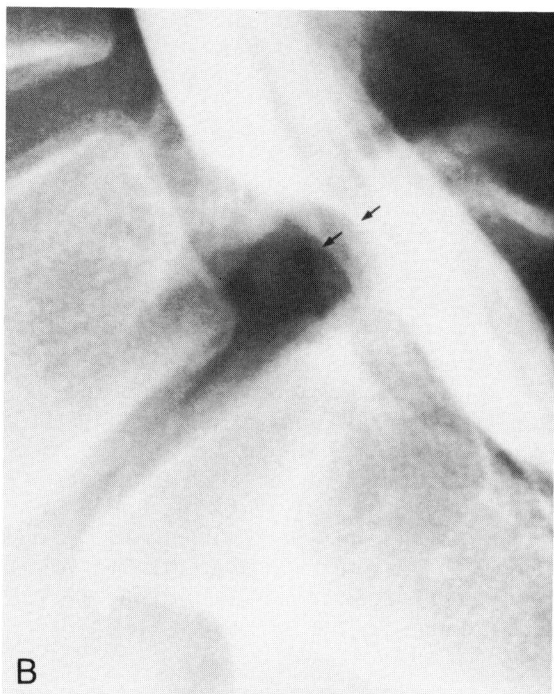

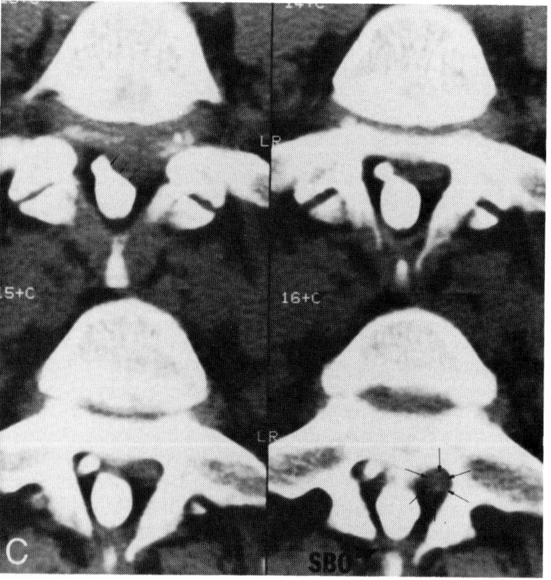

Figure 27–23. Radiographic studies of a 38-year-old male with low back and left leg pain. *A,* Lateral roentgenogram demonstrating Grade I isthmic spondylolisthesis (slip shown between arrows). *B,* Myelogram demonstrates a "double-density" sign (thinned dye column seen between arrowtips) in addition to the olisthesis at the L5–S1 level. *C,* Axial postmyelography CT images of the olisthetic level demonstrate the characteristic disc space appearance. They also provide excellent bone and soft tissue detail, in this case illustrating a left herniated nucleus pulposus, a swollen S1 nerve root, and incidental spina bifida. MRI, as demonstrated in Figure 27–2*D,* also gives excellent detail of soft tissue and bone and of the neutral canal, and is a most useful adjunctive study.

even more useful than the unenhanced CT to evaluate for disc herniation at another level (or same level) in a patient where surgery is planned. MRI demonstrates neural canal anatomy and sources of neural impingement, and allows disc signal comparison at other potentially symptomatic levels (see Fig. 27–14).

Provocative discography at adjacent levels may reproduce a portion of the pain pattern as the disc is injected. If a disc adjacent to an intended fusion level leads to a pain response reproducing the symptoms, consideration may be made to include that level (usually L4–L5) in the fusion.

NONOPERATIVE TREATMENT

Clinical Follow-up

Wiltse has proposed the following guidelines for continued evaluation of young patients with spondylolysis-spondylolisthesis:[138, 140]

1. Pars defect discovered very early (less than ten years): radiographs every four months initially; later, semiannually to 15 years of age; then at one- to two-year intervals until completion of growth.
2. Up to 25 per cent isthmic spondylolisthesis in an asymptomatic child: no limitation of activity; recommend an occupation avoiding heavy labor.
3. Up to 50 per cent slip in an asymptomatic child: radiographs semiannually until skeletal maturity; recommend activity modification and refraining from contact sports; advise an occupation avoiding heavy labor.
4. Up to 50 per cent slip in a symptomatic patient: initiate conservative therapy (exercises, corset, brace, limitation of activities). Recommend semiannual radiographs until 15 years of age and annually thereafter until age 17 or 18; advise a vocation avoiding heavy labor.
5. Greater than 50 per cent slip: consider surgical treatment.

In general, we agree with these guidelines; however, in asymptomatic children with an incidental pars defect, we lean toward Fredrickson's advice that the parents be told of the defect, but that reexamination and a lateral standing radiograph be required only annually, unless the child develops symptoms or gait abnormalities.[42]

Treatment of Congenital and Isthmic Spondylolisthesis

Most children with spondylolysis never develop symptoms; most of those who do can be treated without surgery. Activity modification, including initial bed rest, is a mainstay of effective treatment.[27, 127, 138] Hamstring tightness often improves in response to flexibility and strengthening exercises of the abdominal and gluteal muscle groups and is an excellent clinical guide in evaluating the success or failure of a treatment program.[24, 56, 127] Immobilization by corset, brace, or plaster jacket can reduce symptoms. Some authors advocate a trial of immobilization to provide information concerning the efficacy of future surgical stabilization.[56, 127]

Steiner and Micheli reviewed 67 patients with an average age of 16 years with symptomatic spondylolysis or Grade I spondylolisthesis treated with a modified Boston brace. Patients were followed for an average of 2.5 years after treatment. Seventy-eight per cent reported excellent to good results and returned to full activity. Thirteen per cent remained symptomatic and 9 per cent underwent in situ fusion. Twelve patients with acute, traumatic spondylolysis showed radiographic evidence of pars defect healing after "immobilization" in the orthosis.[121]

The nonoperative treatment of spondylolisthesis is less predictable. Turner and Bianco treated a group of children and adolescents with isthmic defects and slips with full-time, antilordotic brace wear (23 hours a day) for six months and then weaned from the brace over the following six months. Vigorous sports and activities were allowed in the brace as long as patients remained asymptomatic. A physical therapy program emphasizing hamstring stretching, lumbodorsal fascial stretching, and abdominal strengthening was an integral part of the treatment program.[127] These authors reported clinical success in 66 per cent, but poor results in 34 per cent who subsequently had surgery.

Bell and associates reviewed 28 consecutive children treated with an antilordotic brace for low-grade (less than 50 per cent) spondylolisthesis.[9] These patients wore the brace for 23 hours a day for an average of 25 months. In contrast with Turner and Bianco, they claimed that all patients became pain free and without measurable increase in percentage slip.

Pizzutillo and Hummer reviewed their experience with conservative treatment of 82 symptomatic adolescents with spondylolysis or spondylolisthesis. The patients ranged in age from 6.5 to 21 years. Follow-up spanned one to 14.3 years and the duration of treatment averaged 11.5 months. They found nonoperative treatment was effective in two thirds of patients with a slip less than 50 per cent. Flexion exercises and rest were more effective than casting and bracing. In contrast only one of 12 (8 per cent) patients with greater than 50 per cent slip had significant relief.[93]

We emphasize that an adolescent with significant prolonged symptoms should not be psychologically crippled during the socially vital teenage years by an unduly extended conservative treatment plan. The few patients who require surgical stabilization, when appropriately selected, tend to benefit greatly.[1]

SURGICAL ALTERNATIVES

Indications and Goals

The indications for operative intervention in patients with spondylolysis and spondylolisthesis include the following (it should be noted these are prevalently for adolescents and young adults):

1. Persistence or recurrence of major symptoms for at least one year despite activity modification and physical therapy.[13, 56, 63, 68, 70, 84, 112, 127, 130, 133, 138, 140]
2. Tight hamstrings, persistently abnormal gait, or postural deformities unrelieved by physical therapy.[8, 15, 56, 92, 130, 138]
3. Sciatic scoliosis.[127, 130]
4. Progressive neurologic deficit.[13, 70, 84, 127, 130]
5. Progressive slipping beyond 25 to 50 per cent, even when asymptomatic.[13, 56, 63, 70, 84, 112, 114, 127, 130, 133, 138, 140]
6. A high slip angle (40 to 50 degrees) in a growing child, since it is likely to be associated with further progression and deformity.[13]
7. Psychologic problems attributed to shortness of trunk, abnormal gait, and postural deformities characteristic of more severe slips.[14, 30]

The goals of any operative treatment program for spondylolysis or spondylolisthesis include reduction of back and leg pain; prevention of further slip; stabilization of the unstable L5–S1 segment; reversal of neurologic deficit; restoration of more normal spine mechanics, posture and gait; and improved appearance.

Surgical treatments advocated for spondylolisthesis include repair of the defect for spondylolysis, root decompression (Gill L5 laminectomy) for radiculopathy, in situ fusion, and reduction.

Pars Defect Repair

To increase the chance of fusion, techniques have been proposed to reduce and fix low-grade (less than 25 per cent) slips.[16, 22, 23, 48, 80, 86, 90, 128] The major theoretical advantage of this approach is that if the pars defect can be fused and the vertebra stabilized, the L5–S1 and perhaps L4–L5 motion is preserved. The disc at the level of slippage is usually incompetent if the slip is of long duration and may be a source of pain. Hence, the value of preserving that disc can be questioned, especially in adults. Nevertheless several procedures have been described that attempt to reduce low-grade spondylolisthesis and fuse the pars defect. Screws can be inserted across the pars defect for partial reduction and stabilization combined with local grafting.[22, 23, 90, 128] Stainless steel wires or Mersilene tape can be passed under (anterior to) both of the L5 transverse processes in a looped fashion and then twisted and tightened over the L5 spinous process and lamina.[16, 61, 86] With these techniques, theoretically the pars can be roughened and fused; however, reports on these methods include only a limited number of patients with less than ideal results and short follow-up. Direct repair of the pars defect with or without reduction has never become an accepted approach, and is now rarely performed.

Decompression

When radicular pain is the primary symptom, or neurologic deficit is present, Gill and others advocated removal of the L5 lamina and pars fibrocartilage to decompress the L5 and other roots.[8, 13, 27, 28, 46, 54, 70, 73, 79, 84, 85, 92, 99, 101, 112, 113, 118, 127, 130, 138] In recent years, a "Gill" laminectomy without fusion has fallen out of favor because of experience with residual back pain and increased slippage after surgery, particularly in younger patients (under age 40).[3, 28, 89, 130] In the treatment of adolescent spondylolisthesis, the Gill procedure alone is contraindicated since it can lead to increased instability, progression of slip, and increased lumbosacral kyphosis.[8, 12, 15, 56, 70, 79, 89, 127, 138, 140] Others note that fusion alone is often associated with gradual improvement, even with a neurologic deficit in adolescents.[15, 56, 138] At present, decompression alone is not recommended in patients under 40 without concomitant fusion, and is rarely needed in the child and adolescent years.

In Situ Fusion Versus Reduction–Fixation

The present role of in situ fusion versus reduction–fusion is in transition. Until recently, most authors concluded that slips of less than 50 per cent without neurologic deficit were best treated with an in situ posterolateral fusion.[13, 24, 27, 63, 84, 112, 127, 130, 138, 140] With greater understanding of spondylolisthesis biomechanics and improving methods for reduction–fixation, the indications for reduction–fixation are broadening.[19, 30, 32, 37, 120, 136]

IN SITU FUSION

Posterior

Posterior in situ fusion is the oldest surgical treatment described for spondylolisthesis. Posterior fusions must extend from the sacrum to at least L4, since the L5 lamina is detached from the body of L5 in spondylolisthesis. Reported results vary widely; adequate relief of symptoms is reported in 60 to 100 per cent of patients, with solid fusion attained in 40 to 85 per cent.[17, 52] Harris and Weinstein reported on a group of 21 patients all less than 25 years of age, with greater than 50 per cent spondylolisthesis.[52] They were treated by posterior interlaminar fusion and follow-up averaged 24 years. Despite nine (50 per cent) of their study group having one or more neurologic findings, 95 per cent were asymptomatic or mildly symptomatic at follow-up. In contrast, Apel and associates reviewed 12 adults treated for Grade I L5–S1 spondylolisthesis with an average follow-up of 40 years after Hibbs posterior fusions. The pseudarthrosis rate was high (43 per cent). Subsequent attempts at fusion also had a high failure rate. Failure of fusion was closely associated with a poor clinical result and long-term disability.[4]

Posterolateral

Posterolateral in situ fusion is more effective than posterior fusions in relieving symptoms (86 to 100 per cent), obtaining fusion (66 to 100 per cent), and preventing progression after fusion (Figs. 27–24 and 27–25).[12, 13, 52, 55, 63, 70, 91, 96, 98, 100, 125, 127, 140] To achieve successful arthrodesis, fusion from L4 to the sacrum is recommended if the L5 transverse process is small, the L5 horizontal angle is greater than 55 degrees, the slip is 50 per cent or greater, or the L4–L5 disc is incompetent or symptomatic (Figs. 27–22, 27–26, 27–27).[140]

The degree of postoperative immobilization required after in situ fusion remains controversial. When midline structures are preserved, some authors do not recommend postoperative immobilization.[56, 84, 140] Others apply a body cast with leg extension for three

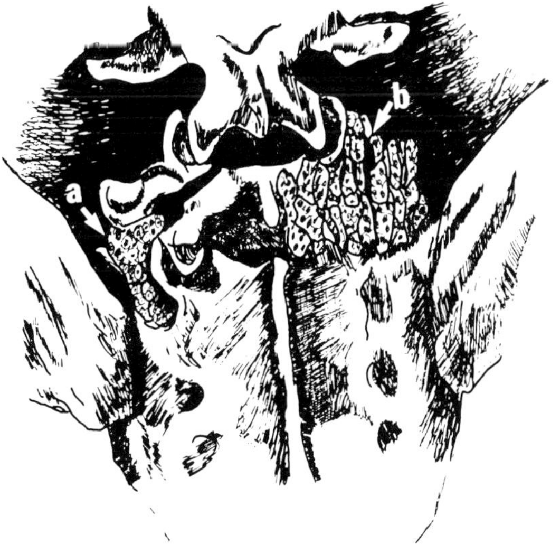

Figure 27–24. Diagrammatic representation of the preparation and extent of bone grafting for a posterolateral in situ fusion. *a* demonstrates a flap of bone that is folded up from the sacral ala. This bridges space between the sacral ala and L5 transverse process. *b* depicts the extent of the graft, including the lateral surface of the superior articular process of L5 to the tips of the transverse process and ala. The L4–L5 facet joint is not violated.

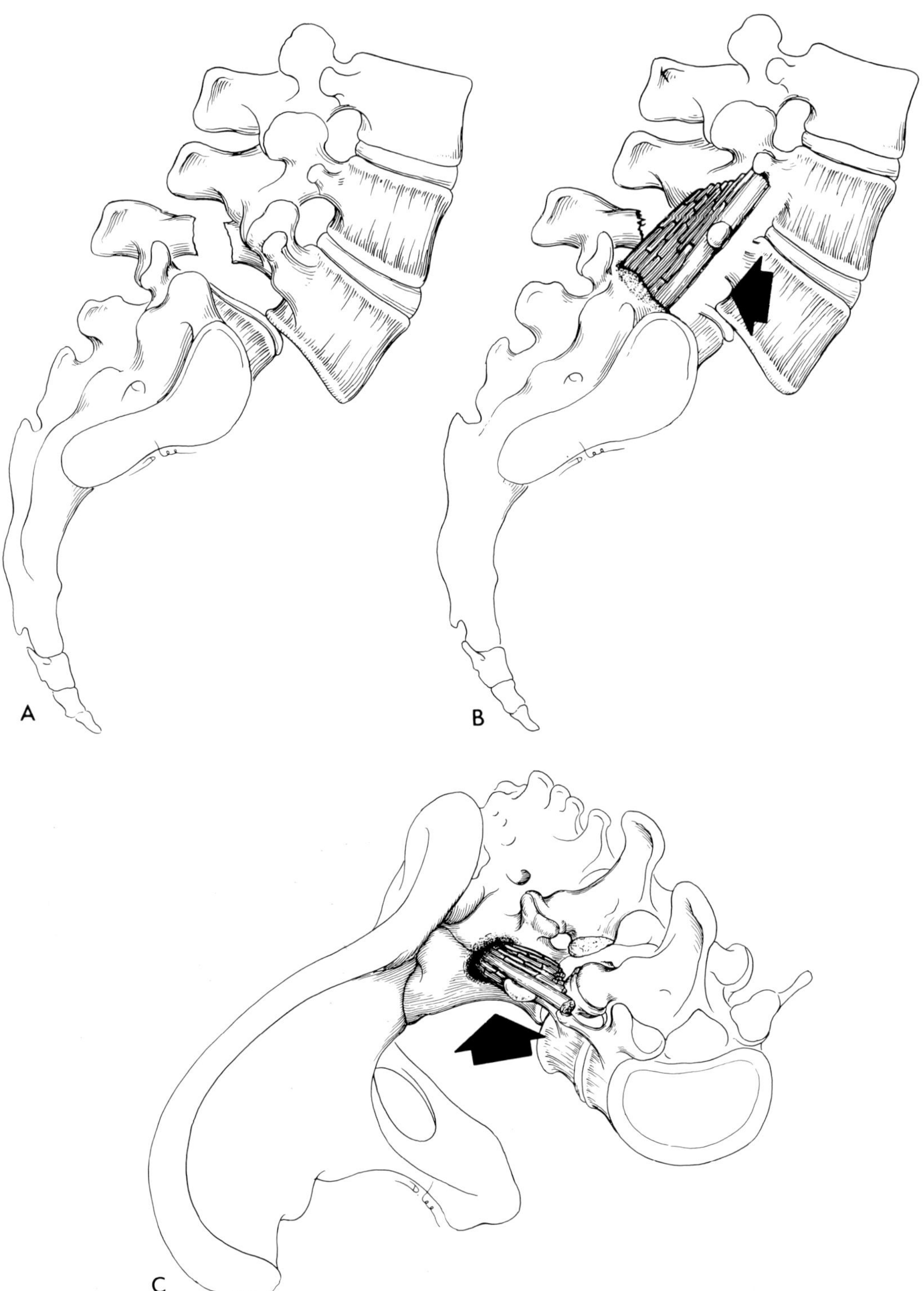

Figure 27–25. *A*, Lumbosacral spine with spondylolysis of the L5 pars interarticularis and spondylolisthesis. *B*, The posterolateral fusion surgical procedure preferred by the authors. A large window has been made in the ala of the sacrum *(arrow)* in which a large piece of cortical-cancellous bone has been flapped down and extends to the transverse process of the proximal vertebra. This forms the floor of the bone graft on which the cancellous portion of the graft is placed. It is important that the graft nearly parallel the forces through the L5–S1 joint. *C*, The graft in place.

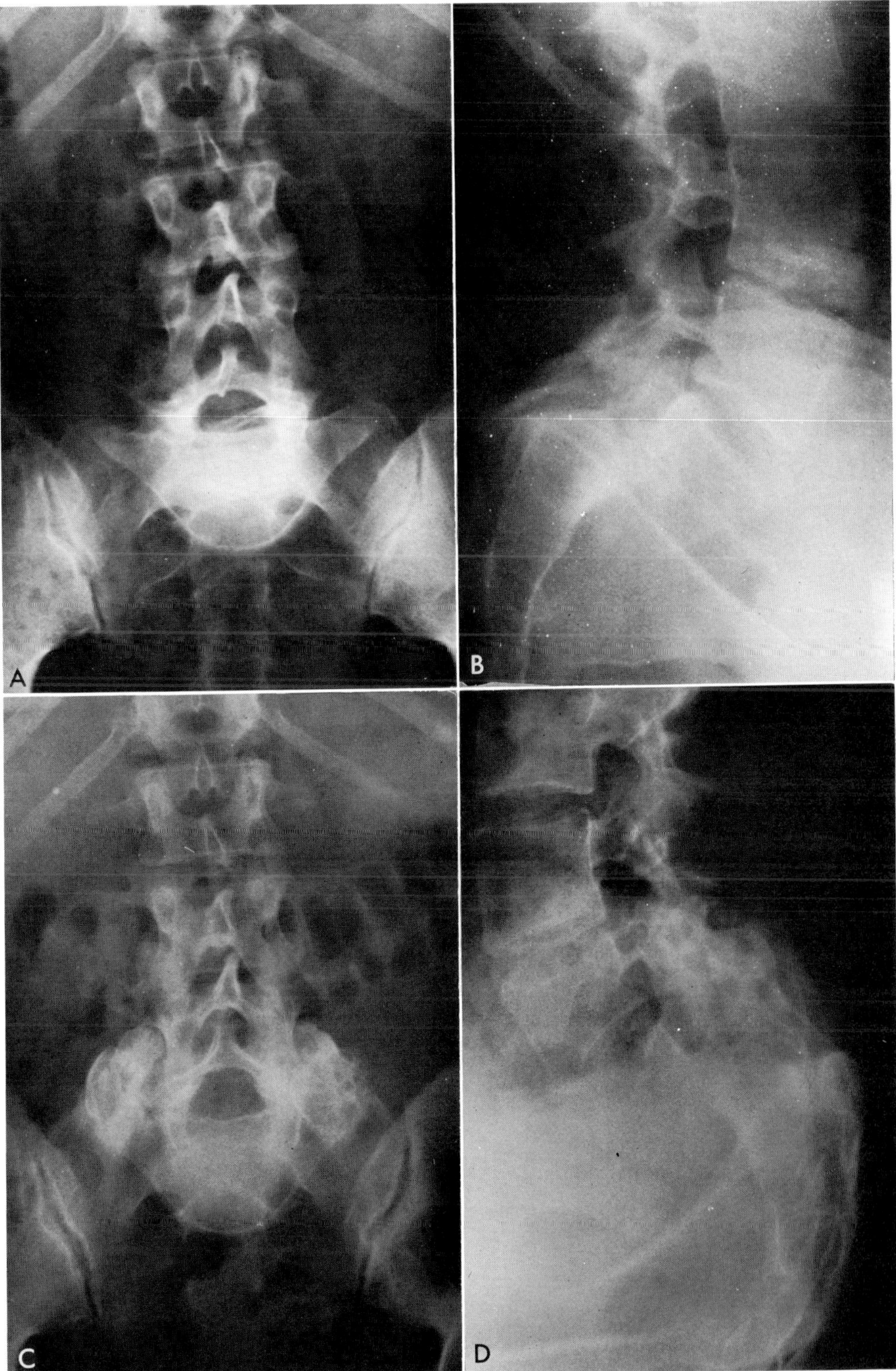

Figure 27–26. A 19-year-old with Grade III spondylolisthesis. *A*, *B*, Preoperative roentgenographic appearance. *C*, *D*, Appearance three years after bilateral-lateral column fusion. There has been no further progression of the spondylolisthesis, and the patient enjoys complete remission of symptoms. This result is to be anticipated when this method is used.

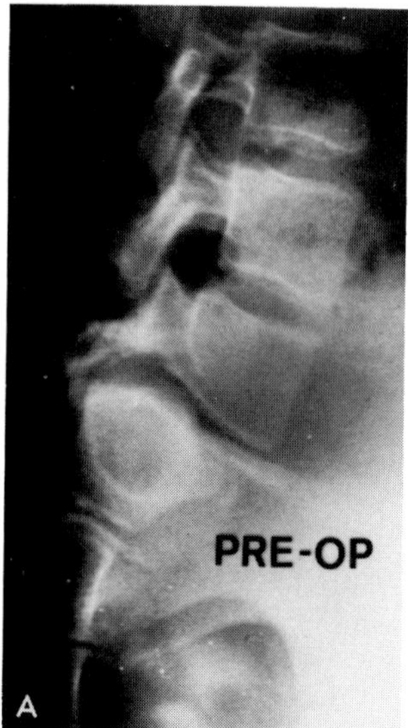

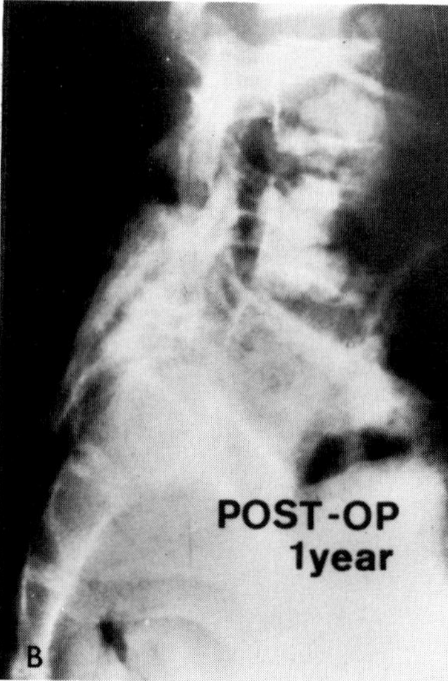

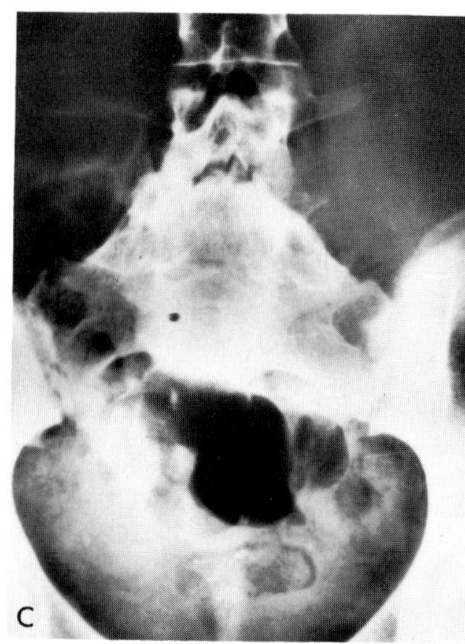

Figure 27–27. *A*, Roentgenographic appearance before bilateral-lateral column fusion, L4 to the sacrum, of an 11-year-old female with Type I dysplastic spondylolisthesis and Grade III spondylolisthesis. *B, C*, Postoperative appearance at age 12, demonstrating a solid fusion and no further progression of the spondylolisthesis. The patient was immobilized in a bilateral pantaloon spica cast for three months after the surgery to prevent further slippage.

months. We use a custom-molded lumbosacral body jacket often with a thigh extension for two to three months in most patients with high-grade slips.[1]

Even slips of greater than 50 per cent can be successfully treated with in situ fusion in children and early adolescents (see Fig. 27–8). Johnson and Kirwan reported on 17 patients with greater than 50 per cent spondylolisthesis.[63] These authors noted significant diminution of back pain, decreased hamstring tightness, improvement in straight-leg-raising restriction, and no progression of slip in 16 of 17 patients who underwent bilateral–lateral fusion. Reynolds and Wiltse reported on 24 adolescent patients with greater than 50 per cent spondylolisthesis.[96] At five years' average follow-up, 17 of 24 patients had excellent and seven had good pain relief. Of 21 patients with preoperative hamstring tightness, 19 resolved over an average of 7.5 months from surgery. There was no change in the average percentage of slip (73 per cent) or slip angle (26 per cent). Indeed, Wiltse reports that for over 30 years he has performed in situ fusions through bilateral muscle splitting incisions without neural decompression for all children with isthmic spondylolisthesis, regardless of grade. He claims most have at least a "good" result, with solid fusions, resolution of pain and hamstring spasm, improvement in preoperative body posture, and minimal complications.[145] Riley and associates evaluated 47 children with greater than 50 per cent spondylolisthesis treated with bilateral-lateral fusion.[98] All had follow-up greater than one year. Twenty-four (51 per cent) had an increase of greater than 10 degrees in sagittal rotation, believed to be due to bending of the fusion mass. Nevertheless, 85 per cent had good to excellent relief of back or leg pain. Complications were negligible in each of the series.

Successful surgical treatment of the adult with symptomatic isthmic spondylolisthesis is more difficult and variable (Figs. 27–28 and 27–29).[28, 54] The reported posterolateral fusion rate in adults varies between 66 and 89 per cent.[2, 13, 41, 98, 119, 125, 145] There are lower average union rates reported for adults than adolescents with the same degree of slip. This appears to be due to smoking, greater forces working against the fusion mass, and reduced healing potential compared with the adolescent. Hanley and Levy analyzed variables affecting results in the treatment of 50 adults with Grade I to III spondylolisthesis.[49] Factors associated with an unsatisfactory outcome included male gender, middle age, smoking, and radicular symptoms. Cigarette smoking has been found to be deleterious to the lumbar

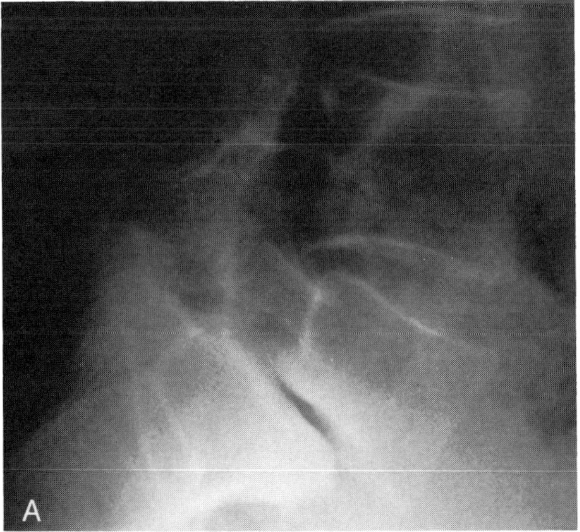

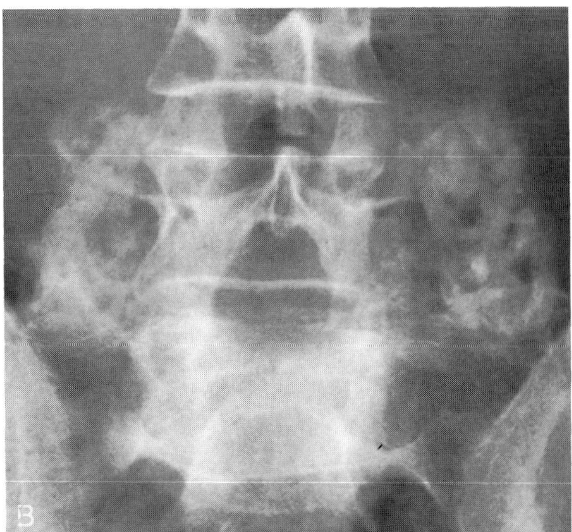

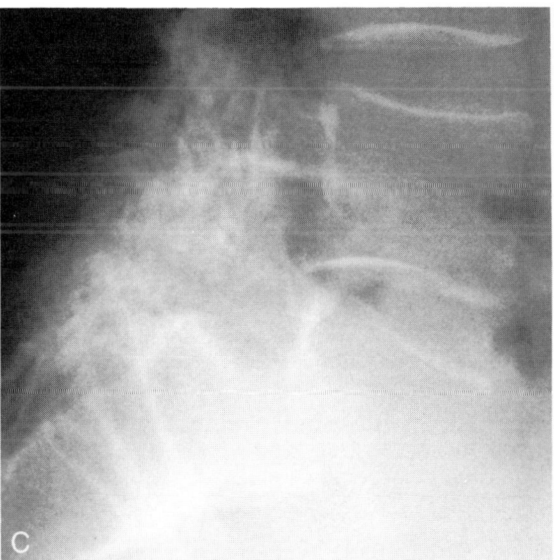

Figure 27–28. Radiographs of a 39-year-old male with a 10- to 15-year history of low back pain who presented with footdrop on the right side. MR and CT scans demonstrated no disc fragment. The neurologic deficit was presumed related to the spondylolisthesis and the fibrocartilaginous bar at the pars detect irritating the L5 nerve root. *A*, Preoperative standing lateral view showing approximately 50 per cent subluxation of L5 on S1. A vacuum phenomenon can be seen. There are no traction spurs and there is limited sclerosis. There is retrolisthesis of L4 on L5. *B*, The patient had laminectomies and decompression of the L5 nerve roots and bilateral-lateral fusion of L4 to the sacrum. The results were excellent and he returned to full activities with no restriction. This anteroposterior view shows the fusion mass from L4 to the sacrum. *C*, Lateral view of the same patient showing perhaps a slightly increased slip of L5 on S1. This has not proved to be a symptomatic problem but emphasizes the need for concomitant fusion when decompression is performed in an individual under 45 or 50 with underlying isthmic spondylolisthesis.

spine fusion rate in other studies as well.[2, 21, 49] The presence of disability issues or development of pseudarthrosis had a profoundly negative effect on clinical results.

To improve the outcome in persistently symptomatic adult spondylolisthesis patients, segmental stabilization with bilateral-lateral fusions is now frequently recommended. For example, Peek and Wiltse claimed excellent results with bilateral fusion alone for eight adult patients with high-grade isthmic spondylolisthesis and sciatica.[91] After five-year average follow-up, all eight cases fused solidly with relief of back pain and sciatica and resolution of neurologic deficits in six of eight patients.

It must be emphasized that it is important, particularly in the adult, to assess adjacent levels with MRI, CT, or provocative discography to ensure that the signs and symptoms are confined to the spondylolisthesis level. Occasionally an adjacent level may be the source of pain (herniated or degenerative disc).

Decompression with In Situ Fusion

Decompression of the canal or roots without fusion is controversial.[28, 76] Many authors have advocated decompression with any neurologic

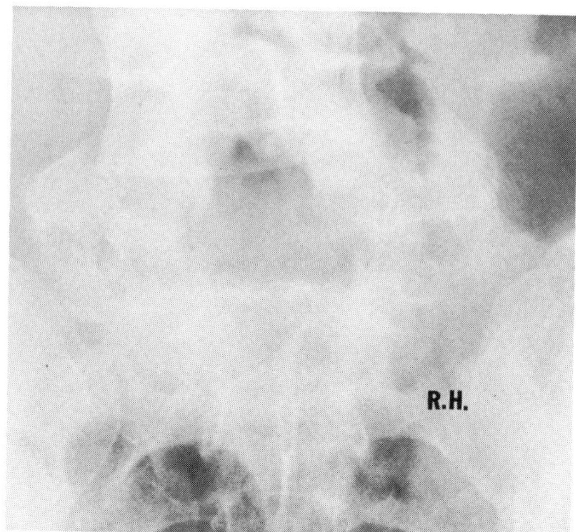

Figure 27–29. Anteroposterior roentgenogram of a successful, solid L5–S1 posterolateral fusion.

deficiency, including reflex, motor, and sensory changes, tight hamstrings, and gait abnormalities.[11, 30, 70, 85, 89, 92, 127, 130, 133] Others believe that decompression is rarely indicated and that neurologic improvement occurs by obtaining a solid fusion.[12, 13, 15, 56, 66, 79, 140] Wiltse and associates suggest that after successful posterolateral fusion, the pseudarthrosis mass at the pars spontaneously decreases in size, thus eventually decompressing the nearby root.

The only absolute indication for root decompression is in patients with bowel and bladder dysfunction, or a motor deficit that interferes with normal walking. In congenital spondylolisthesis with an intact arch, the L5 lamina slides forward and compresses the cauda against the posterosuperior corner of the body of S1. These cases can have severe hamstring tightness that may not resolve after in situ fusion alone and are at risk for a cauda equina syndrome. They should be addressed with decompression and reduction–fixation.

If decompression is performed, there is probably increased risk of slip progression and nonunion (see Fig. 27–28).[12, 52, 98, 125] Accordingly, immobilization with a cast or orthosis or segmental internal fixation should be considered. Amundson and McGuire have reported on a prospective, randomized study of spondylolisthesis patients with significant radiculopathy, treated with decompression, internal fixation and posterolateral fusion compared with decompression and fusion. Although the overall results were good, they could not demonstrate a statistically significant increase in the fusion rate by the addition of posterior plate and pedicle screw fixation.[2]

Decompression with In Situ Fusion for Spondyloptosis

Because of the difficulties in obtaining union without further progression when decompression is necessary in the presence of severe deformity, a number of procedures have been described involving an interbody in situ fusion through an anterior or posterior approach using fibula, tibia, iliac crest, or internal fixation, sometimes combined with anterior sacral decompression (Fig. 27–30).[11, 26, 32, 43, 64, 73, 132] The anterior procedures are then supplemented for the most part with posterior bilateral-lateral fusions. The complications of this approach are substantial and include graft dislodgement, sacral fracture, iliac vessel injury, injury to the presacral plexus, and a necessity for two, if not three, operative procedures.[13, 56]

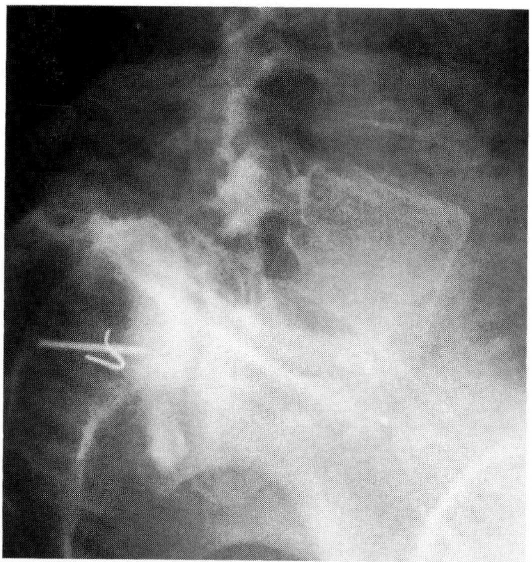

Figure 27–30. A 37-year-old male dancer developed increasing back and radiating leg pain, hamstring tightness and difficulty walking because of pain, deformity, and weakness. This lateral postoperative radiograph demonstrates erosion and beaking of S1. Myelography, CT, and MR scans showed no other evidence of disc abnormality. Because of the beaking and significant deformity, no attempt was made at reduction. A posterior laminectomy, nerve root exploration, and fusion were performed followed by anterior interbody fusion.

To reduce the need for two separate procedures, Bohlman and Cook have described a posterior approach that allows an interbody fusion with graft fixation of high-grade spondylolisthesis.[11] This requires laminectomy and careful retraction of the dura, L5, and S1 roots. A hole is drilled through the posterior aspect of the S1 body directed anteriorly into L5. A fibular dowel graft is then inserted across the L5–S1 disc space, without the necessity of operating anteriorly. A bilateral–lateral fusion is performed at the same time.

Shortcomings of In Situ Fusion

Some authors consider the results of in situ fusion to be highly satisfactory for all grades of adolescent spondylolisthesis without significant further slippage or nonunion.[55, 63, 91, 96, 97, 145] Most surgeons encounter a higher rate of pseudarthrosis, progression, and other problems than is considered acceptable for other spine reconstructive procedures, however, especially when treating older adolescents and adults.

Pseudarthrosis

It is noteworthy that large lumbosacral fusion studies that report union rates according to diagnosis cite a lower union rate for spondylolisthesis fusions (an average of 72 per cent) than other primary conditions (an average of 88 per cent).[25, 41, 119] Evaluation of spondylolisthesis series with over 50 cases treating primarily adults shows that the average union rate for in situ fusions using iliac crest autografts is 75 per cent.[12, 25, 54, 100] Series reporting posterolateral fusions with iliac crest autografting note a higher union rate (81 per cent) than those using only posterior fusions (75 per cent).[12, 13, 25, 54, 70, 98, 100, 125] The average union rate for Grade 3+ slips in adolescents is about the same as for Grade 1 slips in adults.[12, 13, 70, 100, 127] This information is particularly sobering in view of Bradford's observation that of ten symptomatic spondylolisthesis patients thought to have solid in situ fusion radiographically, seven actually had a pseudarthrosis at the time of surgical exploration.[17] Hence, when treating adolescents or adult patients with spondylolisthesis, the true union rate for primary posterolateral in situ fusions is probably in the range of 60 to 70 per cent. Many of the nonunions eventually cause mild to moderate pain.[12, 38, 49]

Loss of Motion Segments

Most in situ fusions for high-grade (III–IV) spondylolisthesis are from L4 to the sacrum, with extension occasionally to L2 or L3 for high-grade slips. Fusion across normal joints above the slip is recommended to improve union rates by placing the fusion mass in a more vertical orientation and providing more graft contact area; however, proximal extension of the fusion reduces lumbar motion segments and concentrates more load than necessary at the first open joint.

Further Slippage

Even when solid fusion is achieved for the unreduced spondylolisthetic deformity, it may fail to arrest slip progression. This is because the same anterior bending and shear forces that dissuade union in the first place persist even after successful fusion. Tension forces working against the graft can bend and elongate the immature fusion. Even when the fusion matures, the substantial flexion moment present in high-grade deformity may lead to fatigue failure of the posterior fusion mass and additional lumbosacral kyphosis.

Many studies of in situ fusion for spondylolisthesis acknowledge progression of deformity despite apparently solid arthrodesis.[12, 27, 52, 63, 70, 84, 89, 131] The reported incidence of slip progression varies from 11 to 72 per cent for an average reported incidence of 33 per cent.[12, 13, 27, 52, 70, 84, 89] The slip angle (LS kyphosis) tends to progress to a greater extent than L5–S1 displacement. For the one third of in situ fusion patients who progress, the average slip angle increase is reported at 15 to 20 degrees.[12, 13, 98]

Slip progression after in situ fusion is encouraged by Gill laminectomy, lack of postoperative immobilization, and a high initial slip angle.[27, 98] Although L5 laminectomy can increase the chance of slip progression, it can occur even when the L5 arch is left in place or when patients are kept supine for several months.[12, 13, 27, 52, 70, 89, 98, 131] Boxall and associates noted that 40 per cent of patients with a slip angle of more than 55 degrees progressed in the presence of an apparent solid arthrodesis.[13]

Dandy found that most progression occurs after the patient begins to ambulate, but within six months of surgery.[27] On the average, however, approximately 2 per cent additional translation and 1 to 2 degrees angulation occur per year for at least several years.[13, 27]

Neurologic Deficit

In situ fusion for adolescent patients with slips exceeding 50 per cent carries the risk of neurologic injury. Dandy reported minor motor or sensory deficits in 12 per cent of patients following posterolateral in situ fusions.[27] Despite using the Wiltse bilateral paraspinous muscle splitting approach, Maurice published results of three cases with postoperative development of a permanent cauda equina syndrome, including reduced perineal sensation and bowel or bladder dysfunction.[74] This serious complication occurs more frequently than once thought. In 1990 Schoenecker and associates identified 12 cases of cauda equina syndrome with loss of bowel and bladder control that developed after in situ fusion in adolescent patients with Grade 3 or 4 spondylolisthesis. Posterolateral fusion was performed through a bilateral paraspinous muscle splitting incision in four and through the midline in eight cases, without known dural injury. The cases were performed by six experienced spinal surgeons who reported a 6 per cent (12 of 189 cases) combined incidence of cauda equina syndrome complications after in situ fusion. Schoenecker and associates postulated that muscle relaxation after general anesthesia and surgical dissection led to additional slippage that stretched sacral roots over the posterosuperior corner of the sacrum. Patients most at risk were those with an initial slip angle of more than 45 degrees.[109]

Residual Deformity

Fusing a high-grade spondylolisthetic deformity in place may leave the patient with abnormal spinal mechanics and a tarnished self-image. Patients with more than 30 degrees of lumbosacral kyphosis must hold their thoracolumbar spine in maximal hyperextension to maintain sagittal balance. This causes muscle fatigue and can lead to facet changes and disc degeneration. Retrolisthesis is reported above the in situ fusion in 24 per cent of cases.[52] Late degenerative changes secondary to abnormal spine mechanics may account for much of the mild but continuous low back and thigh pain experienced by 30 per cent of patients after "successful" in situ fusion.[100, 107]

Wiltse and others have observed improvement in the cosmetic appearance of patients with high-grade slips after successful in situ fusion. This may be due to postarthrodesis relaxation of hamstring tightness, since spine alignment and trunk height are not addressed by in situ fusion. Although some patients will achieve adequate cosmetic improvement with in situ fusion, at this time it is unknown which patients will improve and to what extent.[63, 96]

Patients with higher degrees of lumbosacral kyphosis have the most unsightly appearance. They develop an abnormal waddling gait secondary to the vertical pelvis and hip and knee flexion, which are required for sagittal balance. The combination of protruding ribs from anterior translation and thoracolumbar hyperlordosis, loss of trunk height, flattened buttocks, and crouched stance are unsightly. Unfortunately, most high-grade spondylolisthetic deformities occur in adolescent girls who often find their appearance distressing (Fig. 27–31). Osterman and colleagues observed that despite solid union, eight out of ten girls in this series of in situ fusion for spondyloptosis considered their own result cosmetically poor.[89]

REDUCTION AND FIXATION

Most current reduction techniques use segmental pedicle screw fixation; hence, the advantages of reduction and segmental fixation will be discussed together. Since a procedure using reduction, fixation, and fusion involves more extensive surgery than in situ fusion alone, it must offer clear advantages to be worthy of consideration.

Potential Advantages

1. ***Stops progression of deformity.*** Internal fixation, preferably in a reduced position, eliminates the approximately one-third chance of progression seen despite successful in situ fusion. Reduction increases the likelihood that fixation will remain secure by diminishing the anterior bending forces working against the instrumentation.

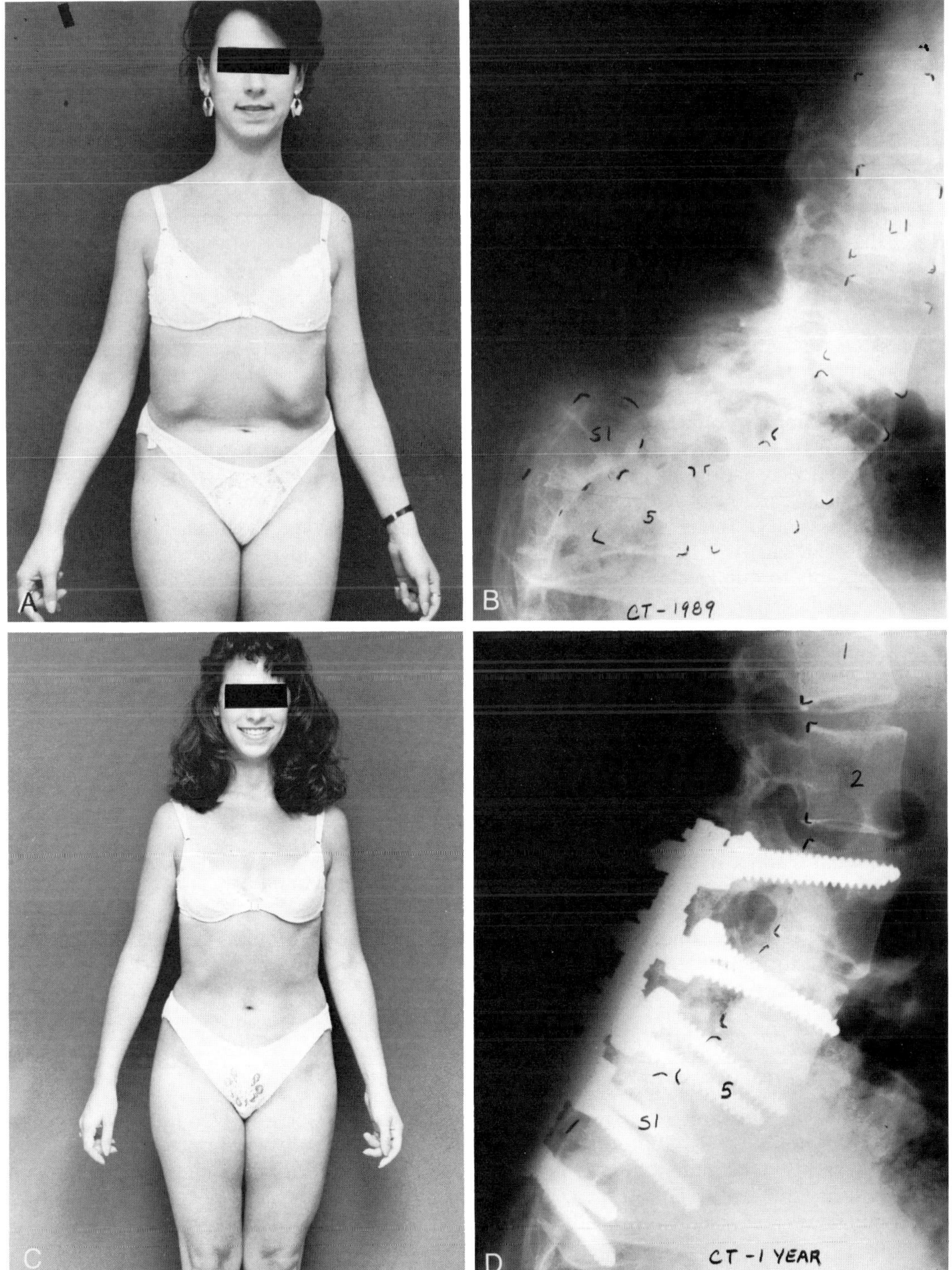

Figure 27–31. *A*, A 23-year-old female with spondyloptosis demonstrating loss of trunk height, protrusion of the rib cage with ribs resting on the iliac crests, lack of waistline, abdominal and flank folds, and hip flexion contracture. *B*, Preoperative standing lateral radiograph demonstrating severe spondyloptosis and compensatory panlumbar hyperlordosis. *C*, View taken one year after instrumented reduction of the deformity. Trunk height is restored with the appearance of a waistline and loss of abdominal folds. Sagittal spine alignment is corrected with elimination of rib cage prominence. *D*, Standing lateral radiograph one year after surgical reconstruction. Reduction was accomplished with the application of corrective forces using the Modular Spinal System; there was no need for disc resection or abdominal release. Disruption of the L3–L4 facets from a previous failed in situ fusion attempt made it necessary to extend instrumentation proximally to L3.

2. ***Lessens postoperative pain.*** Effective fixation blocks anterior shear at the unstable lumbosacral joint to greatly reduce the back pain associated with ambulation during the first weeks after spinal fusion. Edwards has observed that secure internal fixation lowers total analgesic consumption by more than 50 per cent of that required by patients without fixation.

3. ***Permits full nerve decompression.*** Although some authors advise against decompression for radiculopathy in anticipation of eventual remodeling after fusion, most investigators favor root decompression for prompt pain relief and optimum nerve recovery.[12, 13, 27, 28, 46, 52, 54, 70, 73, 79, 85, 92, 98, 101, 113, 118, 124] Root pain or deficit is present in up to 70 per cent of surgical candidates and is most often due to compression of the fifth lumbar root by the pars fibrocartilage.[13, 28, 46, 87] Internal fixation makes it possible to fully decompress all symptomatic L5 roots without fear of residual instability or progressive slippage.

Sacral radiculopathy is caused by stretching of the sacral roots over the posterosuperior corner of the sacrum as the lumbar spine slips forward. Loss of the Achilles reflex and other signs of compression of the first two sacral roots are reported in up to 29 per cent of patients requiring surgery for higher grade spondylolisthesis.[70] S2–S4 root compression, with bowel and bladder dysfunction, generally occurs only in patients with rapidly progressing high-grade slips. Spondylolisthesis reduction is theoretically the ideal treatment for sacral radiculopathy. Restoring the lumbar spine to its proper position over the sacrum relieves anterior pressure from the sacral roots, shortens their course, and hence relaxes the cauda equina.

4. ***Promotes union.*** Arthrodesis can be difficult to achieve in an unreduced spondylolisthesis for three reasons. Rotation of the lumbar spine around the sacrum shifts the body's central axis anterior to the lumbosacral graft. The resulting flexion moment subjects the graft to considerable tensile forces. The slip itself (anterior displacement) first decreases and then eliminates axial loading across the lumbosacral interspace; and without the buttressing effect of the L5 facets posteriorly or the sacral end plate inferiorly, the lumbosacral graft is subjected to considerable anteroinferior shear forces. Reduction addresses each of these biomechanical irregularities to increase the chance of successful union. Correction of the slip angle (kyphosis) restores the body's central axis over the sacrum to greatly reduce the bending moment and tensile stress working against the lumbosacral graft. Correcting the slip itself restores axial loading across the lumbosacral interspace. Pedicular fixation of the aligned spine will then eliminate shear.

5. ***Limits fusion length.*** When normal biomechanics are restored by correction of the deformity, it is possible to restrict instrumentation and fusion to the affected lumbosacral joint in most cases. Even for the most severe cases of spondyloptosis with L4–L5 joint pathology, or associated scoliosis, it is possible to limit the proximal extent of fusion to L4.

6. ***Restores body posture and mechanics.*** Full correction of the spondylolisthesis deformity (lumbosacral kyphosis, loss of height, and anterior translation) restores normal spine mechanics and body posture. Correction of lumbosacral kyphosis eliminates the need for patients to maintain maximum lumbar lordosis, pelvic tilt, or hip flexion for sagittal balance. This leads to spontaneous correction of compensatory lumbar and thoracolumbar lordosis, reduction in muscle fatigue, and a more efficient gait.[19] Restoration of trunk height improves the length-tension relationship of paraspinous and abdominal muscles for more effective spinal function.[43]

7. ***Improves appearance and self-image.*** We agree with DeWald's and Bradford's findings, that many adolescents with high-grade spondylolisthetic deformities are disturbed by their abnormal posture, proportions, body contours, and gait.[19, 30] This results in a poor self-image and perhaps personality disorders. Full reduction of the spondylolisthetic deformity can dramatically improve the patient's self-image. Correction of lumbosacral kyphosis eliminates the crouched posture, waddling gait, and protruding rib cage, and improves buttock contour. Restoration of trunk height eliminates abdominal folds and restores normal waist contours and body proportions. Patients with major preoperative deformity emerge several inches taller and more attractive (Fig. 27–31). Adolescent girls in particular become happier, more outgoing, and generally have more positive family and peer relationships.

The theoretic advantages of spondylolisthesis reduction–fixation are substantial, but two questions remain. Can full reduction be accomplished for most patients? If so, can it be achieved without excessive risk and morbidity, relative to in situ fusion?

Development of a Reduction Capability

Traction–Cast Reduction

The history of reduction of spondylolisthetic deformities began with Richard Scherb, a German surgeon. In 1921 he reported successful reduction of spondylolisthesis in a remarkably flexible 14-year-old girl that was maintained with a panlumbar tibial graft at one year follow-up.[108] Jenkins was the first to actually describe a reduction technique. In 1936 he reduced an adolescent boy with longitudinal traction and a pelvic sling. Interbody fusion with a tibial dowel maintained reduction for more than a year, but it ultimately failed.[62, 77]

In 1951 Harris renewed interest in spondylolisthesis reduction with a preoperative traction technique that combined longitudinal femoral pin traction with anterior traction through anterior iliac crest tongs to flex and translate the sacrum. After performing a posterolateral fusion, he resumed traction in his patient and then incorporated the tongs in a pantaloon cast for three months.[53] Lance first used Steinman pins rather than tongs for improved iliac fixation.[56] Early reports suggest that although traction–cast reduction was occasionally achieved in children, it was rarely maintained during graft consolidation and it sometimes was associated with major neurologic complications.[56, 84, 123]

Two reports in 1976 reactivated some interest in closed-reduction techniques for spondylolisthesis. Scaglietti emphasized the importance of longitudinal traction with hips in maximal extension to flex the pelvis, and thus counteract lumbosacral kyphosis. He placed the patient in an extension double pantaloon Minerva cast with traction maintained on a fracture table. While the plaster hardened, he pushed against the sacrum to achieve additional sacral flexion and improve lumbosacral alignment. Despite four months of preoperative traction-casting and ten months of postoperative cast protection, Scaglietti achieved only about 50 per cent correction; thus, he abandoned the technique in favor of internal fixation.[107] In the same year, Snijder and associates, and later others, reported that preoperative traction was unnecessary.[13, 77, 116] Snijder and associates also reported the successful use of posterior traction wires from the lumbar lamina to an outrigger worn on the patient's back to help maintain reduction during graft consolidation.[116] Ohki and associates combined intraoperative halo-femoral traction with Snijder's spinous process wiring technique.[88]

Despite these attempts, most reports on traction–cast reduction of spondylolisthesis remained negative. It never enjoyed widespread usage because of three concerns. First, neurologic deficit—several authors reported motor deficits in up to one third or more of patients while in traction before or after posterior surgery.[17, 18, 77] Second, unpredictable reduction results—most investigators found traction–cast reductions unpredictable since they relied on the flexibility of the deformity.[73] They generally failed to achieve or maintain satisfactory correction.[13, 40, 73, 84, 107, 113, 123] Third, discomfort and immobility—months of confinement in an extension pantaloon cast, usually in bed, was difficult for the children and their families.

Both Bradford and associates and Garfin and Heller achieved acceptable results with closed reduction by limiting the technique to young patients with intermediate deformity and by synthesizing the most effective elements of previous techniques (Figs. 27–32, 27–33, 27–34).[18, 45] Details of their techniques and results are discussed later under Current Options.

Posterior Distraction Instrumentation

In 1967 Paul Harrington was the first to use *internal* traction for reduction of spondylolisthesis. He placed distraction rods between the lamina of L1 and a transiliac "sacral" bar in a 13-year-old girl. By distracting the spine he was able to correct much of the slippage by ligamentotaxis. After a Gill laminectomy and lateral fusion, the patient was treated in a bilateral spica cast.[50] The use of distraction instrumentation was rapidly embraced by Vidal, Scaglietti, DeWald and others.[30, 107, 133] Scaglietti modified the surgical construct with alar hooks rather than a transiliac rod for distal fixation.[107] Unfortunately the rods tended to rotate into flexion about their single-point of distal hook fixation on the sacrum or the iliac

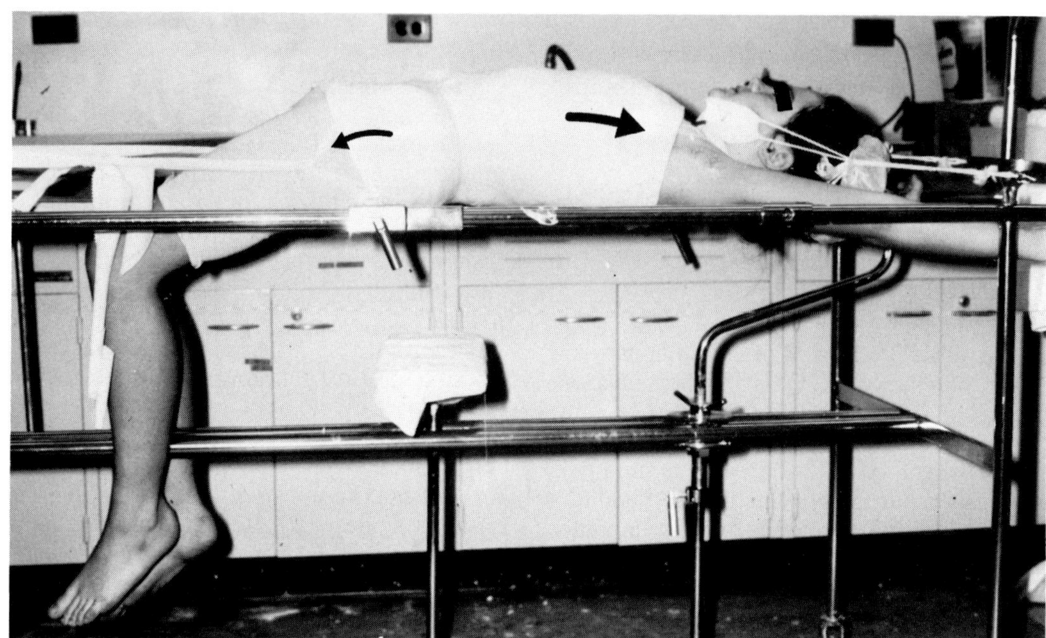

Figure 27–32. Cast reduction of spondylolisthesis. The patient is placed on the cast frame in the supine position. An elongation force is applied to the trunk *(thick arrow)*. The lower extremities hang free or with slight support, hyperextending the hips and allowing the pelvis to pivot *(thin arrow)* on a crossbar. The hip capsule and musculature pulls the pelvis forward, rotating the sacrum beneath L5 to approximate the normal sacral angle. Reduction may be further increased by positioning a localizer against the sacrum. The trunk portion of the cast is completed and molded carefully to maintain the reduction. The lower extremities are returned to a more comfortable position, and the bilateral pantaloon portion is completed.

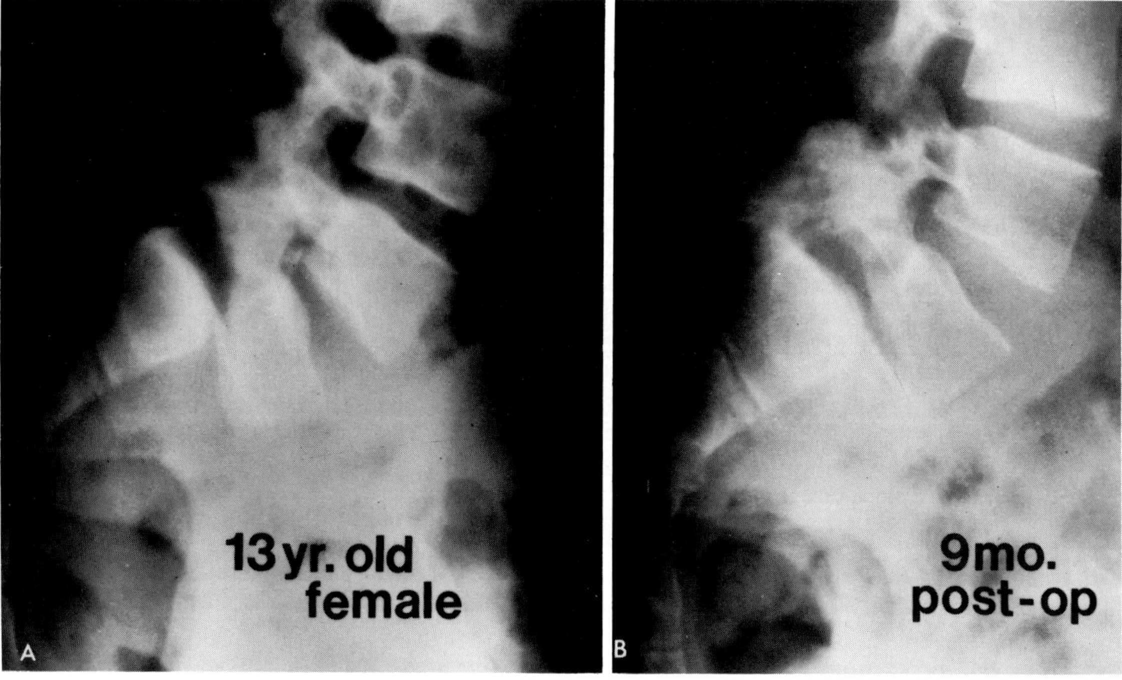

Figure 27–33. A 13-year-old female with isthmic spondylolisthesis (Type II). *A*, Roentgenographic appearance of the spine before surgical stabilization. Note the degree of tangential subluxation and angle of tilt. *B*, Roentgenographic appearance nine months after bilateral-lateral column fusion and cast reduction. There is a slight improvement in "tangential" slip, significant improvement in "angle of tilt," and clinically an excellent improvement in appearance.

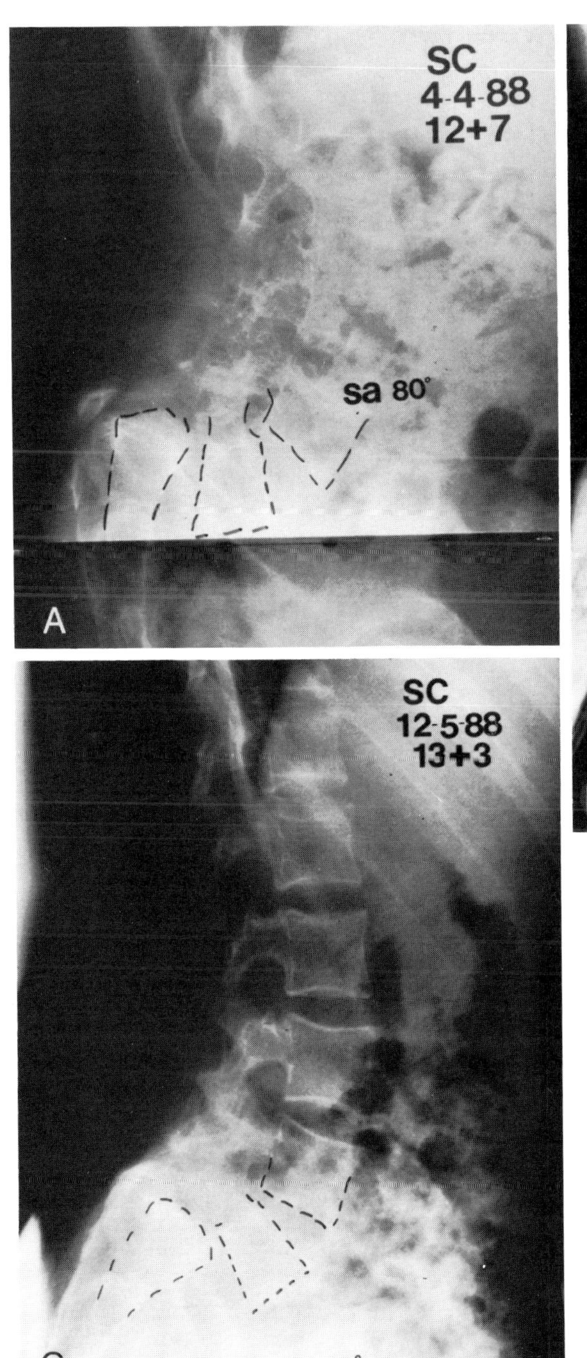

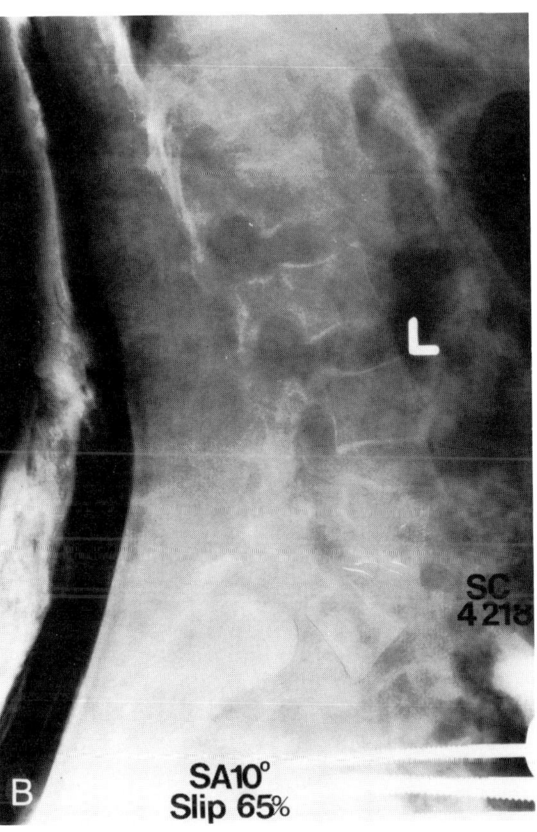

Figure 27–34. *A*, Standing lateral radiograph of a 12-year-old female with progressive and flexible spondyloptosis. *B*, Lateral radiograph after posterior surgery and traction-cast reduction with iliac pins-in-plaster to maintain sacral flexion and reduction of lumbosacral kyphosis. *C*, Lateral radiograph after cast removal. The slip angle has improved from 80 degrees preoperatively to 30 degrees. (Courtesy of David S. Bradford, M.D.)

rod. Resulting progressive loss of reduction was noted by Harrington and other early investigators.[13, 51, 107] In an effort to prevent forward rotation and slippage, Harrington and Vidal bolstered the anterior column with an interbody fusion from the posterior approach and Scaglietti performed a second-stage interbody fusion from the anterior approach.[51, 107, 133]

Reduction results from distraction instrumentation alone were generally unsatisfactory. Final correction of 50 to 60 per cent of the original slip was possible, but there was no improvement in the slip angle or degree of abnormal vertical sacral inclination (L-S kyphosis).[17, 51, 107] Moreover, most of these panlumbar distraction rod fusions caused considerable flattening of normal lumbar lordosis, a major problem for patients with spondylolisthesis, who required lumbar hyperlordosis to maintain sagittal balance.

During the late 1970s efforts were made to reduce the length of the lumbar fusion. Some used long rods but fused only L4–S1, with subsequent rod removal.[13] Others used much shorter rods extending from L3 or L4 to the sacrum.[65, 133, 134] Alignment results were still unsatisfactory. In the largest current series using distraction rods, Kaneda presented 39 cases in which the amount of slippage was corrected from only 26 to 21 per cent, but with a 7-degree *worsening* of the slip angle.[65]

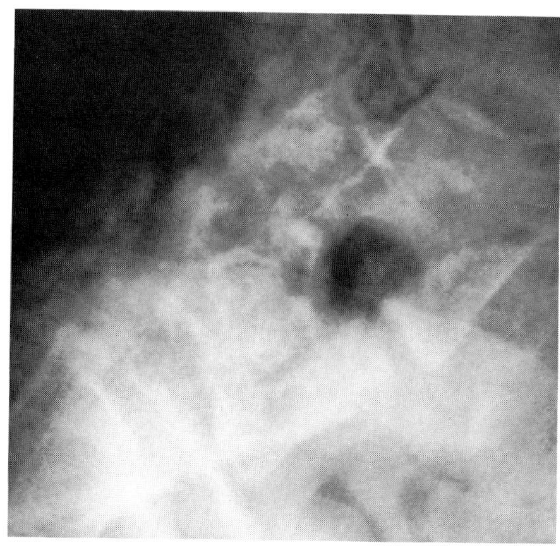

Figure 27–35. Grade IV spondylolisthesis reduced by posterior instrumentation and fusion. Because of a persistent infection, despite multiple debridements, the instrumentation was removed. When the infection cleared an anterior interbody fusion was performed. A graft across L5 into the sacrum can be seen in this lateral radiograph.

Anteroposterior Resection–Reductions

With the limitations of closed reduction techniques and the liabilities of posterior distraction rods, surgeons turned to more extensive operations in the quest for a more effective reduction capability. Combined procedures for spondylolisthesis reduction were first described in 1956 by Denecke (Fig. 27–35).[29] He resected the inferior L5 body anteriorly and sacral dome posteriorly to shorten the spine. From the posterior approach he then inserted a reduction instrument between L5 and S1 to lever L5 back in place on the sacrum. Axial Steinmann pins were used to hold the reduction.

In 1973 DeWald undertook staged anterior and posterior surgery for adolescents with Grades 3 and 4 slips. He began with posterior laminectomy with or without sacral dome resection, posterolateral grafting, and reduction of the deformity by distracting with long Harrington rods, while manually extending the pelvis during surgery. The second stage consisted of anterior discectomy, further reduction, and interbody fusion with large iliac wedge grafts. Patients had three months of bed rest in a pantaloon cast and a third operation for rod removal. He obtained excellent slip correction (86 per cent) and moderate improvement in lumbosacral kyphosis.[30]

In 1979 both McPhee and O'Brien and Bradford reported multistage surgery for correction of Grades 3 and 4 slips without the use of distraction instrumentation.[14, 72] They began with posterior laminectomy and fusion followed by two to three weeks of halofemoral traction in extension. Bradford then obtained additional correction by using an anterior lever between L5 and S1 followed by placement of a dowel graft.[14] McPhee and O'Brien maintained fixation with an anterior screw.[77] Patients were then treated in a bilateral spica extension cast for four months in bed. In a subsequent report Bradford added a third-stage procedure to place posterior Harrington compression or Luque rods for fixation.[17] In 1988 Dick and Schnekel described a four-stage reduction sequence. They began with percutaneous pedicle screws for preliminary distraction, followed by anterior discectomy and grafting. During the third stage they applied an internal fixator and manually reduced the deformity by pulling back, then angulating L4 and S1 screws into lordosis. Patients were ambulated in a brace, but fixator removal was required at one year.

Six major studies have reported the results using the anterior and posterior techniques outlined above.[14, 17, 32, 77, 87, 106] All were essentially confined to adolescents with Grade 3 or 4 slips. Correction of translation (slip) averaged approximately 45 per cent in two series and up to 73 per cent for the others.[14, 17, 32, 77, 87, 106] Correction of lumbosacral kyphosis ranged from 20 degrees to 63-degree improvement in Bradford's most recent series.[17, 32, 106] The complication rate for multistage resection–reduction methods is high with an approximate 30 per cent incidence of neurologic deficit and a 10 to 20 per cent incidence of dislodgement and nonunions.[14, 17, 30, 32] In summary, these series documented substantial reduction for adolescents with spondylolisthesis; however, the clinical indications for resection–reduction are limited by the amount of surgery required, the frequency of complications, and the length of recumbency.

Vertebrectomy

In an effort to improve spinal alignment for patients with true spondyloptosis, a few surgeons have extended the concept of spine shortening to include resection of the entire fifth vertebra. This relaxes surrounding soft tissues and the cauda equina to facilitate reduction and minimize stretch radiculopathy. Gaines and Nichols provided the first description of this procedure in the English literature.[43] They began with anterior resection of the fifth vertebral body. They then removed the posterior elements of L5, and reduced the slip with the aid of Harrington distraction instrumentation between L2 and the ala. They performed an L4-to-sacrum lateral fusion and stabilized the reduction with Harrington compression rods attached from over the lamina of L4 to the first sacral foramina. Their patients were placed at bed rest in a spica cast for five months. Other surgeons have reported five additional cases using this procedure.[17, 20, 60]

Results published to date suggest that L5 vertebrectomy achieves full correction of spine alignment and the slip angle, with moderate correction of the slip from a spondyloptosis to a Grade 1 or 2 anterolisthesis.[17, 20, 60] On the other hand, complications are substantial. Two of seven patients developed residual weakness of L5 innervated muscles and two required additional surgery to repair delayed unions or nonunions.[17, 34, 43] Because of its risk and magnitude, vertebrectomy is now typically reserved for selected spondyloptosis patients with fixed deformities for whom less extensive procedures offer little chance of success.[19]

Pedicle Fixation

The advent of pedicle screw fixation addressed many shortcomings of previous techniques. In 1967 Harrington and others wired L5 pedicle screws to distraction rods to help limit postoperative loss of correction at the completion of reduction.[50, 133, 147] The screws provided little advantage and were soon discontinued, however.[51] Later it was shown that with only one level of sacral fixation, the rods rotate into flexion about this axis of distal fixation with loss of translational correction.[35]

Louis and other Europeans added pedicle fixation to the anteroposterior resection reduction methods to maintain correction and permit early ambulation.[71] Louis resected the anterior disc and reduced the deformity by traction, extension, and by levering L5 on S1; he held open the disc space with fibular struts and blocked translation with an axial fibular dowel or screw across the bodies of L5 and S1. Posteriorly he used an L5–S1 plate and cancellous screws as a tension band to work in conjunction with the anterior graft for stable fixation. He reported 189 Grades 1 to 3 slips with excellent correction of both the slip and kyphosis, and permanent neurologic deficit in only 6 per cent of his cases. Dick also used pedicle fixation as part of a multistage reduction method for higher Grades 3 and 4 slips.[31] He obtained approximately 60 per cent correction of the slip and kyphosis, but had a 20 per cent incidence of residual neurologic deficit.[32]

A third group of surgeons began using pedicle screws to apply *active* posterior translation for low to moderate grade slips. This was made possible by a screw-bolt described by Matthiass and Heine in 1973.[73] The screw-bolt was threaded into L5. A slotted plate was placed over the bolt portion. By tightening a nut over the plate it was possible to pull L5 posteriorly along the sacrum. Active posterior translation with plates and screw bolts was popularized by

Roy-Camille and associates.[103] After posterior release, they used fracture table traction, pelvic extension, distraction forceps, and a plate with L4 and L5 threaded bolts to obtain approximately 55 per cent slip correction in 11 of 12 patients with primarily Grade 3 slips. Their permanent L5 deficit rate was 9 per cent. Sijbrandji combined posterior disc resection, distraction with Harrington rods, and posterior translation with screw-bolts for reduction followed by interbody fusion and tension-band L5–S1 plate fixation in a one-stage posterior procedure.[113, 147] He reported on only three patients using this technique, but achieved over 80 per cent correction of both slip and slip angle.

Posterior Levered Reduction

Since moderate L5–S1 slips are always associated with varying degrees of forward tilt (kyphosis) and loss of height, it became clear that posterior translation from plates and screws alone was often inadequate to correct the spondylolisthesis deformity. To gain the necessary height and lordosis, some used traction and fracture table positioning during surgery; others used temporary distraction rods, and another group of surgeons used manual leverage to achieve height and lordosis.[8, 75, 103, 113] In 1973 Schollner developed and Matthiass published the posterior leverage method employed by many surgeons today using variable screw placement (VSP) (Steffee) slotted plates.[73, 110] Posterior levered reduction is a single-stage operation with five surgical steps: mobilization of the dura with discectomy with sacral dome resection when necessary for shortening;[116] the application of distraction by manually raising L5 with a lever placed in the L5–S1 disc space; posterior translation by shortening a screw bolt on a slotted plate; posterior lumbar interbody fusion (PLIF) for anterior support combined with a posterolateral fusion;[51] and pedicle screw fixation to allow early patient ambulation. The slotted plate employed by Schnoller and Matthiass was affixed to the sacrum by distal flanges that fit into the dorsal foramina of S2.[73, 110] They used a Cobb elevator in the disc space to raise L5 and recommended monitoring nerve conduction during reduction. Matthiass reported on 48 adolescents with lumbosacral spondylolisthesis treated with posterior levered reduction. He obtained good correction of deformity in 47, but one third experienced postoperative neurologic deficits, most of which resolved.[73]

Steffee recently reported results of 14 patients with Grade 3 and 4 slips treated with the Schnollner-Matthiass technique. To gain height he levered a "persuader" within the L5–S1 disc space. For posterior translation, he used screw-bolts in conjunction with his VSP slotted plate. The plates were then contoured for lordosis and reapplied with pedicle screws for fixation. In agreement with Matthiass, Steffee stressed the importance of using a PLIF for anterior support (Fig. 27–36). Good reduction was maintained in 11 patients with both interbody and lateral fusions; however, the three patients *without* interbody fusion lost reduction.[120]

Gradual Instrumented Reduction

The concept of gradual instrumented reduction for spondylolisthesis was developed by Edwards and fellow members of the Spinal Fixation Study Group during the mid 1980s. The goal was to achieve *full* correction of the spondylolisthesis deformity with *less* surgery and morbidity than alternative methods. Four concepts were combined to accomplish this goal: the simultaneous application of three corrective forces; two-point sacral fixation; viscoelastic stress relaxation; and restoration of full anatomic alignment to obviate the need for interbody grafting.

Three Corrective Forces. Since the spondylolisthesis deformity results from anterior slippage, loss of height, and lumbosacral kyphosis, it was postulated that full reduction might be possible by simultaneously applying the opposite forces of distraction, posterior translation of the lumbar spine, and sacral flexion (lordosis).[35] To simultaneously apply the three corrective forces, it is necessary to use instrumentation with three-dimensional adjustability. A modular spinal system that includes finely ratcheted rods for initial distraction and adjustable connectors between the rods and pedicle screws to effect posterior translation of the lumbar spine and flexion of the sacrum is used.

Two-Point Sacral Fixation. To provide lumbosacral *lordosis*, it is necessary to extend the lumbar spine and flex the sacrum. To maximize the necessary rotational force (extension moment) to accomplish this, two-point fixation on

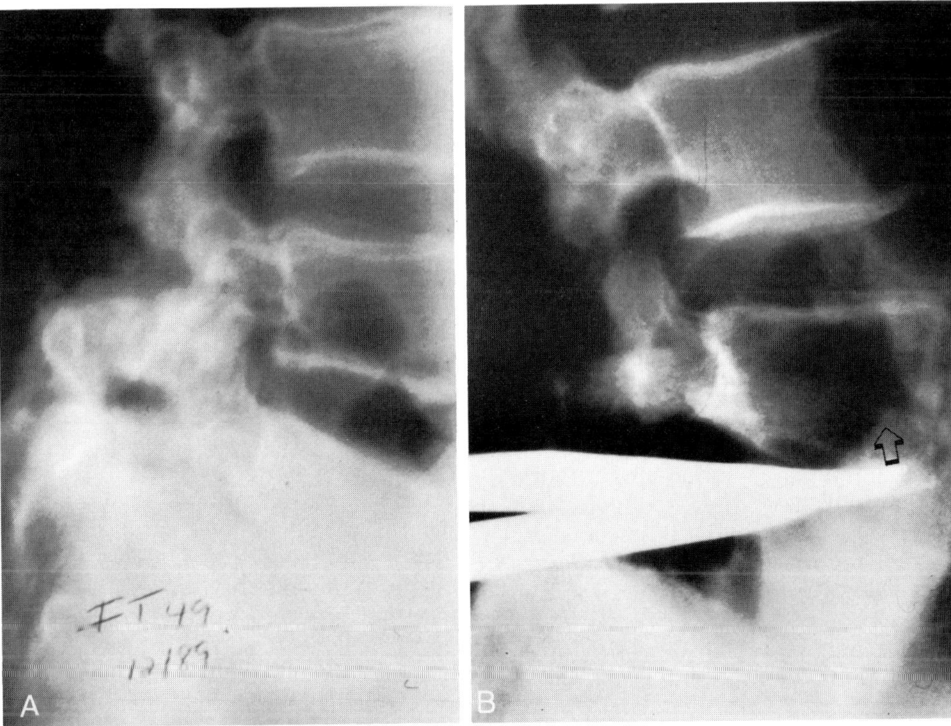

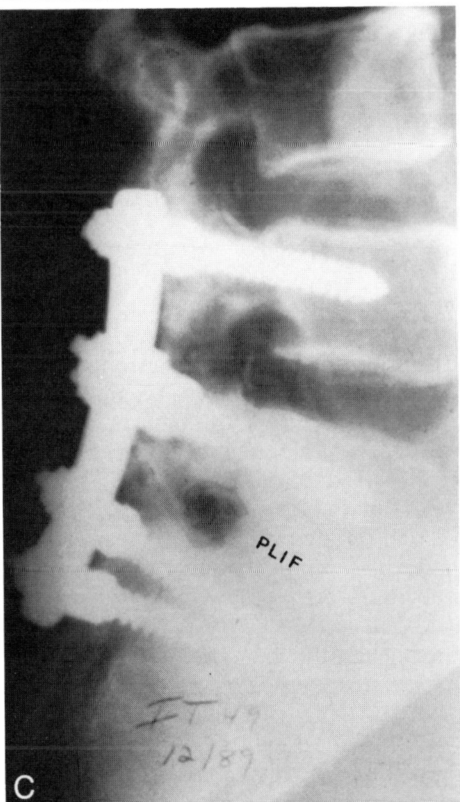

Figure 27–36. *A*, Lateral radiograph of an adult with symptomatic Grade III spondylolisthesis. *B*, Intraoperative radiograph with "persuader" between L5 and the sacrum to restore height before application of plates and screw bolts for reduction of the translational slip. *C*, Lateral postoperative radiograph with variable screw placement (VSP) plates to maintain reduction and posterior lumbar interbody fusion (PLIF) for anterior column support. (Courtesy of Arthur Steffee, M.D.)

the sacrum is required. Accordingly, considerably better maintenance of spondylolisthesis reduction is achieved with screw fixation at both S1 and S2, rather than alone.[35]

Stress Relaxation. To lessen the magnitude of surgery and risk of neurovascular injury, viscoelastic stress–relaxation is employed and manual manipulations are avoided. As symbolized by the crooked tree of Nicholas Andre, the use of corrective forces over time to reduce deformity is a long-standing principle of orthopedics. The earliest traction–cast techniques for reducing spondylolisthesis made use of tissue creep. DeWald and others have recognized the advisability of *gradually* correcting the spondylolisthesis deformity at surgery.[30, 52, 73, 107, 113] It was not known to what *extent* stress–relaxation could be employed at surgery until Edwards reported that even spondylo*ptosis* could be fully reduced in both adolescents *and* adults by applying the three corrective forces over several hours without the need for disc section or anterior release (see Fig. 27–31).[39] Hence, by continuously replenishing the forces of distraction, posterior translation, and sacral flexion, contracted anterior structures gradually lengthen until they return to their original dimensions, resulting in *full* correction of most spondylolisthetic deformities (Fig. 27–37).

Anatomic Alignment. Restoration of normal alignment appears to eliminate the need for anterior grafting. With anatomic alignment, anterior bending forces at the lumbosacral junction are reduced and grafts are not subjected to excessive tensile stress. As a result, lateral fusions can be expected to unite and strengthen with time. Hence, it does not appear necessary to routinely resect the disc and place interbody grafts anterior to the dura.

To test this reduction hypothesis, Edwards conducted a prospective study of 25 consecutive patients. All were treated with a single-stage posterior procedure using corrective forces alone, without discectomy or discotomy, followed by early ambulation in a brace. The procedure maintained 91 per cent slip correction and 88 per cent correction of lumbosacral kyphosis in addition to restoration of normal trunk height. Two patients with spondyloptosis had transient root deficits, but patients with Grade 2 to 4 slips remained completely free of neurologic complications.[37] Successful use of this method has also been reported by Bradford, and West and Bradford.[19, 136] The detailed results of 180 cases documented by members of the Spinal Fixation Study Group will be discussed later in this chapter.

Indications for Reduction–Fixation

Until recently the magnitude and morbidity of the multistage operations required for reduction of most spondylolisthetic deformities inspired restrictive indications for reduction. With the increased advantages associated with *anatomic* alignment and the reduced risk associated with gradual instrumented reduction, however, the indications for spondylolisthesis reduction–fixation are beginning to broaden. Indeed our recent experience and current data from the Spinal Fixation Study Group, indicate that the likelihood of complications from reduction and fixation of Grades 1 to 4 spondylolisthesis in experienced hands is no more than that reported in comparable series from in situ fusion. It should be noted, however, that the difficulty and complication rate for correcting high-grade spondyloptosis is considerable. Accordingly, our discussion of indications will focus on spondylolisthesis and borderline spondyloptosis. We still consider the reduction of higher grade spondyloptosis to be an investigational procedure.

Prerequisites for Reduction

Safe and effective correction of spondylolisthesis is greatly facilitated by lumbosacral mobility and adequate bone stock and complicated by L5–S1 autofusion or surgical arthrodesis. Hence, if preoperative flexion/extension or standing/supine films show no L5–S1 motion, and tomograms or CT suggest arthrodesis, we are reticent to advise attempted reduction.

Adequate bone stock is necessary for instrumented reduction. Since these procedures rely on pedicle screw fixation, the patient's vertebrae must be large enough to accommodate available screw sizes. A preoperative CT scan can be helpful in making this determination. In patients below the age of 10, vertebrae are often too small for pedicle screw reduction–fixation. Good screw purchase requires adequate bone quality. Accordingly, elderly patients or those with severe osteoporosis are poor candidates for reduction techniques.

INSTRUMENTED REDUCTION

EDWARDS' METHOD

GRADUAL APPLICATION OF:

- Distraction
- Posterior translation
- Sacral flexion

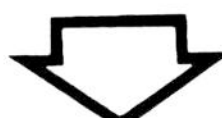

COLLAGEN STRESS-RELAXATION

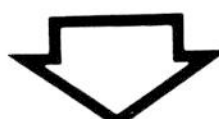

REDUCTION

A *without anterior release*

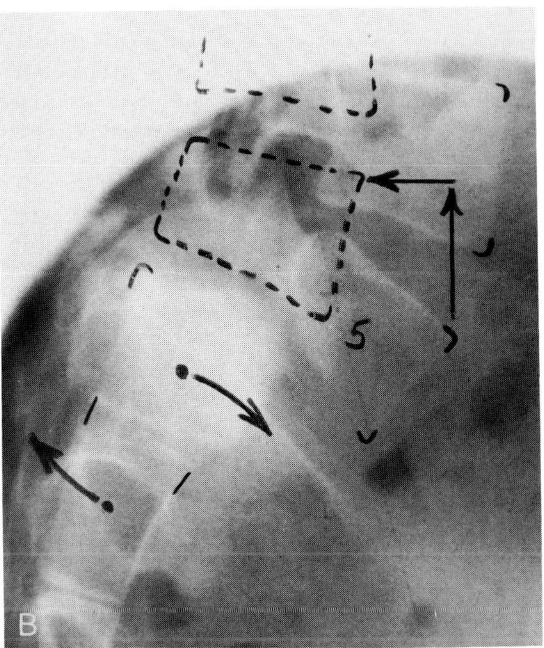

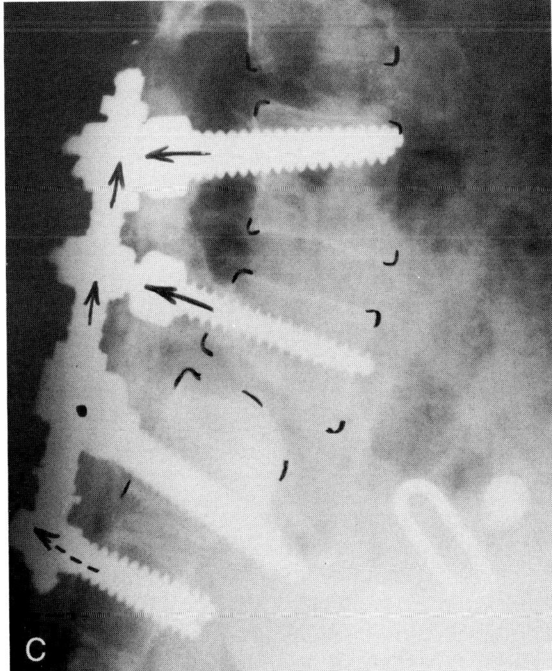

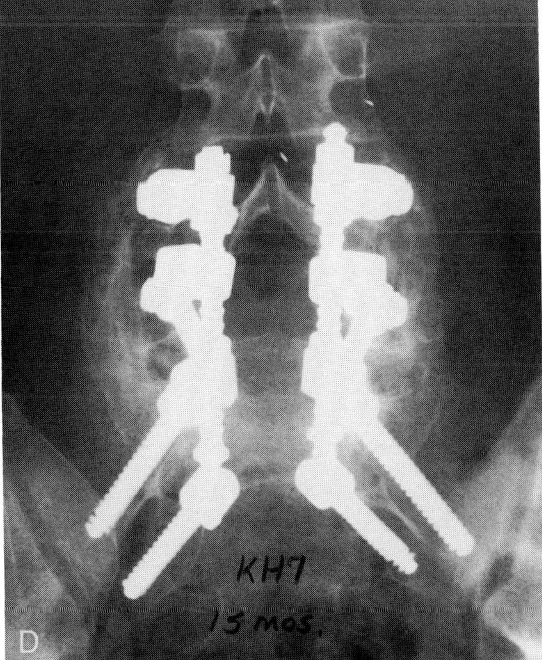

Figure 27–37. *A*, Edwards' method. *B*, Lateral radiograph demonstrating typical Grade IV spondylolisthesis with loss of height, anterior translation, and lumbosacral kyphosis. The opposite corrective forces of (1) distraction, (2) posterior translation, and (3) sacral flexion are indicated by vector arrows and required for reduction. *C*, Postreduction radiograph of the patient in *B* after application of the three corrective forces. Neither disc section nor anterior release was required. *D*, Anteroposterior radiograph 15 months after surgery. The patient proceeded to painless union without neurologic deficit or other complications.

Indications for Reduction

Reduction is indicated where the advantages of reduction are greater and the risk of failure less than in situ fusion with or without root decompression. If the surgeon is well trained in current reduction methods, available data support the following indications:

Cauda Equina Syndrome. Sacral root stretch causing loss of normal bowel and bladder control and/or plantar flexion weakness in the lower extremities is best treated with reduction. Since the sacral roots are tented over the posterior corner of the sacral end plate, restoring canal alignment relaxes the cauda equina and relieves anterior pressure on the sacral roots.

Progressive Slip Surpassing 40 to 50 Per Cent. Laurent correlated age with degree of slip and concluded that a slip of more than 30 degrees in a young person tends to progress.[70] It is well known that most progression occurs in late childhood and early adolescence.[13, 27, 55, 65] Hence, when documented progression surpasses 40 per cent in the child, we recommend reduction–fixation–fusion. As the slip progresses to 50 per cent, the surface contact between the lumbar spine and sacrum is only 38 per cent of normal and then rapidly diminishes with further slip progression.[115] More than 50 per cent slip in the adult suggests unusual instability and a greater likelihood for nonunion, progression, or even cauda equina syndrome after in situ fusion. In these cases the risk of deficit may be greater after in situ fusion than after reduction–fixation with current methods.[37]

Major Deformity Causing Decompensation or Distress. We agree with Bradford that the clinical consequences of major deformity are often great enough to warrant the risk of complications encountered when reducing higher grade spondylolisthesis.[19] Hence, reduction can be indicated for severe deformities with either loss of sagittal compensation or major negative psychologic impact. Restoration of anatomic alignment for these patients can dramatically improve their spinal mechanics, appearance, and self-image.

Major Pain or Deficit Plus Two or More Risk Factors. The likelihood of surgical failure or complications arising from in situ fusion appears to be increased by the eight factors listed below. Conversely, several of these factors simplify reduction and decrease its risks. Therefore it seems reasonable to offer surgical candidates the advantages of reduction when two or more of the risk factors listed below are present.

Risk Factors

The risk factors known to increase the tendency for pseudoarthrosis, slip progression, neurologic deficit, or late symptoms from abnormal spine mechanics after in situ fusion include:

1. *Lumbosacral kyphosis or slip angle greater than 25 degrees.* The slip angle (lumbosacral kyphosis) is measured from the perpendicular to the line describing the posterior cortex of the proximal sacral bodies and either the superior or inferior end plate of L5. In the normal spine there are 5 or more degrees of lordosis at the lumbosacral junction; hence, 25 degrees of kyphosis represents a 30-degree deformity.

2. *Trapezoidal L5.* Trapezoidal deformity (wedging) of the fifth vertebral body may be considered an independent risk factor when the posterior vertebral body height is less than 75 per cent of anterior vertebral body height. Bosworth and associates found that slip progression was proportional to the amount of L5 wedging.[12] During their study, patients with minor wedging slipped 9.5 per cent; those with a 25 per cent difference in anterior versus posterior body height slipped 21 per cent.

3. *Rounded sacral end plate.* Patients with obliteration or rounding of the anterior aspect of the first sacral end plate tend to have progressive slipping.[13, 70, 115, 123] This is probably because the rounded sacral dome provides little support for the anterior column of the lumbar spine. In contrast, patients who form a large sacral beak (osteophyte) anteriorly are less likely to progress (Figs. 27–30 and 27–38).

4. *Hyperlordosis exceeding 50 degrees L2–S1.* Lumbar hyperlordosis increases the vertical inclination of the first sacral end plate. This causes increased vertical shear that most likely delays arthrodesis and promotes further slippage with possible neurologic sequelae.[13]

5. *L5 radiculopathy requiring decompression.* Several investigators have observed an increased rate of pseudarthrosis or nonunion after L5 laminectomy and root decompression.[12, 19, 25] Nevertheless many spondylolisthesis patients coming to surgery have L5 pain or weakness. Full decompression at the time of

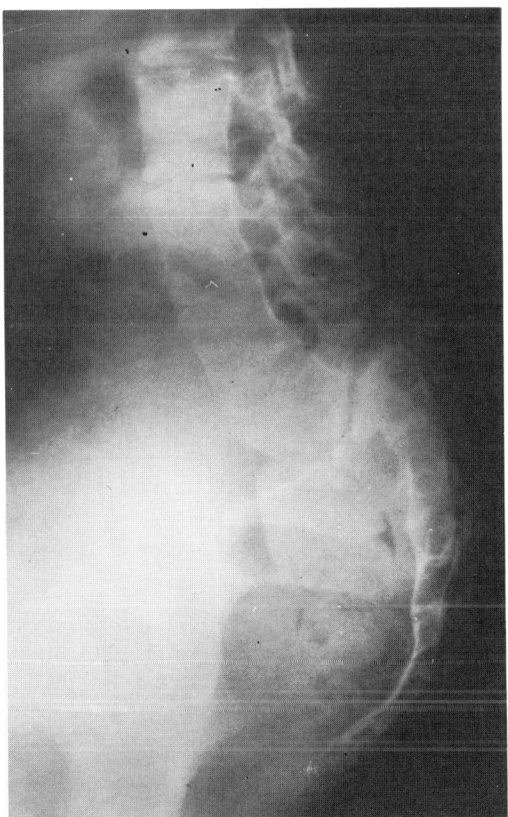

Figure 27–38. In this situation the forward slide of the fifth lumbar body has been slowed by the sclerotic reaction between L5 and the sacrum. The sclerotic buttress forming on the anterior lip of the sacrum is a defensive measure to resist progression of the spondylolisthesis.

surgery is highly desirable, since it can fully relieve their radicular pain and speed root recovery.[13, 27, 28, 46, 54, 70, 73, 79, 85, 92, 101, 113, 118]

6. *Female adolescents with over 40 per cent slips.* Young girls are most likely to slip further and also attach more importance to the cosmetic advantages of reduction than other patient groups. Most progression of deformity occurs during adolescence.[13, 27, 70] During Bosworth's study, girls slipped 25 per cent and boys only 14 per cent.[12] Ostermann studied 87 adolescents with severe slips; he noted that the ten most severe deformities in his series all occurred in girls.[89]

7. *Excess lumbosacral mobility.* Significant slippage is usually associated with disc space narrowing and reduced lumbosacral motion. Thus, more than 3 mm of translation or 10 degrees of angulation between flexion/extension or standing/supine radiographs may represent unusual mobility for a patient with spondylolisthesis. These numbers are only approximate guidelines, since specific correlative studies have not been completed. Nevertheless it is important to assess L5–S1 motion since excess lumbosacral mobility tends to shift the risk-benefit ratio balance toward reduction–fixation. The mobile spine is more difficult to fuse in situ without progression or nonunion, but easier and less risky to reduce than more fixed deformities.

8. *Signs of sacral root stretch.* Schoenecker and associates believed that sacral root signs may be a precursor to the most serious complication of in situ fusion: the cauda equina syndrome.[109] They documented that two thirds of their 12 cases of cauda equina syndrome complicating in situ fusion had at least subtle signs of sacral root dysfunction before surgery. The following findings may indicate early sacral root stretch: a strongly positive Lasègue sign,[70] decreased Achilles reflex, or subtle bowel and bladder dysfunction.

CURRENT METHODS OF SPONDYLOLISTHESIS REDUCTION

When reduction, fixation, and fusion are indicated, the surgeon must select the method offering the greatest potential advantage with the least morbidity for each case. After surveying results from the numerous methods reported for reduction of spondylolisthesis, the authors have identified three techniques that appear to best address the needs of each patient category. These include posterior release followed by extension casting for children with highly flexible deformities; posterior instrumentation for patients in whom reduction–fixation–fusion is indicated; and anterior resection with posterior pedicle fixation for adults with fixed or high-grade spondyloptosis.

Posterior Grafting with Extension Casting

Indications

This approach has evolved from the traction–cast techniques of the past. It is most effective in reducing the kyphotic aspect of a spondylolisthesis deformity, but has little effect on translation. This technique is best reserved for young patients with primarily kyphotic and flexible deformities. It is mainly used for children whose bones may be too small for pedicle screws and who may tolerate months of recumbency in a hyperextension cast better than adolescents or adults.

Technique

One week after standard L4–S1 posterolateral fusion, patients are placed in longitudinal traction on a Risser frame. To reduce lumbosacral kyphosis the legs are extended and anterior pressure is applied directly over the back of the sacrum. A localizer cast including one leg is applied to maintain extension.[18] Serial casting over six weeks can be performed to improve slip angle correction.[44] Some patients can be ambulated, but most are kept supine in the cast for three months.

For patients with higher grade slips and less malleable deformities, Bradford often adds three techniques to improve correction: removal of the posterior arch of L5 to facilitate reduction; insertion of Hoffman half pins into each ilium with incorporation of these into an extension cast to maintain pelvic flexion and lumbosacral extension; and attachment of percutaneous wires from the L2–L4 lamina to an outrigger on the cast to maintain the posterior position of the lumbar spine relative to the sacrum.[7, 18]

Results

Bradford reported 22 children and adolescents with an average 50 per cent slip and a mean slip angle of 33 degrees. He obtained a two-thirds reduction of the slip angle (33 to 12 degrees), but little change in trunk height or the amount of slip (50 per cent preoperatively to 40 per cent slip at fusion). There was slight further improvement in both parameters with time, owing to differential growth of the unfused anterior column and sacral dome remodeling after correction of sagittal alignment. Surgical complications were limited to transient L5 weakness in two patients who were placed in halofemoral traction and nonunion in one patient with complete loss of correction. Partial loss of reduction tended to occur in patients with more than 70 per cent slip, after Gill laminectomy, or when residual deformity left the L4 body anterior to the axial plane of the proximal sacrum, the so-called "stable zone."[18, 19]

Posterior Instrumented Reduction for Spondylolisthesis

The gradual posterior reduction method combines simultaneous and gradated distraction, posterior translation of the proximal spine, and flexion of the sacrum to reduce all aspects of the spondylolisthesis deformity. After reduction the instrumentation counteracts anterior shear forces at L5–S1 and permits axial loading across the graft to promote union (Fig. 27–39).

Indications

Posterior instrumented reduction often provides the best risk-benefit ratio of available methods for patients over the age of 10 with unfused spondylolisthesis or borderline spondyloptosis.[6] It requires pedicle screw–based instrumentation with three-dimensional adjustability and detailed knowledge of the surgical anatomy and technique, however.

Preoperative Planning

Preoperative studies should include a standing lateral radiograph of the entire lumbar spine to assess sagittal alignment, an AP projection to assess pedicle size and possible scoliosis, and bending films to determine the degree of lumbosacral mobility and the amount of fixed thoracolumbar lordosis. In young patients in whom adequate pedicle size (7-mm cortical diameter) cannot be documented on the AP radiograph, CT is helpful. CT and conventional polytomography are also useful tests for delineating the presence and location of an autofusion when no motion can be seen on bending or standing/supine films.

Technique

The deformity is reduced in a single-stage posterior operation. After L5 laminectomy, the fibrocartilage and osteophytes overlying the L5 roots are removed to fully decompress the roots out to the ala and to expose the L5 pedicles. Bicortical screws are inserted into L5

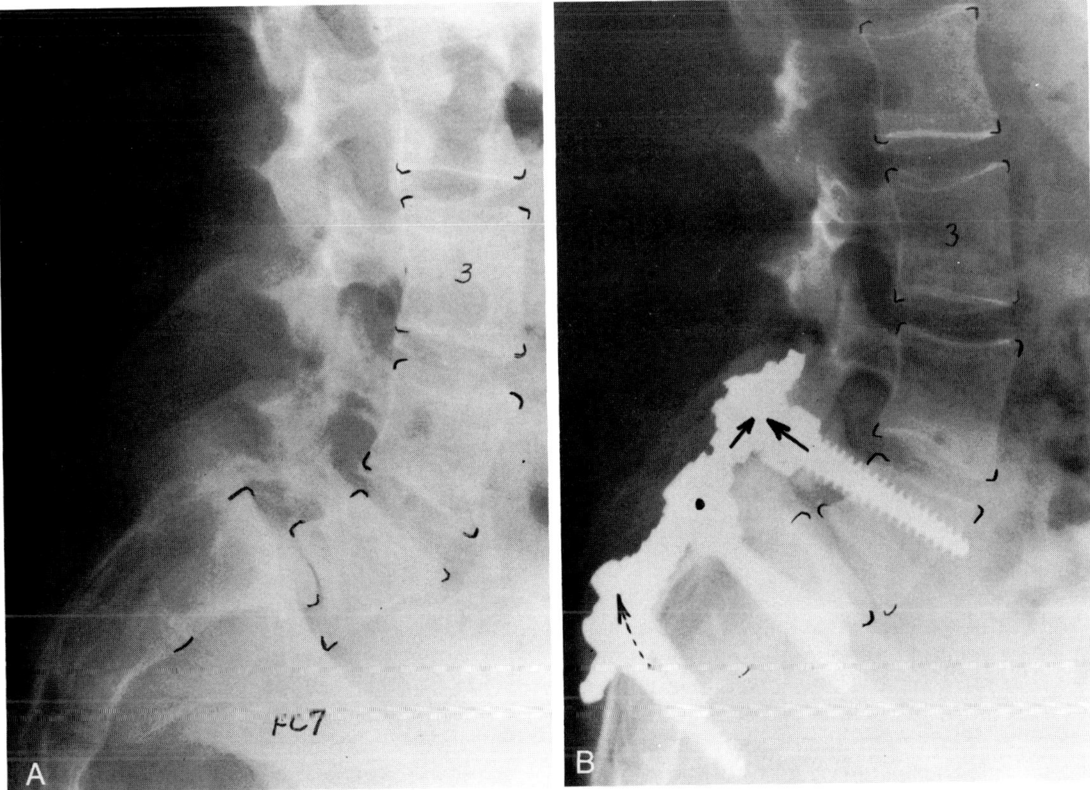

Figure 27–39. *A*, Lateral radiograph of symptomatic slip in a 45-year-old female. *B*, Postoperative radiograph demonstrating full correction of deformity from the gradual application of distraction, posterior translation, and sacral flexion only. Edwards instrumentation crosses only the involved disc space. Arrows indicate the direction of forces used to obtain reduction.

and across the ala at S1 and S2 after probe and guidewire confirmation of position. Extension to L4 is recommended for Grade 4 slips and those Grade 3 slips with substantial lumbosacral kyphosis or scoliosis. This is because the L4–L5 facet overlaps the L5 pedicle and the hyperextended L4–L5 disc is prone to degenerative changes, instability, and retrolisthesis.[32, 70]

Reduction is accomplished by the gradual application of corrective forces with instrumentation. There is no need to cross the canal or disturb the disc. Height is gradually restored by distracting with finely ratcheted rods. Posterior translation of the lumbar spine and flexion of the sacrum is effected by gradually shortening connectors between the L5 screws (and L4 screws if used) and the posterior rods (or plates). Distraction and translational forces are restored every ten minutes; generally 30 to 45 minutes reduction time is required for each grade of deformity. When radiographs document full reduction, all distraction is then released to permit axial loading. The instrumentation is then locked in position and lateral fusion performed. Wake-up testing and somatosensory evoked potential (SEP) peroneal nerve monitoring is employed for Grade 4 spondylolisthesis, or when the slip angle exceeds 45 degrees. If the components required for instrumented reduction are not available to the surgeon, the risks of reduction may increase and must be balanced against the benefits.

Results of Gradual Instrumented Reduction

Results of 25 consecutive patients with L5–S1 spondylolisthesis have been presented by Edwards.[37] Eighteen had Grade 2 to 4 spondylolisthesis and seven had spondyloptosis. Patient age ranged from 12 to 59 with an average age of 25. Slip correction averaged 91 per cent at an average two-year follow-up. The 33 degree preoperative slip angle was reduced to a mean of 4 degrees kyphosis (90 per cent correction). In addition 35-mm (mean) trunk height (L1–S1) was restored with a 43-mm increase for patients with spondyloptosis. Patients ambulated at discharge in a total contact orthosis with one thigh extension. Complications for patients with spondylolisthesis were remarkably few. One patient with borderline spondyloptosis developed unilateral dorsiflexion weakness. There were no dislodgements, there was one donor site infection, and one patient required repair of a nonunion.

Similar results have been reported for 180 L5–S1 spondylolisthesis cases treated by members of the Spinal Fixation Study Group (SFSG), a select group of spinal surgeons trained and monitored in these techniques. Complication rates from the SFSG series include 3 per cent transient radiculopathy, 1 per cent neurologic deficit, 1 per cent infection, and 2 per cent S2 screw pull-out for Grade 1 to 4 spondylolisthesis. Solid fusion was achieved in 88 per cent of patients at one year follow-up. Hence, results to date suggest that instrumented reduction is an effective and relatively safe new alternative for the treatment of spondylolisthesis (Fig. 27–40).

Nevertheless, the concept of reducing spondylolisthesis remains controversial. This is understandable since full reduction with its potential advantages was rarely achieved in the past and the complications associated with attempted reduction were considerably more than with in situ fusions. It appears that with newer methods patients can now obtain a nearly anatomic reduction without excessive risk, however, and in some cases with fewer complications than attempted fusion without reduction. Despite these advances, in situ fusion will properly remain the standard procedure for some time.

Reduction, or even segmental fixation, of spondylolisthesis is a technically challenging operation. It requires hands-on training, case feedback, and a long learning curve to master the planning and reduction techniques necessary for excellent results. The authors strongly caution those without experience in these surgical techniques, and without instrumentation that allows multiplane, gradual correction to defer surgery or perform in situ fusion, where the results are well known and currently accepted.

Staged Posterior Reduction for Spondyloptosis

Both the advantages and risks of reduction are greatest for patients with true spondyloptosis. Correction of deformity increases the distance through which lumbar roots must travel and subjects spinal instrumentation to much greater stresses than during reduction of Grade 2 to 4 spondylolisthesis. Accordingly, the likelihood of lumbar root deficit, fixation failure, and nonunion is increased. With careful preoperative planning, neural monitoring, supplemental traction, limited shortening, and staged reduction, the incidence of these complications can be lowered to acceptable levels, however.

Neural Limits of One-Stage Reduction

In spondyloptosis the lumbar spine slips anteriorly, rotates into flexion, and drops within the pelvis to shorten the distance between the neural foramina and exit of both the femoral and sciatic nerves from the pelvis. With time these nerves contract, eventually limiting the amount of correction that can be obtained without shortening the spine itself.

From our ongoing analysis, it appears that most patients will tolerate about 3 cm of lengthening between L4 and the sacrum in one surgical session. More axial lengthening is possible when the slip has progressed rapidly, in especially flexible deformities, in younger patients, and when the slip angle is low. Less single-stage lengthening is tolerated for those with high slip angles, long-standing deformities, or previously fused or rigid deformities, or for older age groups.

If preoperative radiographs show that more axial lengthening is required than lumbar roots can tolerate according to these guidelines, two courses of action can be followed: shorten the spine by sacral dome osteotomy to permit single-stage lengthening within tolerable limits, or stage the reduction to give lumbar roots more time for stress–relaxation. If 1.5 cm of shortening will suffice, this can be safely accomplished by a sacral dome osteotomy from the posterior approach after L5 laminectomy and mobilization of the dural sac. If additional shortening is required, anteroposterior resection procedures are necessary.

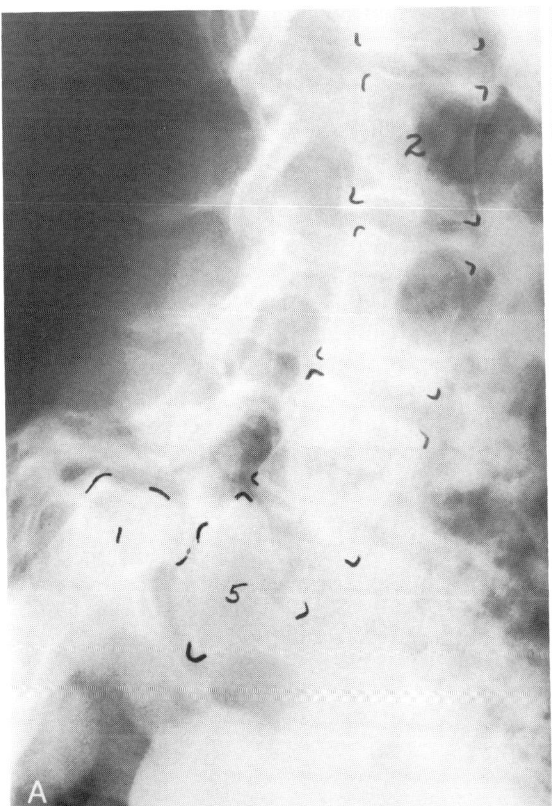

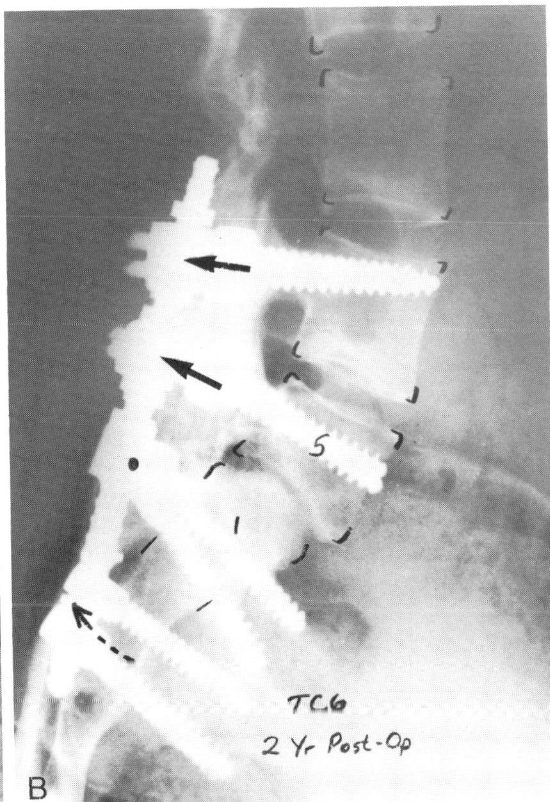

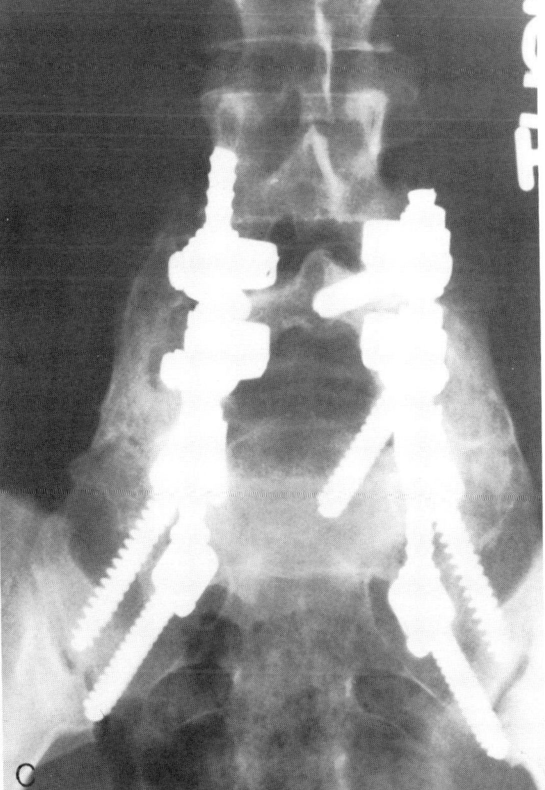

Figure 27–40. *A*, Preoperative radiograph of a 15-year-old female with 100 per cent slip and early rotation of L5 about the rounded sacral dome. This represents almost the maximal deformity that can safely be reduced in a single stage without shortening the spinal column. *B*, Lateral radiograph two years after surgery demonstrating full reduction of the deformity by corrective forces alone without discotomy, traction, or anterior surgery. The patient proceeded to painless union without neurologic deficit or other complications. *C*, Anteroposterior radiograph demonstrating a well-consolidated lateral fusion mass. Arrows indicate the direction of forces used to obtain reduction.

In all cases with borderline or true spondyloptosis, neurologic monitoring should be performed during reduction. In addition, wake-up tests should be performed after any sustained lessening in SEP amplitude or increase in latency. A 30 to 50 per cent drop in amplitude is significant. When performing a wake-up test, the critical action is active ankle dorsiflexion. For patients requiring considerable reduction of kyphosis, wake-up tests should always be performed, including knee extension to assess femoral nerve function.

Staged Reduction

Staging the reduction makes it possible to correct most cases of spondyloptosis without resorting to the more extensive anteroposterior resection procedures. Gradual reduction is continued until there is a significant amplitude drop on SEPs or reduced function on the wake-up test. When correcting spondyloptosis, this typically occurs when about a 50 per cent slip and 30 degrees of slip angle remain. The instrumentation is then locked in place and the wound closed. Patients are log rolled and kept at bed rest for one to two weeks until they return to the operating room to complete the reduction (Fig. 27–41).

After surgery most spondyloptosis patients follow the same regimen as described above for spondylolisthesis. If there is any question about the quality of fixation, however, patients should be kept recumbent in their brace for four to six weeks. If anatomic alignment is not achieved for any reason, secondary anterior grafting should be performed.

Results

One of the authors has been using the techniques outlined above for the treatment of

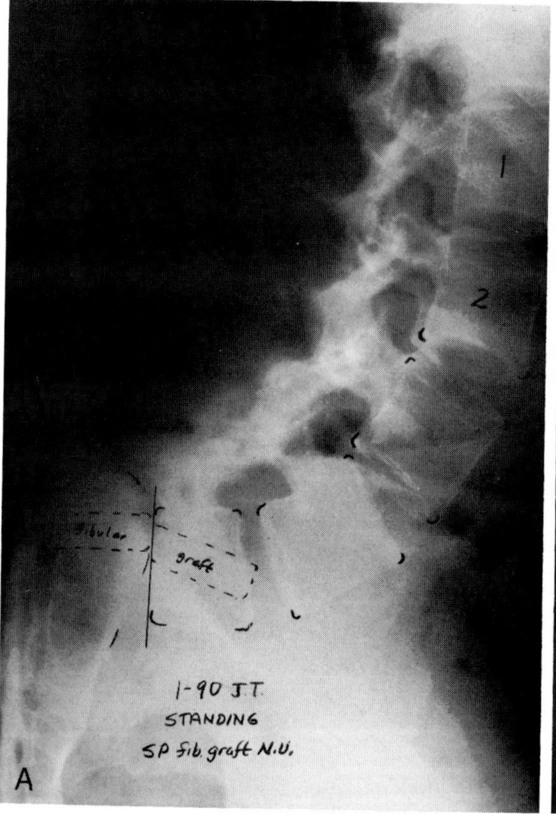

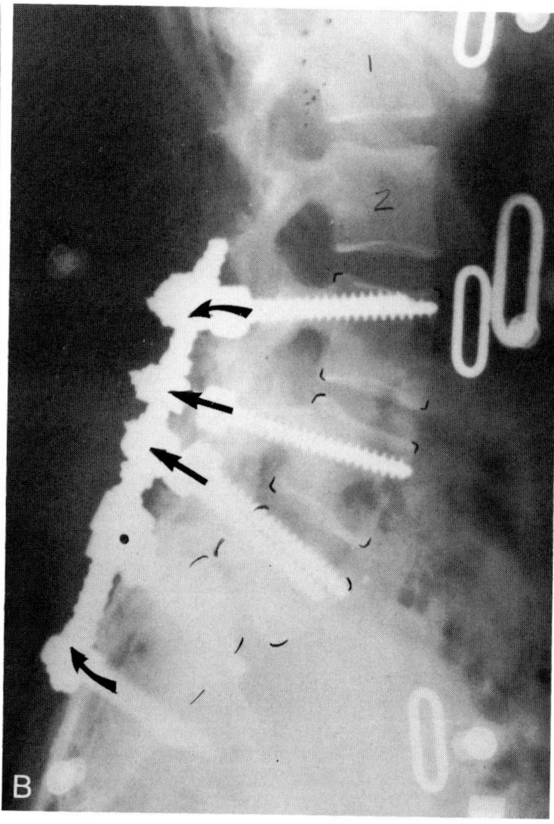

Figure 27–41. *A*, Standing lateral radiograph of a 23-year-old female with progressive deformity and radiculopathy after failed in situ fibular dowel graft fusion after earlier failed L3–S1 lateral in situ fusion. *B*, Standing lateral radiograph in a brace after instrumented reduction. Surgery consisted of mobilization of the dural sac and L5 and S1 roots, sacral dome osteotomy, and two-stage posterior reduction with Edwards instrumentation. It was necessary to extend the fusion to L3 because of L3–L4 facet disruption from previous in situ fusion attempts. After surgery there was early improvement in neurologic function and lessening of back and leg pain. Arrows indicate the direction of forces used to obtain reduction.

low- to intermediate-grade spondyloptosis for the past two years. With careful planning and adherence to the details of gradual posterior reduction, nearly anatomic spinal alignment, a residual 10 to 30 per cent slip, and 5 to 20 degrees of kyphosis can be expected. Complications vary according to the severity and duration of the deformity, amount of previous surgery, and age of the patient. Average expectations are for 15 per cent transient neurologic deficit and perhaps a 10 per cent incidence of lasting radiculopathy. The latter typically involves unilateral weakness of ankle dorsiflexion. We have not seen any case of a cauda equina syndrome or plantar flexion weakness. Failure of fixation at S2 with loosening and partial pull-out after final reduction occurs in approximately 10 per cent of the cases. With restoration of anatomic alignment and axial loading, we expect union rates slightly below the 88 per cent documented for cases of spondylolisthesis treated by SFSG members. Despite the favorable early experience, gradual instrumented reduction for spondyloptosis remains investigational and long-term follow-up is not yet available.

Anteroposterior Resection–Reduction

Indications

Combined anterior and posterior methods require more extensive surgery and present greater risk and morbidity than other current options. Hence, they are best reserved for deformities beyond the scope of extension cast or posterior instrumented reductions. Combined anterior and posterior surgery offers a unique advantage when treating surgical or autofusion of high-grade spondylolisthesis, or chronic high-grade spondyloptosis.

Autofusion between the inferior end plate of L5 and the anterior aspect of the sacrum is suggested when no motion is seen on either standing/supine or flexion/extension motion studies. It is confirmed with tomograms or CT. Initial open anterior osteotomy is presently safer than attempted blind posterior osteotomy of a fused L5–S1 interspace.

We define spondyloptosis as high grade when flexion tilt and loss of height have progressed to the point where the entire fifth vertebral body lies below the dome of the sacrum on standing films. Chronicity of the deformity is suggested by lack of perceptible motion on standing/supine or flexion/extension radiographs. The amount of lengthening that can be tolerated by the lumbar roots during reduction is inversely proportional to the duration of the deformity, the degree of fixed thoracolumbar lordosis, and the amount of lengthening required. Hence, shortening the anterior spinal column can help protect against radiculopathy during reduction of high-grade chronic spondyloptosis. If discectomy and sacral dome resection only are needed, they are best carried out from the posterior approach; however, if additional shortening to remove the inferior portion of L5 or even the entire vertebral body is required, this is best accomplished through an anterior approach (Fig. 27–42).

Technique

Before surgery for reduction of high-grade spondyloptosis, it is important to plan carefully the level and inclination of anterior and posterior osteotomies from preoperative radiographs. The first stage of surgery is anterior osteotomy and grafting. The lumbar spine is approached through the midline, the inferior portion of the L5 body is osteotomized, the disc material is excised, and bone removed from the L5 body is morselized and used as graft.[31]

The second stage is scheduled one to two weeks later. It is best to avoid halofemoral traction during this interval since most reported root complications associated with combined anterior and posterior spondylolisthesis/optosis reductions have occurred during periods of unmonitored traction. To further reduce the risk of root injury, we advise removal of the posterior L5 arch (Gill procedure) with complete dissection and decompression of the L5 and S1 roots. The dura can then be safely mobilized followed by further sacral dome osteotomy (if necessary) and posterior discectomy. Reduction is accomplished over several hours according to the gradual instrumented reduction method.

Results

Edwards, Bradford, Whitesides, and others have performed a number of resection–reductions using the technique described above, although no series have yet been published. Nevertheless, by combining the results with earlier anteroposterior techniques reported by

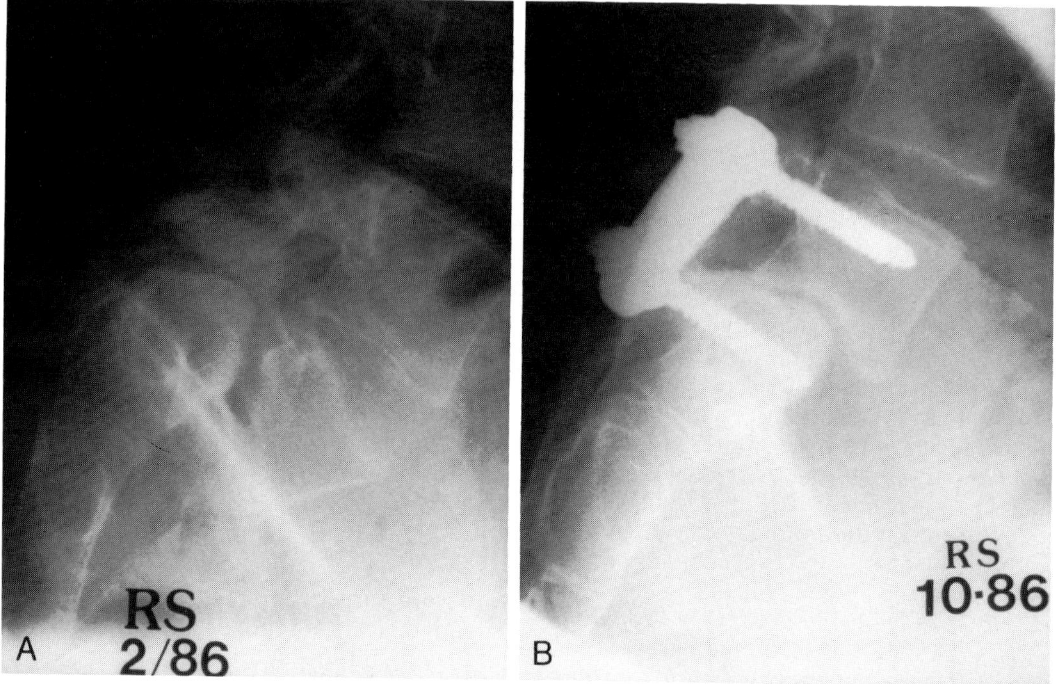

Figure 27–42. *A*, Preoperative lateral radiograph demonstrating spondyloptosis in an adult patient. *B*, Postoperative lateral radiograph after resection of L5 from anterior and posterior approaches. After correcting spinal alignment, the L4 vertebra was affixed to the sacrum with a VSP plate. L4 and L5 roots both exited the L4 foramen. (Courtesy of Robert W. Gaines, M.D.)

Bradford and Gotfried and DeWald and associates, we estimate that an experienced spinal surgeon can expect 80 to 90 per cent correction of slip angle and reduction of translation (slip) to a residual Grade 1 or 2.[17, 30] Complications are frequent but rarely catastrophic if the recommended procedures are carefully followed. Approximately 30 per cent of patients develop root deficits. About half of these eventually resolve. The most common deficit is unilateral foot drop. The nonunion rate is 10 to 15 per cent, with occasional loss of midsacral fixation. In addition, there are the less frequent general complications of posterior surgery including infection, and of anterior surgery including ileus, pulmonary problems, bowel obstruction, iliac vein thrombosis, and sexual dysfunction in men.

TREATMENT OF DEGENERATIVE SPONDYLOLISTHESIS

Degenerative spondylolisthesis usually follows segmental instability with disc and facet degeneration. The facet cartilage erodes and arthritic changes manifest themselves. This allows vertebral displacement and stimulates development of marginal, hypertrophic osteophytes that lead to stenosis and root compression.

The major goals in the treatment of degenerative spondylolisthesis are relief of back and leg pain and maintenance of spine stability. Pain can arise from both root compression and motion across the arthritic joint. Adequate neural decompression can usually be accomplished by partial medial facetectomy with preservation of the pars interarticularis and facet joints.

The role of spinal fusion in degenerative spondylolisthesis is less clear. Most authors agree that fusion should be performed if total facetectomy or iatrogenic instability is produced by neural decompression. Other reported indications for selective fusion include a patient less than 60 or 65 years of age, physiologically active patients, and the absence of associated degenerative disc disease at adjacent levels.[58] Posterolateral fusion should also be considered if preoperative flexion/extension stress radiographs demonstrate greater than 3 to 4 mm AP translation change, or sagittal plane rotation of greater than 10 degrees at any level from L1–L5. At the L5–S1 level, greater than 4 mm translation and 20 degrees of sagittal plane rotation suggest that a fusion should be considered.[81]

When fusion is indicated, an in situ posterolateral fusion can be performed with a high (80 per cent) rate of successful fusion and good clinical results in patients with a collapsed disc and little motion across the interspace. Postoperatively patients are treated with a lumbosacral corset for comfort. If instability is present preoperatively or created intraoperatively, the addition of segmental internal fixation can prevent slip progression with recurrent impingement, stabilize the joint to reduce postoperative pain, and negate shear to facilitate union.

For degenerative slips exceeding 1 cm, reduction with pedicle screws can also restore canal alignment and thereby assist in canal decompression indirectly. Either plates or ratcheted rods from the Modular Spinal System with screw fixation on either side of the slip and one interspace below can achieve good reduction of a low-grade degenerative slip. When degenerative spondylolisthesis is associated with lateralolisthesis, reduction requires distraction and both posterior *and* lateral translation.

SUMMARY

Spondylolysis and spondylolisthesis are the most common causes of back pain in children and adolescents. The onset of symptoms coincides with the adolescent growth spurt, a period during which slips may also progress. Symptoms include back pain and, less commonly, radicular pain or deficit. Unlike adults, children may have postural and gait abnormalities without significant pain. Physical findings, particularly in high-grade slips, include a shortened trunk; square-appearing, flattened buttocks; accentuated lumbar lordosis; hamstring tightness; and a characteristic waddling gait. The severity of the physical findings correlates with the degree of slip.

Symptoms from spondylolysis and spondylolisthesis usually respond to such nonoperative measures as bed rest, activity modification, wearing of a brace or corset, and aspirin or nonsteroidal anti-inflammatory medications. Surgical fusion is indicated for patients with persistent or recurrent symptoms despite activity modification, and those with progressive slips, greater than 50 per cent displacement, neurologic deficit, or persistent postural and gait abnormalities. Because of the high success rate with current methods, the patient with persistent, disabling symptoms should undergo fusion when symptoms persist after a reasonable period of nonoperative care. Although many operative methods exist, most patients requiring surgery predictably respond to posterolateral in situ fusion. For patients with more severe slips or other factors predisposing them to problems with in situ fusion, however, new methods providing instrumented reduction of the deformity and secure fixation appear promising.

References

1. Amundson, G. M., and Wenger, D. R.: Spondylolisthesis: natural history and treatment. Spine *1*:323–338, 1987.
2. Amundson, G. M., and McGuire, R. A.: The use of primary internal fixation in spondylolisthesis with radiculopathy. Presented at the American Academy of Orthopaedic Surgeons meeting, February 7–13, 1990, New Orleans, LA.
3. Amuso, S. J., Neff, R. S., Coulson, D. B., et al.: The surgical treatment of spondylolisthesis by posterior element resection: a long-term follow-up study. J. Bone Joint Surg. *52A*:529–536, 1970.
4. Apel, D. M., Lorenz, M. A., and Zindrick, M. R.: Symptomatic spondylolisthesis in adults: four decades later. Spine *14*:345–348, 1989.
5. Armstrong, G. W. D., and Chen, B. Y.: Sacral configuration in dysplastic spondylolisthesis. J. Bone Joint Surg. *67B*:335, 1985 (abstr.).
6. Baker, D. R., and McHollick, W.: Spondyloschisis and spondylolisthesis in children. J. Bone Joint Surg. *38A*:933, 1956.
7. Balderston, R., and Bradford, D.: Technique for achievement and maintenance of reduction for severe spondylolisthesis using spinous process traction wiring and external fixation of the pelvis. Spine *10*:377, 1985.
8. Barash, H. L., Galante, J. O., Lambert, C. N., and Ray, R. D.: Spondylolisthesis and tight hamstrings. J. Bone Joint Surg. *52A*:1319–1328, 1970.
9. Bell, D. F., Erlich, M. G., and Zaleske, D. J.: Brace treatment of symptomatic spondylolisthesis. Clin. Orthop. *236*:192, 1988.
10. Boachie-Adjei, O.: Conservative treatment of spondylolysis and spondylolisthesis. Semin. Spine Surg. *1*:106–115, 1989.
11. Bohlman, H. H., and Cook, S. S.: One-stage decompression and posterolateral and interbody fusion for lumbosacral spondyloptosis through a posterior approach. J. Bone Joint Surg. *64A*:415–418, 1982.

12. Bosworth, D. M., Fielding, J. W., Demarest, L., and Bonaquist, M.: Spondylolisthesis: a critical review of a consecutive series of cases treated by arthrodesis. J. Bone Joint Surg. *37A*:767–786, 1955.
13. Boxall, D., Bradford, D. S., Winter, R. B., and Moe, J. H.: Management of severe spondylolisthesis in children and adolescents. J. Bone Joint Surg. *61A*:479–495, 1979.
14. Bradford, D. S.: Treatment of severe spondylolisthesis: a combined approach for reduction and stabilization. Spine *4*:423–429, 1979.
15. Bradford, D. S.: Management of spondylolysis and spondylolisthesis. Instructional Course Lectures XXXII. American Academy of Orthopaedic Surgeons. St. Louis, C. V. Mosby Co., 1983, pp. 151–162.
16. Bradford, D., and Iza, J.: Repair of the defect in spondylolysis or minimal degrees of spondylolisthesis by segmental wire fixation and bone grafting. Spine *10*:673–679, 1985.
17. Bradford, D. S., and Gotfried, Y.: Staged salvage reconstruction of Grade IV and V spondylolisthesis. J. Bone Joint Surg. *69A*:191–202, 1987.
18. Bradford, D. S.: Closed reduction of spondylolisthesis: a combined approach for reduction and stabilization. Spine *13*:580–587, 1988.
19. Bradford, D. S., and Boachie-Adjei, O.: Reduction of spondylolisthesis: *In* Evarts, C. M. (ed.): Surgery of the Musculoskeletal System. 2nd ed. New York, Churchill Livingstone, 1990, pp. 2129–2142.
19a. Brailsford, J. F.: Deformities of lumbosacral region. Br. J. Surg. *16*:562–627, 1929.
20. Brown, C. W., Heinig, C. F., Odom, J. A., Donaldson, D. H., and Boyd, B.: A new method of reduction and fusion of symptomatic spondylolisthesis: the "crowbar" procedure. Orthop. Trans. *8*:403, 1984.
21. Brown, C. W., Orme, T. J., and Richardson, H. D.: The rate of pseudarthrosis (surgical non union) in patients who are smokers and patients who are non smokers: a comparison study. Spine *11*:942–943, 1986.
22. Buck, J.: Direct repair of the defect in spondylolisthesis: preliminary report. J. Bone Joint Surg. *52B*:432–437, 1970.
23. Buck, J.: Further thoughts on direct repair of the defect in spondylolysis. J. Bone Joint Surg. *61B*:123, 1979.
24. Bunnell, W. P.: Back pain in children. Orthop. Clin. North Am. *13*:587–604, 1982.
25. Cleveland, M., Bosworth, D. M., and Thompson, F. R.: Pseudoarthrosis in the lumbosacral spine. J. Bone Joint Surg. *30A*:302–312, 1948.
26. Cloward, R. B.: Spondylolisthesis: treatment by laminectomy and posterior interbody fusion: review of 100 cases. Clin. Orthop. *154*:74–82, 1981.
27. Dandy, D. J., and Shannon, M. J.: Lumbosacral subluxation (group I spondylolisthesis). J. Bone Joint Surg. *53B*:578–595, 1971.
28. Davis, I. S., and Bailey, R. W.: Spondylolisthesis: indications for lumbar nerve root decompression and operative technique. Clin. Orthop. *117*:129–134, 1976.
29. Denecke, H.: Reposition der luxierten Wirelsaule bei Spondylolisthese. Ver. Deutsch. Orthop. *44*:404–410, 1956.
30. DeWald, R. L., Faut, M. M., Taddonio, R. F., and Neuwirth, M. G.: Severe lumbosacral spondylolisthesis in adolescents and children. J. Bone Joint Surg. *65A*:619–626, 1981.
31. Dick, W.: The "Fixateur Interne" as a versatile implant for spine surgery. Spine *12*:882–900, 1987.
32. Dick, W. T., and Schnebel, B.: Severe spondylolisthesis: reduction and internal fixation. Clin. Orthop. *232*:70, 1988.
33. Dietrich, M., and Kurowski, P.: The importance of mechanical factors in the etiology of spondylolysis: a model analysis of loads and stresses in human lumbar spine. Spine *10*:532–542, 1985.
34. Dimar, J. R., and Hoffman, G.: Grade 4 spondylolisthesis: two-stage therapeutic approach of anterior vertebrectomy and anterior-posterior fusion. Orthop. Rev. *15*:49–54, 1986.
35. Edwards, C. C.: Reduction of spondylolisthesis: biomechanics and fixation. Orthop. Trans. *10*:543, 1986.
36. Edwards, C. C.: Early results correcting spondylolisthesis. Presented at the 23rd annual meeting of the Scoliosis Research Society, Baltimore, 1988.
37. Edwards, C. C.: Prospective evaluation of a new method for complete reduction of L5–S1 spondylolisthesis using corrective forces alone. Orthop. Trans. *14*:549, 1990.
38. Edwards, C. C., and Weigel, M. C.: A prospective study of 51 low lumbar nonunions. Orthop. Trans. *12*:608, 1988.
39. Edwards, C. C., White, J. B., and Levine, A. M.: One-stage reduction of spondyloptosis using corrective forces alone: a new surgical option. Orthop. Trans. *12*:136, 1988.
40. Fisk, J. R., Moe, J. H., and Winter, R. B: Scoliosis, spondylolysis, and spondylolisthesis: their relationship as reviewed in 539 patients. Spine *3*:14–25, 1978.
41. Flatley, T. J., and Derderian, H.: Closed loop instrumentation of the lumbar spine. Clin. Orthop. *196*:273–278, 1985.
42. Fredrickson, B. E., Baker, D., McHolick, W. J., et al.: The natural history of spondylolysis and spondylolisthesis. J. Bone Joint Surg. *66A*:699–707, 1984.
43. Gaines, R., and Nichols, W.: Treatment of spondyloptosis by two-stage L5 vertebrectomy and reduction of L4 onto S1. Spine *10*:680–686, 1985.
44. Garfin, S. R., and Amundson, G. M.: Spondylolisthesis. Update on Spinal Disorders *1*:3–9, 1986.
45. Garfin, S. R., and Heller, J.: The operative reduction of spondylolisthesis: indications, results, complications. Semin. Spine Surg. *1*:125–132, 1989.
46. Gill, G. G., Manning, J. G., and White, H. L.: Surgical treatment of spondylolisthesis without spine fusion. J. Bone Joint Surg. *37*:493–520, 1955.
47. Gill, G. G.: Long-term follow-up evaluation of a few patients with spondylolisthesis treated by excision of the loose lamina with decompression of the nerve roots without spinal fusion. Clin. Orthop. *182*:215–219, 1984.
48. Hambly, M., Lee, C. K., Gutteling, E., Zimmerman, M. C., Langrana, N., and Pyun, Y.: Tension band wiring-bone grafting for spondylolysis and spondylolisthesis: a clinical and biomechanical study. Spine *14*:455–460, 1989.
49. Hanley, E. N., and Levy, J. A.: Surgical treatment

of isthmic lumbosacral spondylolisthesis: analysis of variables influencing results. Spine *14*:48–50, 1989.

50. Harrington, P. R., and Tullos, H. S.: Reduction of severe spondylolisthesis in children. South. Med. J. *62*:1–5, 1969.
51. Harrington, P. R., and Tullos, H. S.: Spondylolisthesis in children: observations and surgical treatment. Clin. Orthop. *79*:75–84, 1971.
52. Harris, I. E., and Weinstein, S. L.: Long-term follow-up of patients with grade III and IV spondylolisthesis. J. Bone Joint Surg. *69A*:960–969, 1987.
53. Harris, R. I.: Spondylolisthesis. Ann. R. Coll. Surg. Engl. *8*:259–297, 1951.
54. Hendersen, E. D.: Results of the surgical treatment of spondylolisthesis. J. Bone Joint Surg. *48A*:619–642, 1966.
55. Hensinger, R. N., Lang, J. R., and McEwen, G. D.: Surgical management of spondylolisthesis in children and adolescents. Spine *1*:207–216, 1976.
56. Hensinger, R. N.: Spondylolysis and spondylolisthesis in children. *In* Rothman, R. H., and Simeone, F. A. (eds.): The Spine. 2nd ed. Philadelphia, W. B. Saunders Co., 1982, pp. 263–284.

56a. Herbiniaux, G.: Traité sur divers accouchements laborieux et sur les polypes de la matrice. Brussels, J. L. Boubers, 1782.

57. Herring, J. A.: Instructional case: severe spondylolisthesis. J. Pediatr. Orthop. *5*:737–739, 1985
58. Herron, L. D., and Trippi, A. C.: L4–5 degenerative spondylolisthesis: the results of treatment by decompressive laminectomy without fusion. Spine *14*:534–538, 1989.
59. Hodgson, A. R., and Wong, S. K.: A description of a technic and evaluation of results in anterior spinal fusion for deranged intervertebral disk and spondylolisthesis. Clin. Orthop. *56*:133–162, 1968.
60. Huizenga, B. A.: Reduction of spondyloptosis with 2-stage vertebrectomy. Orthop. Trans. *7*:21, 1983.
61. Ibrahim, K.: Repair of the pars defect in spondylolysis with bone graft and figure-of-eight Mersilene tape. Presented at the 23rd annual meeting of the Scoliosis Research Society, Baltimore, 1988.
62. Jenkins, J. A.: Spondylolisthesis. Br. J. Surg. *24*:80–85, 1936.
63. Johnson, J. R., and Kirwan, E. O.: The long-term results of fusion in situ for severe spondylolisthesis. J. Bone Joint Surg. *65B*:43–46, 1983.
64. Jones, A. A. M., McAfee, P. C., Robinson, R. A., et al.: Failed arthrodesis of the spine for severe spondylolisthesis: salvage by interbody arthrodesis. J. Bone Joint Surg. *70A*:25–30, 1988.
65. Kaneda, K., Satoh, S., Nohara, Y., and Oguma, T.: Distraction rod instrumentation with posterolateral fusion in isthmic spondylolisthesis: 53 cases followed for 18–89 months. Spine *10*:383–389, 1985.
66. Kilian, H. F.: Schilderungen neuer Beckenformen and ihres Verhaltens in Leben. Mannheim, Verlag von Bassermann and Mathey, 1854.
67. Klinghoffer, L., and Murdock, M. G.: Spondylolysis following trauma: a case report and review of the literature. Clin. Orthop. *166*:72–74, 1982.
68. LaFond, G.: Surgical treatment of spondylolisthesis. Clin. Orthop. *22*:175–179, 1962.
69. Lance, E. M.: Treatment of severe spondylolisthesis with neural involvement. J. Bone Joint Surg. *48A*:883–891, 1966.
70. Laurent, L. E., and Osterman, K.: Operative treatment of spondylolisthesis in young patients. Clin. Orthop. *117*:85–91, 1976.
71. Louis, R.: Fusion of the lumbar and sacral spine by internal fixation with screw plates. Clin. Orthop. *203*:18–33, 1986.
72. Lowe, J., Schechner, E., Hirschberg, E., et al.: Significance of bone scintigraphy in symptomatic spondylolysis. Spine *9*:653–654, 1984.
73. Matthiass, H. H., and Heine, J.: The surgical reduction of spondylolisthesis. Clin. Orthop. *203*:34–44, 1986.
74. Maurice, H. D., and Morley, T. R.: Cauda equina lesions following fusion in situ and decompressive laminectomy for severe spondylolisthesis. Spine *14*:214–216, 1989.
75. Mazel, C., Roy-Camille, R., Saillant, G., and Bouchet, T.: Spondylolisthesis: treatment and results. Orthop. Trans. *11*:500, 1987.
76. McAfee, P. C., and Yuan, H. A.: Computed tomography in spondylolisthesis. Clin. Orthop. *166*:62–71, 1982.
77. McPhee, I. B., and O'Brien, J. P.: Reduction of severe spondylolisthesis. Spine *4*:430–434, 1979.
78. McQueen, M. M., Court-Brown, C., and Scott, J. H. S.: Stabilization of spondylolisthesis using Dwyer instrumentation. J. Bone Joint Surg. *68B*:185–188, 1986.
79. Monticelli, G., and Ascani, E.: Spondylolysis and spondylolisthesis. Acta Orthop. Scand. *46*:498–506, 1975.
80. Nachemson, A.: Repair of the spondylolisthetic defect and inter-transverse fusion for young patients. Clin. Orthop. *117*:101–105, 1976.
81. Nachemson, A.: The role of spine fusion. Question 8: how do you define instability? Spine *6*:306–307, 1981.
82. Neugebauer, F. L.: A new contribution to the history and etiology of spondylolisthesis. New Syndenham Society Selected Monographs *121B*:1–64, 1888.
83. Newman, P. H.: The etiology of spondylolisthesis. J. Bone Joint Surg. *45B*:39–59, 1963.
84. Newman, P. H.: A clinical syndrome associated with severe lumbosacral subluxation. J. Bone Joint Surg. *47B*:472–481, 1965.
85. Newman, P. H.: Stenosis of the lumbar spine in spondylolisthesis. Clin. Orthop. *115*:116–121, 1976.
86. Nicol, R., and Scott, J.: Lytic spondylolisthesis repair by wiring. Spine *11*:1027–1030, 1986.
87. O'Brien, J. P., Mehdian, H., and Jaffray, D.: Reduction of severe lumbosacral spondylolisthesis. Orthop. Trans. *12*:620, 1988.
88. Ohki, I., Inoue, S., Murta, T., and Mikanagi, K.: Reduction and fusion of severe spondylolisthesis using halo-pelvic traction with wire reduction device. Int. Orthop. *4*:107–113, 1980.
89. Osterman, K., Lindholm, T. S., and Laurent, L. E.: Late results of removal of the loose posterior element (Gill's operation) in the treatment of lytic lumbar spondylolisthesis. Clin. Orthop. *117*:121–128, 1976.
90. Pedersen, A., and Hagen, R.: Spondylolysis and spondylolisthesis treatment by internal fixation and bone grafting of the defect. J. Bone Joint Surg. *70A*:15–24, 1988.
91. Peek, R. D., Wiltse, L. L., Reynolds, J. B., Thomas,

J. C., Guyer, D. W., et al.: In situ arthrodesis without decompression for Grade III or IV isthmic spondylolisthesis in adults who have severe sciatica. J. Bone Joint Surg. *71A*:62–68, 1989.
92. Phalen, G. S., and Dickson, J. A.: Spondylolisthesis and tight hamstrings. J. Bone Joint Surg. *43A*:505–512, 1961.
93. Pizzutillo, P. D., and Hummer, B. A., III: Nonoperative treatment for painful adolescent spondylolysis or spondylolisthesis. J Pediatr. Orthop. *9*:538–540, 1989.
94. Pizzutillo, P. D., Mirenda, W., and MacEwen, G. D.: Posterolateral fusion for spondylolisthesis in adolescence. J. Pediatr Orthop. *6*:311–316, 1986.
95. Reynolds, J. B.: Spondylolisthesis. *In* White, A. H., Rothman, R. H., and Ray, C. D. (eds.): Lumbar Spine Surgery: Techniques and Complications. St. Louis, C. V. Mosby Co., 1987, pp. 279–284.
96. Reynolds, J. B., and Wiltse, L. L.: The treatment of severe spondylolisthesis in the young. Proceedings of the third annual meeting of the North American Spine Society, Colorado Springs, Colorado. St. Louis, C. V. Mosby Co., 1988, p. 122.
97. Reynolds, J. B., and Wiltse, L. L.: The treatment of severe spondylolisthesis in the young. Orthop. Trans. *13*:27, 1989.
98. Riley, P. M., Gillespie, R., and Koreska, J.: Severe spondylolisthesis and spondyloptosis: results of posterolateral fusion in children and adolescents. J. Bone Joint Surg. *68B*:856, 1986.
99. Risser, J. C., and Norquist, D. M.: Sciatic scoliosis in growing children. Clin. Orthop. *21*:137–155, 1961.
100. Rombold, C.: Treatment of spondylolisthesis by posterolateral fusion, resection of pars interarticularis and prompt mobilization of the patient. J. Bone Joint Surg. *48A*:1283–1300, 1966.
101. Rosenberg, N. J.: Degenerative spondylolisthesis: surgical treatment. Clin. Orthop. *117*:112–120, 1976.
102. Rowe, G. G., and Roche, M. B.: The etiology of separate neural arch. J. Bone Joint Surg. *35A*:102–109, 1953.
103. Roy-Camille, R., Saillant, G., and Mazel, C.: Internal fixation of the lumbar spine with pedicle screw plating. Clin. Orthop. *203*:7–17, 1986.
104. Saraste, H.: Prognostic radiologic aspects of spondylolisthesis. Acta Radiol. *25*:427–432, 1984.
105. Saraste, H.: Long-term clinical and radiographic followup of spondylolysis and spondylolisthesis. J. Pediatr. Orthop. *7*:631–638, 1987.
106. Savini, R.: Surgical treatment of severe spondylolisthesis. Orthop. Trans. *10*:11, 1986.
107. Scaglietti, O., Frontino, G., and Bartolozzi, P.: Technique of anatomical reduction of lumbar spondylolisthesis and its surgical stabilization. Clin. Orthop. *117*:164–175, 1976.
108. Scherb, R.: Zur indikation und technik der Albee-de Quervainschen operation. Schweiz. Med. Wochen. *2*:763–765, 1921.
109. Schoenecker, P. L., Cole, H. O., Herring, J. A., Capelli, A. M., and Bradford, D. S.: Cauda equina syndrome after in situ arthrodesis for severe spondylisthesis at the lumbosacral junction. J. Bone Joint Surg. *72A*:369–377, 1990.
110. Schollner, D.: Ein neues Verfahren zur Reposition und Fixation bei Spondylolisthesis. Orthop. Praxis *4*:270–274, 1975.
111. Sevastikoglou, J. A., Spangfort, E., and Aaro, S.: Operative treatment of spondylolisthesis in children and adolescents with tight hamstrings syndrome. Clin. Orthop. *147*:192–199, 1980.
112. Sherman, F. C., Rosenthal, R. K., and Hall, J. E.: Spine fusion for spondylolysis and spondylolisthesis in children. Spine *4*:59–67, 1979.
113. Sijbrandij, S.: A new technique for the reduction and stabilization of severe spondylolisthesis. J. Bone Joint Surg. *63B*:266–271, 1981.
114. Sijbrandij, S.: Reduction and stabilization of severe spondylolisthesis: a report of three cases. J. Bone Joint Surg. *56B*:40–42, 1983.
115. Sijbrandij, S.: A new technique for the reduction and stabilization of severe spondylolisthesis: a report of nine cases. Int. Orthop. *9*:247–253, 1985.
116. Snijder, J. G. N., Seroo, J. M., Snijder, C. J., and Schijvens, A. W. M.: Therapy of spondylolisthesis by repositioning and fixation of the olisthetic vertebra. Clin. Orthop. *117*:149–156, 1976.
117. Speck, G. R., McCall, I. W., and O'Brien, J. P.: Spondylolisthesis: the angle of kyphosis. Spine *9*:659–660, 1984.
118. Stanton, R. P., Meehan, P., and Lovell, W. W.: Surgical fusion in childhood spondylolisthesis. J. Pediatr. Orthop. *5*:411–415, 1985.
119. Stauffer, R. N., and Coventry, M. B.: Posterior lateral lumbar spine fusion. J. Bone Joint Surg. *54A*:1195–1204, 1972.
120. Steffe, A. D., and Sitkowski, D. J.: Reduction and stabilization of grade IV spondylolisthesis. Clin. Orthop. *227*:82–89, 1988.
121. Steiner, M. E., and Micheli, L. J.: Treatment of symptomatic spondylolysis and spondylolisthesis with the modified Boston brace. Spine *10*:937–943, 1985.
122. Stewart, T. D.: The age incidence of neural arch defects in Alaskan natives, considered from the standpoint of etiology. J. Bone Joint Surg. *35A*:937, 1953.
123. Taillard, W.: Etiology of spondylolisthesis. Clin. Orthop. *115*:30–39, 1976.
124. Takeda, M.: A newly devised "three-one" method for the surgical treatment of spondylolysis and spondylolisthesis. Clin. Orthop. *147*:228–233, 1980.
125. Ternes, J. P., Alexander, A. H., and Burkus, J. K.: Treatment of spondylolisthesis with posterolateral fusion. Orthop. Trans. *13*:166, 1989.
126. Tojner, H.: Olisthetic scoliosis. Acta Orthop. Scand. *33*:291–300, 1963.
127. Turner, R. H., and Bianco, A. J., Jr.: Spondylolysis and spondylolisthesis in children and teenagers. J. Bone Joint Surg. *53A*:1298–1306, 1971.
128. Van Der Werf, F., Tonino, A., and Zeegers, W.: Direct repair of lumbar spondylolysis. Acta Orthop. Scand. *56*:378, 1985.
129. Van Rens, J. G., and Van Horn, J. R.: Long-term results in lumbosacral interbody fusion for spondylolisthesis. Acta Orthop. Scand. *53*:383–392, 1982.
130. Velikas, E. P., and Blackburne, J. S.: Surgical treatment of spondylolisthesis in children and adolescents. J. Bone Joint Surg. *63B*:67–70, 1981.
131. Vercanteren, M., De Groote, W., Van Nuffel, J., et

al.: Reduction of spondylolisthesis with severe slipping. Acta Orthop. Belg. *47*:502–511, 1981.

132. Verbiest, H.: The treatment of lumbar spondyloptosis or impending lumbar spondyloptosis accompanied by neurologic deficit and/or neurogenic intermittent claudication. Spine *4*:68–77, 1979.

133. Vidal, J., Fassio, B., Buscayret, C., and Allieu, Y.: Surgical reduction of spondylolisthesis using posterior approach. Clin. Orthop. *154*:156–165, 1981.

134. Waters, P. M., Emans, J. B., and Hall, J. E.: Technique for maintenance of reduction of severe spondylolisthesis using L4–S4 posterior segmental hyperextension fixation. Orthop. Trans. *11*:499, 1987.

135. Watkins, M. B.: Posterolateral bone-grafting for fusion of the lumbar and lumbosacral spine. J. Bone Joint Surg. *41A*:388–396, 1989.

136. West, J. L., and Bradford, D. S.: Grade IV spondylolisthesis. Orthop. Consult *9*:1–7, 1988.

137. Wiltse, L. L.: Etiology of spondylolisthesis. Clin. Orthop. *10*:48–60, 1957.

138. Wiltse, L. L.: Spondylolisthesis in children. Clin. Orthop. *21*:156–165, 1961.

139. Wiltse, L. L.: Spondylolisthesis: Classification and etiology. Symposium on the Spine. American Academy of Orthopaedic Surgeons. St. Louis, C. V. Mosby Co., 1969, pp. 143–168.

140. Wiltse, L. L., and Jackson, D. W.: Treatment of spondylolisthesis and spondylolysis in children. Clin. Orthop. *117*:92–100, 1976.

141. Wiltse, L. L., Newman, P. H., and McNab, I.: Classification of spondylolysis and spondylolisthesis. Clin. Orthop. *117*:23–29, 1976.

142. Wiltse, L. L., Widell, E. H., and Jackson, D. W.: Fatigue fracture: the basic lesion in isthmic spondylolisthesis. J. Bone Joint Surg. *57A*:17–22, 1975.

143. Wiltse, L. L.: Spondylolisthesis and its treatment. *In* Finneson, B. E. (ed.): Low Back Pain. 2nd ed. Philadelphia, J. B. Lippincott Co., 1980, pp. 451–493.

144. Wiltse, L. L., and Winter, R. B.: Terminology and measurement of spondylolisthesis. J. Bone Joint Surg. *65A*:768–772, 1983.

145. Wiltse, L. L., and Rothman, S. L. G.: Spondylolisthesis: classification, diagnosis, and natural history. Semin. Spine Surg. *1*:78, 1989.

146. Wynne-Davies, R., and Scott, J. H. S.: Inheritance and spondylolisthesis: a radiographic family survey. J. Bone Joint Surg. *61B*:301–305, 1979.

147. Zielke, K., and Stempel, A. V.: Posterior lateral distraction spondylodesis using the twofold sacral bar. Clin. Orthop. *203*:151–157, 1986.

148. Zindrick, M. R., and Lorenz, M. A.: The nonreductive treatment of spondylolisthesis. Semin. Spine Surg. *1*:116–124, 1989.

INDEX

Note: Page numbers in *italics* refer to illustrations; page numbers followed by (t) refer to tables.

B

D

E

G

I

J

K

L

N

P

Q

S

T

U

V

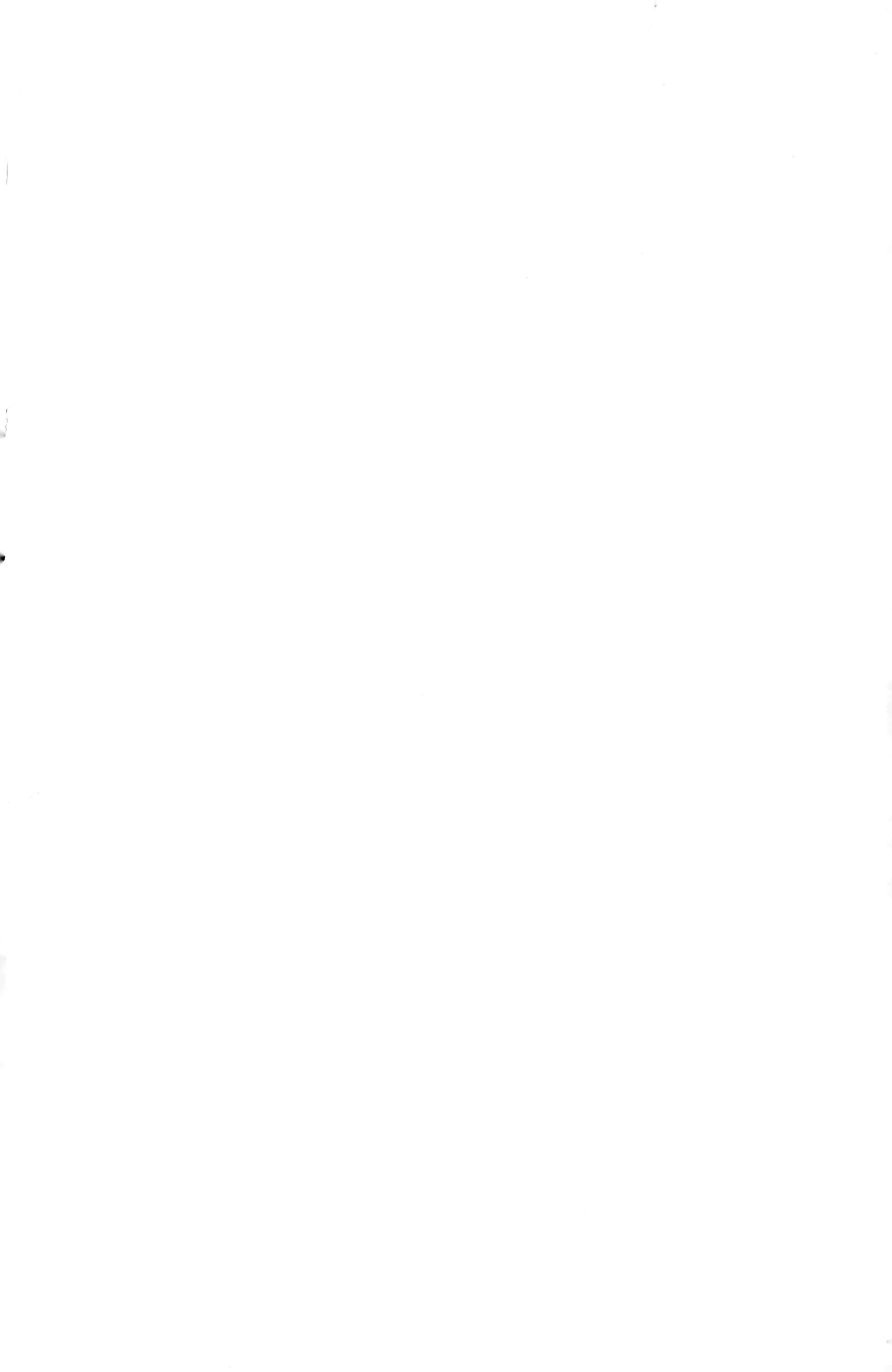